# Yearbook

of
Medical Informatics

## Quality of Health Care: The Role of Informatics

## *Impressum*

The Yearbook of Medical Informatics gives an overview of the latest outstanding research contributions in the field of Health and Medical Informatics.
The Yearbook includes original reviews, reports on research and educational programmes in Health and Medical Informatics, information about IMIA activities and member societies as well as original papers which have been selected as best papers of the recent year. These papers are selected based on an international review process, taking into account their significance, their quality, their originality, and their clarity and organization. The Yearbook of Medical Informatics 2003 covers papers which appeared in refereed journals between April 2001 and March 2002.

Suggestions for high-quality papers for the Yearbook of Medical Informatics 2004 are welcome. They must have been published between April 2002 and March 2003. Suggestions should be sent to the Editorial Office before May 1, 2003.

The publication of the IMIA Yearbook of Medical Informatics is a joint project of the International Medical Informatics Association (IMIA) and Schattauer GmbH, Stuttgart – New York. The copyright on the Yearbook remains vested in IMIA and Schattauer. The Yearbook is published annually in March and is thereafter delivered to IMIA's Member Societies and other interested parties.

The regular price of the Yearbook is EUR/US$ 95,00 per copy including VAT and surface shipping, the student price is EUR/US$ 12 per copy including VAT and surface shipping. Special price for single orders by members of IMIA Societies: EUR /US$ 30,00 per copy including VAT and surface shipping. Discounts are given if the Yearbook is ordered in larger quantities. The Yearbook will be offered to IMIA Member Societies for a special price if ordered in quantities of at least 50 copies.

Requests for orders of placement of advertisements should be directed to Schattauer GmbH before September 1st for the next Yearbook. For any other suggestions or questions, please contact the Editorial Office.


*Schattauer GmbH*
   Verlag für Medizin und Naturwissenschaften
   P.O. Box 104543
   D-70040 Stuttgart
   Germany
   Tel:    +49 711 229 870
   Fax:   +49 711 229 8750
   Homepage: http://www.schattauer.com

*IMIA Yearbook Editorial Office*
   Martina Hutter
   Dept. of Medical Informatics
   University of Heidelberg
   Im Neuenheimer Feld 400
   D-69120 Heidelberg
   Germany
   E-mail: martina_hutter@med.uni-heidelberg.de
   Homepage: http://www.yearbook.uni-hd.de

ISBN 3-7945-2263-X
ISSN 0943-4747

# *Table of Contents*



## *Information on IMIA*



## *In Memoriam Professor Jean-Raoul Scherrer*

## *IMIA Code of Ethics*

*From:*

> *Artificial Intelligence in Medicine*
> *Bioinformatics*
> *Briefings in Bioinformatics*
> *CMAJ: Canadian Medical Association Journal*
> *Current Opinion in Genetics and Development*
> *IEEE Transactions on Biomedical Engineering*
> *International Journal of Medical Informatics*
> *JAMA : The Journal of the American Medical Association*
> *Journal of Advanced Nursing*
> *Journal of Autism and Developmental Disorders*
> *Journal of Biomedical Informatics*
> *Journal of Chemical Information and Computer Sciences*
> *Journal of Magnetic Resonance Imaging*
> *Journal of Telemedicine and Telecare*
> *Journal of the American Medical Informatics Association*
> *Medical & Biological Engineering & Computing*
> *Medical Decision Making*
> *Medical Image Analysis*
> *Methods of Information in Medicine*
> *Molecular and Biochemical Parasitology*
> *Radiographics*
> *Social Science & Medicine*
> *The Journal of Urology*
> *The New England Journal of Medicine*
> *Ultrasound in Medicine & Biology*

# American Health Information Management Association
## 75 Years of Quality Healthcare through Quality Information

The American Health Information Management Association (AHIMA) is the dynamic professional association that represents more than 44,000 specially educated health information management (HIM) professionals who work throughout the healthcare industry. HIM professionals serve the healthcare industry and the public by managing, analyzing, and using data vital for patient care—and making it accessible to healthcare providers when it is needed most.

AHIMA members hold many diverse roles, yet all share a common purpose: providing reliable and valid information that drives the healthcare industry. They are specialists in administering information systems, managing medical records, and coding information for reimbursement and research.

AHIMA produces and publishes many educational resources for HIM professionals:

**In Print**
Journal of the American Health
Information Management Association
AHIMA Advantage
In Confidence
Professional Publications

**Face-to-Face**
Getting Practical with Privacy and
Security Seminars
AHIMA National Convention
Specialty Advancement Institutes
Coding Roundtables

**Online**
Communities of Practice
FORE: HIM Body of Knowledge
Electronic Newsletters
E-learning Courses

**Everywhere**
Legislative advocacy
Certification
FORE

**Contact Us For More Information**
American Health Information
Management Association
233 N. Michigan Ave., Suite 2150
Chicago, IL 60601
USA

Telephone: 011-1-(312) 233-1100
E-mail: info@ahima.org
Website: www.ahima.org

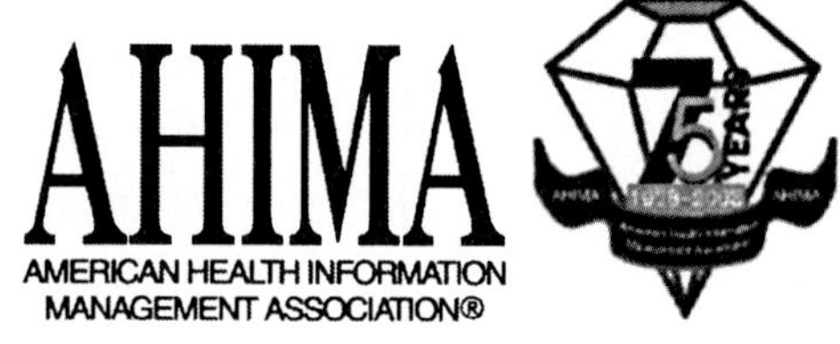


**The 14th Congress of International
Federation of Health Records Organizations**
October 9 - 14, 2004
Washington, DC, USA
Email: ifhrocongress@ahima.org

**Roger A. Côté**

Faculty of Medicine
Université de Sherbrooke
Sherbrooke, Quebec, Canada

# Preface

## *Quality health care requires quality patient data*

The problems with the underlying information basis of the health care system have been under discussion and under review for a number of years, but have not yet been solved. The papers selected for the 2003 Yearbook of Medical Informatics should add to the discussion and hopefully lead to some solution.

According to the Institute of Medicine of the National Academy of Sciences in Washington, D.C., few issues are more central to the ongoing debate on health care in the United States than quality of care. [1]

In 1990, the Institute of Medicine developed a definition which is still widely accepted today: "Quality of care is the degree to which health services for individuals and populations increase the likelihood of desired health outcomes and are consistent with current professional knowledge." [2]

Numerous quality of care studies were done using ICD-9-CM coded data. In a study of complication occurrence in medical inpatients by Geraci et al. [3], it was found that "ICD-9-CM codes in administrative data were poor measures of in-hospital complication occurrence in our study population".

A more recent similar report by McCarthy et al. [4] within the Complications Screening Program is equally critical of the ICD-9-CM codes. In their conclusions, the authors state: "These findings highlight concerns about the clinical validity of using ICD-9-CM codes for quality monitoring."

Most studies to evaluate quality of care in recent years that relied on ICD-9-CM coded data have found this statistical international classification inadequate. Furthermore, the ICD-9-CM coding problems were carried over into the diagnosis-related groupings (DRGs). When the reimbursement of hospitals by Medicare under the prospective-payment system began, the first requirement was that the system be based on the patient's diagnoses at discharge. These were then aggregated into DRGs and these were used for hospital payment following the relative weight of the DRG multiplied by a standard amount adjusted for certain hospital-specific factors.

Although the DRGs have nothing to do with quality, these studies serve to demonstrate further the inadequacy of the ICD-9-CM. One such study on Medicare Prospective Payment by MacMahon and Smits [5] reviewed the ICD-9-CM and its deficiencies. They conclude that the goal of the DRGs was to segregate distinct patient types in terms of use of hospital resources and the goal of the Medicare prospective payment system was to provide hospitals with an incentive to be efficient in the treatment of clinically distinct types of patients. Both of these goals are severely compromised by the lack of specificity of the ICD-9-CM which serves as the foundation of DRGs and the prospective payment system. They also suggest that if the system cannot be revised to allow necessary clinical distinctions among patients, then a new coding system should be developed.

In 1996, with the Health Insurance Portability and Accountability Act (HIPAA), the U.S. Congress transformed the National Committee on Vital and Health Statistics (NCVHS) into the nation's primary external advisory group for health information policy. By October 1998, this committee had prepared a concept paper [6] to assure a health dimension for the national information infrastructure.

This comprehensive report has a section on tasks for the health information infrastructure. It deals with population-based data, computer-based health records, knowledge management and decision support and telemedicine. Following this discussion, there is a section on standards and measures. A paragraph deserves quoting:

*"A high priority is the development of standards and nomenclature for capturing the state of knowledge in medicine and health care. Standards of terminology must be developed, maintained, and made accessible at minimal cost to users. These forms of standardization are critical to the linkages and comparisons needed to assess both the quality of care and the health status of the population.*
*The Unified Medical Language System of the National Library of Medicine is a good start for this process, but it is not sufficiently encompassing. Clinical records need to reflect primarily clinical realities and not focus on financial and billing procedures and terms. Care will be most easily delivered in a cost-effective and high quality manner if the language used for care delivery and a variety of management purposes most accurately reflects medical conditions and treatments."*

The NCVHS was and still is the guardian of the ICDs needed for health statistics, yet, it has finally realized as a high priority that nomenclature and standards of terminology are critical to assess quality of care and the health status of the population. There is of course no mention that such a standardized nomenclature, which is now a sine qua non for their informatics base, was presented to Doctor Theodore Cooper, Assistant Secretary for Health at Health Education, and Welfare on June 9, 1976 in Washington. His staff attending the meeting rejected the concept on the grounds that the ICD was adequate for their needs. The time for a nomenclature of medicine had not yet arrived.

By October, 1998 when the concept paper was presented, a multiaxial nomenclature for the medical record existed but was not mentioned, however the Unified Medical Language System of the National Library of Medicine was mentioned as a good start, but not sufficiently encompassing.

In spite of the predominant use of statistical classifications by government agencies, it has now become a high priority that, to assure quality care, a standard nomenclature be developed to capture medical data where it is generated at the patient's bedside or during an encounter in a clinic or doctor's office. Many research papers have demonstrated that statistical classifications were not intended or designed to measure the quality of care given to individual patients because of their lack of granularity and specificity.

If one returns to the 1998 report by the National Roundtable on Health Care Quality [1] there are interesting comments in the last paragraph.

*"The burden of harm conveyed by the collective impact of all of our health care quality problems is staggering."*
*"Meeting this challenge demands a readiness to think in radically new ways about how to deliver health care services and how to assess and improve their quality. Our present efforts resemble a team of engineers trying to break the sound barrier by tinkering with a Model T Ford. We need a new vehicle. The only unacceptable alternative is not to change."*

Over the last 25 years, the focus of the governments and medical associations has been to expand the ICD using different extensions to gather better statistics and to develop from the ICD the Diagnosis-Related Groups (DRGs) to reimburse hospitals. The American Medical Association developed a series of editions of the Current Procedural Terminology (CPT) to pay for physician services. There was no plan to develop a nomenclature for the basic clinical information of a specific patient that could be used to assess the quality of care given. In that environment it was taken for granted that quality care was being given, until patients and consumer groups began seriously questioning the system. Now there is a crisis.

The delivery of health care can always be improved by informatics, but the quality of health care cannot be improved unless there is an underlying basis of a standardized multilingual medical terminology to specify the data.

Such a standard exists, but it has yet to be recognized by government agencies and is far from being implemented. In 1993, Marion Ball, then President of IMIA, wrote the Foreword to SNOMED International [7]. Here are a few quotes:

*"SNOMED International offers a predefined structured vocabulary, only a few years ago considered an unobtainable goal."*

*"A comprehensive nomenclature, it can serve as the clinical nucleus for a Composite Clinical Data Dictionary ($C^2D^2$) and provide the infrastructure for computerizing the patient record."*

*"As we work towards global health through informatics, standard nomenclature will give us the foundation – the infrastructure – upon which our future health care delivery system will rest. The work contained in these volumes will take us well into the 21$^{st}$ century and lead the way to information when, where, and how ($W^2H$) we need it. I recommend it to you."*

After 1993, there were numerous papers treating the subject of standard nomenclature and some official bodies stated their position.

In a 1997 position paper by the Board of Directors of the American Medical Informatics Association [8], it was stated that a national health information strategy should focus on a series of objectives one of which was standards development.

*"The potential of computer and communications technologies cannot be realized for health care unless a universal language or vocabulary is developed, kept updated and made accessible at minimal cost."*

If it is now recognized that a standard nomenclature reflecting primarily the clinical realities is essential for the delivery of quality care, this same standardized terminology will soon be recognized as essential to the proponents of evidence-based medicine. In a recent white paper (2001) on Clinical Decision Support Systems for the Practice of Evidence-based Medicine [9], the authors propose five central areas of activity, the first being the "capture of both literature-based and practice-based research evidence into machine-interpretable formats suitable for CDSS use."

Although many scientists and scientific societies have now recognized the need for the specificity of a nomenclature for health care, official government agencies have been reluctant to sanction its development. One exception is the National Health Service of the United Kingdom which acquired the Read Codes which were designed for the primary care physician and his practice.

In the United States, nomenclature development began in 1965 with the publication of the Systematized Nomenclature of Pathology (SNOP) by the College of American Pathologists (CAP). The basic multi-axial structure was widely accepted and SNOP was translated into multiple modern languages. The success of this approach was the impetus that led to its extension to all of medicine and the publication of several editions of the Systematized Nomenclature of Medicine.

By 1998, the CAP, with a new team of physicians, nurses and knowledge base experts began developing SNOMED into a reference terminology for the computerized health care record. In 1999, the CAP formed a strategic alliance with the U.K. National Health Service to merge SNOMED with the Clinical Terms derived from the Read Codes into a single English language master edition called SNOMED-CT.

To all those government agencies and scientific associations who have repeatedly stated the need for a nomenclature as a basis for the delivery of quality health care, they should now realize that one has existed for a number of years and that it has now been refined into a computer-compatible health care reference terminology. This terminology is the foundation of the pyramid of documentation (Figure 1) in the health care setting, where over 90% of the data gathered is patient-related.

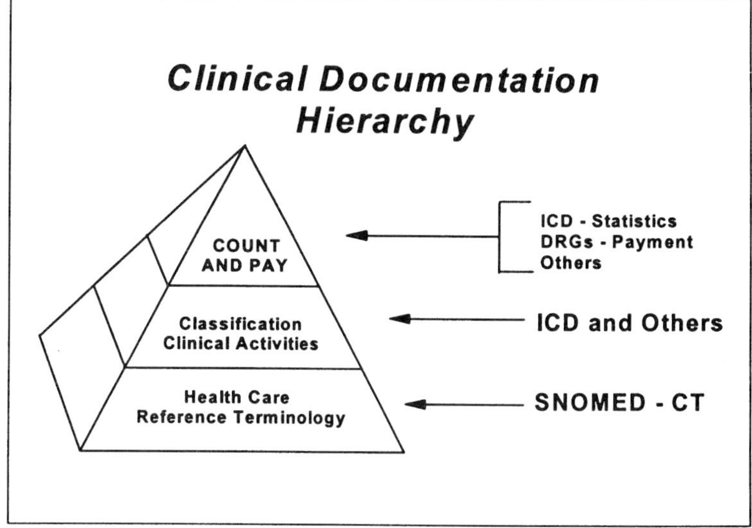


Fig. 1. The pyramidal representation of clinical documentation shows the nomenclature base provided by a controlled clinical terminology. All administrative activities and classifications are derived from solid patient information.

In summary, the computer-capture of coded specific patient information will provide the quality data needed for the delivery of quality health care. Hopefully, the papers gathered in this 2003 Yearbook will further discuss the role of informatics in our collective search for quality health care.

## References


1.  Chassin, MR, Galvin RW and the National Roundtable on Health Care Quality. The Urgent Need to Improve Health Care Quality. JAMA 1998 280(11).
2.  Lohr KN, ed. Medicare: A Strategy for Quality Assurance. Washington, DC. National Academy Press 1990.
3.  Geraci JM, Ashton CM, Kuykendall DH, Johnson ML, Wu L. International Classification of Diseases, 9th Revision, Clinical Modification Codes in Discharge Abstracts are Poor Measures of Complication Occurrence in Medical Inpatients. Med Care 1997;35:589-602.
4.  McCarthy EP, Iezzoni LI, Davis RB, Heather Palmer RH, Cahalane M, Hamel MB, Mukamal K, Phillips RS, Davies DT. Does Clinical Evidence Support ICD-9-CM Diagnosis Coding of Complications? Medicare Care 2000;38:868-876.
5.  McMahon LF, Smits HL. Can Medicare Prospective Payment Survive the ICD-9-CM Disease Classification System? Annuals of Internal Medicine 1986;104:562-566.
6.  National Committee on Vital and Health Statistics. Assuring a Health Dimension for the National Information Infrastructure. Presented to the US Department of Health and Human Services Data Council, 1998 Oct 14.
7.  Côté RA, Rothwell DJ, Palotay JL, Beckett RS, Brochu L. The Systematized Nomenclature of Human and Veterinary Medicine – SNOMED International. College of American Pathologists. Northfield, Illinois 1993 April.
8.  Board of Directors of AMIA. Position Paper: A Proposal to Improve Quality, Increase Efficiency, and Expand Access in the US Health Care System. JAMIA 1997;4:340-341.
9.  Sim I, Gorman P, Greenes RA, Haynes RB, Kaplan B, Lehmann H, Tang PC. Clinical Decision Support Systems for the Practice of Evidence-based Medicine. JAMIA 2001;8:527-534.



Address of the author:

Roger A. Côté, M.D.
President
Secrétariat francophone international
de nomenclature médicale (SFINM)
3001, 12e Avenue Nord
Sherbrooke, Quebec
Canada J1H 5N4
E-mail: Roger.A.Cote@USherbrooke.ca

**Reinhold Haux[1]**
**Casimir A. Kulikowski[2]**
*Editors*

[1] UMIT - University for Health
Informatics and Technology Tyrol
Institute for Health Information Systems
Innsbruck, Austria
Reinhold.Haux@umit.at
[2] Department of Computer Science
Rutgers - The State University
of New Jersey
New Brunswick, New Jersey, USA
kulikows@cs.rutgers.edu

# Editorial

# *Quality of Health Care: The Role of Informatics*

In the Recommendations of the International Medical Informatics Association (IMIA) on Education in Health and Medical Informatics it is stated that:

1 progress in information processing and information and communication technology is changing our societies;

2 the amount of health and medical knowledge is increasing at such a phenomenal rate that we cannot hope to keep up with it, or store, organize and retrieve existing and new knowledge in a timely fashion without using a new information processing methodology and information technologies;

3 there are significant economic benefits to be obtained from the use of information and communication technology to support medicine and health care;

4 similarly the quality of health care is enhanced by the systematic application of information processing and information and communication technology;

5 it is expected, that these developments will continue, probably at least at the same pace as can be observed today"[1].

Following this development we have chosen as topic for the 2003 edition of the IMIA Yearbook of Medical Informatics „Quality of care: The Role of Informatics".

As modern information processing methodology and information and communication technology has strongly influenced our societies, including their health care, we wanted to place strong emphasis on this change. As a consequence of this change, medical informatics as a discipline has taken a leading role in the further development of health care. This involves developing information systems that enhance opportunities for global access to health services and medical knowledge. Informatics methodology and technology will facilitate continuous quality of care in ageing societies, and will decrease the possibilities of health care errors. It enables the dissemination of the latest medical and health information on the web to consumers and health care providers alike.

This year's preface to the Yearbook on „quality health care requires quality patient data" has been prepared by Roger Côté from the University of

---

[1] http://www.imia.org, Methods Inf Med 2000;39:267-77, reprint in IMIA Yearbook of Medical Informatics 2001, 133-143.

Sherbrooke, Canada, the founder of SNOMED. The editors highly appreciate that one of the leaders of our field accepted to write the preface which is devoted to the topic of this Yearbook.

## About the IMIA Yearbook of Medical Informatics

The Yearbook of Medical Informatics of the International Medical Informatics Association (IMIA) is distributed through IMIA's Member and Corresponding Member Societies worldwide. For the 2003 Yearbook we expect that over 7,000 copies will reach the memberships of 44 Member and 13 Corresponding member societies. The Yearbook editors appreciate the contributions of distinguished researchers in medical informatics who have prepared 4 invited review papers, 5 research and education papers, and 9 synopses of papers included in the different disciplinary fields covered. In addition we owe a debt of gratitude to the 67 reviewers who assisted in the selection of papers from the recent refereed literature.

The present Yearbook includes papers selected from the literature for the period April 2001 to March 2002. The criteria for selection include: significance, representativeness and coverage of research in a given subfield, subject to appropriately high levels of quality in presentation and results. A more detailed description of these quality criteria can be downloaded from http://www. Yearbook.uni-hd.de/quality_criteria.pdf. The referees score and rank the papers, and the final selection is made by the editors with the advice of the managing editors from each of the specialty areas.

## In Memoriam Professor Jean-Raoul Scherrer

In 2002 one of the leaders of our field, Professor Jean-Raoul Scherrer,

passed away. A section of this yearbook has been devoted to him in honor of his outstanding contributions to medical informatics.

## IMIA Code of Ethics

After several years of discussion and preparation, the IMIA code of ethics for health informatics professionals was adopted by the IMIA General Assembly at its meeting in Taipei on October 4, 2004.

## Reviews

As is customary, the 2003 Yearbook includes a number of original review articles, which focus primarily on this year's theme. In particular the papers of Marion Ball et al. and Arie Hasman et al. focus on various aspects of the informatics foundations for quality of care. In addition the papers of Grigore Burdea and of Giuseppe Riva survey virtual reality approaches for diagnosis, therapy and rehabilitation.

## Research and Education in Medical Informatics

The Yearbook provides an opportunity for highlighting an international selection of current education, training, and research programs in Medical Informatics. In this 2003 edition authors from Bethesda, Geneva, Osaka, Rotterdam and Thessaloniki summarize their educational and research approaches.

## Challenges in Medical Informatics

In April 2002, an IMIA working conference on challenges in medical informatics took place in Madrid. Selected papers, published as outcome

from this conference, are reprinted here. Mark Musen and Jan van Bemmel, the organizers of this meeting, invite the readers of the Yearbook to comment on these papers.

## Guest Editors

After the selection of papers to be included in the Yearbook was completed, guest editors were asked to write Synopses reviewing the papers in the different sections. The special section on Quality of Health Care was edited by Thomas Bürkle of the University of Münster. The section on Health and Clinical Management was edited by Zhu Ling of Golden Medicine Commodities Network Co., Beijing; that on Patient Records by Johan van der Lei of the Erasmus University of Rotterdam; that on Health Information Systems by Lincoln de Assis Moura Jr. of Atech Foundation, São Paulo; that on Image Processing by Heinz Handels, University of Lübeck; that on Signal Processing by Bernhard Tilg of the University for Health Informatics and Technology Tyrol, Innsbruck; that on Knowledge Processing and Decision Support by Yuval Shahar of Ben Gurion University, Beer Sheva and that on Bioinformatics by Hiroshi Tanaka of Tokyo Medical and Dental University.

## Information on IMIA

The Yearbook contains detailed information about IMIA, its Member Societies, Regional Groups, Working Groups, and Special Interest Groups. Preparation of the general pages describing IMIA activities received considerable assistance from Steve Huesing, the Executive Director. The section on IMIA Working Groups and Special Interest Groups was greatly aided by contributions from Nancy Lorenzi. For the second time a more detailed report on the activities of IMIA regions is included with the help of Regional Editors. We would like to thank Arie Hasman (for EFMI), Sedick Isaacs (for Helina), Jochen Moehr and Charles Safran (for the North American IMIA Member Societies), Chun Por Wong (for APAMI) and Lincoln de Assis Moura, Jr. (for IMIA-Lac) for their support. The IMIA representatives from the individual countries provided the material for their own national societies.

## The 2004 IMIA Yearbook

The theme of the 2004 Yearbook will center around the potential of bioinformatics, in conjunction with medical informatics, to contribute to novel diagnostic and therapeutic approaches in what is often referred to as molecular medicine. The issue will concentrate on clinical implications of research, with the purpose of documenting accomplishments, and encouraging interdisciplinary approaches to the new field of clinical bioinformatics.

## Acknowledgements

The editors gratefully acknowledge the contributions of the Referees and Guest Editors. They would also like to thank the writers of the critical Review Papers and the contributors to the Research and Education Section.

They are most appreciative of the considerable skill, time, and effort devoted by the Managing Editors, especially the Executive Managing Editor Elske Ammenwerth (UMIT - University for Health Informatics and Technology Tyrol, Innsbruck, Austria), and by the Section Managing Editors, Andreas Bohne (German Cancer Research Center, Heidelberg, Germany), Ralf Brandner (University of Heidelberg, Germany), Birgit Brigl (University of Leipzig, Germany), Gerald Fischer (UMIT), Sebastian Garde (University of Heidelberg), Petra Knaup (University of Heidelberg), Franz Ruderich (University of Applied Sciences, Heilbronn, Germany), Rainer Schubert (UMIT), Reiner Singer (University of Applied Sciences, Heilbronn) and Astrid Wolff (University of Heidelberg). Last, but not least, we especially want to thank the Editorial Assistant, Martina Hutter, from the Department of Medical Informatics at the University of Heidelberg, without whose untiring efforts the Yearbook would not have been completed.

The Editors also wish to thank the members of the Advisory Board for their invaluable contributions to the planning of this Yearbook. They are: Marion Ball, Vice-President of Healthlink, Inc. of Baltimore, MD, USA, Jan H. van Bemmel, Rector of Erasmus University Rotterdam, The Netherlands, and Alexa McCray, Director of the Lister Hill Center of the National Library of Medicine, Bethesda, MD, USA.

The referees who contributed to the selection of articles in the 2003 Yearbook of Medical Informatics were:
Jos Aarts, The Netherlands
Ameen Abu-Hanna, The Netherlands
Udo Altmann, Germany
Dominik Aronsky, USA
Suzanne Bakken, USA
Kay Bartholomew, USA
Riccardo Bellazzi, Italy
Marc Berg, The Netherlands
Knut Bernstein, Denmark
Andreas Beß, Austria
Helmar Burkart, Switzerland
Thomas Bürkle, Germany
P.A. de Clercq, The Netherlands
Nicolette de Keizer, The Netherlands
Martin Denz, Switzerland
Jens Dørup, Denmark,
Martin Dugas, Germany

Andrej Fandak, Slovak Republic
Carol Friedman, USA
Dragan Gamberger, Croatia
Antoine Geissbühler, Switzerland
Reda R. Gharieb, Egypt
W.T.F. Goossen, The Netherlands
Stefan Gräber, Germany
Andrew Grant, Canada
James E. Gray, USA
Carolyn J. Green, Canada
Jane Grimson, Ireland
Heinz Handels, Germany
Wilhelm Hasselbring, Germany
Monique Jaspers, The Netherlands
Bonnie Kaplan, USA
Ron Kikinis, USA
György Kozmannn, Hungary
Andy H. Lee, Australia
Thomas Lehmann, Germany
Richard Lenz, Germany
Yu-Chuan (Jack) Li, Taiwan
Ya-bin Liu, Japan
Margarethe Lorensen, Norway
Christian Lovis, Switzerland
Nicos Maglaveras, Greece
John Mantas, Greece
Victor Maojo, Spain
Fernando Martin Sánchez, Spain
Wendy McPhee, Australia
Silvia Miksch, Austria
Peter Moorman, The Netherlands
Peter Murray, United Kingdom
Karl-Peter Pfeiffer, Austria
Andreas Pommert, Germany
Soumya Raychaudhuri, USA
Assa Reichert, Israel
Jeffrey Soar, Australia
Mario Stefanelli, Italy
Robert Stevens, United Kingdom
Selma Supek, Croatia
Ian Symonds, New Zealand
Wilfried Thoben, Germany
Toomas Timpka, Sweden
Mark van Gils, Finland
Michael Vannier, USA
Max Viergever, The Netherlands
Vivian Vimarlund, Sweden
Judith Wagner, Switzerland
Alfred Winter, Germany
Ulrich Woermann, Switzerland

# Central Queensland University
Faculty of Informatics and Communication

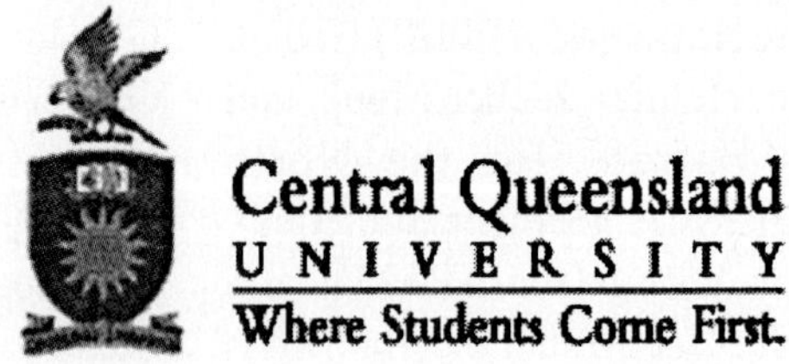


## Locations

Rockhampton, Gladstone, Mackay, Bundaberg, Gold Coast, Brisbane, Melbourne, Sydney, Hong Kong, Singapore, Malaysia, Fiji.

## Vital Statistics

- Central Queensland University was the first Australian University to provide health professionals with timely, educational programs specializing in Health and Nursing Informatics.

- The Graduate Certificate, Diploma and Master of Health Informatics are designed for clinicians, administrators and policy makers to enhance existing skills in information management to improve overall health care performance. Upon completion of graduate health programs, GPs can apply for individual CPD points.

- The Nursing Informatics (post registration) program is specifically tailored to educate and train registered nurses in new technologies to support their areas of practice.

- CQU is an academic institutional member of the International Medical Informatics Association (I.M.I.A). Each Health Informatics degree utilizes IS courses that are part of our existing (ACS accredited) IS programs. Exercises and problem workings are modified for health students to enable them to choose exercises and assignments that have relevance to their industry.

- The Nursing Informatics (Post Registration), Graduate Certificate, Diploma and Master of Health Informatics are available by distance education, which means you can study anywhere in the world.

- CQU's Program Director, Associate Professor Evelyn Hovenga, is leading IMIA's education working group to establish a virtual health, medical and nursing informatics University.

- Due to CQU's participation in various Government and Standards Committees we are able to provide cutting edge learning materials.

## The Overall Picture

Computer, information and telecommunication technologies are increasingly important in the provision of health services. This is because the uses of technologies, including electronic health records, have the potential to improve the efficiency, safety and quality of patient care. The health and nursing informatics programs available through the Faculty of Informatics and Communication provide all health professionals with a sound foundation for expanding their knowledge of the implementation of these technologies to support contemporary health practices.

Individual courses include: Electronic Health Records and Standards, Performance Measurement in Health Care, Health Planning, Policy and Program Evaluation, Health Information Science, Management of Health Services, Advanced Nursing Informatics.

**NB:** The Health and Nursing Informatics programs include courses from other disciplines, enabling students to access specialization in relevant fields.

For further details please visit: http://www.infocom.cqu.edu.au or call 1300 360 444. Intakes commence in March, July and November.

# Information on IMIA

## *International Medical Informatics Association*

### IMIA BOARD
*President*:
K.C. Lun, Singapore,
2002-2004
*Secretary*:
Ian Symonds, New Zealand,
2000-2003
*Treasurer*:
Batami Sadan, Israel
2002-2004

*Vice Presidents*:
MedInfo
Patrice Degoulet, France (2001-2004)
Services
Reinhold Haux, Germany (2002-2005)
Membership
Branko Cesnik, Australia (1999-2003)
Working & Special Interest Groups
Nancy Lorenzi, Canada (2002-2003)
Special Services
Charles Safran, United States (2000-2004)
*IMIA Executive Director:*
Steven A. Huesing, Canada

IMIA Web site: www.imia.org

## *Regional Groups*

*EFMI: European Federation for Medical Informatics*
*Liaison*:
Rolf Engelbrecht, Germany

*IMIA-LAC: Federation of Health Societies in Latin America*
*President*:
Lincoln de Assis Moura, Brazil

*APAMI: Asian Pacific Association for Medical Informatics*
*President*:
C.P. Wong, Hong Kong

*African Region:*
*Coordinator*:
Sedick S. Isaacs, South Africa

**WELCOME TO IMIA!**

### General

The International Medical Informatics Association is an independent organization established under Swiss law in 1989. The organization was established in 1967 as Technical Committee 4 of the International Federation for Information Processing (IFIP). In 1979, it evolved from a Special Interest Group of IFIP to its current status as a fully independent organization. IMIA continues to maintain its relationship with IFIP as an affiliate organization.

The organization also has close ties with the World Health Organization (WHO) as a NGO (Non Government Organization).

The working language of IMIA is English.

### Purpose, Goals, Objectives

IMIA plays a major global role in the application of information science and technology in the fields of healthcare and research in medical, health and bio informatics. The basic goals and objectives of the association are to:

- promote informatics in health care and research in health, bio and medical informatics;
- advance and nurture international cooperation;
- to stimulate research, development and routine application;
- move informatics from theory into practice in a full range of health delivery settings, from physician's office to acute and long term care;
- further the dissemination and exchange of knowledge, information and technology;
- promote education and responsible behaviour; and
- represent the medical and health informatics field with the World Health Organization and other international professional and governmental organizations.

In its function as a bridge organization, IMIA's goals are:

- moving theory into practice by linking academic and research informaticians with care givers, consultants, vendors, and vendor-based researchers;
- leading the international medical and health informatics communities throughout the 21st century;
- promoting the cross-fertilization of health informatics information and knowledge across professional and geographical boundaries; and
- serving as the catalyst for ubiquitous worldwide health information infrastructures for patient care and health research.

### Membership

IMIA membership consists of National, Institutional and Affiliate Members and Honorary Fellows.

*National Members* represent individual countries. A member is a society, a group of societies, or an appropriate body, which is representative of the medical, and health informatics activities within that country. Where no representative societies exist, IMIA accommodates involvement through "Correspondent" members within developing countries.

National IMIA members may organize into regional groups. Currently, such regions exist for Latin America and the Caribbean (IMIA LAC), Europe (EFMI), Asia/Pacific (APAMI) and Africa (Helina).

*Institutional Members* consist of corporate and academic members. Corporate members include vendor, consulting, technology firms as well as national professional organizations. Academic members include universities, medical centres, research centres and like institutions.

*Affiliate Members* consist of international organizations that share an interest in the broad field of health and medical informatics, and in addition to the WHO and IFIP includes the International Federation of Health Records Organizations (IFHRO).

*Honorary Fellows* are individuals who have earned exceptional merit in furthering

<table><tr><td>

*International Medical Informatics Association (Continued)*

</td><td>

the aims and interests of the IMIA; fellowship is conferred for life. In 2002 the honour of fellowship was awarded to Prof. Jan H. van Bemmel, immediate past president of IMIA for his many years of meritorious service to IMIA and the medical informatics community in general.

**Governance**

IMIA is governed by its General Assembly that consists of one representative from each IMIA National and Institutional member, Honorary Fellows, Chairs of IMIA's Working Groups and a representative from IFIP, the World Health Organization, and each of IMIA's Regions. Only National Members have full voting rights. The General Assembly meets annually.

The Board of IMIA, elected by the General Assembly, conducts the association's affairs. The day-to-day operations are supported by the IMIA's Executive Director who is also responsible for IMIA's electronic services.

The officers of the Board and IMIA's vice presidents vigorously pursue IMIA's mission to:

- Monitor the range of special interest areas and focus support on new developments.
- Capitalize on the synergies and collective resources of IMIA's constituents.
- Minimize fragmentation between scientific and professional medical informaticians.
- Ensure successful adaptation to changes in the medical informatics marketplace and discipline.
- Raise the profile and awareness of IMIA within and outside of the IMIA organization.
- Encourage cooperation between the scientific and commercial health informatics communities.
- Equitably balance support to emerging and existing IMIA members.
- Establish and maintain cooperation and harmony with organizations that emerge to address medical informatics issues.
- Continue to position IMIA as the gatekeeper for medical informatics issues in the international community.

</td><td>

**Activities**
### *MEDInfo's*

IMIA organizes the internationally acclaimed tri-annual "*World Congress on Medical and Health Informatics*", MEDInfo. MEDInfo 2001, held in London, UK, September 2 - 5, 2001 at the newly developed Docklands area was hosted by the British Computer Society: Health Informatics Specialist Group. It was a highly successful scientific event.

MedINFO 2004 will be held at the Hilton Hotel in San Francisco, USA on September 7 – 11, 2004. Potential participants and exhibitors are encouraged to visit their web site at www.medinfo2004.org. The American Medical Informatics Association (AMIA) is the hosting society for MedInfo 2004.

Bids for MedInfo 2007 are currently being solicited.

Previous MedInfos have been held in Stockholm (1974), Toronto (1977), Tokyo (1980), Amsterdam (1983), Washington (1986), Beijing/Singapore (1989), Geneva (1992), Vancouver (1995) and Seoul (1998).

### *Working and Special Interest Groups*

The IMIA family includes a growing number of Working and Special Interest Groups, which consist of individuals who share common interests in a particular focal field. The groups hold Working Conferences on leading edge and timely health and medical informatics issues.

Current and future activities of the Working and Special Interest Groups are posted on the IMIA Website at www.imia.org

**Activities and Initiatives**

IMIA code of Ethics

IMIA reached a major milestone by the adoption of the "IMIA Code of Ethics for Health Information Professionals". The approval of the code was the culmination of years of ongoing effort on the part of IMIA's Working Group on Data Protection in Health Information Systems under the leadership of Prof. Ab Bakker (The

</td></tr></table>

## International Medical Informatics Association (Continued)

Netherlands). The primary author of the code, based on the contributions of a multiplicity of individuals, agencies and organizations, is Dr. Eike-Henner W. Kluge (Canada). The code, currently being translated into several languages is freely available to the public at IMIA's website www.imia.org.

IMIA-UMIT Medical Informatics Award of Excellence

Through the generosity of TILAK, one of IMIA's Corporate Institutional members, IMIA approved the creation of the IMIA-UMIT Medical Informatics Award of Excellence. The Award will given every three years jointly by IMIA and the Private University of Health Informatics and Technology Tyrol (UMIT) to an individual whose personal commitment and dedication to Medical Informatics has made a lasting contribution to medicine and health care through her or his achievements in research, education, development or application in the field of medical informatics. The Award includes a Diploma, a cash prize and the opportunity to give the IMIA/UMIT Medical Informatics Award Lecture at a plenary session at MedInfo 2004.

HELINA 2003- Communication and Information Technology in the Fight against HIV/AIDS in Africa

HELINA 2003 conference in South African in the fall of 2003 will primarily focus on communication and information technologies in the fight against HIV/AIDS. Under the leadership of Dr. Charles Safran, IMIA VP of Services, IMIA, the South African Health Informatics Association, Harvard Medical International, the National Library of Medicine (USA), the Medical Research Council of South Africa, and the Center for Disease Control and Prevention (USA) will jointly sponsor the conference.

This conference is in accordance with the focal vision of IMIA president KC Lun for IMIA to focus on "bridging the knowledge gap" by facilitating and providing support to developing nations. Specific goals include supporting the ongoing development of the African Region, and, on a broader basis, the development of the "Virtual University", an ongoing initiative of IMIA's working group on Health and Medical Informatics Education.

IMIA continues to develop its communication capabilities through its web-site www.imia.org. The site now contains profiles on its members, working groups and activities. The site uses a dynamic database to facilitate user-friendly communications for news, announcements, and an events calendar for the public, and access to e-mail communications, minutes, reports and association information for its members.

In addition, IMIA has reached an agreement with one of its corporate members, Schattauer GmbH, whereby *Methods of Information in Medicine,* publishes IMIA news and a Calendar of events in each issue of the journal.

IMIA is constantly striving to further the services it provides to its members and the informatics community in general by promoting free interaction among and between its member network and the medical and health informatics community at large.

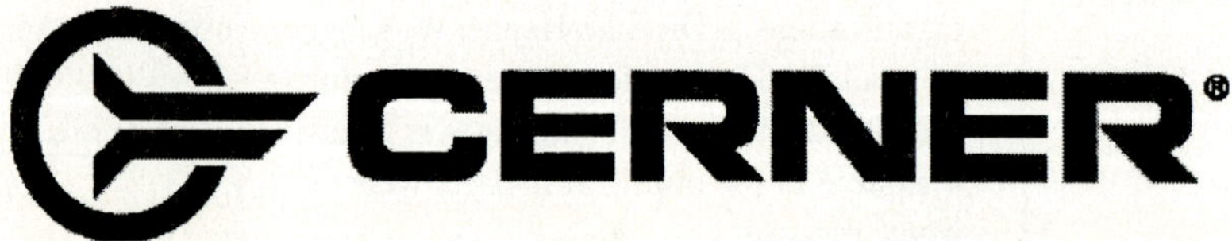

Cerner Corporation is an information technology company that is transforming health care across the globe. Our sophisticated software helps health care professionals speed diagnosis, eliminate medical errors, reduce variance and improve revenue tracking. We equip caregivers with the critical information they rely on to make smarter decisions. We empower consumers to more easily access the health care system, manage their records and diseases, and contribute to a healthier community. Simply put, our innovations save time, save money and, most importantly, save lives.

Clients around the world realize significant returns on their investment in Cerner products. Our solutions eliminate millions of dollars in waste and inefficiencies, helping clients reduce their costs and increase profitability, all while improving the quality of care.

Cerner believed so strongly in the vision for health care transformation that we overhauled the foundation of our product line in the mid-1990s. With the passion of entrepreneurs, Cerner has invested seven years and more than $400 million to create Cerner Millennium.™

Today Cerner Millennium is the only architecture on the market that can seamlessly deliver clinical and financial information to virtually every point in the health care system. Our vision is transforming the way health systems care for you today and will care for you for generations to come.

# Progress Report by the President of IMIA

*President:*
Kwok Chan Lun
Professor and Vice Dean
School of Biological Sciences
Nanyang Technologcial University
Singapore
E-mail: kclun@ntu.edu.sg

This report of the President of IMIA covers the period between the General Assembly meeting held during MEDINFO 2001 in London, September 2001 and the General Assembly held in Taipei, China in October 2002.

## Report of the President

A year has passed since I assumed the IMIA Presidency at the Closing Ceremony of MEDINFO 2001 in London last September. I am happy to present to you my first President's Report to the General Assembly.

### 1. *In Memoriam* – Professor Jean-Raoul Scherrer

In March this year, the international medical informatics community was saddened by news of the passing of Professor Jean-Raoul Scherrer of Geneva, Switzerland. Jean-Raoul was a very dear and outstanding IMIA colleague and friend. I was proud to have been acquainted with this extraordinarily knowledgeable friend since 1989. Those of us who knew Jean-Raoul and had the privilege of working with him on medical informatics projects and IMIA activities would, no doubt, feel the deep sense of loss of a caring friend and loyal IMIA colleague. Jean-Raoul would be best remembered for his key contributions to medical informatics including DIOGENE, the HON Foundation, the EFMI Presidency and his IMIA contributions as Chair of MEDINFO 92 OC, representative of EFMI, IFIP and VP Working Groups and SIGs.

### 2. MEDINFO 2001

IMIA has just received the final account statement from the MEDINFO 2001 Organizing Committee and I am happy to report to you that Conference had been a success. Over 1300 delegates from some 74 countries attended the congress. In support of encouraging more participants from developing countries to attend the Conference, the OC disbursed some $38,000 for bursaries, about $18,000 more than originally budgeted. Under the contractual arrangements made with the London OC, IMIA will receive $62,745.35 covering profit-sharing arrangements for registration fees, tutorials, and exhibitions.

All of the members of the Organizing Committee, chaired by Jean Roberts, the Scientific Program Committee co-chaired by Arie Hasman and Hiroshi Takeda and the Editorial Committee chaired by Vimla Patel and comprising Ray Rogers and Reinhold Haux deserve our warmest congratulations on a job well done. We also wish to express our heartfelt thanks and appreciation to all, including the delegates, exhibitors and volunteers, who had contributed to the success of MEDINFO 2001.

As all of you know, shortly after the London conference came the terrible September 11 terrorist attacks in the USA that left a very lasting impact on the world economy and caused upheavals in travel activities and work plans. We were indeed fortunate that MEDINFO took place before September 11, as otherwise the impact on the conference would have been disastrous.

### 3. MEDINFO 2004

Preparations for MEDINFO 2004 in San Francisco are already making very good progress. Appointments of the OC chair, the SPC co-chairs and the EC have already been made. VP (Medinfo) Dr Patrice Degoulet, in consultation with the MEDINFO Steering Committee, the MEDINFO 2004 OC and SPC chairs, various WG and SIG chairs as well as national representatives, have completed the full composition of the SPC and the EC. These appointments have been given the full endorsement of the IMIA Board.

The MEDINFO contract between IMIA and AMIA has also been signed. I have no doubt that with their track record and experience with organizing the AMIA conferences, the AMIA secretariat and the MEDINFO 2004 OC will give us a memorable and highly successful MEDINFO. We can confidently look forward to a good conference in San Francisco in 2004.

### 4. Bridging the Medical Informatics Divide

In my inaugural address in London last September, I had pledged to work towards the bridging of the medical informatics divide during the tenure of my presidency.

*Progress Report by the President of IMIA (Continued)*

Key initiatives will include: (a) HELINA 2002 and the African regional group and (b) the Virtual University of Medical Informatics.

### (a) Helina 2002

Highest priority of these initiatives was the convening of HELINA 2002 and initiation of efforts to form the African regional group to intensify the promotion of our IMIA activities in Africa. Prior to the last MEDINFO meeting in London, I had contacted Omar El Hattab of Egypt to provide the local organization for Helina 2002 in Cairo and this was followed by some very enthusiastic discussions during MEDINFO at the WG9 workshop on Health Informatics for Development. Unfortunately, events following the Conference such as the September 11 attacks and the continuing political crises in the Middle East made it virtually impossible to organize Helina 2002 in Cairo, as originally planned.

Under the leadership of Dr Charles Safran, VP (Special Affairs) IMIA is now sponsoring an initiative to incorporate a Helina meeting within a 3-day conference in South Africa in 2003 on the use of IT in the global fight against HIV/AIDS. The initiative will be driven by IMIA in association with the South African Health Informatics Association (SAHIA), the Harvard Medical School and Harvard Medical International. Already, Dr Safran has secured sponsorship from the National Library of Medicine and the CDC and other international organizations.

### (b) Virtual University

In my Inaugural Address I expressed my commitment to supporting the Virtual University initiative, spearheaded by WG1 and its two co-chairs, Dr. Evelyn Hovenga and Dr. John Mantas. There was an active workshop to discuss the initiative at MEDINFO but little progress appears to have been made since then. A website to facilitate the establishment of the planned Virtual University is expected to be announced soon.

### (c) e-Lectures in Medical Informatics

In parallel with the Virtual University initiative by WG1, I am also working on a project to launch "e-Lectures in Medical Informatics". This project is modeled after the University of Pittsburgh "Supercourse" (http://www.pitt.edu/~super1/) on Epidemiology, the Internet and Global Health which features a global academic faculty to develop and freely share their best and most passionate lectures in the area of public health and Internet on the Web so as to give teachers and students in developing countries an opportunity to access information and knowledge which would not normally be available to them.

For this initiative, we will invite experts in our field, particularly from among the resources within our own organization, to contribute their lectures on a full range of medical informatics topics. These will be stored on a server from where users can freely access them as 'lecture-on-demand' if they have the bandwidth. Alternatively, just like the Supercourse, a CD of the lectures will be cut and distributed FOC worldwide.

The Taiwan Association of Medical Informatics (TAMI) under the leadership of Professor Prof. Jack Li is very keen to assist IMIA spearheading this project and will provide the resources and manpower to digitize and disseminate lectures without charge.

### 5. Promoting IMIA internationally

We continue to maintain our relationship with the World Health Organization as an NGO and were invited by WHO to attend the World Health Assembly in Geneva as well as assemblies of its regional offices. Wherever possible, IMIA makes arrangements for its national representatives in the countries where these meetings are held to represent the President and IMIA as observers.

We also continue to maintain our traditionally strong ties with IFIP and appointed Mr. Gilles Laporte, the newly-elected Director of COACH: Canada's Health Informatics Association, to represent IMIA at the IFIP General Assembly in Montreal in September 2002.

### 6. Changes in the Nomination Process for IMIA Executive Board Membership

In deference to the wishes of IMIA national members, I have recommended to the Nominations Committee, beginning at this General Assembly, that they allow our members to be consulted in the selection process of filling vacancies on the IMIA

## Progress Report by the President of IMIA (Continued)

Board. Prior to the convening of this General Assembly, the Executive Director's office had sent out notices on behalf of the Nominating Committee to all national representatives to invite nominations of individuals to fill these posts. We were encouraged by the response. The list of nominees received was scrutinized by the Nominating Committee and short-listed individuals will be presented at this General Assembly, based on their professional and/or scientific experience in health and medical informatics and a working knowledge on operational aspects of IMIA.

### 7. Code of Ethics for Health Information Professionals

The Code of Ethics to be presented at this General Assembly meeting for final review and approval represents yet another landmark achievement on the part of IMIA working groups.

At the last meeting of the IMIA General Assembly in London, IMIA Working Group 4 on Data Protection in Health Information submitted a draft Code of Ethics for Health Information Professionals. There was general concurrence that the Group continue to review the document and seek additional comments and input from IMIA's National member societies and other interested parties. That process has now been completed. In addition to the "code", a detailed handbook of explanations that go along with the principles and clauses of the code will be presented. Plans are already underway for translation of the code into several languages.

Dr. Eike-Henner W. Kluge, Professor, Department of Philosophy, University of Victoria, Victoria, BC, Canada, will make the presentation to the General Assembly on behalf of the Working Group, and the many individuals and organizations who have contributed to the code. It is my privilege to thank Dr. Kluge, Prof. Ab Bakker, the Chair of WG4, and their colleagues for this outstanding contribution to our field.

### 8. IMIA Guidelines for Conference/Meeting Support or Sponsorship

From time to time, IMIA receives requests from within the organization (e.g. Working Groups/SIG, regional groups) as well as outside the organization for support or sponsorship of meetings/conferences. As we need clear guidelines to decide on the degree and extent of support of these activities, I have asked Mr. Steven Huesing, our Executive Director, to draw up a set of guidelines that will be presented for discussion at this General Assembly.

### 9. Congratulations to Dr Marion Ball

On behalf of the IMIA community, I would like to extend our heartiest congratulations to Dr Marion Ball, our former IMIA President (1992-95) for being chosen as the 2002 recipient of the Morris F. Collen Award of Excellence. The award is given annually by the American College of Medical Informatics (ACMI) to an individual who has "shown leadership and made significant contributions to medical informatics".

### 10. Working with the Executive Director and the Secretariat

Over the past 12 months of my presidency, I have been maintaining close contact with Steven Huesing, our Executive Director and the IMIA secretariat via emails. I have also implemented a monthly teleconference with Steven to discuss matters that could not be easily done over a few lines of email. This has proven to be very effective.

Finally, I wish to thank our Executive Director, Board Members as well as IMIA colleagues and friends for your support to enable me to complete the first 12 months of my term and to achieve some of the early goals that I have outlined for the tenure of my presidency. I look forward to your continued support so that, together, we can continue to build IMIA as a truly international organization in support of health and medical informatics.

# HiMSS®

## *Healthcare Information and Management Systems Society*

The Healthcare Information and Management Systems Society (HIMSS) provides leadership in healthcare for the advancement and management of information technology. Headquartered in Chicago, HIMSS provides services to more than 13,000 members, including IT healthcare corporations, firms and professionals from around the globe. Through the collaboration of over 40 chapters and 20 special interest groups, HIMSS directs and shapes the healthcare industry, encourages emerging technology and promotes public policies that will improve healthcare delivery.

HIMSS focuses on the following:

- **Industry Intelligence**

  As the central source for healthcare management and technology intelligence, HIMSS provides the resources and tools to efficiently provide healthcare information. Through its premier Annual Conference, a Web-based solutions tool, and collaborative industry research, HIMSS provides industry intelligence that assists organizations and companies in reaching their strategic goals.

- **Industry Affairs**

  By actively advising the government on issues and policies related to healthcare information, HIMSS is the recognized expert on legislation, regulations, policies, standards and practices.

- **Professional Development**

  HIMSS provides career development programs and services to educate, advance, and recognize professionals in the healthcare IT industry. Web-based education, publications, and certification programs help executives and healthcare professionals succeed in their careers.

- **Community Affiliations**

  HIMSS is the organization that links its members to the industry. Through member relations, Chapters and Special Interest Groups, HIMSS helps build prominent networks and brings the healthcare community closer.

**For more information, visit HIMSS at <u>www.himss.org</u>.**

# *National and Corresponding Members*

*National Members*

| | |
|---|---|
| Argentina | Argentine Association of Medical Informatics |
| Australia | Health Informatics Society of Australia Ltd. |
| Austria | Austrian Computer Society Working Group Medical Informatics |
| Belgium | Belgian Society for Medical Informatics |
| Bosnia & Herzegovina | Society for Medical Informatics of Bosnia and Herzegovina |
| Brazil | Brazilian Society of Health Informatics |
| Canada | COACH: Canada's Health Informatics Association |
| China | China Medical Informatics Association |
| Croatia | Croation Society for Medical Informatics |
| Cuba | Cuban Society of Medical Informatics |
| Czech Republic | Czech Society for Biomedical Engineering and Medical Informatics |
| Denmark | Danish Society for Medical Informatics |
| Finland | Finnish Social and Health Informatics Association |
| Georgia | Georgian Association of Medical Informatics and Biomedical Engineering (Observer Status) |
| France | Association pour les Applications de l'Informatique à la Médecine |
| Germany | German Association for Medical Informatics, Biometry and Epidemiology |
| Hong Kong | Hong Kong Society of Medical Informatics |
| Hungary | Biomedical Section of John von Neumann Society for Computing Sciences |
| Ireland | Healthcare Informatics Society of Ireland |
| Israel | The Israeli Association for Medical Informatics |
| Italy | Italian Medical Informatics Society |
| Japan | Japan Association for Medical Informatics |
| Kazakstan | Kazakstan MedPharmInfo Association |
| Korea | The Korea Society of Medical Informatics |
| Mexico | Assucion Mexicana de Informatica Medica (Observer Status) |
| Netherlands | VMBI, Society for Healthcare Informatics |
| New Zealand | Health Informatics New Zealand |
| Norway | The Norwegian Society for Medical Informatics |
| Peru | Peruvian Health Informatics Association (Observer Status) |
| Philippines | Philippine Medical Informatics Society, Inc. |
| Poland | Polish Society of Medical Informatics |
| Romania | Romanian Society for Medical Informatics |
| Singapore | Association of Informatics in Medicine |
| Slovak Republic | Slovak Society for Biomedical Engineering and Medical Informatics |
| Slovenia | Slovenian Medical Informatics Society |
| South Africa | South African Health Informatics Association |
| Spain | Spanish Society of Health Informatics |
| Sweden | Swedish Federation for Medical Informatics |
| Switzerland | Swiss Society for Medical Informatics |
| Turkey | Turkish Medical Informatics Association |
| Ukraine | The Ukrainian Association for Computer Medicine (Observer Status) |
| United Kingdom | British Computer Society Health Informatics Committee |
| Uruguay | Uruguay Society of Medical Informatics |
| USA | American Medical Informatics Association |

*Corresponding Members*

Armenia, Botswana, Chile, Egypt, India, Iran, Malaysia, Moldova, Saudi Arabia, Syria, Tanzania, United Arab Emirates, Venezuela

# *Institutional Members*

## CORPORATE MEMBERS

**American Health Information Management Association (AHIMA)**
Chicago, IL - USA                    *Advertorial see page X*

**Cerner Corporation**
Kansasa City, MO - USA               *Advertorial see page 12*

**Covansys** (Formerly Complete Business Solutions, Inc.)
Farmington Hilss, MI - USA

**DynCorp**
Reston, VA - USA

**Elsevier Science, Health Sciences Division (Provisional)**
London - UK

**Healthcare Informatics, McGraw-Hill Healthcare Information Group**
Minneapolis, MN - USA

**Healthcare Information & Management Systems Society (HIMSS)**
Chicago, IL - USA                    *Advertorial see page 16*

**HISCOM - Health Information Solutions**
Leerbroek - The Netherlands

**Lippincott Williams & Wilkins**
Philadelphia, PA - USA

**Schattauer GmbH**
Stuttgart - Germany

**Siemens Medical Solutions**
Erlangen - Germany

**TILAK Tiroler Landeskrankeanstalten GmbH**
Innsbruck - Austria                  *Advertorial see page 24*

**Wolters Kluwer International Healthcare Publishing**
Philiadelphia, PA - USA

## ACADEMIC MEMBERS

**Academic Medical Center (AMC)**
Amsterdam - The Netherlands

**Central Queensland University**
Rockhampton, NSW - Australia         *Advertorial see page 8*

**Centre for Health Information, Research and Development**
Winchester - UK

**Centre for Healthcare Informatics, University College Dublin**
Dublin - Ireland

**Erasmus University Rotterdam**
Rotterdam - The Netherlands

**Galil Center for Telemedicine and Medical Informatics**
Haifa - Israel

**Georg-August-University Goettingen**
Goettingen - Germany

**Medical Informatics Foundation (Fundacion de Informatica Medica)**
Buenos Aires - Argentina

**Monash University**
Victoria, Australia

**National and Kapodistrian University of Athens**
Athens - Greece

**National Cancer Institute**
Bethesda, MD - USA

**NHS Information Authority - England**
United Kingdom

**Oregon Health & Science University (Provisional)**
Portland, OR - USA

**Stanford University School of Medicine**
Stanford, CA - USA

*Institutional
Members
(Continued)*

**Taiwan Association for Medical Informatics**
Taipei -Taiwan

**Tasmanian University Department of Rural Health**
Launceston, Tasmania - Australia

**University for Health Informatics and Technology Tyrol (UMIT)**
Innsbruck - Austria                    *Advertorial see page 58*

**University of Heidelberg**
Heidelberg - Germany                   *Advertorial see page 106*

**University of Maryland**
Baltimore, MD - USA

**University of Sydney**
Sydney - Australia                     *Advertorial see page 20*

**University of Victoria, School of Health Information Science**
Victoria, BC - Canada

**University of Waterloo**
Waterloo, ON - Canada

**University of Wollongong**
Wollongong, NSW - Australia


**Yearbook Advertorial**

IMIA Institutional Member are offered the opportunity to publish an advertorial, i.e. a corporate description of their institute's or company's activities linked to Medical Informatics in the IMIA Yearbook. The number of the page on which you can find an advertorial of an institutional member is indicated on the list of institutional members (see above).

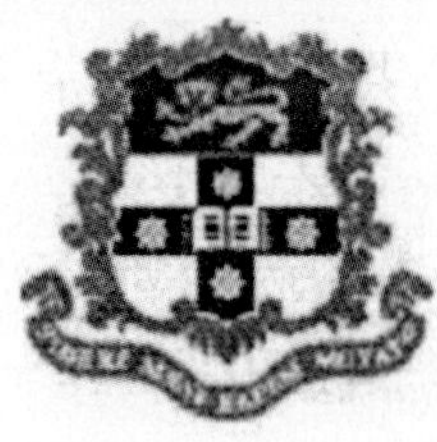

# The University of Sydney

# Master of Health Science (Health Informatics)

## Why Health Informatics?
The field of health informatics is one of the fastest growing areas within the health sector. Exciting career opportunities are emerging for health professionals with knowledge and skills in information technology, management and health care systems. In response to industry demands, The University of Sydney has developed a Master of Health Science in Health Informatics.

## About the Course
The Master of Health Science (Health Informatics) is designed to provide graduates with a theoretical and practical understanding of the role of information and communication technologies in health care and the skills required for the successful integration of such technologies into the health system. The course focuses on three central knowledge areas:
- Principles and applications of health informatics
- Database management systems and the classification of data
- Managing the integration of health informatics within the health care environment

## Course Structure and Delivery
The course is offered on a one-year full-time basis over two semesters, or a two-year part-time basis covering four semesters. The units of study in the program are delivered flexibly with most units offered in 3 - 4 day on-campus workshop format. The option of an additional Honours year is available.

## Who Should Consider this Course?
The course is suitable for health professionals who wish to enhance their understanding and ability to work effectively with information and information technologies. The course is also designed for those graduates who wish to pursue a career as a health informatics specialist. In order to qualify for admission applicants should have:

i)      a bachelor's degree from an Australian tertiary institution or equivalent; or
ii)     experience and/or qualifications as deemed appropriate by the Head of School.

## Contact us for More Information

**School of Health Information Management**
Faculty of Health Sciences
The University of Sydney
PO Box 170
Lidcombe  NSW  1825, Australia

Phone: +61 2 9351 9494
Fax: +61 2 9351 9672
Email: himinfo@fhs.usyd.edu.au
**www.fhs.usyd.edu.au/him**

# Publications

## MEDINFO Proceedings


Anderson J, Forsythe JM, editors. MEDINFO 74. Amsterdam: North-Holland; 1974

Shires DB, Wolf H, editors. MEDINFO 77. Amsterdam: North-Holland ; 1977.

Lindberg DAB, Kaihara S, editors. MEDINFO 80. Amsterdam: North-Holland; 1980.

Van Bemmel JH, Ball MJ, Wigertz O, editors. MEDINFO 83. Amsterdam: North-Holland; 1983.

Salamon R, Blum BI, Jørgensen M, editors. MEDINFO 86. Amsterdam: North-Holland; 1986.

Barber B, Cao D, Qin D, Wagner G, editors. MEDINFO 89. Amsterdam: North-Holland; 1989.

Lun KC, Degoulet P, Piemme TE, Rienhoff O, editors. MEDINFO 92. Amsterdam: North-Holland; 1992.

Greenes RA, Peterson HE, Protti DJ, editors. MEDINFO 95. Amsterdam: North-Holland; 1995.

Cesnik B, McCray AT, Scherrer J-R, editors. MEDINFO 98. Amsterdam: IOS Press; 1998.

Patel V, Rogers R, Haux R, editors. MEDINFO 01. Amsterdam: IOS Press; 2001


## Yearbooks of Medical Informatics


Van Bemmel JH, McCray AT, editors. 1992 Yearbook of Medical Informatics: Advances in an Interdisciplinary Science. Stuttgart: Schattauer; 1992.

Van Bemmel JH, McCray AT, editors. 1993 Yearbook of Medical Informatics: Sharing Knowledge and Information. Stuttgart: Schattauer; 1993.

Van Bemmel JH, McCray AT, editors. 1994 Yearbook of Medical Informatics: Advanced Communications in Health Care. Stuttgart: Schattauer; 1994.

Van Bemmel JH, McCray AT, editors. 1995 Yearbook of Medical Informatics: The Computer-based Patient Record. Stuttgart: Schattauer; 1995.

Van Bemmel JH, McCray AT, editors. 1996 Yearbook of Medical Informatics: The Integration of Information for Patient Care. Stuttgart: Schattauer; 1996.

Van Bemmel JH, McCray AT, editors. 1997 Yearbook of Medical Informatics: Computing and Collaborative Care. Stuttgart: Schattauer; 1997.

Van Bemmel JH, McCray AT, editors. 1998 Yearbook of Medical Informatics: Health Informatics and the Internet. Stuttgart: Schattauer; 1998.

Van Bemmel JH, McCray AT, editors. 1999 Yearbook of Medical Informatics: The Promise of Medical Informatics. Stuttgart: Schattauer; 1999.

Van Bemmel JH, McCray AT, editors. 2000 Yearbook of Medical Informatics: Patient-centered Systems. Stuttgart: Schattauer; 2000.

Haux R, Kulikowski C, editors. 2001 Yearbook of Medical Informatics: Digital Libraries and Medicine. Stuttgart: Schattauer; 2001.

Haux R, Kulikowski C, editors. 2002 Yearbook of Medical Informatics: Digital Libraries and Medicine. Stuttgart: Schattauer; 2002.


## Conference Proceedings


Peterson HE, Isaksson AI. Communication networks in health care. Amsterdam: North Holland; 1982 ISBN0444865136

Scholes M, Bryant Y, Barber B. *The Use of Computers in Nursing.* London, UK; 1982. ISBN-0-444-866-825

Cote RA, Protti DJ, Scherrer JR. Role of informatics in health data coding and classification systems. Amsterdam: North Holland; 1985 ISBN0444876820

Hannah KJ, Guillemin EJ, Conklin DN. *Nursing Uses of Computers and Science,* Calgary, Canada. Amsterdam: Elsevier North Holland; 1985. ISBN-0-444-87904-8

Van Bemmel JH, Gremy F, Zvarova J. Medical decision making: diagnostic strategies and expert systems. Amsterdam: North Holland; 1985 ISBN0444878408

Harris EK, Yasaka T. Maintaining a healthy state within the individual. Amsterdam: North Holland; 1986 ISBN 0444702709

Peterson HE, Gerdin-Jelger U, editors. *Preparing Nurses for Using Information Systems* (Working conference) 1986 Stockholm, Sweden. N.Y.: National League for Nursing; 1987. ISBN-0-88737-416-6

Willems JL, Van Bemmel JH, Michel J. Progress in computer/assisted function analysis. Amsterdam: North Holland; 1987 ISBN0444703845

Daley N. and Hannah KJ. *Proceedings of the Third International Symposium on Nursing Use of Computers and Information Science.* 1988 Dublin, Ireland. St. Louis: Mosby; 1988. ISBN-0-8016-3258-8

Bakker AR, Ball MJ, Scherrer JR, Willems JL, editors. *Towards new hospital information systems.* Amsterdam: North-Holland; 1988.

Hayes GM, Robinson N, editors. *Primary Care Computing.* Amsterdam: Elsevier Science Publ (North Holland); 1990.

Ozbolt JG, Vandewal D, Hannah KJ. *Decision Support Systems in Nursing.* (Working conference) 1988 Dublin, Ireland. St. Louis Mosby; 1990. ISBN-0-8016-3236-6

Hovenga EJS, Hannah KJ, McCormick KA, Ronald JS. *Nursing Informatics '91.* Melbourne, Australia, Berlin: Springer-Verlag; 1991. ISBN-3-540-53869-0 / ISBN-0-387-53869-0

Marr PB, Axford RL, Newbold SK. *Health Care Information Technology; Implications*

# *Publications (Continued)*


*for Change.* (Post conference) Melbourne, Australia, 1991. Berlin: Springer-Verlag; 1991. ISBN-3-540-54124-1 / ISBN-0-387-54124-1

Turley J. P and Newbold S. K. *Nursing Informatics '91: Preconference Proceedings* (Preconference) Melbourne, Australia 1991. Berlin: Springer-Verlag; 1991.

Van Bemmel JH, Zvárová J, editors. *Knowledge, Information and Medical Education.* Amsterdam: Elsevier Science Publ (North-Holland); 1991.

Timmers T, Blum B, editors. *Software Engineering in Medical Informatics.* Amsterdam: Elsevier Science Publ (North-Holland); 1991.

Duisterhout JS, Salamon R, Hasman A, editors. *Telematics in Medicine.* Amsterdam: Elsevier Science Publ (North-Holland); 1991.

Bakker AR, Ehlers CT, Bryant JR, Hammond WE, editors. *Hospital Information Systems: Scope-Design-Architecture.* Amsterdam: Elsevier Science Publ (North-Holland); 1992.

Williams BT, Collen MF, Schmidt RM, editors. *Special Issue on International Health Evaluation* (IHEA/IMIA). Meth Inform Med 1993;32:187-264.

Haux R, Leven FJ, Moehr JR, Protti D, editors. *Special issue on Health and Medical Informatics Education.* Heidelberg/Heilbronn, Germany. Methods Inf Med 1993;34/3.

Mandil SH, Moidu K, Korpela M, Byass P, Forster D, editors. *Health Informatics in Africa - HELINA '93.* Amsterdam: Elsevier Science Publ (North Holland); 1993.

Van Gennip EMSJ, Bakker A. *Challenges and opportunities for technology assessment in medical informatics - Case Study: PACS.* Med Inform 1993;18:209-18

Ball MJ, Silva JS, Douglas JV, Degoulet P, Kaihara S, editors. *The Health Care Professional Workstation.* Special Issue of Int J Biomed Comput 1994;34:1-415.

Barber B, Bakker AR, Bengtsson S, editors. *Caring for Health Information: Safety, Security and Secrecy.* Amsterdam: Elsevier Science Publ (North-Holland); 1994.

Grobe SJ, Pluyter-Wenting ESP. *An International Overview for Nursing in a Technological Era.* (San Antonio, Texas, USA, 1994). Amsterdam: Elsevier North-Holland; 1994.

Roger France FH, Noothoven van Goor J, Staer Johansen K, editors. Case-based telematic systems towards equity in health care. Amsterdam: IOS Press; 1994

Henry S, Holzemer W, Tallberg M, Grobe SJ. *The Infrastracture for Quality Assessment and Improvement in Nursing.* 1994 Austin, Texas, USA (postconference). 1995.

Van Bemmel JH, Rosenfalck A, Saranummi N, eds. Special Issue on *Biosignal Interpretation.* Proceedings of a IMIA/IFMBE Working Conference. Methods Inf Med 1994;33:1-160.

Bakker AR, Barber B, Tervo-Pellikka R, Treacher A, editors. (IMIA WG4). *Communicating Health Information in an Insecure World :* (Proceedings of the Helsinki Working Conference 1995). Amsterdam: Elsevier Publishing Co; 1995. 43:1, 2:1-s (also Special Issue of the Int J Biomed Comput, Vol. 43).

McCray AT, Scherrer J-R, Safran C, Chute CG, editors. *Concepts, Knowledge, and Language in H ealthcare Information Systems.* Methods Inf Med 1995;34: 1-231.

Hammond WE, Bakker AR, Ball MJ, editors. *Information Systems with fading Boundaries.* Special issue of Int J Biomed Comput 1995;39:1-192.

PAHO and Koop Foundation Meeting: *Telecommunications in Health and Healthcare for Latin America and the Caribbean,* November 12-15, 1996, Washington DC, USA.

1st Argentine Symposium of Nursing Informatics, December 4-6, 1996, Buenos Aires, Argentina.

Gerdin U, Tallberg M, Wainwright P. *Nursing Informatics: the impact of nursing knowledge on health care informatics.* Stockholm, Sweden 1997. Amsterdam: IOS Press; 1997.

Van Bemmel JH, Saranummi N, Yana K, Sato S, editors. *Biosignal Interpretation.* Proceedings of an IMIA/IFMBE Working Conference. Methods Inf Med 1997;36:235-375.

Haux R, Swinkels W, Ball MJ, Knaup P, Lun KC, editors : Special Issue on *Health and Medical Informatics Education : Transformation of Healthcare through innovative use of Information Technology.* Int J Med Inf 1997;44.

Bakker AR, Barber B, Ishikawa K, Yamamoto K, editors. *Common Security Solutions for Communicationg Patient Data.* Int J Med Inf. Special Issue; 1998;49.

Chute CG, Baud RH, Cimino JJ, Patel WL, Rector AL, editors. *Special Issue on Coding and Language Processing.* Methods Inf Med 1998;37.

Ehnfors M, Grobe SJ, Tallberg M. *Nursing Informatics: Combining Clinical Practice Guidelines and Patient Preferences Using Health Informatics* (postconference). Stockholm: SPRI 1998.

Kay S, editor. Special Issue on *Health Informatics: Challenges to Progress.* Methods Inf Med 1999;38.

Safran C, Degoulet P, Cesnik B, editors. Special Issue on Medinfo '98, Med Inform 1999; 53.

Talmon JL, Lorenzi N, van Gennip EMSJ,

## *Publications (Continued)*


Nykänen P, editors. *Organisational issues and technology assessment in health informatics*. Int J Med Inform 1999, Vol. 56.

Van der Lei J, Moorman PW, Musen M. Special Issue on *Electronic Patient Records in Medical Practice*. Methods Inf Med 1999;38.

Bakker AR, Barber B, Moehr J, editors. *Security of the Distributed Electronic Patient Record* (EPR). Int J Med Inf. Special Issue; 2000;60.

Hasman A, Blobel B, Dudeck J, Engelbrecht R, Gell G, Prokosch HU, editors: Medical Infobahn for Europe. Amsterdam: IOS Press; 2000.

Oliveri N, Sandor T, Lazaro C, Wiese B, Porta C, editors. Informedica 2000: 1st Ibero-American Virtual Congress of Medical Informatics. Proceedings of the Congress. CD Rom Spanish and English Edition. Fundación de Informática Médica. Argentina. 2000.

Saba V, Carr R. Sermeus W, Rocha P. *One Step Beyond: The Evolution of Technology and Nursing*. Auckland, New Zealand: Adis International; 2000. ISBN 0-86471-081-X.

McArthur J, Carr R, Westbrooke L, Honey M, Bakken S, editors. Proceedings of the NI2000 Post Congress Workshop: Rotorua, New Zealand, 3-6 May 2000. Auckland, New Zealand: Premier Print; 2001.

Roger France FH, Mertens I, Closon MC, Hofdijk J, editors. Case Mix: Global views, local actions. Amsterdam: IOS Press; 2001.

Hasman A, Mantas J, editors. Texbook in health informatics. Amsterdam: IOS Press; 2002.

Surjan G, Engelbrecht R, McNair P, editors. Health data in the information society; Proceedings of MIE2002, Amsterdam: IOS Press ; 2002.

# TILAK ...

...(Tiroler Landeskrankenanstalten GmbH)

**...as a public owned health care company responsible for five hospitals**

- 2.100 beds
- a staff of 5.800 persons, including 1.000 physicians
- 91.000 inpatients
- 322.000 outpatients

# TILAK ...

**...as a health care education institution (Ausbildungszentrum West – AZW)**

- 480 graduates in nursing p.a.
- 132 graduates in medical technical services p.a.
- 85 graduates in health- and hospitalmanagement p.a.

# TILAK ...

**... as pioneer for the University for Health Informatics and Technology Tyrol (UMIT)**

# TILAK 's University Hospital in Innsbruck...

**...as a center of excellence for patient care**

- one of three university teaching hospitals in Austria
- 40 medical departments
- 4.000 students

# TILAK ...

**...as user of  highly sophisticated IT-solutions**

- **Cerner HNA Millennium** (Clinical Information System)
- **MEDAS** (Patient Administration and Billing)
- **SAP** (Human Resources, Controlling, Material Management, Datawarehouse)
- hospital wide **PACS- and Advanced Image Management** solutions

# TILAK 's affiliated companies...

**...in search of IT solutions**

- **H.I.T.T.** (Health Information Technolgies Tirol)
- **ITH** – hospital information systems
- **icoserve** – advanced image management
- **AT solution partner** – SAP solutions in healthcare

**For detailed Informations contact...**

**Dr. Georg Lechleitner** – georg.lechleitner@tilak.at

www.tilak.at          www.hitt.at          www.k-m-t.at          www.umit.at

# Addresses of IMIA Member Societies

## Argentina

Argentine Association of Medical Informatics
Asociación Argentina de Informática Médica (AAIM)
http://www.aaim.org.ar

*National Office:*
Guido 1948 1 B
Buenos Aires 1119, Argentina
Tel:    +54 11 4807 5923
Fax:    +54 11 4807 5982

*President:*
Carlos Hugo Leonzio
Fundacion Favaloro
Buenos Aires
Tel:    +54 11 4378 1200 Int 4438
Fax:    +54 11 4378 1311
E-mail: hleonzio@aaim.org.ar

*Vice-President:*
Dr. Carlos Porta
Circulo Medico de Moron
Buenos Aires
E-mail: cporta@aaim.org.ar

*IMIA Representative
and Secretary:*
Tomas A. Sandor
Ministerio de Salud de la Nacion
Buenos Aires
Tel:    +54 11 4309 5479
Fax:    +54 11 4309 5400
tsandor@aaim.org.ar

## Australia

Health Informatics Society of Australia Ltd. (HISA)
http://www.hisa.org.au

*HISA Executive Director:*
Ms. Joan Edgecumbe
Health Informatics Society of Australia
413 Lygon Street
Brunswick East 3057
Victoria, Australia
Tel:    +61 3 9388 0555
Fax:    +61 3 9388 2086
E-mail: hisa@hisa.org.au

*President:*
Paul Cohen
Knowledge Manager
Medibank Private
Melbourne
E-mail: Paul_Cohen@
            medibank.com.au

*Secretary:*
Ms. Robyn Cook
Clinical Informatics Co-ordinator
South Eastern Sydney Area
Health Service, Zetland NSW
E-Mail: CookR@
            sesahs.nsw.gov.au

*IMIA Representative:*
Prof. Jeffrey Soar
University of Wollongong
School of Information Technology
and Computer Science
Tel:    +61 2 4221 5321
Fax:    +61 2 4221 4170
E-mail: jeffrey@uow.edu.au

*Treasurer:*
Steve Tipper
University of South New Wales
Centre for Health Informatics
Kensington NSW
E-mail: s.tipper@unsw.edu.au

## Austria

Austrian Computer Society
Working Group Medical Informatics
Österreichische Computergesellschaft
Arbeitskreis Medizinische Informatik
http://www.kfunigraz.ac.at/imiwww/ak/

*President and IMIA
Representative:*
Prof. Bernhard Tilg
University for Health Informatics
and Technology Tyrol (UMIT)
Innsbruck, Tyrol, Austria
Tel:    +43 512 586 734-0
Fax:    +43 512 586 734 850
E-mail: Bernhard.Tilg@umit.at

*Secretary/Treasurer:*
Dr. Andreas Holzinger
Graz University
Institute of Medical Informatics,
Statistics and Documentation
Engelgasse 13
A-8010 Graz, Austria
Tel:    +43 316 385 3883
Fax:    +43 316 385 3590
E-mail: andreas.holzinger@
            kfunigraz.ac.at

## Belgium

Belgian Medical Informatics Association
http://www.bmia.be

*President:*
Dr. Etienne De Clercq
Ecole de Santé Publique - SESA
Université Catholique de
Louvain
Clos Chapelle aux Champs, 30.41
1200 Brussels
Tel:    +32 2 764 3262
Fax:    +32 2 764 3031
E-mail: declercq@sesa.ucl.ac.be

*IMIA Representative:*
Prof. Francis H. Roger France
Université Catholique de
Louvain
Brussels
Tel:    +32 2 764 4711
Fax:    +32 2 764 4717
E-mail: roger@infm.ucl.ac.be

*Secretary:*
Dr. P. Piette
E-mail: p.piette@hopiteaux-
            gilly.be

## Bosnia and Herzegovina

Society for Medical Informatics of Bosnia and
Herzegowina

*President and IMIA
Representative:*
Prof. Dr. Izet Masic
Medical Faculty
Center for Medical Informatics
Mose Pijade 6, 71000 Sarajevo
Tel/Fax: +387 71 444 714
E-mail: imasic@utic.net.ba

## Brazil

Brazilian Society of Health Informatics
Sociedade Brasileira de Informática em Saúde - SBIS
http://www.sbis.org.br

*SBIS Office Address:*
Rua Afonso Braz 656 - sala 12
PO Box 20397 -CEP: 04041-990
São Paulo SP - Brazil

*President :*
Dr. Lincoln de Assis Moura Jr.
Atech Foundation
São Paulo SP
Tel:     +55 11 3089 6745
Fax:     +55 11 9182 7495
E-mail: lincoln@atech.br

*IMIA Representative:*
Dr. Umberto Tachinard
InCor - São Paulo Heart Institute
Tel:     +55 11 3069 5477
Fax:     +55 11 3069 5311
E-mail: tachinardi@incor.usp.br

*Secretary/Treasurer:*
Ms. Fabiane Bizinella Nardon
System Analyst
Summa Technologies
São Paulo SP
Tel:     +55 11 3846 1622
Fax:     +55 11 3845 3514
E-mail: fabiane@summa-tech.com

## Canada

COACH, Canada's Health Informatics Association
http://www.coachorg.com

*Secretariat:*
Andrew Parr (executive director)
1304 - 2 Carlton Street
Toronto, Ontario M5B 1J3
Tel:     +1 416 979 5551
Fax:     +1 461 979 1144
E-mail: info@coachorg.com

*President:*
Mr. Gil Sampson
Consultant
Feronia Group
Tel:     +1 250 283 9190
Fax:     +1 250 283 9197
E-mail: gsampson@island.net

*Secretary/Treasurer:*
Ms Shelagh Maloney
VP Clinical Information Services
& Chief Privacy Officer
THiiNC Information
Management Inc.
Tel:     +1 416 203 5904
Fax:     +1 416 203 1148
E-mail: shelagh.maloney@
        thiincimi.com

*IMIA Representative:*
Prof. Jochen Moehr
University of Victoria
School of Health Information
Science
Tel:     +1 250 721 8581
Fax:     +1 250 472 4751
E-mail: jmoehr@uvic.ca

*Executive Director:*
Ms. Elizabeth Di Chiara
COACH: Canada's Health
Informatics Association
Tel:     +1 416 979 5551 Ext. 242
Fax:     +1 416 979 1144
E-mail: info@coachorg.com

## China

China Medical Informatics Association (CMIA)
China Medical Informatics Association of Chinese
Institut of Electronics
http://www.cmia.net

*CMIA Office Address:*
17 Zhengjue Jiadao
Xinjiekou, Xicheng District
Beijing 100035
P.R. China

*President:*
Prof. Debing Wang
Peking University
Tel:     +86 10 6275 7072
Fax:     +86 10 6275 1207
E-mail: wdb@pku.edu.cn

*Secretary/Treasurer:*
Mr. Ying I. Liang
China Medical Informatics
Association
Tel:     +86 10 6615 3078
E-mail: medinfo@cmia.net

*IMIA Representative:*
Dr. Ling Zhu
Marketing Director
Beijing Lianshi Technology
Co. Ltd.
Tel:     +86 10 8048 2626
Fax:     +86 10 8048 2627
E-mail: lzhu_md@yahoo.com

## Croatia

Croatian Society for Medical Informatics (CSMI)
Hrvatsko drustvo za medicinsku informatiku
http://www.snz.hr/wnew/csmi.html

*President:*
Prof. Dr. Gjuro Dezelic
Medical School
University of Zagreb
Tel:     +385 1 468 4440
Fax:     +385 1 468 4441

*Secretary:*
Mira Hercigonja-Szekeres
Polimedika, Ltd., Zagreb
Tel:     +385 1 663 6500
E-mail: mira.hercigonja-
        szekeres1@zg.tel.hr

*IMIA Representative:*
Prof. Dr. Josipa Kern
Andrija Stampar School of
Public Health
Medical School
University of Zagreb
Tel:     +385 1 468 4440
Fax:     +385 1 468 4441
E-mail: jkern@snz.hr

## Cuba

Cuban Society of Medical Informatics
Sociedad Cubana de Informática Médica
http://www.cedisap.sld.cu

*Office Address:*
CEDISAP
Calle 23 No. 177 entre N y O,
Vedado, Plaza
Ciudad de la Habana, Cuba

*President:*
Prof. Dr Esperanza O'Farrill
Center of Cybernetics Applied
to Medicine (CECAM)
Ciudad de la Habana
Tel:     +537 21 1354
E-mail: espe@cecam.sld.cu

*IMIA Representative:*
Dr. Athos Sanchez Mansolo
E-mail: Athos@cecam.sld.cu

*Secretary/Treasurer:*
Ms. Maria Vidal
Ministry of Public Health
Centro de Desarollo Informatico
de Salud Publica
Ciudad de la Habana
Tel:     +537 55 3325
Fax:     +537 55 2222
E-mail: swmedic@infomed.sld.cu

## Czech Republic

Czech Society of Biomedical Engineering
and Medical Informatics
Ceska spolecnost biomedicinskeho inzenyrstvi a
lekarske informatiky
http://www.cls.cz/

*Office Address:*
Sokolska 33
Prague, Czech Republic

*President:*
Dr. Jaromir Cmíral
Institute of Aviation Medicine
Generála Piky 1
160 60 Prague 6
Tel:     +420 2 2020 8120
Fax:     +420 2 2431 1934
E-mail: ulz@telecom.cz

*Secretary/Treasurer:*
Jiri Holcik
Technical University Brno
Tel:     +420 5 4114 9546
Fax:     +420 5 4114 9542
E-mail: holcik@
        dbme.fee.vutbr.cz

*IMIA Representative:*
Prof. Dr.  Jana Zvárová
Charles University and
Academy of Sciences
Prague 8
Tel:     +420 2 6605 3097
Fax:     +420 2 6897 013
E-mail: zvarova@euromise.cz

*Executive Director:*
Dr. Alexander Stozicky
Czech Medical Society HJ.E.
Purkyne
Prague
Tel:     +420 2 2426 6223
Fax:     +420 2 2426 6226

## Denmark

The Danish Society for Medical Informatics
Dansk Selskab for Medicinsk Informatik
http://www.dsmi.dk

*Office Address:*
Dansk Selskab for Medicinsk
Informatik
St. Kongensgade 59 A
Copenhagen
Denmark

*President:*
Prof. Ole Hejlesen
Aalborg University
Medical Informatics Group
Tel:     +45 9635 8808
E-mail: okh@mi.auc.dk

*Secretary/Treasurer:*
Karsten Niss
TIANI Nordic Aps
DK-9920 Aalborg
Tel:     +45 7214 6614
Fax:     +45 9635 4599
E-mail: karsten.niss@tiani.com

*IMIA Representative:*
Dr. Knut E. Bernstein
Danish Centre for Health
Telematics
Heden 18
DK-5000 Odense C
Tel:     +45 6613 3066
Fax:     +45 6613 5066
E-mail: kbern@inet.uni2.dk

## Finland

Finnish Social and Health Informatics Association
(FinnSHIA)
Sosiaali - ja terveydenhuollon tietojenkäsittely
-yhdistys ry ry
http://www.oskenet.fi/tty

*President and IMIA
Representative:*
Dr. Mikko Korpela
University of Kuopio
Computing Centre
P.O. Box 1627
FIN-70211 Kuopio
Tel:     +358 17 16 2811
Fax:     +358 17 282 5566
E-mail: mikko.korpela@uku.fi

*Treasurer:*
Kauko Hartikainen
Association of Finnish Local and
Regional Authorities
Helsinki
Tel:     +358 9 771 2647
Fax:     +358 9 771 2291
E-mail: Kauko.Hartikainen@
       Kuntaliitto.fi

*Executive Director:*
Ms. Ursula Cornér
National Research and
Development Centre for
Welfare and Health (STAKES)
Helsinki
Tel:     +358 9 3967 2329
Fax:     +358 9 3967 2443
E-mail: Ursula.Corner@stakes.fi

## France

French Medical Informatics Association (AIM)
Association pour les Applications de l'Informatique
à la Médecine

*IMIA Representative:*
Prof. Patrice Degoulet
Pompidou University Hospital
Hospital Informatics Department
Paris
Tel:     +33 1 5609 2030
Fax:     +33 1 5609 2052
E-mail: patrice.degoulet@
       egp.ap-hop-paris.fr

## Georgia

Georgian Association of Medical Informatics and
Biomedical Engineering (GAMIBE)

*IMIA Representative:*
Prof. Gaioz S. Vasadze
51 Iv. Javakhishvili str.
380002 Tbilisi, Georgia
Tel:     +995 32 953 418
Fax:     +995 32 960 300
E-mail: aiha@nilc.org.ge

## Germany

German Association for Medical Informatics, Biometry
and Epidemiology
Deutsche Gesellschaft für Medizinische Informatik,
Biometrie und Epidemiologie (GMDS) e.V.

GMDS-Geschäftsstelle
Schedestrasse 9
D-53113 Bonn, Germany
Tel:     +49 228 24 222 24
http://www.gmds.de

*President:*
Prof. Walter Lehmacher, PhD
Cologne University Hospital
Institute of Medical Statistics,
Informatics and Epidemiology
Tel:     +49 221 478 6501
Fax:     +49 221 478 6520
E-mail: Walter.Lehmacher
       @Medizin.Uni-Koeln.de

*IMIA Representative:*
Prof. Dr. Herbert Witte
Institute of Medical Statistics
and Computer Sciences
Friedrich Schiller University Jena
Jahnstr. 3
D-07740 Jena
Germany
Tel:     +49 3641 933 133
Fax:     +49 3641 933 200
E-mail: iew@imsid.uni-jena.de

## Hong Kong

Hong Kong Society of Medical Informatics
http://www.hksmi.org

*Office Address:*
c/o Dr.CP Wong

*President and IMIA Representative:*
Dr. Chun Por Wong
Chief of Integrated Medical Services
Ruttonjee Hospital
266 Queens's Road East
Wanchai, Hong Kong
Tel:     +852 2291 1345
Fax:     +852 2291 1335
E-mail: cpwong@ha.org.hk

*Secretary/Treasurer:*
Anthony Cheung
Senior Systems Manager
IT Division, Hospital Authority
147B Argyle Street
Kowloon, Hong Kong
Tel:     +852 2300 6538
Fax:     +852 2300 5395

## Hungary

Biomedical Section of John von Neumann Society for Computing Sciences
http://www.njszt.iif.hu

*President and IMIA Representative:*
Prof. Dr. Attila Naszlady
Polyclinic of Hospitaller Bros
Budapest
Tel:     +36 1 4388 432
Fax:     +36 1 212 5378
E-mail: naszlady.attila
            @irgalmas.hu

## Ireland

Healthcare Informatics Society of Ireland
Cumann Riomheolais Sláinte
http://www.hisi.ie

*Office Address:*
58 Eccles Street
Dublin 7
Republic of Ireland

*President:*
Prof. Jane Grimson
Trinity College, Dublin
Tel:     +353 1 608 1780
Fax:     +353 1 608 2512
E-mail: jane.grimson@tcd.ie

*Executive Director:*
Gerard Hurl
Institute of Healthcare Informatics
Dublin
Tel:     +353 1 830 7958
Fax:     +353 1 830 7728
E-mail: ghurl@mater.ie

*IMIA Representative:*
Diarmuid UaConaill
Biochemistry Laboratory
Mater Misericordiae Hospital
Eccles Street, Dublin 7
Tel:     +353 1 803 2423
Fax:     +353 1 803 4781
E-mail: duaconaill@mater.ie

*Secretary:*
Ms. Ann Sheridan
Eastern Regional Health Authority
Dublin
Tel:     +353 1 620 1731
Fax:     +353 1 620 1625
E-mail: ann.sheridan@erha.ie

## Israel

The Israeli Association for Medical Informatics

*Office Address:*
P.O. Box 50006
Tel Aviv, Israel

*President and IMIA Representative:*
Dr. Batami Sadan
MDG Medical Inc., Or Yehuda
Tel: +972 3 634 0404 x216
Fax: +972 3 634 0411
E-mail: sadanba@netvision.net.il

*Secretary/Treasurer:*
Ms. Dorit Shaul
ILA/The Israeli Association for
Medical Informatics, Tel Aviv
Tel:     +972 3 514 0503
Fax:     +972 3 514 0077
E-mail: ILA@kenes.com

## Italy

Italian Medical Informatics Society (AIIM)
Associazione Italiana di Informatica Medica
http://www.aiim.it

*Office address:*
c/o MGA
Viale Mazzini, 145
Rome, Italy

*President and IMIA Representative:*
Prof. Angelo A.S. Serio
Università di Roma "La Sapienza"
Facoltà die Medicina
Tel:     +39 6 4991 2542
Fax:     +39 6 3973 0337
E-mail: angelo.serio@tiscalinet.it

## Japan

Japan Association for Medical Informatics
http://jami.umin.ac.jp

*Office Address:*
Medical Information Systems Development Center
2-3-4 Akasaka
Minato-ku
Tokyo, Japan

*President:*
Dr. Michitoshi Inoue
President
Osaka National Hospital,
Japan
Tel:    +81 6 6946 3500
Fax:    +81 6 6946 8031
E-mail: inoue@onh.go.jp

*Secretary:*
Prof. Kiyomu Ishikawa
Chief, Dept. of Hospital
Systems Management
Hiroshima University
Tel:    +81 82 257 5080
Fax:    +81 82 257 5084
E-mail: kiyomu@
        hiroshima-u.ac.jp

*IMIA Representative:*
Prof. Ken Toyoda
Director
BearingPoint Co.
Healthcare Group
Tel:    +81 3 3266 8512
Fax:    +81 3 3266 7839
E-mail: kent105@attglobal.net

## Kazakstan

Medical Pharmaceutical Information Association
(MedPharmInfo)
http://www.med.kz

*Office address:*
47 Mynbaev Street
Almaty
Republic of Kazakstan 480008

*President :*
Prof. Azat Abdrakmanov
Tel:    +7 3272 4575 78
Fax:    +7 3272 4575 78
E-mail: azat@med.kz

*Executive Director:*
Dr. Aliya Kusherova
MedPharmInfo Association
Tel:    +7 3272 4790 54
Fax:    +7 3272 4575 78
E-mail: aliya@ean.kz

*IMIA Representative:*
Prof. Temirhan Bekbosinov
Vice President
MedPharmInfo Association
Tel:    +7 3272 4534 04
Fax:    +7 3272 4559 32
E-mail: temir@med.kz

## Korea

The Korean Society of Medical Informatics (KOSMI)
http://www.kosmi.org

*Office address:*
Chongno-gu Myungryun-dong 2 ga 237
Anam Apt #301-204
Seoul, Korea

*President:*
Prof. Jung Ho Park, RN, PhD
College of Nursing
Seoul National University
Tel:    +82 2 740 8818
Fax:    +82 2 745 0617
E-mail: nurspjh@snu.ac.kr

*Secretary:*
Dr. Jinwook Choi, MD
Assistant Professor
Seoul National University
College of Medicine
Dept. of Biomed. Engineering
Tel:    +82 2 760 3421
Fax:    +82 2 745 7870
E-mail: jinchoi@snu.ac.kr

*IMIA Representative:*
Prof. Hune Cho
Associate Professor
Kyungpook National University
School of Medicine
Dept. of Medical Informatics
Tel:    +82 53 420 6051
Fax:    +82 53 420 6059
E-mail: hunecho@knu.ac.kr

## Mexico

Mexican Medical Informatics Association
Assucion Mexicana de Informatica Medica (AMIM)

*IMIA Representative:*
Dr. Cesar Colina Ramirez
Universidad Nacional Autonoma
de Mexico
Tel:    +52 623 24 85
Fax:    +52 623 24 80
E-mail: ccolina@
        drbaz.fmedic.unam.mx

## The Netherlands

Society for Healthcare Informatics
Vereniging voor informatieverwerking in de zorg
(VMBI)
http://www.vmbi.nl

*Office Address:*
Postbus 986
Zeist, Utrecht, The Netherlands

*President and IMIA Representative:*
Prof. Dr. Arie A. Hasman
Dept of Medical Informatics
Maastricht University
PO Box 616
6200 MD  Maastricht
The Netherlands
Tel:      +31 43 388 2242
Fax:      +31 43 388 4170
E-mail: hasman@mi.unimaas.nl

*Secretary:*
Hans H. Maring
University Medical Centre Utrecht
Corporate I & A
Tel:      +31 30 250 6822
Fax:      +31 30 250 6822
E-mail: h.maring@azu.nl

*Treasurer:*
Dr. Peter P.J. Branger
Deloitte & Touche
Management and ICT
Consultants
Tel:      +31 20 495 2323
Fax:      +31 20 495 2345
E-mail: pbranger@deloitte.nl

## New Zealand

Health Informatics New Zealand

*Office Address:*
PO Box 62-578
Kalmia Street PO Boxes
Auckland, New Zealand

*President:*
Ms. Ann C. Browett
Mercy Hospital and Health
Services
Clinical Services
Tel:      +64 9 623 5700
Fax:      +64 9 623 5701
E-mail: annb@mercy.co.nz

*IMIA Representative:*
Ian H. Symonds
Wellington Pathology Ltd.
Tel:      +64 4 801 5111
Fax:      +64 4 801 5432
E-mail: ihs@welpath.co.nz

*Secretary/Treasurer:*
Ms. Anne Andrews
Waitemata Health Ltd.
Child Disability Service
Tel:      +64 9 489 9134
E-mail: andrewsp@whl.co.nz

## Norway

Norwegian Society for Medical Informatics
Forum for Databehandling i Helsesektoren (FDH)
http://www.fdh.no

*President:*
Prof. Margarethe J. Lorensen
University of Oslo
Institute of Nursing Science
E-mail: m.j.lorensen@
              sykepleievit.uio.no

*IMIA Representative:*
Ms. Irma Iversen
Pasientombudet for Akershus
Fylkeskommune
Tel:      +47 221 70491
Fax:      +47 221 75270
E-mail:irma.iversen@po.ah.no

## Peru

Peruvian Health Informatics Association
Asociacion Peruano de Informatica en Salud (APIS)
http://www.apisnet.org

*Office Address:*
Av. Brasil 1008
Brena, Lima
Peru

*President and IMIA Representative:*
Dr. Crisogono Rubio Nieto
Telefonica Data Peru S.A.A,
Lima
Tel:      +51 1 210 4592
Fax:      +51 1 422 0591
E-mail: crubio@tp.com.pe

*Secretary/Treasurer:*
Dr. Jorge Ballon Echegaray
Unversidad Nacional San Agustin
Arequipa
Tel:      +51 54 233 803
E-mail: jballon@viabcp.com

## Philippines

**Philippine Medical Informatics Society, Inc.**

http://www.pmis.org

*Office Address:*
UP College of Medicine
Medical Informatics Unit
547 Pedro Gil Street
Ermita, Manila, Philippines

*President:*
Dr. Herman D. Tolentino,
UP College of Medicine
Medical Informatics Unit
Manila
Tel:    +63 2 526 4254
Fax:    +63 2 874 6992 0918
         +63 2 874 9040 294
E-mail: hermant
         @cm.upm.edu.ph

*IMIA Representative:*
Dr. Alvin Marcelo
UP College of Medicine, Manila
Tel:    +1 301 435 3278
Fax:    +1 603 452 3657
E-mail: amarcelo@cm.upm.edu.ph

Secretary:
Dr. Alex C. Yu
University of the Philippines
Manila
Tel:    +63 2 526 0371
Fax:    +63 2 526 0371
E-mail: alexcyou@eudoramail.com

## Poland

**Polish Society of Medical Informatics**

*President and IMIA
Representative:*
Prof. Dr. Edward Kacki
Technical University of Lódz
Tel:    +48 42 329 757
Fax:    +48 42 303 414
E-mail: ekacki@ics.p.lodz.pl

## Romania

**Romanian Society of Medical Informatics
Societatea Romana de Informatica Medicala**

http://medinfo.umft.ro/rsmi/

*Office Address*:
Spl. T. Vladimirescu 14, Timisoara, Romania

*President and IMIA
Representative:*
Prof. Dr. George I. Mihalas
Univ. Medicine and Pharmacy
Timisoara
Tel:    +40 256 190 288
Fax:    +40 256 190 288
E-mail:mihalas@medinfo.umft.ro

*Secretary:*
Ms. Mariana Bazavan
Center for Health Computing
Statistics and Medical
Documentation
Bucharest
Tel:    +40 21 314 0890
Fax:    +40 21 311 2998
E-mail: mbazavan@yahoo.com

## Singapore

**Association for Informatics in Medicine, Singapore
(AIMS)**

http://www.aims.org.sg

*Office Address*:
School of Biological Sciences
Nanyang Technological University
1 Nanyang Walk, Block 5, Level 3, Singapore

*President and IMIA Representative:*
Prof. Kwok-Chan Lun
Nanyang Technological University
School of Biological Sciences
Tel:    +65 6790 3726
Fax:    +65 6896 8032
E-mail: kclun@ntu.edu.sg

*Treasurer*:
Ms. Swee Wah Chew-Goh
National University of Singapore
Computer Centre
Tel:    +65 874 2480
Fax:    +65 778 0198
E-mail: ccegohsw@nus.edu.sg

## Slovak Republic

**Slovak Society for Biomedical Engineering
and Medical Informatics**

http://www.fmed.uniba.sk/~biofyzika/engin.html

*President:*
Prof. Peter Kneppo
Slovak Institute of Metrology
Bratislava
Tel:    +421 7 6542 6208
Fax:    +421 7 6542 9592
E-mail: pkneppo@smu.gov.sk

*Secretary:*
Dr. Milan Tyšler
Slovak Academy of Science
Bratislava
Tel:    +421 7 5477 5950
Fax:    +421 7 5477 5043
E-mail: umertyssl@savba.sk

*IMIA Representative:*
Dr. Mikuláš Popper
Comenius University
Faculty of Mathematics,
Physics and Informatics
Bratislava
Tel:    +421 2 6542 7469
E-mail: popper@fmph.uniba.sk

## Slovenia

Slovenian Medical Informatics Society (SMIS)

*President and IMIA Representative:*
Dr. Marjan Premik
Institute for Social Medicine
Ljubljana
Tel/Fax: +386 61 131 4210
E-mail: premik@
    ibmi.mf.uni-lj.si

## South Africa

South African Health Informatics Association

*President*:
Dr. Sedick S. Isaacs
Groote Schuur Hospital/
University of Capetown
Observatory Western Cape
Tel:    +27 21 404 2058
Fax:    +27 21 404 2070
E-mail: seisaacs@
    pawc.wcape.gov.za

*IMIA Representative*:
John D. Tresling
Meditech SA, Halfway House
Tel:    +27 11 805 1631
Fax:    +27 11 805 1430
E-mail: jtresling@meditech.co.za

*Secretary/Treasurer*:
Ms. Lyn A. Hanmer
Medical Research Council
Tygerberg Western Cape
Tel:    +27 21 938 0343
Fax:    +27 21 938 0315
E-mail: lyn.hanmer@mrc.ac.za

## Spain

Spanish Society of Health Informatics
Sociedad Española de Informática de la Salud (SEIS)
http://www.seis.es

*Office Address*:
CEFIC (SEIS Secretary)
C/Olimpo, 33 1° C

28043 Madrid, Spain
*President*:
Prof. Luciano Saez-Ayerra
Institute of Health "Carlos III"
Dept. of Health Informatics
Tel:    +34 91 387 7835
Fax:    +34 91 387 7790
    +34 62 937 1639
E-mail: lsaez@isciii.es

*Secretary:*
Dr. Salvador Arribas
Hospital Universitario La Paz
Tel:    +34 91 350 2600 ext. 1156
E-mail: sarribas@hulp.insalud.es

*IMIA Representative*:
Dr. Fernando J. Martin-Sanchez
Institute of Health "Carlos III"
Dept. of Health Informatics
Tel:    +34 91 509 7027
Fax:    +34 91 509 7917
E-mail: fmartin@isciii.es

## Sweden

Swedish Federation for Medical Informatics
Svensk Förenig för Medicinsk Informatik
http://www.sfmi.org

*Office Address*:
21 Slatbaksvagen
Arsta, Sweden

*President:*
Dr. Magnus Fogelberg
Sahlgrenska University Hospital
Department of Neurology
Tel:    +46 31342 2326
Fax:    +46 31342 2383
E-mail: magnus.fogelberg@
    vgregion.se

*Secretary/Treasurer:*
Claes Schonqvist
Uppsala County Council
Tel:    +46 18 611 6055
Fax:    +46 18 611 6299
E-mail: claes.schonqvist@
    it.ck.lul.se

*IMIA Representative:*
Hans Adolfsson
Swedish Society for Medical
Information
Tel:    +46 855 670 155
Fax:    +46 855 670 155
E-mail: hans.adolfsson@
    telia.com

## Switzerland

Swiss Society for Medical Informatics (SSMI)
Schweizerische Gesellschaft für Medizinische
Informatik
Société Suisse d'Informatique Médicale
http://www.sgmi-ssim.ch/

*SSMI Secretariat:*
SGMI / SSIM
PO Box 229, Daelhoelzliweg 3
Bern 6, Switzerland

*President:*
Dr. Judith Wagner
H+ die Spitaeler der Schweiz
Medical Informatics and
Statistics Department
Tel:    +43 41 31 306 6130
Fax:    +43 41 31 306 6110
E-mail: judith.wagner@bluewin.ch

*Executive Director:*
Ms. Anita Eymann
Sekretariat SGMI c/o VSAO
Tel:    +43 31 436 4499
Fax:    +43 31 436 4498
E-mail: admin@sgmi.ssim.ch

*IMIA Representative:*
Prof. Dr. Antoine Geissbuhler
Geneva University Hospital
Division of Medical Informatics
Tel:    +43 41 22 372 6201
Fax:    +43 41 22 372 6255
E-mail: antoine.geissbuhler
        @hcuge.ch

*Secretary:*
Dr. Ruedi Tschudi
Spital Thurgau AG
Tel:    +43 41 71 686 4550
Fax:    +43 41 71 686 4549
E-mail: ruedi.tschudi@kttg.ch

## Turkey

Turkish Medical Informatics Association (TURKMIA)
TIP BILISIMI DERNEGI
http://www.turkmia.org

*Office Address:*
Gazi Universitesi Tip
Fakultesi Nukleer Tip AD
Besevler, Ankara, Turkey

*President:*
Mehmet T. Kitapci
Gazi University School of
Medicine, Ankara
Tel:    +90 312 214 1000/6161
Fax:    +90 312 215 6456
E-mail: mkitapci@yahoo.com

*MIA Representative:*
Dr. K. Hakan Gülkesen
Akdeniz University, Antalya
Tel:    +90 532 775 7910
E-mail: gulkesen@turk.net

*Secretary:*
Dr. Tamer Calikoglu
Oncology Hospital
Tel:    +90 312 435 5343
Fax:    +90 312 435 4006
E-mail: tamer@pleksus.net.tr

## Ukraine

The Ukraine Association for "Computer Medicine"
(UACM)
http://www.uacm.cit-ua.net

*IMIA Representative:*
Prof. Oleg Y. Mayorov, Ph.D.,
M.D., Dr.Sc.
Ministry of Healthcare
Kharkiv
Tel:    +380 57 711 8032
Fax:    +380 57 262 8179
E-mail: snd@ic.kharkov.com

## United Kingdom

British Computer Society Health Informatics
Committee
http://www.bcshic.org

*Office Address:*
Chair, British Computer Society HIC
1 Sanford Street
Swindon, Wiltshire, UK

*Chair:*
Dr. Glyn Hayes
Torex Health, Bromsgrove
E-mail: glyn@
        online.demon.co.uk

*Treasurer:*
Prof. Graham Wright
Centre for Health Information,
Research and Development
Winchester Hampshire
Tel:    +44 1980 863 953
E-mail: g.wright@wkac.ac.uk

*IMIA Representative:*
Peter Murray
Telematics Consultancy
Lincoln, Lincolnshire
Fax:    +44 870 056 0424
E-mail: imiaukrep@btinternet.com

## Uruguay

Uruguayan Society of Medical Informatics
Sociedad Uruguaya de Informática en la Salud
http://www.suis.org.uy

*IMIA Representative:*
Dr. Alvaro Margolis
Tel:    +598 2 401 4701
Fax:    +598 2 402 6170
E-mail: margolis@mednet.org.uy

*Office Address:*
Bvar. Artigas 1515
Montevideo

## USA

American Medical Informatics Association (AMIA)
http://www.amia.org

*AMIA Office:*
4915 St. Elmo Avenue, Suite 401
Bethesda, MD 20814 USA

*President:*
Dr. W. Ed Hammond
Duke University
Durham NC
Tel:    +1 919 684 6421
Fax:    +1 919 684 8675
E-mail: hammo001@mc.duke.edu

*Secretary:*
Dr. William R. Hersh
Oregon Health and Science
University
Portland OR
Tel:    +1 503 494 4563
Fax:    +1 503 494 4551
E-mail: hersh@ohsu.edu

*IMIA Representative
and Treasurer:*
Dr. Nancy M. Lorenzi
Vanderbilt University Medical
Center
Nashville TN
Tel:    +1 615 936 1423
Fax:    +1 615 936 1427
E-mail: nancy.lorenzi@
          mcmail.vanderbilt.edu

*Executive Director:*
Dennis J. Reynolds
American Medical Informatics
Association
Tel:    +1 301 657 1291
Fax:    +1 301 657 1296
E-mail: dennis@mail.amia.org

## EFMI (IMIA Europe)

European Federation for Medical Informatics
http://www.hiscom.nl/efmi

*President:*
Dr. Assa Reichert
SAREL, Supplies & Services for
Medicine
Zone south Netanya POB 8466
Netanya, Israel
Tel:    +972 9 892 2005
Fax:    +972 9 892 2123
E-mail: reichert@sarel.co.il

*Vice President:*
Dr. Robert Baud
Hospital of Geneva
Div. Informatique Médicale
Rue du Crest
CH-1211 Geneva 14
Switzerland
Tel:    +41 22 372 6203
Fax:    +41 22 372 6255
E-mail: robert.baud@dim-hcuge.ch

*Vice President - IMIA:*
Dr. Rolf Engelbrecht
MEDIS - Institut
GSF-National Research Center
for Environment and Health
Ingolstädter Landstr. 1
D-85764 Oberschleißheim
Germany
Tel:    +49 89 3187 4138
Fax:    +49 89 3187 3008
E-mail: engel@gsf.de

*Treasurer:*
Patrick Weber
Nice Computing
Rte de Fey
CH-1414 Rueyres
Tel:    +41 21 887 6031
Fax:    +41 212 887 6031
E-mail: patrick.weber@
          nicecomputing.ch

*Secretary:*
George Mihalas
University of Medicine and
Pharmacy
Dept. of Medical Informatics
P-ta Eftimie Murgu 2
1900 Timisoara, Romania
Tel:    +40 56 193 082/ 190 288
Fax:    +40 56 190 626/ 190 288
E-mail:  mihalas@medinfo.umft.ro

*Executive Officer:*
John Bryden
Bryden Consulting Ltd.
Public Health & Health
Information consultant
34 Sherbrooke Drive
Glasgow C41 5AA
Tel:    +44 141 427 2959
Fax:    +44 709 201 2511
E-mail: jsbry@healthinfo.win-
uk.net

*Information Officer:*
Dr. Jacob Hofdijk
HISCOM
Schipholweg 97
NL-2316 XA Leiden
Netherlands
Tel:    +31 71 525 6708
Fax:    +31 71 521 6675
E-mail: Jacob@hiscom.nl

*Publication Officer:*
Prof. Dr. Arie Hasman
University Maastricht
Dept. of Medical Informatics
P.O. Box 616
NL-6200 MD Maastricht
The Netherlands
Tel.:    +31 43 3882 240
Fax:    +31 43 367 1052
E-mail: hasman@mi.unimaas.nl

## IMIA-LAC (Latin America)
Federation of Health Societies in Latin America

*President and IMIA Representative:*
Dr. Lincoln de Assis Moura Jr.
Atech Foundation
São Paulo SP
Tel:     +55 11 3089 6745
Fax:     +55 11 9182 7495
E-mail: lincoln@atech.br

## APAMI (IMIA Asia Pacific)
Asia Pasific Association for Medical Informatics

http://www.apami.net

*IMIA Representative:*
Dr. Chun Por Wong
Chief of Integrated Medical Services
Ruttonjee Hospital
Tel:     +852 2291 1345
Fax:     +852 2291 1335
E-mail: cpwong@ha.org.hk

## Helina (African Region)

*IMIA Representative*:
Dr. Sedick S. Isaacs
Groote Schuur Hospital/
University of Cape Town
Observatory, Western Cape
Tel:     +27 21 404 2058
Fax:     +27 21 404 2070
E-mail: seisaacs@
            pawc.wcape.gov.za

# Information on IMIA Societies

## Argentina

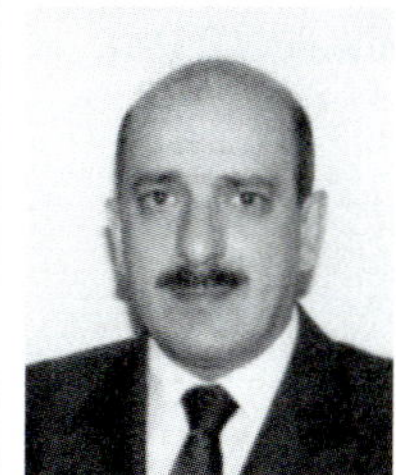

Carlos Hugo Leonzio, President

The Argentine Association of Medical Informatics "AAIM" is an academic institution born as an encompassing organization created to fulfill the needs related to the development and application of Medical/Health Informatics in Argentina.

AAIM is open to all representatives of business and academic groups, and independent profetionals, which produce developments in the field of Medical/Health Informatics all over the country.

The "AAIM" is a Non Profit organization, funded in 1995, as a response to requirements for projects and knowledge interchange between the members, definition of standards, international relationships, scientific and technical developments and implementation programs.

Since 1996, AAIM is the national Representative of IMIA: International Medical Informatics Association.

All activities of AAIM are performed in coordination with the Regional Medical Informatics Association (IMIA LAC), in particular, the Annual Virtual Congress on Internet, Informedica 2000, 2002, etc.

Objectives of AAIM are:
- Promote the development and application of Medical Informatics in the scope of improving patient health care.
- Implement teaching programs in the Health area
- Develop Health care Administration programs and investigation projects
- Promote the knowledge interchange between national and international academic Centers, Business firms, and Health Institutions.
- Transmit and expand the Health Informatics knowledge
- Represent all associates into national and internacional institutions

## Australia

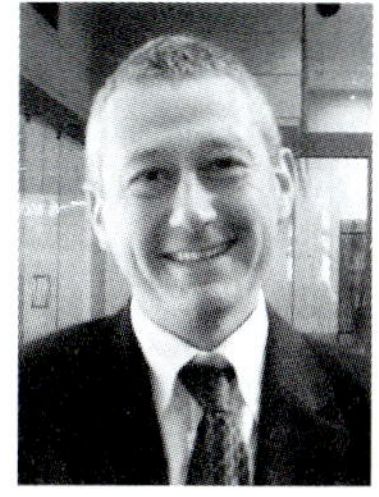

Paul Cohen, President

*HISA Mission Statement*

HISA is a member-friendly, professional organisation, focussing on healthcare informatics with benefits for practitioners, disciplines and sectors of healthcare in any geographic region of Australia and the world.

Member services are developed with the aim of value-adding knowledge for the individual member and enhancing networking opportunities between members.

*HISA Objectives*
- A national focus for health informatics in Australia Management and administration of HISA
- National assistance to members and others
- Publishing through print and electronic media
- Information collection, analysis and distribution
- Research promotion, support and co-ordination

## Austria

Computers have become more important for medicine. At the edge of the 21st Century, informational technology, computer science, knowledge management and communications engineering are of increasing importance as Interfaces between humans and machines. Improved medical technology has helped doctors to raise the level of health care.

Teaching and learning technology has proved to be equally valuable in the education and training of medical students. We aim to achieve an improved inter-disciplinary cooperation between medical and technological personnel.

Topics:
- Information Systems
- Internet - Intranet
- Knowledge Management
- Knowledge Technology
- Multimedia in Medicine
- Telemedicine
- PACS
- Human - Computer - Interaction
- Quality Management
- Standards

## Belgium

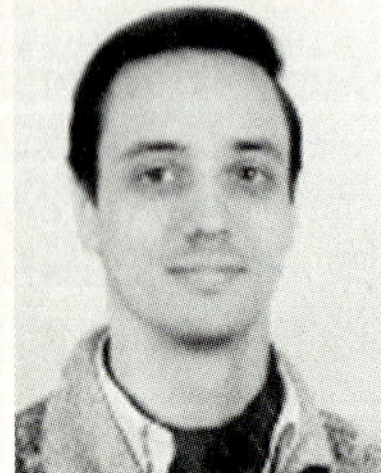

Etienne De Clercq, President

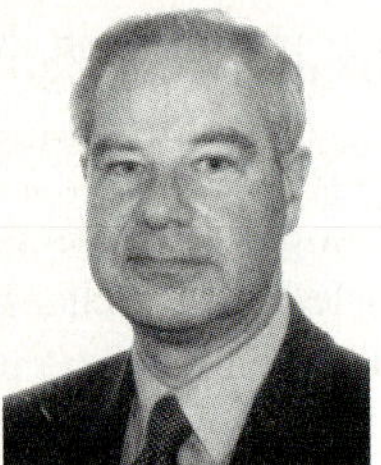

Francis H. Roger France,
IMIA Representative

The Belgian Society for Medical Informatics ("MIM") was established in 1974 to promote and develop medical information science and technology in Belgium. It is a national bilingual (French and Dutch) society consisting of about 300 members, all involved or interested in the use of computers and telematics in the health-care environment. The administrative board includes 15 members (physicians, engineers and computer specialists) from academic institutions, hospitals, computers and the software industry.

The MIM is a scientific society. Its major activities focus on improving communication among researchers and developers in the field of medical computing and telematics. It is also the place of choice where problems related to the role of medical informatics in society and its ethical aspects are discussed.

International related medical informatics societies:

- The MIM is the Belgian member of EFMI (European Federation for Medical Informatics) and of IMIA (International Medical Informatics Association). As such, the MIM is involved in the setting up of whose congresses, scientific events and publications.
- The MIM cooperates closely with the Dutch (VMBI), French (AIM) and Swiss (SSIM) medical informatics societies to organize annual scientific meetings: the «Medish Informatica Congres» (MIC) and the «Journées Francophones d'Informatique Médicale» (JFIM).

## Bosnia and Herzegovina

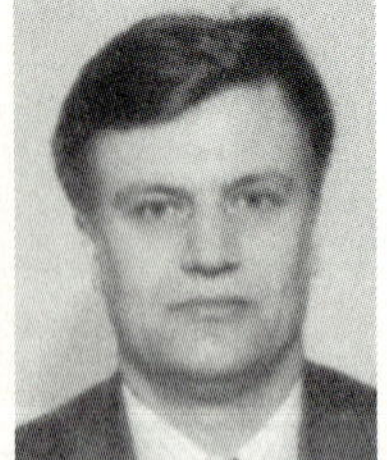

Izet Masic, President

The Society of Medical Informatics of the Republic of Bosnia and Herzegovina (DMI BiH) was founded in 1998, and has now over 80 members. The Society has its statutory bodies - the Administrative Board and Committees. The members of the administrative Board are the President of the Society, two Vice-Presidents, a Secretary, a Treasurer and four additional members. The current president is Prof.Dr. Izet Masic, the founder of the Society. Prof. Masic is also the official representative of the Society in EFMI and IMIA.

The society became an official member of EFMI and IMIA in 1994.

The Society carries out the following activities:

a) Promotion and improvement of informatics within the health-care system, health insurance and bio-medical research,
b) Engagement of experts in the field of medical informatics in B&H on development and establishment of health care information systems
c) Assistance in research, development and professional work in the field of medical informatics in B&H
d) Distribution and development of technical information in the field of medical informatics in B&H
e) Assistance in education of medical informatics experts
f) Exchange of professional experience on national and international level
g) Publishing activities in the field of medical informatics

The society edits its own professional journal-ACTA INFORMATICA MEDICA, and has organized four scientific and professional symposia during wartime in BIH. In November 1992, the Society has organized the First Symposium of Medical Informatics in BIH about Nomenclatures and classification systems in Bosnia and Herzegovina. Next Symposium was organized in 1993 with the theme:

Health Information Systems in Bosnia and Herzegovina. In 1994 the Society of Medical Informatics prepared new Symposium: Medical informatics according to the War medicine. Several books and monographs in the field of Medical Informatics have been published. Our experts have taken part in various scientific and professional gatherings and symposia at home and aboard on EFMI and IMIA Congresses and workshops during last eight years. They also participate in development and realization of information system health care, at regional as well as national levels.

## Bosnia and Herzegovina (Continued)

In this way the Society contributes considerably to the improvement of health care in Bosnia and Herzegovina.

The First congress of Medical informatics in B&H that was held in Sarajevo on November 5 & 6, 1999 gave us the opportunity to discuss the experiences in the current state of this science and its practical use in the world and our country. The Congress attracted over 100 participants, who attended seven very attractive sessions.

## Brazil

The Brazilian Health Informatics Association - SBIS - aims at improving the quality and reducing the costs of healthcare via the use of Health Informatics techniques, concepts and technologies, by:

- Stimulating educational activities related to Health Informatics;
- Stimulating scientific research and technical development in Health Informatics;
- Organising conferences, symposiums, courses, seminars, and other activities that lead to experience and knowledge exchange;
- Joining individuals, groups and organizations together;
- Cooperating with sister societies;
- Contributing to the construction of healthcare policies;
- Promoting of Health Informatics as a means to reduce costs and improve the quality of healthcare services;
- Promoting the use of standards for healthcare information.

## Canada

COACH: Canada's Health Informatics Association, founded in 1975, represents a strong community of over 900 members from a broad range of health care related backgrounds who are committed to advancing the practice of health informatics. The Association's mandate is to 'promote the understanding and effective utilization of information and information technologies within the Canadian health care industry through education, information, networking and communication'.

Key activities include a newly launched professional development series consisting of three workshops focusing on Information Management, Security and Privacy and the Electronic Health Record, the publication of resource information such as the Guidelines for the Protection of Health Information and partnering with the Canadian Institute for Health Information (CIHI) in the development of e-Health, a major national conference on health informatics.

COACH provides an excellent opportunity for networking among members and with other related organizations locally, nationally and internationally.

## China

The China Medical Informatics Association (CMIA), established in 1980, is an academic organization constituted by physicians, researchers, technologists, and administrators who are researching how to utilize computer science and information science in health care field. CMIA is a National Member in International Medical Informatics Association (IMIA), and is the only representative of China in IMIA. There are more than 5,700 members, 31 professional committees and 22 regional branches in CMIA.

The development of CMIA, also named as China Medical Informatics Association of Chinese Institute of Electronics, has won support from Ministry of Information Industry, Ministry of Health, State Economy and Trade Commission, State Drug Administration, etc. CMIA has built up broad relationship with hospitals, universities, academic institutions and industries.

Medical informatics is developed with a rapid speed in today's China. CMIA's goals and objectives are to advance the understanding and use of information technologies in China health care; to support the development of medicine and pharmacy; to build up the bridges among researchers, scientists, practitioners, suppliers, managers in health care field.

## Croatia

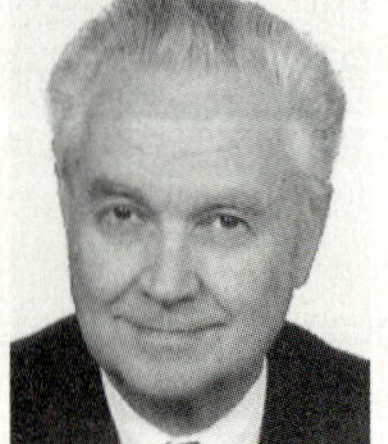

Gjuro Dezelic, President

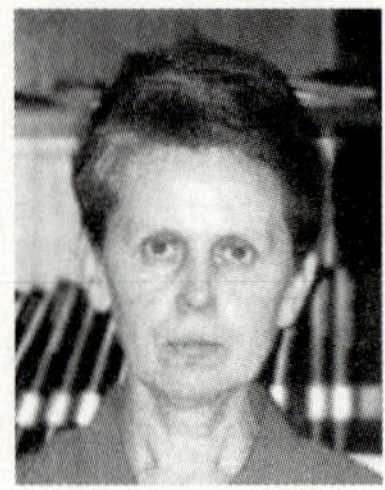

Josipa Kern, IMIA Representative

The Croatian Society for Medical Informatics is a non-profit organization concerned with the scientific field of medical informatics, which comprises the theory and practice of information science and technology within health care and health care science. The basic objectivities of the CSMI are as follows:

(1) to advance dissemination of information in the field of MI in Croatia,
(2) to promote high standards in the application of work in this field,
(3) to promote research and development in this field,
(4) to encourage high standards in education in this field,
(5) to advance international cooperation in this field.

CSMI organizes professional and scientific meetings biannually. Recently, two working groups were established:

WG1 - standardization in medical informatics
WG2 - data protection and data security.

The Society publishes a bulletin with papers of the CSMI members, and relevant information two times a year.

## Cuba

The Cuban Society of Medical Informatics groups specialists of different fields working on Medical and Health Informatics throughout the country. Health Research Centers, Medical Sciences Faculties, Specialized Informatics Centers working on Medical and Health Computerized Applications are also involved. The main goal of the Society is to develop and widespread scientific and updated informatic knowledge in all medical and health fields supporting the Health Policy of the National Health System. A major movement towards generalizing Medical Informatics is being developed through the creation in Provincial and Municipal Health Administrative Levels as well as in most Health Institutions of Health Informatics Groups. These groups are in charge of training the current staff of health organizations and institutions on the use of computers and the application of specific Medical and Health Informatics Systems performed. A National Policy on Health Informatics is ongoing with the active support of the Society.

## Czech Republic

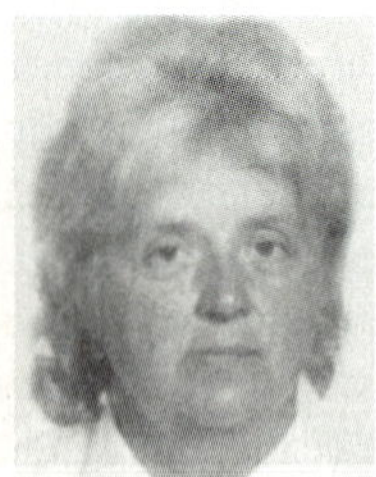

Jana Zvárová, IMIA Representative

The Czech Society of Biomedical Engineering and Medical Informatics is one of the medical societies gathered in the Czech Association of Medical Societies of J.E. Purkyne. The Medical Informatics Section of the Czech Society of Biomedical Engineering has been established in 1978. Through this section the activities in the field of medical informatics has been developed. Nowadays the Society is mostly concerned with activities in three sections: "Medical Informatics","Clinical Engineering" and "Biophysics". The Czech Society of Biomedical Engineering is the member of International Medical Informatics Association (IMIA), European Federation for Medical Informatics (EFMI) and International Federation for Medical and Biological Engineering (IFMBE).

The Society is ruled by the genral board of eleven elected society members. The president of the Czech Society of Biomedical Engineering and Medical Informatics is J. Cmíral, the Medical Informatics Section is headed by J. Zvárová (IMIA representative), the Clinical Engineering Section by V. Grospic and Biophysics Section by Z. Grossman. The Czech Society of Biomedical Engineering and Medical Informatics has issued the journal Physician and Technology, edited by J. Zvárová. The journal is published bimonthly and basic information about the journal can be found at the www address: lat.euromise.cz. The Society has structural links with other medical societies J.E. Purkyne and co-operates with other Czech scientific societies in this field, mainly Society for Cybernetis and

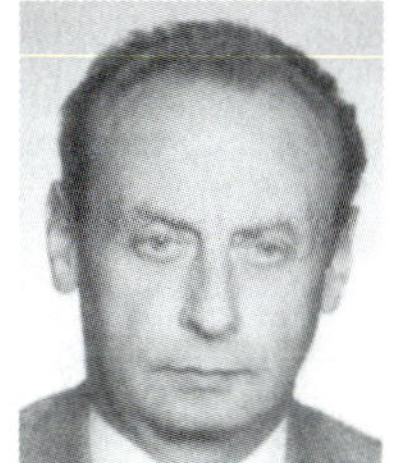

## Czech Republic (Continued)

Jaromir Cmíral, President

Informatics and Czech Scietific and Technical Society. The Society has close contacts with scientific societies in Hungary, Bulgaria, Poland and Austria.

The main activities of the Czech Society of Biomedical Engineering and Medical Informatics developed in the past together with Slovakia, were seminars, conferences and congresses, namely three international biomedical engineering conferences held in Mariánské Lázne (1983), Bratislava (1987) and in Prague (1991). The Society has co-sponsored the international conference System Science in Health Care in Prague 1992 and has been involved in Biosignal international conferences in Brno each year. The last conference Biosignal was held in Brno, June 21st - 23rd , 2000.

## *Denmark*

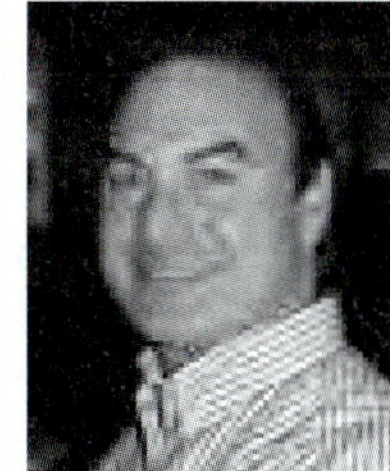

Knut Bernstein, IMIA Representative

The interest in medical informatics, or more appropriate - health care informatics - is increasing in the Danish community. The awareness among health care professionals is growing, the topic is clearly on the political agenda, and the marketplace is expanding.

It is interesting to note, that

- the Government has published its IT strategy - where health care has a very high priority. An agreement has been reached with the Counties (which runs the hospitals) for a strategy and the financing of an expansion of IT use in hospitals.
- the national health care network programme (MedCom) has been made a permanent activity. More than 1,5 million health care messages are sent via the network every month. (www.health-telematics.dk/)
- the Ministry of Health is supporting 10 project regarding the development of Danish electronic patient records. An increasing number of hospitals are starting to use electronic health care records. (www.hep.dk/)
- the National Panel for Standardisation of Medical Informatics has published a popular booklet on standardisation of electronic health care records.
- the use of Internet in health care is increasing. The Danish Medical Association has established a medical Intranet and supplies all Danish doctors with free Internet access. (A public part is on www.dadl.dk)
- the post graduate education in health care informatics is running at Aalborg University for the forth year, graduating Masters of Information Technology. DSMI has once again supported some of

the students with grants. (www.v-chi.dk/)
- the number of members in The Danish Society for Medical Informatics is increasing. (www.dsmi.dk)

The Danish Society for Medical Informatics - Dansk Selskab for Medicinsk Informatik (DSMI) was established in 1966. It is an independent society with an associated status to the Danish Medical Societies. The aim of the society is to compile and disseminate theoretical and practical knowledge in medical informatics, and to stimulate research and the use of medical information systems. The 350 members are physicians, nurses and others who work with theoretical or practical aspects of medical information technologies.

DSMI organises meetings, conferences and courses to pursue the goals of the society. One of the largest efforts for the Society was the organisation of MIE'96 in Copenhagen. More that 1000 participants participated in the high quality scientific programme and the large exhibition.

Other meetings have been successfully organised on electronic patient records, classification and semantics, clinical databases, resource management, the information highway etc.

The Society is represented in various groups, i.e. the Ministry of Health's advisory group and the Danish Standardisation Committee. The Society publishes a newsletter with abstracts of the meetings, papers, book reviews, announcements of international conferences and other relevant information. The DSMI homepage is playing a large role in the communication with the members: www.dsmi.dk.

## Finland

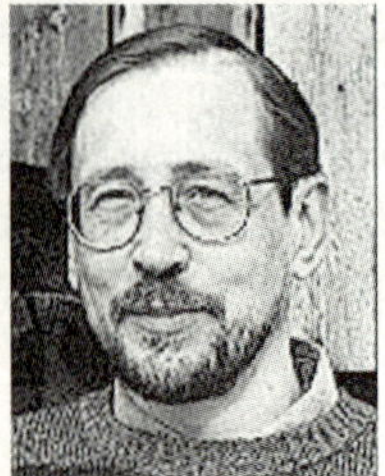

Mikko Korpela, IMIA Representative

The Finnish Social and Health Informatics Association was founded in 1974 and it organised the MIE conference in 1985. After that the association's activities decreased and it became dormant by the mid 1990s.

Since research, education and development projects in health informatics have been increasing strongly in Finland recently, the association was re-vitalised in May 2000. The scope of the association was expanded to social services informatics in June 2001.

The activities of the association focus on international relations (IMIA, EFMI and HUSITA), expanding the membership base, and maintaining a web site and an e-mail list for information dissemination. The main event of the association is the annual national Social and Health Care Informatics Research Days (SoTeTiTe-tutkimuspäivät), the sixth of which will be held in May 2003.

## France

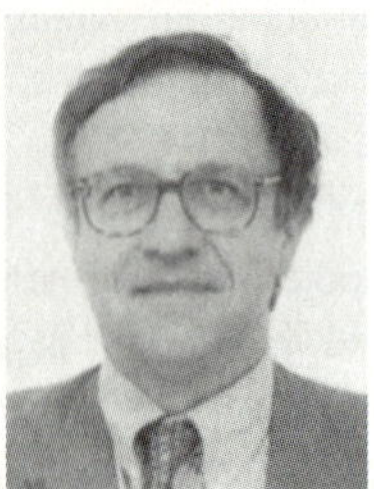

P. Degoulet, IMIA Representative

AIM, the acronym for the Association pour les Applications de l'Informatique en Médecine , was created in 1968. Since its beginning, the association has been involved in the promotion of computer applications in health care through the organization of scientific meetings, publications and various educational efforts. In the early seventies, AIM was directly involved in the organization of the Journées d'Informatique Médicale de Toulouse, which were among the first international meetings devoted to medical informatics. AIM is the official representative of France within the IMIA and EFMI boards and counts approximately 500 affiliate members. AIM currently organizes one or two meetings per year.

## Germany

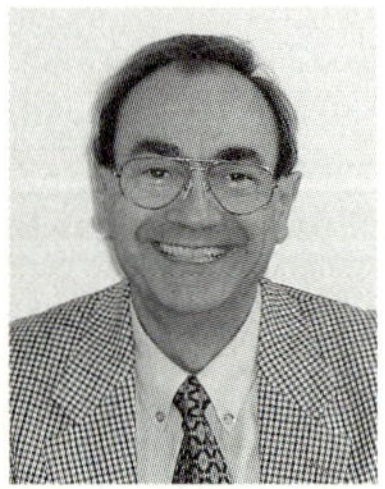

Walter Lehmacher, President

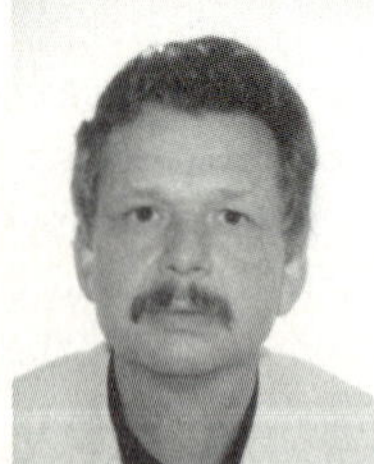

Herbert Witte, IMIA Representative

The GMDS, Deutsche Gesellschaft für Medizinische Informatik, Biometrie und Epidemiologie (German Association for Medical Informatics, Biometry and Epidemiology) is the only scientific organization in this field and as such the official national member within EFMI and IMIA. It closely cooperates with two professional organizations: the Berufsverband Medizinischer Informatiker (BVMI) and the Deutsche Verband Medizinischer Dokumentare (DVMD).

The scientific association GMDS was founded in the Fifties and is with more than 1600 members one of the largest scientific societies in this field in the world.

The basic structure of the GMDS consists of four divisions (medical informatics, medical biometry, epidemiology and medical documentation), with a wide variety of working groups. The management board of the GMDS is led by its president (Prof. Klar, Freiburg, 1999-2001; Prof. Lehmacher, Köln 2001-2003, Prof. Wichmann, Oberschleißheim, 2003-2005). The full structure of the GMDS and its work is described in www.gmds.de.

The GMDS issues a national scientific journal: Biometrie, Informatik und Epidemiologie in Medizin und Biologie (Gustav Fischer Verlag, Stuttgart, Eugen Ulmer Verlag, Stuttgart). The journal includes a newsletter of the national society.

Besides a spring congress on Hospital Information Systems and some smaller working conferences, the GMDS annually organizes one large national meeting with about 700 to 900 participants. The 2002 GMDS congress was held in Berlin. The 2003 congress will be held in Münster (Sept. 14th-18th; http://www.gmds2003.de). All national congresses have been published in proceedings volumes.

As education is a main concern of GMDS it has published a national strategic plan for education in medical informatics as well as for medical biometry. The GMDS is also actively involved in the definition of the medical curriculum and of the content of CME for physicians and for certified further professional qualification of medical informaticians, biometricians, epidemiologists and medical documentalists.

## Hong Kong

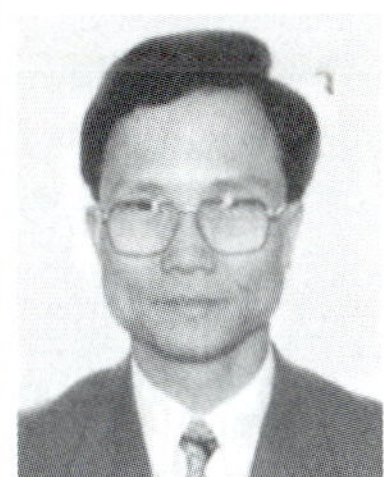

Chun Por Wong, President
and IMIA Representative

The Hong Kong Society of Medical Informatics was founded in April 1987 by a group of medical practitioners with special interests in medical informatics and computing. It expanded rapidly and now encompasses all workers in the health care information technology industry. In 2000, the Society had more than 1000 members.

The specific objectives of the Society are:

1. To promote applications of computers and information technology in medicine, and to maintain knowledge on information science and computer basics for health care workers in Hong Kong.
2. To provide a forum for the exchange of ideas and experience in medical computing among its members.
3. To hold lectures, seminars, exhibitions and conferences on subjects related to medical informatics.
4. To liaise with overseas medical informatics organizations, in order to capture first-hand information on the development of medical informatics.

The most important projects undertaken by the Society were the hosting of the series of five Hong Kong Asia-Pacific Medical Informatics Conferences since 1990. The Society has also acted as the technical organizer in the Medical Informatics Pavilions of various computer exhibitions in Hong Kong.

Hong Kong is now the President of the APAMI for the year 2000-2003. We look forward to a joint effort in Asia Pacific countries to further promote the standing of Medical Informatics in the region to a more prominent level in the global scene, and more importantly, to assist under-developed countries to develop and improve the medical informatics development in their region.

## Ireland

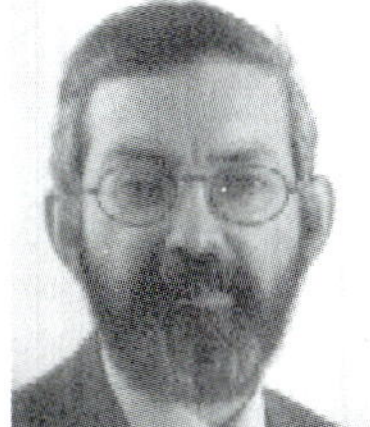

Diarmuid UaConaill, IMIA Representative

From 1976 to 1996, Healthcare Informatics interests in the Republic of Ireland were represented by the Health Care Specialist Group of the Irish Computer Society. This group represented Ireland at the European Federation for Medical Informatics (EFMI) and the International Medical Informatics Association (IMIA). It hosted the European Medical Informatics conference, MIE 82, and was associated with the IMIA Working Group 8 international symposium on Nursing Informatics held in Dublin in 1988.

In May 1996 the members of the Health Care Specialist Group formed a new society, the Healthcare Informatics Society of Ireland (Cumann Ríomheolais Sláinte), in order to broaden the base of membership and increase the range of services offered. By formal agreement with the Irish Computer Society, the Health Care Specialist Group was disbanded, and its functions, assetts and liabilities transferred to the new Society, which then became affiliated to the Irish Computer Society.

The Healthcare Informatics Society of Ireland was inaugurated formally at its First Annual Conference in the Burlington Hotel, Dublin, on Thursday 10th October 1996. The new society incorporates the Healthcare Informatics section of the Royal Academy of Medicine in Ireland. Thus the Healthcare Informatics Society is in a position to build bridges between computer professionals interested in health care, and health care professionals interested in computing, while supporting and embracing the new professionals of health care informatics. There are currently some 270 members, drawn from information technology, medicine, nursing, other professions allied to medicine, education, government and industry.

The officers of the Society are:

President: Prof. Jane Grimson, Trinity College, Dublin.

Chair: Mr. Gerard Hurl, Mater Misericordiae Hospital, Dublin.

Secretary: Ms. Ann Sheridan, St. John of God Hospital, Dublin.

Treasurer: Mr. Diarmuid UaConaill, Mater Misericordiae Hospital, Dublin.

The objectives, as set out in the Constitution, are:

1. To develop and disseminate knowledge of the use of informatics in health care.
2. To promote research and education in health care informatics.
3. To participate internationally with bodies of similar interests.

In pursuit of the third objective, the Healthcare Informatics Society of Ireland has been accepted as a member of the European Federation for Medical Informatics, and the International Medical Informatics Association.

For further information, see our website at: http://www.mater.ie/hisi/hisi.htm or http://hisi.ie.eu.org/hisi.htm

## Israel

The Israeli Association of Medical Informatics(IAMI) was established in 1983 with the following goals:

- To promote knowledge of Medical Informatics by organizing scientific and professional conferences, seminars courses and exhibitions.

- Advance cooperation among health professionals in the field of Medical Informatics.
- Provide forums for exchange of information and ideas.
- Present the interest of health professionals in goverment committees and other bodies.

## Italy

The Italian Association for Medical Informatics (AIIM) was founded 1975 to promote the applications of informatics in the different areas of medicine.

The objectives of the AIIM are the dissemination and exchange of information on medical informatics, for support patient care, teaching, research and health care administration; to advance international cooperation in medical informatics; to promote medical informatics education and to organize courses for health services personnel.

AIIM is a Member of the European Federation for Medical Informatics (EFMI)and the International Medical Informatics Association (IMIA).

The Membership categories are:

(a) Regular members including physicians, nurses, dentists, teachers, researchers, biomedical engineers, health services administrators, other health care professionals who have a strong interest in medical informatics;

(b) Honorary members: very important persons in the field of medical informatics;

(c) Correspondent members, including representatives of other Organizations and Associations having similar aims (European Society for Medical Decision Making; National Association for Informatics in Neuroscience, Italian Telematics Forum, etc).

The President of AIIM and the national council (10 members), are elected every four years by the membership.

At present, AIIM organize a National Congress every two years, and annually other meetings and workshops on specific topics. The previous AIIM National Congresses have been held in Parma (1997), Catania (1985), Firenze (1988), Como (1989), Cassino (1990), Catania (1991), Genova (1992), Roma (1994), Venezia (1996), Taranto(1998) and Padova (2001); furthermore AIIM organized in Rome the Seventh European Congress on Medical Informatics (MIE 1987): about 1,000 participants coming from 32 countries all over the world took part in the Congress.

The proceedings of the national congresses published by AIIM are an important source of information for the knowledge of medical informatics progress in Italy.

At present, the following Working Groups are operating in AIIM:

- Data Protection and Security in Health Information Systems,Bio-Ethics
- Standards in Health Information Systems
- Computerized Medical Records, Cards
- Telemedicine and Health Telematics
- Decision-Support Systems

AIIM cooperates with governmental bodies as an adviser in the field of medical informatics.

Guidelines on Telemedicine and Telematics in Health Care and on Health Cards, were approved during the national Congress in Venice(1996) with the participation of representatives of governmental and military health organizations, health professionals and scientific associations,researchers, telecommunication and information technology companies and industries, national research council, and citizens associations.

# *Japan*

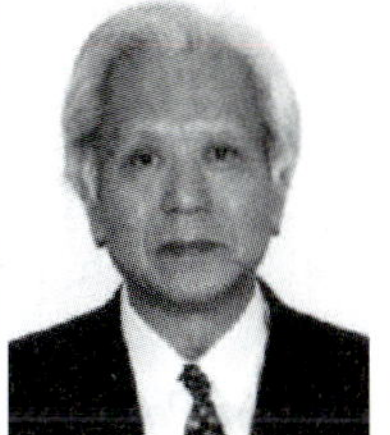

Michitoshi Inoue, President

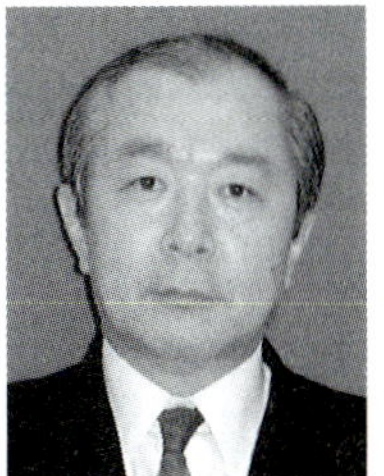

Ken Toyoda, IMIA Representative

Activities of the Japan Association for Medical Informatics (JAMI) are mainly performed through 5 commitees and 15 research groups supported by 2,107 members.

The president of JAMI is Dr. Inoue, President of Osaka National Hospital and Professor Emeritus of Osaka University.

Six issues of „Iryo Jouhou Gaku" (Japan Journal of Medical Informatics), the official journal of JAMI, have been published in 2002 (Volume 22). Included are two supplements for „The JAMI Symposium" and „The 22nd Joint Conference on Medical Informatics".

The „JAMI Symposium 02" entitled „Evaluation and Practice of Medical Information Systems" was held at KOKUYO-hall at Tokyo on June 1. There were two sub-themes, „Health Information as Common Property" and „Privacy and Security".

„The 22nd Joint Conference on Medical Informatics" was held on November 14-16 at Fukuoka city. The chairperson of the organization committee was Prof. Yoshiaki Nose, Kyusyu University. The main theme was „Focus on Medical Needs in Social Environment". More than 2,000 members participated and about 500 papers were presented.

The 4th China-Japan-Korea Joint Symposium on Medical Informatics" (CJKMI'01) was held on August 3 at Beijin, China.

The JAMI Symposium 2003, entitled „Care Management and Medical Information" will be held at Kiyakyusyuu-city on June 13,14,2003.

The 23rd Joint Conference on Medical Informatics will be held at Makuhari on November, 2002. The chairperson of the organization committee is Mr. Ken Toyoda, Bearing Point.

For more information about JAMI, contact the home page of JAMI (http://jami.umin.ac.jp/) or MEDIS-DC by telefax: 81-3-3505-1996 or by phone: 81-3-3586-6321.

# *Kazakstan*

MedPharmInfo Association (medical - pharmaceutical information) was established in March, 2000 on the basis of The Information Center and Institute of Standardization, Metrology and Certification jointly with an inquiry-information bureau under private company ZdravTechStandard. Besides mentioned organizations founders of the Association include several non-governmental medical centers, pharmaceutical companies, educational and scientific institutions.

The need for such association was due to an absolute necessity of an operational and professional information for specialists engaged in various healthcare organizations. First and foremost, this provides an opportunity to obtain the full code of laws and standard Acts, regulating public healthcare activity, production and supply of medicines and medical products etc. In the course of professional activities medical men quite often search for specialized information covering different fields of medical sciences as well as practical issues. Population lacks accessible sources of popular information as to preventive methods, diseases, treatment and so forth. The list of problems can be extended further.

Taking into account the aforesaid grounds, founders of the Association set a goal to create a public organization uniting all the concerned medical and pharmaceutical organizations, scientific institutions, chemists, institutes of higher education and colleges, industrial enterprises etc., which are in need of access to contemporary information technologies. The Association initiated the creation of a large specialized informational center, which already comprises highly qualified specialists (doctors, pharmacists, marketing and information experts, computer programmers, electronics engineer etc.).

Modern material and logistic support is being created, new communication and technological solutions are in the process of implementation. This Center is meant for a large-scale information support in the field of healthcare in Kazakhstan, medical achievements and rendering various information to both specialists and vast population strata.

**Activities**: In the sake of the users large marketing and analytical research of the pharmaceutical market is being conducted in Kazakhstan, wholesale and retail prices

## Kazakstan (Continued)

for medications and medical equipment are being monitored. The Center has developed unique schemes for gathering and processing of information concerning wholesale and retail pricing in Almaty and other regions of Kazakhstan.

A free of charge round-the-clock phone inquiry office Medicines and Medical Services is successfully working under the jurisdiction of the Association. Every month more than 70000 citizens use its services by multi-line telephone (3272) 50-50-60. This number is constantly growing.

The Center regularly publishes information bulletins: „Wholesale Prices for Medicines in Almaty, Kokshetau, Karagandy, Petropavlovsk and Shymkent"(twice a month), „Average Retail Process for Medicines in Almaty City» (monthly), and „Cost of Medical Services in Almaty" (at request). The bulletins are being distributed at pharmacists and clinics, in large pharmaceutical companies in Almaty, Astana, Aktyubinsk, Atyrau, Karagandy, Kokshetau, Kostanai, Pavlodar, Petropavlovsk, Semipalatinsk, Taraz, Ust-Kamenogorsk, Shymkent.

The Center's information database has been updated every day. Electronic versions of any information are available at the first request. Analytical data as to the population's requests allow obtaining extra information on the demand for certain medications.

For the first time in Kazakhstan The Center is publishing information materials on diverse healthcare issues in the Internet - on the website http://www.med.kz, which enlarges possibilities of the users to get necessary information such as code of laws and standards Acts on pharmaceutical and medical undertakings in the Republic of Kazakhstan; medical equipment producers and manufacturers; wholesale pharmaceutical companies; pharmacists in Almaty; medicines registered in Kazakhstan, wholesale and retail prices; international conferences and exhibitions, and many other aspects.

Since August 2000 there was launched a project „Telemedicine in Kazakhstan" http://www.tele.med.kz, within which framework the Association started to implement educational projects - monthly seminars Contemporary Internet technologies in the healthcare sphere (for free), and quarterly 3-day computer courses for medical specialists.

The Association is intended to widen up its services in the future for local and foreign organizations. It's planned to establish international co-operation in informational support for the healthcare system.

**Conferences**: Conferences and meetings are being held on the regular basis. Conference Achievements of Internet Technologies in Healthcare was arranged.

## Korea

The Korean Society of Medical Informatics (KOSMI) was founded in 1987 with a specific aim to promote and collaborate multidisciplinary specialities in medicine and health care. For the last 15 years since then, the research activities in medical informatics are rapidly increased to become a major focus of attention from medical community. Domestic KOSMI conferences have been carried out biannually. Due to increasing number of paper submission, biannual publication of the Journal of KOSMI has been promoted to quarterly.

During the 1990s, tremendous efforts were put into the development and implementation of hospital information systems for major hospitals, and a great amount of funding support was provided simultaneously. As a result, Korea is probably regarded as one the most well-informatized country in the globe at the present time. Network infrastructure is well-established enough to support not only electronic commerce in general but also small business unit such PC chamber (or PC-bang in Korean). As applications of e-Commerce appear to be in its continuous expansion, e-Health is expected to settle in seamlessly in the foreseeable future.

In addition to clinical applications of medical informatics, two major topics of medical informatics are of interest: education and standardization.

There are 41 medical schools (including 10 national universities) in Korea, and most schools are now considering education reform. Because patient needs are constantly on the rise, lecture based medical education methods are found to be inefficient as societal and clinical environmental

## Korea
### (Continued)

changes pervade. MEDINFO'98 in Seoul is found to be a great momentum for promoting medical informatics in many respects in Korea. Medical education for example, the first academic department of medical informatics was inaugurated at Kyungpook National University School of Medicine in 1999. Medical informatics has been gradually recognized as a standard curriculum in many medical schools. Also recently, nursing informatics is launched as a graduate study program in College of Nursing, Seoul National University.

In 3 consecutive joint symposia with the Korean Society of Medical Education in 2001-2002, the suggestions of Medical School Objectives Project (MSOP) by American Association of Medical Colleges (AAMC) and IMIA WG1 are highly regarded, and therefore medical informatics is strongly recommended to be included in the regular medical curriculum. Although medical education curriculum is in transition, the role of medical informatics should be more than computer literacy to play a critical role in the medical education reform.

Standardization is another major thrust in medical informatics. Due to rapid spread of computer technology in both hospitals and medical practices throughout the world, developers and implementers are concerned about incorporating information technology into networked healthcare environments to exchange and share medical information such as Electronic Medical Record (EMR). In this regard, Health Informatics Standardization committee was formed in KOSMI since 1999 in order to actively participate not only in the international standardization (ISO TC215, Health Informatics) but also in the national informatics standardization with the government support from Korean Agency for Technology and Standards (KATS), the Ministry of Commerce, Industry and Energy (MOCIE). HL7 (Health Level Seven) is also incorporated to facilitate standardization of messaging and communication of medical information. A number of international standardization activities have been organized with KOSMI such as ISO Technical Committee 215 Conference.

Asian-specific on-going issues of health informatics standardization will be discussed in APAMI to be held in Taegu . Oct 29-31, 2003 (Dr. Yun Sik Kwak, Organizing Chair). Especially, KOSMI Fall Conference will celebrate the 15th anniversary in in Seoul Nov. 29, 2002 (Dr. Young Moon Chae, Organizing Chair)

All members of KOSMI are determined to accomplish multidisciplinary objectives that we all face up to now, and we have no double that the spirit of KOSMI will continue and prosper.

## The Netherlands

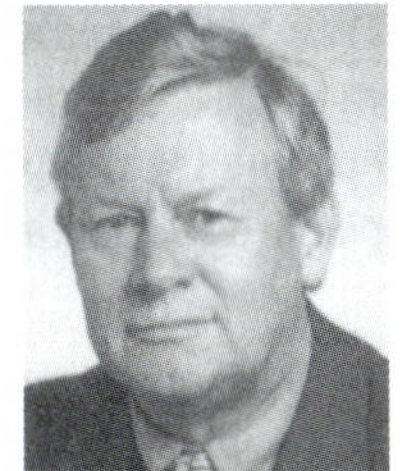

Arie Hasman, President and IMIA Representative

The goal of the VMBI, the Dutch Society for Health Care Informatics, is to promote research, development, and applications in medicine and health care, and in the biological sciences.

The Society is a meeting place for people in medical informatics in the broadest sense, i.e. physicians, nurses, informaticians, physicists, hospital administrators, and health care managers.

All hospitals in The Netherlands have systems installed to support administration, communication and patiënt care. In primary care, over 85% of GPs, all retail pharmacists, dentists, and the majority of physiotherapists have systems in use. An increasing numberv of systems are interconnected by EDI and networks. Development of computer-based patient records has much attention in R&D institutions. The Dutch professional medical societies play a major role in the promotion of information systems in healthcare. Most universities offer some training in medical informatics as part of the curriculum. This dynamic activity is a very healthy environment for the VMBI.

The activities of the VMBI include monthly meetings (lecturers, demonstrations) in Utrecht, in the center of the country, most of them in the late afternoon / early evening, annual two-day Conferences (called MIC, Medical Informatics Conference), together with the Belgian Society for Medical Informatics MIM, where about 400 people meet around lecturers, workshops and a large exhibition, an which is alternately held in The Netherlands and Belgium. The VMBI publishes a quarterly called I& (Informatie & Zorg, in english: Information & Care).

---

## The Netherlands (Continued)

Over the past years, several IMIA Working Conferences have been organized in The Netherlands on subjects such as Telematics in Health Care, Hospital Information Systems, Electronic Patient Records in Medical Practice and Software Engineering in Health Care.

The VMBI developed a strategy to reinforce the relationships with professional medical societies and to increase its membership of practicing physicians. A working group has been established to develop concrete plans to widen the scope of the Society.

## New Zealand

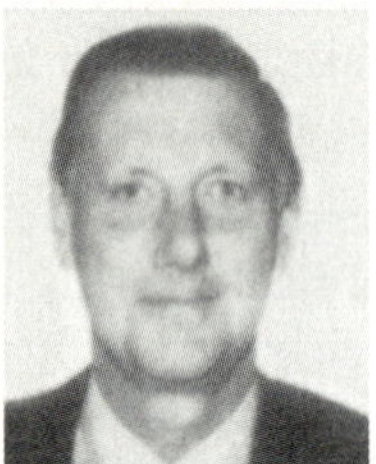

Ian H. Symonds, IMIA Representative

Health Informatics New Zealand is a national group open to anyone interested in Health Informatics We also have international members. Membership can be Individual or Corporate, (which allows unlimited members), Honorary or an affiliate. Health informatics relates to information technology in all areas of health care: clinical practice, administration, research, and education. It is the use of computers, information systems and other technologies which will provide better outcomes for patients who require health interventions.

We exist to :

- Promote and contribute to the growth of knowledge in Health Informatics
- Participate in the development of health information technologies and their use
- Lobby government on related health informatics issues to ensure informed input into decisions which affect health care outcomes in New Zealand
- Network and support those people interested in the use and application Health informatics Network with related national and international health informatics groups

Benefits for our members:

- Regular newsletters
- Bi annual conferences
- Study days/seminars
- Travel/conference funding/grants
- Website

## Norway

The Norwegian Society for Medical Informatics - Forum for Databehandling i Helsesektoren (FDH) was established in 1972 as a special interest group of The Norwegian Informatics Society - Den Norske Dataforening (DND). Since 1989 FDH has been an independent society with primary interest in medical informatics and an associated status to DND. FDH has a long-established membership in EFMI and IMIA.

The society has both individual and institutional members. Most of the individual members are health care workers.

FDH organizes meetings, seminars and courses to share knowledge and information with the members as well as to promote involvement of medical informatics in the Norwegian health care system.

FDH arranges seminars and meetings regularly on topics like EPR, Data Security, Trusted Third Parties, Legal Issues and Healthcare Legislation, Healthcare Politics.

## Romania

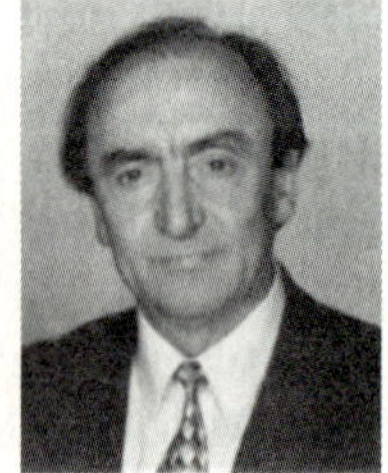

George I. Mihalas, President and IMIA Representative

The Romanian Society for Medical Informatics, RSMI, is a scientific, professional, non-governmental organisation aimed to promote the activities in the development of medical informatics in Romania and to represent the activities in the country and abroad.

RSMI was founded in 1990 and has now almost 200 members: physicians, computer scientists, engineers, mathematicians and other professionals working in the field of medical informatics. It continues the tradition of a group of specialists who started to work in this field in 1977.

The activities of RSMI concern stimulation and co-ordination of the activities of its members in promoting medical informatics in the country and to support international co-operation in this field, which implies:

- organising scientific and professional conferences, symposia, courses and exhibitions and collaboration in such activities with related organisations;
- publishing scientific, professional and educational publications in the field of medical informatics;
- promoting scientific and professional contacts with similar societies at the

---

<table>
<tr><td>

*Romania*
*(Continued)*

</td><td>

international level;

- collaboration with the Romanian Academy and with the Academy of Medical Sciences in medical informatics research;
- collaboration with medical universities in developing education in medical informatics.

RSMI members serve in several professional and scientific committees and also in various expert groups of the Ministry of Health and the Ministry of Education.

During 2001 and 2002 RSMI members participated in international events: MEDINFO2001 in London (5 participants) and MIE2002 in Budapest (12 participants with a generous support of EFMI). The Romanian Society of Medical Informatics expressed its gratitude to all those who helped the contacts of their members either as sponsorship for participation to meetings and/or direct collaboration in international projects; the society aims to increase its efforts in this line.

Romania was represented as a correspond-

</td><td>

ing member in IMIA since 1986 and RSMI has become a full member in 1994, having now representatives in several active working groups of IMIA. In the same year 1994 RSMI also joined EFMI.

The 24th National Conference on Medical Informatics, organised by the Romanian Society of Medical Informatics, was held in Bucharest 7-9 June 2001 joint to MIE2001 Special Topic Conference "Healthcare Telematics in Transition Countries"; EFMI Council Meeting was held in Bucharest immediately after the Conference. The jubiliar 25th National Conference on Medical Informatics, MEDINF2002 "Trends in Romanian e-Health" was held in Timisoara 14-16 June 2002.

The 26th Conference will be held in co-operation with European Society for Engineering and Medicine Society for the Internet in Medicine as the 1st MEDINF International Conference on Medical Informatics & Engineering "MEDINF2003' will be held in Craiova, 9-11 October 2003.

</td></tr>
</table>

<table>
<tr><td>

*Singapore*

</td><td>

The Association for Informatics in Medicine, Singapore (AIMS) was established in 1986 with the following aims:

- promote the growth, development and usage of information science and information technologies as applied to health care and to the education of health professionals in Singapore;
- advance cooperation among health professionals in the field of medical informatics;
- provide a forum for the dissemination, exchange and analysis of information through education and participation of its members;
- offer recommendations to international or governmental agencies and other appropriate bodies concerning the need for, and the structure of eductional programs in the field of medical informatics. Attention will be given to the mechanisms for implementing such educational programs in informatics;
- represent the interests of health professionals in the promotion and pursuit of

</td><td>

informatics with international or governmental agencies and other bodies.

AIMS (www.aims.org.sg) currently has about 100 members who are mainly health, medical or IT professionals. AIMS promotes its activities in a variety of ways including organizing local conferences and seminars, the publication of a newsletter and an annual Medical Informatics Lecture. The Association was also instrumental in assisting IMIA to stage MEDINFO 89 Part II in Singapore on short notice.

Nationally, the Association works closely with the governmental IT agencies, health and medical professional associations and the IT and healthcare industries while internationally, the Association is a member of IMIA and actively supports the international organization in its activities. AIMS was instrumental in helping IMIA to establish the Asia Pacific Association of Medical Informatics (APAMI) which was inaugurated in Singapore on November 10, 1994. APAMI (www.apami. org) currently has 13 national members.

</td></tr>
</table>

## Slovak Republic

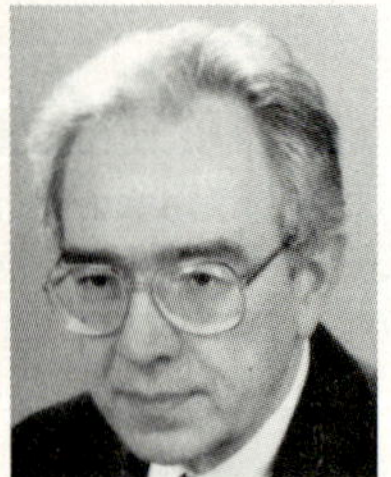

Peter Kneppo, President

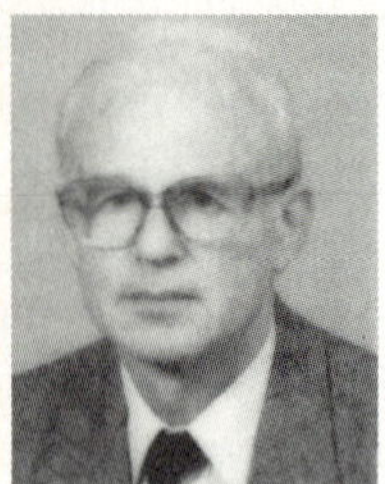

Mikulas Popper,
IMIA Representative

For the year 2001 the following major activities are planned regarding medical informatics:

- Seminar on Developments in Medical Informatics - as an accompanying action of the SLOVMEDICA EXHIBITION (September-October)
- Conference on Hospital Information Systems NIS'2001 (October/November)
- Seminar on Developments in Bionics (preliminary tittle, the approx. date is to be specified)

The steering board of our Society meets 3-4 times in a year (i.e. approx. quarterly)

## South Africa

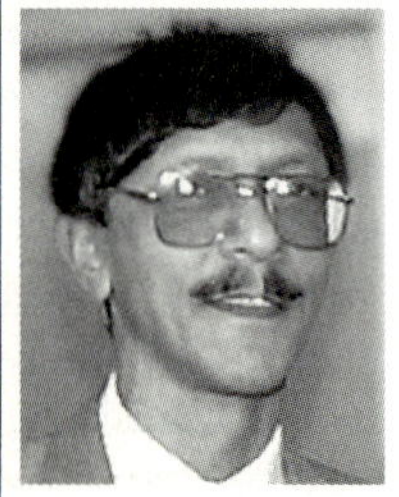

Sedick Isaacs, President

The South African Health Informatics Association (SAHIA) was formed to promote the professional application of Health Informatics in South Africa.

The goals of the organisation include:

- to represent South African Health Informatics nationally and internationally
- to promote and uphold the status of the Health Informatics profession

- to stimulate the advancement of Health Informatics in South Africa, and
- to promote the interests of members.

The focus of SAHIA activities is in the HISA (health informatics for Southern Africa) conferences, which will be held annually from 2000. Members are involved in a wide range of Health Informatics activities in both the public and private sectors.

## Spain

The Spanish Society of Health Informatics is a non-profit scientific society, built up in 1976 and joining today more than five hundred professionals, technicians or health scientists with interest in the promotion of the use of Information and Communications Technologies in the health environment. In this way it arises as a common debate forum for the professional of medicine, informatics, pharmacy, nursery, biology, and all the other Health Sciences, as well as for the students of any related career.

Among the multiple activities and projects developed by our society in the recent years, outstands the National Congress on Health Informatics that, in a biannual basis, has had three editions until date.

In addition to this general congress (INFORSALUD), the society organises more specific congresses targeted to professional sectors (Pharmacy and Informatics, Medical Informatics, Nursery and Informatics, Bio-informatics) or technological aspects (Internet in Health, medical data protection, ...).

## Sweden

The Swedish Federation for Medical Informatics is an association of persons with an interest in issues of medical informatics. Anyone working in health care and dental care is welcome as a member regardless of profession. The Federation is also a section of The Swedish Society of Medicine founded in 1807; the oldest organisation for the medical profession in Europe.

Our main objective is to create a platform for discussion and information exchange in the Medical Informatics field. We arrange an annual Conference „IT in Health Care" and a scientific seminar at the annual general meeting for doctors.

## Switzerland

Before February, 1985, the date of the creation of the Swiss Society for Medical Informatics (SSMI), most of the medical activities related to the application of computer sciences, were held within the Swiss Society for Biomedical Engineering where, as expected, most of the professionals were engineers. The SSMI, on the contrary, has been set up and led, since its creation, by a majority of health-care professionals: physicians as well as nurses. Already from its first year the SSMI became a member of the Swiss Federation for Informatics, which regroups all the other Swiss informatics Societies being the Swiss national society and a member of IFIP.

Naturally, the SSMI became an IMIA and EFMI member, within the Swiss IFIP Chapter, and the former place of TC4 (Technical Committee 4) is held by the IMIA representative delegated by the SSMI. It follows that our IMIA national society is associated with all the other computer science activities handled by the IFIP special interest groups as well as its technical committees.

More information on the society and its various activities can be found on its website: http://www.sgmi-ssim.ch

## Turkey

TURKMIA is a nonprofit membership organization, dedicated to guiding development and organisation of health and medical informatics in Turkey.

TURKMIA was founded in 1999 in Ankara. It organized First Medical Informatics Symposium in November 1999.

Aims of TURKMIA include:

- to collect, process and distribute information about the activities related to health and medical informatics of companies, governmental and non-governmental organizations.
- to stimulate all the professionals related to health and medical informatics to reach the contemporary level of knowledge and skills, prepare the background for communication and interaction between the professionals in the field, promote multidisciplinary study.
- to determine the problems related to health and medical informatics domain in Turkey, suggest solutions to these problems, collaborate with other organizations to realize the projects, announce the results of the projects or applications.
- to enhance the knowledge of health care providers and demanders about health and medical informatics, organize meetings and publish materials to shape public opinion.
- to inform, sensitize and stimulate the decision making and administrating people and organizations about the issues related to medical informatics.

Activities of TURKMIA:

- TURKMIA started SBS 2000 (Health Information Strategies of Turkey in the New Millenium) project in June 2000 by a meeting in Ankara. Preliminary reports of the study groups discussed in the First Congress of Medical Informatics which was held in 28-29th April 2001 in Istanbul. Final reports were collected in a book and in press. This book will be presented to the governmental and civil organizations, healthcare institutions, professional associations, commercial companies and non governmental organizations which are active in the healthcare sector in order to establish

## Turkey
## (Continued)

# *Ukraine*

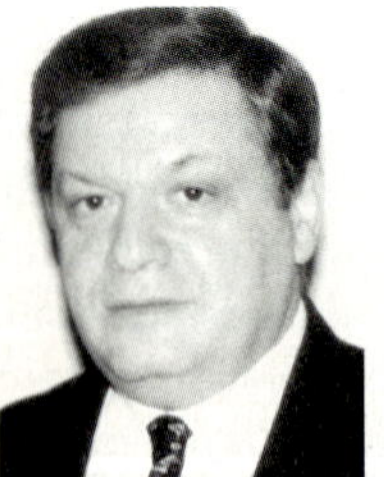

Oleg Mayorov, IMIA Representative

---

the health information vision, goals, strategy and politics of Turkey

· TURKMIA is in collaboration with Turkish Informatics Foundation (Turkiye Bilisim Vakfi) for informatics projects in healthcare domain.

· A study group is founded to prepare guidelines for electronic medical journals in Turkey.

· TURKMIA organizes regular monthly meetings in Istanbul, the largest city of Turkey, to bring together people responsible of and/or interested in hospital information systems.

---

UACM was set up in August 1992 in Kharkiv, where the IVth World Congress of WFUPS (World Federation of Ukrainian Physicians Societies) was taking place.

UACM became a national member of International Medical Informatics Association (IMIA) in September 1993 (Kyoto, Japan).

In May 1994 UACM was adopted as a National Member of European Federation of Medical Informatics (EFMI) at the IVth European Congress on Medical Informatics in Lisbon (Portugal).

It unites 78 scientific research institutes, universities, scientific societies, enterprises and hospitals. Over 900 scientists are individual members of the UACM.

The structure of the UACM has Scientific Council including 68 leading scientist-experts in medical informatics, medicine, radio-electronics from Ukraine, NIS, USA, UK, Canada, France, Japan, Israel and Turkey.

This Council's terms of reference cover:

· elaboration and discussion of complex computerisation programmes in various fields of healthcare;

· analysis and sharing of experience of computer technologies usage according to the situation in Ukraine;

· consideration of foreign proposals dealing with introduction and selling of computer technologies in the field of medicine to Ukraine and making proposals to the Ministry of Healthcare of Ukraine to buy them;

· progressive directions on elaborating and consideration of possible joint projects;

· carrying out expert estimations for receiving state licences.

A Regulation on certification information technologies in Healthcare was worked out with the help of the UACM Scientific Council and was approved by the Ministry of Healthcare and the State Committee for Standards. Committee on certification was set up under the Ministry of Healthcare.

Starting from 1998 its work will be based on the Ukrainian Institute of Public Health. All programme products for medical application will be forwarded to this Institute for certification. Since 1998 all medical software used in Healthcare of Ukraine must receive the certificate from the mentioned Committee.

Purposes:

Working out new medical software and biotechnical systems. Carrying out independent expert control and preparing materials to receive certificate.

Putting the best Ukrainian and foreign systems into medical practice.

Organising educational activity to train for new and postgraduate education; patent search; author's rights protection. Contacts with IMIA and EFMI members, foreign scientific societies, universities. Participation in state and foreign programs of Informatization of Healthcare in Ukraine. Organising symposia, forums, exhibitions and competitions.

The UACM experts has worked out the Concept of State Policy of Informatization of the Ukraine Healthcare adopted by the Ministry of Healthcare, agreed with Academy of Medical Sciences (http://www.uacm.cit-ua.net (Ukr. Radiological Journal 1996. №2.p. 115-118). The National Program of Healthcare Informatization to be put into practice has created.

National healthcare network of direct access UkrMedNet is being set up. The Concept of creation of the direct access State National Healthcare Network (UkrMedNet) has been developed by UACM experts (http://www.uacm.cit-ua.net).

The Information Analytical System (its medical part) for emergency situations within Cabinet of Ministers of Ukraine is under development.

The project of the system of medical information exchange in the NIS is worked out.

## *Ukraine (Continued)*

The UACM is an initiator of the National Program Hospital Information Systems.

The fact that the UACM joins the Internet plays an important role in its development. In 1996 the UACM has created of its own WWW-server in 3 languages: Ukrainian, Russian and English (http://www.uacm.cit-ua.net). The UACM members have the possibility to use data bases and scientific information on medical informatics world-wide and Europe-wide in Ukrainian and Russian (WWW-servers of EFMI, IMIA, WHO, EHTO European Observatory on Telemedicine), UNESCO and different WWW-servers of IMIA/EFMI (WG's and SIGs). The UACM has received an offer and has created affiliate Web-EHTO-UKRAINE server in Ukraine (http://www.ehto-ukr.cit-ua.net).

In 1996 the United Commission on Telemedicine of the Ministry of Healthcare and the Academy of Medical Sciences has been created. The Commission co-operates with the UN International Telecommunication Union (ITU) and European Commission on Telemedecine (DGXIII). In June 1997 the UACM specialists took part in the 1st World Symposium on Telemedecine for developing countries and made a report. The Symposium took part in Lisbon, Portugal, under the patronage of UN and WHO. In July 1998 the UACM specialists took part in the Conference "Telemedecine International Medical Care Networks" in Visby (Sweden) for co-operation and efficient use of resources by building networks within the Baltic Region. In 1998 under the initiative of UACM started the Ukrainian-American project on monitoring of birth defects in Ukraine.

The annual scientific conferences, exhibitions and sales of medical software are carried out with the participation of leading foreign firms and Ukrainian enterprises within the Programme of Health Care Informatization.

Since a 1993 UACM conducts annual International Conference Computer Medicine.

## *United Kingdom*

The British Computer Society, through its Health Informatics Committee (HIC), is the internationally recognised body for health informatics in the UK. HIC is a body formed to co-ordinate the work of the BCS specialist groups involved in healthcare computing - Nursing, Primary Health Care, London Medical, Northern Medical, and Scotland Medical. We also have a newly-established South West regional group and an Allied Health Professions group will be formed in the very near future.

HIC, which has been established for over 30 years, has a threefold role: to assist its constituent groups; to act for the BCS in all aspects of health and healthcare matters; and to run its own activities. The most important of its activities is the annual Healthcare Computing Congress, the largest such event in Europe, attracting over 1200 conference attendees and approaching 5000 exhibition visitors, and held annually in March in Harrogate; the twentieth event will be held on 24-26 March 2003. Each of the HC conferences results in a book (or recently CD-ROM) of Proceedings, carrying the full text of all the papers presented. HIC has also published a series of books on the field of health informatics, with multi-authorship.

Through the BCS, HIC appoints the UK representatives to the two relevant international bodies - the International Medical Informatics Association (IMIA) and the European Federation of Medical Informatics (EFMI). The current representatives are Dr Peter J. Murray at IMIA and Dr. John Bryden at EFMI.

European Federation of Medical Informatics (EFMI). The current representatives are Dr Peter J. Murray at IMIA and Dr. John Bryden at EFMI.

The Specialist Groups also organise their own conferences and meetings, details of which can be found on their own websites or through the HIC site.

In keeping with HIC's role of acting for the BCS on healthcare matters, it has recently provided expert opinion and commentary on important issues affecting health informatics and the health services in the UK. Among recent activities, HIC has commented on The Wanless Report , a report commissioned by the Chancellor of the Exchequer to help inform the Government's Spending Review. HIC has also been involved in evaluating the proposals for the NHS University.

## United Kingdom (Continued)

## USA

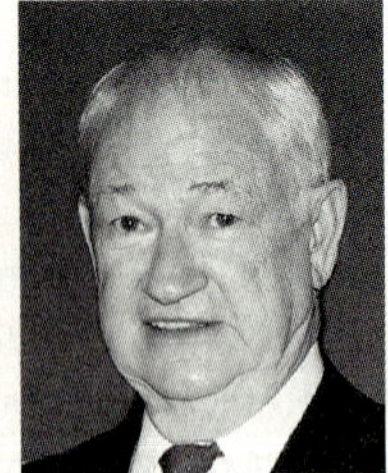

W. Ed Hammond, President

HIC recently established a think tank on innovative ways to move forward informatics in support of health; called 'Radical Steps'. After an invited workshop, wide consultation has been invited on key themes such as confidentiality, information governance, implementation management, standards, procurement, partnership with industry, ensuring capacity and coordinating change.

HIC is involved in leading a recent initiative to explore the creation of an umbrella organisation to bring together existing professional bodies and interest groups. It is envisaged that partnership working will commence by the end of 2002 to look at how best to move towards voluntary registration and regulation for health informatics professionals throughout the UK.

Full and latest information on HIC is available through its website: www.bcshic.org

The American Medical Informatics Association (AMIA) was incorporated in the District of Columbia in 1988 following more than a year of discussions among the boards of directors of the American Association for Medical Systems and Informatics, the American College of Medical Informatics, and the Symposium on Computer Applications in Medical Care (SCAMC). It brings together a professional association solely devoted to medical informatics, the organization responsible for the major annual meeting in the field, and the College of recognized leaders who have made major contributions to the field.

The oldest of the three organizations was the Symposium on Computer Applications in Medical Care. The Symposium was first conducted in 1977 as a regional effort in the Washington-Baltimore area. Two years later, SCAMC expanded its horizon, and quickly grew to a meeting attracting more than 2,000 participants. The name of the meeting was eventually changed to the AMIA Annual Symposium. Now over 100 organizations/companies and 2,000+ attendees participate in the Annual Symposium featuring scientific paper presentations, panel discussions, tutorials, workshops, system demonstrations, posters and commercial product exhibits. The Proceedings of the Annual Symposium reflects the body of work that is accomplished each year in medical informatics in the United States and abroad and is indexed by the National Library of Medicine.

The American Association for Medical Systems and Informatics (AAMSI) was formed in 1981 through a merger of the Society for Computer Medicine and the Society for Advanced Medical Systems. This union of two organizations with nearly 500 members each resulted in the largest membership society in the country at that time, with a principal interest in the advancement of medical informatics. A tradition was established of a spring meeting held annually on the West Coast, known as the AAMSI Spring Congress.

In response to a perceived need for the recognition of experts and leaders in the medical informatics field, the American College of Medical Informatics was established in 1985. Candidates are proposed by the Fellows and elected by mail ballot. ACMI meets three times each year, which includes an ACMI Symposium and meetings held in conjunction with the AMIA Annual Symposium and the AMIA Spring Congress.

By 1987 it had become clear that the leadership of the three organizations created an interlocking directorate. It appeared to many that the interests of the organizations and of the field would best be served by a merger. Early in 1988 representatives of the three organization began meeting and in November, 1988 they formed the American Medical Informatics Association (AMIA), a society that can speak with one voice to the United States and to the international medical informatics community.

### Purpose

The purpose of AMIA is to advance the public interest through charitable, scientific, literary and educational activities and by promoting the development and application of medical informatics in the support of patient care, teaching, research and health care administration.

*USA*
*(Continued)*

AMIA contributes to the advancement of medical systems and informatics by:

- Serving as an authoritative body in the field of medical informatics and providing representation with respect to such matters in international forums;
- Fostering liaisons between disciplines involved in health care, computers, information, communications, systems sciences, engineering and technology;
- Promoting training and development of professional and allied health personnel necessary to support medical informatics;
- Planning and conducting scientific, technical, and educational meetings and programs;
- Publishing and distributing educational materials through various media;
- Coordinating medical informatics activities with other national and international organizations to advance the public's interest; and
- Carrying on other activities as are necessary, suitable, and proper for the fulfillment of the Association's charitable, scientific, literary and educational purposes.

These objectives are accomplished through a variety of activities and services that AMIA offers:

- Holding scientific, technical and educational meetings;
- Publishing and disseminating reports, digests, proceedings and other pertinent documents and contributing to the professional literature;
- Publishing a journal, the Journal of the American Medical Informatics Association (JAMIA);
- Sponsoring Working Groups (WGs) and Special Interest Groups (SIGs);
- Providing a communications network via telematics (information systems databases, computer and telecommunications);
- Providing a focus for the development of standards, terminology and coding systems;
- Stimulating, conducting and sponsoring research into the application and evaluation of technical systems as they apply to health care and health sciences;
- Representing the United States in the international arena of medical systems and informatics; and
- Advising and coordinating matters of mutual interest to its members.

In late 1999, the Board of Directors and members of AMIA undertook a strategic planning exercise to re-define the vision, mission and goals of the association. As of the fall of 2000, these are the draft statements.

*Vision*

The American Medical Informatics Association is the premier organization to advance discovery and innovation in the use of information in health and biomedicine.

*Mission*

The mission of the American Medical Informatics Association is to improve healthcare through innovation in the use of information by advancing the field, fostering scientific exchange, educating professionals and the public, and influencing decision makers and policy makers.

*Goals*

I. Be the premier membership and peer communication organization in medical informatics.
II. Promote and integrate medical informatics as a field.
III. Expand and maintain multiple forums for interchange and dissemination of advances in the field.
IV. Promote research, development, and diffusion of medical informatics to solve healthcare problems and improve health quality.
V. Foster cooperation and establish relationships with relevant organizations.
VI. Foster and ensure an effective governance and management foundation to enable the American Medical Informatics Association to achieve all of its goals.

*Membership Categories*

- Regular Member: Physicians, nurses, dentists, biomedical engineers, educators, medical librarians, researchers and other health care professionals who have a strong interest in medical informatics. Regular members receive JAMIA (both print and on-line

## USA
## (Continued)

versions), Access AMIA, AMIA Alert, AMIA Yearbook & Directory and the IMIA Yearbook of Medical Informatics at no extra charge. Regular members also receive membership in two working groups as part of their membership fee. Discounts for AMIA Annual Symposium, Spring Congress and Site Visits apply. $250/year

- Institutional Member: Nonprofit organizations, nonprofit associations, nonprofit universities, nonprofit hospitals and libraries. All regular member benefits apply for one individual designated as the AMIA contact person. Additional benefits include JAMIA online access, conference publications and promotional opportunities offering support and exposure. $450/year
- Corporate Member: For-profit corporations that are supporters of the medical informatics community. Numerous corporate membership benefits apply at the four levels of membership—bronze, silver, gold, and platinum. Corporate members have representatives that receive all the benefits of regular members plus additional advertising and sponsorship opportunities. $1,500, $3,500, $7,500 or $12,500/year
- Retired Member: Retirees at least 60 years of age who have been members of AMA for the past two years or longer. All benefits of regular membership apply. $100/year
- Student Member: Persons currently enrolled full-time in a degree-granting program or in an academic program such as a medical residency or post-doctoral fellowship. A certified letter attesting to the student's full time status at an academic institution is required along with membership application. JAMIA is not included in student membership fees, but students may subscribe at a special rate of $35 for a year's subscription (6 issues) and on-line access. Students are automatic members of the student working group at no additional charge. Special conference discounts apply. $35/year
- Associate Member: Individuals may join one working group or special interest group for one year only. No regular member benefits apply. No journals or conference discounts will be given. $30/year

*Member Services*

Membership in AMIA provides a means of staying abreast of the rapid changes in medical systems and informatics, and is open to anyone with interest in the field. AMIA offers a growing array of services designed to meet professional needs:

- Meetings & Conferences: AMIA's meetings and conferences offer the best in panels, tutorials, paper presentations, workshops and exhibits. By joining AMIA, you will receive significant discounts to meetings and conferences. AMIA holds two major meetings each year, the AMIA 2003 Spring Congress being held May 28-30 in Philadelphia, Pennsylvania and focused on bridging the digital divide and the AMIA 2003 Annual Symposium being held November 8-12, 2003 in Washington, DC. AMIA 2003, Biomedical and Health Informatics: From Foundations to Applications, is expected to draw 2,000+ attendees interested in the multidisciplinary arena of medical informatics.
- Working Group Program: AMIA members are encouraged to join and participate in the association's working groups and special interest groups. The working groups conduct programs and activities and produce products to benefit AMIA and the medical informatics community. Working groups are also important in helping members develop personal networks within specific professional or topic areas.
- Continuing Education Credits: By attending the AMIA Annual Symposium and Spring Congress, members may earn valuable continuing medical education credits and nursing contact hours.
- Job Exchange: Members can learn "who's looking" and "what's available" for various positions within the medical informatics field.
- President's Club – AMIA's Member-Get-A-Member Campaign: Any AMIA member can participate in the campaign. Each new member who signs-up for membership and indicates the name of the AMIA member who sponsored his/her membership, will earn the current AMIA member one point toward the campaign. All current AMIA members earning at least one

point in the campaign will be invited to the President's Club Reception held at the Annual Symposium where awards are given. The more points accumulated during the campaign, the more prestigious the award.

- Web Site – AMIA's web site provides valuable information to members and prospective members about the association and member services. The site also has a resource center which contains information about academic and training programs, conferences and meetings, publications of interest, the health IT marketplace, public policy and news developments and research and grant information. Be sure to visit the site at www.amia.org.

### Publications

AMIA members have the opportunity to subscribe at discounted rates to numerous publications. We also offer the following periodical publications when you join:

- JAMIA – The Journal of the American Medical Informatics Association: AMIA's timely and informative journal is the primary source of information for professionals in medical informatics. All regular, institutional, corporate and retired members receive JAMIA bi-monthly and receive 24 hour on-line access. Students may order JAMIA at a special student member rate (which also includes on-line access).
- Access AMIA and AMIA Alert: Two monthly e-mail alerts letting you know about what's going on at your association's headquarters, new services on the horizon, messages from AMIA's leaders and the latest information about the field.
- AMIA Yearbook & Directory: This valuable networking tool, available exclusively to AMIA members for noncommercial purposes, provides completed address, phone, fax and e-mail information for each AMIA member. It also provides an overview of the current year, and lets you know what's in store for the following year.
- IMIA Yearbook of Medical Informatics: Published by the International Medical Informatics Association, this annual publication includes the best papers in medical informatics from an international arena.

### JAMIA

AMIA's own journal is called JAMIA, the Journal of the American Medical Informatics Association. This peer-reviewed specialty journal is the official publication of AMIA and is published by Hanley & Belfus. The content of the regular issues emphasizes the publication of peer-reviewed, original and unsolicited full-length manuscripts dealing with hypotheses and findings that are relevant to medical informatics in all arenas of health care delivery, biomedical education and biomedical research. Also included are brief technical notes, abstracts or full-length papers submitted for presentation at meetings of AMIA, state-of-the-art papers, refereed discussion forums, invited editorials and news and announcements of the association. An occasional regular issue may be dedicated to a collection of invited full-length manuscripts on a single topic. The Proceedings of the AMIA Annual Symposium are published as a supplement to JAMIA. Those who pay full registration to the Annual Symposium receive a CD-ROM copy of the Proceedings. The Proceedings may also be purchased independently of the meeting in either print form or on CD-ROM.

JAMIA is regarded by investigators as the premier vehicle for the archival publication of peer-reviewed papers containing original hypotheses and findings. Submitted material is judged on the originality and quality of work. The journal is reviewed as relevant by the many constituencies that make up AMIA's membership. Each issue contains one or more practical papers addressing the problems facing individuals in the biomedical and health profession who are interested in informatics but do not consider themselves to be researchers. State-of-the-art papers and refereed discussion forums can meet this need while outlining the issues in the field that are controversial or require further investigation.

JAMIA is owned, copyrighted and sponsored by AMIA and is an automatic member benefit to most AMIA members. When subscribing to JAMIA, members also receive access to the on-line version of the journal available at www.jamia.org. Outside subscriptions are also available.

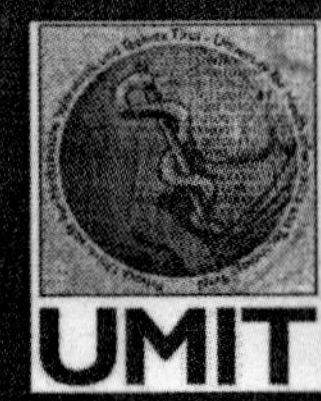

# University for Health Informatics and Technology Tyrol
## Private Universität für Medizinische Informatik und Technik Tirol
### Innsbruck, Austria

Informatics expertise in medicine, biology, and health care is in high demand and short supply. UMIT is the first university in Europe and possibly the world, concentrating entirely on medical informatics and the novel integration of disciplines that it requires.

Located in an outstanding intellectual and physical environment, encompassing multiple health care institutions in the Tyrol, UMIT is building a comprehensive curriculum for biomedical and health informatics, drawing from top-tier international research faculty and their resources world wide.

In the academic year of 2002/2003 the following educational programs are offered:

## Medical Informatics - Full time Study

Bachelor of Science
Master of Science
Doctoral (PH.D.) Studies

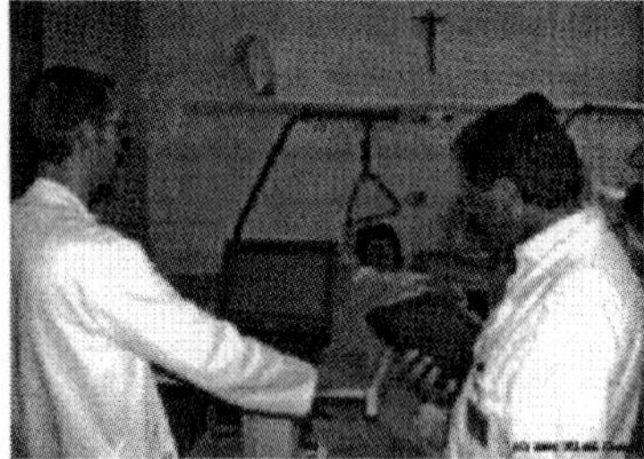

## Medical Informatics - Part time Study

Master of Science
Doctoral (PH.D.) Studies

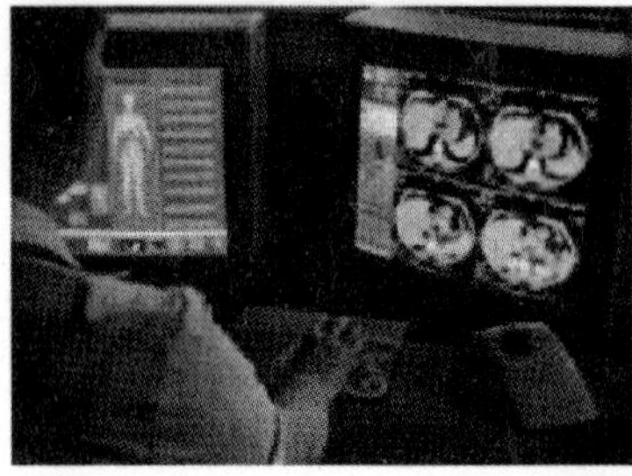

**For further information please visit www.UMIT.at**

---

### Mission Statement
The University for Health Informatics and Technology Tyrol sets for itself the following goals:

- To explore opportunities and practical applications of information and communication technologies, so as to contribute to high-quality, efficient health care that does justice to the individual and to society, and to contribute to progress in medical and health sciences research.
- To respect the freedom of science and its teachings in a community of students and teachers, who engage in open scholarly inquiry following principles of good scientific practice, always striving towards the highest quality in research and education.
- To promote the development and intellectual growth of the students, so that upon graduation they are well prepared for professional and related social responsibilities.
- To seek cooperation with other universities and research institutions, in particular with the LEOPOLD-FRANZENS-University of Innsbruck, and with health care institutions and other health related enterprises.

(from the Constitution of the University for Health Informatics and Technology Tyrol)

---

UMIT, Innrain 98, A-6020 Innsbruck, Austria / www.UMIT.at / info@UMIT.at / Tel. +43/512/586734-0

**Nancy M. Lorenzi,**
*Guest-editor*

Vanderbilt University,
Medical Center,
Nashville, Tennessee, USA

# IMIA's Working Groups and Special Interest Groups:

# *Quality and IMIA Working Group Efforts*

In addition to the exponential growth of medical information, clinicians face problems posed by system failures. A review of current biomedical literature outlined sources of medical error, including: harm as a result of medication withdrawal; missing data resulting in prescription of a "contraindicated drug;" possible interaction of multiple prescriptions for a patient; "inaccuracies in program inputs or program logic which could lead to erroneous recommendations;" and knowledge gaps of the clinician-user that directly pertain to decision support system recommendations.[1] A "medical imperative" exists to promote patient safety by redesigning systems "to make errors difficult to commit and create a culture in which the existence of risk is acknowledged and injury prevention is recognized as everyone's responsibility".[2] A majority of accidents in complex systems result from the combined effect of smaller failures, "each necessary but only jointly sufficient to produce the accident."

In a June 2002 issue of the *Annals of Internal Medicine*, a case of surgery performed on the wrong patient cited 17 independent "active" medical errors—none of which could have been singularly responsible for harming the patient—that interacted with system failures to produce the adverse event. The patient had a similar sounding name to the correct patient but initial mistaken identity was only one of several factors contributing to the error.[3] According to the authors of the report, the most significant system features contributing to the error were lack of communication—a problem inherent in most large healthcare organizations—teamwork, and identity verification. "Perhaps the most striking feature of this case—that will be familiar to all clinicians who have worked in large hospitals—is the frighteningly poor communication it exemplifies. Physicians failed to communicate with nurses, attending physicians failed to communicate with residents and fellows, staff from one unit failed to communicate with those from others, and no one listened carefully to the patient."[4] Other issues at hand included: an illegible patient record with little documentation of patient history; "a patchwork of homegrown information mini-systems" that failed to effectively

---

[1]  Goldstein MK, Hoffman BB, Coleman RW et al. Patient Safety in Guideline-Based Decision Support for Hypertension Management: ATHENA DSS. Proc AMIA Symp 2001.

[2]  Leape LL, Woods DD, Hatlie JD, et al. Promoting patient safety by preventing medical error. *JAMA* 1998; 280:1444-7.

[3]  Chassin MR, Becher EC. The wrong patient. Ann Intern Med 2002;136:826-33.

[4]  Ibid.

interact; lack of standardized procedure for patient identification-verification; and a "culture of low expectations" involving an expectation of incomplete communication. Furthermore, the medical literature and reported incidents of similar errors involving invasive procedures and patient misidentification, as well as the problems with coordination and communication in healthcare, are incomplete/under-documented at best.[5]

### Quality

The IMIA Special Interest and Working Groups are either directly or indirectly working on tasks that will improve the capabilities of informatics to support the health care and research systems. Some working groups target their work for better concept representation to enable better understanding of complex topics and yet others work on the areas of data security and protection. Some groups work on subjects that directly apply to health information systems and others focus on the technical side of information systems, e.g. biosignal processing, biostatistics, standards, e-health—telematics—etc. Working groups who focus their efforts for disciplines (e.g. dentistry, mental health, nursing, primary care) often integrate the information from other working groups into their efforts. Some of the working groups directly focus on organizational and quality improvement issues. One working group focuses its efforts on quality and informatics for the developing world. The work of the IMIA working groups is significant for improving and enhancing the multiple topics that surround the health care and health related research.

As a brief overview, in the last three and a half years the working group chair organized and held ten working conferences. At least two others are currently in the planning stages.

- Intelligent Data Analysis and Data Mining (WG 3)
- Security of the Distributed EPR (WG 4)
- Medical Concept Representation (WG 6)
- Biosignal Interpretation (WG 7)
- Informatics in the Mental Health Area (WG 8)
- Health Information Systems (WG 10)
- Organizational Issues and Assessment (WG 13 and WG 15)
- Computerized Patient Record (WG 17)
- E-Health: High-tech Medicine, Community Medicine (WG 18)
- Nursing International Conference (Nursing)

A number of special efforts have been accomplished. The following is only a small sample to reflect the intellectual capital that working groups bring to IMIA:

- Developed a Code of Ethics.
- Created a list of IMIA recommendations for Health and Medical Informatics. Education (Translated into Spanish, Chinese, Italian, Turkish, Croatian, Czech, and Japanese)
- Created outstanding web pages (e.g., Dental Informatics as a worldwide model.)
- Created a virtual worldwide university for informatics educators.
- Worked on a better understanding of the relationships between predictive data mining and evidence-based medicine.

---

[5] Ibid.

In addition to the above, the working groups held planning sessions and workshops, sponsored world-wide dialogue and offered support to people interested in informatics no matter where they are in the world. Developing and organizing a working conference is a major accomplishment and serves the health care world at large. The chairs personally assume much of the overall coordination for the conference. Developing and sustaining a worldwide effort in an all-volunteer organization for the special accomplishments listed above and the many other activities is also a major accomplishment. On behalf of the significant efforts of the working group chairs, I am happy to present the Special Interest and Working Groups 2003 Yearbook report.

## *Nursing Informatics (Special Interest Group 1)*

**Chair:**
Dr. Virginia K. Saba
Distinguished Scholar, Adjunct
Georgetown University
Professor, Adjunct
Uniformed Services University
2332 South Queen Street
Arlington, VA 22202, USA
Tel:      +1 703 521 6132
Fax:      +1 703 521 3866
E-mail:    vsaba@worldnet.att.net

**Objectives:**
- To foster collaboration among nurses and others interested in nursing informatics.
- To explore the scope of nursing informatics and implications for information handling activities.
- To support the development of nursing informatics in member countries.
- To conduct informatics conferences and meetings.
- To encourage publication and dissemination of research and development materials.
- To develop recommendations, guidelines, tools, and courses.

**General Information**
NI-SIG meets annually—International Conference held every three years (Medinfo) or at other IMIA and/or Nursing Informatics-related meetings. It currently has 30 official members, including its officers, from 27 IMIA member countries, organizations and/or universities. It has been integrated into the new IMIA Web Site: http://www.imia.org/ni/index/html/.

NI-SIG Executive Committee:
Chair, Virginia K. Saba, USA
Vice-Chair/Treasurer, Heather Strachan, UK
Secretary, Robyn Carr, NZ.

NI-SIG has several working groups addressing different nursing informatics activities:
- Concept Representation:  Virginia Saba, USA
- Reference Terminology Model:  Suzanne Bakken, USA
- International Nursing Minimum Data Set: Connie Delaney, USA
- Research:  Heather Strachan, UK
- Management:  Robyn Carr, NZ
- Education:  Margareta Ehnfors, SW and Diane Skiba, USA
- Data Standards:  Kathleen McCormick, USA
- History: Marianne Tallberg, FN
- Evidenced-Based Practice:  Connie Weaver, USA
- Consumer Health:  Betty Chang, USA
- Telematics:  Paula Proctor, UK
- Web Site:  Peter Murray, UK

| *Nursing Informatics (Special Interest Group 1) (Continued)* |
|---|

**Recent Activities:**

- NI-SIG hosted its Annual Meeting at Medical Informatics Europe (MIE) Conference in Budapest on August 24-26, 2002. There they also:
  - Hosted a one-day tutorial where the working group chairs presented the focus and status of their activities.
  - Participated in a workshop on selected nursing informatics topics.
  - Proposed a Nursing Informatics Certificate Program for all NI member experts in their member countries. The Certificate will be based on the member's portfolio demonstrating expertise in Nursing Informatics.
  - Working group reports were posted on the Web Site.
- NI-SIG has been actively involved in the development the "Integration of a Reference Terminology Model for Nursing" within the International Standards Organization (ISO) Technical Committee (TC) 215.
  - The New Work Item Proposal (NWIP) was submitted in 1999 via theWorking Group 3 – Concept Representation – US TAG Regional Technical Advisory Group, ISO/TC215 by Chris Chute. It continues to progress through the various ISO/TC215 stages.
  - The NWIP #142 was prepared by NI-SIG and co-sponsored by the International Council of Nursing (ICN). It has been reviewed and discussed at numerous national and international informatics meetings.
  - The RT Model is being overseen by: Steering Committee: Chaired– Virginia Saba, Kathleen McCormick, Amy Coenen, and Evelyn Hovenga— who are responsible for the coordination and final preparation of the submission of the drafts.
- Work Item Task Group: Facilitator–Suzanne Bakken, USA and an International Technical Advisory Group
- Expert Committee: Selected ISO members and other national and international experts who review the prepared documents.

**Future Activities:**

- Continue to support the RT Model through the ISO/TC 215 stages.
- Support the activities of the NI-SIG Working Groups.
- Conduct workshops at all IMIA-related conferences and/or meetings such as AMIA in November 2002.and assist in the planning, reviewing papers, and finalizing the program for the conference.
- International Congress Nursing Informatics to be held in Rio de Janeiro, Brazil in June 2003. The NI 2003 is chaired by Heimar Marin, Professor, Federal University, Sao Paulo, Brazil.

Homepage: http://www.imia.org/ni/index/html/

# *WG 1 - Health and Medical Informatics Education*

**Chair:**
Dr. Evelyn J.S. Hovenga RN
School of Mathematical and Decision Sciences
Informatics and Communication
Central Queensland University
Blg 18, Room G20
Rockhampton CQMC 4702, Australia
Tel:       +61 749 309 839
Fax:       +61 749 309 871
E-mail:    e.hovenga@cqu.edu.au

**Co-chair:**
Prof. Dr. John Mantas
University of Athens, Dept. of Nursing
Laboratory of Health Informatics
PO Box 77313
GR-17510 Athens, Greece
E-mail:    jmantas@dn.uoa.gr

## Objectives:

- To disseminate and exchange information on Health and Medical Informatics (HMI) programs and courses.
- To promote the IMIA HMI database on programs and courses on HMI education.
- To produce international recommendations on HMI programs and courses.
- To support HMI courses and exchange of students and teachers.
- To advance the knowledge of: (1) how informatics is taught in the education of health care professionals around the world, (2) how in particular health and medical informatics is taught to students of computer science/informatics, and (3) how it is taught within dedicated curricula in health and medical informatics.

## Recent Activities:

- The recommendations of the IMIA on Education in Health and Medical Informatics have now been translated into Spanish, Chinese, Italian, Turkish, Czech and Japanese. Anyone undertaking further translations must (1) formally seek permission from Schattauer, the publisher of the recommendations, (2) notify Dr. Reinhold Haux at (Reinhold.Haux@umit.at) and (3) forward the URL to Dr. Evelyn Hovenga (e.hovenga@cqu.edu.au) so that a link can be established on the WG 1 website.
- IMIA HMI has a mailing list and anyone interested is able to join this list by sending a message to majordomo@cqu.edu.au and subscribe to imia-wg1@cqu.edu.au or to Dr. Evelyn Hovenga.
- Web pages are accessible via the IMIA homepage at http://www.imia.org.

## Future Activities:

- The recommendations of the IMIA on Education in Health and Medical Informatics will be reviewed and updated.
- A Global (Virtual) University initiative is being undertaken. A steering committee consisting of Dr. John Mantas, Dr. Jim Turley, Dr. Umberto Giani, Dr. William Hersh and Dr. Yu-Chuan (Jack) Li was established at the last meeting held during Medinfo 2001 in London. A glossary of terms describing the many data elements used to describe various aspects of programs and courses is being compiled. Approximately 20 issues needing exploration from which recommendations can be made have been identified. A number of members are contributing to this effort. It is expected that the results of this work will be published in a textbook. One of the objectives is to meet educational needs of developing countries.
- The next meeting will be held October 5-6 2002 in Taipei, in conjunction with the Taiwan Association of Medical Informatics' (TAMI) "Medical Informatics Symposium of Taiwan" (MIST2002).

WWW site and IMIA HMI database on health/medical informatics:
http://www.imia.org/wg1

## *WG 2 - Consumer Health Informatics*

**Chairs:**

Alejandro (Alex) R. Jadad, MD DPhil
University of Toronto  and
Toronto General Hospital
Eaton Wing, EN 6-242
Toronto, Ontario M5G 2C4, Canada
Tel        +1 416 340 4800 Ext. 6823
Fax:        +1 416 340 3595

Betty L. Chang, DNSc (2000-2003)
School of Nursing, Box 956918
University of California, Los Angeles
Los Angeles, CA 90095-6918, USA
Tel:        +1 310 206 3834
Fax:        +1 310 206 0914

Gunther Eysenbach, MD (2000-2003)
University of Toronto
Toronto General Hospital
R. Fraser Elliott Building, 4th Floor
Room #4S435
190 Elizabeth Street
Toronto, ON M5G 2C4, Canada
Tel:        +1 416 340 4800 Ext. 6427
Fax        +1 416 340 3595

## Objectives:

- To provide a forum to enhance collaboration, share experiences, and promote research in Consumer Health Informatics (CHI.)
- To increase communication with other working groups at IMIA and other informatics organizations relevant to CHI.
- To establish itself as a group for funding agencies to consult on issues related to information technology projects in health care.

## Recent Activities:

- The Consumer Health Informatics Working Group (CHIWG) became an official IMIA Working Group in 2000. The CHIWG is concerned with electronic information related to health care available to the public (e.g. Internet, wireless, standalone electronic media). For its purposes, it defines Consumer Health Informatics as "the use of modern computers and telecommunications to support consumers in obtaining information, analyzing unique health care needs and helping them make decisions about their own health" (U.S. General Accounting Office, 1996, p.1.), in which the consumer interacts with the applications directly with or without the presence of health care professionals. The group's interests focus on, but are not limited to, world wide web sites that offer advice about healthy living, research findings, and recommendations on specific disease conditions, descriptions of products, medications, and self-care health programs available to the public. Issues of concern may be the evaluation of the quality of information, education of the public, ethical issues related to electronic information and its effect on a person's health care and relationship with health care providers.
- The working group has a new web site: http://www.jmir.org/imia-chi.
- The working group sponsored a panel, "Leveling the playing field: international initiatives to promote consumer health informatics" at the Medinfo conference. The organizer of the workshop is Alex Jadad and the moderator is Betty Chang. The speakers were Alex Jadad, Gunther Eysenbach, and extensive audience participation. In this workshop, participants had the opportunity to listen to and exchange ideas with a group of speakers that discussed the opportunities and challenges of promoting the development of consumer health informatics around the world. The presenters described international projects designed to help consumers use information technology and the best available knowledge to guide their health-related decisions. The discussion focused on the following aspects of consumer health informatics at an international level: how much we know; practical lessons from completed and ongoing efforts; ethical, social, methodological and political challenges for international projects; international efforts and opportunities for collaboration with other countries; and the need for a clear agenda to promote meaningful and effective efforts on consumer health informatics worldwide.
- Since the initial proposal, the CHIWG has been seeking opportunities to collaborate with other working groups or associations in related areas. Some example areas include the examination of computerized patient care records in hospitals, clinics, or physicians' offices, the ethical aspects of public participation in the development and evaluation of health informatics tools, and the impact of the Internet in consumer education and participation in health care decisions. The IMIA CHI WG is collaborating with the IMIA Nursing Sig in presenting opportunities for collaboration in Consumer Health Informatics at the Med Info Europe (MIE 2002) held in Budapest, sponsored by the European Federation of Medical Informatics. Betty Chang will be presenting

## Consumer Health Informatics (IMIA WG2) (Continued)

possible ideas for international exploration/collaboration, at the MIE 2002.

- The group held a business meeting at Medinfo 2001. During the meeting, they explored ways in which participants can share activities and experiences related to CHI.
- The American Medical Informatics Association, CHI-WG has co-sponsored a post conference on *Critical Issues in Consumer Health Informatics* following the AMIA Fall 2001 meeting—Nov 7th and 8th, 2001.

## *WG 3 - Intelligent Data Analysis and Data Mining*

**Chair:**
Dr. Riccardo Bellazzi (2000-2003)
Dipartimento di Informatica e Sistemistica
Università di Pavia
via Ferrata 1
27100 Pavia, Italy
Tel:        +39 0382 505511
Fax:        +39 0382 505373
E-mail:     Riccardo.Bellazzi@unipv.it

**Co-chair:**
Assist. Prof. Dr. Blaz Zupan (2000-2003)
Faculty of Computer and Information Sciences
University of Ljubljana
Trzaska 25
SI-1000 Ljubljana, Slovenia
and Department of Human and Molecular Genetics
Baylor College of Medicine,
Houston, Texas, USA
Tel:        +386 1 4768 402
Fax:        +386 1 4264 647
E-mail:     blaz.zupan@fri.uni-lj.si

**Objectives:**

- To increase the awareness and acceptance of intelligent data analysis and data mining methods in medical community.
- To foster scientific discussion and disseminate new knowledge on AI-based methods for data analysis and data mining techniques applied to medicine. To promote the development of standardized platforms and solutions.
- To provide a forum for presentation of successful intelligent data analysis and data mining implementations in medicine, and for discussion of best practices in introduction of these techniques in medical and health-care information and decision support systems.

**Recent Activities:**

- During AMIA 2001, members of the working group organized an evening workshop to disseminate their activity.
- During the European Conference on Artificial Intelligence 2002 in Lyon, a full-day scientific workshop on the working group topics was organized (IDAMAP 2002; Chair: Peter Lucas, co-chairs: Lars Asker and Silvia Miksch.)
- Fifteen papers have been presented; they are available at the working group web site: http://www.idamap.org. The results of the workshop will be also presented in a workshop at AMIA 2002.
- A joint effort to disseminate the results and practice of DM methodologies has been planned with the Special Interest Group on Data Mining and Knowledge Discovery of AMIA (chair: J. Holmes.) The web site of the group contains new pages on temporal data mining. (Access web site through http://www.idamap.org.)

**Future Activities:**

- The working group will focus on specific topics of interest for the scientific community. In particular, the following issues will be explored:
  - Relationships between predictive data mining and evidence based medicine
  - Knowledge-based functional genomics and temporal data mining
- The working group's web site will be further enriched, in order to offer a list of most relevant publications, technical notes and recent results to the general audience.
- The WG is planning the organization of the IDAMAP 2003 workshop.

## WG 4 - Data Protection in Health Information Systems

**Chair:**
Prof. Ab R. Bakker
Atjehweg 10
2202 AP Noordwijk
The Netherlands
Tel:        +31 71 362 1984
Fax:        +31 71 361 7500
E-mail:     abakker@addabit.demon.nl

Other contact person:
Kees Louwerse (secretary)
LUMC Central Information
Processing Department
PO Box 9600, 2300 RC Leiden
The Netherlands
Tel:        +31 71 526 3240
Fax:        +31 71 524 8240
E-mail:     c.p.louwerse@lumc.nl

### Objectives:

To examine the issues of data protection and security within the health-care environment. The Data Protection in Health Information Systems Working Group addresses state-of-the-art security of distributed electronic patient records (EPR.)

### Recent Activities:

- Working conference "Security of the Distributed EPR," Victoria Canada, June 21-24 2000. Proceedings published as special issue of the *International Journal of Medical Informatics*, Vol. 60, No. 2 CD-ROM with presentations during the conference available through Jochen Moehr (email: jmoehr@uvic.ca.)
- As a follow-up to the recommendations of this working conference the IMIA AGM asked this working group to develop a draft for an Ethical Code of Practice and a draft for a Security Policy Framework. Two working teams were created to prepare the drafts. Eike Kluge (Canada) is leading the team for the Ethical Code of Practice; Barry Barber (UK) is leading the team for the Security Policy Framework.
- A workshop was organized at Medinfo2001 to discuss a draft of the Ethical Code of Practice
- An updated draft of the Ethical Code of Practice was sent to the IMIA members in January 2002, asking them for comments. The draft of the Ethical Code of Practice is on the agenda of the IMIA AGM 2002 (at Taipei) for endorsement.
- A panel session was organized at Medinfo 2001 to discuss the approach to arrive at a draft for the Security Policy Framework.
- In January 2002 the working team for the draft Security Policy Framework met at Leiden, The Netherlands to discuss its approach.

### Future activities:

- Preparation of a draft Security Policy Framework, progress has been limited. The working team will meet again on August 29 in Budapest, in conjunction with MIE2002.
- A business meeting of the working group will be held on August 29 in Budapest.
- The next working conference: *"Designing Security into the Electronic Patient Record"* is being prepared. It will take place at Varenna, Italy, May 31-June 3 2003. The SPC will meet August 29 in Budapest.
- The "Informatics Ethical Code of Practice" was endorsed by the IMIA General Assembly in Taipei, Taiwan in October 2002. The Code will be available on the IMIA web site and within the Yearbook of Medical Informatics. It will be translated by September 2004 into Spanish, Portuguese, Japanese, Chinese, and Czech through the assistance of volunteers.

# WG 5 - Primary Health Care Informatics

**Co-chairs:**
Dr. Michael Kidd, M.D.
Head Department of General Practice
The University of Sydney
37A Booth Street
Balmain 2041, Sydney, Australia
Tel:        +61 2 9818 1400
Fax:        +61 2 9818 1343
E-mail:     michael.kidd@
            med.usyd.edu.au

Dr. H. C. "Moon" Mullins, M.D.
Crozer Keystone Health Systems
PO Box 545
Montrose, AL 36559, USA
Tel:        +1 334 928 0905
Fax:        +1 334 928 0106
E-mail:     hmullins@
            jaguar1.usouthal.edu

**Objectives:**

To promote primary care computing by:

- Acting as a forum for exchange of ideas between its members.
- Providing information to its members to assist them in progressing primary care computing in their own country.
- Increasing the understanding of primary care computing issues with a view to publishing the results of these discussions.

**Recent Activities:**

- The working group consolidated its work plan for the next three years at the Medinfo 2001 meeting.
- Radcliffe Medical Press has launched the new journal, Informatics in Primary Care, with endorsement from IMIA WG5 and involvement of members of the working group on the Editorial Board. Full text available at: www.radcliffe-oxford.com/ipc.
- Members of the working group continue to liaise at an international level on key local and regional initiatives in primary care informatics. Our key international partners include EFMI Working Group 7 (Primary Care), Informatics Working Party of WONCA (The World Organization of Family Doctors), and the American Medical Informatics Association's Primary Care Informatics Working Group.

**Future Activities**

- Continued development of recruitment plan for working group.
- Continued development of work plan to deliver our stated objectives.
- Continued collaboration with Informatics in Primary Care journal.
- Website presence through the IMIA web site.
- Sharing outcomes from each nation and region.

# WG 6 - Medical Concept Representation

**Chair:**
Dr. Christopher G. Chute
Department of Health Sciences
Research, Mayo Foundation
Rochester, MN 55905, USA
Tel:        +1 507 284 5541
Fax         +1 507 284 1516
E-mail:     chute@mayo.edu

**Co-chair:**
Dr. Werner Ceusters, Director R&D
Language & Computing
Hazenakkerstraat 20a
B-9520 Zonnegem, Belgium
Tel:        +32 53 62 95 45
Fax:        +32 53 62 95 55
http        www.landc.be

**Objectives:**

To provide a forum for state of the art dialogue and collaboration on natural language processing and concept representation in healthcare applications. IMIA's Medical Concept Representation Working Group is the international forum for issues related to informatics in the classification and coding of health data. The working group is charged with:

1) Reviewing health data nomenclature and classification needs for the world community.
2) Evaluating information processing technology in meeting these defined needs.
3) Recommending methods for future classification and nomenclature systems.

**Recent Activities:**

- This Working Group sponsored a conference on Natural Language and Medical Concept Representation in Jacksonville, Florida in 1997.
- The Proceedings of the working conference were published in *Methods of Information in Medicine* in 1998, issues 4 and 5.
- The Working Group on Medical Concept Representation held its triennial conference on Natural Language Processing and Medical Concept Representation in late 1999, in Phoenix, Arizona, USA. This fifth conference, spanning a 15-year history, provided a forum for presentation and discussion of the state of the art in health terminology issues relevant to informatics research and applications.
- The working group had several papers and meeting at the Medinfo 2001 conference in London.

<table>
<tr><td>

*Medical Concept Representation (IMIA WG 6) (Continued)*

</td><td>

**Future Activities:**
- Planning for content and foci are underway for the 6th Triennial meeting, to be held in Belgium, in late 2003.
- The European Commission is offering possibilities for European research groups to involve USA, Japanese, Australian, etc., experts within the 6th Framework Program that begins in 2002.

Homepage: http://www.mayo.edu/imia-wg6

</td></tr>
</table>

## WG 7 - Biomedical Pattern Recognition

**Chair:**
Dr. Christoph Zywietz
Medizinische Hochschule Hannover
Biosignalverarbeitung - 8440 -
Carl-Neuberg-Strasse 1
30625 Hannover, Germany
Tel:      +49 511 532 4412
Fax:      +49 511 532 4295
E-mail:   zywietz.christoph@
          MH-Hannover.de

**Objectives:**
- To explore the field of biosignal interpretation, model-based biosignal analysis, interpretations and integration, extending existing signal-processing technology for the effective use of biosignals in a practical environment.
- To provide a forum for discussion and collaboration on problems of biosignal processing, biomedical pattern recognition and on quality assurance in this field. This includes the following topics:
  - Measurement and interpretation of physiological signals
  - Signal-based modeling and simulation in biomedicine
  - Biological control systems, e.g., the human autonomous regulation system
  - Quality assurance and evaluation of physiological analysis systems

**Recent Activities:**
- The working group held the IMIA 4th International Workshop on Biosignal Interpretation on June 24-26, 2002 in Villa Olmo, Como, Italy. Program Committee members included: Metin Akay, Dartmouth, College, Hanover, USA; Sergio Cerutti (Chairman), Polytechnic University of Milan; Bin He, University of Illinois, Chicago, USA; Shunsuke Sato, Osaka University, Japan; and Christoph Zywietz, Medizinische Hochschule of Hannover, Germany. Approximately 130 scientists from all over the world participated. The conference program consisted of 10 plenary sessions on a broad spectrum of topics and two poster sessions. The topics of the 10 main sessions included:
  - Session S1: *Data Processing in Genomic and Proteinomics*
    First keynote speaker Prof. Dr. Alain Arneodo introduced the session with a presentation entitled "*Fractal Analysis of DNA Sequences Using Wavelet Techniques.*"
  - Session S2*: Time-frequency and Wavelets Analysis*
  - Session S3: *Non-Linear, Fractal and Chaotic Analysis*
  - Session S4: *EMG Signal Analysis*
  - Session S5: *Myocardial Signal Analysis and Modeling*
  - Session S6: *Heart Rate Variability Signal*
  - Session S7: Panel Discussion: *Cardiovascular variability signals: advanced tools of signal processing and physiological interpretation* (Panel: S. Akselrod (chair), S. Cerutti, D. Eckberg, A. Malliani, P. Persson)
  - Session S8: *Processing of Electrical Signals in the Brain*
    This session began with the second keynote speaker Prof. Dr. Jose Pricipe on "Signal Processing Techniques in Neuroscience and Brain-Machine Interface."
  - Session S9: *Analysis of EEG Signal and Neuronal Activity*
  - Session S10: *Medical Decision Making*

<table><tr><td>

## *Biomedical Pattern Recognition (IMIA WG 7) (Continued)*

</td><td>

- In addition to the oral presentations there were two posters sessions with approximately 40 posters in each session. Awards were presented for the three best posters. The first prize was given to M. Bucolo, L. Fortuna, M. Fraska, et al's poster *"A Non-linear Circuit Architecture for Magneto-Encephalographic Signals Analysis."*
- Information on the 4th International Workshop on Biosignal Interpretation is still available at the web site: http://www.BSI2002.polimi.it.

**Future Activities:**
- A Special Issue of *Methods of Information in Medicine* will feature 25-30 papers selected from the conference. The guest editors of the Special Issue will be S. Cerutti, Donna Hudson and Chr. Zywietz. The material for the Special Issue will be completed by end of 2002.

</td></tr></table>

<table><tr><td>

## *WG 8 - Mental Health Informatics*

**Chair:**
Michael Rigby
Centre for Health Planning and
Management
Darwin Building, Keele University,
Keele, Staffordshire, ST5 5BG, UK
Tel:      +44 1782 583193
Fax:      +44 1782 711737
E-mail:   hma10@keele.ac.uk

**Co-chair:**
Ann Sheridan
Assistant Director
Nursing and Midwifery Planning &
Development Unit
Eastern Regional Health Authority
Stewarts Hospital
Mill Lane
Plamerstown, Dublin 20, Ireland
Tel:      +353 1 620 1731
Fax:      +44 406 5611
E-mail:   sheridanaj@eircom.net

</td><td>

**Objectives:**
- This group was established at the IMIA Board meeting in August 2000 with formal confirmation being received in October 2000. The proposal was triggered by an increasing recognition of the need to consider the special information and informatics needs of this domain, which represents some 10% of all healthcare activity. The domain has special information-handling requirements, and a range of challenges commencing with the longer-term, multi-site nature of much mental health care and the emphasis on qualitative and attitudinal data. At the same time, it is hoped that techniques to assist with these particular needs in health informatics will enrich more biophysical care domains as well.

**Recent Activities:**
- An open forum was held at the Medinfo 2001 and drew representatives from three continents.
- As planned, the working group held its first inaugural scientific meeting on 14-15 November 2001 in Dublin, linked to the Health Informatics Society of Ireland (HISI) conference. Financial support from the Nuffield Trust, London, made this possible. The theme was "Critical Success Factors in Mental Health Electronic Patient Record Systems." International speakers included Cheryl Plummer (Chief Information Officer, Riverview Hospital, Port Coquitlam, British Columbia, Canada, *Organizational, Provincial and National Issues of Mental Health EPRs*); Bosse Ivarsson Consultant Psychiatrist (Boras Psychiatric Unit, Western Sweden, Electronic Records, *Challenges in Addressing the Clinical Culture*); Per Lund (Chief Executive Officer, Skt. Hans Hospital, Copenhagen, Denmark, *The Organizational and Managerial Issues of Implementing a Mental Health EPR*); and Walter Gulbinat (Executive Secretary, International Consortium for Mental Health Policy and Service formerly Head Scientist, Mental Health Division, WHO.)
- The inaugural meeting also gave opportunity for delegates to brainstorm possible themes for follow-up, and these are now being considered. Unfortunately, some participants have been unable to initiate the intended collaborative work because of resource pressures in the mental health sector and the unwillingness of organizations to commit to anything other than core tasks.
- In line with IMIA policy to collaborate with IFHRO, the chair and co-chair had active roles in the 10th European Health Records Conference in August 2002.

</td></tr></table>

## *Mental Health (IMIA WG 8) (Continued)*

In particular, the co-chair led a workshop on the theme of consent in medical records, with particular reference to the interests of patient self-determination at times when illness temporarily restricts mental competence.
- Liaison continues with the World Psychiatric Association's IT special interest group. The psychiatrists are considering the development of an ethical protocol to address the issues of remote virtual service delivery, and the IMIA group has proposed a joint approach to involve the clinical and informatics aspects and communities.

**Future Activities:**
- The initial advances listed above will be the foundation for future activities. Awareness, not least through the IMIA web site, has led to a number of expressions of interest, or requests for guidance, from individuals in several countries, indicating the need in this domain.
- Identification of resources, linked to individual topics, will continue to be a priority to facilitate the Working Group.

## *WG 9 - Health Informatics for Development*

**Chair:**
Nora Oliveri
Medical Informatics Foundation
801 Brickell Bay Drive,
Box 4, PMBC 134,
Miami, FL, 33131, USA
Tel:    +17864253818/+13057101528
Fax:    +15097525912
E-mail: norao@fim.org.ar

**Objectives:**
- To find out how health care informatics could improve live conditions in developing regions and implement programs in that direction.
- Organization of forums to exchange of experiences of colleagues working in the field of health informatics.
- Making a list of the needs and resources in medical informatics for each country.
- Organization of educational activities in developing regions, especially through the implementation of professors' exchange.
- Organizing workshops and seminars with international experts participation

**General Information**
- Information about activities, publication, how to join the WG9 and links to web sites related are available at www.fim.org.ar/wg9/ URL: www.mifound.org/WG9.
- To facilitate communication between members and all professionals interested in IMIA-Health Informatics for Developing Countries goals. Language: English and Spanish. To subscribe, send a message to: IMIA-WG9@pccorreo.com.ar. Subject: Subscribe. Body: name last name e-mail contact data.
- Related Mailing Lists:
  HELINA-List: HELINA-L@uku.fi, Contact: Mikko Korpela;
  International Network for the Availability of Scientific Publications: INASP_Health@compuserve.co, Contact: Neil Pakenham-Walsh;
  SUPERCOURSE: super3+@pitt.edu, Contact: Ron Laporte;
  WG94 : wg94-l@uku.fi

**Recent Activities:**
- This Working Group held a day workshop during Medinfo 2001 on Issues for Health Informatics for Developing Countries: Globalization and Development. The workshop on September 4, 2001 had 110 participants and the administrative workshop had 28 participants on September 5, 2001. The agenda and presentations can be found: www.mifound.org/WG9/ Representatives of Africa, Asia, Eastern Europe and Latin America informed the participants about the situation in each region. Presentation of the Super-course promoted

*Health Informatics for Development (IMIA WG 9) (Continued)*

by the University of Pittsburgh and invitation to collaborate with its diffusion worldwide. The IMIA headquarters was asked to support the electronic publication of documents from this conference (see the IMIA web site).

- During year 2001 this working group collaborated with Informedica 2000's First Iberoamerican Virtual Congress of Medical Informatics. Oct 30, 2000-April 30, 2001. [www.informedica.org] / [www.informedica.org.ar]
- This working group maintains a valuable exchange of ideas and experiences with IMIA's Health and Medical Informatics Education Working Group and the European Federation of Medical Informatics working group on Health Informatics for Development.
- Dr. Marcelo Sosa-Iudicissa was appointed like secretary of WG9 during Medinfo 2001.
- Dr. Lincoln deAssis Moura, Jr was elected as the head of IMIA-LAC. (He is also the president of the Brazilian Health Informatics Society)
- There was a Health Informatics for Developing Countries, Workshop titled, "Difficulties in Implementing Healthcare Informatization Strategies in Transition Countries: How a Good Project Can Fail" during MIE 2002, Budapest. George Mihalas: mihalas@ms.ro

**Future Activities:**
- To develop a close collaboration and action program with IMIA-LAC (Latin America), the African Region and APAMI (Asian Pacific Association of Medical Informatics.)
- To improve access to information for health care workers.
- To support next HELINA Conference (date is tbd.) Contact Omar El Hattab: ohattab@hotmail.com.
- To hold a Virtual Meeting during Informedica 2002.
- Development of new initiatives in Internet applications: Virtual library of MI conferences: Invitation to good lectures in medical informatics and making up available on the Net and/or on CD for developing countries.
- To support Informedica 2002: 2nd Virtual Iberoamerican Congress of Medical Informatics in Internet, November 4 – 30, 2002. Contact Nora Oliveri: Nora_Oliveri@mifound.org. Informedica intends to become a virtual library of medical informatics conferences for Iberoamerican countries in Spanish and Portuguese languages. We invite members of IMIA societies to send lectures in medical informatics to Nora Oliveri and she will make them available on the web or on CD. Informedica 2002 will be held virtually since all activities will be available through the web/internet.
- During 2003 this working group is planning to hold a working meeting during the Nursing Informatics 2003 meeting in Rio de Janeiro, Brazil.
- A new publication about Medical Informatics and Developing Countries is under discussion.

Homepage: http://www.fim.org.ar/wg9/

# *WG 10 - Health Information Systems*

**Chair:**
Dr. Klaus A. Kuhn
Professor of Medical Informatics
Philipps-University Marburg
Bunsenstr. 3
D-35037 Marburg, Germany
Tel: +49 6421 286 6205
Fax: +49 6421 286 3599
E-mail: kuhn@mailer.uni-marburg.de

**Co-chair:**
Dr. Dario A. Giuse
Informatics Center
Vanderbilt University Medical Center
Eskind Biomedical Library
Nashville, TN, 37232-8340, USA
Tel: +1 615 936 1435
Fax: +1 615 936 1427
E-mail: Dario.Giuse@vanderbilt.edu

**Objectives:**
- To provide a forum for collaboration among world members, and to promote systematic development and research in the field of health information systems.
- To identify and assess problems and success factors of health information systems and to provide intensive feedback between the scientific community, healthcare professionals, and the health IT industry. This implies a "horizontal" orientation with close contact to other working groups.

**Recent Activities:**
- A successful working conference was held in Heidelberg, Germany, from April 8-10, 2002, in close cooperation with GMDS, the German Association for Medical Informatics, Biometry, and Epidemiology. In the first part of the working conference, five topics were covered by presentations of international HIS experts and by discussion groups which actively involved all participants:
    - (1)    The basic bottlenecks - HIS recommendations revisited
    - (2)    Pathways to open architectures
    - (3)    Patient empowerment
    - (4)    Socio-technical issues of HIS
    - (5)    HIS outcomes/metrics.

  In the second part of the conference, commercial systems were presented by scientists in close cooperation with the HIS industry.
- Approximately 100 persons participated in the first part of the conference; more than 200 participated in the second part. The IMIA conference was accompanied by an industrial exhibition and followed by the German GMDS HIS conference (April 11-12.) Altogether, 580 persons participated in the conference.
- The conference proceedings will appear as special issues in the International Journal of Medical Informatics (conference part 1) and in Methods of Informatics Medicine (conference part 2.)

**Future Activities:**
- The conference has resulted in a WG agenda to be published in the proceedings; the WG will follow this agenda by circulating (white) papers and by holding further workshops and conferences.

# *WG 11 - Dental Informatics*

**Chair:**
Dr. Wook-Sung Yoo
Computer and Information Sc. Dept.
Gannon University
109 University Square
Erie, PA 16506 USA
Tel:        +1 814 871 7692
Fax:        +1 814 871 7616
E-mail:     yoo@gannon.edu

**Co-chair:**
Dr. John Eisner
School of Dental Medicine
University of Buffalo
315 Squire Hall
Buffalo, NY 14214, USA
Tel:        +1 716 829 2057
Fax:        +1 716 833 3517
E-mail:     jeisner@buffalo.edu

**Objectives:**
To bring the small, but rapidly growing, community of dental informaticians around the world into closer contact.

**Recent Activities:**
- More members have joined this working group. There are currently 76 list members and 43 web members.
- The Dental Informatics working group home page (http://www.ecs.gannon.edu/IMIA) has been updated and more dental informatics related literature information was entered to the "Dental Informatics Literature Survey" site.

**Future Activities:**
- The next addition to the home page will be a "News" page identifying current dental informatics activities in countries and posting summaries or links to news items or web-sites related to these activities.
- "Technology Fair and Expo" will be held at the Annual Session of American Dental Education Association (ADEA), in March 2003. Many members of this IMIA working group are expected to attend the meeting.

# *WG 12 - Biomedical Statistics and Information Processing*

**Chair:**
Dr. Jana Zvárová
EuroMISE Center, Charles University
and Academy of Sciences
Pod vodarenskou vezi 2
182 08 Prague
The Czech Republic
Tel:        +420 2 6605 3097
Fax:        +420 2 8658 1453
E-mail:     zvarova@euromise.cz

**Co-Chair:**
Dr. Leon Bobrowski
Institute of Biocybernetics and
Biomedical Engineering,
Polish Academy of Sciences,
Trojdena 3, Warsaw, Poland
Tel:        +48 2 2 659 9143 (Ext 416)
Fax:        +48 2 2 659 7030
E-mail:     Leon.Bobrowski@ibib.waw.pl

**Objectives:**
- Statistical methodology plays a great role in many tasks of information processing. It contributes to both biomedical research and healthcare applications. There is no possibility of critically analysing papers in biomedical journals without understanding principles of statistics.
- Papers published in reviewed journals should guarantee both a scientific quality and practical significance of published results. However, we can often find wrong statistical analyses of collected data that lead to misleading conclusions. It is clear that often we need to generalize findings received only from samples drawn from populations under consideration. In this case statistical inductive reasoning makes it possible to calculate the degree of confidence of generalized conclusions objectively. Therefore, statistical methodology concerns itself with different aspects of data collecting (sampling methods) and data processing (computational statistics) using statistical tools for estimation of unknown population parameters and hypotheses testing. Statistical methods are often used in a broad field of biomedical applications, e.g. clinics, epidemiology, genetics, pharmacology, and other areas of healthcare. The Working Group will focus on a broad scope of statistical methods in medicine and health care including their contribution to the topics of clinical trials, meta-analysis, data mining, and decision support.

**Recent Activities:**
- The WG members have been active in the past in different conferences and workshops connected with statistics in biomedicine and healthcare. Every two years, workshops on Statistics in clinics have been organized at the Institute of Biocybernetics and Biomedical Engineering and the Polish Academy of Sciences. The most recent workshop was held in June 2000. These workshops combine education and research in the field of clinical statistics. The working group seeks to organize sessions at these conferences, as well as in the future MIE, IMIA conferences. It intends to establish closer co-operation in this field with IMIA

## *Biomedical Statistics and Information Processing (IMIA WG 12) (Continued)*

member countries as well as with international societies and other bodies in the field of biomedical and health statistics, e.g. Biometric Society, International Society for Clinical Biostatistics, and International Society for System Science in Health Care.

- On June 4th, 2002 during The Fifth International Seminar on Statistics and Clinical Practice in Warsaw, Poland the Panel Discussion on initial and future activities of the IMIA Working 12 was held. The discussion was chairing by Jana Zvárova, Norbert Victor and Leon Bobrowski. The conclusion was to prepare a workshop on topics of statistical methods in clinical studies in terms of the conference MIE 2003 in Saint Malo, France. The meeting on the occasion of MIE 2002 in Budapest, Hungary was held. The workshop took place on August 26th, 2002 at the EFMI Meeting Eötvös Loránd University, Congress Centre Pázmány Péter sétány 1/a, Budapest, Hungary. The main goal of the workshop has revealed interactions between the field of biomedical statistics and data mining. The invited contributions stimulated discussions of the following topics.
  - Introduction (Zvárová J.)
  - Data Mining in Cardiology (Rauch J., Tomeèkova M., Mrázek V., Štochl J.)
  - Data Mining in Hybrid Decision Support Systems (Nykanen P.)
  - The Application of Data Mining Algorithms to Small Data Sets (Sharp M.)
  - Special Tools for Mining Clinical Data (Moisil I.)
  - Discussion.
- More than 60 participants attended this meeting. The meeting was co-chaired by J. Zvarova and I. Moisil. The presented lectures were highly appreciated and broadly discussed by the participants of the workshop. All these contributions will be published in English with the Czech translation in the Czech journal Physician and Technology in 2003.
- The participants supported the idea to organize the conference of the working group in Prague on April 12-14, 2004.
- The membership of the IMIA WG 12 is open to all interested in more active contributions to the filed of biomedical statistics and information processing. To the end of August 2002 there were 27 active members.

### Future Activities:

- The next meeting and workshop are scheduled to be held at MIE2003 Saint Malo, 4.-7 May, 2003 http://www.med.univ-rennes1.fr/mie2003. The proposal for organizing the IMIA WG 12 conference in Prague, April 12-14, 2004, is under preparation.

## *WG 13 – Organizational and Social Issues*

**Chair:**
Dr. Bonnie Kaplan
Center for Medical Informatics
Yale University, School of Medicine
59 Morris Street
Hamden, CT 06517, USA
Tel:       +1 203 777 9089
Fax:       +1 203 777 9089
E-mail:    bonnie.kaplan@yale.edu

### Objectives:

- To investigate organizational, social, ethical, and individual behavioral issues surrounding the introduction and use of informatics applications.
- To determine strategies for product design and technological change to support health care delivery through information and communication technologies.
- To incorporate organizational change management and human concerns into information technology projects.

### Recent Activities:

- *IMIA Yearbook*
  - An invited review paper on People, Organizational, and Social Issues was published in the IMIA 2002 Yearbook.
  - Papers were submitted for consideration for a new section on Organizational and Social Issues in the 2003 Yearbook.

<table>
<tr>
<td>

*Organizational and Social Issues (IMIA WG 13) (Continued)*

</td>
<td>

- *MEDINFO 2001 Activities*
  - WG13, together with the AMIA People and Organizational Issues WG, presented two panels and a workshop on alternatives to the randomized controlled clinical trials as a model for evaluation.
  - The chair of WG13 taught a tutorial on Organizational Readiness For Clinical Information Technologies: "Culture, Change Management And Evaluation."
  - A business meeting was held.
- *AMIA SYMPOSIUM Activities*
  - "Evaluating the Impact of Health Care Information Systems", presented by the chair of the AMIA Quality Improvement WG and the chair of IMIA WG13, was accepted as a tutorial for the AMIA Fall Symposium 2002.
  - Joint panels with AMIA WGs were accepted for the AMIA 2002 Symposium:
    - "When Technology Is Not Enough: Barriers & Drivers to Adoption of Technology" - Co-sponsored with AMIA Genomics WG and People and Organizational Issues WG
    - "Incorporating The Social Into Medical Informatics" - Co-sponsored with AMIA People and Organizational Issues WG and AMIA Ethical, Legal, and Social Issues WG
    - "Bio-medical Informatics: Perspectives on Gender" - Co-sponsored with AMIA People and Organizational Issues WG
    - "Socio-technical Approaches In Health Informatics: Results of the Rotterdam Conference" - Co-sponsored with: EFMI WG9: Human and Organizational Issues and AMIA People and Organizational Issues WG
    (The latter two were chosen as plenary sessions.)
- *Outreach And Collaborative Activities*
  The chair's activities to raise awareness of organizational and social issues in medical informatics included:
  - Keynote speaker at e-Health 2002, the annual meeting of COACH (Canada's Health Informatics Association) and CIHI (the Canadian Institute for Health Information) and also a tutorial there on culture, change management and evaluation in Vancouver, April 2002.
  - Panel presenter for the IFIP 8.2 Conference on Global and Organizational Discourse about Information Technology, in Barcelona December 12-14, 2002.
  - Program Chair for the IFIP 8.2 2004 conference in Manchester, England.
- *Continuing Collaborative Projects*
  - Together with AMIA People and Organizational Issues WG, a bibliography of key papers is being developed. The first version will be posted on the People and Organizational Issues web site. For further information, contact Annette Valenta at valenta@uic.edu.
  - Papers were nominated for the Diana Forsythe Award of the AMIA People and Organizational Issues WG, and the chair served again on the Awards Committee.

**Future Activities:**
- JoAnne Callen (jcallen@cchs.usyd.edu.au) is coordinating the project to collect curricula and cases related to social and organizational issues and to develop recommendations for curriculum guidelines.
- Under the leadership of Vivian Vimarlund (vivvi@ida.liu.se) the WG is developing criteria for writing and reviewing papers on social and organizational issues.

</td>
</tr>
</table>

## WG 15 - Technology Assessment and Quality Improvement (TAQI)

**Chair:**
Dr. Jan Talmon (2001-2004)
Dept. Medical Informatics
Maastricht University
PO Box 616
6200 MD Maastricht
The Netherlands
Tel:       +31 43 388 2243
Fax:       +31 43 388 4170
E-mail:    talmon@mi.unimaas.nl

**Co-chair:**
Jytte Brender
Dept. of Health Science and Technology
Aalborg University and Virtual Centre
for Health Informatics
Fredrik Bajers Vej 7d
DK-9220 Aalborg East, Denmark
Tel:       +45 4541 0124
Fax:       +45 4541 0150
E-mail:    jytte.brender@v-chi.dk

**Objectives:**
- To promote comprehensive assessments of healthcare information technologies.
- To demonstrate the value of assessment methods in healthcare information technologies.
- To promote international cooperation toward developing methodological issues.

**Recent Activities:**
- A workshop was organized at the MIE 2002 conference in Budapest with quite an active audience. Presentations were given by Jytte Brender (DK) and Arjen Stoop (NL) on national initiatives to develop toolboxes for assessment. Elske Ammenwerth presented a new EFMI working group on evaluation. It was agreed that the Dutch and Danish initiatives will provide input to IMIA and EFMI and the Evaluation Working Group in EFMI and TAQI of IMIA will closely collaborate and share results.
- The chairman of TAQI attended the IMIA WG10 working conference in Heidelberg. Evaluation issues were high on the agenda. WG10 would welcome a generally available resource on evaluation and technology assessment.

**Future Activities:**
- In the next year the collaboration with the EFMI working group on evaluation will be further detailed.
- Further collaboration with other working groups will be established. The website that will be developed in the Netherlands will also be made available for the IMIA working group. Members of TAQI and from other interested working groups will be contacted to provide feedback.

## WG 16 - Standards in Health Care Informatics

**Chair:**
Michio Kimura, M.D., Ph.D.
Board member of Japan Association
of Medical Informatics
Professor and Director
Medical Informatics Department
Hamamatsu University
School of Medicine
1-20-1 Handa, Hamamatsu,
431-3192 Japan
Tel:       +81 53 435 2770
Fax:       +81 53 435 2769
E-mail:    kimura@mi.hama-med.ac.jp

**Objectives:**
- To advise about standards from an academic perspective.
- To promote the mutual identification of needed standards world-wide.
- To share information to facilitate mutual coordination of standards development in health informatics.

**Content areas that will be worked on by the Working Group:**
- WG 16 itself does not create a new standard but promotes mutual identification and coordination by posting and maintaining an inventory of health informatics standard activities.
- Usually, standard development activities are by volunteers, vendors, and immediate users. It is quite natural and fine for them to devote efforts to acquire fruitful outcomes. Sometimes, however, potential future users' profit could be underrated.
- IMIA is an academically oriented and worldwide organization which has connections with countries currently participating less in existing standard development activities, so WG 16 will input thoughtfulness for future users and for multi-cultural environments, as advisory to standard development activities.

## *Standards in Health Care Informatics (IMIA WG 16) (Continued)*

## *WG 17 – Computerized Patient Records*

**Chair:**
Dr. Johan van der Lei
Institute of Medical Informatics
Medical Faculty
Erasmus University
P.O. Box 1738
NL-3000 DR Rotterdam
The Netherlands
Tel:      +31 10 408 7050
Fax:      +31 10 408 9447
E-mail:   vanderlei@mi.fgg.eur.nl

**Co-Chair:**
Dr. Mark A. Musen
Section of Medical Informatics
Stanford University
School of Medicine
Medical School Office Building
Room X-215, Route 5
Stanford, CA 94305-5479
USA
Tel:      +1 650 723 3390
Fax:      +1 650 725 7944
E-mail:   musen@stanford.edu

**Future Activities:**
- Post and maintain an inventory of health informatics standard activities, for the purpose of promoting mutual identification between activities, as well as proliferation to users.
- Provide advising from academy side to activities and ISO/TC215 and CEN TC 251. (IMIA is already a liaison of ISO/TC 215.)
- Supply advice to activities for them to be worldwide, with thoughtfulness of multi-cultural environment. Virtually, initial mission is to highlight differences of health and personal information handling caused by each country's health and medical cultural differences.

**Objectives:**
- To support studies of the electronic patient record in the clinical environment.
- To study the electronic patient record in relation to evidence-based medicine.
- To stimulate the infrastructure required by an electronic patient record by supporting development and testing of the definition (1) of medical terms, (2) specific data sets, and (3) standards for electronic data exchange.

**Recent Activities:**
- The working group held its first conference on October 8-10, 1998 in Rotterdam. The Proceedings of this conference appeared in a special issue of *Methods of Information in Medicine* (1999; 38).
- During the MEDINFO 2001, the WG had a workshop discussing the role of academia in the development of electronic patient records. Although an increasing number of vendors have initial versions or partial implementations of electronic patient records on the market, members of the WG believed there was still a significant role for academia.
- The issue of merging with other working groups was raised, but no decisions were made.

**Future Activities:**
- The working group will schedule its a major meeting at the Medinfo 2004 meeting. In preparing that meeting, collaboration with other WGs will be sought.
- The working group also is considering hosting a workshop that would explore requirements for management of genomic information with electronic patient records.

# WG 18 - Telematics in Healthcare

**Chair:**
Dr. Regis Beuscart
Professor of Medical Informatics
The University of Lille
1, Place de Verdun
59045 Lille, France
Tel:        +33 3 2052 6970
Fax:        +33 3 2052 1022
E-mail:     rbeuscart@chru-lille2.fr

**Objectives:**

To explore the rationale and perspective of Health Telematics

- To promote the design and development of open architecture and inter-operability tools
- To promote the analysis, design and development of methodologies and applications to support collaborative work in healthcare information systems
- To share experiences on E-health, Telemedicine and Professional Healthcare networks.

**Recent Activities:**

- Workshop "Telematics in Healthcare" (London, September 2001)
  During this meeting, presentations by leaders of the domain (from USA, Australia, France, Italy, Denmark) allowed a tour d'horizon of the field, drawing the state of the art of the discipline. The workshop agenda included:
  - Introduction Régis Beuscart (France)
  - From Hospital Information Systems to Healthcare Information Systems Patrice Degoulet (France)
  - Telematics to support the educational and emotional needs of patients: The Baby CareLink Experience Charles Safran(USA)
  - Health Telematics activities in Australia Branko Cesnik (Australia)
  - Towards coherent Telematics network for Health in Denmark Knut Bernstein (Denmark)
  - E-Healthcare: Predictions and Trends for the next 5 years Mario Steffanelli (Italy)
  - Discussion: 9 recommendations for the development of Telematics in Heathcare Régis Beuscart

  This workshop demonstrated that Telematics is not only penetrating the activities of the Healthcare professionals but involves more and more patients, patients organizations, and people, giving access to medical information that is not available elsewhere.

- "E-Health: High-tech Medicine, Community Medicine" Workshop, January 23-24 2002 in Lille, France, organized by the IMIA WG XVIII (Telematics in Heathcare) and the French Association for Medical Informatics (AIM) with the support of the French Ministry of Research and the Région Nord-Pas-de-Calais. It was organized to draw a broad view of the development of Telemedicine Applications and particularly the use of Telematics for a closer contact between Healthcare providers and patients.
  - Day one: new high-tech technologies were presented that can improve the community-based healthcare delivery:
    · Fundoscopy interpretation
    · Ambulatory surgery
    · Telemedicine bag
    · New technologies in cardiology integrated in homecare
    · IT and emergency teleconsultation
    · Telediagnosis in Psychiatry
    · French-speaking Virtual University
  - We explored also the economic challenge of Telemedicine, the legal risks, and humanitarian issues. The Vice-President of the Region Nord-Pas-de-Calais, Mr. Galametz discussed the political framework of the dissemination of telematics application in healthcare.
  - Thirteen companies from Europe demonstrated their commercial products and it was really fascinating to see how up-to-date ideas were incorporated

<table>
<tr>
<td valign="top">

*Telematics in Healthcare (IMIA WG 18) (Continued)*

</td>
<td valign="top">

in ready-to-use and working products. .
- Day Two's introduction was by Jean-Claude Healy, from the European Commission (Brussels). He explained that after 10 years of programs focused on "Information for Health Care", it is time for supporting projects devoted to "Knowledge for Healthcare" and particularly on the themes of "IT", "Genomics", "Neuro and Social Sciences" for Health Care.
- Presentations:
  - Telemedicine and Home monitoring,
  - Teledialysis
  - Dietetics on line
  - Medical Home automation
  - Remote sensors and telemonitoring
  - Homecare and Networks
  - Telemedicne in Denmark (Lars Hulboek Fog and K Bernstein)
  - Telemedicine in Spain (E. Gomez)
  - Telemedicne in Poland (M. Duplaga)
  - Homecare in Belgium (E. Saliez)
  - Telemedicine in France (H. Faure-Poitout)

**Future Activities:**
It becomes obvious that technology is no longer the main obstacle to develop services. The main problems are organizational, legal and of political nature. It is time to define business models for telemedical services if we want to disseminate successful applications or experiments. We must also convince decision makers and politicians that the wide-scale implementation of these applications will bring benefits in terms of improvement of the patients' quality of life and essential savings in the budget for healthcare.

</td>
</tr>
</table>

# *Open Source Health Informatics Working Group (New)*

**Chair:**
MUDr. ing. Jan Vejvalka
Dept. of Applied Informatics
2nd Medical Faculty, Charles
University
V uvalu 84, 15006
Praha 5, Czech Republic
Tel:        +420 2 5721 0345, ext. 272
Fax:        +420 2 2443 5820
E-mail:
jan.vejvalka@lfmotol.cuni.cz

**Co-Chair:**
Prof. Graham Wright
CHIRAD (Centre for Health
Informatics Research and
Development)
41 Firs Road
Firsdown Salisbury SP5 1SJ

**Objectives**:

The open source approach is growing rapidly, and interest in the possible application of open source solutions within health and healthcare organizations is gaining pace. The IMIA (International Medical Informatics Association - www.imia.org) Open Source WG aims to provide a forum for discussion and for a collaborative, non-judgemental work environment to explore, and where appropriate promote and facilitate, the application of open source solutions within health, healthcare and health informatics.

The IMIA Open Source Health Informatics WG will bring together experts and interested individuals from a wide range of health professions and with a range of interests in the potential application of open source solutions within their domains of expertise. The WG will explore the implications of the open source approach for all aspects of IMIA's areas of interest. It will work with other Working and Special Interest Groups to explore the appropriate use of open source solutions and applications. Through close interaction with, and cross-membership with, many other open source groups outside IMIA, the WG will facilitate both the use of other groups' expertise in the areas under consideration, and the input of IMIA views to those other groups' work and discussions.

At present, the Working Group can see the benefits of the open source approach to the development and use of applications within health, healthcare, and health informatics to be centred around (but not limited to) the following points:

* Transparency of solutions, facilitating peer review and better quality assurance
* Re-use of components, stress on collaborative development, and resource sharing
* User needs being a driving force behind the development of solutions
* Flexibility in development processes, taking account of a need for and ability to react to changing needs
* Developments not being controlled by any single organization, enterprise, or vested interest
* Rapid spread of innovation
* Encouraging accessibility to products in developing countries
* Flexibility in distribution of solution costs, giving users more options e.g. for improved support and training
* Creation of new business niches based on services supported by open source solutions
* Usable, rather than purely esoteric, results being developed.

However, many of these proposed benefits remain to be demonstrated at any large scale, as is the general sustainability of open source projects in the field of healthcare applications. The Working Group does not seek to uncritically adopt the open source approach, but will critically examine the implications, and where appropriate make recommendations for or against an open source approach to solving particular problems.

## Recent and Future Activities:

The working group was given provisional status by IMIA Board in April 2002 and approved by the IMIA General Assembly in October 2002. Further information on the WG's current state and activities can be reached through the WG's web site, as linked from www.imia.org.

# *EFMI*

Regional Editor: Arie Hasman

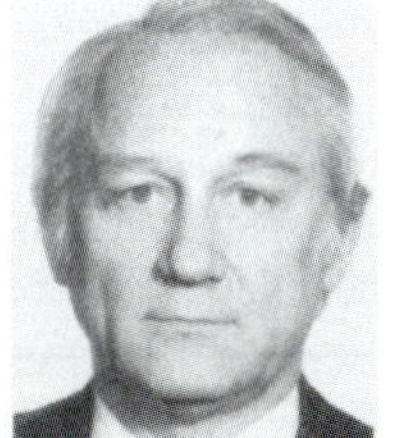

Attila Naszlady, IMIA Representative

## Structure

The constitutional bodies of EFMI are

* The EFMI-Council, a General Assembly of all members, officers and working group chair persons.
* The Board of officers, treasurer, vice presidents and president
* Working Groups organised by a chairperson (see also the EFMI-homepage, addresses, member societies)

## Objectives

The objectives of the European Federation for Medical Informatics (EFMI) founded in 1976 are:

* To advance international co-operation and dissemination of information in Medical Informatics on a European basis;
* To promote high standards in the application of medical informatics;
* To promote research and development in medical informatics;
* To encourage high standards in education in medical informatics;
* To function as the autonomous European Regional Council of IMIA

## Activities

All European countries are entitled to be represented in EFMI by a suitable Medical Informatics Society. The term medical informatics is used to include the whole spectrum of Healthcare Informatics and all disciplines concerned with Healthcare and Informatics. The organisation operates with a minimum of bureaucratic overhead and each national society supports the Federation by sending and paying for a representative to participate in the decisions of the Federation's Council. Also, and again to reduce overhead, English has been adopted as the official language, although simultaneous translation is often provided for congresses in non-English speaking countries.

## Countries

Currently, 26 countries have joined the Federation, and are named as

Austria, Belgium, Bosnia and Herzegovina, Bulgaria, Croatia, Cyprus, Czech Republic, Denmark, Finland, France, Germany, Greece, Hungary, Ireland, Israel, Italy, The Netherlands, Norway, Poland, Portugal, Romania, Slovenia, Spain, Sweden, Switzerland, Ukraine and United Kingdom. Application are open to representative societies in countries within the European Region of WHO. The EFMI council and board normally meets twice a year. Furthermore, it is represented by a Vice President (Europe) at meetings of the Board and the annual General Meetings of the International Medical Informatics Association (IMIA).

## Congresses and Publications

So far 16 general congresses (Medical Informatics Europe – MIE) have been organised by EFMI. These have taken place in Cambridge (1978), Berlin (1979), Toulouse (1981), Dublin (1982), Brussels (1984), Helsinki (1985), Rome (1987), Oslo (1988), Glasgow (1990), Vienna (1991), Jerusalem (1993), Lisbon (1994), Copenhagen (1996), Thessaloniki (1997), Ljubljana (1999), Hannover (2000) and Budapest (2002).

EFMI has started a new series of meetings: the Special Topic Conferences. It's concept has the following components:

* Organization by a member society in combination with its annual meeting
* EFMI council meeting is integral part
* Topic defined to the needs of the member society
* Relevant EFMI Working groups are engaged for the content
* Contributions mostly on invitation
* Small 2-day conference with 100+ participants

The first conferences took place in Bucharest/Romania 2001 and Nikosia/Cyprus 2002. The conferences were a big success and this type of Special Topic Conferences will continue with the 2003 conference on Electronic Patient Record in Copenhagen/Denmark under the chairmanship of the Swedish and the Danish Society for Medical Informatics in October 2003. For 2004 Munich/Germany is envisaged.

The proceedings of these congresses were usually published by Springer in the series *"Lecture Notes in Medical Informatics"* and by IOS Press in the series *"Studies in Health Technologies and Informatics"*.

A selection of the best papers from the MIE-conferences were published in a special volume of the International Journal of Medical Informatics. The next MIE congress will take place in St Malo, France in 2003.

To date four official journals adopted by the Federation are: *Methods of Information in Medicine, Medical Informatics, and Health Informatics Europe, International Journal of Medical Informatics*.

*EFMI (Continued)*

*Working Groups*

The following EFMI-Working Groups are operating:

## MCMS

### MBDS, Case Mix and Severtiy of Cases

Chair:
Prof. F.H. Roger France,
Centre for Medical Informatics
University of Louvain
10 av. Hippocrate, Box 3718
B-1200 Brussels
Tel. +32-2-7644709
Fax: +32-2-7644717
roger@infm.ucl.ac.be

Co-chair/Secretary:
J. Hofdijk
HISCOM, Schipholweg 97
NL-2316 XA LEIDEN, The Netherlands
Fax: +31-71-216675
jacob@bazis.nl

**Objectives**:
The organisation of special topic conferences, workshops, Teaching sessions in the European Region on MBDS, Case Mix and Severity of cases and their applications to Resource management and outcomes of care.

The communication of up to date experiences and/or references between members, including national uniform data sets, terminology, coding system and patient classification methods for resource management and quality of care.

The dissemination of results about informatics tools and telematics systems in this specific area among EFMI and IMIA affiliated members and participants to their meetings.

**Recent activities**:
Special Topic Conference 2001 in Collaboration with PCS-E, Patient Classification Systems Europe. "Case Mix: Global Views, Local Actions" Bruges, 10-13 October 2001.

Workshop during MIE 2002: Case mix and outcome measurements: experience in Hungary and the situation in 20 countries.

**Publications**:
Roger France F.H., De Moor G., Hofdijk J., Jenkins L. (Eds.) Diagnosis Related Groups in Europe, Ghent, Goff BVBA, ISBN 90-73045-01-0, 259 p., 1990
Roger France F.H., Noothoven van Goor J., Staehr Johansen K. (Eds) Case-Based Telematics Systems towards Equity in Health Care, IOS Press, Amsterdam, ISBN 90-51991-82-7, 207 p., 1994
Roger France F.H., Mertens I., Closon M.C., Hofdijk J. (Eds) Case Mix: Global Views, Local Actions – Evolution in Twenty Countries, IOS Press, Amsterdam, No 86, in press (2001)

## DPS

### Data Protection and Security in Health Information Systems

- suspended -

## IPAM

### Information Planning and Modelling in Health Care

Chair:
Bryan Manning
bryan.manning@btinternet.com

**Objectives**:
To develop generic approaches across an ever-widening range of health and linked social care domains

To develop working links to other National and International bodies

**Recent activities**:
This year we have been focusing on Risk and Security Modelling and presented some of these concepts at a two day Conference "Making Medical Informatics Work" held in Manchester in the Spring. These types of event have proved are an ideal vehicle for disseminating the results of our work more widely at no cost other than the time involved.

**Future activities**:
Our aim is to set up a Working Conference with a core theme of:

"Joining-up Healthcare Services in the 21$^{st}$ Century: Modelling the Best Practice"

Its aim will be to examine how to identify Best Clinical and Health Management Practice through:

- the use of appropriate workflow analysis and modelling techniques to provide in-depth mappings of the range of Service Provision Pathways used in delivering care across the spectrum of patient need
- the use of these Pathways as a "backbone" upon which to attach clinical/

## EFMI (Continued)

management protocols, guidelines, check-lists, decision support tools [including risk analysis], etc.

- the interactive use of these Pathways for case planning and semi-automatic record generation for transfer in to full multimedia record databases.
- the integration of diagnostic and bio-medical data into these records
- the use of summary data extracts from multimedia record databases to:
- establish resource profiles/parameters for planning/rostering
- support to clinical governance
- monitor service efficacy, effectiveness, efficiency and economy
- the application of domain-based security modelling and other techniques to determine the varying levels of security required both within agencies and between agencies, and similarly between the professionals involved
- the impacts of the use of semi-secure intranets communicating over public networks and the introduction of public key infrastructure [PKI] controls on clinical practice
- the use of Telemedicine and Telecare
- the opportunities and lessons learnt form e-commence in improving and optimising supply chains

### NURSE

### Nursing Informatics in Europe

Chair:
Patrick Weber
Nice Computing
Ch. De Maillefer 37
CH-1052 Le Mont-sur Lausanne
Switzerland
patrick.weber@nicecomputing,ch
Co-chair:
Paula M. Procter
School of Nursing & MIdwifery
The University of Sheffield
301 Glossop Road
UK-Sheffield S10 2HL
United Kingdom
p.procter@sheffield.ac.uk

Secretary:
Thomas Bürkle
Institut für Medizinische Informatik
und Biomathematik

Universität Münster
Domagkstr. 9
D-48129 Münster
Germany
Thomas.Buerkle@mednet.unimuenster.de

**Objectives**:

To support nurses and nursing organisations in the European countries with information and contacts and the field of informatics

To offer nurses opportunities to build contact networks within the informatics field. This could be accomplished by arranging sessions, workshops and tutorials in connection with the Medical Informatics European (MIE) conferences or by arranging separate meetings.

To support the education of nurses with respect to informatics and computing.

To support research and developmental work in the field and promote publishing of achieved results.

**Recent activities**:
Working group meeting at MEDINFO 2001.

Active presentation at the MIE STC 2002.

Workshop and tutorial during MIE 2002.

**Future activities**:
All information is published at the Website (www.nicecomputing.ch/nieurope).

### EDU

### Education in Health Informatics

Chair:
Prof. John Mantas
Health Informatics Laboratory
University of Athens, Greece
Tel:     +30 10 7461 1459/60
Fax:     +30 10 7461 461
Email: jmantas@cc.uoa.gr

Co-chair/Secretary:
Prof. Arie Hasman
Dept. of Medical Informatics
University Maastricht, The Netherlands
Email: hasman@mi.unimaas.nl

**Objectives**:
To organize workshops and possibly tutorials dedicated to the WG topics at each MIE conference, and other events.

To cooperate with IMIA WG 1 regarding Recommendations about Health Informa-

## EFMI (Continued)

tics Curricula and other subjects involving education and training in health informatics.

To disseminate knowledge about education and training in health informatics by various activities, such as conferences, educational events, publications and electronic means.

To encourage individuals to publish their research and other work in journals.

To provide a forum for discussion and debate.

**Recent activities:**
At the MIE special topic conference in Bucharest a workshop was organized in which five speakers from Rumania presented work in the area of Training and Education in Medical Informatics.

At the MIE special topic conference in Nicosia, Cyprus an update of the current events in Health Informatics education was presented by a number of speakers.

At MIE2002 the working group organised a Workshop on Education focused on the idea of a Virtual University in Health Informatics.

**Future activities:**
A workshop will be organized at MIE 2003.


## PCI

### Primary Care Informatics

Chair:
Dr. N.T. Shaw
E-mail: nikki.shaw@dial.pipex.com


**Objectives:**
To organize workshops and tutorials dedicated to WG topics at each MIE conference, and other events and to provide a forum for discussion and debate.

To establish networks of people involved in primary care informatics throughout Europe, and to learn about new developments and their activities.

To represent EFMI at IMIA WG5; to represent EFMI at MEDINFO; to represent EFMI at WONCA Informatics (the group has recently agreed to act as a European arm of WONCA Informatics); to collaborate with AMIA and other National Organisations.

To disseminate knowledge about primary care informatics issues by various activities, such as conferences, educational events, publications and electronic means.

To encourage individuals to publish their research and other work in journals.

**Recent activities:**
Members of the group participated in leading and organising a workshop during MEDINFO 2001 discussing the need for a global strategy for the use of IT in Primary Care in conjunction with IMIA WG5, WONCA, the Australian GPCG, and AMIA PCI WG.

Members of the group ran a workshop during the British Computer Society's Primary Health Care Specialist Group Annual Conference discussing the potential for international ground level collaboration in primary care informatics focusing on achievability and sustainability.

At MIE 2002 a tutorial and a workshop were organized.

**Future activities:**
 At the current time the group is concentrating on rebuilding a critical mass and is therefore not intending to initiate any large undertakings.

PCI built and publish an updated and current web site (follow link from http:// www.efmi.org) and established an email List group for members (details on the website).

**Publications:**
Shaw N. T. (2001) Going Paperless: A Guide To Computerisation In Primary Care, Radcliffe Medical Press.


## NLU

### Natural Language Understanding

Chair
Robert Baud
Division d'Informatique Médicale
Hôpitaux Universitaires de Genève
CH-1211 GENEVA 14 Switzerland
robert.baud@dim.hcuge.ch

**Objectives:**
To organize workshops dedicated to the WG topics at each MIE conference, and other events.

To organize special topic conferences on Natural Language related subjects.

To have personal connections with people involved in NLP in the medical domain, especially in Europe, and to learn about their

*EFMI (Continued)*

current developments and activities. To develop connections with experts in the general NLP domain and to participate to related events (ACL, COLING, ELSNET …).

To represent EFMI at IMIA WG6; to represent EFMI at AMIA new SIG on NLP. In general, to participate to events of those entities.

To develop a website with information on NLU topics and links to linguistic resources

**Recent activities:**
Tutorial at MEDINFO 2001 on multilingual lexicons given by R Baud.

A workshop is organised at Medinfo 2001 with known persons in NLP, ontologies and knowledge representation.

Organisation of the Special Topic Conference on NLPBA (Natural Language Processing for Biomedical Applications) at MIE STC 2002. Selected papers are published in the International Journal of Medical Informatics.

The Chairman R Baud of NLU, as well as R Engelbrecht as EFMI representative, are participating to the EU-IST BIOINFOMED Study with the stated objective to carry out a *prospective analysis on the relationships and synergy between medical informatics and bioinformatics*. The EU-sponsored meetings were held in Brussels (November 2001), Heraklion (June 2002) and Valencia (November 2002).

A workshop on NLU was held at the MIE 2002 conference. A round table on the subject of bridging between Medical Informatics and Bio-Informatics was organised, with a representative of DG XIII of the EU and different experts of the domains.

**Future activities:**
A new chairperson for IMIA WG6 has been proposed at Medinfo, London: Dr Werner Ceusters from Belgium. Dr Chris Chute, who was the past chairperson, remains active as co-chair. It has been decided to organize a WG6 working conference on invitation in 2003 or 2004 elsewhere in Europe. The NLU will be closely associated to the organisation.

## OIMI

Organisational Impact of Medical Informatics

Chair:
Jos Aarts
Dept. Of Health Policy and Management
Erasmus University Rotterdam
PO Box 1738, 3000 DR Rotterdam
j.aarts@bmg.eur.nl

**Objectives:**
To organize workshops and tutorials dedicated to the WG topics at MIE conferences and other events.

To establish networks of people involved in human and organisational issues in the healthcare domain, and to learn about new developments and their activities.

To disseminate knowledge about human and organisational issues by various activities, such as conferences, educational events, publications.

To encourage individuals to publish their research and other work in journals.

**Recent activities:**
The highlight of the past period was the Working Conferences 'Sociotechnical Approaches in Health Informatics' held in conjunction with MedInfo2001 and supported by the Royal Netherlands Academy of Arts and Sciences (KNAW), the Netherlands Organization for Scientific Research (NWO) and EFMI on September 6 and 7, 2001.

It was a successful conference with 130 participants, 66 presentations and 30 papers accepted for publication in a special issue of Methods of Information Medicine. The special issue will be published early 2003. Participants came from all five continents and represented the domains of medical informatics, information systems research and social studies of science and technology. The abstracts have been published in the conference proceedings.

The participants enjoyed the informal atmosphere of the conference and exchange of ideas and views from very different scientific domains. There was general agreement that a conference like this should be repeated. Details of the conference can

---

## EFMI (Continued)

be found on website http://www.bmg.eur.nl/smw/ithc.

A joint workshop with IMIA Working Group 13 on organizational issues at MedInfo2001

A presentation at the special topic MIE conference in Cyprus.

During the MIE2002 conference in Budapest two tutorials and one workshop were organized.

A panel consisting of presenters of the Rotterdam conference participated in the opening activity of the AMIA 2002 Fall Conference in San Antonio in November 2002.

**Future activities:**
At MIE2003 tutorials and workshops will be organized.


### MICIT

Medical Informatics in Countries in Transition

Chair:
Prof. Dr. George I. Mihalas
University of Medicine and Pharmacy
P-ta Eftimie Murgu 2
1900 Timisoara, Romania
Tel + Fax : +40-256-190288
mihalas@medinfo.umft.ro

Co-chair/Secretary:
Dr. Marcelo Sosa-Iudicissa
European Parliament
Brussels, Belgium
Email: MSosa@europarl.eu.int

**Objectives:**
To promote exchange of information between actors in Europe, developing regions and world-wide, for improved access and use of data and knowledge.

To investigate the needs, opportunities and obstacles for health information systems, informatics and telematics in developing regions.

To disseminate European and world-wide results and experiences across developing regions and professionals.

To facilitate access to European groups and their facilities and outcomes by students, medical practitioners, nurses, health managers and any other person from developing regions interested in learning and working together with partners in Europe and other industrialised countries.

To analyse and promote the use of Internet resources and applications to bridge gaps between north and south and between west and east, to act as a clearinghouse of information on resources of all kinds of mutual interest to health informatics and telematics participants in Europe and developing regions.

**Recent activities:**
Workshop organized by the WG at MIE2000, Hannover, Germany, entitled: *"Let's face reality: differences between expectations and achievements".*

Organizer of the working conference entitled *MIE2001 Special Topic Conference "Healthcare Telematic Support in Transition Countries", Bucharest, June 7-9, 2001,* in co-operation with Romanian Society of Medical Informatics and other EFMI working groups (esp. the EFMI working group on Human and Organisational issues).

Organisation of the workshop: *"Difficulties in implementing healthcare informatization strategies in transition countries"* at MIE 2002.

**Future activities:**
Establish an Internet based discussion group concerning implementation of healthcare information systems, to attract experts from consulting companies to express their opinions on some cases.


### EHR

**Electronic Health Record**

Chair:
PD Dr. Bernd Blobel
University Hospital Magdeburg
Institute of Biometry and Medical Informatics
Leipziger Str. 44
D-39120 Magdeburg, Germany
Tel: +49 391 671 3542
Fax: +49 391 671 3536
bernd.blobel@mrz.uni-magdeburg.de

Co-chair:
David Lloyd
University College London
Centre for Health Informatics &
Multiprofessional Education

## EFMI (Continued)

Highgate Hill, London, England
Tel: +44 171 288 3364
Fax: +44 171 288 3322 (Please mark FAO:
David Lloyd
D.Lloyd@chime.ucl.ac.uk

**Objectives**:
The working group deals with the issue of
electronic health records at different levels.
Such levels concern the case level,
organisational level, regional level, national
level, and international level. In that context,
the Working Group supports:

studies on specification, implementation,
and promotion of standards for EHR,

the modelling of its architecture and its
interoperability, as well as

the education on that topic.

The Working Group

· organises workshops dedicated to the
WG's topics,
· supports contacts to the scene,
· represents EFMI to corresponding
structures within IMIA as well as other
organisations dealing with the topic.

The Working Group especially deals with
the

· analysis of different EHCR approaches,
harmonising tools and methods for
specification, presentation, implementation and use for common views,
· consideration and evaluation of the
single model versus the dual model
approach, especially,
· population of CEN prENV OCC with
KR and Archetypes,
· harmonisation of terminology used,
· correction, refinement and harmonisation of UML models defined in different
approaches,

The Working Group strongly co-operates
with the EUROREC initiative and its
supporting institutions as well as with
global EHR activities.


The Working Group co-operates strongly
with the EFMI WGs "Security" and
"Communications and Interoperability".

**Recent activities**:
Organisation of a set of workshops for
providing insight in and understanding of
the methodologies developed and applied

around the globe such as, e.g., an
international workshop on EHCR standards
in Göttingen, Germany, 23 February 2001

Organisation of a workshop and a tutorial
at, as well as active contribution to, the 4th
Eurorec Conference in Aix-en-Provence,
4-6 November 2001.

Promotion of modelling and tooling for
advanced EHR.

Moving the structure-based models to real
components specifying structure and
functionality.

Contribution to activities within ISO TC
215 and CEN TC 215 for representing the
Working Group interests.

Official partner of the global openEHR
initiative.

MIE Special Topic Conference "The e-
volution of IT in Health Care Systems".
Nicosia, Cyprus, 8-10 March 2002.


### MIP

### Medical Image Processing

Chair:
PD Dr. Dr. Alexander Horsch
Dept. of Medical Statistics and
Epidemiology
Technical University of Munich
Ismaninger Str. 22
D-81675 Munich, Germany
alexander.horsch@imse.med.tu-muenchen.de

**Objectives**:
To establish a reference image database
for medical image processing R&D groups
(RID-MIP) within the EFMI member
countries.

To establish a Web-based Information
System (IS) about European Image
Processing Groups (EIPG) and their current
activities.

To create and maintain a Working Group
Website providing public information and
(in a protected subarea) WG-internal
documents and work plans.

To organize workshops dedicated to the
WG topics at the MIE conferences and
other events.

To build and maintain close relationship
with persons, groups, organisations and

| |
|---|
| *EFMI (Continued)* |

standardisation bodies working on the MIP field and medical domains involved.

**Recent activities:**

At the 1st WG meeting, held on 6-7 June 2002 in Munich, the draft version 0.13 of a concept for the RID-MIP was thoroughly discussed and extended. This resulted in the RID-MIP Preliminary Concept 1.00 which was editorially finished by the chairperson immediately after the meeting and distributed among the WG members on 11th of June.

At July 11, the first version of the WG website has gone online on the domain www.efmi-wg-mip.net. The website shall be linked from the working group page on EFMI website. It contains a public and an internal area (access for members only). The public area informs about news, work, meetings, activities and cooperation, and it provides reports and finished documents for download. The internal area contains the list of members with contact information, actual work lists with current status, and internal protocols, reports, working drafts and other documents for download.

At MIE2002 in Budapest a workshop was held on the RID-MIP topic entitled "Reference Image Datasets for Medical Image Processing Research and Development". At the workshop, the actual state of the WG's RID-MIP work was presented to the participants and then discussed.

On 4 April 2002, the WG chair has met representatives of the CEN TC251 EHRcom (Electronic Health Record communication) task force in London. The topic "integration of medical imaging in the electronic health record" was thoroughly discussed on the background of a possible co-operation. An exchange of documents, mutual input whenever appropriate or necessary was agreed.

In September 2002, a meeting with the CARS (Computer Assisted Radiology and Surgery). organizer is scheduled. At this meeting, concrete co-operation and possibilities for a presence and participation of the WG at the next CARS conference in June 2003 in London will be negotiated.

**Future activities:**

Meetings will be held at MIE2003 in Saint Malo and/or at CARS2003 in London. The final decision has do be made at the next WG meeting.

It is intended that the WG creates spin-offs wherever it makes no sense to continue an initiative by the modest resources inside the WG. This will especially apply to the RID-MIP initiative, where after a starting and piloting phase funding and migration to a project will be necessary to bring the idea into broad exploitation. The 6th Framework of the European Commission is considered as suitable.

# *APAMI*

Regional Editor: Chun Por Wong

---

*Regional President's Report - CP Wong*

### 1. Membership of APAMI

To date, medical informatics societies of 13 countries are members of the APAMI (Australia, the People's Republic of China, Hong Kong, Indonesia, Japan, South Korea, Malaysia, New Zealand, Pakistan, the Philippines, Singapore, Taiwan and Thailand). Sri Lanka and Vietnam have been observer members. Bangladesh, India, Pakistan and Kazahstan are correspondence members.

CJK (China-Japan-Korea Medical Informatics Association) is still working in close linkage to APAMI countries.

### 2. AGM of the APAMI

The last AGM of the APAMI was held in 4th September 2001 in London. Ten countries (Philippines, Japan, New Zealand, Malaysia, Vietnam, Singapore, Korea, PR China, Taiwan and Hong Kong) were represented. Kazahstan was in attendance.

In the AGM the following were resolved:

a. The Annual Report and the Financial Report were received and adopted.

b. Report of the 2000 APAMI Conference in Hong Kong was received and adopted.

c. Reports of activities of medical informatics in various regions (China, Hong Kong, India, Korea, Taiwan and Vietnam) were reported.

d. Date of next AGM will be held in October in Taipei in conjunction with the IMIA GA.

e. Korea announced the next APAMI Conference to be held in South Korea in October 2003.

f. The possibility of holding the APAMI Conference every 2 years instead of 3 years was suggested and to be discussed in future meetings.

### 3. APAMI Conference 2003

The APAMI Conference 2003 will be held in Daegu, South Korea scheduled on 29-31 October 2003. A preparatory meeting was held in Seoul on 13th June 2002. It was suggested that the APAMI Conference will be held in conjunction with CJK 2003 and KOSMI. Furthermore, meetings of the ISO and HL7 working groups will be invited to be host in the same region around the same time.

### 4. Regional Activities

a. The President of APAMI attended the Medical Informatics Society of Taiwan (MIST) Conference in Tao Yuan near Taipei on 27-28th October 2001. A presentation of "The Current Status of Development of Medical Informatics in the Asia Pacific Region" was delivered during the Conference. The President of IMIA, Prof KC Lun, also attended the Conference as the key note speaker.

b. The President also gave a similar talk in KOSMI in Seoul on 14th June 2002.

c. A preparatory meeting for the organization work was held on 13th June 2002 in Seoul. Prof Michio Kimura was also invited in the meeting. Prof Jungho Park will chair the Steering Committee, Prof Yun Sik Kwak heads the Organizing Committee with Prof Hune Cho at the Scientific Committee chair. Members from each member societies will be invited to join the Scientific Committee.

*Members' Activities 2001-2002*

### China (from Dr Ling Zhu)

China remained active in medical informatics. The CJK (China-Japan-Korea) Medical Informatics Group has just held the Annual Event in Beijing in August 2002.

The China Government has strong devotion and support to medical informatics. The Golden Health Project, a 15-year plan from 1995 to 2010 consists of 9 main targets in setting standards, building databases, administration automation, statistical and policy support systems, drug inventory systems, manufacture and enterprise resource planning, pharmaceutical e-commerce, networking of research and education services, and medical informatics service structure.

## APAMI (Continued)

### Hong Kong (from Dr CP Wong)

The Hospital Authority in Hong Kong is actively augmenting its Clinical Management System and Electronic Patient Records projects in recent 2 years. The 44 public hospitals and institutions which serve the 6.7 million population are all networked into one single system. Enhancements like Generic Clinical Requests, Generic Results Reporting, Clinical Data Format, Medication Decision Support, Clinical Data WareHouse, etc are superimposing on the HIS established about 12 years ago. A government project of setting up a Health Information Infrastructure (HII) is now in the Project Definition Stage. It will be launched in 5 years to link all public and private sectors in health care and as a Life Long Investment in Health strategic direction of the government. It facilitates the establishment of Life Long Health Records for all citizens in Hong Kong.

The Hong Kong Society of Medical Informatics in Hong Kong remains active. The membership has trimmed down to include only those actively involved in IT in health. The next Hong Kong International Medical Informatics Conference will be held on 23-25 January 2003. Details could be found at our website at http://www.hksmi.org.

### Japan (from Prof Michio Kimura)

Japan remained one of the most advanced countries in the development of Medical Informatics. The Ministry of Health has unveiled the Grand Design of IT policy in late 2001. Action plans will be targeted with more than 60% of hospitals submitting claims electronically by 2004, and more than 60% hospitals with 400+ beds would have EMR by 2006. For this purpose, standardization activities will be greatly supported, particularly in the areas of HL7 and DICOM.

The government of Japan provides very favorable funding subsidies to assist hospitals to install Hospital Information Systems and Medical Networks. record were hosted by TAMI. TAMI is also actively involved in the planning of multi-million US dollar knowledge-based healthcare project starting 2002.

### Korea (from Dr Hune Cho)

In addition to clinical applications of medical informatics, two major topics are being emphasized in Korea: education and standardization.

There are 41 medical schools (including 10 national universities) in Korea, and most schools are now considering education reform. The first academic department of medical informatics was inaugurated at Kyungpook National University School of Medicine in 1999. Medical informatics has been gradually recognized as a standard curriculum in many medical schools. Also recently, nursing informatics is launched as a graduate study program in College of Nursing, Seoul National University.

In 3 consecutive joint symposia with the Korean Society of Medical Education in 2001-2002, the suggestions of Medical School Objectives Project (MSOP) by American Association of Medical Colleges (AAMC) and IMIA WG1 are highly regarded, and therefore medical informatics is strongly recommended to be included in the regular medical curriculum.

Standardization is another major thrust in medical informatics. In this regard, Health Informatics Standardization committee was formed in KOSMI since 1999 in order to actively participate not only in the international standardization (ISO TC215, Health Informatics) but also in the national informatics standardization with the government support from Korean Agency for Technology and Standards (KATS), the Ministry of Commerce, Industry and Energy (MOCIE). HL7 (Health Level Seven) is also incorporated to facilitate standardization of messaging and communication of medical information. A number of international standardization activities have been organized with KOSMI such as ISO Technical Committee 215 Conference.

Asian-specific on-going issues of health informatics standardization will be discussed in APAMI to be held in Taegu Oct 29-31, 2003 (Dr. Yun Sik Kwak, Organizing Chair). Especially, KOSMI Fall Conference will celebrate the 15th anniversary in in Seoul Nov. 29, 2002 (Dr. Young Moon Chae, Organizing Chair).

*APAMI (Continued)*

**Malaysia** (from Dato Dr Ajai Mohan and Dr Mohamad Azrin Zubir)

Malaysia is very aggressively building its Multimedia SuperCorridor Flagship MSC since 1998 in Kuala Lumpur. The 7 Flagship Applications include TeleHealth, Smart Schools, Electronic Government, Multi-purpose Cards, R & D Clusters, WWW Manufacturing and Borderless Marketing or e-Commerce. The Lifetime Health Plan (LHP), Continuing Medical Education (CME), Mass, Customized, Personalised Health Information & Education (MCPHIE), and TeleConsultation (TC) were the Telehealth flagship applications.

Selayang Hospital is the first hospital in Malaysia to implement a Total Hospital Information System with the aim to provide a total paperless and filmless hospital environment since 1999. It is comprised of clinical, imaging, administrative and financial information system fully integrated through a Health Level Seven and DICOM standard protocol. Encouraging results and satisfactory feedbacks were achieved.

**Singapore** (from Prof KC Lun)

The President of AIMS (Association for Informatics in Medicine, Singapore) Prof KC Lun is now also the President of IMIA.

There were active activities in Singapore. AIMS was one of the sponsors of the Interoperability Medical Registry Systems (IMRS) Conference organized by the NUS Bioinformatics Centre on 19 January 2001. The 1-day conference, which was held at the Tan Tock Seng Hospital Auditorium, was a tremendous success, thanks to the leadership of Assoc Prof Tan Tin Wee and the efforts put in by his BIC staff and postgraduate students. Some 200 participants attended the conference in which a total of 13 papers were presented.

AIMS continued to be actively involved in the activities of IMIA and APAMI. Our members presented 5 papers at APAMI 2000 in Hong Kong and will support the next APAMI conference which will be held in Daegu, South Korea in 2003. We also expect to send delegates to the MEDINFO 2004, the 11th World Congress on Medical Informatics which will be held in San Francisco in September 2004.

The Association continues to maintain strategic international alliances with the Asia Pacific Advanced Network (APAN) consortium, largely through the active involvement of Assoc Prof Tan Tin Wee.

The AIMS is cognizant of the rising prominence of bioinformatics and its increasing convergence with medical informatics. Originally, a conference on Clinical Bioinformatics, to be hosted by AIMS and sponsored by IMIA, is now being planned.

**Taiwan** (from Prof Jack Li)

The progress of clinical information systems in Taiwan accelerates rapidly after the announcement of the new generation Health Information Network (HIN 2.0) in 1999. It consists of a collection of sub-projects which address the issues of life-long electronic health record (EHR), inter-hospital clinical data exchange through a Medical Information Exchange Center (MIEC), medical information standards, public health information systems, Certificate Authority for health professionals (HCA), security and privacy of health information, health insurance smart card and even related legislation. In July 2002, the NHI started to send out health insurance smart cards to the entire population of Taiwan. These smart cards will initially carry only health insurance information. By the year 2005, some personal health information including vaccination records, drug allergy history, recent medication history and reports of medical examinations/tests will also be stored securely in them. The HIN 2.0 also funded eight major hospitals in Taiwan for a trial of electronic medical record that can lead to the goal of a paperless hospital.

The Taiwan Association of Medical Informatics (TAMI) which was established in 1991 quickly gained recognition as the prestigious national association in the field of medical informatics. TAMI has since assisted the Department of Health and other healthcare organizations on issues involving computer applications in medicine and healthcare. TAMI also helped the founding of medical information standards organizations such as HL7 Taiwan and DICOM Taiwan in 2000.

## APAMI (Continued)

One of the largest events TAMI hosts routinely is the annual Medical Informatics Symposium in Taiwan (MIST), which typically attracts around 500 attendees from academia and healthcare industry in the three-day conference. In MIST 2002, we will also host the International Medical Informatics Association General Assembly Meeting and the Asia-Pacific Association of Medical Informatics Annual General Meeting in Taipei from October 3rd to 5th.

Besides governmental efforts and industrial interests, the growing community of medical informatics in Taiwan is strongly supported by academic research. In 1998, the Graduate Institute of Medical Informatics was established in Taipei Medical University. A graduate program for health informatics was offered in National Yang Ming University since 1997 and subsequently became the Institute of Health Informatics and Decisions. Tzu Chi University started an undergraduate program in 2002 under the newly established department of Medical Informatics, which is the first undergraduate program for this multi-disciplinary field. In addition to these formal degree-granting programs, there are many research groups involved in medical informatics projects. Distinguished researchers in the Section on Medical Informatics in National Taiwan University, the Health Informatics and Management Center in National Chung Cheng University and the Institute of Information Science in Academia Sinica are only a few examples of such research groups.

# Helina - African Region

Regional Editor: Sedick Isaacs

*Regional Representative's Report*

As a result of the problems in the Middle East, the Conference (Helina2002) could not take place in Egypt in October 2002. South Africa has agreed to host the conference as an interim measure. Namibia has tentatively offered to host the next Helina.

Discussions are in progress to finalise the linking of Helina2003 to the Aids/HIV conference. A local organising committee as well as a programme is in the process of been established.

It was also learnt that a conference on Routine Health Information systems is also been planned in South Africa for 2003 and discussion with the organizers are been planned to see how we can mutually support one another. They have been thinking of having the conference in Cape Town but this will add about $50 travel cost per delegate.

Helina2003 Conference is taking place in October 2003 in Midrand, South Africa.

**National Health/Medical Informatics Associations**

The development of national organizations is still in progress in Kenya, Nigeria, Zambia, Tanzania, and Egypt. These are all English speaking countries and contact is needed with other language African countries. The formation of the African Union may provide new opportunities.

Dr. Sedick Isaacs
Department of Information Management
Groote Schuur Hospital
Observatory
7925 South Africa
E-mail: seisaacs@pawc.wcape.gov.za
Tel:    +27 21 404 2058
Fax:    +27 21 404 2070

# IMIA-LAC
# The Latin-America and Caribbean Federation of Health Informatics

Regional Editor:
Lincoln A. de Assis Moura Jr.

*Regional President's Report*
*Lincoln A. de Assis Moura Jr.*

## 1. Conferences:

- NI'2003 - See under Brazil, below.

- Support Informedica 2002: 2nd Virtual Iberoamerican Congress of Medical Informatics in Internet. October 15- to November 15, 2002.

- Brazilian Conference on Health Informatics, September 29 to October 02, 2002, Natal, Brazil.

## 2. From the Member Countries:

*Brazil*

In Brazil there are several interesting initiatives going on:

1. SBIS web-site (*www.sbis.org.br*) is undergoing major rebuilding work, as it is to be the preferred means of communication with members and the community as well. SBIS has managed to get a grant from de Brazilian Government to develop 3 products that will be available on the site. They are:

   a. The Health Care Software Catalog
   b. Dynamic Survey on the Use of IT by Health Care Providers
   c. Dynamic Survey on the Use of IT by MCOs (Payors)

   These products will be offered via the Web, on a self-service approach. The idea is to have enough information to influence vendors, investor, authorities and so on. The project began in May and the site and the Health Informatics Survey and Database will be launched during the Brazilian Conference, in October.

   Members will have full access to the Surveys. Non-members will have to pay a fee (big enough to make them consider becoming a member!

2. The Brazilian Conference on Health Informatics (CBIS'02) will be held in Natal, Rio Grande do Norte, Brazil, from September 29 to October 02. Professors Ed Hammond and Branko Cesnik are among the keynote speakers.

3. Dr. Esperanza O'Farrel has been invited to deliver a speech at the Conference which will allows us to have an IMIA-LAC Board Meeting during the Conference.

4. Several regional Health Care Informatics meetings took place in Brazil with SBIS's support. Among them are: a) The 3rd Telemedicine Conference of Fortaleza (InfoSol), in the Northeastern state of Ceará; b) Informatics in Hospitals and Clinics, promoted by the Federation of Hospitals and Clinics of Rio de Janeiro, but organized by SBIS; c) One-day Seminar on Health Care Informatics within CONIP'02 (the National Conference on Public Information Systems). SBIS is also taking part in the 2nd Virtual Iberoamerican Congress of Medical Informatics in Internet.

5. The Brazilian Medical Council has launched a set of regulations stating what requirements Health Information Systems must meet to be certified by the Council. Organizations with certified systems will be released from keeping the information on paper. SBIS will be the certifying body, which is bound to open up a whole set of opportunities for SBIS.

## 3. Contact information:

President: Dr. Lincoln A. Moura Jr., Brazil

Secretary: Dr. Esperanza O'Farrel, Cuba

Mailing List:
Imia_Lac@Yahoogroups.Com

URL: www.imia-lac.org

Email: lamoura@uol.com.br
or lincoln@atech.br

# *North American Medical Informatics (NAMI)*

Regional Editors:
Jochen Moehr, Charles Safran

## North American Medical Informatics (NAMI)

Although IMIA's North American members COACH and AMIA have not yet agreed on forming an official North American region, there is a wealth of activity to report.

## Health Informatics in Canada

The following is a description of a selection of Canadian societies and organizations devoted to health informatics in a wide sense. The selection follows a n approach initiated in 2002. Appropriate representatives designated by their organizations prepared the statements. While most important organizations are likely represented, this is not a complete listing of all health informatics related institutions and initiatives. This is partly in the nature of health informatics and its yet to be defined boundaries, partly because further organizations exist at other levels, such as that of different Provinces, professional groups, etc. We will, in the years to come, endeavor to come to a comprehensive and systematic overview, and hope that the presented information is of use in the meantime[1].

### Canada's Health Informatics Association (COACH) (http://www.coachorg.com)

COACH, formerly known as the Canadian Organization for the Advancement of Computers in Health, has evolved over the 27 years of its history. It now represents a strong community of over 900 members committed to advancing the practice of health informatics.

Last year COACH re-affirmed its mission to *"promote the understanding and effective utilization of information and information technologies within the Canadian health care industry through education, information, networking and communication"*. Four key priorities were established to address a number of issues identified:

1) confirmation of our role through enhancing our understanding of who we are and what our relationships should be with others;
2) enhancing the value of COACH to our members through a clear focus on quality, professional development, and products and services;
3) influencing the improvement of health informatics practices; and
4) strengthening our governance through a transition to a "policy governance" board.

Over the past year, a number of achievements have supported these priorities. For the third consecutive year, COACH and the Canadian Institute for Health Information (CIHI) collaborated on the successful delivery of e-Health 2002 *A New Era of Health Care Delivery* in Vancouver, British Columbia. Attended by over 1,400 delegates from a variety of backgrounds in health informatics, the conference focused on how health care planning, delivery, health practices and decision-making are enhanced through e-health innovations and collaborations. Topics included security and privacy, the electronic health record, telehealth and patient safety as well as information management and emerging trends in health care delivery. Building on 2002, planning is well under way for e-Health 2003 *A Catalyst for Change* to be held May 24-27, 2003 at the Westin Harbour Castle Hotel in Toronto, Ontario.

This year, COACH initiated a new *Professional Development Series* designed to provide opportunities for affordable and accessible professional development in health informatics in three streams: Health Information Management, Security and Privacy, and the Electronic Health Record (EHR). The first two streams were successfully launched in the spring and the EHR stream is in progress, expected for early 2003. Additional sessions are scheduled for the fall and early 2003 for members in the western, central and eastern regions of Canada. Details and registration information can be found on the COACH web site.

Another first was a special *Canada Health Informatics Executive Forum* held at the

---

[1] We hope that this publication is an incentive for those Canadian organizations not represented yet to contact the Canadian IMIA Representative, Dr. Jochen Moehr, jmoehr@uvic.ca.

## North American Medical Informatics (NAMI) (Continued)

time of e-Health 2002 for the purpose of providing a forum for open dialogue among the industry's key stakeholders. Discussion of major issues facing the industry included the need for a common definition of "health informatics", the challenge of integrating health care and IT skills in the delivery of health care, and issues related to the electronic health record, funding and accountability. A second forum is planned for e-Health 2003.

COACH released its *Guidelines for the Protection of Health Information* in the spring of 2001 to a very positive response. This new version of COACH's earlier 1995 publication, *Security and Privacy Guidelines for Health Information Systems*, provides health informatics professionals the framework necessary to implement security and privacy programs in the current environment under the parameters of new legislation. Further information can be found on the COACH web site.

*Building strategic relationships* has been a major focus of COACH. One example is the *new Patron program* launched this past year to support the need to build relationships with the health informatics community. The seven Patrons who have joined to date are recognized as leaders in health informatics and have lent their name and support to assist COACH in developing health informatics in Canada in return for special Patron benefits. In addition, COACH has built and continues to develop excellent relationships with many organizations who share a common interest in the advancement of the industry both within Canada and on the international front, through organizations such as IMIA and the Healthcare Information and Management Systems Society (HIMSS).

As an organization, COACH is looking toward a bright future in *providing leadership and guidance* to those professionals committed to addressing the challenges of integrating professional skills with information and communication technology in order to ensure accountability and quality in the delivery of health care in Canada.

## Société québécoise d'informatique biomédicale et de la santé (SoQibs) (www.soqibs.org)

In Canada, in the province of Quebec, a new society, SoQibs, was officially inaugurated in November 2001. SoQibs is the Société québécoise d'informatique biomédicale et de la santé. By specifying biomedical and health (santé) informatics it intends to act as a unifying place for the various aspects of informatics that have application in the health system. As part of its mission it will enable scientific exchange and the promotion of expertise and learning as well as aim to influence Quebec research, development and application strategies. It will also actively associate with other provincial, national and international activities in health informatics.

In May 2002 it hosted the 9th 'Journées Francophones d'Informatique Médicale (JFIM)' for the first time in North America. This bi-annual francophone event has set to date a very high standard with regular publication of its proceedings as a published monograph, a tradition which was reinforced in May. 200 participants contributed 39 oral presentations, 23 poster presentations, 5 plenary discussion sessions and an industrial exhibition. The presentation abstracts are available on the web-site. The society will be proactive in enabling debates on complex major issues such as patient confidentiality and the law as well as leading initiatives to document health informatics activities in Quebec. It will encourage the activities of special interest groups such as nursing informatics and telehealth and enable a forum of communication across interest groups.

## Canadian Institute for Health Information (CIHI) (http://secure.cihi.ca/cihiweb/)

Created in 1994, the Canadian Institute for Health Information (CIHI) is an independent, pan-Canadian, not-for-profit organization working to improve the health of Canadians and the health care system by providing quality health information.

<table>
<tr><td>

**North American Medical Informatics (NAMI)**
*(Continued)*

</td></tr>
</table>

At CIHI, we:

- Identify and respond to health information needs and priorities;
- Support the development of national health indicators;
- Coordinate and promote the development and maintenance of national health information standards for collecting, processing and sharing health information;
- Develop and manage health databases and registries;
- Analyze information, conduct special studies, and participate in, or support, health care system research;
- Fund and facilitate population health research and analysis, conduct policy analysis and develop policy options;
- Contribute to the development of population health information systems and infrastructure;
- Publish reports on health and health care and share the key findings with Canadians; and
- Offer education programs for our clients and participate in or co-sponsor conferences on emerging key issues in health care.

CIHI is committed to respecting personal privacy, safeguarding the confidentiality of health information and providing a secure environment for information systems under its management. We have a comprehensive Privacy Program in place that includes principles based on Schedule 1 of the Personal Information Protection and Electronic Documents Act as well as stringent privacy and confidentiality policies and guidelines.

Among its many initiatives, is the Partnership for health information standards (www.cihi.ca/partship/partner1.shtml). Created in 1996, the Partnership is a forum that brings together the public and private sectors to share, connect and map the future of health information standards in Canada. It has established interest groups for its members on key health informatics standards topics including identifiers, imaging/devices, modeling/architecture, security, vocabulary, telehealth and electronic health record. In addition, the Partnership also organizes two annual events focusing on major Canadian and international health information standards activities.

Additionally, CIHI is the sponsoring agency for HL7 Canada, the forum for Canadian health information stakeholders to decide how HL7 is adopted and adapted for use in Canada. HL7 Canada is a recognized international affiliate and a voting member of the HL7 International Committee. HL7 Canada is organized to identify and support the unique requirements of its member groups - health information system users, vendors, and administrators.

Among the projects currently under way at CIHI is the development of strategies for the unique identification of clients, providers and health care facilities; the development of an HL7 based client registry message specification to enable various registries to communicate to one another and the development of an HL7 based national electronic health claims standard.

CIHI has also worked on a number of PKI-related documents, produced to assist in the establishment of a health PKI within and across jurisdictions. These documents provide a framework and guidelines for the secure electronic communication of health information.

On the international front, CIHI has also been actively involved in standards development activities within the ISO community, including support of Canadian leadership on standards for country identifiers, a conceptual health indicators framework, a health informatics profiling framework, interoperability of telehealth and telelearning systems, and guidelines on data protection to facilitate trans-border flow of personal health information.


**Canadian Society of Telehealth (CST)**
(http://www.cst-sct.org/)

The Canadian Society of Telehealth (CST) is the first Canadian non-profit health association devoted to Telehealth. The organization promotes all aspects of telehealth, also termed e-Health, which is the use of information and communications technologies to deliver health care over large and small distances. The CST is proud to be the acknowledged Canadian leader in multi-disciplinary and inter-sectoral education and, discourse in telehealth. Launched in 1998, past CST conferences have attracted more than 350 delegates,

## North American Medical Informatics (NAMI) (Continued)

and the 5th conference, in Vancouver, October 3-5, 2002, promises to be even bigger!

The vision of CST is to be the nation's leader in the promotion of Telehealth and an advocate for its integration into the healthcare system to improve the health of all Canadians.

Our objectives are:

1. To serve as a forum for the collection, exchange and dissemination of information related to telehealth;
2. To work, cooperate, and liaise with other organizations, institutions, governments, governmental organizations, individuals, societies, and corporations involved or concerned with the development and implementation of telehealth activities, health care and health care services, and to encourage cooperation among them;
3. To assist in the education of individuals, organizations, corporations, and society with respect to telehealth;
4. To promote the advancement of telehealth opportunities and technologies, and their application for the benefit of Canadians and others;
5. To promote and encourage the use of telecommunications and related technologies in the delivery of health care and health education;
6. To promote the use of telehealth in order to improve the health care system, assist in the improvement of access to health care delivery, and to benefit the participants in the health care system;
7. To encourage telehealth research; and
8. To undertake such other activities as may be incidental and conducive to the foregoing objects and not inconsistent therewith.

Membership in the Canadian Society of Telehealth is open to individuals and organizations interested in telehealth. CST members come from a wide variety of backgrounds including clinical providers, program managers, healthcare researchers, students, institutional administrators, health informatics professionals, telehealth service consultants, government, and technology providers.

## Canadian Healthcare Information Technology Trade Association (CHITTA) (www.chitta.ca)

The Canadian Healthcare Information Technology Trade Association (CHITTA) is in the process of being formulated; it is anticipated that the organization will be fully functional by December 31, 2002. CHITTA is the first Trade Association in Canada specific to the broad spectrum of the industrial sector serving the healthcare and medical community in Canada.

### Mission

The mission of CHITTA is to strengthen the competitiveness of Canada's Healthcare Information and Communications Technology (ICT) industry through cooperative efforts among and between members and through direct contact with all levels of Government and associated agencies.

### Goals and Objectives

1. To increase market share for Canadian healthcare ICT companies both nationally and internationally.
2. To increase the size of the healthcare ICT market through promoting the Industry's value as an integral component of health systems to healthcare professionals, government, and the consumer of health services
3. To catalogue, monitor and report on the industry and the companies therein.
4. To establish an "image of excellence" and quality assurance in the industry through the promotion of standards and certification processes.
5. To facilitate collaboration among and between Canadian ICT companies, governments, healthcare delivery providers and scientific, research and educational institutions.
6. To present a unified industry voice and consultation vehicle for government, policy and investment decision makers.

### Membership

Membership is available to companies, partnerships, proprietorships, associations, and educational institutions that are engaged, in whole or in part, in the business of providing products and/or services to the Canadian Healthcare marketplace.

<table>
<tr><td valign="top">

*North American Medical Informatics (NAMI) (Continued)*

</td><td valign="top">

## Health Informatics Activities in the United States

### American Medical Informatics Association AMIA

The American Medical Informatics Association (AMIA) was formed in 1990 through a merger of three medical informatics organizations, the Symposium on Computer Applications in Medical Care (SCAMC), the American Association for Medical Systems and Informatics (AAMSI), and the American College of Medical Informatics (ACMI).

Today, AMIA has more than 3,500 members including individuals, institutions, and corporations. A Board of Directors that includes 16 elected and 2 ex-officio members govern it. The business of the Association is conducted through a division of responsibility among the Board, 14 standing and ad hoc committees, 18 Working Groups and Special Interest Groups, and a headquarters office with a staff of 12. AMIA holds two meetings per year – the Spring Congress in May, and the Annual Symposium in the autumn – publishes a scholarly journal and several electronic bulletins, engages in public policy initiatives both on its own and in collaboration with other organizations, and carries out a number of other programs.

### Highlights of 2002

#### *AMIA 2002 Annual Symposium*

AMIA hosted the 26th Anniversary meeting on medical informatics, having spent the first 14 of those years predating AMIA as the Symposium on Computer Applications in Medical Care (SCAMC). The AMIA 2002 Annual Symposium, with the theme, *Bio*medical Informatics: One Discipline*, took place November 9-13, 2002 in Washington. The Scientific Program Committee for this meeting was Isaac Kohane, MD, PhD of Boston Children's Hospital and Harvard University.

The AMIA Annual Symposium is renown for its high quality programming, but in 2002 the programming extended into many evolving sub-disciplines of informatics including bioinformatics. The goal, to bring together an international blend of individuals from the many sub-disciplines of informatics to find common bonds, share

</td><td valign="top">

tools and techniques, and confront the challenges of health care delivery together, became a reality with the successful attendance. Self-described informaticians are, and will continue to be, involved in endeavors as varied as medical records implementation, genomics, clinical decision support, image compression, and legal aspects of medical privacy. Nonetheless, a shared mandate argues powerfully for an inclusive discipline. All the sub-disciplines of informatics have as their shared goal the furthering of health care through the creation and use of biomedical knowledge. It was the hope and success of this meeting to engage those in different disciplines to identify strengths and systems from each other to grow stronger collaborative bonds.

Tutorials and presentations on subjects varying from evaluating, building and working with clinical information systems, to utilizing microarrays and SNP analysis for gene study were scheduled in the four main tracks of: Bioinformatics: Computation for the Genome Era, Clinical Informatics: Applications for Research and Clinical Care, Technology Transfer: Disseminating and Generalizing Innovation, and Education and Training: Creating and Enhancing Learning and Learning Environments.

There were many new program additions to the AMIA 2002 Annual Symposium. *Partnerships in Innovation* were designed specifically to illustrate cases of how industry and their clients can collaborate in research, development, and application for the purpose of solving problems in informatics or through the use of informatics. And the AMIA 2002 Scientific program committee developed many special presentations including a panel on *Careers in Medical Informatics*, an update on *Informatics Activities at the Federal Level*, and a presentation on *Federal Funding Opportunities for Informatics*.

#### *AMIA 2002 Spring Congress*

The AMIA 2002 Spring Congress was held in Scottsdale, Arizona on May 20-22, 2002. The theme for this meeting was, *A Drug By Any Other Name: The Role of Informatics From Drug Development Through The Point-Of-Care*. Daniel Z. Sands, MD, MPH, of Harvard University and Beth Israel Deaconess Medical Center was the Chair of the program committee. The National

</td></tr>
</table>

## North American Medical Informatics (NAMI) (Continued)

Library of Medicine made funding available for this meeting, but AMIA also received outstanding corporate support. In addition the Congress held the endorsements of several US pharmaceutical and drug associations, and brought together representatives from both the informatics community and the pharmaceutical/drug discovery community to discuss ways in which medical informatics can assist in the discovery, testing, regulations, prescribing, and administration of medications in the United States. The meeting involved four major tracks of discussion which included Clinical Trials in Drug Development, Vocabulary Building: Explaining Drugs to Computer, Behind the Scenes: From Clinic to Pharmacy, and Point-of-care Technology. The Scientific Program Committee, plenary speakers, track facilitators, and invited experts then took the information gathered to produce a series of recommendations on the role of informatics in pharmaceuticals for publication in AMIA's journal, JAMIA. The slide presentations that were presented at this meeting were also made available at the conclusion of the meeting on the AMIA Web site.

### JAMIA – the Journal of the American Medical Informatics Association

AMIA's scholarly journal continued to excel through its rigorous publishing schedule of 6 issues per year. During 2003, the formal transition of Dr. Randolph Miller as new editor of JAMIA took place. Dr. Miller is Professor and Chairman of the Department of Biomedical Informatics at Vanderbilt University. Dr. Miller has served as an Associate Editor of JAMIA since 1993. He is a past president of the association, and has served on many of the working groups and committees within the AMIA structure. In addition, he was on the Board of Directors for SCAMC, the Symposium on Computer Applications in Medical Care and was the Program Chair for SCAMC in 1990. Dr. Miller has served on many advisory boards and panels for other prestigious publications including Artificial Intelligence in Medicine, Methods of Information in Medicine, and Annals of Internal Medicine. He is currently the President-Elect of ACMI, the American College of Medical Informatics. He received his undergraduate education at Princeton. He did his medical education and residency at University of Pittsburgh, after which he worked at University of Pittsburgh from 1979-1994.

Elsevier purchased Hanley & Belfus, the Philadelphia-based medical publisher that has published JAMIA since its inception. In its capacity as a subsidiary, Hanley & Belfus continues to be the publisher of JAMIA.

In addition, past editions of JAMIA were made available to the general public on a six-month lag through PubMed Central in 2002.

### AMIA On-line – AMIA's Web Site and Other On-line Publications

AMIA continued to increase their on-line presence by affording the members the ability to fully experience their membership virtually. Members in 2002 were able to renew their membership on-line, purchase AMIA publications and other special discounted publications, search the AMIA member directory, download copies of programs for the 2002 meetings, search the on-line program for the AMIA Annual Symposium, receive JAMIA table of contents, read JAMIA on-line, and much more. In addition, the e-publications were refined to deliver members a bi-monthly newsletter of the trends in the industry with references to current news development articles in the areas of general informatics, public policy and legislation, bioterrorism, and research and grants.

### Task Forces – Exploring Leading Strategic Issues and Priorities

The AMIA Board of Directors approved the formation of five task forces and one exploratory initiative that each examined an area of strategic importance to AMIA and its future, and was designed to address either current activities, possible future activities, or important structural and program priorities. Building on the goals and objectives developed during the strategic planning process under immediate past-President Patricia Flatley Brennan, RN, PhD, the AMIA Board Executive Committee under new AMIA President William E. Hammond, PhD, met in early February of 2002 and identified the key areas for the new Task Forces. Each of the Task Forces was chaired by one of the members of the AMIA Board Executive Committee, and

<table>
<tr><td>

*North American Medical Informatics (NAMI)*
*(Continued)*

</td><td>

each was very successful in pursuing valuable initiatives throughout *2002*.

*Member Initiatives – Reflecting Trends in Medical Informatics*

The role of AMIA, as an association, as a conduit to developments in the field of medical informatics is nowhere so evident as in AMIA's Working Group structure. In 2002, AMIA added two Special Interest Groups in the areas of *Knowledge Discovery & Data Mining*, and *Mobile Computing*. In addition, the *Prevention and Public Health Special Interest Group* was elevated to an AMIA Working Group increasing the AMIA lists to 15 Working Groups and 5 Special Interest Groups. In 2002, many groups held programs at the AMIA Annual Symposium and carried out other activities throughout the year. As examples of some of the leading efforts of these groups, AMIA's Primary Care Working Group continued to spearhead a multi-organizational National Alliance for Primary Care Informatics, bringing together representatives from a variety of associations to set forth an agenda to develop a primary care infrastructure in the US with information technologies playing a central role. The Clinical Trials Working Group sponsored a special poster session showcasing some of the latest research gathered from on-going trials.

*Public Policy Initiatives*

For the past several years, AMIA has been closely involved in advocating for a measured approach to medical privacy that both protects citizens and provides opportunities for meaningful use of aggregate data by researchers and in applied settings. These efforts have taken on added significance as the US government has sought to deal with the electronic generation and flow of medical information through changes to the Health Insurance Portability and Accountability Act (HIPAA). Many of AMIA's efforts on medical privacy advocacy have been through its participation in the Coalition on Health Information Policy (CHIP), a four member collaborative.

*The AMIA Board*

The new AMIA President, W. Ed Hammond, PhD, took his position in January of 2002. His first initiatives included

</td><td>

the previously mentioned AMIA Task Forces, which included a special President's Commission on the Electronic Health Record, and the development of the 2002-2003 members of the AMIA committees.

**The Healthcare Information and Management Systems Society**

Founded in 1961, The Healthcare Information and Management Systems Society (HIMSS) is a non-for-profit professional membership association that provides leadership in healthcare for the management of technology, information, and change through member services, education and networking opportunities, and publications. Based in Chicago with an office in Ann Arbor, Mich, HIMSS has more than 13,000 individual members, and nearly 100 corporate members working in healthcare organizations throughout the world. Individual members include healthcare professionals in hospitals, corporate healthcare systems, clinical practice groups, HIT supplier organizations, healthcare consulting firms, and government settings in professional levels ranging from senior staff to CIOs and CEOs. HIMSS corporate members include leading software and hardware suppliers, consultants, executive recruiters, publishers, telecommunications firms, ehealth, and other key players in the industry. Together, HIMSS members are responsible for developing many of today's key innovations in healthcare delivery and administration, including clinical information systems, portable/wireless healthcare computing, and telemedicine. HIMSS' Web site is www.himss.org.

Highlights of 2002

The last half of year 2001 and the year 2002 so far has been an active period for HIMSS. The following are just some of the highlights of this period:

*2002 HIMSS Annual Conference and Exhibition*

The 2002 HIMSS Annual Conference and Exhibition, the Society's educational cornerstone, took place January 27-31 in Atlanta. Over 19,000 industry leaders attended the event, which included more than 600 vendors who showcased a wide variety of state-of-the-art healthcare information technology-related products and services.

</td></tr>
</table>

*North American Medical Informatics (NAMI) (Continued)*

Keynote speakers included former Department of Health and Human Services Secretary Donna Shalala, Former Vice-President Albert Gore, Jr., and Entertainer Ben Vereen. The Conference also featured 150-plus education sessions and interactive workshops on a variety of topics, all geared at intermediate and advanced level professionals, including management.

Among other highlights:

A US Department of Defense/Military Health System Demonstration area highlighting leading-edge military healthcare management and information systems technologies.

A Research, Development, and New Technology Center featuring the latest developments in future healthcare technology. Year three of the Integrating the Healthcare Enterprise (IHE) exhibit, which demonstrates how patient care workflow in radiology can be integrated from scheduling to reporting.

*Professional Services*

Recognizing the need to elevate the professional stature, recognition, and credibility of healthcare information management and systems professionals, HIMSS established a professional certification program. The Certified Professional in Healthcare Information and Management Systems (CPHIMS) designation can only be attained upon passage of a national exam that tests candidates on core competencies of the profession. In development, the Certified in Healthcare Security (CHS) designation focuses on healthcare security competencies and is part of a joint venture with the American Health Information Management Association (AHIMA), who is developing a companion certification of healthcare privacy professionals (CHP). A combined certification designation covering both privacy and security competencies (CHPS) will be available in early 2003.

HIMSS also increased efforts to promote the profession's voice in the public policy arena. The Society now has a significant say on healthcare-related regulatory issues and has broadened member awareness of issues that affect the industry. As part of the Coalition for Health Information Policy (CHIP), HIMSS has regularly supplied issue reports and communicated with policy-makers about HIPAA and other legislation.

*Professional Education*

The Society has provided expanded, timely education on a broader range of topics this year. A key part of that effort was programs offered through WebU – an online educational resource featuring interactive tutorials, lectures, resource guides, and quizzes. Courses are continually developed to keep users in step with the latest issues and core body of knowledge in the field. Topics include career development, clinical information systems, customer relations management, e-health, leadership, error reduction, and security and privacy.

Education opportunities have also been provided through audio conferences – on timely topics such as computerized physician order entry. Several high-level industry leaders who have first-hand knowledge of each topic teach each audio conference.

*Publications*

HIMSS released several new book titles in 2002, including two publications on topics of immense importance to the industry – The Wireless Web in Healthcare by Bryan Bergeron and The Impact of Information Technology on Patient Safety by Rusty Lewis.

In 2002, HIMSS also unveiled the redesigned *Journal of Healthcare Information Management* in time for the Society's Annual Conference. The goal behind the redesign was to enhance the content and physical appearance of the journal, as well as ensure that the journal remained comprehensive, timely, and inviting to readers. Topics featured in the quarterly Journal so far this year included patient safety, HIPAA, and E-health.

## North American Medical Informatics (NAMI) (Continued)

**Medical Records Institute and TEPR**

TEPR 2002 was held May 12-16, 2002 in Seattle, Washington. A faculty of 451 speakers addressed 3,361 attendees. Highlights were the documentation challenge, the awards in 13 categories of Health IT to system developers. The conference consisted of four parts, Health IT, Mobile Health, Security, and Measurable Benefits. The Mobile Healthcare Field is the most growing part. The Medical Records Institute will hold a dedicated Mobile Health Conference October 16-18, 2002 in Las Vegas, NV. See http://www.medrecinst. com/conferences/wireless/index.shtml.

This year the Medical Records Institute has conducted its Fourth Annual Survey of EHR Trends and Usage. A total of 1131 individuals responded to the survey. The Survey focuses on the experience and the attitudes of healthcare providers. After removing responses from payers, vendors and consultants, the total number of provider respondents was determined to be 761. The Survey includes responses from April 15th through May 16th, 2002.

*EHR TRENDS*

One of the interesting observations from this years Survey is that the data reveals that provider motivations to implement EHRs has shown a steady increase over the last four years. Question 6 from the Comprehensive Version of the EHR Survey shows these trends. (See the Table below)

**What are the major clinical factors that are driving the need for EHR Systems?** *(Respondents were asked to select all that apply.)*

| TRENDS | | | | |
|---|---|---|---|---|
| | **2002** | **2001** | **2000** | **1999** |
| Improve the ability to share patient record information among healthcare practitioners and professionals within the enterprise | 90.0% | 83.0% | 85.0% | 73.0% |
| Improve quality of care | 85.3% | 83.0% | 80.0% | 72.0% |
| Improve clinical processes or workflow efficiency | 83.6% | 83.0% | 81.0% | 67.0% |
| Improve clinical data capture | 82.4% | 78.0% | 68.0% | 61.0% |
| Reduce medical errors (improve patient safety) | 81.7% | n/a | n/a | n/a |
| Provide access to patient records at remote locations | 70.7% | 73.0% | 71.0% | 59.0% |
| Facilitate clinical decision support | 70.0% | 69.0% | 66.0% | 58.0% |
| Improve employee/physician satisfaction | 63.0% | n/a | n/a | n/a |
| Improve patient satisfaction | 60.4% | 59.0% | 54.0% | 40.0% |
| Improve efficiency via pre-visit health assessments and post-visit patient education | 40.2% | 38.0% | 36.0% | n/a |
| Support and integrate patient healthcare information from Web-based personal health records | 30.4% | 28.0% | 29.0% | n/a |
| Retain health plan membership | 9.3% | 9.0% | 7.0% | n/a |
| OTHER | 0.3% | 4.0% | 1.0% | 3.0% |
| Responses to this Questions | 729 | 293 | 296 | 358 |

## North American Medical Informatics (NAMI) (Continued)

EHR COMPONENTS AND FUNCTIONS

The MRI Survey of EHR Trends and Usage recognizes the reality that there is no consensus in the industry regarding the definition of an EHR or which components or functions make up an EHR. The Survey addresses this problem by collecting data on all nine components/functions that broad definitions of an EHR have included.

The nine components/functions include:

- Clinical Workstations
- Clinical Data Repositories
- Medical Record Document Imaging Systems
- Master Patient Index for a Single System or Site of Care
- Master Person Index or Enterprise Directory to Support Multiple Facilities
- Integration/Interface Engines
- Networks
- Data Warehouses
- Web-based Personal Health Records

The Survey continues to delineate specific functions or capabilities within each of these nine areas to reveal a comprehensive picture of the status of EHR implementations and near-term plans.

The nine tables that follow come from Question 7 of the Overview Version of the Fourth Annual Survey of EHR Trends and Usage.

**What functions or components of an EHR system do you have in use or planned for implementation?** *(Respondents were asked to select all that apply.)*

Preface:

- The total number of respondents to the eleven sections within Question 7 is 717.
- The first row of results for each subsection is expressed as percentages of 717.
- The second row of results for each subsection is expressed as a percentage of the number of respondents that answered that subsection.

| | Number of Respondents | In Use Today | 1 Year | 2 Years | 3 Years | 4 or More Years |
|---|---|---|---|---|---|---|
| **7-1. Clinical Workstations that support:** | | | | | | |
| Nurse or Staff Order Entry | 717 | 25.0% | 14.1% | 6.7% | 2.1% | 1.0% |
| [Based on all respondents selecting clinical workstations] | 512 | 35.0% | 19.7% | 9.4% | 2.9% | 1.4% |
| Physician Order Entry without clinical decision support | 717 | 10.7% | 9.2% | 5.7% | 2.2% | 1.1% |
| [Based on all respondents selecting clinical workstations] | 512 | 15.0% | 12.9% | 8.0% | 3.1% | 1.6% |
| Physician Order Entry with clinical decision support | 717 | 7.4% | 13.2% | 12.1% | 4.6% | 2.9% |
| [Based on all respondents selecting clinical workstations] | 512 | 10.4% | 18.6% | 17.0% | 6.4% | 4.1% |
| Results Reporting | 717 | 32.1% | 8.1% | 5.2% | 1.7% | 1.0% |
| [Based on all respondents selecting clinical workstations] | 512 | 44.9% | 11.3% | 7.2% | 2.3% | 1.4% |

<table>
<tr><td>

*North American Medical Informatics (NAMI) (Continued)*

</td><td>

**What functions or components of an EHR system do you have in use or planned for implementation?** *(Respondents were* *asked to select all that apply.)*

Note: The total number of respondents to the eleven sections within Question 7 was 717.

</td></tr>
</table>

| | Number of Respondents | In Use Today | 1 Year | 2 Years | 3 Years | 4 or More Years |
|---|---|---|---|---|---|---|
| **7-2. Clinical Data Repositories that support:** | | | | | | |
| Storage of EHR data, text and reimbursement codes (ICD and CPT codes) | 717 | 21.6% | 9.8% | 6.3% | 1.5% | 1.5% |
| [Based on all respondents selecting clinical data repositories] | 436 | 35.6% | 16.1% | 10.3% | 2.5% | 2.5% |
| Also storage of clinical codes (LOINC, MEDCIN, SNOMED, etc.) | 717 | 10.9% | 7.4% | 4.6% | 1.4% | 2.8% |
| [Based on all respondents selecting clinical data repositories] | 436 | 17.9% | 12.2% | 7.6% | 2.3% | 4.6% |
| If you plan to use SNOMED as a structured terminology, do you expect to use it for: | | | | | | |
| Problem lists | 717 | 0.8% | 3.2% | 2.9% | 1.3% | 0.4% |
| [Based on all respondents selecting clinical data repositories] | 436 | 1.4% | 5.3% | 4.8% | 2.1% | 0.7% |
| Lab results | 717 | 3.1% | 2.2% | 1.8% | 0.6% | 0.3% |
| [Based on all respondents selecting clinical data repositories] | 436 | 5.0% | 3.7% | 3.0% | 0.9% | 0.5% |
| Radiology results | 717 | 1.4% | 1.3% | 2.1% | 0.4% | 0.4% |
| [Based on all respondents selecting clinical data repositories] | 436 | 2.3% | 2.1% | 3.4% | 0.7% | 0.7% |
| Other uses for SNOMED | 717 | 0.3% | 1.3% | 0.8% | 0.1% | 0.1% |
| [Based on all respondents selecting clinical data repositories] | 436 | 0.5% | 2.1% | 1.4% | 0.2% | 0.2% |
| Also storage of voice or sound | 717 | 2.8% | 3.2% | 3.2% | 1.8% | 2.5% |
| [Based on all respondents selecting clinical data repositories] | 436 | 4.6% | 5.3% | 5.3% | 3.0% | 4.1% |
| Also storage of clinical images | 717 | 9.9% | 7.8% | 7.0% | 2.5% | 2.8% |
| [Based on all respondents selecting clinical data repositories] | 436 | 16.3% | 12.8% | 11.5% | 4.1% | 4.6% |
| | | | | | | |
| ***7-3. Medical Record Document Imaging Systems*** | | | | | | |
| Interim to a clinical data repository | 717 | 4.5% | 3.6% | 2.0% | 0.6% | 0.6% |
| [Based on all respondents selecting Medical Record Document Imaging)] | 358 | 8.9% | 7.3% | 3.9% | 1.1% | 1.1% |
| Supplemental to a clinical data repository | 717 | 8.8% | 6.3% | 3.5% | 1.1% | 0.3% |
| [Based on all respondents selecting Medical Record Document Imaging)] | 358 | 17.6% | 12.6% | 7.0% | 2.2% | 0.6% |
| | | | | | | |
| **7-4. Master Patient Index for a single system or site of care** | 717 | 22.7% | 4.6% | 1.5% | 0.8% | 0.8% |
| [Based on all respondents selecting Master Patient Index] | 209 | 74.4% | 15.1% | 5.0% | 2.7% | 2.7% |
| | | | | | | |
| **7-5. Master Person Index or Enterprise Directory to support multiple facilities** | 717 | 9.8% | 2.8% | 2.0% | 0.3% | 0.0% |
| [Based on all respondents selecting Master Person Index] | 106 | 66.0% | 18.9% | 13.2% | 1.9% | 0.0% |

| | Number of Respondents | In Use Today | 1 Year | 2 Years | 3 Years | 4 or More Years |
|---|---|---|---|---|---|---|
| **7-6. Integration/Interface Engine to connect the Data Repository to Clinical Workstations and departmental systems** | 717 | 22.2% | 6.0% | 2.0% | 0.7% | 0.4% |
| [Based on all respondents selecting Integration/Interface Engines] | 168 | 65.5% | 22.6% | 7.7% | 2.4% | 1.8% |
| [Based on hospital respondents selecting Integration/Interface Engines] | 114 | 75.4% | 15.8% | 5.3% | 1.8% | 1.8% |
| | | | | | | |
| **7-7. Network connecting the Data Repository to Clinical Workstations and departmental systems** | 717 | 20.9% | 7.0% | 3.3% | 1.8% | 1.3% |
| [Based on all respondents selecting networks] | 246 | 61.0% | 20.3% | 9.8% | 5.3% | 3.7% |

## North American Medical Informatics (NAMI) (Continued)

| | | | | | |
|---|---|---|---|---|---|
| **7-8. A Data Warehouse or secondary database of patient information to support retrospective analysis of outcomes, utilization, and clinical processes** | 717 | 6.4% | 3.8% | 2.1% | 1.5% | 1.0% |
| [Based on all respondents selecting Data Warehouse or secondary database] | 106 | 43.4% | 25.5% | 14.2% | 10.4% | 6.6% |

| | | | | | |
|---|---|---|---|---|---|
| **7-9. Web-based Personal Health Records** | 717 | 2.5% | 2.4% | 1.0% | 0.8% | 0.7% |
| [Based on all respondents selecting Web-based Personal Health Records] | 53 | 34.0% | 32.1% | 13.2% | 11.3% | 9.4% |

| | | |
|---|---|---|
| **7-10. Other** | 717 | 3.50% |

| | | |
|---|---|---|
| **7-11. We do not have any components installed, and do not have time frame for implementation** | 717 | 11.70% |

## DATA SECURITY GUIDELINES, STANDARDS, AND FEATURES

The MRI Survey of EHR Trends and Usage also reveals the status of provider data security implementations and plans. The following data is excepted from Question 16 of the Overview Version of the EHR Survey.

**What is the status of the data security guidelines, standards, or features within your organization?** *(Respondents were asked to select all that apply.)*

<u>Preface:</u> The total number of respondents for Question 16 is 550.

| Security Guidelines, Standards or Features | Percentage of Respondents Selecting this Option | In Use Today | 1 Year | 2 Years | 3 Years | 4 or more Years |
|---|---|---|---|---|---|
| **Access Controls** | | | | | | |
| Passwords | 95.1% | 90.4% | 2.9% | 0.7% | 0.0% | 1.1% |
| User access by role/class/location | 87.5% | 77.3% | 6.5% | 1.8% | 0.7% | 1.1% |

| Security Guidelines, Standards or Features | Percentage of Respondents Selecting this Option | In Use Today | 1 Year | 2 Years | 3 Years | 4 or more Years |
|---|---|---|---|---|---|
| **Authentication of users** | | | | | | |
| Electronic signatures | 62.2% | 34.2% | 15.6% | 8.0% | 2.7% | 1.6% |
| Digital certificates | 32.9% | 10.0% | 10.5% | 6.5% | 3.5% | 2.4% |
| Biometric Technologies | 32.0% | 2.4% | 10.2% | 10.0% | 3.5% | 6.0% |
| | | | | | | |
| **Protection of data over networks** | | | | | | |
| Virus detection | 90.7% | 87.5% | 2.0% | 0.5% | 0.0% | 0.7% |
| Firewalls | 86.4% | 82.7% | 2.2% | 0.7% | 0.2% | 0.5% |
| Data Encryption | 68.0% | 53.6% | 8.9% | 3.8% | 0.9% | 0.7% |
| | | | | | | |
| **Protection of data within the enterprise** | | | | | | |
| Policies and practices | 83.1% | 76.2% | 4.9% | 1.3% | 0.4% | 0.4% |
| Backup and recovery procedures | 86.4% | 82.7% | 2.5% | 0.2% | 0.0% | 0.9% |
| Audit logs | 74.0% | 60.9% | 9.5% | 2.4% | 0.7% | 0.5% |
| | | | | | | |
| **Other data security policies, practices, or techniques** | 4.4% | 2.0% | 0.9% | 1.1% | 0.2% | 0.2% |

The Overview Version of the MRI Survey of EHR Trends and Usage is available for review or download on the MRI Website (<u>www.medrecinst.com</u>).

# Department of Medical Informatics
## University of Heidelberg

### Research

*Information infrastructures for health care* are investigated with special emphasis on fully electronic medical records, authentication and digital signature, records shared among institutions and professions.

*Medical documentation* research concentrates on registries, quality assurance of records, ontology-based electronic data capture (EDC) for multi-center clinical trials, and usage of speech recognition for note taking.

*Knowledge based decision support* spans from basic decision theoretic investigation to implementing guidelines in clinical pathways.

Projects are normally run in close cooperation with clinical partners. In several cases they include health technology assessment activities. The conjoint Department of Medical Biometry becomes involved whenever experimental investigations of new methods are aimed at.

### Education

Education covers the full from graduate, post-graduate and Ph.D. academic curricula to vocational classes for radiology and laboratory assistants. In cooperation with the University of Applied Sciences Heilbronn, the department is responsible for the only German Master's (Diploma) program in Medical Informatics and a post-graduate program for physicians on Information Management in Medicine. The Akademie Medizinische Informatik (akadeMIe) offers several courses for IT career development in the health care sector. Online courses have just been started.

### Professional organizations and international contacts

International education and career development is supported through a cooperation with other leading curricula in Amsterdam, NL, Minneapolis, MN, and Salt Lake City, UT which constitute the IΦE (International Partnership in Health Informatics Education). Besides serving in several national organizations such as GMDS (German Society for Medical Informatics, Biometry and Epidemiology) or GI (Association for Informatics), the department is involved in editing the Methods of Information in Medicine and the IMIA Yearbook of Medical Informatics.

*Contact*: Thomas Wetter, University of Heidelberg, Department of Medical Informatics, Im Neuenheimer Feld 400, D-69120 Heidelberg, Germany, Thomas_Wetter@med.uni-heidelberg.de

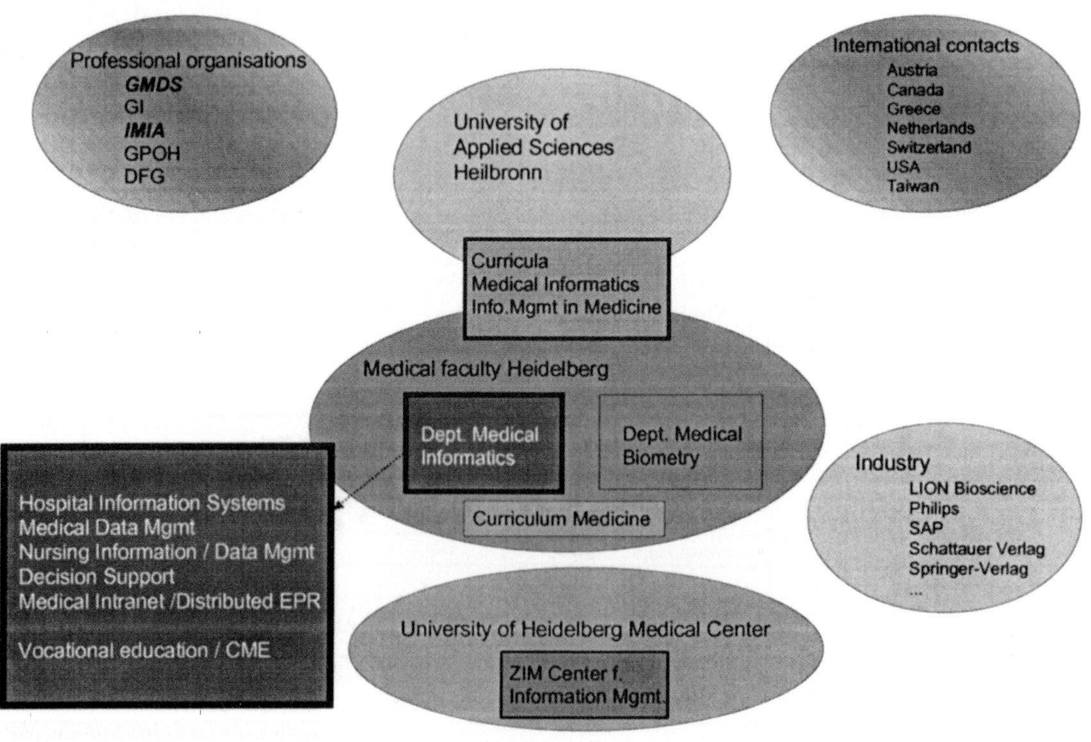

# *In Memoriam Professor Jean-Raoul Scherrer*

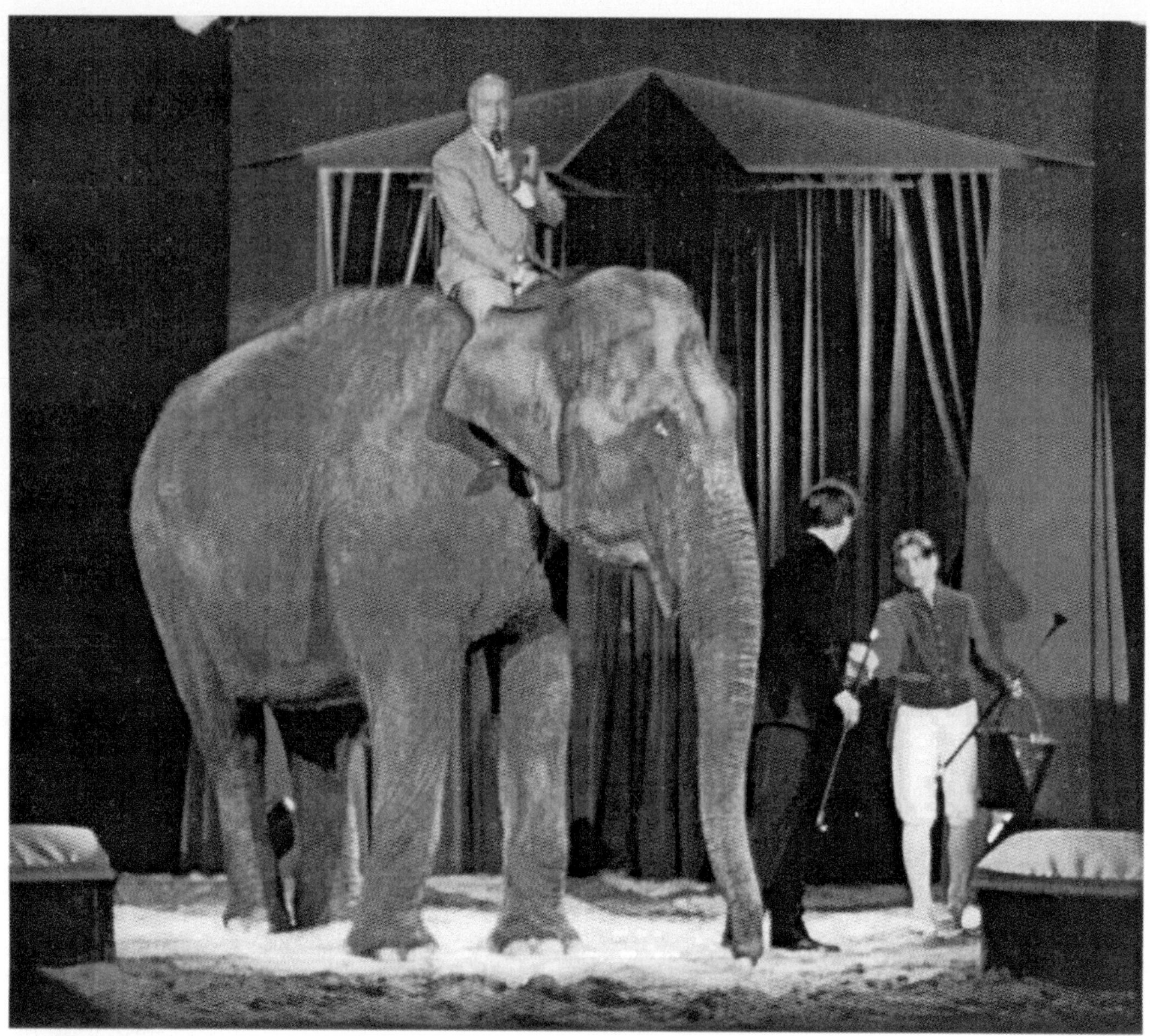

Jean-Raoul Scherrer at Medinfo 1992 in Geneva

**K.C. Lun**

IMIA President

# In Memoriam

## *Jean-Raoul Scherrer – intellectual, renaissance man and dear IMIA colleague*

On 19 March 2002, the international medical informatics community was deeply saddened by the passing of a warm and well-loved colleague, Professor Jean-Raoul Scherrer of Geneva, Switzerland, after a short illness.

I had the privilege of having JRS as a close friend since 1989 when he participated in MEDINFO '89 Part II in Singapore. Immediately we struck up a warm friendship that lasted until his untimely departure.

Jean-Raoul's contributions to the International Medical Informatics Association (IMIA) were outstanding. He was one of the early pioneers involved in growing the international organization from an IFIP Technical Committee (TC4) in 1979. For many years, he represented the Swiss Medical Informatics Association and the European Federation of Medical Informatics at IMIA meetings, including his term as EFMI President. He also served as IMIA representative to IFIP and WHO general assemblies. JRS also left a lasting impact on his contributions to IMIA, having served as the Chair of the Organizing Committee for MEDINFO 92 in Geneva as well as VP for Working Groups and SIGs. Everyone who was at the circus treat during MEDINFO 92 would have fondly remembered JRS making a grand entrance atop an elephant!

To many of us who knew him within IMIA, JRS was more than just an IMIA colleague. He was a renaissance man, equally comfortable in talking about issues in the sciences, arts and humanities, politics and music. He was a wine connoisseur and I learnt a great deal about the subject during a dinner conversation I had in his Geneva home together with his dear wife, Monique. JRS had widely-read and widely-travelled. When we were together at MEDINFO 98 in Seoul, he stumped me with the revelation that the Great Wall of China actually terminated in Korea!

JRS was always caring for his family and friends, generous with his advice and help, and unselfish in the sharing of his vast knowledge. Everyone in IMIA who knew him felt a deep sense of loss of a caring friend and a loyal colleague. We were deeply saddened by his loss and will always cherish the wonderful times we had together with him.

**Assa Reichert**

EFMI President

# In Memoriam

## *Prof. Jean-Raoul Scherrer, a professional leader*

On the 11th of March the EFMI council, in its Spring meeting held in Cyprus, unanimously resolved that the former EFMI president, a scientist and one of the leading pioneers in global medical informatics – Prof. J. R. Scherrer would be nominated as an Honorary Fellow of EFMI.

It was thus easy to understand the great surprise and deep shock of the EFMI family, when 8 days later the sad news of his untimely passing away was announced. He was, to his last days, a scientist who continue to be so involved, so active, so full of future plans, and above all: so energetic that this sad news to all of his acquaintances was shared with many other colleagues, all over the world, who did not know him personally, but knew his unusually remarkable achievements in the field of health informatics.

With the death of Prof. Scherrer, one remembers moments shared together with happiness, and the sorrow that they will never be repeated. Many remember his special sense of humour, his warm smile and the special way he phrased his ideas.

His vast knowledge in fields unrelated to his profession was always impressive and astonishing to his friends and colleagues. I can recall a conversation during his visit to the Holy Land in the early 90's, when he asked some questions concerning the birthplace of Christianity and the life of Jesus. Questions that of course nobody could reply; he then presented, with that famous smile on his face, a wealth of historical facts demonstrating his vast knowledge of ancient history.

We were always astonished of his ability to go on with his scientific work, even when, in the winter of 1990, a cruel fate took away two of his sons in a terrible avalanche in the Himalayan mountains. It seems that he did not allow this terrible tragedy to interfere with his work. His friends in the EFMI council met with him that year in the MIE-1990 in Glasgow where he received our condolences with a strong handshake and a modest smile.

During the MEDINFO held in Washington, we attended a lecture on an innovative HIS initiated in the Cantonal hospital in Geneva. Already then, in the summer of 1986, the room was completely full, due to the interest aroused by this innovative System. Prof. Scherrer came up to the podium and gave an outstanding presentation, of what was later known as the famous DIOGENE System that paved the way to many future Hospital Information Systems to come.

As a scientist, Prof. Scherrer's name appears on 119 published articles, covering his professional activities from 1965 till last year. His unusual organizational abilities were very well demonstrated when he chaired the MEDINFO 1992, and his special sense of humor was demonstrated when he entered the arena at that MEDINFO 1992 riding on an elephant.

The world of health informatics saluted Prof. J.R.S. in November 2000 by awarding him the highest distinction in the domain of medical informatics, the Morris F. Collen AWARD.

With his death the world lost that Scientist – a man small in physical height but a giant in charisma, leadership and professional pioneering, who led the way to many colleagues and friends..

The untimely death of J.R.S. is a loss, not only to his family, but also to the entire EFMI and IMIA community, and his colleagues and friends in all continents.

Sometimes, we need a light to guide us in a given direction; once this light is seen we can then head in that direction and keep on going even if the light goes out.

That light for many of us was Jean Raoul Scherrer. He was the lighthouse showing the way that can now be followed by his successors. They will wisely use the light emitted from his scientific inheritance and follow the footsteps of this great man.

**Jan H. van Bemmel**

Institute of Medical Informatics,
Erasmus University Medical Center,
Rotterdam, The Netherlands

# In Memoriam

# *Medical Information Systems in the Age of Jean-Raoul Scherrer* [1]

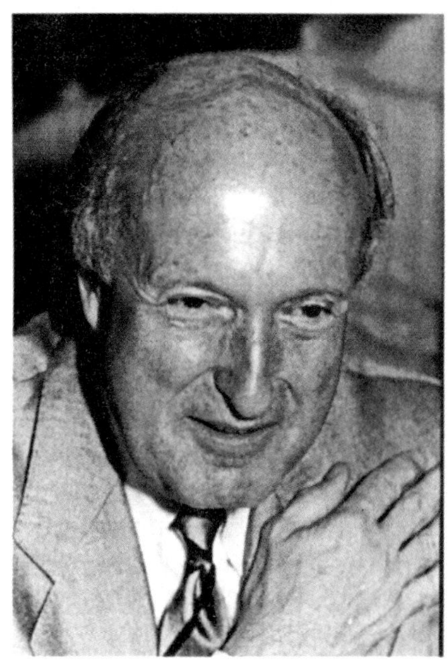

Jean-Raoul Scherrer
(photograph by Anne Angelillo-Scherrer)

## Introduction

It was less than four years ago, on September 29th 1998, that I presented a lecture on the occasion of the retirement of our dear friend Jean-Raoul Scherrer (1932-2002) during his Farewell Symposium in Geneva. But was it really a retirement? After his 'official abdication' he remained as busy as ever in his exploration of new frontiers, stimulating others about his plans, and searching for resources to realize his ideas. During his many active years, chairing Medical Informatics in Geneva, Jean-Raoul could be compared with an explosive container, full of innovative ideas. Who has not seen him defending his case, supporting his words with his characteristic gesticulations? We met on numerous occasions all over the world, but perhaps most often in Geneva. The last time I went to this beautiful city with its famous *'jet d'eau'*, was on March 25th 2002 – only a few months ago – to pay tribute to Jean-Raoul at what was the final farewell, in the small church of Vésenaz, where Jean-Raoul lived, close to Geneva. For all these reasons, this contribution will be a personal impression of some aspects of the professional life of and my friendship with Jean-Raoul Scherrer.

Many of his colleagues will remember the way to Jean-Raoul's office. Very appropriately, it was not too far from the *Boulevard des Philosophes,* the area where Jean-Raoul carried out his many projects. With his 70 years of age, professor Scherrer had lived a very fruitful life. He was a man gifted not only with a clear mind, but also with a warm heart; not only a professional in the discipline in which he matured over the years, Medical Informatics, but also in many other areas of life, such as art and history, philosophy and religion, good food and wine tasting. During our many personal meetings, it was a great pleasure to talk together and discuss the future of our profession, as well as exchanging personal opinions and views, generally ending in a conversation about life itself. Both of us are admirers of the great French philosopher, physicist and mathematician Blaise Pascal. Thus it was not a coincidence that on the announcement that informed us of Jean-Raoul's unexpected death, a part was cited from the *Mémorial* of Pascal: *Dieu d'Abraham, Dieu d'Isaac, Dieu de Jacob, non des philosophes et des savants. Certitude. Certitude. Sentiment. Joie. Paix* [2]. Such words were characteristic of the sensitive, but at the same time razor-sharp thinker Pascal, but no less so of Jean-Raoul.

---

[1]  Based on a keynote lecture, presented on August 25th 2002 at the conference MIE 2002 in Budapest, organized by the European Federation of Medical Informatics.

[2]  It translates as: *God of Abraham, God of Isaac, God of Jacob, not of philosophers and scientists. Certainty. Certainty. Emotion. Joy. Peace.*

In this contribution I do not intend to offer a scientific, let alone complete review of Jean-Raoul's professional accomplishments – a book would then be more appropriate. Besides, his closest colleagues and collaborators in Geneva have already written a concise review, entitled: *A Humanist's Legacy in Medical Informatics: Visions and Accomplishments of Professor Jean-Raoul Scherrer*, that recently appeared in Methods of Information in Medicine [1]. Here, I would like to describe some aspects of Jean-Raoul as a Prize Winner, an Explorer, a Diogenist, a Decision Supporter, a Scientist, an Image Processor, a Bio-informatician, an HONest Person, and a Networker.

## The Prize Winner

When can a person be called a prize winner? When speaking to young researchers I sometimes compare the way we conduct our research with the Olympic games. All participants are equals, and often are even close friends, but only very few win the gold, silver and bronze medals. Science, too, is full of competition. Jean-Raoul, himself a sportsman, knew how to exercise and to prepare himself for the competition. In many cases he won. He received, for instance, many substantial grants from both the Swiss government and the State of Geneva. In addition, he was extremely successful in obtaining substantial support from the European Union, although the final bill was most often presented to the Swiss government. The last project that was granted to him was the WRAPIN project (*World –Wide Reliable online Advice to Patients and Individuals*), in June 2001.

One of the medals awarded to him was the *Morris Collen Award of Excellence*, bestowed on him in 2000 by the American Medical Informatics Association. The medal was given to him for the many accomplishments that he realized in his professional life, a few of which I will mention in this contribution.

## The Explorer

Jean-Raoul was continuously exploring the new frontiers of our profession. Because he often had to travel considerable distances, he combined professional activities with other types of enterprises, such as visiting cultural events or exploring nature. For instance in 1995, right after MEDINFO 95 in Vancouver, we made an expedition together to the island of San Juan where, under the supervision of my colleague Astrid van Ginneken, we studied the Orcas, also called killer whales. Astrid is the brain behind the ORCA (Open Record for CAre) system for computer-based patient records [2] that was developed by our team. Jean-Raoul was part of the group that visited the killer whale research station on San Juan Island (where Astrid is the co-principal investigator), in between Vancouver Island and the coast of British Columbia. He enjoyed it tremendously.

In all our professional projects, international collaboration is essential in order to remain at the forefront of R&D. Many of Jean-Raoul's projects dealt with international projects in the area of medical communication and information. Particularly successful were the European projects SYNAPSES and SYNEX, in which he played a key role. The SYNAPSES project was based on middleware, a concept that was strongly promoted by Jean-Raoul, because he and many others realized that the existing heterogeneous legacy information systems could never be integrated into a functional network until the software became available to interconnect those systems [3]. The subsequent SYNEX project was in a way a continuation of the SYNAPSES project, because also the European Commission realized that to have proper competition between the scattered European health-care industry it was necessary to offer a system concept that would enable exchange of patient data between systems from different companies. Therefore, in SYNEX (that was started in 1999) different R&D centers, such as the one in Geneva and our own in Rotterdam, collaborated with several European industrial partners. Projects such as SYNAPSES and SYNEX highlighted the complexity of the health-care domain, especially if one intends to introduce one overall model for the support of patient care.

Over the past many, say, 30 years, Medical Informatics has been both a function of developments in technology and challenges in medicine and health care. Our profession has responded to new challenges and opportunities in both domains. In technology, for instance, we have seen – after the wave of the large mainframes – the advent of minicomputers, workstations, personal computers, large storage capacity and networking, 'intelligence' built into medical equipment and instrumentation, the Internet, the explosion of filmless Radiology, and fully automated laboratories – to mention only a few. These developments are also reflected in the evolution of the information systems in Geneva.

The current key challenges in health care to which our profession has to respond are, for instance: the increase in diseases and new infections; cancer and cardiovascular diseases that are still the main causes of mortality; the growing insight in genetic causes of diseases and the related early prediction of diseases. We can also mention that health-care costs are an ongoing source of concern in all countries (partly due to the growing population of elderly persons), that patient associations and professional health-care organizations are demanding continuous assessment of the quality of care, and that there is a shift towards ambulatory and primary care. Thus on all levels of health care there is a need for better accessibility to data and knowledge. Health care is considered to be too scattered and patients want to be more involved in their own care and bear greater responsibility. There is no medical informatics department that does not respond to changes such as these. This was and is also true for the center that Jean-Raoul has built in Geneva. I would like to review some of these developments.

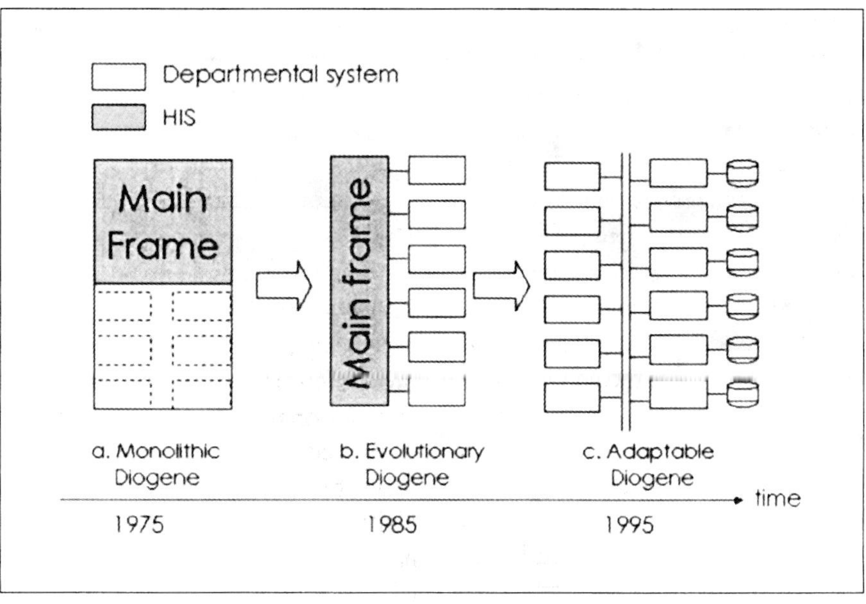


Fig. 1. Evolution of the Diogene hospital information system, as it has been developed in Geneva under the supervision of Jean-Raoul Scherrer.

## The Diogenist

Amongst all his other achievements, the accomplishment by which Jean-Raoul is perhaps best known is the DIOGENE system [4, 5](see Fig. 1). This is the reason why I would like to characterize him as a '*Diogenist*'.

Starting in 1971, the Geneva University Hospital offered Jean-Raoul the opportunity to begin the development of a hospital information system that became known as the DIOGENE system. Over the years it underwent several changes, mainly due to the developments sketched above. During the ensuing 30 years, Jean-Raoul enjoyed being in the driver's seat of the development of DIOGENE.

Summarized below is a list of requirements, compiled by Shortell, that a well-organized information system should fulfill [6]. It is an interesting exercise to verify whether the information systems in one's own environment meet the requirements of Shortell:

· Does the system meet the health needs of the population?

· Does the service capacity it offers match the needs of health care?
· Does it provide coordination across the continuum of health care?
· When in use, does it provide information on cost, quality, and other parameters?
· Have financial considerations been used as incentives; and does the system align to the needs of the users?
· Does the system allow for the improvement of health care on a continuous basis?
· Does the system stimulate collaboration with other parties to satisfy all objectives?
· Does the information system interlink patients and providers across the continuum of health care?

I guess that the DIOGENE system met most, if not all of these conditions; but we will take a closer look at the DIOGENE system as it has evolved over the years. Many hospitals in Western countries use hospital information systems (HISs) to support patient registration, administration, billing, and internal communication. Some hospitals may sometimes have installed a very extensive HIS, as well as a wide variety of other information systems, such as for the clinical laboratory, the hospital pharmacy, radiology, intensive care, and so on. This is also the case in Geneva.

The first generation of DIOGENE, long before the advent of the first personal computer, was built on a mainframe (Fig. 1a), as was the case in most other centers in the world at that time. Its goal was to support care by providing access to the system from over 100 nursing stations. A special characteristic of DIOGENE was the assistance provided by an intermediate person between the system and the nurse. The nurse on the ward spoke by telephone to an intermediate person (also a trained nurse) instead of typing the data herself on a keyboard, but also had immediate visual feedback, originally via a video connection to the system. This first generation system could be characterized as a 'monolithic' approach, because of its centralized system architecture.

The next generation of DIOGENE was built at the end of the 1980s, still around a mainframe, now under UNIX, but integrated with PCs and work-stations [7] (Fig. 1b). It is an example of a gradual evolution towards an integrated network of separate computers, each with its own task but interconnected in an overall system's approach. The last and present generation consists of a true network of workstations and PCs, without a mainframe computer (Fig. 1c). This development started around 1995 and allows for a continuous adaptation to new requirements.

The development of the HIS in Geneva, under the directorship of Jean-Raoul Scherrer, is a beautiful example of an ideal situation. It was only achievable because of the vision and driving force of a director that was trusted by the Hospital Board and who was able to obtain ample resources to realize his ideas. That scenario is probably very scarce in the world, but one now sees that in-house built systems are rapidly being replaced by industrial solutions. The latter, however, lack the versatility and adaptability of a system that has been developed by one's own team.

## The Decision Supporter

My next characterization of Jean-Raoul is one as a 'decision supporter'. Research in the field of decision support takes place in many medical informatics research centers all over the world. In Geneva it was mainly focused on natural language understanding [8], which was seen as the key to understand and interpret the huge amount of data contained in patient records. However, although Jean-Raoul and his team paid much attention to this line of research, it was in my opinion never at the top of their interest. Yet, because our own team in Rotterdam has put an enormous amount of effort in this domain, and in order to present a balanced overview of the main

research areas in our field, I would like to make a few comments on medical decision-support systems from outside the Geneva setting.

The main reasons for offering medical decision support by computer are the following:

· People sometimes make errors or mistakes (e.g., in routine cases as well as in complex cases);
· Clinicians cannot keep up with the ever-increasing medical knowledge;
· It may be more efficient to automate decision making when dealing with large numbers of routine decisions (e.g., when many standard laboratory tests must be assessed or when many ECGs must be interpreted);
· Health-care organizations may mandate the use of certain clinical practices both to improve the quality of care and to lower the cost of care.

In health care, in contrast to areas governed by strict rules, specific issues may hamper computer-supported decision making:

· Medical knowledge is ever expanding, but is limited in the human brain;
· Patient data are sometimes only partly available;
· The problem of a specific patient may be new and unique.

Computers require a structured approach to problem solving; this holds for both data and knowledge. In teaching computers to assist in solving a decision problem, it is important to collect enough and reliable patient observations and knowledge. With the help of those data and based on such knowledge, a decision model may be "trained" to arrive at the best decisions. Once the decision model has been trained, it should be tested by a sufficiently large and representative test set of patient data. Only when the results of this assessment are accepta-

ble, a computer may be used to assist in clinical decision making in real practice. Let me give an example from our own research that was based on formalized knowledge, also known as medical evidence.

We investigated in several projects whether computer-based patient records contain sufficient data to generate critiques and to support decision making. I will mention one system only, because it has drawn much attention in the clinical literature. In this system we use patient data from the computer-based patient records in primary care as input to a system that intends to change blood test-ordering behavior of physicians. The effects of two different approaches for changing blood test-ordering behavior were assessed for a group of Dutch general practitioners. These two approaches were each incorporated in a decision-support system and integrated with the CPR systems, operational in Dutch General Practice.

The two different versions of the decision-support system for blood test ordering, called *BloodLink*, were assessed in a large clinical trial [9]. The two decision-support systems consisted of (1) a version with a reduced number of tests, called *BloodLink-Restricted*, and (2) a version based on guidelines of the Dutch College of General Practitioners, called *BloodLink-Guideline*. A total of 44 primary care practices, including 60 general practitioners, were randomly assigned to either *BloodLink-Restricted* or *BloodLink-Guideline*. We monitored the use of *BloodLink* in primary care for one full year and compared the blood test orders with all received requests for blood tests in the laboratory.

The clinical trial revealed that general practitioners who had access to *BloodLink-Guideline* ordered on average significantly fewer tests than those using *BloodLink-Restricted* (5.5 tests versus 6.9 tests, respectively). Both the *BloodLink-Restricted* and *BloodLink-Guideline* intervention group showed a significant decrease in the average number of tests ordered per form, when comparing the intervention period with the two years preceding the intervention: 7.7 versus 6.8, respectively. Our conclusion is that both *BloodLink-Restricted* and *BloodLink-Guideline* are able to change test-ordering behavior. We also observed that the use of *BloodLink-Guideline* shows a greater reduction in ordered tests per order form than *BloodLink-Restricted* (5.5 tests versus 6.9 tests per form). We concluded, therefore, that decision-support systems could be effective for introducing guidelines into clinical practice.

In Geneva, a different line was taken in decision-support research. Attempts to represent knowledge were carried out by participating in the GALEN project [10]. Besides paying attention to natural language processing, the Geneva team also developed the ARCHIMED system [11], primarily a data warehouse of patient data, to be used for quality assessment, economic studies in health care, data mining, and knowledge acquisition.

## The Scientist

As remarked above, Jean-Raoul loved to participate in philosophical discussions, including deliberations on the scientific basis of our profession. He was invited a few times to participate in a PhD defense at our university; he loved the scientific debate and Jean-Raoul could from time to time be fairly passionate in his argumentation. On the other hand, his argumentation was deeply rooted in his broad philosophical and cultural upbringing and education.

Jean-Raoul is living proof of the fact that Medical Informatics is a multidisciplinary field. He had a classical education in Fribourg, specializing in mathematics; became an M.D. at the Geneva Medical School, where he got his diploma in 1959. Thereafter he was a postgraduate assistant in human physiology and completed his PhD thesis on the acetyl cholinesterase activity of human erythrocytes as a function of temperature. He completed his specialization in Internal Medicine in 1966 in Geneva and subsequently followed education and training in physics with a special emphasis on informatics, resulting in a diploma in 1968. From 1967 to 1969 he did research in the Medical Physics Division of the Medical Department of Brookhaven National Laboratory in the USA, before returning to Geneva and accepting his chair in Medical Informatics.

The question is often addressed whether medical informatics is a science in its own right. In the absence of a generally accepted underlying theory, however, it is difficult to give a description of medical informatics as a scientific discipline. If our underlying theory is to be borrowed from tradi-tional computer science, from physics or from statistics, we are still left with the question of what might remain at the core of medical informatics that we can claim to be our own discipline. I have already given some examples of medical informatics research, and many other examples can be found in the *Handbook of Medical Informatics* [12]. Whether medical informatics is a scientific discipline in its own right, remains an open question that challenges us not only now, but will for many years to come. Several major discussions have taken place on this subject that have been well documented in the literature [13]. Jean-Raoul played an active part in these deliberations.

## The Image Processor

Imaging and image processing have always been a substantial activity of the Geneva team. The same holds for many other medical informatics institutes, including our own. We must realize, however, that the field of medical imaging has ripened to such a degree that we can no longer claim that it still belongs to the inner core of medical informatics. In fact, Radiology has taken over most of the imaging and image processing research and applications, and industry is very successful in offering indispensable systems for clinical use.

The Geneva team has pioneered many of the systems that are in use not only in the Geneva clinics, but also at many centers all over the world. For instance, the image presentation system OSIRIS was an early realization of a practical system for both research and clinical applications. Many of the applications developed by the team in Geneva were distributed worldwide; OSIRIS was distributed to over 5,000 centers. The team also developed an in-house *Picture Archiving and Communications System* for use in the University Hospital of Geneva. With the advent of the worldwide web, the medical imaging applications were also made available via the Internet.

## The Bio-informatician

An important new research area is undoubtedly the field of bio-informatics or computational biology. Jean-Raoul Scherrer was at the root of developments in bio-informatics as well. He can also be considered as one of the founding fathers of SWISSPROT, a database used by many centers in the world for proteomics research [14]. Bio-informatics is an area that is in rapid development. Although this research domain shares many of its methods with medical informatics, it is particularly oriented toward:

- The conversion of biomolecular information into biochemical and biophysical knowledge;
- The construction and usage of protein and genomic databases;
- Database searching and data mining;
- Database integrity and reliability, and the development of standards for data interchange;
- Pattern recognition and matching;
- Functional genomics and gene expression;
- Biomolecular modeling and visualization.

Bio-informatics is viewed by some researchers as only marginally linked to medical informatics. Jean-Raoul Scherrer, however, considered the field of bio-informatics as an essential part of our profession. Therefore, he stimulated bio-informatics research from its very onset. Research in Geneva started with the Melanie project, intended for the analysis of protein maps [15]. Nowadays, the field of Proteomics ranks high among other exciting biomedical research areas. The Melanie system is still used by many researchers worldwide. Collaboration with centers elsewhere resulted in the SwissProt protein sequence database. Another system in this domain is the ExPASy website in Geneva, the first biomedical website, launched in 1993, with seven mirror sites elsewhere. The bio-informatics research that was started in Geneva also gave rise to the Swiss Institute of Bioinformatics, at present employing over 100 scientists.

## An HONest person

Jean-Raoul strongly believed in the value of providing reliable information to health professionals and to patients and their relatives, using the Internet.

That is why I consider him as a very HONest person.

Much health-related information on the Internet is of dubious reliability. This was the reason for Jean-Raoul to start the *Health-on-the-Net* project, over the years very substantially supported by the State of Geneva [16]. HON intends to be the intermediate in providing freely available, reliable, trustworthy, and regularly updated health information to patients and professionals.

The Health On the Net Foundation is the leading organization for promoting and guiding the deployment of such useful and reliable online medical and health information and its appropriate and efficient use. HON is an independent and neutral organization, recently (July 2002) granted NGO status from the Economic and Social Council of the United Nations. Since its creation in 1995, HON has attempted to solve two major bottlenecks of the Internet: the accessibility of health-related data and their reliability.

At present, HON has over 14,000 visitors a day. In April 2002, over 300,000 visitors from over 80 countries viewed 2 million HON web pages. In Google, the query "health" brings HON in a second position between the NIH and WHO. Since 1996 HON has published a voluntary self-regulated code of practice for medical and health online information, the HON Code of Conduct (HON code), also called Code of Good Behavior [17]. Other codes developed since then are based on the same principles. HON is the only organization since 1997 that enforces its code by a formal application process and accreditation mechanism, strengthened by online and dynamic certification. Up to July 2000, 3,300 websites from 66 countries, on all five continents, have already been accredited. The HON code is based upon three principles:

- Never use an anonymous document;
- Clearly discern between scientific, editorial and commercial information;
- Each document should state references to external source references.

In summary, the HON Code contains eight principles:

1. *Authority*
   Information should only be provided by medically qualified professionals
2. *Complementarity*
   Information on the Web should only support, not replace, the relationship with a physician
3. *Confidentiality*
   Confidentiality of individual patient data should be respected
4. *Attribution*
   Information should be supported by references to source data
5. *Justifiability*
   Any claims of the Website owner related to possible benefits should be clarified
6. *Transparency of authorship*
   Webmasters should display their full e-mail address for feedback
7. *Transparency of sponsorship*
   The identities of sponsors of the web site should be clearly identified
8. *Honesty in advertising and editorial policy*
   If advertising is a source of funding it should be clearly stated as such.

The last visionary project of Jean-Raoul was WRAPIN (Worldwide online Reliable Advice to Patients and Individuals), a EU project granted in June 2001, involving seven European partners and partly financed by the Swiss government. The WRAPIN project aims at offering an evaluation system, using a semi-automatic editorial policy tool applicable to any medical and health online document, to assess the trustworthiness of this tested information against published reliable scientific documents.

## The Networker

Jean-Raoul was not only a computer network builder, but also a human networker. He must have known hundreds of people from visiting virtually all conferences that were organized in our field. Jean-Raoul participated in the foundation and the development of the Swiss Society for Medical Informatics and of the European Federation of Medical Informatics (EFMI), both belonging to the family of IMIA. From 1996 to 1998 he was the Executive President of the European Federation of Medical Informatics, inspiring the field with his enthusiasm and energy. One of the highlights in Jean-Raoul's career was the organization of the 7th World Conference of Medical Informatics, MEDINFO 92, in Geneva.

## Concluding remark

I hope that I have given some good impressions of Jean-Raoul as a Prize Winner, an Explorer, a Diogenist, a Decision Supporter, a Scientist, an Image Processor, a Bio-informatician, an HONest person, and a true Networker. Above all, I hope that everyone who knew him will share the belief of Jean-Raoul, expressed in his last message to us: *God of Abraham, God of Isaac, God of Jacob, not of philosophers and scientists. Certainty. Certainty. Emotion. Joy. Peace.*


## References

1. Geissbühler A, Lovis C, Spahni S, Appel RD, Ratib O, Boyer C, et al. A humanist's legacy in Medical Informatics: visions and accomplishments of Professor Jean-Raoul Scherrer. Methods Inf Med 2002;41:237-42.
2. Van Ginneken AM, Stam H, Van Mulligen EM, De Wilde M, Van Mastrigt R, Van Bemmel JH. ORCA: the versatile CPR. Methods Inf Med 1999;38:332-8.
3. Spahni S, Scherrer JR, Sauquet D, Sottile PA. Towards specialised middleware for healthcare information systems. Int J Med Inf 1999;53:193-201.
4. Borst F, Appel R, Baud R, Ligier Y, Scherrer JR. Happy birthday DIOGENE: a hospital information system born 20 years ago. Int J Med Inf 1999;54:157-67.
5. Scherrer JR, Lovis C, Baud R, Borst F, Spahni S. Integrated computerized patient records: the DIOGENE 2 distributed architecture paradigm with special emphasis on its middleware design. Stud Health Technol Inform 1998;56:15-31.
6. Shortell S, Becker S, Neuhauser D. The effects of management practices on hospital efficiency and quality of care. In: Shortell S, Brown M, eds. *Organizational Research in Hospitals, an Inquiry Book.* Chicago IL: Blue Cross Association, 1976.
7. Scherrer JR, Baud RH, Hochstrasser D, Ratib O. An integrated hospital information system in Geneva. MD Comput 1990;7:81-9.
8. Rassinoux AM, Miller RA, Baud RH, Scherrer JR. Modeling concepts in medicine for medical language understanding. Methods Inf Med 1998;37: 361-72.
9. Van Wijk MAM, Bohnen AM, Van der Lei J. Analysis of the practice guidelines of the Dutch College of General Practitioners with respect to the use of blood tests. J Am Med Inform Assoc 1999;6:322-31.
10. Rector AL, Nowlan WA and the GALEN Consortium. The GALEN project. Comput Methods Programs Biomed 1993;45:75-78.
11. Thurler G, Borst F, Breant C, Campi D, Jenc J, Lehner-Godinho B, et al. ARCHIMED: a Network of Integrated Information Systems. Methods Inf Med 2000;39:36-4
12. Van Bemmel JH, Musen MA, editors. *Handbook of Medical Informatics.* Heidelberg: Springer Verlag 1997.
13. Musen MA, Van Bemmel JH, editors. Challenges for Medical Informatics as an Academic Discipline. Methods Inf Med 2002;41:1-63.
14. Bairoch A., Apweiler R. The SWISS-PROT protein sequence database and its supplement TrEMBL in 2000. Nucleic Acids Res 2000;28:45-48.
15. Appel RD, Hochstrasser DF, Funk M, Vargas R, Pellegrini C, Muller AF, et al. The MELANIE project - From a Biopsy to Automatic Protein Map Interpretation by Computer. Electrophoresis 1991;12, 722-35.
16. http://www.hon.ch/
17. Boyer C, Selby M, Scherrer JR, Appel RD. The Health On the Net Code of Conduct for medical and health Websites. Comput Biol Med 1998;28:603-10.



Address of the author:

Jan H. van Bemmel,
Institute of Medical Informatics
Erasmus University Medical Center
P.O. Box 1738
3000 DR Rotterdam
The Netherlands
E-mail: vanbemmel@mi.fgg.eur.nl

# A Humanist's Legacy in Medical Informatics: Visions and Accomplishments of Professor Jean-Raoul Scherrer *


A. Geissbühler[1], C. Lovis[1], S. Spahni[1], R. D. Appel[2], O. Ratib[3], C. Boyer[4], D. F. Hochstrasser[5], R. Baud[1]

[1]Division of Medical Informatics, Geneva University Hospitals, [2]Swiss Institute of Bioinformatics and Geneva University, [3]Department of Radiology, University of California in Los Angeles, USA, [4]Health-On-the-Net Foundation, Geneva, [5]Geneva Proteomics Center, Central Clinical Chemistry Laboratory, Department of Pathology, Geneva University Hospital and Geneva University, Switzerland



## Summary

*Objective:* To report about the work of Prof. Jean-Raoul Scherrer, and show how his humanist vision, his medical skills and his scientific background have enabled and shaped the development of medical informatics over the last 30 years.

*Results:* Starting with the mainframe-based patient-centered hospital information system DIOGENE in the 70s, Prof. Scherrer developed, implemented and evolved innovative concepts of man-machine interfaces, distributed and federated environments, leading the way with information systems that obstinately focused on the support of care providers and patients. Through a rigorous design of terminologies and ontologies, the DIOGENE data would then serve as a basis for the development of clinical research, data mining, and lead to innovative natural language processing techniques. In parallel, Prof. Scherrer supported the development of medical image management, ranging from a distributed picture archiving and communication systems (PACS) to molecular imaging of protein electrophoreses. Recognizing the need for improving the quality and trustworthiness of medical information on the Web, Prof. Scherrer created the Health-On-the-Net (HON) foundation.

*Conclusions:* These achievements, made possible thanks to his visionary mind, deep humanism, creativity, generosity and determination, have made of Prof. Scherrer a true pioneer and leader of the human-centered, patient-oriented application of information technology for improving healthcare.

## Keywords

Hospital information systems, bioinformatics, e-health


Methods Inf Med 2002; 41: 237–42

It takes a visionary mind, global intelligence, and relentless perseverance to pave the way for a new discipline, in particular when this discipline, medical informatics, is at the crossroads of medicine, science and technology. Professor Jean-Raoul Scherrer, combining his clinical skills in internal medicine, his research background in physiology, and his experience in computer science, shaped the field of medical informatics over the last 30 years, from the early days of mainframe computing applied to the patient-centered hospital information system, to the current challenges of taming the internet and help improve its potential to deliver useful medical information for patients.

Professor Scherrer also was a man of amazing erudition, with a profound sense of humanism that transpired in all his projects. A true Renaissance man, he applied classical and renaissance principles of humanism, multidisciplinarity and sharing in his works in medical informatics.

Putting the human – and the patient in particular – at the center of the computer-enabled solutions: the DIOGENE wheel (Fig. 1) which illustrated the concept of the Hospital Information System built at the Geneva Cantonal Hospital in the seventies clearly set the patient as the organizing principle and the finality of the information and communication system. The same concern still prevailed at the creation of the

---

*Dedicated in memoriam to Prof. J.-R. Scherrer

Health-On-the-Net (HON) foundation in 1995, when it became clear that the Internet could become a useful tool for promoting health and for informing patients, provided that the quality of its information could be enhanced and validated.

Fostering creativity across disciplines and in multiple directions has been the hallmark of Prof. Scherrer's research and development groups: an abundance of applied and research projects that emulated and nurtured each other, open to innovative experiments and out-of-the-box creations, in topics as diverse as systems architecture, natural language processing, knowledge representation, picture archiving and communication systems (PACS), biomedical imaging, and bioinformatics.

Setting up networks to connect people was very important to Prof. Scherrer, who participated in the foundation and the development of the Swiss Society for Medical Informatics (SSMI) and the International Medical Informatics Association (IMIA). Believing in collaboration across borders well in advance of his nation's attitude, he developed and drove many important European Union research projects in medical informatics, most of which dealt with aspects of communication and information sharing, ranging from knowledge representation in the GALEN project to federated electronic health care records of SYNAPSES and SYNEX.

Recognized as a pioneer and leader in the field, he was awarded the Morris Collen award by the American College of Medical

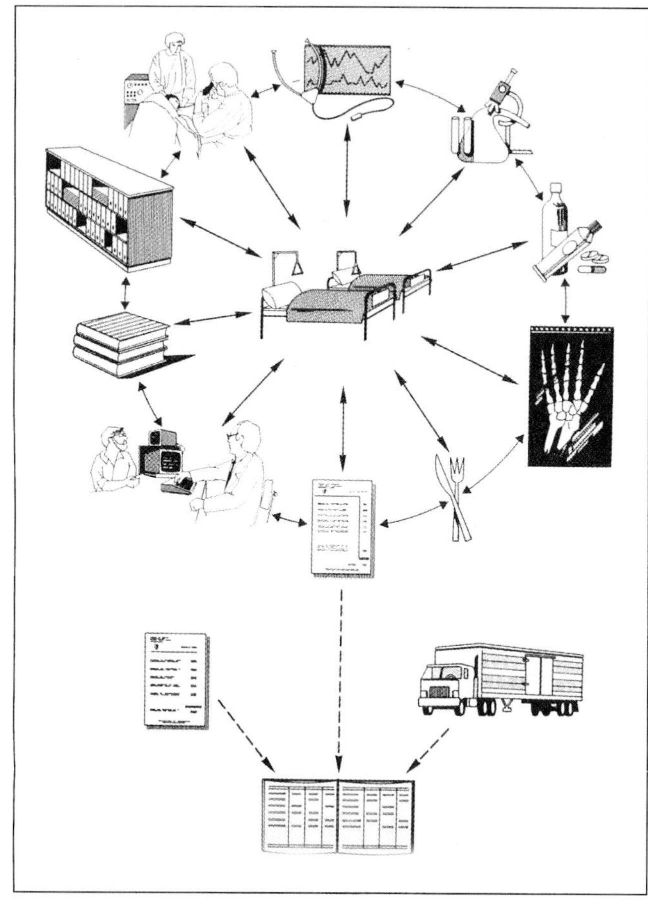

**Fig. 1**
The DIOGENE wheel, a conceptual model of the DIOGENE hospital information system, circa 1975

Informaticians in 2000, a distinction regarded as the "Nobel Prize" of medical informatics, of which he was the first non-American recipient. Prof. Scherrer passed away in March of 2002. He was 69 years old.

This paper attempts to summarize his accomplishments over more than 30 years of activity in the field of medical informatics, and to render some of his visions that still inspire and guide us today.

# Patient-centered Systems Architectures, from the Mainframe to the Internet

As early as 1971, Prof. Scherrer was able to hire a team for the tremendous task of building a hospital information system centered around the patient: this was the DIOGENE project. He still was 25 years

later a recognized leader, when promoting Natural Language Processing and Knowledge Representation techniques, with a unique and consistent goal: to better serve the patient through medical applications.

The DIOGENE system was first presented under the form of a wheel (see Fig. 1): applications on the periphery and a bed at the center (and later also a waiting room representing ambulatory care). Computing resources being limited, the leading idea was to give priority to the applications for care-providers, mainly the nurses and the physicians. Without terminals and 15 years before the advent of personal computers, the challenge was to create a convivial man-machine interface – easy to use, comprehensive and fast –, granting access to the care providers in more than one hundred nurses stations with only 64 terminal connections available in the system. The design of a pool of phone operators who mediated the interaction between profession-

als and the mainframe computer, sending direct visual feedback through video cables, was an exemplary solution, the so-called "Geneva solution" (1) (see Fig. 2), to an ergonomical, organizational and technical problem that can still be found in today's solutions (2, 3).

At the end of the eighties, the central system was a success, providing a set of services for more than 2000 registered users. The palette of applications was broad and the computer acquaintance was improved year after year. Professor Scherrer early recognized that the way to better applications and services is to be discovered one step at a time. The true benefit comes not from a single spectacular application, but most probably from a slow, persuasive and never-ending integration of multiple processes, either from the regular workflow of the hospital or computer-mediated. A design team was in charge of promoting new architectures and applications and a "thinking team" was responsible to advise for better solutions. In 1987, the decision to migrate to the Unix and PC environment was made (4-6), and mainframes were decommissioned in 1995.

Middleware was an important topic for applied research. The SYNAPSES European project helped Prof. Scherrer to promote this approach (7, 8). Started in January 1996, SYNAPSES aimed at standardizing mechanisms for describing a Federated Healthcare Record (FHCR) and its associated servers, and for integrating such concepts into existing environments. SYNAPSES was seen from the beginning as one element of the healthcare-specific middleware (9). In this project, the vision of Prof. Scherrer was a key success factor: having gone through the (r)evolution towards distributed systems, it was unthinkable for him to consider that a central healthcare record repository was a realistic long-term solution. For him, the FHCR server had to be integrated into existing environments, federating sources of heterogeneous information, relying on lower level middleware components for exchanging data with already existing components. The strong relationship between the R&D and the operation of the University Hospitals of Geneva made possible the development of a true

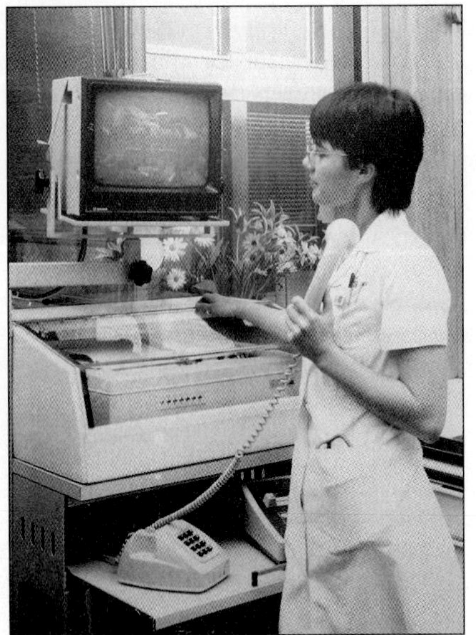

a)

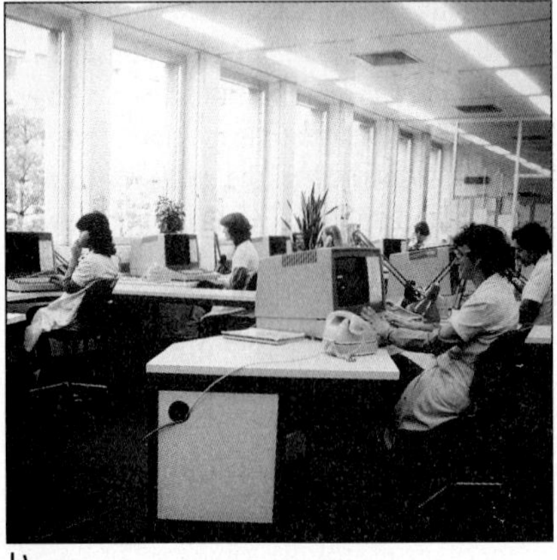

b)

**Fig. 2** The DIOGENE I telestation, a phone-operated terminal, with video feedback and a printer (a), connected to a pool of operators (b).

SYNAPSES-based record server for validating the results of the project.

Year 1998 saw the kick-off of the SYNEX – SYNergy on the EXtranet – European project, of which Prof. Scherrer was one of the initiators and then the leader of the steering board of the consortium. SYNEX was a continuation of SYNAPSES: while SYNAPSES focused on the access to the medical data inside one organization, SYNEX focused on the sharing of such data between organizations. Therefore, one could find among the main goals of this quite ambitious project the defini-

tion and the promotion a common middleware framework for medical applications as well as the set-up of a portal enabling the sharing of data between organizations of different nature. Indeed, as middleware was one of the strategic R&D axes of Prof. Scherrer, it is not surprising that the SYNEX project, which focused on state of the art solutions, had a very strong use of this concept (10-12).

SYNEX was not an easy project to manage and to make reach its goals: with 27 partners coming from nine countries, industrials, hospitals as well as academic entities, reaching a consensus on major strategic issues like the using the middleware approach or building all data exchanges on protocols like HTTP and XML was not an easy task. But his enthusiasm as well as his convictions on the way to go forward forced the way to the success. Finally, SYNEX ended not only with true demonstrators but also with pre-products and products, which is not so common in large R&D projects. SYNEX proved to be a very innovative project: apart from the strategic aspects of the middleware approach, concrete implementations have been realized and a prototype of a regional healthcare infrastructure was demonstrated in Geneva. Such a concrete realization, implying not only the hospitals of Geneva but also private practitioners, enabled a better understanding of the challenges as well as the potential problems encountered when moving from the theory to the practice for implementing shared care.

# Knowledge Representation and Natural Language Processing

Besides systems architecture and middleware, Prof. Scherrer developed a research line focusing on knowledge representation and natural language processing. Natural language understanding was viewed as an indispensable step to deal with the enormous amount of information and knowledge contained in medical texts (13). Underlying this effort, expertise in the ability to represent knowledge was developed

by participating to the GALEN projects (14, 15). Ten years later, both activities are still very active, giving contributions to the latest software developments (16, 17) and improving the man-machine dialog.

In parallel, the use of common terminologies for representing the concepts used in the hospital information system, as well as an obstinate belief that data encoding should primarily serve clinical purposes, enabled the creation of a rich clinical data warehouse, ARCHIMED (18), that would serve as a basis for quality assessment, identification of patient populations, medico-economical studies, and the development of data-mining and knowledge-acquisition techniques.

# Digital Medical Imaging

Management and communication of medical images in an electronic medical record environment has always been a major technical and strategic challenge. Very early on Prof. Scherrer pioneered the innovative concept of integrating images and graphical documents in a multi-media medical record as part of the essentials component supporting medical decision-making. As part of a major overhaul of the Geneva Medical Informatics Infrastructure, with the new phase of DIOGENE II, Prof. Scherrer created a dedicated Medical Imaging Unit in 1988. The mission of this division was to develop and implement innovative concepts in image management and communication for medical applications. The vision of the division was far beyond the traditional paradigm of managing and transmitting images from radiological devices, but was intended as generic support for all images in medicine and biology.

Almost 20 years ago Prof. Scherrer had already envisioned that molecular imaging and other biological imaging techniques would play a major role in modern clinical application and today's patient management. The Digital Imaging Unit rapidly acquired a major reputation in Europe and internationally by developing and promoting new concepts and tools for image management both in molecular imaging and electrophoreses, as well as in traditional medical imaging of radiological modalities. Supported by several grants, the members of the Digital Imaging Unit participated under the leadership of Prof. Scherrer into several major European multi-centric projects funded by the European Economic Community (EEC) (19,20). Among several projects, two large multicentric projects are worth mentioning: The TELEMED project, one of the first EEC-funded project on telemedicine and teleradiology including 12 centers from 7 different European countries and the MIMOSA project, another large European project setting the foundation for standardization in medical image management and communication.

At that early stage of medical imaging developments around the world, the University of Geneva took the leadership in development of software applications for display and management of medical images. The group was also heavily involved in standardization effort at that early stage of adoption of standard such as ACR/NEMA and DICOM standards in Europe and in the United States. Prof. Scherrer always promoted the concept of software sharing and open source for software being developed in Geneva. Many of the applications developed by the Digital Imaging Unit were distributed worldwide to other institutions. One of the most famous was the software named OSIRIS, which was one of the first available image display and manipulation software running on multiple computer platforms such as Macintosh, UNIX workstations, and Windows-based personal computers. The OSIRIS software was one of the most widely used and recognized image viewers supporting the DICOM standard. A survey conducted in 1997 showed that over 5000 centers around the world were using the OSIRIS software for research or clinical applications. The Digital Imaging Group was also responsible for developing an enterprise-wide Picture Archiving and Communications System (PACS) at the University Hospital of Geneva. This was one of the first clinical implementations in Europe demonstrating the feasibility of a distributed storage and archiving architecture using standard commercial components that were integrated together using homegrown image management and database software (20). A special emphasis was put on demonstrating the usefulness of image distribution in critical clinical wards such as intensive care units and emergency rooms. This system, developed in Geneva, and its architecture were often referred as a reference for recent developments and commercial applications of enterprise-wide data management and complex environments such as university hospitals. A close collaboration with manufacturers and the industry led to a wide adoption of some of the concepts developed in Geneva. Thanks to Prof. Scherrer's effort in collaboration and involvement in several European and international research groups the Medical Imaging Unit became well recognized among the academic and scientific community, hosting one of the first NATO symposiums on PACS and medical imaging in 1991 (21). This two-week symposium is well recognized as one of the landmark events in the recent history of developments of Picture Archiving and Communications Systems. The Digital Imaging Unit also became very active in European initiatives and hosted the EuroPACS meeting in 1994, in Geneva, Switzerland. Prof. Scherrer strongly supported and encouraged academic and research activities of the Digital Imaging Unit, which had a double mission to develop and implement a clinically usable system but also to explore and develop new and innovative concept and research projects.

With the rapid development of the worldwide web by colleagues from CERN in Geneva, the members of the Digital Imaging Unit enthusiastically adopted the concept and the tools of the worldwide web, rapidly deploying an experimental web-based support for medical record and medical imaging application environment.

# Molecular Imaging and Bioinformatics

Prof. Scherrer not only was a promoter of informatics developments that could immediately be applied for the patient's direct care. He also supported work whose relationship with health was sometimes harder to guess, but which he believed would eventually bring its own substantial contributions to healthcare and medicine. Many of these visionary projects developed into successful scientific ventures. While bioinformatics is regarded by some as being only remotely linked to medical informatics, Prof. Scherrer always considered it as an essential tool for medical information technology. Thus he promoted bioinformatics research in Geneva since its early days and fostered the development of two major bioinformatics research areas.

It first started in 1987 with the Melanie project for the analysis of protein map images by computer (22,23). The study of protein expression and its automated analysis by computer were at that time regarded by science policy-makers as basic tool development with little scientific interest. Prof. Scherrer, anticipating the way medical informatics would develop by the end the of millennium, supported the scientists and allowed them to carry out their work within the Medical Imaging Unit that he had just created at the Medical Informatics Center. Thirteen years later one can conclude that Prof. Scherrer was right is his vision: not only does the study of protein expression represents today one of the major components of proteome analysis (known as proteomics [24]), but the group then supported by him developed into an internationally recognized center of excellence in this field. Also, the Melanie software for the analysis of 2-DE images, now in its fourth generation, has been distributed since 1994 and is now used by hundreds of people world-wide (see [25] and http://www.expasy.org/melanie/). The development of a molecular scanner provides a new tool to analyze complex protein mixture, to do imaging by mass spectrometry and therefore large scale proteomic studies (26-28).

The second bioinformatics project facilitated by Prof. Scherrer's visionary policy started in July 1993. The Melanie project had produced a number of protein 2-DE reference maps (29) that needed to be published so that other members of the 2-DE scientific community could use them. The maps formed a collection of images linked to a database, called Swiss-2Dpage (30), containing textual information related to the maps. Collaborations started, resulting in the linkages with the Swiss-Prot annotated protein sequence database (31) and the Swiss-3Dimage database (32). The advent of the World-Wide Web provided a good mean of publishing these databases. In July 1993 the first biomedical Web server, called ExPASy ([33, 34] and http://www.expasy.org) was built. As this technology, then little known, was a big consumer of network bandwidth, the project generated quite some opposition among the local IT people. Prof. Scherrer immediately recognized the power of the World-Wide Web for Life Sciences and made sure that the server could be developed. It eventually became one of the main bioinformatics data provider over the Web. Prof. Scherrer actively promoted this new technology by publicly advertising his belief that combining databases with the type of data access made possible through Web technology represented a new paradigm, not only in bioinformatics, but also in Health and Life Sciences in general. Nearly ten years later, the ExPASy Web service is still alive and active: besides the main Web site located in Geneva, seven mirror sites are currently active on the American, European and Asian continents and are being accessed about 7 million times per month.

In 1998 the bioinformatics activities supported by Prof. Scherrer, linked to several other such activities in the Geneva region, gave birth to a new institution, the Swiss Institute of Bioinformatics (SIB – http://www.isb-sib.ch), which now employs more that 100 scientists. There is no doubt that Prof. Scherrer's vision of medical informatics and openness to novelty greatly helped in making Switzerland one of the centers in this exciting field.

## Health-On-the-Net (HON)

In 1993, only a few people realized the impact that Internet would have on our society, especially in the medical field. Prof. Scherrer was one of those: he was already convinced at that time that the new facilities offered by the Web would play an important role in the relationship between the patient and the physician in the healthcare system (35). Two years later, he organized the Constituent assembly for promoting the creation of the Health On the Net Foundation (HON) (36). HON was founded on the initiative of the Geneva Ministry of Health headed by Guy-Olivier Segond. Prof. Scherrer was elected president in 1998 when he retired from the Geneva University Hospitals where he had been director of the Medical Informatics division for more than 25 years.

HON's main objective has been to serve individuals (patients and healthcare professionals) throughout an open system of freely available, reliable, trustworthy, and regularly updated health information. For Prof. Scherrer, one of the major problems of our times is due to the loneliness of the citizen faced with the power of the State (37): individuals and citizens are progressively losing confidence in the State, in the healthcare system as well as the confidence they used to have in their private physician who is not listening enough. These individuals look for new authorities to get information and answer their questions.

HON claims the right to be considered one of these authorities. It first offers medical information search tools such as the MedHunt full text medical search engine powered by MARVIN (Multi-Agent Retrieval Robot on Information Network) (38, 39) and HONselect, a multilingual encyclopedia of 33000 medical terms (40).

HON also pioneered the e-Health field by creating ethical guidelines in 1996: the HON Code of Conduct (HONcode) (41). The HONcode is based upon three pillars: a) never consider an anonymous document, b) the distinction between scientific editorial and commercial content must be clearly identifiable, and c) each document must state external references in order to allow comparison. The trustworthiness of any document or information appears to be a major concern for the users. HON has made it a priority to improve patient searches and the quality of medical and health Web sites (42).

In order to extend the HON services capabilities, Prof. Scherrer launched the WRAPIN project in 2001, a project financed by the European Union. WRAPIN stands for a World-wide online Reliable Advice to Patients and INdividuals. The ambition of this project is to help in the formulation of more efficient medical queries and facilitate the access to multiple knowledge sources. With a more efficient sharing of reliable knowledge, WRAPIN will help the citizen/individual to make appropriate judgments on medical information found on the Web. This is the last enterprise of a humanist who wanted to give to all access to the most advanced power of information technology.

## Conclusion

Prof. Jean-Raoul Scherrer's vision of the human-centered, patient-oriented, application of information and communication technology for improving healthcare, based on multidimensional collaborative research and development, creativity, generosity and obstination, has been demonstrated through several generations of implemented systems, and is still very much alive and influential in the teams that he lead, inspired and trained, in Geneva and throughout the world.

## References


1. Coiera E. When Conversation Is Better Than Computation. J Am Med Informatics Ass 2000; 7: 277-86.
2. Scherrer JR, Baud RH, Hochstrasser D, Ratib O. An integrated hospital information system in Geneva. MD Computing 1990 Mar-Apr; 7 (2): 81-9.
3. Borst F, Appel R, Baud R, Ligier Y, Scherrer JR. Happy birthday DIOGENE: a hospital information system born 20 years ago. Int J Med Informatics 1999 Jun; 54 (3): 157-67.
4. Scherrer JR. Communications-future needs and present solutions. Int J Biomed Comput 1995 Apr; 39 (1): 47-52.
5. Scherrer JR, Lovis C, Baud R, Borst F, Spahni S. Integrated computerized patient records: the DIOGENE 2 distributed architecture paradigm with special emphasis on its middleware design. Stud Health Technol Informatics 1998; 56: 15-31.
6. Spahni S, Scherrer JR, Sauquet D, Sottile PA. Towards specialised middleware for healthcare

information systems. Int J Med Informatics 1999 Feb-Mar; 53 (2-3): 193-201.

7. Scherrer JR, Spahni S. New opportunities for processing the OSI-7 layer protocols using parallel processing (transputers). Int J Biomed Computing 1994 Jan; 34 (1-4): 387-98.

8. Spahni S, Scherrer JR, Sauquet D, Sottile PA. Middleware for healthcare information systems. Medinfo 1998; 9 Pt 1: 212-6.

9. Scherrer JR, Spahni S. Healthcare information system architecture (HISA) and its middleware models. Proceedings of the AMIA Symposium 1999: 935-9.

10. Andany J, Bjorkendal C, Ferrara FM, Scherrer JR, Spahni S. Authorization & security aspects in the middleware-based healthcare information system. Stud Health Technol Informatics 1999; 68: 315-20.

11. Spahni S, Scherrer JR, Andany J, Labussiere S, Sauquet D. "THE PILOT": a tool for connecting existing HIS to an extranet quickly, easily and smoothly. Medinfo 2001; 10 (Pt 1): 53-7.

12. Xu Y, D'Alessio L, Jaulent MC, Sauquet D, Spahni S, Degoulet P. Integrating medical applications in an open architecture through generic and reusable components. Medinfo 2001; 10 (Pt 1): 63-7.

13. Lyman M, Sager N, Tick L, Nhan N, Borst F, Scherrer JR. The application of natural-language processing to healthcare quality assessment. Med Decision Making 1991 Oct-Dec; 11 (4 Suppl): S65-8.

14. Rassinoux AM, Miller RA, Baud RH, Scherrer JR. Modeling concepts in medicine for medical language understanding. Methods Inf Med 1998 Nov; 37 (4-5): 361-72.

15. Wagner JC, Rogers JE, Baud RH, Scherrer JR. Natural language generation of surgical procedures. Medinfo 1998; 9 Pt 1: 591-5.

16. Lovis C, Michel PA, Baud R, Scherrer JR. Word segmentation processing: a way to exponentially extend medical dictionaries. Medinfo 1998; 9 Pt 1: 591-5.

17. Baud R, Lovis C, Rassinoux AM, Michel PA, Scherrer JR. Automatic extraction of linguistic knowledge from an international classification. Medinfo 1998; 9 Pt 1: 581-5.

18. Thurler G, Borst F, Breant C, Campi D, Jenc J, Lehner-Godinho B, Maricot P, Scherrer JR. ARCHIMED: a Network of Integrated Information Systems. Methods Inf Med 2000 Mar; 39 (1): 36-4.

19. Aubry F, Chameroy V, Giron A, Di Paola R, Gibaud B, Bizais Y, et al. MIMOSA: Conceptual modelling of Medical Image Management in an Open System Architecture. In: Laxminarayan SaC, J.-L. eds, editor. 14th Annual International Conference of the IEEE Engineering in Medicine and Biology Society. vol. 3/7. Paris: IEEE-EMBS; 1992, p. 1199-201.

20. Ratib O, Ligier Y, Hochstrasser D, Scherrer JR. Hospital Integrated Picture Archiving and Communication System (HIPACS) at the University Hospital of Geneva. In: Schneider R, Jost G, Dwyer III S, editors. Medical Imaging V: PACS design and Evaluation. vol. 1446. San-Jose: SPIE; 1991, p. 330-8.

21. Huang HK, Ratib O, Bakker AB, Witte G. Picture Archiving and Communication System (PACS) in Medicine. Berlin Heidelberg: Springer-Verlag; 1991.

22. Hochstrasser DF, Appel RD, Vargas R, Perrier R, Ravier F, Funk M, Pellegrini Ch, Muller AF, Scherrer J-R. Clinical molecular scanner: The Melanie project. MD-Computing, 8, 85-91, 1991.

23. Appel RD, Hochstrasser DF, Funk M, Vargas R, Pellegrini Ch, Muller AF, Scherrer J-R. The MELANIE project – From a Biopsy to Automatic Protein Map Interpretation by Computer. Electrophoresis, 12, 722-35, 1991.

24. Herbert BR, Sanchez JC, Bini L. Two-Dimensional Electrophoresis: The State of the Art and Future Directions. In: Proteome research: new frontiers in functional genomics, Wilkins MR, Williams KL, Appel RD, Hochstrasser DF (Eds), Springer Verlag Berlin Heidelberg 1997, pp. 13-33.

25. Appel RD, Palagi P, Walther D, Vargas JR, Sanchez JC, Pasquali C, Ravier F, Hochstrasser DF. Melanie II: a third generation software package for analysis of two-dimensional electrophoresis images – I. Features and user interface. Electrophoresis 1997; 18: 2724-34.

26. Muller M, Gras R, Appel RD, Bienvenut WV, Hochstrasser DF. Visualization and analysis of molecular scanner peptide mass spectra. J Am Soc Mass Spectrom 2002 Mar; 13 (3): 221-31.

27. Binz PA, Muller M, Walther D, Bienvenut WV, Gras R, Hoogland C, Bouchet G, Gasteiger E, Fabbretti R, Gay S, Palagi P, Wilkins MR, Rouge V, Tonella L, Paesano S, Rossellat G, Karmime A, Bairoch A, Sanchez JC, Appel RD, Hochstrasser DF. A molecular scanner to automate proteomic research and to display proteome images. Anal Chem 1999 Nov 1; 71 (21): 4981-8.

28. Bienvenut WV, Sanchez JC, Karmime A, Rouge V, Rose K, Binz PA, Hochstrasser DF. Toward a clinical molecular scanner for proteome research: parallel protein chemical processing before and during western blot. Anal Chem 1999 Nov 1; 71 (21): 4800-7.

29. Hochstrasser D, Frutiger S, Paquet N, Bairoch A, Ravier F, Pasquali C, Sanchez J-C, Tissot J-D, Bjellqvist B, Vargas R, Appel R, Hughes G. Human liver protein map: a reference database established by microsequencing & gel comparison. Electrophoresis 1992; 13 (12): 992-1001.

30. Hoogland C, Tonella L, Sanchez JC, Binz P-A, Bairoch A, Hochstrasser DF, Appel RD. The '99 SWISS-2DPAGE database update. Nucleic Acids Res 2000; 28: 286-8.

31. Bairoch A, Apweiler R. The SWISS-PROT protein sequence database and its supplement TrEMBL in 2000. Nucleic Acids Res 2000; 28: 45-8.

32. Peitsch MC, Stampf DR, Wells TNC, Sussman JL. The Swiss-3DImage collection and PDB-Browser on the World-Wide Web. Trends in Biochemical Sciences 1995; 20: 82-4.

33. Appel RD, Bairoch A, Hochstrasser DF. A new generation of information retrieval tools for biologists: the example of the expasy WWW server. Trends Biochem Scienc TiBS (222), 1994; 19, (6): 258-60.

34. Hochstrasser DF, Appel RD, Golaz O, Pasquali C, Sanchez J-C, Bairoch A. Sharing of World-wide Spread Knowledge Using Hypermedia Facilities & Fast Communications Protocols (Mosaic & World-Wide Web): The Example of ExPASy. Methods Inf Med 1995; 34: 75-8.

35. Boyer C, Appel RD, Griesser V, Scherrer JR. Internet for physicians: a tool for today and tomorrow. Revue Medicale Suisse Romande 1999 Feb; 119 (2): 137-44.

36. http://www.hon.ch/

37. Hannah Arendt in "The origin of totalitarism" New York 1955.

38. Boyer C, Baujard O, Baujard V, Aurel S, Selby M, Appel RD. Health On the Net automated database of health and medical information. Int J Med Informatics 1997 Nov; 47 (1-2): 27-9.

39. Baujard O, Baujard V, Aurel S, Boyer C, Appel RD. MARVIN, multi-agent softbot to retrieve multilingual medical information on the Web. Medical Informatics (Lond). 1998 Jul-Sep; 23 (3): 187-91.

40. Boyer C, Baujard V, Griesser V, Scherrer JR. HONselect: a multilingual and intelligent search tool integrating heterogeneous web resources. Int J Med Informatics 2001 Dec; 64 (2-3): 253-8.

41. Boyer C, Selby M, Scherrer JR, Appel RD. The Health On the Net Code of Conduct for medical and health Websites. Comput Biol Med 1998 Sep; 28 (5): 603-10.

42. Fallis D, Fricke M. Indicators of accuracy of consumer health information on the Internet: a study of indicators relating to information for managing fever in children in the home. J Am Med Informatics Ass 2002 Jan-Feb; 9 (1): 73-9.

**Correspondence to:**
Prof. Antoine Geissbühler, MD
Division of Medical Informatics
Geneva University Hospitals
Hopital Cantonal
24, rue Micheli-Du-Crest
1211 Geneva 14
Switzerland
E-mail: antoine.geissbuhler@hcuge.ch

*These authors describe a fully integrated computing system, which even includes physician encoding of diagnoses, in a 1600-bed hospital in Geneva.*

# AN INTEGRATED HOSPITAL INFORMATION SYSTEM IN GENEVA

JEAN-RAOUL SCHERRER, M.D., ROBERT H. BAUD, PH.D.,
DENIS HOCHSTRASSER, M.D., AND OSMAN RATIB, M.D., PH.D.

The DIOGENE (Division Informatique Hôpital Genève) hospital information system (HIS) at the University Hospital of Geneva was designed, in accordance with the requirements of the government of Geneva, to provide the hospital with ways of reducing the average length of stay and to improve its operations [1–4]. The hospital comprises 5 buildings and has 1600 beds, 35,000 inpatients per year, 450,000 outpatients per year, and 5500 employees (including physicians). The DIOGENE project was approved in 1973, with a budget of 25 million Swiss francs over a period of 10 years.

The system was introduced for administrative applications, including personnel management, in 1974. Invoicing was added in 1977, patient admissions in 1978, and general accounting in 1979. The system was progressively extended to all the wards in 1979 and 1980. Extensions to the radiology department and laboratories occurred from 1979 to 1982. Interactive medical encoding by interns and residents was added in 1985. The system soon included new emergency laboratories (1986), monthly and yearly medical statistics on patients (1987), the pharmacy (1987), integrated outpatient clinics in surgery (1987) and medicine (1988), and the medical bacteriology laboratory (1988).

## SYSTEM DESIGN

It is not possible to build a hospital information system simply by combining several smaller systems that were originally unrelated. Use of a patient-oriented system is essential. But the multiplicity of physical areas simultaneously providing services to the patient poses problems. A sound ADT (ad-

## ABSTRACT

*Since the initial design phase from 1971 to 1973, the DIOGENE hospital information system at the University Hospital of Geneva has been treated as a whole and has retained its architectural unity, despite the need for modification and extension over the years. In addition to having a centralized patient database with the mechanisms for data protection and recovery of a transaction-oriented system, the DIOGENE system has a centralized pool of operators who provide support and training to the users; a separate network of remote printers that provides a telex service between the hospital buildings, offices, medical departments, and wards; and a three-component structure that avoids barriers between administrative and medical applications.*

*In 1973, after a 2-year design period, the project was approved and funded. The DIOGENE system has led to more efficient sharing of costly resources, more rapid performance of administrative tasks, and more comprehensive collection of information about the institution and its patients.*

[KEYWORDS: *hospital information system, computer systems, networks, telecommunications, medical record coding, Europe, Switzerland*]

mission, discharge, and transfer) system including all the basic information describing the patient—identity, location, length of stay, and services received—is therefore paramount. Any local copy of this information will rapidly become out of date. Hence, a substantial part of the data must be centralized.

### The Common Database
The fully integrated database function is undoubtedly of foremost importance in the hospital information system. All other functions revolve around it. To protect sensitive personal data and permit them to be viewed only by authorized persons, the access-control function is available. In addition, backup and recovery functions guarantee that information will not be lost.

## APPLICATIONS
Like other large hospital information systems [5–11], DIOGENE supports many applications throughout the hospital (Table 1) [12]. In an effort to avoid barriers between the administrative and medical programs, the system was built around three elements: the patients, the personnel, and the suppliers (Fig. 1). The patient element (including both inpatients and outpatients) is the central component of the system. The patient application programs (described in detail elsewhere [1]) are for ADT, the ward units, the central laboratories (clinical chemistry, hematology, biology, medical bacteriology, and anatomy-pathology), the radiology department, the pharmacy, and the medical records department. Most of the application programs have facilities for multiple views, with one view for each main category of users: medical, hospital, management, and nursing.

### Admissions
The admissions system, the cornerstone of the DIOGENE system, captures essential data on the patient's identity at the time of admission. The nurses keep the list of inpatients updated in real time with use of the "telestations" installed on each ward [1].

### Laboratories
The integrated laboratory applications, which handle requests as issued by the wards, provide for printing of laboratory test results as soon as they are available. A cumulative report is printed out on the ward where the patient is located, regardless of where the test was requested. All the results related to a patient since the day of admission can be viewed at a terminal, and a copy of the results sheets can be obtained at any time. Manual transcription of data has thus been reduced to a mini-

## THE DIOGENE HOSPITAL INFORMATION SYSTEM

**Table 1**

| | |
|---|---|
| **Use of telestations** | |
| No. of ward telestations | 118 |
| Calls per year | 300,000 |
| Calls per peak hour | 60 |
| Average seconds per call | 115 |
| Frames available on terminals | 6,100 |
| **Operator pool** | |
| Operators | 18 |
| User training (course hours per year) | 150 |
| **Patient database** | |
| Active patients | 2,000 |
| Patients in database | 300,000 |
| Employees | 10,000 |
| Volume of storage | 700 MB |
| Authorized users | 2,450 |
| Modifications of database per day | 27,000 |
| **Peripheral hardware** | |
| Interactive terminals | 245 |
| Printers and plotters | 220 |
| Intersat network nodes | 350 |
| **No. of documents printed** | |
| Per day | 6,500 |
| Per peak day | 7,500 |
| Per peak hour | 800 |
| **Use of medical records application** | |
| Services using manual coding sheets | 8 |
| Services using interactive data entry | 8 |
| Services not yet registering diagnoses | 9 |
| **Discharge summaries per year** | |
| Manual coding (by physicians) for 581 beds | 25,867 (58.9%) |
| Interactive coding (by physicians) for 530 beds | 13,516 (30.8%) |
| Unrecorded (by physicians) for 454 beds | 4,500 (10.3%) |
| Diagnoses per patient (average) | 2.4 |
| Procedures per patient (average) | 1.5 |

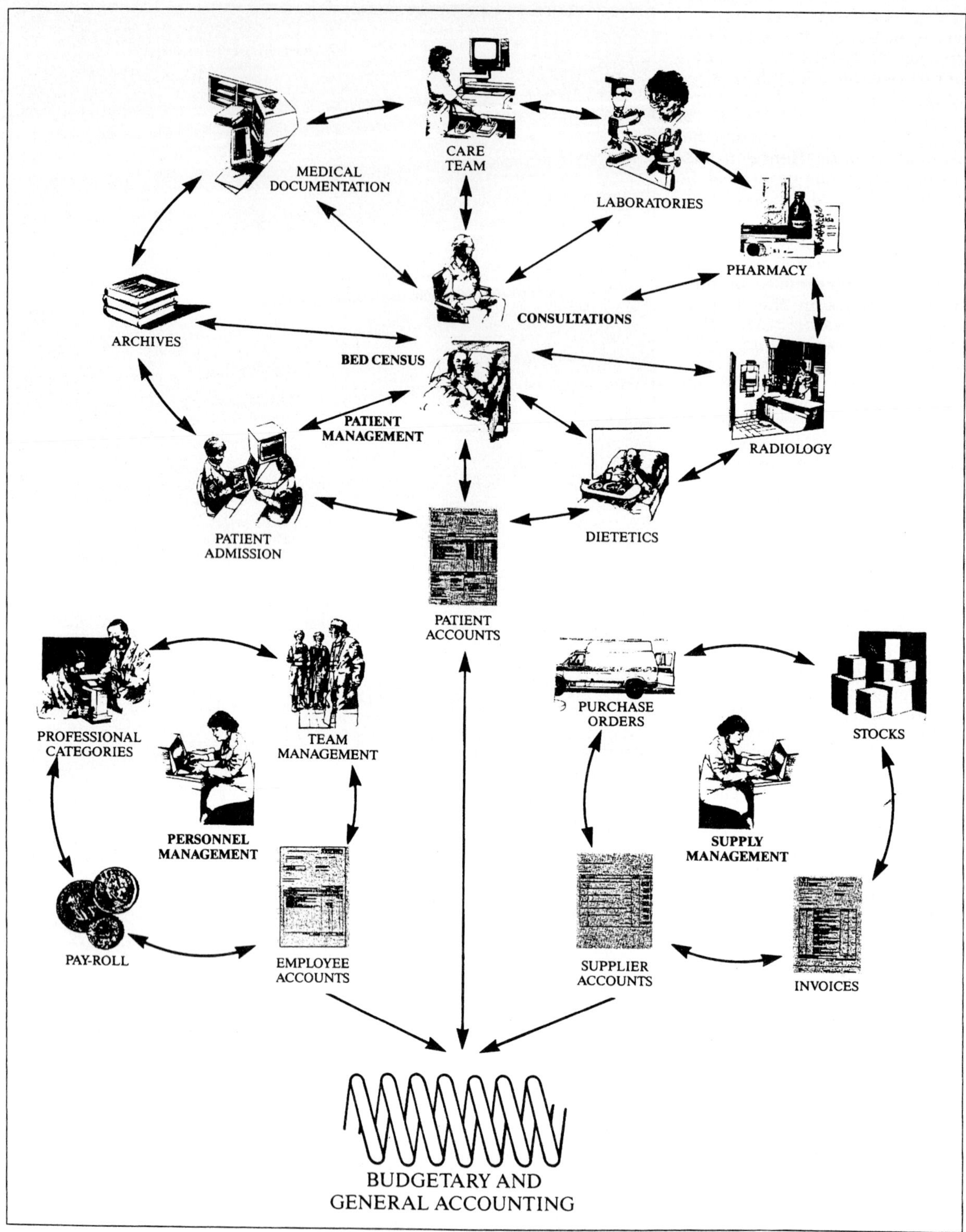


**Figure 1. The main elements of the DIOGENE hospital information system. The system is built up around three nuclei: the patient nucleus, the personnel nucleus, and the supplier nucleus. The three nuclei provide up-to-date information for daily operations and various accounting and statistical needs. This information is shared between medical and administrative services.**

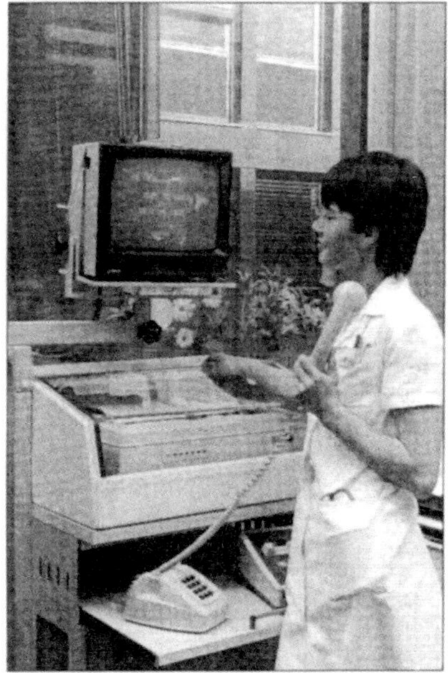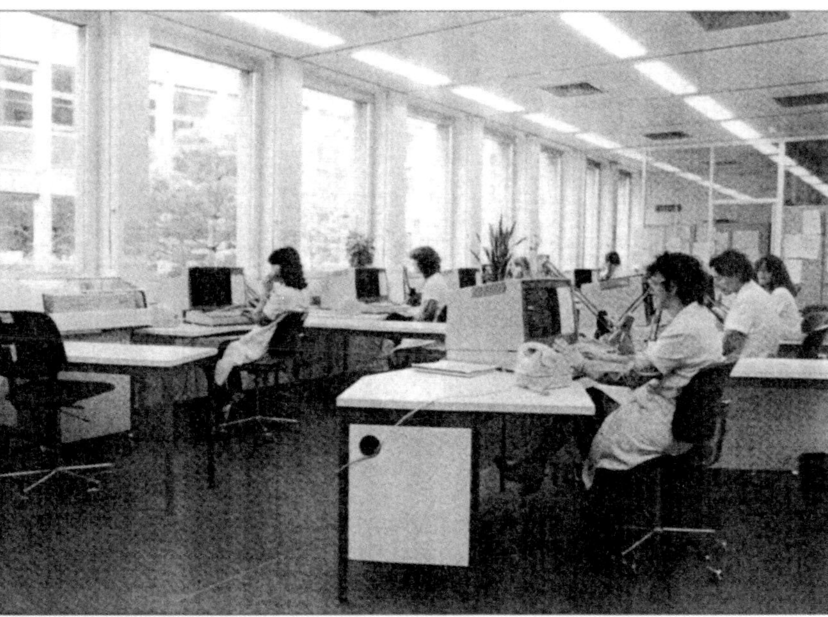

**Figure 2. A DIOGENE telestation. The telestation consists of a telephone linked to an operator pool, a television monitor to visualize the transaction, an identification-badge reader for access control, and a printer. These photographs show a nurse using her telestation in a ward and the operator pool working on DIOGENE terminals. The video monitor in the ward reproduces the image of the operator's terminal, and transactions are executed under the nurse's visual control.**

mum, saving time and lessening the possibility of human error.

*Radiology*
The radiology information system, developed locally and in use since 1979, detects duplicated requests for examinations, reviews previous results for comparative studies, generates an examination file for the radiologist or assistant performing the test, and prints out nominative labels. The examiners use stickers printed by the HIS for identification of x-ray films and complete coded cards for subsequent interpretation by an optical card reader. This procedure initiates the preparation of the diagnostic report. The system also provides a cumulative report of x-ray examinations for each patient, daily activity reports, treatment records and invoicing, stock management, and monthly and annual statistics.

*Pharmacy*
The pharmacy system helps in managing pharmaceutical stocks and monitoring and studying drug consumption. Personnel in the wards transmit their daily orders to the central pharmacy, which obtains all supplies and records do

liveries. Deliveries are made either from the central pharmacy or from one of the satellite pharmacies.

*Finance*
To ensure that the hospital's finances and budget are well managed, an organizational charts-management system has been implemented. All the costs (there are more than 500 different accounts for working costs alone) and income centers (there are 320 centers of working costs) have been identified and may be approached according to a matrix structure given by the charts and their history [13]. The centers, called cells, also include properties independent of the hospital, such as real estate to be managed. Depending on the kinds of queries or actions to be taken, it is appropriate to have several charts simultaneously involved. Every DIOGENE transaction, whether for a patient or not, will necessarily make reference to the different charts. For example, let us suppose that a patient transferred to a given ward is under new medical care (a new medical hierarchy) and also under new nursing care (a new nursing hierarchy). The ap-

propriate cost and revenue cells are charged on the basis of the management charts. These can be changed if necessary. In addition, these structural modifications require appropriate access rights.

## THE OPERATOR POOL AND THE DIOGENE TELESTATION

From the ward, the nurses communicate with the hospital information system through a telestation (Fig. 2). The telestation consists of a telephone linked to the operator pool, a television monitor to visualize transactions, an identification-badge reader for access control, and a printer. The nurse orally transmits instructions to an operator, who then executes the transaction. The nurse follows the transaction's progress by watching the television monitor in the ward. The advantages of telestations in the wards are the following: ease of use, even for newcomers and occasional users; reductions in initial and follow-up training times; permanent user support; use of simple and familiar equipment (a telephone and TV screen); control of transactions at the ward level; and protection of data confidentiality by positive and selective user identification.

The operator pool ensures that a person with knowledge of the computing system is present for the support of users on a 24-hour basis. At peak periods, up to 9 operators answer calls from as many as 120 wards. The operators also perform various supervisory and data-updating tasks [1,4]. Instead of forcing all users to learn a highly specialized language that permits dialogue with the computer, the system has a human operator perform the translation from natural language. In our experience, this approach gives users a degree of freedom they would not have otherwise. The operator pool offers continuous training (when personnel are new or when there are changes in procedures) as well as information capture and updating of access rights.

The importance of the user-support function is often underestimated during the design of information systems. If this function is neglected, however, good software may not be used. At our hospital the support of the operator pool is particularly valued during interruptions of services, changes in software characteristics, the introduction of new applications, and the training of newcomers. The operators concentrate particular attention on the emergency center and the laboratories, given the critical importance of time in their activities.

Any user of the hospital information system, including users of the interactive terminals, can reach an operator at any time to draw attention to a fault in the system (whether it is related to the software or the hardware). The operator will either solve the problem directly on the telephone or, if necessary, mobilize the appropriate resources. The function of supervising the network allows the operator on duty to check the conditions of printers, ensuring early detection of equipment failure. The communication of daily events to the operators allows them to distribute important information to other sectors of the hospital. Over short periods, the operator pool is also able to provide qualified personnel to certain users who need assistance with research and data entry. The services of the op-

erator pool are those of a team that is responsible for maintaining regular contacts with users and ensuring their preliminary and on-going training.

## HOSPITAL COMPUTING FACILITIES

The computing center is built around two Control Data Corporation mainframe computers: a CYBER 180/845 (upgraded to 180/855 in 1988) with 8 MB of RAM, and a CYBER 180/840 with 16 MB of RAM. The system also contains 24 disk drives (16 GB), 6 magnetic tape drives (1600/6250 bytes per inch), 4 front-end processors to link the mainframe computers to the network, 9 satellite computers operating under UNIX (4 SUN machines, 4 HP-9000/825–845s, and 1 VAX-750), 113 ward unit stations, 454 connected personal computers and terminals, 202 remote printers (beside the ward unit stations), 8 remote fast printers, and 237 asynchronous lines of communication.

### The Network

The Intersat network [14] links every computer in the DIOGENE system with every other computer and with every terminal and printer (Fig. 3). Various types of computers are connected on the network, including large computers (CYBERs), UNIX machines (VAX and SUN), personal workstations (IBM personal computers and compatibles), and small, low-cost network nodes (Micro-1). The nodes are made up of microprocessor-based systems that act as interfaces between the network and groups of terminals and printers. There is no hierarchy among the elements that make up the network. The communication protocol permits communication between any two elements, such as two terminals or a terminal and a program.

### Language

The BABEL language, developed locally, allows communication between applications distributed among different computers in the

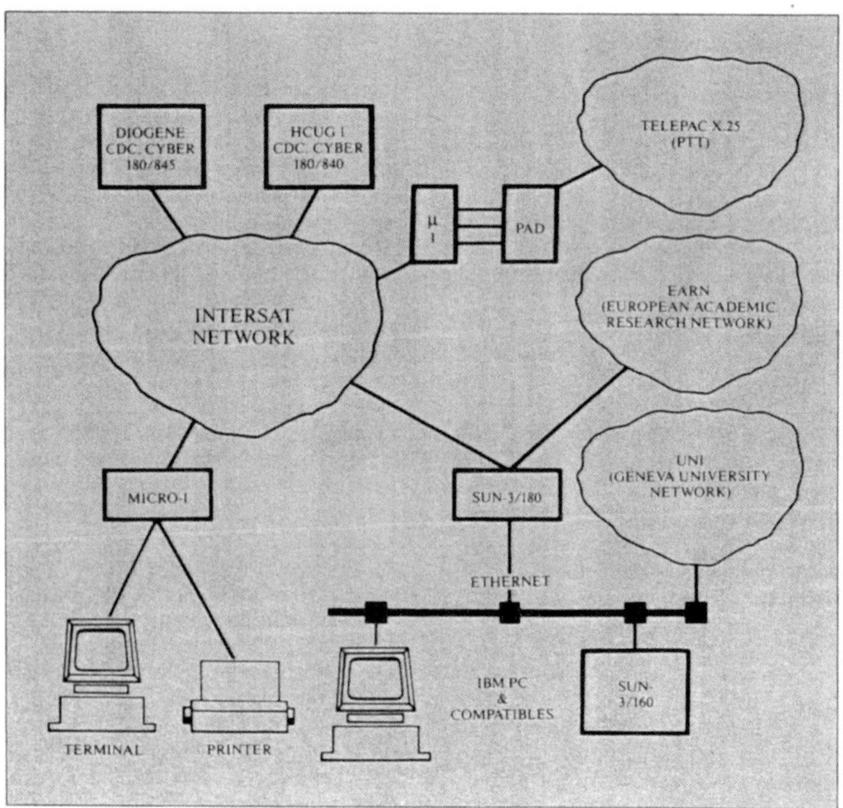


**Figure 3. The Intersat network.**

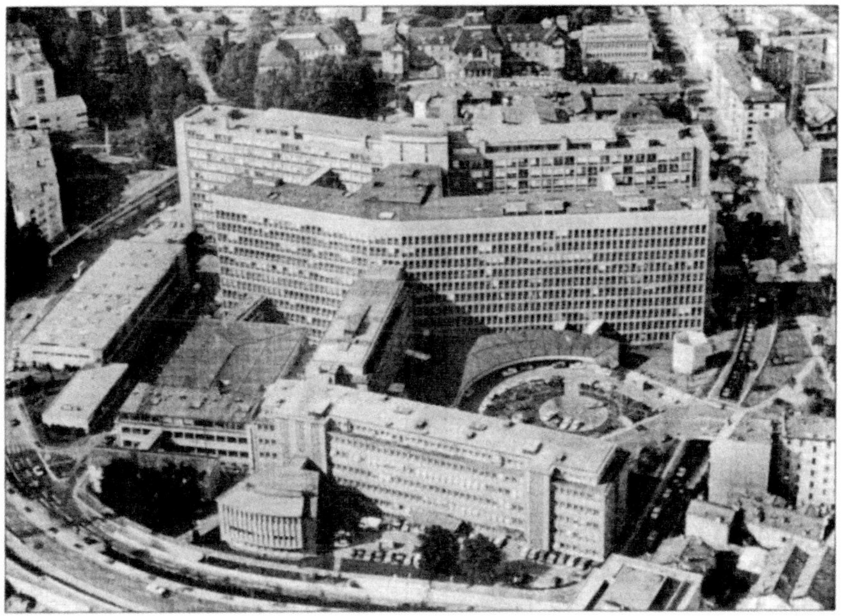

**The University Hospital in Geneva.**

network. The format of the messages exchanged is largely derived from the basic terms of PROLOG. A version for UNIX machines and personal computers written in C is also used. BABEL versions for the CYBER machines and the FORTRAN language are currently being developed. The Intersat network is being extended in two ways: by enlarging the available bandwidth and by introducing high-level mechanisms for the exchange of information between distributed applications.

## TRANSACTIONS

The architecture of DIOGENE is primarily determined by the fact that it is a transactional system. We believe that in the perpetually changing context of a hospital, only a real-time transactional mode can be appropriate. It must be stressed that during the first 2 days of a stay in our hospital, the patient is the object of more than 50 actions performed with the hospital information system. Moreover, these actions are interdependent.

Through a unique path of access, the transaction function channels all actions related to a database, controls their progress, and ensures their coherence when several users are working simultaneously. The principal characteristic of the transactional system is the breakdown of all actions that might modify the database into small parcels of requests that are logical, coherent entities with respect to the database. A logical entity thus defined is known as a transaction. It corresponds to an action that is visible to a user at a terminal. The principle that is always respected is that the database should remain coherent between any two transactions, but not necessarily during a transaction.

### Access to the System

The terminals of various medical departments can provide identical functions. However, these functions involve different groups of patients, depending on where the terminal is located. The profile of access rights of each user is registered in the database. A link exists between this file and that of the hospital's employees. Only the programs for the validation of rights permit access to this privileged sector of the database. Updating of the list of authorized users and their rights is centralized and takes place through interactive dialogue. A list of default rights is attributed to each category of personnel and to each department. When rights are provided to an employee, the list is modified according to the employee's job in the hospital.

A user can be denied access to the system at any time. The user's card or password can be invalidated immediately or as of a stipulated date. This happens when there is a change of post, when an employee leaves, when a card is lost, and sometimes, when the system is abused. The system checks access rights at the beginning of every session of work at a terminal. A check also takes place when a transaction is requested with the help of the menu-selection system, as well as during the execution of an application program.

### Protection of Data

The access-control function defines the authorized domains for each user and ensures that the limits thus defined are respected. The system not only safeguards data against untimely loss but also ensures that information concerning a patient is available only to those with a right to it and that only duly authorized users may update it. Every user has a card providing access to the system; he or she may begin working either by using the card or by entering a personal password. The card gives access to a list of terminals and a list of transactions defined in the user's profile.

A strict protocol for access to data avoids collisions during transactions while maintaining the multi-user characteristics of the system. This protocol guarantees the sequential execution of conflicting requests for access and allows for parallelism in normal circumstances. The process is almost invisible to the user, except in some rare instances when response time is slightly longer than usual. In the course of a transaction, requests to the database are "locked" when a user wishes to have exclusive use of data in order to make modifications. Locking continues throughout the transaction. This approach requires that transactions be made in sequence. The risk of a mutual and perpetual block of two transactions exists (and deadlocks occur, on average, once a day). When deadlocks occur, however, they are automatically detected and resolved by cancellation of one of the two blocked transactions.

## REPORTS

The application programs generate documents for distribution in the hospital after transactions are executed automatically or by users. A central program, known as Impex, is responsible for the distribution of printed material within the hospital. Each day, the program prints 6500 to 8000 documents [14]. In general terms, the program is responsible for the delivery of documents without concern for their contents. Impex can be used for the transfer of images, text, programs, or any other information as long as the volume concerned is compatible with the bandwidth of the network.

Certain documents are considered particularly valuable, either because they have legal importance or because they cannot be reproduced (when the database has been modified since their creation). For this type of document, Impex produces a backup copy to be used if the first copy is destroyed. Backup copies are stored on magnetic tape for 6 months.

Documents waiting to be printed by a malfunctioning printer may be rerouted to another printer.

The function of document distribution is, for historical reasons, carried out on the same computer as the database function and transactions. In the future, this function will be implemented on a dedicated processor to permit an increase in the volume of documents.

## MEDICAL ENCODING BY PHYSICIANS

The medical records application captures the diagnoses and procedures for each patient during the course of hospitalization. Succinct medical summaries provide data on the activities of the various medical services and facilitate clinical research [1]. A pilot interactive system for recording diagnoses and procedures was installed in two medical departments in 1985. Interactive capturing of data at different terminals is progressively replacing the traditional manual method, which used preprinted coding sheets.

Physicians have interactive terminals in their offices. After finding a patient's name on the list of patients in the ward, the physician registers the diagnoses.

Three strategies for the establishment of diagnoses have been tried. The first involves surveying the list of the most frequently used terms for a specific service (up to 400 such terms are organized, according to the user's needs, in groups of up to 10 terms). The second involves choosing the code that corresponds to the appropriate diagnosis for a particular patient within a comprehensive alphabetical directory (comprising 7600 terms), and then entering this code at the terminal so as to check its translation into full text. The third strategy involves surveying, on the terminal screen, the complete tree of the International Classification of Diseases in order to identify the appropriate diagnosis. The same method is used to capture surgical procedures (2100 related terms defined). For each procedure, the physician also enters the date and the name of the surgeon.

Because the medical record includes demographic information supplied by the admissions service, as well as the history of the patient's stay provided by the nurses, a summary of the patient's stay can be made available (Fig. 4). Such summaries, in narrative form, contain information that will subsequently be made available for statistical and scientific investigation (e.g., calculation of case mix and retrieval of all cases with certain characteristics). The physician responsible for a medical service automatically receives a list of discharged patients who were under his or her care and whose summaries are not yet complete. Physicians are authorized to obtain an exhaustive coding of data on all patients. When signing the letter of discharge, the chief physician can check whether the coded information corresponds to the contents of the letter of discharge.

The aims of the documentation system are as follows: statistical analyses of diagnoses and surgical procedures, monitoring and comparing the activities of the medical services, retrieval of cases for inclusion in retrospective studies, case presentation for teaching, analyses of health care costs with respect to disorder, and etiologic study.

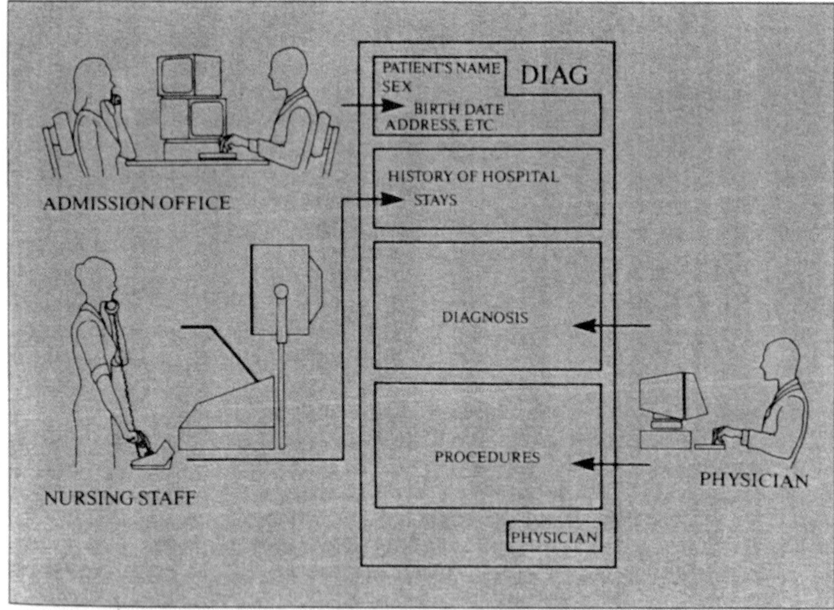



**Figure 4. Development of the medical summary describing the patient's stay. The admissions office enters the patient's identifying information, the nurses notify the operators of transfers, and the physicians enter the diagnoses and procedures.**

# THE FULLY INTEGRATED DATABASE FUNCTION IS UNDOUBTEDLY OF FOREMOST IMPORTANCE IN THE HOSPITAL INFORMATION SYSTEM.

## DISCUSSION

The change from traditional coding on forms to a system of interactive capture of information in text form has resulted, as would be expected, in considerable improvement in the quality and availability of information at our hospital. An interesting result has been the reaction of the medical personnel. After the introduction of the HIS, the doctors spontaneously rebelled against the imprecise terms found in the available classification systems, with the aim of replacing them with terms specific to nosologic entities, either general (large mesh), or detailed (fine mesh), according to the specialty or field concerned. Several aspects of the evolution of this application are notable: the replacement of the International Classification of Diseases, ninth revision, with a nomenclature more appropriate to the hospital's needs; the transcodification of this nomenclature back to existing international classifications, both documentary and statistical; and the extension of interactive methods of data entry to the description of clinical situations and important events occurring during a patient's stay.

The use of the DIOGENE system has been accompanied by a reduction in the average length of stay in the hospital—one of the original goals of the project—but this effect is probably the result of the large increase in outpatient consultations.

Now that the HIS has been in place for 11 years, we are more convinced than ever of the usefulness of such a system in a large university hospital. The success of the project from the users' standpoint has been demonstrated by continual requests for more features and a resulting need to enlarge the system. Indeed, integrated centralized systems will not last long unless they can evolve and grow toward distributed and open architectures.

The DIOGENE system is built around a central mainframe computer housing a unique database. Except for a proliferation of personal microcomputers, generally not connected to other computers, the DIOGENE system, with a single team of computer scientists, is responsible for all the computer-based functions and information in the hospital. The need for growth is critical, and migration to a second-generation hospital information system has been under study since 1986. New hardware, including the new generation of RISC machines, and new software have been selected, and a financial plan, together with a description of the objectives of the DIOGENE 2 system, has been submitted to the government of Geneva. The project was approved, with a 4-year budget, in May 1989.


## REFERENCES

1. Scherrer JR, Baud R, Brisebarre A, et al. A hospital information system in continuous operation and expansion. In: Orthner HF, Blum BI, eds. Implementing health care information systems. New York: Springer-Verlag, 1989:100-22.
2. Scherrer JR. The integrated real-time hospital information system: DIOGENE. World Hospital 1983; 19(4):8-11.
3. Berney JP, Baud R, Scherrer JR. Towards the use of a tree branching logic in the environment of a hospital information system. Methods Inf Med 1980; 19(4):187-94.
4. Assimacopoulos A, Baud RH, Rivollet R, et al. A computer station for the ward-unit adapted to routine work as well as to the permanent support and training of users. In: Lindberg DAB, Kaihara S, eds. MEDINFO 80: proceedings of the Third Conference on Medical Informatics. Amsterdam: North-Holland, 1980:1084-8.
5. McDonald CJ, Murray R, Jeris D, Bhargava B, Seeger J, Blevins L. A computer-based record and clinical monitoring system for ambulatory care. Am J Public Health 1977; 67:240-5.
6. Pryor TA, Gardner RM, Clayton PD, Warner HR. The HELP system. J Med Syst 1983; 7:87-102.
7. Simborg DW, Chadwick M, Whiting-O'Keefe QE, Tolchin SG, Kahn SA, Bergan ES. Local area networks and the hospital. Comput Biomed Res 1983; 16:247-59.
8. Stead WW, Hammond WE. Computerized medical records: a new resource for clinical decision making. J Med Syst 1983; 7:213-20.
9. Bakker AR. The development of an integrated and co-operative hospital information system. Med Inf 1984; 9:135-42.
10. Bleich HL, Beckley RF, Horowitz GL, et al. Clinical computing in a teaching hospital. N Engl J Med 1985; 312:756-64.
11. Whiting O'Keefe QE, Whiting A, Henke J. The STOR clinical information system. MD Comput 1988; 5(5):8-21.
12. The DIOGENE hospital information system. Geneva: Hôpital Cantonal Universitaire de Genève, 1983.
13. Scherrer JR. Organisation matricielle dynamique de l'hôpital. Journées d'informatique médicale francophones de Montpellier, Rennes: Editions Ecole Nationale de la Santé Publique, 1989:272-5.
14. Rouge A, Baud RH, Scherrer JR. An integrated network of telex printers within DIOGENE hospital information system. In: van Bemmel JH, Ball MJ, Wigertz O, eds. MEDINFO 83: proceedings of the Fourth Conference on Medical Informatics. Amsterdam: North-Holland, 1983:1159-62.



JEAN-RAOUL SCHERRER, M.D.
*Dr. Scherrer is an internist who received his M.D. from the Geneva University Medical School in 1959. From 1967 to 1969, he collaborated in research in physics at Brookhaven National Laboratory in New York. He became lecturer on medi-*

cal informatics at the Geneva University Medical School in 1971, and professor at the same medical school in 1979. He is now director of the Center for Informatics of the University Cantonal Hospital of Geneva. He has participated in the development of the DIOGENE system since the design stage in the 1970s. Dr. Scherrer is also interested in mathematical modeling and automatic encoding of clinical narratives.

### ROBERT H. BAUD, PH.D.

*Dr. Baud received a doctoral degree in physics at the University of Geneva in 1971. A visiting scientist at the European Center for Nuclear Research from 1967 to 1971 and a member of the staff of the DIOGENE HIS at the University Cantonal Hospital of Geneva since 1971, he is now vice-director of the Center for Informatics at the hospital. His chief interests are in software engineering, artificial intelligence in medicine, natural-language processing, and knowledge representation.*

### DENIS HOCHSTRASSER, M.D.

*Dr. Hochstrasser obtained his M.D. at the Geneva University Medical School. His residency was at the University of North Carolina at Chapel Hill, and he was a fellow in internal medicine at the University Cantonal Hospital of Geneva. He was a guest researcher in biochemical genetics at the National Institutes of Health for one year and is now attending physician on the medical ward at the University Cantonal Hospital of Geneva. Dr. Hochstrasser leads a group on numeric imaging at the hospital.*

### OSMAN RATIB, M.D., PH.D.

*Dr. Ratib is a certified cardiologist who received his M.D. at the Geneva University Medical School in 1979. He has been working in the field of medical imaging for the past 10 years and has written numerous articles on digital cardiac imaging. He received a Ph.D. in medical imaging at UCLA in 1989 and is now in charge of the development of a radiologic picture archiving and communication system at the University Cantonal Hospital of Geneva.*

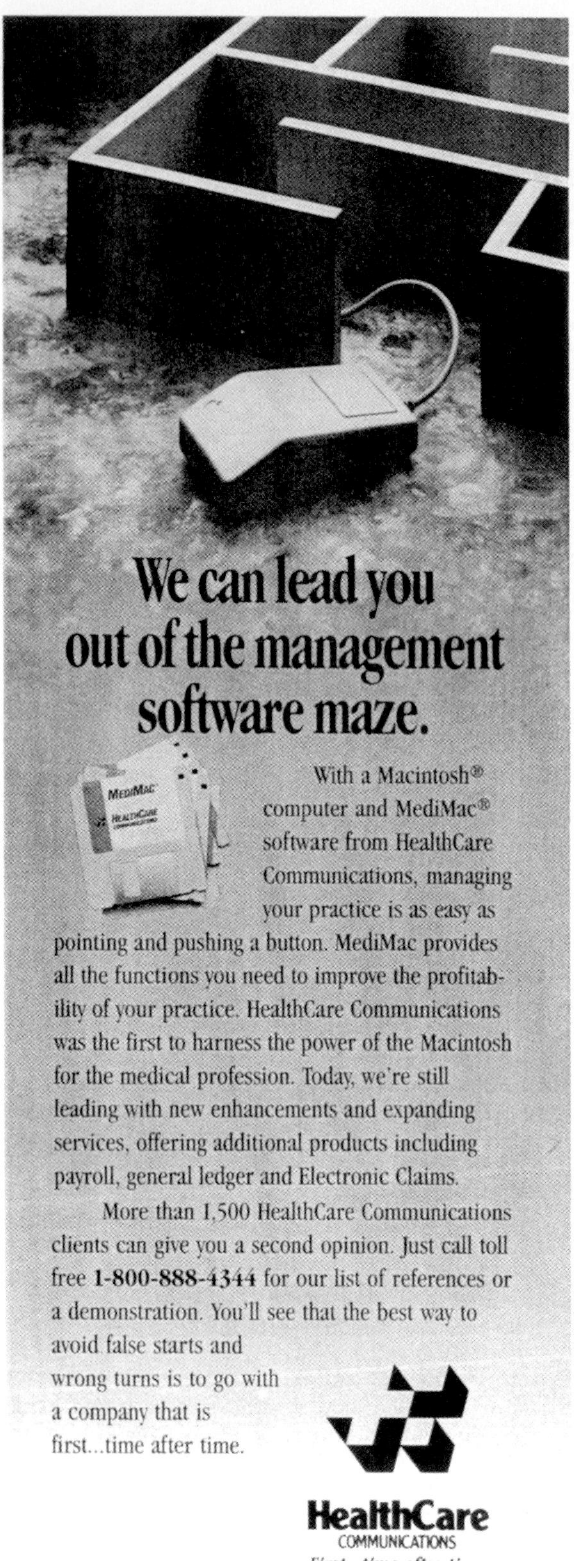

**CIRCLE NO. 18 ON READER SERVICE CARD**

# *IMIA Code of Ethics*

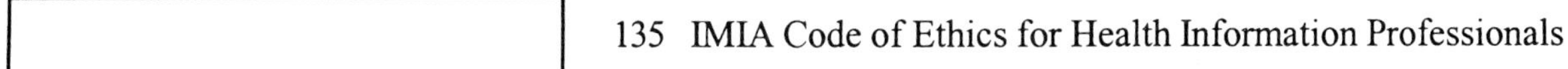

135   IMIA Code of Ethics for Health Information Professionals

**History**: This Code was developed by Working Group 4 as part of its mandate of dealing with policy matters in medical informatics that affect security and confidentiality. Initial work on the Code was begun in 1996 in Heemskerk under the direction of Ab Bakker as Chair of the Working Group, with Eike-Henner Kluge taking the lead in the development of the Code itself. Aspects of the Code were presented and discussed at WG4's meeting in 1998 in Helsinki, and the full draft was presented and finalized in 2000 at WG4's meeting in Victoria. The Code was then presented for comment and consideration at MedInfo 2001 in London, England. It was then posted on the IMIA website for further consideration and comments. WG4 also solicited comments from interested parties. The amended Code was adopted by the IMIA General Assembly at its meeting in Taipei on October 4, 2002. Like any Code, the IMIA Code of Ethics for Health Information Professionals is a living document subject to emendation, and WG4 has been given the mandate to exercise a watching brief in this regard.

# IMIA Code of Ethics for Health Informatics Professionals

## Preamble

Codes of professional ethics serve several purposes:

1. to provide ethical guidance for the professionals themselves,
2. to furnish a set of principles against which the conduct of the professionals may be measured, and
3. to provide the public with a clear statement of the ethical considerations that should shape the behaviour of the professionals themselves.

A Code of Ethics for Health Informatics Professionals (HIPs) should therefore be clear, unambiguous, and easily applied in practice. Moreover, since the field of informatics is in a state of constant flux, it should be flexible so as to accommodate ongoing changes without sacrificing the applicability of its basic principles. It is therefore inappropriate for a Code of Ethics for HIPs to deal with the specifics of every possible situation that might arise. That would make the Code too unwieldy, too rigid, and too dependent on the current state of informatics. Instead, such a Code should focus on the ethical position of the Health Informatics specialist as a professional, and on the relationships between HIPs and the various parties with whom they interact in a professional capacity. These various parties include (but are not limited to) patients, health care professionals, administrative personnel, health care institutions as well as insurance companies and governmental agencies, etc.

The reason for constructing a code of ethics for HIPs instead of merely adopting one of the codes that have been promulgated by the various general associations of informatics professionals is that HIPs play a unique role in the planning and delivery of health care: a role that is distinct from the role of other informatics professionals who work in different settings.

Part of this uniqueness is centred in the special relationship between the electronic health record (EHR) and the subject of that record. The EHR not only reveals much about the patient that is private and should be kept confidential but, more importantly, it functions as the basis of decisions that have a profound impact on the welfare of the patient. The patient is in a vulnerable position, and any decision regarding the patient and the EHR must acknowledge the fundamental necessity of striking an appropriate balance between ethically justified ends and otherwise appropriate means. Further, the data that are contained in the EHR also provide the raw materials for decision-making by health care institutions, governments and other agencies without which a system of health care delivery simply could not function. The HIP, therefore, by facilitating the construction, maintenance, storage, access, use and manipulation of EHRs, plays a role that is distinct from that of other informatics specialists.

At the same time, precisely because of this facilitating role, HIPs are embedded in a web of relationships that are subject to unique ethical constraints. Thus, over and above the ethical constraints that arise from the relationship between the electronic record and the patient, the ethical conduct of HIPs is also subject to considerations that arise out of the HIPs' interactions with Health Care Professionals (HCPs), health care institutions and other agencies. These constraints pull in different directions. It is therefore important that HIPs have some idea of how to resolve these issues in an appropriate fashion. A Code of Ethics for HIPs provides a tool in this regard, and may be of use in effecting a resolution when conflicting roles and constraints collide.

A Code of Ethics for HIPs is also distinct from an account of legally conferred duties and rights. Unquestionably, the law provides the regulatory setting in which HIPs carry out their activities. However, ethical conduct frequently goes beyond what the law requires. The reason is that legal regulations have purely juridical significance and represent, as it were, a minimum standard as envisioned by legislators, juries and judges. However, these standards are formulated on the basis of circumstances as they obtain here and now; they are not anticipatory in nature and therefore can provide little guidance for a rapidly evolving discipline in which new types of situations constantly arise. HIPs who only followed the law, and who only adjusted their conduct to legal precedent, would be ill equipped to deal with situations that were not envisioned by the lawmakers and would be subject to the vagaries of the next judicial process.

On the other hand, a Code of Ethics for HIPs is grounded in fundamental ethical principles as these apply to the types of situations that characterize the activities of the Health Informatics specialist. Consequently such a Code, centring in the very essence of what it is to be an HIP, is independent of the vagaries of the judicial process and, rather than following it, may well guide it; and rather than becoming invalidated by changes in technology or administrative fashion, may well indicate the direction in which these developments should proceed. Therefore, while in many cases the clauses of such a Code will be reflected in corresponding juridical injunctions or administrative provisions, they provide guidance through times of legal or administrative uncertainty and in areas where corresponding laws or administrative provisions do not exist. At a more general level, such a Code may even assist in the resolution of the problems posed by the technological imperative. Not everything that can be done should be done. A Code of Ethics assists in defining the ethical landscape.

The Code of Ethics that follows was developed on the basis of these considerations. It has two parts:

### 1. Introduction
This part begins with a set of *fundamental ethical principles* that have found general international acceptance. Next is a brief list of *general principles of informatic ethics that* follow from these fundamental ethical principles when these are applied to the electronic gathering, processing, storing, communicating, using, manipulating and accessing of health information in general. These general principles of informatic ethics are high-level principles and provide general guidance.

### 2. Rules of Ethical Conduct for HIPs
This part lays out a detailed set of ethical rules of behaviour for HIPs. These rules are developed by applying the general principles of informatic ethics to the types of relationships that characterize the professional lives of HIPs. They are more specific than the general principles of informatic ethics, and offer more particular guidance.

The precise reasoning that shows how the *Principles of Informatic Ethics* follow from the *Fundamental Ethical Principles,* and that indicates how the *Principles of Informatic Ethics* give rise to the more specific *Rules of Ethical Conduct for HIPs* is contained in a separate *Handbook* and may be consulted there for greater clarity.

It should also be noted that the *Code of Ethics* and the accompanying set of *Rules of Ethical Conduct* do not include what might be called "technical" provisions. That is to say, they do not make reference to such things as technical standards of secure data communication, or to provisions that are necessary to ensure a high quality in the handling, collecting, storing, transmitting, manipulating, etc. of health care data. This is deliberate. While the development and implementation of technical standards has ethical dimensions, and while these dimensions are reflected in the *Code* and the *Rules* as ethical duties, the details of such technical standards are not themselves a matter of ethics.

# Part I.

## *Introduction*

### A. Fundamental Ethical Principles

All social interactions are subject to fundamental ethical principles. HIPs function in a social setting. Consequently, their actions are also subject to these principles. The most important of these principles are:

1. *Principle of Autonomy*
   All persons have a fundamental right to self-determination.

2. *Principle of Equality and Justice*
   All persons are equal as persons and have a right to be treated accordingly.

3. *Principle of Beneficence*
   All persons have a duty to advance the good of others where the nature of this good is in keeping with the fundamental and ethically defensible values of the affected party.

4. *Principle of Non-Malfeasance*
   All persons have a duty to prevent harm to other persons insofar as it lies within their power to do so without undue harm to themselves.

5. *Principle of Impossibility*
   All rights and duties hold subject to the condition that it is possible to meet them under the circumstances that obtain.

6. *Principle of Integrity*
   Whoever has an obligation, has a duty to fulfil that obligation to the best of her or his ability.

### B. General Principles of Informatic Ethics

These fundamental ethical principle, when applied to the types of situations that characterize the informatics setting, give rise to general ethical principles of informatic ethics.

1. *Principle of Information-Privacy and Disposition*
   All persons have a fundamental right to privacy, and hence to control over the collection, storage, access, use, communication, manipulation and disposition of data about themselves.

2. *Principle of Openness*
   The collection, storage, access, use, communication, manipulation and disposition of personal data must be disclosed in an appropriate and timely fashion to the subject of those data.

3. *Principle of Security*
   Data that have been legitimately collected about a person should be protected by all reasonable and appropriate measures against loss, degradation, unauthorized destruction, access, use, manipulation, modification or communication.

4. *Principle of Access*
   The subject of an electronic record has the right of access to that record and the right to correct the record with respect to its accurateness, completeness and relevance.

5. *Principle of Legitimate Infringement*
   The fundamental right of control over the collection, storage, access, use, manipulation, communication and disposition of personal data is conditioned only by the legitimate, appropriate and relevant data-needs of a free, responsible and democratic society, and by the equal and competing rights of other persons.

6. *Principle of the Least Intrusive Alternative*
   Any infringement of the privacy rights of the individual person, and of the individual's right to control over person-relative data as mandated under *Principle 1*, may only occur in the least intrusive fashion and with a minimum of interference with the rights of the affected person.

7. *Principle of Accountability*
   Any infringement of the privacy rights of the individual person, and of the right to control over person-relative data, must be justified to the affected person in good time and in an appropriate fashion.

These general principles of informatic ethics, when applied to the types of relationships into which HIPs enter in their professional lives, and to the types of situations that they encounter when thus engaged, give rise to more specific ethical duties. The *Rules of Conduct for HIPs* that follow outline the more important of these ethical duties. It should be noted that as with any ethical rules of conduct, the *Rules* cannot do more than provide guidance. The precise way in which the *Rules* apply in a given context, and the precise nature of a particular ethical right or obligation, depends on the specific nature of the relevant situation.

# Part II.

### *Rules of Ethical Conduct for HIPs*

The rules of ethical conduct for HIPs can be broken down into six general rubrics, each of which has various sub-sections. The general rubrics demarcate the different domains of the ethical relationships that obtain between HIPs and specific stakeholders; the sub-sections detail the specifics of these relationships.

## A. Subject-centred duties

These are duties that derive from the relationship in which HIPs stand to the subjects of the electronic records or to the subjects of the electronic communications that are facilitated by the HIPs through their professional actions.

1. HIPs have a duty to ensure that the potential subjects of electronic records are aware of the existence of systems, programmes or devices whose purpose it is to collect and/or communicate data about them.

2. HIPs have a duty to ensure that appropriate procedures are in place so that:
   a. electronic records are established or communicated only with the voluntary, competent and informed consent of the subjects of those records, and
   b. if an electronic record is established or communicated in contravention of **A.2.a**, the need to establish or communicate such a record has been demonstrated on independent ethical grounds to the subject of the record, in good time and in an appropriate fashion.

3. HIPs have a duty to ensure that the subject of an electronic record is made aware that

a. an electronic record has been established about her/him,
b. who has established the record and who continues to maintain it,
c. what is contained in the electronic record,
d. the purpose for which it is established,
e. the individuals, institutions or agencies who have access to it or to whom it (or an identifiable part of it) may be communicated,
f. where the electronic record is maintained,
g. the length of time it will be maintained, and
h. the ultimate nature of its disposition.

4. HIPs have a duty to ensure that the subject of an electronic record is aware of the origin of the data contained in the record.

5. HIPs have a duty to ensure that the subject of an electronic record is aware of any rights that he or she may have with respect to
   a. access, use and storage,
   b. communication and manipulation,
   c. quality and correction, and
   d. disposition
   of her or his electronic record and of the data contained in it.

6. HIPs have a duty to ensure that
   a. electronic records are stored, accessed, used, manipulated or communicated only for legitimate purposes;
   b. there are appropriate protocols and mechanisms in place to monitor the storage, accessing, use, manipulation or communication of electronic records, or of the data contained in them, in accordance with section **A.6.a**;
   c. there are appropriating protocols and mechanisms in place to act on the basis of the information under section **A.6.b** as and when

the occasion demands;
d. the existence of these protocols and mechanisms is known to the subjects of electronic records, and
e. there are appropriate means for subjects of electronic records to enquire into and to engage the relevant review protocols and mechanisms.

7. HIPs have a duty to treat the duly empowered representatives of the subjects of electronic records as though they had the same rights concerning the electronic records as the subjects of the record themselves, and that the duly empowered representatives (and, if appropriate, the subjects of the records themselves) are aware of this fact.

8. HIPs have a duty to ensure that all electronic records are treated in a just, fair and equitable fashion.

9. HIPs have a duty to ensure that appropriate measures are in place that may reasonably be expected to safeguard the
   a. security,
   b. integrity,
   c. material quality,
   d. usability, and
   e. accessibility
   of electronic records.

10. HIPs have a duty to ensure, insofar as this lies within their power, that an electronic record or the data contained in it are used only
    a. for the stated purposes for which the data were collected, or
    b. for purposes that are otherwise ethically defensible.

11. HIPs have a duty to ensure that the subjects of electronic records or communications are aware of possible breaches of the preceding duties and the reason for them.

## B. Duties towards HCPs

HCPs who care for patients depend on the technological skills of HIPs in the fulfilment of their patient-centred obligations. Consequently, HIPs have an obligation to assist these HCPs insofar as this is compatible with the HIPs' primary duty towards the subjects of the electronic records. Specifically, this means that

1. HIPs have a duty
   a. to assist duly empowered HCPs who are engaged in patient care in having appropriate, timely and secure access to relevant electronic records (or parts of thereof), and to ensure the usability, integrity, and highest possible technical quality of these records; and
   b. to provide those informatic services that might be necessary for the HCPs to carry out their mandate.

2. HIPs should keep HCPs informed of the status of the informatic services on which the HCPs rely, and immediately advise them of any problems or difficulties that might be associated or that could reasonably be expected to arise in connection with these informatic services.

3. HIPs should advise the HCPs with whom they interact on a professional basis, or for whom they provide professional services, of any circumstances that might prejudice the objectivity of the advice they give or that might impair the nature or quality of the services that they perform for the HCPs.

4. HIPs have a general duty to foster an environment that is conducive to the maintenance of the highest possible ethical and material standards of data collection, storage, management, communication and use by HCPs within the health care setting.

5. HCPs who are directly involved in the construction of electronic records may have an intellectual property right in certain formal features of these records. Consequently, HIPs have a duty to safeguard
   a. those formal features of the electronic record, or
   b. those formal features of the data collection, retrieval, storage or usage system in which the electronic record is embedded
in which the HCP has, or may reasonably be expected to have, an intellectual property interest.

## C. Duties towards institutions/ employers

1. HIPs owe their employers and the institutions in which they work a duty of
   a. competence,
   b. diligence,
   c. integrity, and
   d. loyalty.

2. HIPs have a duty to
   a. foster an ethically sensitive security culture in the institutional setting in which they practice their profession,
   b. facilitate the planning and implementation of the best and most appropriate data security measures possible for the institutional setting in which they work,
   c. implement and maintain the highest possible qualitative standards of data collection, storage, retrieval, processing, accessing, communication and utilization in all areas of their professional endeavour.

3. HIPs have a duty to ensure, to the best of their ability, that appropriate structures are in place to evaluate the technical, legal and ethical acceptability of the data-collection, storage, retrieval, processing, accessing, communication, and utilization of data in the settings in which they carry out their work or with which they are affiliated.

4. HIPs have a duty to alert, in good time and in a suitable manner, appropriately placed decision-makers of the security- and quality-status of the data-generating, storing, accessing, handling and communication systems, programmes, devices or procedures of the institution with which they are affiliated or of the employers for whom they provide professional services.

5. HIPs should immediately inform the institutions with which they are affiliated or the employers for whom they provide a professional service of any problems or difficulties that could reasonably be expected to arise in connection with the performance of their contractually stipulated services.

6. HIPs should immediately inform the institutions with which they are affiliated or the employers for whom they provide a professional service of circumstances that might prejudice the objectivity of the advice they give.

7. Except in emergencies, HIPs should only provide services in their areas of competence; however, they should always be honest and forthright about their education, experience or training.

8. HIPs should only use suitable and ethically acquired or developed tools, techniques or devices in the execution of their duties.

9. HIPs have a duty to assist in the development and provision of

appropriate informatics-oriented educational services in the institution with which they are affiliated or for the employer for whom they work.

## D. Duties towards society

1. HIPs have a duty to facilitate the appropriate
   a. collection,
   b. storage,
   c. communication,
   d. use, and
   e. manipulation

of health care data that are necessary for the planning and providing of health care services on a social scale.

2. HIPs have a duty to ensure that
   a. only data that are relevant to legitimate planning needs are collected;
   b. the data that are collected are de-identified or rendered anonymous as much as possible, in keeping with the legitimate aims of the collection;
   c. the linkage of data bases can occur only for otherwise legitimate and defensible reasons that do not violate the fundamental rights of the subjects of the records; and
   d. only duly authorised persons have access to the relevant data.

3. HIPs have a duty to educate the public about the various issues associated with the nature, collection, storage and use of electronic health-data and to make society aware of any problems, dangers, implications or limitations that might reasonably be associated with the collection, storage, usage and manipulation of socially relevant health data.

4. HIPs will refuse to participate in or support practices that violate human rights.

5. HIPs will be responsible in setting the fee for their services and in their demands for working conditions, benefits, etc.

## E. Self-regarding duties

HIPs have a duty to
1. recognize the limits of their competence,
2. consult when necessary or appropriate,
3. maintain competence,
4. take responsibility for all actions performed by them or under their control,
5. avoid conflict of interest,
6. give appropriate credit for work done, and
7. act with honesty, integrity and diligence.

## F. Duties towards the profession

1. HIPs have a duty always to act in such a fashion as not to bring the profession into disrepute.

2. HIPs have a duty to assist in the development of the highest possible standards of professional competence, to ensure that these standards are publicly known, and to see that they are applied in an impartial and transparent manner.

3. HIPs will refrain from impugning the reputation of colleagues but will report to the appropriate authority any unprofessional conduct by a colleague.

4. HIPs have a duty to assist their colleagues in living up to the highest technical and ethical standards of the profession.

5. HIPs have a duty to promote the understanding, appropriate utilization, and ethical use of health information technologies, and to advance and further the discipline of Health Informatics.

# *Review Section*

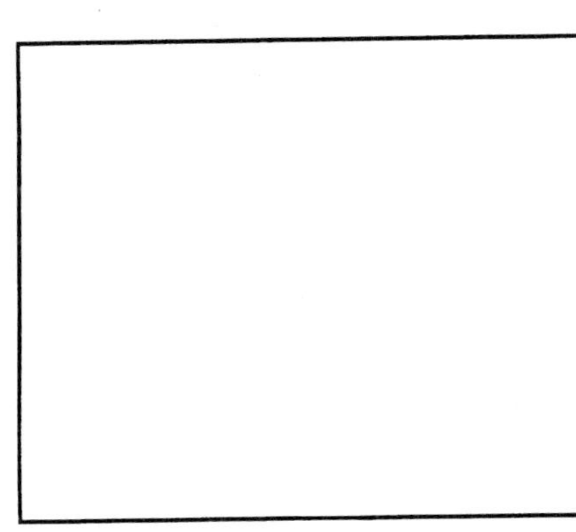

**A. Hasman[a], C. Safran[b],
H. Takeda[c]**

[a] Department of Medical Informatics
University Maastricht
The Netherlands

[b] Harvard Medical School
Boston, MA
and Clinician Support Technology
Newton, MA, USA

[c] Department of Medical Information
Science, Graduate School of Medicine
Osaka University, Japan

# Review

# *Quality of health care: informatics foundations.*

**Abstract**: In this article we will discuss in what ways computer systems can contribute to the quality of healthcare and on which principles of informatics successful systems are founded. Section 2 presents an overview of studies that investigate the usefulness of decision support, and Section 3 discusses factors that determine the success of decision support systems. The foundations of guideline systems are presented in Section 4. Section 5 offers a brief review of physician order entry, and Section 6 presents a discussion of medical risk management and the results of Japanese studies in this area.

## 1. Background

In the past, clinical information systems were used in healthcare mainly for administrative purposes and for recording medical patient data. The medical data concerned medication, clinical laboratory results, EKG analyses and radiology reports, for example. Narratives, including medical history, results of physical examination and progress notes were often only recorded on paper.

Other groups were developing decision support systems (DSS) in order to raise the quality of healthcare. These were usually stand-alone systems designed to help physicians solve a diagnostic or therapeutic problem. Solving therapeutic problems mainly concerned dosage determinations. Diagnostic problems usually were differential diagnosis problems. The physician or nurse had already limited the search space to a few hypotheses that were further analysed by the decision support system. The decision support systems used statistical meth-

ods (Bayes' rule, regression, pattern recognition methods like linear discriminant analysis, etc.), fuzzy logic or decision trees.

Later, artificial intelligence (AI) approaches (symbolic reasoning) were introduced. Instead of statistical programs, where physicians made decisions on the basis of calculated probabilities that were difficult to interpret, now the programs were able to explain their decisions by showing the reasoning steps that led to the solution. Related to AI research is research concerning neural networks and genetic algorithms. These approaches are also used in some diagnostic systems.

A number of diagnostic systems covered a broad range of diseases: Internist [1], QMR [2], Iliad [3] and Dxplain [4]. Diseases that explain the entered findings are displayed and hints are given to ask for other findings in order to reduce the number of possible diagnoses. The main disadvantage of these systems was that they were usually slow and because the systems

were stand-alone, the physician or nurse had to evoke the program and had to enter a large amount of data.

Blois [5] argued that computer support makes most sense at the end of the clinical judgment process. He compared this process with a funnel, with its large diameter at the onset of the process and its small end at the conclusion. The decreasing diameter of the funnel represents the shrinking cognitive span required by the physician. For situations at the beginning of the process, the totality of possibilities must be confronted; whereas for situations at the end of the process, the task domain is already structured through previous human effort, an abstraction is available, and only a little common sense knowledge may be required. Physicians can readily deal with the first type of broad and unstructured situation. They also perform well in more structured settings, although there are a growing number of specific and computable processes that may enable a computer to outperform physicians here.

Decision support programs such as protocol systems and reminder systems not only help in decision-making but also support therapy decisions and management of the patient.

The question is whether computerized decision support makes the healthcare process more efficient and/or leads to better patient outcomes. And if so, does this imply that physicians or nurses will automatically use these systems, or are there also other factors that influence the success of a decision support system?

Medical risk management is another area where the use of Information and Communication Technology (ICT) can be very useful. Compared to other industries, quality management of health care services has not been successful. A 1999 Institute of Medicine (IOM) report estimates that between 44,000 to 98,000 hospital patients die each year due to medical errors [6].

Risk management is a process of identifying, assessing and evaluating risks that have adverse effects on the quality, safety and effectiveness of service delivery, and taking positive action to eliminate or reduce these effects. Medical record review, clinical incident reporting and other methods can detect adverse events. Incidents are events that produce, or have the potential to produce, unexpected or unwanted outcomes that affect the safety of patients, users or other persons. However, if the documents are paper-based, it will take time and consume health care resources to communicate, archive them and later feed the results back [7].

Risk management is also important to ICT applications. Information systems can contain wrong code, standards for communication can be incorrectly applied, knowledge in decision support systems can be wrong,

etc. Therefore, and especially for decision support systems, it should be clear that the systems are not hazardous instead of providing useful advice [8].

The primary objective of the quantitative approach of medical risk management is to electronically collect data on incidents and to evaluate the possible causes of these incidents is [9]. Incident reports (IR) are analyzed to determine latent and active errors and to rank the incidents in order of risk severity. Action is then planned and implemented to prevent the event from recurring. Effective actions include simplifying systems, standardizing procedures, introducing constraints, using reminders and checklists, providing timely information, and facilitating small-group interactive education.

Incident-reporting systems may produce potentially valuable information, but seriously underestimate the true level of incidents [10]. Deming [11] suggested 14 principles for the transformation of quality management in medical service. Among them, he listed, "Require statistical evidence of quality of incoming materials, such as pharmaceuticals, serums and equipment. Inspection is not the answer. Inspection is too late and unreliable. Inspection does not produce quality. The quality is already built in and paid for." The importance of applying industrial quality management science to health care was already pointed out a decade ago [12]. However, only advanced ICT is able to acquire and integrate the care process data.

A suitably designed electronic patient record system (EPR) will be a potent tool for directly identifying sources of health care incidents, errors and accidents and will provide quantitative information. The EPR can be used on the site of health care for quick and easy safety checks. For

example, by scanning the identification bracelet on a patient's wrist that patient's EPR will appear on the computer screen. Then the bar code on the drug to be given at that time, ordered by the patient's doctor, is scanned. If all is fine, the computer gives no alert and instantly changes the medical record to show that the treatment was given.

The EPR database provides a quantitative basis for risk and quality management, since the medical record includes information about the process and outcome of a patient's health care. If the methodology is established, quality management in health care will reach the same level as that of the production of goods. Quality management would be enhanced if a quality manager were allowed to link EPR data within an institution. Institutional or patient permission should be obtained for accessing these data for quality management purposes provided a security policy guideline is followed.

## 2. Do decision support systems help?

The debate over health system reform and the intensive search for cost-effective methods repeatedly highlight the need for adequate technology assessment of clinical information systems. Initially DSS were largely conceived as oracles, with clinicians seen as passive recipients of the system's advice. Early evaluation studies therefore focused on the accuracy of information generated by the computer system (e.g. [2-4]). Not all studies describe the performance using similar metrics and consequently it is difficult to compare the results. Berner et al. examined the performance of four DSS on a common set of cases and proposed a set of scores to describe different aspects of their performance [13].

The question of primary interest nowadays is the extent to which the system improves the diagnostic hypotheses of clinicians, not the extent to which its advice is correct. Since most broad-based, general DSS produce a list of diagnoses for each case, their effect on the process of care is not directly evident, even if we have determined the performance of the system. In addition as Elstein et al. [14] indicate, the issue is not how well the DSS reasons to a conclusion given a complete database. Rather, given the necessarily incomplete database that a puzzled clinician might have assembled in the workup of a diagnostically challenging case, to what extent does the DSS improve the quality of the differential diagnosis and/or suggest the relevant clinical findings needed to reach a more definitive conclusion. Friedman et al. [15] showed that "hands-on" use of diagnostic DSS can influence the diagnostic reasoning of clinicians. The overall increase in diagnostic quality scores due to a DSS was shown to be between the effect size typically considered small and medium in magnitude.

Balas et al. [16] systematically reviewed randomised controlled clinical trials of computer interventions and demonstrated significant improvements in the process and outcome of care due to these interventions. The most frequently studied and most successful interventions included patient and physician reminders, computer-assisted patient education and computerized treatment planners. Since the authors employed the vote-counting method for evaluating success rates, the magnitude of the effect could not be determined.

Shea et al. [17] carried out a meta-analysis of studies that investigated (via randomised controlled trials) the potential of reminder systems to improve preventive services in ambulatory settings. Sixteen separate randomised controlled studies were identified. The preventive services were grouped into six categories (vaccinations, breast cancer screening, colorectal cancer screening, cardiovascular risk reduction, cervical cancer screening and other preventive services). The studies showed that in four out of six categories, computer reminders increased preventive practices compared with a control group. The overall increase in the odds ratio attributable to computer generated reminders compared with the control condition across different preventive services was found to be 77%. The interpretation of this effect in terms of an absolute increase in delivery of preventive services to patients depends on the baseline prevalence of compliance with the recommended preventive service. For example, if the baseline is 50%, this increase in odds ratio implies an increase to 64%.

The findings imply that the physicians and other providers accepted the recommendations implicit in the alerts. The authors indicate that preventive services are an area where despite many areas of ongoing controversy a consensus exists regarding a substantial number of practices. They conclude that it is more important that users reach a consensus on appropriate guidelines than that they accept the computer as a way of delivering reminders (since manual reminders were also effective, although less than computer reminders). Austin et al. [18] analysed trials that assessed the effects of computer-based reminder systems on cervical cancer screening and tetanus immunization. This meta-analysis demonstrated a beneficial effect in both cases.

Johnston et al. [19] reviewed evidence from controlled trials of the effects of computer-based clinical decision support systems on clinical performance and patient outcome. Four different types of support were identified: drug dose determination, diagnosis, enhancing quality of preventive and active medical care. Of the 28 studies, ten studied patient outcome and only three of them showed statistically significant benefits. This small number may be due to small sample sizes. DSS for dose determination and diagnosis hardly were effective. Again reminders and feedback generally had positive effects on the process but effects on patient outcomes could hardly be shown.

In a follow-up review (Hunt et al. [20]) it was concluded that given the new evidence it is now reasonable to use decision support systems for potentially toxic, intravenously administered medications. These medications can be more effectively titrated than without using a decision support system. No new clinical trials of diagnostic decision aids were found. The authors concluded that decision support systems can enhance clinical performance for drug dosing, preventive care, and other aspects of medical care, but not convincingly for diagnosis.

Balas et al. [21] studied whether prompting physicians improved preventive care. They concluded that prompting leads to a significant improvement in health maintenance: the cumulative health maintenance rate difference (defined as the ratio of the number of preventive care actions to the number of eligible physician-patient encounters) was 13.1%. The method of presenting the prompt (attachment to the record, computer monitor display, tagged progress notes) did not have an effect on the clinical response. Also the method by which the prompts were generated (computerized or not) did not lead to significant differences.

Oxman et al. [22] determined the effectiveness of different types of interventions in improving health professional performance and health outcomes. They emphasize that several interventions (educational material, conferences, outreach visits, local opinion leaders, patient mediated interventions, audit and feedback, reminders, etc.) have been found to improve provider performance and to a lesser degree health outcomes. They drew an analogy between trials of interventions to improve the performance of healthcare professionals and drug trials. There are no wonder drugs; often several medications are needed, along with lifestyle and environmental changes, to effect clinically important changes in health status. It is the same with the alteration of health professional performance: many interventions have modest or negligible practical effects when used alone. However, when coupled with other strategies the effects may be cumulative and significant.

Clinical practice guidelines are systematically developed statements to assist practitioner and patient decisions about appropriate healthcare for specific clinical circumstances [23]. Studies have shown the benefits of using clinical guidelines in the practice of medicine [24]. Although the importance of guidelines is widely recognized, health care organizations typically pay more attention to guideline development than to guideline implementation for routine use in daily care. Implementing guidelines in computer-based DSS promises to improve the acceptance and application of guidelines. According to the IOM, DSS are in fact crucial elements in long-term strategies that promote the use of guidelines [25].

## 3. What factors determine the success of decision support systems?

Clinicians complain that they have less time available than in the past because of increasing patient volumes, greater demands for documentation and the complexity of modern practice. To be successful, decision support systems therefore have to be faster than the current way of working. According to Payne [26], advice based on guidelines is most useful if the recommendations are based on each patient's data. These data should be available in machine-processible form instead of having to be entered by the user, which costs more time.

Decision support systems can be passive, containing heavily indexed information that must be searched by the users. Passive display of guideline documents in the literature, on the Web, or on other electronic media for example is not always an effective or reliable method for obtaining decision support since it takes time to retrieve the guideline and find the relevant information and because it is not always directly clear what the quality of the guideline is.

The success of active decision support systems depends to a large extent on the direct availability of patient data. Current electronic patient records provide a repository of patient data that can be used by the DSS. These data can only be used when they are stored in the same format as needed by the DSS and when the semantics of the data is the same. Standardisation of terminology is therefore very important.

Additionally, the systems should be incorporated into the workflow of the clinic. Healthcare delivery is a complex effort with labour divided among many professions. Decision support systems should be designed to fit into this workflow as smoothly as possible, because changing the workflow of many professionals is difficult.

Decision support systems sometimes come under criticism as examples of cookbook medicine because they appear to provide knowledge of a clinical nature, to show initiative, and to correct physician behaviour. Questions may arise about whether they might increase malpractice liability if a clinician chooses to ignore a suggestion from the system [27]. However, it should be made clear to the user that the system functions as an active partner, providing important information at the right time so that the clinician can make the right decision about a patient's care.

## 4. Informatics foundations of decision support systems

Reggia and Tuhrim [28] documented many of the early approaches to computer-assisted medical decision-making. Artificial intelligence approaches are described in Miller [29]. The approaches can be characterized by the way the knowledge is represented and by the type of reasoning (inference method) that is carried out. Reggia and Tuhrim discern a number of methodologies:

- **conventional programming methods** (formulas and branching logic as knowledge representation and calculation with formulas or traversal of branching logic as inference method),
- **statistical pattern classification** (prior and conditional probabilities or discriminant functions as knowledge representation and calculation of posterior probabilities, calculation of discriminant scores as inference method),
- **production rules** (rules as knowledge representation and deduction as inference method) and cognitive models (frames, semantic networks as knowledge representation and hypothesize and test (abduction) as inference method).

The reminder systems that were described in the studies Shea et al. [17] investigated shared the above-mentioned design philosophy: an expert system monitors the clinical database and makes use of a knowledge base in which the logic that triggers the reminders is represented. The reminders are data-generated rather than sought by the user.

The knowledge usually is elicited from experts. Knowledge discovery techniques (data mining, machine learning) are also used to extract knowledge from existing databases. The knowledge, however obtained, has to be represented in a way that the DSS can reason with it. Knowledge editors are usually available to enter knowledge in the right format.

We will focus here on issues concerning the representation of guidelines. Implementation of guidelines in DSS is not easy. Guidelines are usually in narrative form and have to be formalized before they can be used in DSS. Also the terminology used in the guidelines can impede implementation, especially when they have to be integrated with electronic patient records, because the terminology that is used in both is likely to be different. To facilitate the (re-)use of a guideline among different institutions, the representation should support the use of standard medical terminology.

In order to alleviate the problem of disseminating guidelines to other institutions a formal guideline model is needed. A formal and expressive guideline model will provide 1) an in-depth understanding of the clinical procedures addressed by the guideline; 2) a precise and unambiguous description of the guideline; and 3) a means for automatic parsers to execute guidelines. The representation formalism must be able to represent relatively simple guidelines that model independent modular rules, but also complex ones that use notions such as temporal abstraction and scheduling.

Guidelines contain decisions and actions as individual steps. Decisions are expressed by means of logical expressions and therefore the guideline representation formalism must support some form of (temporal) logic and uncertainty handling. Entry points (depending on the patient state) have to be used as an entrance into a complex guideline for a specific patient. In a similar way exit points have to be defined. Although the format of these expressions is similar to the logical expressions used in decisions, in complex guidelines they should be distinguished from these normal decision points.

Actions refer to clinical interventions and information gathering. Again these actions must be expressed in terms of domain-specific concepts. Since guidelines describe a process, the representation formalism must allow the representation of the order in which actions and decisions have to be carried out. In this section we will describe a number of published guideline models.

The Arden syntax [30] was developed as a response to the inability to share medical knowledge among different institutions. The representation encodes modular guidelines as Medical Logic Modules (MLM). Each MLM contains a production rule that relates a set of input conditions to a particular set of actions to take. Most MLMs are triggered by clinical events. Since the guidelines are modelled as independent modular rules, the syntax is usually used for representing simple guidelines, like the ones providing alerts in feedback systems. The Arden syntax does not support standard terminologies. Therefore sharing of MLMs among institutions is not that easy. Since MLMs are modular rules there are no concepts that correspond to entry points. Instead MLMs contain an evoke slot in which events are specified that will fire an MLM.

The Guideline Interchange Format (GLIF) was developed to model guidelines in terms of a flowchart that consists of structured scheduling steps, representing clinical actions and decisions. The intended purpose of GLIF is to facilitate sharing of guidelines between various institutions by modelling guidelines in such a manner that the guidelines are understandable by human experts as well as by automatic parsers used in different clinical decision support systems. GLIF is an object-oriented representation, consisting of a set of classes that describe characteristic guideline entities (e.g. actions and decisions), attributes for those classes and data types for the attribute values.

The first published version of GLIF [31] distinguishes a number of guideline steps (action, conditional, branch and synchronization). Conditional steps model decision points and direct flow from one guideline step to another. Branch steps direct flow to multiple guideline steps. Attributes of the branch step specify whether all, some or only one of these steps should actually be carried out and in which sequence. Synchronization steps are used in conjunction with branching steps. The multiple guideline steps that follow a branch step always converge in a corresponding synchronization step.

In GLIF2 most of the attributes were text strings that were not easily interpretable by parsers. To address this and other issues a new version, GLIF3 [32], is now under development. It includes among others a more formal expression syntax and a number of new guideline steps.

PROforma [8, 33] is a knowledge composition language supported by acquisition and execution tools with the goal of supporting guideline dissemination in the form of expert systems that assist patient care through active decision support and workflow management.

PROforma addresses two aspects of the guideline development and implementation process. First it defines an abstract model that represents the general clinical decision-making process, called the domino model. The model assumes that a trigger may lead to the recognition of some kind of clinical problem, which requires a solution. The next step is to apply some kind of problem solving process to identify possible solutions to the problem. These possible solutions are then evaluated to determine the strengths and weaknesses of each solution. Based on the outcome of the evaluation, a care provider can decide to adopt a certain solution by selecting the corresponding care plan. Alternatively, a care provider can decide that additional data (for example based on new patient data) are required to select the most favourable solution. Once a care plan has been adopted, the sequence of clinical actions needed to execute the plan is scheduled and carried out. Finally, executing a care plan may involve new clinical actions that require additional clinical patient data such as relevant symptoms and additional lab data.

To represent the domino model PROforma defines a task ontology that contains all concepts required to model various types of guidelines. Each guideline is modelled as a plan consisting of a sequence of tasks (plans, decisions, actions and enquiries). Guidelines are stored using the Red Representation Language, a time-oriented knowledge representation language [8].

Asbru is a guideline representation formalism, developed at Stanford University and the Vienna University of Technology and is part of the Asgaard project, which focuses on the application of time-oriented clinical guidelines [34]. The Asbru language is a plan representation language that represents clinical guidelines as time-oriented skeletal plans.

EON, also developed at Stanford University, is a component-based architecture used to build decision-support systems that reason about guideline-directed care [35]. Similar to GLIF, the guideline model of EON, called Dharma, is object-oriented and consists of classes that describe guideline entities as a sequence of structured temporal steps. Besides the Dharma guideline model, the EON architecture also contains a number of run-time components, used to construct execution-time systems.

When a guideline model is available, tools can be designed that support the specification of guidelines. Some examples of knowledge editors are described in the literature [33], [36] and [37].

---

# 5. Physician Order Entry

Computer programs to improve quality in healthcare work best when integrated into the background of clinical workflow. As McDonald and many others have shown [38], physicians can get an A on factual tests, but sometimes get B's or C's in real life settings when their performance is compared against quality measures. The major problem seems to be a failure to attend to a situation rather than a lack of knowledge. The attention of physicians is diverted by increasing workloads, increasing complexity of care management, increasing demands for documentation and the resulting decrease in time for each clinical encounter. Clinical computing systems that have alerts and reminders, clinical checklists, and clinical practice guidelines as active components seem to be effective and generally well accepted.

Curiously, the wide practice variation that results from non-adherence to these types of rules rarely can be shown to affect patient outcomes such as long-term survival. One area of computer-based crosschecking that has shown the most promise in the past several years has been Physician Order Entry (POE).

POE is not new. The very first hospital-wide systems like the Technicon system at El Camino Hospital in California in the early 1970's had POE. These systems in recent years have been shown to dramatically cut down on medication errors and have the potential to reduce costs as well. In the United States, influential business groups like Leapfrog have backed such systems as well. In the coming years, POE is likely to be the informatics application with the greatest impact on healthcare quality.

The physicians' direct order entry system implemented in the Osaka University Hospital [39] saved human power and increased the efficiency of the hospital functions. All orders and reports except the pathological examination orders and the corresponding reports were electronically exchanged. There has been a great deal of discussion about ways to implement an EPR, including a computerized physician order entry system [40]. Because of the improved man-machine interface, most Japanese physicians and nurses are now in favor of direct order entry [41]. However, data input and output covering the same content as a paper-based medical record still are a major problem for physicians. An integrated design with dynamic templates for structured data entry, the possibility of multiple display modes and a dynamic problem oriented system may provide a solution.

## 6. Medical risk management

Osaka University Hospital, a Japanese national university hospital, reengineered its paper-based incident reporting system into a computerized integrated reporting, notification, and tracking system [42]. An on-line Incident Reporting System (OIRS) was developed to collect anonymous IR via a reporting form available on the Intranet Web. By using a template, the process to write an IR was simplified and the IR is much easier to complete. Instead of writing a narrative report, now it is mainly a matter of checking off boxes. An example of the data input screen is shown in Figure 1. The structured data entry of incidents also facilitates root cause analysis. However, some data elements, including a detailed description of the case, causes, and possible ways to prevent similar incidents still have to be reported in free-text.

In July 2001 the medical quality management department of the Osaka University Hospital started to operate the OIRS to decrease the time needed to complete an incident report, to collect more precise data about the incident and to provide members of the hospital committee for risk management with instant access to all IR generated by the hospital staff. IR are stored in a database and available for future root cause analyses. The organizational structure is illustrated in Figure 2.

Anonymity and freedom from punitive action are essential for increasing the number of reports. Reports of potential errors provide valuable insight into the system's vulnerabilities, whereas timely input and review of reports by means of information technology enables a rapid systematic PDCA (Plan-Do-Check-Act) cycle for preventing medical errors and providing a valuable link between the risk, quality, and safety functions of the organization. The new system was designed to streamline the error-reporting process and reduce the occurrence of future medical errors, with a goal of increasing patient safety and encouraging better reporting.

A non-random sample of hospital employees including physicians, nurses and other medical staff submitted incident reports anonymously. From July 2000 through December 2001, 1550 incidents were reported. Nurses reported 73%, physicians including

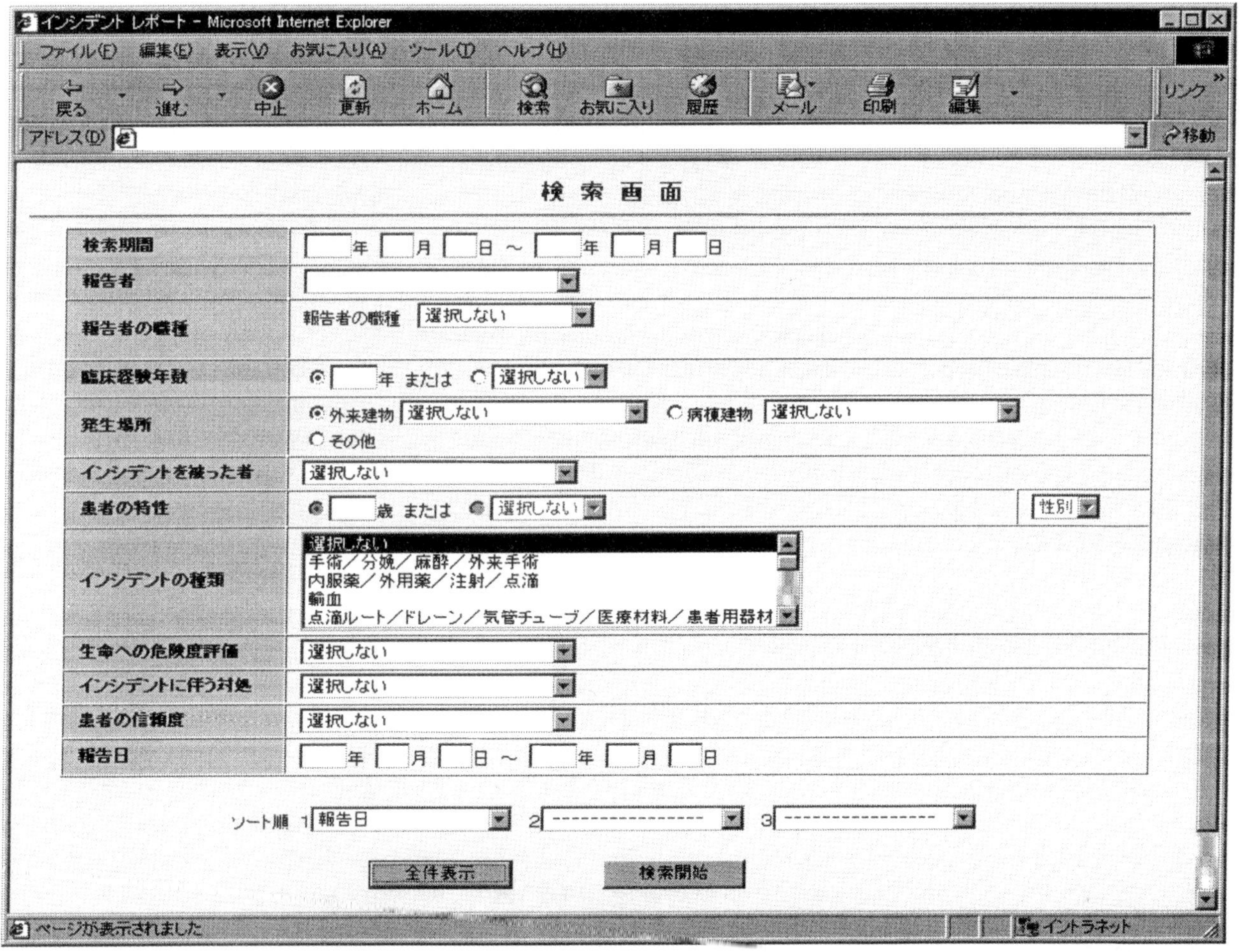

Fig. 1 A sample of structured data entry in the On-line Incident Report System (OIRS) in the Osaka University Hospital

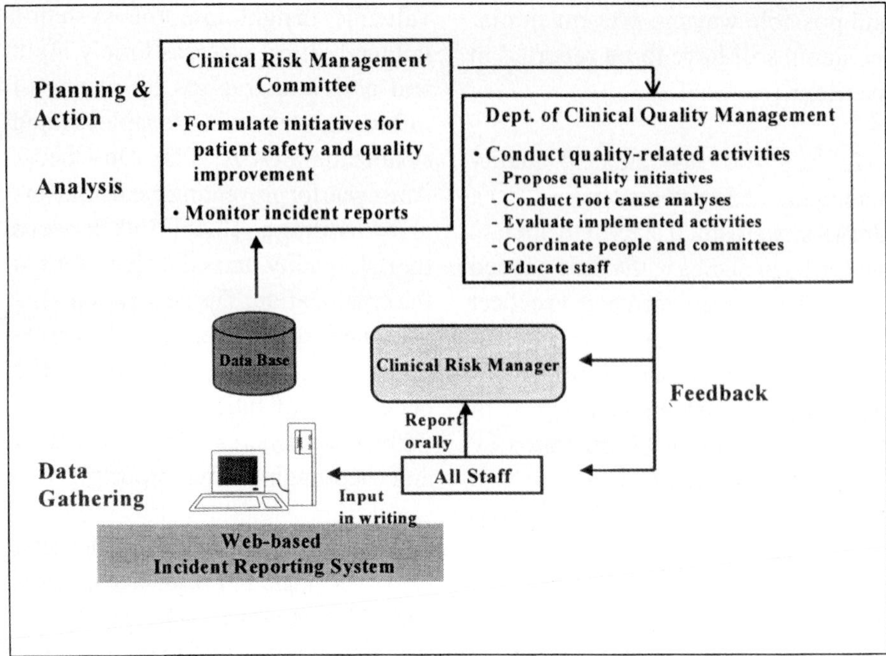

Fig. 2. The organization and the process from data gathering to feedback in the

trainees 16%, and pharmacists 7% of the reports. Drug prescription and medication related errors comprised 43% of the total number of incidents. The relatively high reporting rate of physicians may indicate that the OIRS has been well accepted by the hospital staff as an efficient tool for the prevention of medical errors. From the reported IR the true rate of incidents cannot be inferred, however.

Because of the successful operation of the above-mentioned ordering and reporting system, an electronic patient record system (EPROU) was installed in January 2001 in the Osaka University Hospital [43]. The EPROU features 1) physicians' direct structured data entry, 2) multi-modal output of registered clinical data and 3) a dynamic problem-oriented system. To increase the operability and the utility of the EPR, the system made use of structured data entry using dynamic templates [44]. The EPROU viewer provides an integrated view of information of each patient [45].

The EPROU database stores medical event data. A 'medical event'

is an abstract concept which includes information from the records of healthcare providers, ordering and processing data, examination reports, image header data, and so on. All these data are transferred to the EPROU database [46].

The EPROU database only contains one database file. One record corresponds to one medical event. Medical event ID, patient ID, medical event type, department, transaction time, validate time, user ID, and several other items are stored. No deletion or editing is allowed. Data protection is essential. EPROU has a mechanism for making a message digest for each record. Thus illegal changes of the record can be detected. When the data is transferred from the server to the client, the data is encoded to avoid theft or change during transmission. The files stored in PCs are also encoded to protect the data.

One study using EPROU data concerned the determination of the distributions of the length of stay (LOS) of in-patients in the hospital as a function of diagnosis procedure combinations

(DPC), the Japanese version of diagnosis related group (DRG). Information about 10,687 patients discharged during the period from April 2000 to March 2001 was analyzed. The average LOS value in the fiscal year 2000 was 31.7 days (including patients from the department of psychiatry, with an average LOS of 78.8 days). In total 51.2% of the patients could be classified into 80 DPC categories (Japanese DPC version 1.0). The low percentage is due to the immaturity of the DPC system. DPC-specific LOS distributions were determined and the mean, median and standard deviation for each DPC were calculated.

The results showed that most DPC-specific distributions were not normal but rather similar to log-normal distributions and that some distributions were multi-modal. For all DPCs the mean values and standard deviations were larger than corresponding data obtained from other national hospitals. The study showed that DRG or DPC specific distributions of length of hospital stay, extracted from an EPR, provide statistical evidence of medical quality. As the principle of quality control clearly indicates, the larger standard deviation should be made smaller and the long mean LOS should be reduced by quality management interventions such as application of evidence-based guidelines and critical pathways. The concept is shown in Figure 3.

## Conclusion

It is apparent from the literature that DSS that are mainly developed for the purpose of diagnosis do not have a large impact on the process and outcome of health care. Despite the many publications concerning diagnostic systems, their use in clinical practice seems to be rather limited. This may be partly due to the fact that many of these systems start with a differential diagnosis

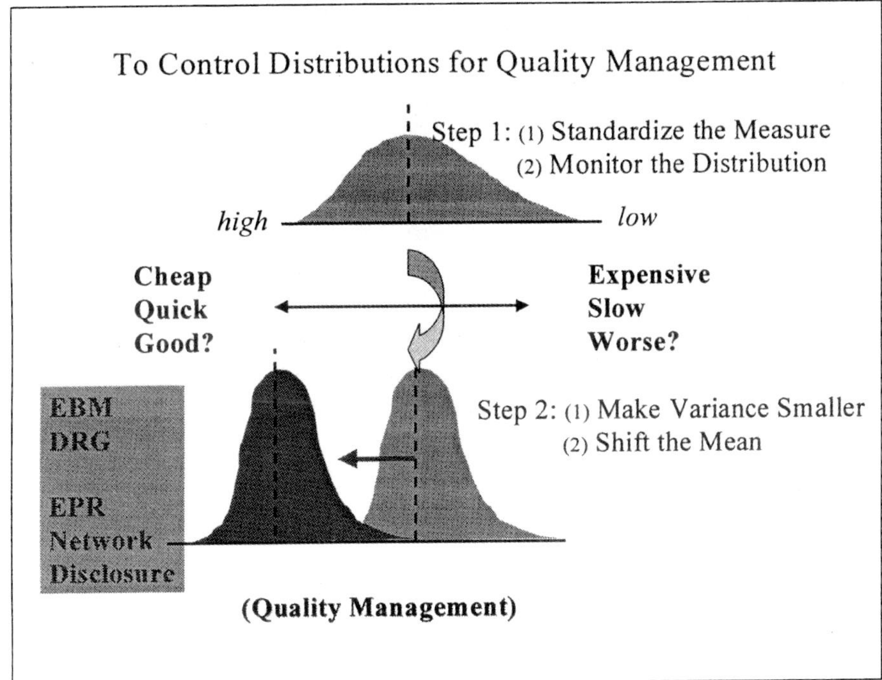



Fig. 3. Conceptual illustration of the controlling distributions for the quantitative management of health care.

and then try to determine the patient's disease or condition, which does not save the physician significant amounts of time. Reminder systems, on the other hand, do appear to have an impact on health outcomes.

Guideline systems can be useful in supporting the physician or nurse in managing patients, but a standard guideline model must be developed so that guidelines can be effectively shared across systems. A great deal of promising research is currently being carried out with respect to guideline models and tools for entering guidelines into DSS.

Finally, medical risk management can be aided by electronic patient records and physician order entry systems, which can not only provide guidance but also produce valuable data about errors and their causes.

## References


1. Miller RA, Pople HE, Myers JD. INTERNIST-1, an experimental computer-based diagnostic consultant for general internal medicine. N Engl J Med 1982;307:468-76.
2. Berman L, Miller RA. Problem area formation as an element of computer aided diagnosis: a comparison of two strategies within Quick Medical Reference (QMR). Methods Inf Med 1991;30:90-5.
3. Lau LM, Warner HR. Performance of a diagnostic system (Iliad) as a tool for quality assurance. Comput Biomed Res 1992;25:314-23.
4. Feldman MJ, Barnett GO. An approach to evaluating the accuracy of Dxplain. Comput Methods Programs Biomed 1991;35:261-6.
5. Blois MS. Information and medicine. The nature of medical descriptions. Berkeley, CA: University of California Press, 1984.
6. Kohn LT, Corrigan JM, Donaldson MS, editors. To Err Is Human: Building a Safer Health Care System. Committee on Quality of Health Care in America, Institute of Medicine. Washington DC: National Academy Press, 1999.
7. Staender S, Davies J, Helmreich B, Sexton B, Kaufmann BM. The anaesthesia critical incident reporting system: an experience based database. Int J Med Inf 1997; 47:87-90.
8. Fox J, Das S. Safe and sound: artificial intelligence in hazardous applications. Menlo Park, CA: AAAI Press/ The MIT Press, 2000.
9. Kobus DA, Amundson D, Moses JD, Rascona D, Gubler KD. A computerized medical incident reporting system for errors in the intensive care unit: initial evaluation of interrater agreement. Mil Med 2001;166:350-3.
10. Stanhope N, Crowley-Murphy M, Vincent C, O'Connor AM, Taylor-Adams SE. An evaluation of adverse incident reporting. J Eval Clin Pract 1999;5:1-4.
11. Deming W. Out of the Crisis. Boston: MIT Press, 1982.
12. Blumenthal D, Scheck AC. Improving Clinical Practice. San Francisco: Jossey-Bass, 1995.
13. Berner ES, Webster GD, Shugerman AA et al. Performance of four computer-based diagnostic systems. N Engl J Med 1994;330:1792-6.
14. Elstein AE, Friedman CP, Wolf FM et al. Effects of a decision support system on the diagnostic accuracy of users: a preliminary report. J Am Med Inform Assoc 1996;3:422-8.
15. Friedman CP, Elstein AE, Wolf FM et al. Enhancement of clinician's diagnostic reasoning by computer based consultation. A multi-site study of 2 systems. J Am Med Inform Assoc 1999;282:1851-6.
16. Balas EA, Austin SM, Mitchell JA, Ewigman BG, Bopp KD, Brown GD. The clinical value of computerized information services. A review of 98 randomized clinical trials. Arch Fam Med 1996;5:271-6.
17. Shea S, Dumouchel W, Bahamonde L. A meta-analysis of 16 randomized controlled trials to evaluate computer-based clinical reminder systems for preventive care in the ambulatory setting. J Am Med Inform Assoc 1996;3 (6):399-409.
18. Austin SM, Balas EA, Mitchel JA, Ewigman BG. Effect of physician reminders on preventive care: meta-analysis of randomised clinical trials. J Am Med Inform Assoc 1994;1(suppl):121-4.
19. Johnston ME, Langton KB, Haynes RB, Mathieu A. Effects of computer-based clinical decision support systems on clinical performance and patient outcome. Ann Intern Med 1994;120:135-42.
20. Hunt DL, Haynes RB, Hanna SE, Smith K. Effects of computer-based clinical decision support systems on physician performance and patient outcomes. JAMA 1998;280:1339-46.
21. Balas EA, Weingarten S, Garb CT, Blumenthal D, Boren SA, Brown GD. Improving preventive care by prompting physicians. Arch Intern Med 2000;160: 301-8.
22. Oxman AD, Thomson MA, Davis DA, Haynes RB. No magic bullets: a systematic review of 102 trials of interventions to improve professional practice. Can Med Assoc J 1995; 153 (10):1423-31.
23. Field MJ, Lohr KN, eds. Clinical practice

guidelines: directions for a new program. Washington DC: National Academy Press, 1990.

24. Grimshaw JM, Russel IT. Effects of clinical guidelines on medical practice: a systematic review of rigorous evaluation. Lancet 1993; 342: 1317-1322.

25. Field MJ, Lohr KN, eds. Guidelines for clinical practice guidelines: from development to use. Washington DC: National Academy Press, 1992.

26. Payne TH. Computer decision support systems. Chest 2000;118:47S-52S.

27. Teich JM, Wrinn MM. Clinical decision support systems come of age. MD Comput 2000;17(1):43-6.

28. Reggia JA, Tuhrim S. Computer-assisted medical decision making. Volumes 1 and 2. New York: Springer Verlag, 1985.

29. Miller PL. Selected topics in medical artificial intelligence. New York: Springer Verlag, 1988.

30. Hripcsak G, Ludemann P, Pryor TA, Wigertz OB, Clayon PD. Rationale for the Arden Syntax. Comput Biomed Res 1994;27(4):291-324.

31. Ohno-Machado L, Gennari JH, Murphy S, Jain NL, Tu SW et al. The Guideline Interchange Format: A model for representing guidelines. J Am Med Inform Assoc 1998;5 (4):357-72.

32. Peleg M, Boxwala A, Ogunyemi O, Zeng Q, Tu SW, et al. GLIF3: the evolution of a guideline representation format. In: Proc. AMIA Annual Symposium; 2000. p. 645-9.

33. Fox J, Johns N, Lyons C, Rahmanzadeh A, et al. PROforma: a general technology for clinical decision support systems. Comput Methods Programs Biomed 1997;54 (1-2):59-67.

34. Shahar Y, Miksch S, Johnson P. The Asgaard project: a task specific framework for the application and critiquing of time-oriented clinical guidelines. Artif Intell Med 1998;14 (1-2):29-51.

35. Musen MA, Tu SW, Das AK, Shahar Y. EON: a component based approach to automation of protocol-directed therapy. J Am Med Inform Assoc 1996;3 (6):367-88.

36. Grosso WE, Eriksson H, Fergerson RW, Gennari JH, Tu SW, Musen MA. Knowledge Modeling at the Millennium (The Design and Evolution of Protégé-2000). Twelfth Workshop on Knowledge Acquisition, Modeling and Management (KAW'99). 1999.

37. De Clercq PA, Hasman A, Blom JA, Korsten HHM. Design and implementation of a framework to support the development of clinical guidelines. Int J Med Inf 2001;64 (2-3):285-318.

38. McDonald CJ, Overhage JM, Tierney WM, et al, The Regenstrief Medical Record System: a quarter century experience. Int J Med Inf 1999;54 (3):225-53.

39. Matsumura Y, Takeda H, Inoue M. Implementation of the totally integrated hospital information system (HUMANE) in Osaka university hospital, In: Greenes RA, Peterson HA, Protti DJ, editors. Medinfo '95, North-Holland, Amsterdam; 1995. p. 590-3.

40. Sittig DF, Stead WW. Computer-based physician order entry: the state of the art. J Am Med Inform Assoc 1994;1:108-23.

41. Haruki Y, Ogushi Y, Okada Y, Kimura M, Kumamoto I, Sekita Y. Status and perspective of hospital information systems in Japan. Methods Inf Med 1999;38:200-6.

42. Nakajima K, Kuwata S, Matsumura SY, Oshima H, Takeda H. Operation and effects of computerized incident reporting system for prevention of medical adverse events. J Japanese Med Inform Assoc. 2001;21:77-82.

43. Takeda H, Matsumura Y, Okada T, Kuwata S, Inoue M. A Japanese approach to establish an electronic patient record system in an intelligent hospital. Int J Med Inform 1998;49:45-51.

44. Matsumura Y, Takeda H, Okada T, Kuwata S, Hiroaki N, Hazumi N, et al. Devices for structured data entry in electronic patient record. In: Cesnik B, McCray AT, Scherrer JR, editors. Medinfo '98. IOS Press, Amsterdam; 1998. p. 85-8.

45. Matsumura Y, Kuwata S, Kusuoka H, Takahashi Y, Onishi H, Kawamoto T, et al. Dynamic Viewer of Medical Events in Electronic Medical Record. In: Patel VL, Rogers R, Haux R, editors. Medinfo '2001. IOS Press, Amsterdam; 2001. p. 648-52.

46. Kondoh H, Takeda H, Matsumura Y, Kuwata S, Yoshimua H, Narumi Y, et al. PACS linked to EPR. In: Patel VL, Rogers R, Haux R, editors. Medinfo '2001. IOS Press, Amsterdam; 2001. p. 915-8.

Address of the authors:
Arie Hasman
Department of Medical Informatics
University of Limburg
P.O. Box 616
NL-6200 MD Maastricht
The Netherlands
E-mail: hasman@mi.unimaas.nl

Charles Safran
Harvard Medical School
Boston, MA
and Clinician Support Technology
One Wells Avenue, Suite 201
Newton, MA 02459, USA
E-mail: csafran@cstlink.com

Hiroshi Takeda
Department of Medical Information Science,
Graduate School of Medicine
Osaka University
2-2, Yamada-oka Suita City
Osaka 565-0871, Japan
E-mail: takeda@hp-info.med.osaka-u.ac.jp

**M.J. Ball[1], D.E. Garets[2], T.J. Handler[3]**

[1] Healthlink Inc., Baltimore, MD, USA
[2] Healthlink Inc., Snohomish, WA, USA
[3] Gartner Inc., Woodbridge, CT, USA

# Review

# *Leveraging IT to Improve Patient Safety*

**Abstract**: Medical errors and issues of patient safety are hardly new phenomena. Even during the dawn of medicine, Hippocrates counselled new physicians " to above all else do no harm." In the United States, efforts to improve the quality of healthcare can be seen in almost every decade of the last century. In the early 1900s, Dr. Ernest Codman failed in his efforts to get fellow surgeons to look at the outcomes of their cases. In the 1970s, there was an outcry that the military allowed an almost blind surgeon to continue to practice and even transferred him to the prestigious Walter Reed Hospital. More recently, two reports by the Institute of Medicine caught the attention of the media, the American public, and the healthcare industry. *To Err Is Human* highlights the need to reduce medical errors and improve patient safety, and *Crossing The Quality Chasm* calls for a new health system to provide quality care for the 21st century.

## Healthcare Has a Problem

The IOM is not the only source indicating that the delivery of healthcare has significant shortcomings. A Rand Corporation report describes the U.S. healthcare system as "substandard" and medical errors as "rife." Only 60% of the chronically ill receive the care they need. Of the care given to the chronically ill, about 20% is "unnecessary and potentially harmful" [1]. According to a Kaiser study, 71% of consumers - who are increasingly involved in making their own healthcare decisions - are concerned or very concerned about patient safety [2]. 61% fear being given the wrong medication, 56% fear complications in a medical procedure [3]. Furthermore, more than half of U.S. physicians believe that their ability to deliver quality care has decreased in the past five years, and 30% rate their hospitals as fair or poor at finding and addressing medical errors [4]. In a Robert Wood Johnson Foundation survey, *Pursuing Perfection*, four of five providers believe that "funda-

mental" changes are needed to ensure patient safety. Seventy-eight percent feel that their organization should take responsibility for developing solutions to the quality challenge. Fewer than 10% find the system close to error-free. The percentage of physicians (95%), nurses (89%), and administrators (82%) who report having witnessed a serious medical mistake is appalling [5].

And then there are the numbers. According to the IOM, medical errors account for an estimated 44,000 to 98,000 deaths per year in U.S. hospitals, making it a leading cause of death in the United States. Although some have questioned the validity of these numbers, the reality is that people are dying from medical errors. One study of 182 deaths of patients hospitalized for CVA (stroke), pneumonia, or heart attack found that at least 14% and potentially as many as 27% of the deaths might have been prevented [6]. If morbidity and the outpatient environment is considered, the numbers may be far worse than the IOM suggests. A

growing number of studies in the peer-reviewed literature document the problem. Just over one-fifth of these studies define errors and adverse events, while 65% are medication related. Only recently did a small number of studies begin to examine costs involved [7].

## Looking Just at Medication Related Errors

According to the Agency for Healthcare Research and Quality, adverse drug events cause 777,000 injuries and deaths a year [8]. Medication related deaths in the United States increased 2.37-fold in hospitalized patients and 8.48-fold among outpatients between 1983 and 1993. This equated to one out of 854 inpatient deaths and one out of 131 outpatient deaths in 1993 [9]. Researchers found 5.5 adverse drug events per 100 outpatients coming for care. Of these, 38% were preventable and 23% were serious. Even these numbers must be considered suspect as there is general consensus that errors are underreported for a host of reasons. One study indicated that while 92% of hospital CEOs reported that they were knowledgeable about the frequency of medication errors in their facilities, only 8% said that they had more than 20 per month, when probably all of them did [10]. In another recent prospective study of surgical units, almost 80% of the errors identified by trained observers were not officially recognized or recorded [11].

## The Challenge in Medicine Today: To Apply What We Know

It is not surprising that healthcare is experiencing difficulty. We are at a time of unprecedented discovery. All told, "the science and technologies involved in healthcare - the knowledge, skills, care interventions, devices, and drugs - have advanced more rapidly than our ability to deliver them safely, effectively, and efficiently" [12]. For example, in 1998 the FDA approved 90 new drugs, 30 new molecular entities, and 124 new uses for already approved drugs [13]. Furthermore, new medical technologies are at an all time high, and our medical knowledge is growing exponentially. In 1995, over 10,000 articles were published on randomized clinical trials, our best source of data for evidence-based care, one hundred times as many as in 1966 [14]. Except for rare and exceptional clinicians, it is just not possible to keep up to date on advances in medical knowledge.

## The Nature of Medical Errors

Analysis of the nature and causes of medical errors has made it clear that they arise from a variety of causes and impact virtually all medical activities. Furthermore, they do not readily point to a common set of causes. More often than not, errors result from a combination of a series of latent errors that are

built into the system. A recent prospective study could identify the individual who "might" be responsible in only 37.8% of the cases. In more than one third of the cases, it was "simply not possible to assign any responsibility." More than 60% of all errors were in the system. Even when an individual could be identified, the person was acting within the system [11]. This complex and pervasive nature of medical errors means that they cannot be eliminated by efforts that are simplistic or narrowly focused.

## Taking Action to Improve Patient Safety

The push to improve patient safety remains slowgoing, although definite efforts continue to arise. The Joint Commission on Accreditation of Healthcare Organizations made its new patient safety standards effective July 1, 2001. They call for internal reporting of medical errors, design of remedial steps to prevent future occurrences of these errors, prospective analysis and redesign of vulnerable patient care systems, and, finally, telling patients and their families when they have been hurt by a medical error [15]. The American Hospital Association offers its members educational materials to use in creating "a culture of safety." The Leapfrog Group is bringing the influence of private sector employers to bear upon the issue. The government has also taken steps. In 2001, Congress allocated $50 million to establish the national Center for Quality Improvement and Patient Safety within the Agency for Healthcare Research and Quality (AHRQ). Through 2003, AHRQ expects to award up to $25 million annually to establish centers for safety research and practice and to support research and education in key areas, including best practice guidelines. The states have also taken some initial steps to improve patient safety. California legislation requires hospitals to imple-

ment a formal plan for eliminating or substantially reducing medication-safety related errors by 2005. Other states have also passed laws related to medical errors. For example, fifteen states have mandatory reporting from hospitals for adverse events. Five states and the District of Columbia have voluntary reporting.

## Making Patient Safety Happen

To reach the goal of patient safety, each healthcare organization needs:

· Its own vision for patient safety that is clear, realistic, achievable, and measurable
· An understanding of what constitutes "best in class performance" outside its walls
· A carefully selected and limited set of strategies and unambiguous measures for each
· Organization-wide deployment and development of leadership across the organization to align its daily work with the vision

Each and every one of these components is essential to developing a "culture of safety"— and none can succeed without leadership and commitment of the medical staff, nursing, and other leaders. Several steps can be taken to ensure that the process of improving patient safety is ultimately successful. The <u>education</u> component brings all participants to a common level of understanding and recognition of the possibilities. The <u>diagnostic</u> component allows a healthcare organization to gain an overview of and clearly define the scope of patient problems within the organization. <u>Process improvement</u> is critical to providing safer patient care and better outcomes. Applying what is known about "best practices" to clinical processes is the first step in continuous quality improvement. Healthcare organizations gain real value from access to an up-to-date, wide-reaching knowledge base of what actually works in other organizations similar to theirs. <u>Evaluation</u> follows on an ongoing basis. Every process change and every new tool must be evaluated to determine whether it does indeed improve care. By gathering and analyzing its own data and comparing those data to national benchmarks when appropriate, healthcare organizations can create their own evidence-based practices. In such an environment, evaluation and process improvement are concurrent and continuous.

## Educate

- Understand the problems associated with patient safety and the solutions that have been tried elsewhere and proven effective.
- Benefit from the experience of other institutions in identifying types of medical errors and applying clinical solutions.
- Understand the tools available to assist in the process and the cultural dimensions involved in creating a culture of safety.
- Establish a patient safety advisory team, including information technology staff, clinicians, and administrative staff, to advise on clinical solutions.

## Diagnosis

- Involve the patient safety advisory team throughout the assessment process, eliciting their input to strengthen "buy-in" across the organization.
- Identify a proven methodology to assess the extent of the problem across the organization.
- Apply the methodology to generate an evidence-based picture of patient safety across the organization.
- Create an inventory of all sources of medical errors in all areas to be studied.
- Review the evidence to develop a prioritized listing of problems.
- Identify strategies and tools to address prioritized problems.

- Evaluate and select specific problem or problems for action.
- Provide an accurate projection of the hospital's return on investment resulting from an investment of resources and a reduction in medical errors.

## Process improvement

- Continue to work with the patient safety advisory team to ensure that the implementation runs smoothly.
- Develop a detailed plan for education and training, using multiple modalities and providing ongoing support to ensure that the clinician's job becomes easier.
- Install selected software solution.
- Be sure the mission of the safety team is part of the strategy and is part of the overall strategic plan.

## Evaluate

- Analyze data to measure effectiveness of the solution implemented.
- Monitor data on an ongoing basis to determine problem areas for which there are identifiable solutions.
- Continue to work with the advisory team to provide constant surveillance of patient safety and ensure continuous improvement of clinical care.

---

## Using Technology as Enabler

It is clear that achieving substantial (50% or greater) reductions in preventable medical errors is a difficult task. However, there is consensus: IT can improve healthcare. In its report to the President, PITAC outlines the role the federal government must play in using IT to transform healthcare [16]. In addition to calling for a national vision and a national information infrastructure, PITAC charges the federal government with coordinating its own cross-agency activities - which are numerous and far reaching in scope - and establishing pilot projects and Enabling Technology Centers. The President's Information Technology Advisory

Committee concluded that "information technology tools can provide the healthcare sector with unprecedented productivity and quality of care if there is a strategic vision and adequate research to ensure success" [16]. The IOM's call for action reviews the medical literature, adds the insights of experts, and reiterates the need, first set forth in *The Computer-based Patient Record*, to make use of information technology as an "enabler" in the service of patient care [12, 17]. It is our position that in order to achieve the goal of significant error reduction, a computer-based patient record (CPR) is essential. The use of a CPR is mandatory because of the wide variety of medical errors that can occur and the broad set of tools and capabilities needed to enable a care delivery organization (CDO) to detect, correct, and compensate for them across this diverse environment.

CPR offerings can be defined by five separate generations of CPR systems based on the progressive capabilities they offer. *First-generation CPRs* are simple systems that provide a site-specific encounter solution to the need for access to clinical data. *Second-generation CPRs* are basic systems that allow clinicians to document care adequately. *Third-generation CPRs* include episodic as well as encounter coverage and must work in ambulatory and acute-care settings. *Fourth-generation CPRs* are more complex, with integrated documentation, workflow and decision support, and must cover more than just the ambulatory and acute-care settings. *Fifth-generation CPRs* are complex, fully integrated systems crossing the continuum of care and designed to be used by healthcare providers and healthcare consumers. Currently, vendors are predominately delivering Generation 2 products.

Since different CPRs offer different sets of capabilities, it is reasonable to ask, "What degree of error reduction should one expect to be able to achieve with various generations of CPRs?" Figure 1 gives a high-level answer to this question. Each of the five generations of CPR is plotted on a graph. On the horizontal axis is the anticipated time when such a system will become available and on the vertical axis is the projected efficacy of that generation in reducing medical errors. Note that the vertical axis deals with preventable errors, not total errors. The 1999 IOM report estimated that roughly 70% of medical errors are preventable. Thus, it is important to note that no CPR system, no matter how sophisticated, can ever be expected to eliminate errors completely.

In order to estimate the error reduction potential of different CPR generations, the types of errors reported in the IOM report were analyzed and combined with the minimal features required for each CPR generation.

**Generation 1** CPRs are relatively simple systems that create a clinical data repository where information from a wide variety of sources (such as laboratory and pharmacy systems) can be consolidated. The creation of a single comprehensive location for clinical information makes possible the elimination of approximately 15% of preventable medical errors by ensuring that needed information can be located efficiently and reliably.

**Generation 2** CPRs make an additional 25% reduction in errors possible by adding the capability to handle on-line documentation of clinical activities including physician order entry. A major differentiator from Generation 1 systems is the inclusion of basic clinical decision support systems (CDSS). CDSS with its associated rules engine is a key capability for eliminating errors by

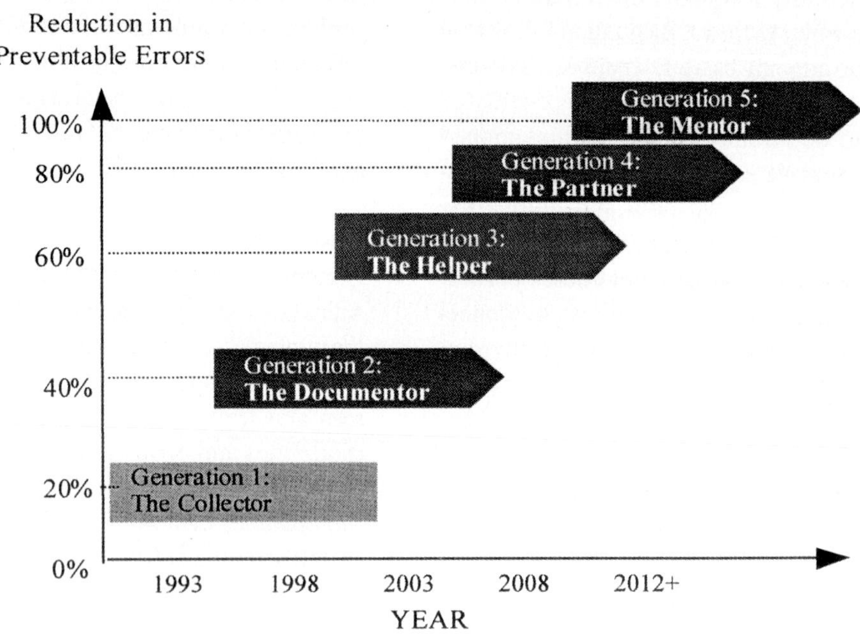


Fig. 1. Error Impact of CPR Generations Source: Gartner, Inc.

permitting the CDO to implement a wide variety of checks to ensure that mistakes are avoided and serious situations are rapidly brought to the attention of caregivers. The combination of these capabilities means that Generation 2 CPRs can achieve roughly an overall 40% reduction in preventable errors.

**Generation 3** CPRs will make possible the single largest incremental improvement in error reduction over a previous generation and is expected to result in the potential for over 70 percent reduction in preventable errors. The combination of improved CDSS, operation across the continuum of care (inpatient and ambulatory), use of a controlled medical vocabulary to normalize medical concepts, and POE to better manage the ordering process will produce dramatic results. These systems are also seeing the emergence of workflow capabilities that will become progressively important as tools to support the optimal delivery of medical care. When workflow is combined with CDSS, an even more powerful error reduction capability emerges.

Generation 3 CPRs also have the basic infrastructure needed to assess the incidence of potential errors, to measure the effectiveness of interventions to prevent these errors, and to document the improved outcomes that result. Since Generation 3 CPRs are now beginning to emerge and will become more capable after 2003, we believe that CDOs now have viable automation options that can help them realistically hope to achieve the IOM goal of at least a 50% reduction in preventable medical errors.

It is expected that around 2007, there will be general availability of **Generation 4** CPRs. With more sophisticated clinical decision support than was included in earlier generations of CPRs, these systems will be aware of the detailed context of each individual patient. Formal workflow capability will be an integral part of these systems and will ensure that the proper balance occurs between the medical practice consistency needed to ensure optimal outcomes and the individual variations needed to treat each individual patient appropriately, given their unique set of circumstances. The combination of context awareness, clinical protocols, knowledge management, and formal workflow should lead to an additional 20% reduction in preventable errors.

The final step in CPR evolution is predicted to occur some time after 2010 with the advent of **Generation 5** systems. These complex systems will have sophisticated clinical decision support that is not only aware of the individual context of each patient, but has knowledge regarding the experience of the clinician as well as an understanding of the capabilities of the specific CDO site where the patient is being treated. It will also utilize sophisticated clinician interfaces to ensure that caregivers always have a full and up-to-date picture of the status of each of their patients and will be equipped to efficiently and effectively deal with multiple concurrent medical conditions in the same patient. It will also support interfaces to mobile personal monitoring devices that can provide an up-to-the-minute picture of the person's medical status. True evidence-based medicine will be possible using these systems since they will automatically track the outcomes experience of each episode of care as well as relevant new results as they become available in the medical literature. A Generation 5 CPR should provide the entire basic infrastructure needed to address preventable errors. Of course, the specific CPR implementation at a CDO site will determine how close that site comes to actually achieving this ideal.

## Evidence to Support the Use of Technology

While the CPR is the best technology to use for overall error reduction, there is evidence that components of the CPR can result in definite improvement in patient safety.

### Physician order entry

A POE system can reduce the potential for error in increasingly complex CPR environments by ensuring that orders are more legible, complete, and appropriate. When combined with clinical decision support, they also help identify serious potential complications including drug-drug interactions, potentially life threatening allergies, and conditions that require different treatment options (e.g. an alternative antibiotic if the patient's lab values indicate renal failure and the prescribed medication is renally excreted).

Evidence:

| Institution | Documented Results |
|---|---|
| Brigham and Women's Hospital, Boston (Included decision support features) | 88% drop in serious medication errors<br>55% reduction in error rates |
| LDS Hospital, Salt Lake City | 70% in adverse drug events |
| Ohio State University Medical Center, Columbus (pilot) | Average length of stay down by 2 days<br>Turnaround for pharmacy orders 2 hours faster<br>Pharmacy charges down $910 per admission |
| Montefiore Medical Center, New York | Medication errors down 50%<br>Turnaround for pharmacy orders 2 hours faster |
| Wishard Memorial Hospital, Indianapolis | Average length of stay down 0.9 days<br>Average hospital charges down 13% |

### Computerized Alerting Systems

Alerting systems are a type of clinical decision support. By notifying physicians about likely adverse events at the time those events actually occur, online alerts can improve the timeliness of response. The end results: fewer errors, improved quality of care, and better patient outcomes. The challenge has been to deliver the message in real time to the physician responsible for the patient to take timely and appropriate action. Messages on computer terminals, email, flashing lights - they have all been tried - and can be effective.

Evidence:

Email alerts to physicians on markedly abnormal lab values in patients receiving drugs affecting kidney function resulted in medications being adjusted or discontinued 21.6 hours earlier than when no email was delivered [18].

Paging clinicians about "panic" lab values decreased time to therapy by 11% and mean time to resolution of an abnormality by 29% [19].

### Medical Error Reporting Systems

Medical error reporting systems link hospital-based systems to larger data repositories, allowing individual hospitals to benchmark their performance against other provider organizations and to determine how much errors cost and affect patient outcomes.

Case Study: Iowa Health System, Des Moines, OH [20].

A 10,000-patient pilot project at this 11-hospital delivery system is using a data analysis system to electronically flag patients who are at risk from drug/drug interactions or other adverse events. Iowa Health transmits data every week to Active Health Management's databases, which process the data using more than 600 clinical rules. The medical directors at Iowa Health review the analysis and contact the primary care physicians of patients who have been identified. In potential emergency situations, such as drug/drug interactions, Active Health notifies the medical directors immediately. Thus far, they have identified 250 "intervention opportunities" and are developing a "Top 5" list of situations warranting immediate intervention.

## Conclusion

The current situation regarding patient safety is unacceptable. In addition to the high mortality and morbidity associated with medical errors, there are numerous 'secondary' costs as well. Clinical outcomes are poor because of the complications and injuries associated with medical mistakes. This clearly leads to patient dissatisfaction but also yields dissatisfaction on the part of caregivers who are unable to provide the quality of medical care they desire because of the limitations of inadequate healthcare automation systems. In addition, serious errors can lead to malpractice suits with the concomitant risk of financial losses as well as injury to the institution's reputation. The challenge of patient safety is twofold. On the one hand more adverse events must be identified, including those without dire consequences, and the number of preventable adverse events that result from such errors must be reduced. Although much of a patient safety initiative will involve process changes, technology must be employed as well. The technology has been shown to work, the time is ripe to actually implement the necessary systems.

## References


1. Romano M. Woe is us: Stinging reports criticize health industry. Mod Healthc 2001 May 14;31(20):4-5, 12.
2. Kaiser Family Foundation. National Survey on Americans as Health Care Consumers: An Update on the Role of Quality Information. December 2000, http://www.ahrq.gov/qual/kffhigh00.htm.
3. American Society of Health Systems Pharmacists. ASHP Patient Concerns National Survey Research Report. Bethesda, MD; September 1999.
4. Blendon RJ, Schoen C, Donelan K, Osborn R, DesRoches CM, Scoles K, et al. Physicians' views on quality of care: a five-country comparison. Health Aff (Millwood). 2001 May-Jun;20(3):233-43
5. www.ihi.org/pursuingperfection. Accessed 7/26/02.
6. Dubois RW, Brook RH. Preventable deaths: Who, how often, and why? Ann Intern Med. 1988 Oct 1;109(7):582-9.
7. Kohn LT, Corrigan JM, Donaldson MS, editors. To Err Is Human: Building a Safer Health System. Institute of Medicine. Washington DC: National Academy Press; 1999.
8. Agency for Healthcare Research and Quality. Reducing and Preventing Adverse Drug Events to Decrease Hospital Costs. 2001. http://www.ahrq.gov/qual/aderia/aderia.htm. Accessed 7/25/02.
9. Phillips DP, Cristenfeld N, Glynn LM. Increase in US medication error death rates between 1983 and 1993. Lancet 1998;351(9103):643-4.
10. Bruskin Goldring Research. February 1999. A Study of Medication Errors and Specimen Collection Errors. Commissioned by Becton-Dickinson and College of American Pathologists. http://www.bd.com/bdid/whats_new/pdfs/whitepaper.pdf Accessed 7/25/02.
11. Krizek TJ. Surgical error: Ethical issues of adverse events. Arch Surg 2000 Nov;135(11):1359-66.
12. Committee on Quality Health Care in America. Institute of Medicine. Crossing the Quality Chasm: A New Health System for the 21st Century. Washington DC: National Academy Press; 2001.
13. www.fda.gov/cder/index.html. Accessed 8/6/02.
14. Chassin M. Is health care ready for six sigma quality?. Milbank Q. 1998;76(4):565-91, 510.
15. www.jcaho.org. Accessed 7/26/02.
16. President's Information Technology Advisory Committee. Transforming Health Care Though Information Technology. Washington DC: PITAC; February 2001.
17. Institute of Medicine. The Computer-Based Patient Record: An Essential Technology for Health Care, Revised Edition;1997.
18. Kuperman GJ, Boyle D, Jha A, Rittenberg E, Ma'Luf N, Tanasijevic MJ, et al. How promptly are inpatients treated for critical laboratory results? J Am Med Inform Assoc 1998 Jan-Feb; 5(1):112-9.
19. Kuperman G, Sittig DF, Shabot M, Teich J. Clinical decision support for hospital and critical care. Journal of Healthcare Information Management 1999;13(4):81-96.
20. Gillespie G. IT paints a different picture. Health Data Management; 2001 Jun;9(6): 26-8. www.healthdatamanagement.com



Address of the authors:
Marion J. Ball, Ed.D.
Vice President, Clinical Informatics Strategies
Healthlink, Inc.
2 Hamill Road
Quadrangle 359 West
Baltimore, MD 21210
Tel: +1 410 433 7110
Fax: +1 410 433 7419
Office e-mail: marion.ball@healthlinkinc.com
Home e-mail: marionball@earthlink.net
www.healthlinkinc.com
www.marionball.com

David E. Garets
Executive Vice President
Healthlink, Inc.
5031 113th Ave. SE
Snohomish, WA 98290
Tel: +1 360 563 5780
Fax: +1 360 563 0811
E-mail: dave.garets@healthlinkinc.com

Thomas J. Handler, M.D.
Research Director
Gartner, Inc.
14 Old Quarry Road
Woodbridge, CT 06525
Tel: +1 203 393 0032
E-mail: thomas.handler@gartner.com

## G. Riva, Ph.D.

Applied Technology
for Neuro-Psychology Lab.
Istituto Auxologico Italiano
Milan, Italy

# Review Paper

# *Medical Applications of Virtual Environments*

**Abstract**: Technologies that were hardly used ten years ago, such as the Internet, e-mail, and video teleconferencing are becoming familiar methods for diagnosis, therapy, education and training. However, the possible impact of virtual reality (VR) on health care is even higher than the one offered by the new communication technologies. In fact, VR is a technology, a communication interface and an experience: a communication interface based on interactive 3D visualization, able to collect and integrate in single real-like experience different inputs and data sets.

The first health care applications of VR started in the early '90s with the need for medical staff to visualize complex medical data, particularly during surgery and for surgery planning. A couple of years later, the scope of VR applications in medicine has broadened to include neuropsychological assessment and rehabilitation.

This paper intends to investigate the role of VR in medicine, presenting some of the most interesting applications actually developed in the area. Moreover, it discusses the clinical principles, technological devices and safety issues associated with the use of virtual reality in medicine.

## 1 Introduction

As recently noted by Satava and Jones [1], the advantages of virtual environments (VEs) to health care can be summarized in a single word: revolutionary. Since the development of methods of electronic communication, clinicians have been using information and communication technologies in health care: telegraphy, telephony, radio and television have been used for distance medicine since the mid 19th century [2]. However, rapid and far-reaching technological advances are changing the ways in which people relate, communicate, and live. Technologies that were hardly used ten years ago, such as the Internet, e-mail, and video teleconferencing are becoming familiar methods for diagnosis, therapy, education and training. However, the possible impact of virtual reality (VR) on health care is even higher than the one offered by the new communication technologies. In fact, VR is a technology, a communication interface and an experience. This is why research in the virtual reality field is moving fast. If we check the two leading clinical databases – MEDLINE and PSYCINFO – using the "virtual reality" keyword we can find 829 papers listed in MEDLINE and 693 in PSYCINFO (all fields query, accessed Aug. 8, 2002).

From the analysis of the retrieved papers we can find that the first health care applications of VR started in the early '90s with the need for medical staff to visualize complex medical data, particularly during surgery and for surgery planning [3]. Actually, surgery-related applications of VR fall mainly into three classes: surgery training, surgical planning and augmented reality for surgery sessions in open surgery, endoscopy, and radiosurgery. A couple of years later, the scope of VR applications in medicine has broadened to include neuropsychological assessment and rehabilitation [4, 5].

In recent years, VR has generated both great excitement and great confusion. These factors are evident in the extensive material published in both scientific and popular press, and in the unrealistic expectations on the part of the health care professionals. In this paper we try to outline the current state of research and technology that is relevant to the development of VEs in medicine. Moreover, we discuss the clinical principles, technological devices and safety issues associated with the use of virtual reality in medicine.

## 2 The role of VR in health care

### 2.1 The two faces of VR in health care

For many health care professionals VR is first of all a technology. Since 1986, when Jaron Lamier used the term for the first time, VR has usually been described as a collection of technological devices: a computer capable of interactive 3D visualization, a head-mounted display and data gloves equipped with one or more position trackers. The trackers sense the position and orientation of the user and reports that information to the computer that updates (in real time) the images for display.

However, the analysis of the different VR applications clearly shows that the focus on technological devices is different according to the goals of the health care provider.

For instance, Rubino et al. [6], McCloy and Stone [7], and Székely and Satava [8] in their reviews share the same vision of VR: "a collection of technologies that allow people to interact efficiently with 3D computerized databases in real time using their natural senses and skills" [7]. This definition lacks any reference to head mounted displays and instrumented clothing such as gloves or suits. In fact, less than 20% of VR health care applications in medicine actually use any immersive equipment.

However, if we shift our attention to behavioral sciences, where immersive devices are used by more than 50% of the applications, VR is described as "an advanced form of human-computer interface that allows the user to interact with and become immersed in a computer-generated environment in a naturalistic fashion" [9]. In fact, to achieve the feeling of "being there" the VR applications use specialized devices such as head-mounted displays, tracking systems, earphones, gloves, and sometimes haptic-feedback devices.

These two definitions underline two different visions of VR. For physicians and surgeons, the ultimate goal of VR is the presentation of virtual objects to all of the human senses in a way identical to their natural counterpart [8]. As noted by Satava and Jones [1], as more and more of the medical technologies become information-based, it will be possible to represent a patient with higher fidelity to a point that the image may become a surrogate for the patient – the *medical avatar*. In this sense, an effective VR system should offer real-like body parts or avatars that interact with external devices such as surgical instruments as close as possible to their real models.

For clinical psychologists and rehabilitation specialists the ultimate goal is radically different [10, 11]. They use VR to provide a new human-computer interaction paradigm in which users are no longer simply external observers of images on a computer screen but are active participants within a computer-generated three-dimensional virtual world. Within the VE the patient has the possibility of learning to manage a problematic situation related to his/her disturbance. The key characteristics of virtual environments for these professionals are both the high level of control of the interaction with the tool without the constraints usually found in computer systems, and the enriched experience provided to the patient [9]. Virtual environments are highly flexible and programmable. They enable the therapist to present a wide variety of controlled stimuli, such as a fearful situation, and to measure and monitor a wide variety of responses made by the user. This flexibility can be used to provide systematic restorative training that optimizes the degree of transfer of training or generalization of learning to the person's real world environment [12].

Moreover, virtual reality systems open the input channel to the full range of human gestures: in rehabilitation it is possible to monitor movements or actions from any body part or many body parts at the same time. On the other side, with disabled patients feedbacks and prompts can be translated into alternate and/or multiple senses [13].

### 2.2 VR as communication interface

As we have just seen, if we consider VR mainly as a technology, we have two different visions of VR related to the final goal of the health care professional. But what do these two visions have in common?

The starting point for answering to this question is a definition of VR presented by Heim. According to this author [14], VR is "an immersive, interactive system based on computable information... an experience that describes many life activities in the information age" (p.6). In particular, he describes the VR experience around its "three I's": immersion, interactivity and information intensity. Developing this position, Bricken [15] identifies the core characteristic of VR in the inclusive relationship between the participant and the virtual environment, where direct experience of the immersive environment constitutes communication. According to this position, VR can be considered as the leading edge of a general evolution of present communication interfaces like television, computer and telephone [16, 17]. The main characteristic of this evolution is the full immersion of the human sensorimotor channels into a vivid and global communication experience [18].

Following this approach, it is also possible to define VR in terms of human experience [19] "a real or simulated environment in which a perceiver experiences telepresence," where telepresence can be described as the "experience of presence in an environment by means of a communication medium" (pp.78-80).

This position better clarifies the possible role of VR in medicine: a communication interface based on interactive 3D visualization, able to collect and integrate different inputs and data sets in a single real-like experience. It is up to the health care provider to decide if the VR application will be more focused on the integration of different data sets or on the realism of the virtual experience (or "sense of presence"). Considering VR as a communication interface also helps health care developers to focus their efforts.

Most of the work in this area is trying to improve the efficacy of a VE by providing the user with a more "realistic" experience, such as adding physical qualities to virtual objects or improving graphical resolution. But is this focus on the graphical characteristics really so important for the effectiveness of a medical VE?

Probably, apart from some high-end surgical applications, the answer is no. More than the richness of available images, the sensation of presence depends on the level of interaction/interactivity which actors have in both "real" and simulated environments [20]. According to Sastry and Boyd [20] a VE, particularly when it is used for real world applications, is effective when "the user is able to navigate, select, pick, move and manipulate an object much more naturally (pp.235). In this sense, emphasis shifts from quality of image to freedom of interaction, from the graphic perfection of the system to the affordances provided to the users in the environment [21].

This approach has recently received the status of international standard, through the International Organization for Standardization's ISO 13407 "Human centered design for interactive systems". According to the ISO 13407 standard [22], human-centered design requires:

- the active involvement of users;
- clear understanding of use and task requirements;
- appropriate allocation of function;
- the iteration of design solutions;
- a multi-disciplinary design team; and it is based around the following processes:
- Understand and specify the context of use;

- Specify the user and organizational requirements;
- Produce designs and prototypes;
- Carry out user-based assessment.

A sample of VE developed using the ISO 13407 guidelines is the IERAPSI surgical training system [7, 23].

## 3 Applications of Virtual Reality in Medicine

### 3.1 Medical education

The teaching of anatomy is mainly illustrative, and the application of VR to such teaching has great potential. Through 3-D visualization of massive volumes of information and databases, clinicians and students can understand important physiological principles or basic anatomy. For instance, VR can be used to explore the organs by "flying" around, behind, or even inside them. In this sense VEs can be used both as didactic and experiential educational tools, allowing a deeper understanding of the interrelationship of anatomical structures that cannot be achieved by any other means, including cadaveric dissection.

A significant step towards the creation of VR anatomy textbooks was the acquisition of the Visible Human male and female data made in August of 1991 by the University of Colorado School of Medicine [24]. The Visible Human female data set contains 5189 digital anatomical images obtained at 0.33-mm intervals (39 Gbyte). The male data set contains 1971 digital axial anatomical images obtained at 1.0-mm intervals (15 Gbyte). [25]. Actually, the US National Library of Medicine in partnership with other US government research agencies has begun the development of a tool kit of computational programs capable of automatically performing many of the basic data handling functions required for using Visible Human data in applications [26].

The National Library of Medicine made the data sets available under a

no-cost license agreement over the Internet. This allowed the creation of a huge number of educational VEs. In their recent edited book, Westwood and colleagues [27] report more than ten different educational and visualization applications.

In the future we can expect the development of different VR dynamic models illustrating how various organs and systems move during normal or diseased states, or how they respond to various externally applied forces (e.g., the touch of a scalpel).

### 3.2 Surgical simulation and planning

Surgeons know well that in training there is no alternative to hands-on practice. However, students wishing to learn laparoscopic procedures face a tough path [28]: usually they start using laparoscopic cholecystectomy trainers consisting of a black box in which endoscopic instruments are passed through rubber gaskets. After, the students begin practicing these techniques on inanimate tissues, when cost and availability allow. Obviously, there is a substantial difference for students between training with artificial or inanimate tissues and supervised procedures on real patients. This is why in the early 1990s, different research teams tried to develop VE simulators [29, 30]. The science of virtual reality provides an entirely new opportunity in the area of simulation of surgical skills using computers for training, evaluation, and eventually certification [31]. However, the first simulators were limited by low-resolution graphics, the lack of tactile input and force feedback and the lack of realistic deformation of organs. In the last years a new generation of simulators has appeared that has showed improved training efficacy over traditional methods. For instance, a randomized trial using the Minimally Invasive Surgery Training-Virtual Reality (MIST-VR) trainer [32] showed that

Virtual reality simulation was effective in training the novice to perform basic laparoscopic tasks (see Figure 1).

Another typical use of visualization applications is the planning of surgical and neuro-surgical procedures [33-35]. The planning of these procedures usually relies on the studies of series of two-dimensional MR (Magnetic Resonance) and/or CT (Computer Tomography) images, which have to be mentally integrated by surgeons into a three-dimensional concept. This mental transformation is difficult, since complex anatomy is represented in different scanning modalities, on separate image series, usually found in different sites/departments. A VR-based system is capable of incorporating different scanning modalities coming from different sites providing a simple to use interactive three-dimensional view. Within the Virtual Collaborative Clinic project, NASA researchers developed Cyberscalpel, a typical VR based surgical system for planning and practice [36]. To plan the operation of a patient with cancer of the jaw, the upper and lower jaws were reconstructed using Cyberscalpel starting from a CT scan. The scan was reduced to 20000 polygons and the final model was used to prove how fibular bone could be sectioned to mimic and replace the jaw pieces.

## 3.3 Virtual Endoscopy

Every year the screening for cancer requires the performance of over 2 million video colonoscopic procedures. However, these procedures are not perfect:
- all endoscopic procedures are invasive;
- the patients are subject to complications such as perforation, bleeding, etc.
- the cost for a typical colonoscopy is significant.

To overcome these problems, different researchers are investigating the possibility of virtual endoscopy [6, 37]. Virtual endoscopy is a new procedure that fuses computed tomo-

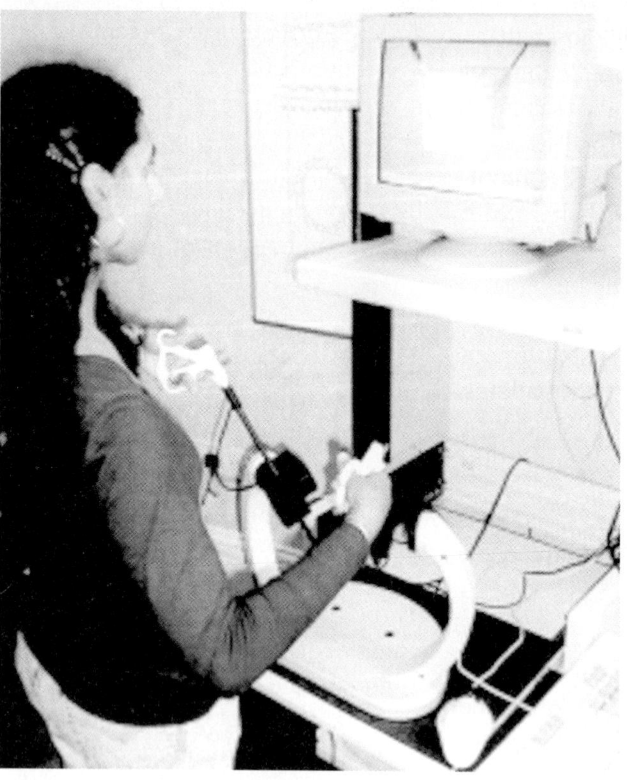

Fig. 1. Minimally Invasive Surgery Training-Virtual Reality (MIST-VR) trainer (Mentice Medical Simulation AB, Gothenburg, Sweden).

graphy with advanced techniques for rendering three-dimensional images to produce views of the organ similar to those obtained during "real" endoscopy. A virtual endoscopy is performed by using a standard CT scan or MRI scan [1], reconstructing the organ of interest into a 3-D model, and then performing a fly through it. Typical examples include the colon, stomach, esophagus, tracheo-bronchial tree (bronchoscopy), sinus bladder, ureter and kidneys (cystoscopy), pancreas or biliary tree.

Virtual endoscopy is completely non-invasive and thus without known complications. The actual cost is less than traditional endoscopy, since it is performed in the same place and manner as all imaging modalities, utilizes the same staff, and has no consumable materials.

## 3. 4 VR in neuro-psychological assessment and rehabilitation

VR is starting to play an important role in clinical psychology [38, 39], which is expected to increase in the next years. According to a recent posi-tioning paper on the future of psycho-therapy [40], the use of VR and computerized therapies are ranked respectively 3rd and 5th out of 38 psychotherapy interventions that are predicted to increase in the next 10 years.

In most VEs for clinical psychology, VR is used to simulate the real world and to assure the researcher full control of all the parameters implied. VR constitutes a highly flexible tool, which makes it possible to program an enormous variety of procedures of intervention on psychological distress. The possibility of structuring a large amount of controlled stimuli and, simultaneously, of monitoring the possible responses generated by the user of the virtual world offers a considerable increase in the likelihood of therapeutic effectiveness, as compared to traditional procedures [17]. In particular, a key advantage offered by VR is the possibility for the patient to manage a problematic situation related to his/her disturbance successfully. Using VR in this way, the patient is more likely not only to gain an awareness of his/her need to do something to create change but also to experience a greater sense of personal efficacy.

In general, these techniques are used as triggers for a broader empowerment process. In psychological literature *empowerment* is considered a multi-faceted construct reflecting the different dimensions of being psychologically enabled, and is conceived as a positive additive function of the

following three dimensions [41]
- *perceived control*: includes beliefs about authority, decision-making skills, availability of resources, autonomy in the scheduling and performance of work, etc;
- *perceived competence*: reflects role-mastery, which besides requiring the skillful accomplishment of one or more assigned tasks, also requires successful coping with non-routine role-related situations;
- *goal internalization*: this dimension captures the energizing property of a worthy cause or exciting vision provided by organizational leadership.

Virtual reality can be considered the preferred environment for the empowerment process, since it is a special, sheltered setting where patients can start to explore and act without feeling threatened. In this sense the virtual experience is an "empowering environment" that therapy provides for patients. As noted by Botella [42], nothing the patient fears can "really" happen to them in VR. With such assurance, they can freely explore, experiment, feel, live, and experience feelings and/or thoughts. VR thus becomes a very useful intermediate step between the therapist's office and the real world.

Even if the clinical rationale behind the use of VR is now clear, much of this research growth, however, has been in the form of feasibility studies and pilot trials. As a result there is still limited convincing evidence available from controlled studies (see Table 1), of the clinical advantages of this approach. Up to now the clinical effectiveness of VR was only verified in the treatment of these four psychological disorders: acrophobia, body image disturbances, binge eating disorders (see Figure 2, next page) and fear of flying.

In the cognitive rehabilitation area the situation is even worse. Even if different case studies and review papers suggest the use of VR in this area [9, 12, 43-47] there are no controlled clinical trials to support this position. A better situation can be found in the assessment of cognitive functions in persons with acquired brain injuries. In this area VR assessment tools are effective and characterized by good psychometric properties [48-52]. A typical example of these applications is ARCANA. Using a standard tool (Wisconsin Card Sorting Test - WCST) of neuropsychological assessment as a model, Pugnetti and colleagues have created ARCANA: a virtual building in which the patient has to use environmental clues in the selection of appropriate choices (doorways) to navigate through the building. The doorway choices vary according to the categories of shape, color, and number of portholes. The patient is also required to refer to the previous doorway for clues to appropriately make his/her next choice. After the choice criteria are changed, the patient must shift the cognitive set, analyze clues, and devise a new choice strategy. The parameters of this system are fully adjustable so that training applications can follow initial standardized assessments.

## 4 VR Hardware and Software

For many years one of the main obstacles to the development of VR applications was the price of the equipment: a typical VR system required a costly fridge-size Silicon Graphic workstation in the range of 150000 US$ and up. Even if high-end applications still require powerful workstations such as SGI Origin or

Table 1. Controlled Trials with more than 10 patients/users included in Medline/PsycInfo.

| Workstation | Indicative Prices (as 01 Aug 02) | |
|---|---|---|
| SGI Origin 3200, R12K Graphic Card, 8x400MHz processors, 8 Gbyte RAM, 220 Gbyte Hard Disk | US$ | 5000 |
| SGI Octane2, V12 Graphic Card, 2x400MHz processors, 512 Mbyte Ram, 18 Gbyte Hard Disk | US$ | 23000 |
| Xeon branded PC, 2x2.7 Ghz processors, 512 Mbyte Ram, 80 Gbyte Hard Disk and 17" monitor | US$ | 3800 |
| Pentium IV or Athlon XP branded PC, 2.7 Ghz processor, 512 Mbyte Ram, 80 Gbyte Hard Disk and 17" monitor | US$ | 2200 |
| **Consumer graphic cards** | | |
| GeForce  NV30 128 Mbyte Vram AGP | US$ | 400 |
| Radeon 9700 128 Mbyte Vram AGP | US$ | 400 |
| **Professional graphic cards** | | |
| Quadro4 900XGL 128 Mbyte Vram AGP | US$ | 1200 |
| Fire GL X1 256 Mbyte Vram AGP | US$ | 1200 |
| **Tracking system** | | |
| Polhemus Fastrak | US$ | 7000 |
| Ascension PC Flock of Birds | US$ | 2200 |
| Intersense Intertrax 2 | US$ | 1100 |
| **3D Shutter Glasses** | | |
| StereoEyes Wireless | US$ | 320 |
| Elsa 3D Revelator IR | US$ | 180 |
| VRex Cordless | US$ | 100 |
| **Head Mounted Display** | | |
| Kaiser Proview XL 40/50 (XGA  resolution – 3D, wide fov) | US$ | 50000 |
| N-visor Datavisor Hi-res (XGA resolution – 2D, wide fov) | US$ | 35000 |
| Daeyang I-Visor DH4400 VP 3D (SVGA resolution – 3D) | US$ | 1900 |
| Olympus Eye-Trek FMD-700 (SVGA resolution – 2D) | US$ | 1300 |
| Daeyang I-Visor DH4400 VP (SVGA resolution – 2D) | US$ | 1200 |
| Olympus Eyetrek 250 W (Video output only – 2D) | US$ | 600 |
| Sony Glasstron PLM-A35 (Video output only – 2D) | US$ | 500 |
| **VR Gloves** | | |
| Pinch Glove | US$ | 2000 |
| 5DT Right Hand | US$ | 650 |

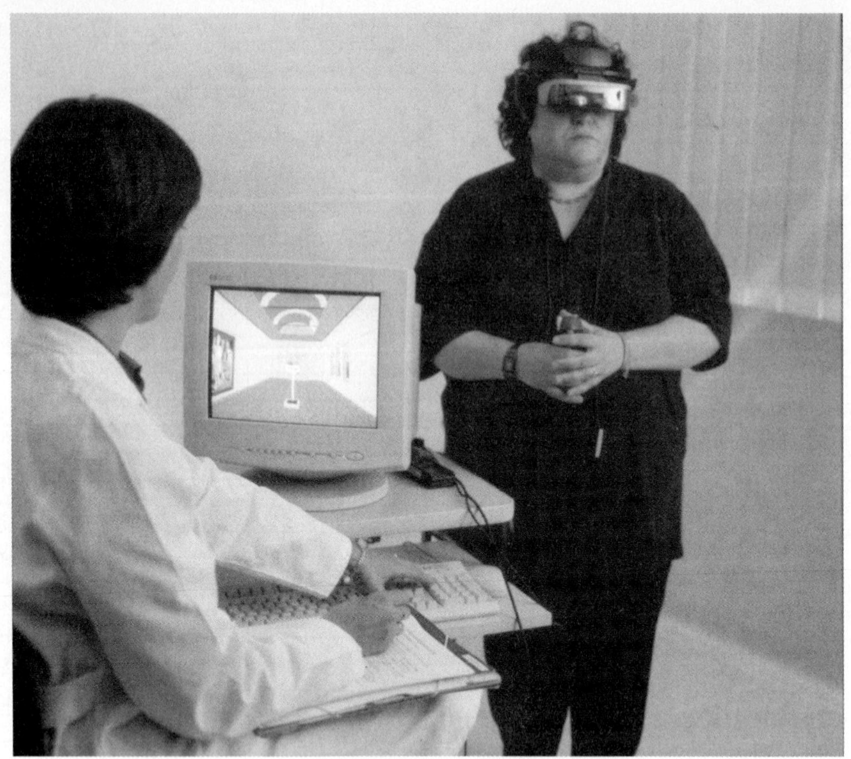

Fig.2. The Virtual Reality for Eating Disorders Modification - VREDIM (Istituto Auxologico Italiano I.R.C.C.S., Milan, Italy).

Octane (see Table 2), during the last two years about 60% of the VR applications for health care were developed for use on PC platforms.

The significant advances in PC hardware that have been made over the last five years are transforming PC-based VR into reality. The cost of a basic desktop VR system has gone down by many thousand dollars since that time, and the functionality has improved dramatically in terms of graphics processing power. A simple immersive VR system now may cost less than 6000 US$ (see Table 1).

The availability of powerful PC engines based on such computing work-horses as Intel's Xeon and IBM G4/G5 processors, and the emergence of reasonably priced Direct 3D and OpenGL-based 3D accelerator cards allow high-end PCs to process and display interactive 3D simulations in real time.

While a standard Celeron/Duron processor with as little as 64 Mbytes of RAM can provide sufficient processing power for a simple VR simulation, a fast Pentium IV/Athlon XP-based PC (2.2 Ghz or faster) with 256 Mbytes of RAM, can transport users to a convincing virtual environment, while a dual Xeon configuration (2.4 Ghz or faster) with 1 Gbyte of RAM, OpenGL acceleration and 128 Mbytes of VRAM running Windows XP Pro rivals the horsepower of a mid-level graphics workstation.

The graphics card landscape is also evolving quickly. In particular, two advancements are interesting for VR users: the inclusion of a VGA-to-TV converter and tuner, the Accelerated Graphics Port (AGP) and the new faster 3D chips (GeForce NV30/35, Radeon 9700/9800) with 128 Mbytes or more of dedicated video Ram (VRam).

- *Accelerated Graphics Port (AGP):* The accelerated graphics port is a high-speed, point-to-point connection between the system chip set and the graphics chip. AGP provides a high-speed pipeline between the graphics accelerator and the PC's system memory: using an AGP connection, a graphics chip is able to access system memory directly through the system chip set at memory-bus speeds, reducing latency and substantially increasing performance versus standard PCI-memory transfers. The graphics card gains access to system RAM to store and execute texture bitmaps, which allows more detailed textures of unlimited size while speeding 3-D rendering. When textures are large, AGP can make the difference between smooth or choppy frame rates in 3-D rendering.

- *Faster 3D cards*: In VR, performance is critical. VEs gave mainstream 3-D acceleration its start, and developers have been adding a sense of realistic depth to their creations for years. However, the addition of a $z$-axis in rendering, as opposed to simply drawing on an $x, y$-coordinate plane, requires more sophisticated horse-power. In addition, VR applications contain more complex objects and complex *textures*: bitmap renderings of detailed surfaces (bricks, sand, or transparent water) that heighten realism. To exploit this potential, a fast graphics card with a lot of video Ram is a must. Happily, the new chip sets (GeForce NV30/35 and Radeon 9700) included in consumer graphics cards have 8 times more video Ram and 3,5 times more 3-D acceleration than the first generation of chips (GeForce and Radeon VE) for a price tag of less than US$500. Also, professional graphics cards received a significant speed bump. New Open GL cards such as the Quadro 4 900XGL or the FireGLX1 offer graphics power that rival the one provided by Unix graphic workstations.

- *VGA-to-TV converter*: One welcomed feature of the new graphics cards is the inclusion of a VGA-to-TV (NTSC or PAL) converter and TV tuner right on the card. This feature lets you display computer data on a standard

Table 2. VR Hardware.

| Authors | Paper | Sample |
|---|---|---|
| Emmelkamp, P.M.G., Bruynzeel, M., Drost, L., & van der Mast, C.A.P.G. | (2001) Virtual reality treatment in acrophobia: A comparison with exposure in Vivo, *Cyberpsychol Behav, 4*(3), 335-339. | 10 acrophobia patients |
| Ali, M.R., Mowery, Y., Kaplan, B., DeMaria, E.J. | (2002) Training the novice in laparoscopy. *Surg Endosc, 16 (8), 1, 1210-1216.* | 27 high school students |
| Emmelkamp, P.M.G., Krijn, M., Hulsbosch, A.M., de Vries, S., Schuemie, M.J., van der Mast, C.A.P.G. | (2002) Virtual reality treatment versus exposure in vivo: a comparative evaluation in acrophobia, *Behav Res Ther,* 40, 509–516. | 33 acrophobia patients |
| Grundman, J. A., Wigton, R. S., & Nickol, D. | (2000). A controlled trial of an interactive, web-based virtual reality program for teaching physical diagnosis skills to medical students. *Acad Med, 75*(10 Suppl), S47-49. | 121 medical students |
| Hoffman, H. G., Patterson, D. R., & Carrougher, G. J. | (2000). Use of virtual reality for adjunctive treatment of adult burn pain during physical therapy: a controlled study. *Clin J Pain, 16*(3), 244-250. | 12 burn patients |
| Riva, G., Bacchetta, M., Baruffi, M., & Molinari, E. | (2001). Virtual reality-based multidimensional therapy for the treatment of body image disturbances in obesity: a controlled study. *Cyberpsychol Behav, 4*(4), 511-526. | 28 obese patients |
| Riva, G., Bacchetta, M., Baruffi, M., & Molinari, E. | Virtual reality-based multidimensional therapy for the treatment of body image disturbances in binge eating disorders: A preliminary controlled study *IEEE Transactions on Information Technology in Biomedicine, in press, 2002.* | 20 binge eating patients |
| Rothbaum, B. O., Hodges, L. F., Kooper, R., Opdyke, D., & et al. | (1995). Effectiveness of computer-generated (virtual reality) graded exposure in the treatment of acrophobia. *American Journal of Psychiatry, 152*(4), 626-628. | 17 college students |
| Rothbaum, B. O., Hodges, L., Smith, S., Lee, J. H., & Price, L. | (2000). A controlled study of virtual reality exposure therapy for the fear of flying. *J Consult Clin Psychol, 68*(6), 1020-1026. | 49 fear of flying patients |
| Torkington, J., Smith, S. G., Rees, B. I., & Darzi, A. | (2001). Skill transfer from virtual reality to a real laparoscopic task. *Surg Endosc, 15*(10), 1076-1079. | 30 medical students |
| Wiederhold, B.K., Jang, D.P., Kim, S.I., & Wiederhold, M.D. | (2002). Physiological monitoring as an objective tool in virtual reality therapy, *Cyberpsychol Behav. 5*(1) 77-82. | 36 fear of flying patients, 22 non-phobics |
| Wiederhold, B.K., Jang, D.P., Kim, S.I., & Wiederhold, M.D. | (2002). A controlled trial comparing physiological responses during virtual reality exposure and imaginal exposure in flight phobics. *IEEE Transactions on Information Technology in Biomedicine, in press, 2002.* | 30 fear of flying patients |

television without the need for an external scan converter (usually US$100 or more). Business users can then give PC-based presentations with TVs as large-screen monitors, and home users can play computer games on their TV sets. However this feature is also useful for VR users: thanks to the converter it is possible to use - without any extra hardware - the new low-cost DVD oriented head-mounted displays from Olympus (EyeTrek, 600 US$) or Sony (Glasstron PLM-A35, 500 US$).

On the software side, an interesting low cost solution is the use of 3D engines included in commercial 3D games for developing simple virtual environments. Many 3D games (US$ 50 each), such as Quake 3 or Unreal, include level editors that allow the user to customize the environments and the avatars. Moreover, Discreet has released the free software, *gmax™*, which allows the professional customization of 3D games. Intended to be a fully capable 3D level editing, modeling, animation, and texture-mapping tool, *gmax* ships with a full suite of professional 3D content and animation features. Discreet approved game developers can publish *gmax* "game packs", which customize the downloadable version of *gmax* into a fully featured level editor for supported game titles. Using this software, it is possible to edit and create 3D environments, materials, 3D objects, weapons, images and lights.

Obviously, level editing does not allow full control of the environment. In particular, the user interaction with the 3D objects is usually very limited. To overcome this limitation, now there are different VR development toolkits available for PCs, ranging from high-end authoring toolkits that require significant programming experience to simple "hobbyist" packages. Despite the differences in the types of virtual worlds these products can deliver, the various tools are based on the same VR-development model: they allow users to create or import 3D objects, to apply behavioral attributes such as weight and gravity to the objects, and to program the objects to respond to the user via visual and or audio events. Ranging in prices from free (http://www.alice.org) to US $5000 (Virtools Dev 2.1 or Sense 8 WorldUp R5), the toolkits are the most functional of the available VR software options. While some of them rely exclusively on C or C++ programming to build a virtual world, others offer simpler point-and-click operations to develop a simulation. Using VR toolkits, it is also possible to bring in files from a wide array of software packages, such as Wavefront, 3D Studio, EDS Unigraphics, Pro Engineer, and Intergraph EMS, and they can also import VRML and Multigen databases as well as animation scripts and sounds.

---

# 5 Challenges and Open Issues

## 5.1 Technical challenges

Even if the significant advances in computer and graphic technology drastically improved the characteristics of a typical VE, VR is still limited by the maturity of the systems available. Even today, no off-the-shelf solutions are available. So, the set up of a VR system usually requires a lot of patience for dealing with conflicting hardware or lacking drivers. Nearly every VR system requires a dedicated staff member or at least a computer technician to keep the system running smoothly. Moreover, much VR technology is still uncomfortable or unpleasant to use. In particular here are some current VR technology limitations for users [53]:

- Virtual acoustic displays that require a great deal of computational resources in order to simulate a small number of sources;
- Force and tactile displays, still in their infancies, with limited functionality;
- Image generators that can't provide low-latency rendering of head tracked complex scenes, requiring severe trade-offs between performance & scene quality;
- Position trackers with small working volumes, inadequate robustness, and problems of latency and poor registration.
- HMDs with limited field of view, and encumbering form factor;

As we have seen, a typical area for VR applications is surgery. However, there have been few developments in the area of tactile feedback. The ability to feel tissue is important. Procedures that require palpitation, such as artery localization and tumor detection, are extremely difficult when the only form of haptic exploration is in the form of forces transmitted through long, clumsy instruments. As noted by Moline [54], "The ability to remotely sense small scale shape information and feel forces that mesh with natural hand motions would greatly improve the performance of minimally invasive surgery and bring a greater sense of realism to virtual trainers" (p. 21).

## 5.2 Safety Issues

The introduction of patients and clinicians to VEs raises particular safety and ethical issues [28]. In fact, despite developments in VR technology, some users still experience health and safety problems associated with VR use [55]. The key concern from the literature is VR-induced sickness, which could lead to problems [56] including:
- symptoms of motion sickness;
- strain on the ocular system;
- degraded limb and postural control;
- reduced sense of presence;
- the development of responses

inappropriate for the real world, which might lead to negative training.

The improved quality of VR systems is drastically reducing the occurrence of simulation sickness. For instance, a recent review of clinical applications of VR reported instances of simulation sickness are few and nearly all are transient and minor [4]. In general, for a large proportion of VR users these effects are mild and subside quickly [55].

Nonetheless, patients exposed to virtual reality environments may have disabilities that increase their susceptibility to side effects. Precautions should be taken to ensure the safety and well being of patients, including established protocols for monitoring and controlling exposure to virtual reality environments.

Strategies are needed to detect any adverse effects of exposure, some of which may be difficult to anticipate, at an early stage. According to Lewis & Griffin [56] exposure management protocols for patients in virtual environments should include:
- Screening procedures to detect individuals who may present particular risks.
- Procedures for managing patient exposure to VR applications to ensure rapid adaptation with minimum symptoms.
- Procedures for monitoring unexpected side effects and for ensuring that the system meets its design objectives.

Finally, the effect of VEs on cognition is not fully understood. In a recent report, the US National Advisory Mental Health Council [57] suggested that "Research is needed to understand both the positive and the negative effects [of VEs]... on children's and adult's perceptual and cognitive skills." Such research will require the merging of knowledge from a variety of disciplines including (but not limited to) neuropsychology, neuroimaging, educational theory and technology, human factors, medicine, and computer science.

## 5.3 Research and clinical issues

In the last five years there has been a steady growth in the use of virtual reality in health care due to the advances in information technology and to the decline in costs [58]. As we have seen, using the "virtual reality" keyword we can find 829 papers listed in MEDLINE and 693 in PSYCINFO (accessed Aug. 8 2002). Much of this growth, however, has been in the form of feasibility studies and pilot trials.

The "best" evidence in evaluating the efficacy of a therapy/approach is the results of randomized, controlled clinical trials. However, if we check the available literature we can find only twelve controlled trials (see Table 2).

Three tested the training possibilities offered by VR: in surgical training and in teaching physical diagnosis skills. Eight verified the effectiveness of VR in the treatment of four psychological disorders: acrophobia, body image disturbances, binge eating disorders and fear of flying. The final study analyzed the use of VR in the treatment of adult burn pain.

Why there are so few controlled trials in VR research? There are three possible answers .

First, the lack of standardization in VR devices and software. To date, very few of the various VR systems available are interoperable. This makes their use in contexts other than those in which they were developed difficult.

Second, the lack of standardized protocols that can be shared by the community of researchers. If we check the two clinical databases, we can find only four published clinical protocols: for the treatment of eating disorders [59], fear of flying [60], fear of public speaking [61] and panic disorders [62].

Finally, the costs required for the set-up trials. As we have just seen, the lack of interoperable systems added to the lack of clinical protocols force most researchers to spend a lot of time and money in designing and developing their own VR application: many of them can be considered "one-off" creations tied to proprietary hardware and software, which have been tuned by a process of trial and error. According to the European funded project VEPSY Updated [63], the cost required for designing a clinical VR application from scratch and testing it on clinical patients using controlled trials may range between 150000 and 200000 US$. As noted by a recent report prepared by the US National Research Council [64], "the government support has been the single most important source of sustained funding for innovative research in both computer graphics and VR. Beginning in the 1960s with its investments in computer modeling, flight simulators, and visualization techniques, and continuing through current developments in virtual worlds, the federal government has made significant investments in military, civilian, and university research that laid the groundwork for one of today's most dynamic technologies. The commercial payoffs have included numerous companies formed around federally funded research in graphics and VR." (p. 227). In Europe, the most important source of funding for health care VR applications was the European Commission through its Information Society Technology programme. However, in the last five years the funds for VR research coming from the European Commission has been between one-third and one-fifth of the total amount distributed by the US government.

---

# 6. Conclusions

In general, the review of current applications show that VR can be considered a useful tool in diagnosis, therapy, education and training. However, several barriers still remain. The PC-based systems, while inexpensive and easy-to-use, still suffer from a lack of flexibility and capabilities necessary to individualize environ-

ments for each patient [65]. On the other hand, in most circumstances the clinical skills of the therapist remain the most important factor in the successful use of VR systems. It is clear that building new and additional virtual environments is important so therapists will continue to investigate applying these tools in their day-to-day clinical practice [4]. Further, many of the actual VR applications are in the clinical investigation or laboratory stage, as clearly shown by the lack of controlled trials.

Significant efforts are still required to move VR into commercial success and therefore routine clinical use. Possible future scenarios will involve multi-disciplinary teams of engineers, computer programmers, and therapists working together to treat specific clinical problems. Finally, communication networks have the potential to transform VEs into shared worlds in which individuals, objects, and processes interact without regard to their location. In the future, such networks will probably merge VR and telemedicine applications allowing us to use VE for such purposes as distance learning, distributed training, and e-therapy.

It is hoped that by bringing together this community of experts, further stimulation of interest from granting agencies will be accelerated. Information on advances in VR technology must be made available to the health care community in a format that is easy-to-understand and invites participation [66]. Future potential applications of VR are really only limited by the imaginations of talented individuals.

## Acknowledgments

The present work was supported by the Commission of the European Communities (CEC), in particular by the IST programme (Project VEPSY UPDATED, IST-2000-25323, http://www.psicologia.net; http://www.e-therapy.info).

## References

1. Satava RM, Jones SB. Medical applications of virtual reality. In: Stanney KM, editor. Handbook of Virtual Environments: Design, Implementation, and Applications. Mahwah, NJ: Lawrence Erlbaum Associates, Inc.; 2002. p. 368-91.
2. Wootton R. Telemedicine: an introduction. In: Wootton R, editor. European Telemedicine 1998/99. London: Kensington Publications Ltd; 1999. p.10-2.
3. Chinnock C. Virtual reality in surgery and medicine. Hosp Technol Ser 1994;13(18):1-48.
4. Riva G, Wiederhold B, Molinari E, editors. Virtual environments in clinical psychology and neuroscience: Methods and techniques in advanced patient-therapist interaction. Amsterdam: IOS Press. Online: http://www.psicologia.net/pages/book2.htm; 1998.
5. Beolchi L, Riva G. Virtual reality for health care. In: Akay M, Marsh A, editors. Information Technologies in Medicine. Toronto: John Wiley & Sons; 2001. p. 39-83.
6. Rubino F, Soler L, Marescaux J, Maisonneuve H. Advances in virtual reality are wide ranging. BMJ 2002;324(7337):612.
7. McCloy R, Stone R. Science, medicine, and the future. Virtual reality in surgery. BMJ 2001;323(7318):912-5.
8. Székely G, Satava RM. Virtual reality in medicine. BMJ 1999;319(7220):1305.
9. Schultheis MT, Rizzo AA. The Application of Virtual Reality Technology in Rehabilitation. Rehabil Psychol 2001;46(3):296-311.
10. Riva G, Rizzo A, Alpini D, Attree EA, Barbieri E, Bertella L, et al. Virtual environments in the diagnosis, prevention, and intervention of age-related diseases: A review of VR scenarios proposed in the EC VETERAN project. Cyberpsychol Behav 1999;2(6):577-91.
11. Rizzo AA, Wiederhold B, Riva G, Van Der Zaag C. A bibliography of articles relevant to the application of virtual reality in the mental health field. Cyberpsychol Behav 1998;1(4):411-25.
12. Rizzo AA, Buckwalter JG. Virtual reality and cognitive assessment and rehabilitation: the state of the art. In: Riva G, editor. Virtual reality in neuro-psycho-physiology. Amsterdam: IOS Press; 1997. p. 123-46.
13. Riva G, Alcañiz M, Anolli L, Bacchetta M, Baños RM, Beltrame F, et al. The VEPSY Updated project: Virtual reality in clinical psychology. Cyberpsychol Behav 2001;4(4):449-55.
14. Heim M. Virtual Realism. New York: Oxford University Press, 1998.

15. Bricken W. Virtual reality: Directions of growth. Seattle, WA: University of Washington, 1990.

16. Riva G, Mantovani G. The need for a socio-cultural perspective in the implementation of virtual environments. Virtual Reality 2000(5):32-8.

17. Riva G, Davide F, editors. Communications through Virtual Technologies: Identity, Community and Technology in the Communication Age. Amsterdam: Ios Press. Online: http://www. emergingcommunication.com/volume1.html, 2001.

18. Biocca F, Levy MR, editors. Communication in the age of virtual reality. Hillsdale, NJ: Lawrence Erlbaum Associates, 1995.

19. Steuer JS. Defining virtual reality: Dimensions determining telepresence. Journal of Communication 1992;42(4):73-93.

20. Sastry L, Boyd DRS. Virtual environments for engineering applications. Virtual Reality: Research, development and applications 1998;3(4):235-44.

21. Satava RM, Ellis SR. Human interface technology. An essential tool for the modern surgeon. Surg Endosc 1994;8(7):817-20.

22. ISO. ISO/IEC 9126 - Software engineering — Product quality — Part 1: Quality model. Geneva: International Organization for Standardization, 2001.

23. John NW, Thacker N, Pokric M, Jackson A, Zanetti G, Gobbetti E, et al. An integrated simulator for surgery of the petrous bone. Stud Health Technol Inform 2001;81:218-24.

24. Ackerman MJ. The Visible Human Project. J Biocommun 1991;18(2):14.

25. Spitzer V, Ackerman MJ, Scherzinger AL, Whitlock D. The visible human male: a technical report. J Am Med Inform Assoc 1996;3(2):118-30.

26. Ackerman MJ, Yoo T, Jenkins D. From data to knowledge—the Visible Human Project continues. Medinfo 2001;10(Pt 2):887-90.

27. Westwood JD, Hoffman HM, Mogel GT, Stredney D, editors. Medicine meets virtual reality 2002. Amsterdam: IOS Press, 2002.

28. Durlach NI, Mavor ASE. Virtual reality: scientific and technological challenges. Washington, D.C.: National Academy Press. Online: http://www.nap.edu/books/0309051355/html/index.html, 1995.

29. Satava RM. Surgery 2001: A Technologic Framework for the Future. Surg Endosc 1993;7:111-3.

30. Satava RM. Virtual reality surgical simulator. The first steps. Surg Endosc 1993;7(3):203-5.

31. Satava RM. Surgical education and surgical simulation. World J Surg 2001;25 (11):1484-9.

32. Ali MR, Mowery Y, Kaplan B, DeMaria EJ. Training the novice in laparoscopy. Surg Endosc 2002.

33. Dammann F, Bode A, Schwaderer E, Schaich M, Heuschmid M, Maassen MM. Computer-aided surgical planning for implantation of hearing aids based on CT data in a VR environment. Radiographics 2001;21(1):183-91.

34. Xia J, Ip HH, Samman N, Wong HT, Gateno J, Wang D, et al. Three-dimensional virtual-reality surgical planning and soft-tissue prediction for orthognathic surgery. IEEE Trans Inf Technol Biomed 2001;5(2):97-107.

35. Herfarth C, Lamade W, Fischer L, Chiu P, Cardenas C, Thorn M, et al. The effect of virtual reality and training on liver operation planning. Swiss Surg 2002;8(2):67-73.

36. Ross MD, Twombly IA, Bruyns C, Cheng R, Senger S. Telecommunications for health care over distance: the virtual collaborative clinic. Stud Health Technol Inform 2000;70:286-91.

37. Halligan S, Fenlon HM. Virtual colonoscopy. BMJ 1999;319(7219):1249-52.

38. Vincelli F. From imagination to virtual reality: the future of clinical psychology. Cyberpsychol Behav 1999;2(3):241-8.

39. Vincelli F, Molinari E, Riva G. Virtual reality as clinical tool: immersion and three-dimensionality in the relationship between patient and therapist. Stud Health Technol Inform 2001;81:551-3.

40. Norcross JC, Hedges M, Prochaska JO. The face of 2010: A Delphi poll on the future of psychotherapy. *Prof Psychol Res Pr* 2002;33(3):316-22.

41. Menon ST. Psychological Empowerment: Definition, Measurement, and Validation. Canadian Journal of Behavioural Science 1999;31(3):161-4.

42. Botella C, Perpiña C, Baños RM, Garcia-Palacios A. Virtual reality: a new clinical setting lab. Stud Health Technol Inform 1998;58:73-81.

43. Riva G. Virtual environments in neuroscience. IEEE Trans Inf Technol Biomed 1998;2(4):275-81.

44. Rose FD, Brooks BM, Attree EA, Parslow DM, Leadbetter AG, McNeil JE, et al. A preliminary investigation into the use of virtual environments in memory retraining after vascular brain injury: indications for future strategy? Disabil Rehabil 1999;21(12):548-54.

45. Gourlay D, Lun KC, Lee YN, Tay J. Virtual reality for relearning daily living skills. Int J Med Inf 2000;60(3):255-61.

46. Riva G. Virtual reality in rehabilitation of spinal cord injuries. Rehabil Psychol 2000;45(1):81-8.

47. Sisto SA, Forrest GF, Glendinning D. Virtual reality applications for motor rehabilitation after stroke. Topics in Stroke Rehabilitation 2002;8(4):11-23.

48. Zhang L, Abreu BC, Masel B, Scheibel RS, Christiansen CH, Huddleston N, et al. Virtual reality in the assessment of selected cognitive function after brain injury. Am J Phys Med Rehabil 2001;80(8):597-604; quiz 605.

49. Wald J, Liu L. Psychometric properties of the driVR: a virtual reality driving assessment. Stud Health Technol Inform 2001;81:564-6.

50. Pugnetti L, Mendozzi L, Motta A, Cattaneo A, Barbieri E, Brancotti A. Evaluation and retraining of adults' cognitive impairment: which role for virtual reality technology? Comput Biol Med 1995;25(2):213-27.

51. Broeren J, Bjorkdahl A, Pascher R, Rydmark M. Virtual reality and haptics as an assessment device in the postacute phase after stroke. Cyberpsychol Behav 2002;5(3):207-11.

52. Piron L, Cenni F, Tonin P, Dam M. Virtual Reality as an assessment tool for arm motor deficits after brain lesions. Stud Health Technol Inform 2001;81:386-92.

53. Gross D. Technology Management and User Acceptance of VE Technology. In: Stanney KM, editor. Handbook of Virtual Environments: Design, Implementation, and Applications. Mahwah, NJ: Lawrence Erlbaum Associates, Inc., 2002.

54. Moline J. Virtual reality in health care: a survey. In: Riva G, editor. Virtual reality in neuro-psycho-physiology. Amsterdam: IOS Press, 1997:3-34.

55. Nichols S, Patel H. Health and safety implications of virtual reality: a review of empirical evidence. Appl Ergon 2002;33(3):251-71.

56. Lewis CH, Griffin MJ. Human factors consideration in clinical applications of virtual reality. In: Riva G, editor. Virtual reality in neuro-psycho-physiology. Amsterdam: IOS Press, 1997:35-56.

57. A report of the U.S. National Advisory Mental Health Council. Washington, D.C.: U.S. Goverment Printing Office, 1995.

58. Riva G. Virtual reality for health care: the status of research. Cyberpsychol Behav 2002;5(3):219-25.

59. Riva G, Bacchetta M, Cesa G, Conti S, Molinari E. Virtual reality and telemedicine based Experiential Cognitive Therapy: Rationale and Clinical Protocol. In: Riva G, Galimberti C, editors. Towards CyberPsychology: Mind, Cognition and Society in the Internet Age. Amsterdam: IOS Press; 2001. p. 273-308.

60. Klein RA. Treating fear of flying with virtual reality exposure therapy. In: VandeCreek L, Jackson TL, editors. Innovations in clinical practice: A source

book, Vol. 17.. Sarasota, FL, US.; 1999. p. 449-65

61. Botella C, Banos RM, Villa H, Perpina C, Garcia-Palacios A. Telepsychology: Public speaking fear treatment on the internet. Cyberpsychol Behav 2000;3(6):959-68.

62. Vincelli F, Choi YH, Molinari E, Wiederhold BK, Riva G. A VR-based multicomponent treatment for panic disorders with agoraphobia. Stud Health Technol Inform 2001;81:544-50.

63. Riva G, Bolzoni M, Carella F, Galimberti C, Griffin MJ, Lewis CH, et al. Virtual reality environments for psycho-neuro-physiological assessment and rehabilitation. In: Morgan KS, Weghorst SJ, Hoffman HM, Stredney D, editors. Medicine Meets Virtual Reality: Global Healthcare Grid. Amsterdam: IOS Press; 1997. p. 34-45.

64. Hughes T, Clark DD, Banks PM, Lineberger WC, editors. Funding a Revolution: Government Support for Computing Research. Washington, DC: National Academy Press. Online: http://stills.nap.edu/html/far/contents.html, 1999.

65. Riva G, editor. Virtual reality in neuro-psycho-physiology: Cognitive, clinical and methodological issues in assessment and rehabilitation. Amsterdam: IOS Press. Online: http://www.psicologia.net/pages/book1.htm, 1997.

66. Riva G, Bacchetta M, Baruffi M, Borgomainerio E, Defrance C, Gatti F, et al. VREPAR Projects: The use of virtual environments in psycho-neuro-physiological assessment and rehabilitation. Cyberpsychol Behav 1999;2(1):69-76.

Address of the author:
Prof. Giuseppe Riva, Ph.D.
Dipartimento di Psicologia
Università Cattolica del Sacro Cuore
Largo Gemelli 1
20123 Milan, Italy
Tel:       +39-02-58216892
Fax:      +39-02-70034918
E-mail:   auxo.psylab@auxologico.it
Web site:  http://www.atnplab.com

**G. Burdea**

CAIP Center, Rutgers University
Piscataway, New Jersey, USA

# Review Paper

# *Virtual Rehabilitation - Benefits and Challenges*[1]

**Abstract**: Virtual rehabilitation represents the provision of therapeutic interventions locally or at a distance, using Virtual Reality hardware and simulations. Such therapy has been applied to various patient populations, including musculo-skeletal, post-stroke, and cognitively- impaired. This article reviews the benefits brought by VR-enhanced and VR-based rehabilitation to the above patient groups. Also discussed are the many challenges in integrating this new technology into the medical care system.

## Introduction

Virtual Reality technology has been commercially available since the late 80's, with the first systems sold by VPL Research. A dramatic improvement in computer technology, coupled with better programming tools have contributed to the "rebirth" of VR in the late 90's. Currently its application domains (with significant cost advantage) range from the oil and gas industry, to manufacturing (especially airplanes and cars), to military and medical care.

Within Medicine, VR has been used in teaching anatomy, training in diagnostic procedures (such as virtual colonoscopy, or virtual bronchroscopy), teaching open and minimally-invasive surgery procedures, and in rehabilitation. Within the scope of this article, we are interested in Virtual Rehabilitation, which can be defined as the provision of therapy using VR hardware and simulations. While newer than other medical VR application domains, it is growing at an incredible pace in the US, Europe and Asia. A testimonial to the ongoing research into what may soon revolutionize the "art" of therapy are several recent conferences focusing on Virtual Rehabilitation.

The present review of Virtual Rehabilitation starts with ways to classify it. Subsequently its many benefits are discussed, looking at therapeutic approaches, medical efficacy and patient's subjective reaction to the technology. Our enthusiasm for this new field of Medicine is tempered by the realization that many challenges exist, from equipment issues, to cost and the attitude of the therapist community towards this new technology. The article ends with a summary of benefits/challenges, some being common to all forms of Virtual Rehabilitation, some being specific to a given patient population. This review is by no means all-encompassing, owing to space and time limitations. Many projects exist, in various stages of development, from concept to prototype, to clinical pilot studies, in addition to those mentioned here.

## Types of Virtual Rehabilitation

There are several ways to classify Virtual Rehabilitation. An obvious one is related to the *specific patient population* it is destined for. Thus we can distinguish musculo-skeletal Virtual Rehabilitation, post-stroke Virtual Rehabilitation, and cognitive Virtual Rehabilitation, among others. Musculo-skeletal (orthopedic) patients are those that suffered a bone or muscle/ligament injury, are younger and more numerous than other patients needing rehabilitation. For example, in the United States, every day 25,000 individuals sprain

---

[1] Based on the Key note address with the same title given at the 1st *International Workshop on Virtual Rehabilitation*, Lausanne, Switzerland, November 7-8, 2002. © Grigore Burdea

---

their ankle, according to the American Association of Orthopedic Surgeons [1]. Post-stroke patients are those that have survived a neural hemorrhage, or blood clot to the brain, resulting in paralysis to half of their body. There are 500,000 such new cases yearly, according to the American Stroke Association [2]. The cognitive patient population groups individuals with various psychological disorders, ranging from attention deficit/ hyperactivity, to eating disorders, to post-traumatic stress and phobias [10].

Another way to classify Virtual Rehabilitation relates to the *rehabilitation protocol*. Here we distinguish VR-augmented and VR-based therapy. In VR-augmented rehabilitation patients receive a mixture of "classical" exercises, done on equipment available in the clinic (or at home), as well as a VR regimen of simulation exercises. Rehabilitation which is VR-based eliminates the classical exercises entirely, and is a newer approach compared to VR-augmented therapy.

Virtual Rehabilitation simulations differ depending on the particular *therapeutic approach*, such as "teaching by example," "video game-like," and "exposure therapy." Teaching by example has been used to treat post-stroke chronic patients by researchers at the Massachusetts Institute of Technology. As shown in Figure 1a [8], motor training of the arm reach motion is done with a "teacher" object (in this case a cube). The required motion trajectory, typical of a frontal reach task, is visualized to help the patients. Their arm motion is tracked and mapped to the motion of another virtual object following the teacher's example. By contrast, Figure 1b [3] shows a video game-like approach, where the patient pilots an airplane through 3-D hoops. Here there is no teacher object, and the patient has a higher cognitive load when performing the exercise.

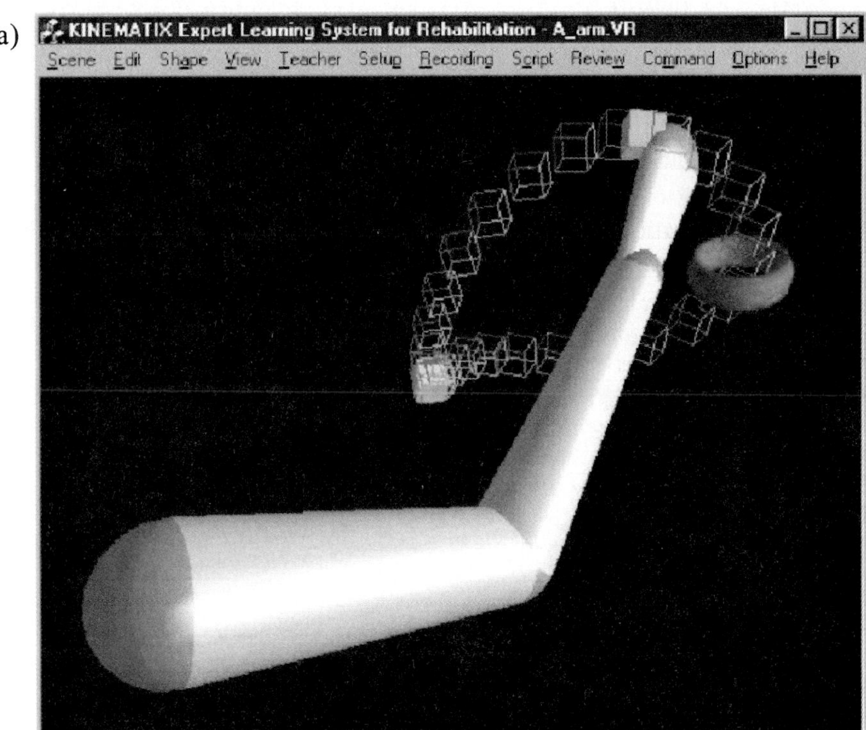


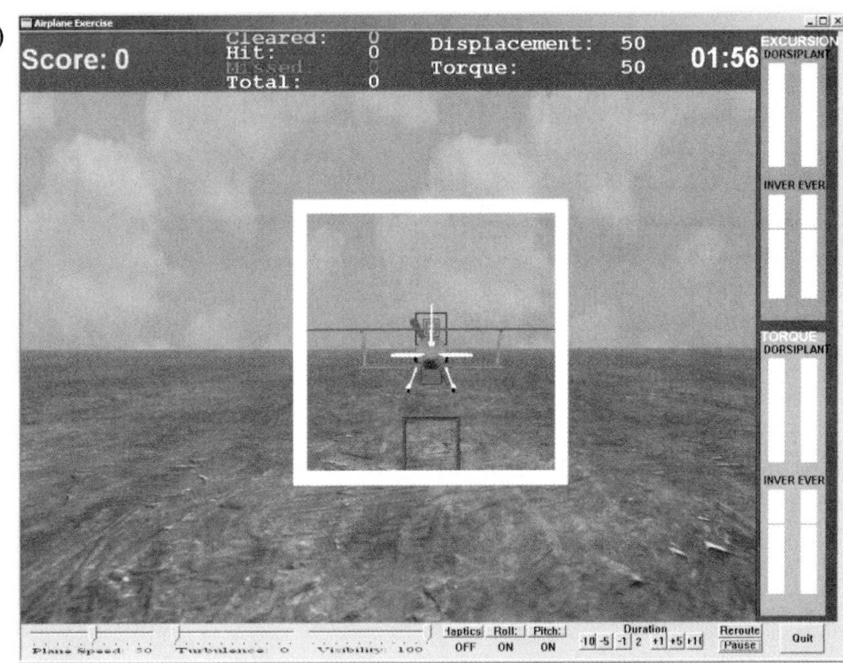


Fig. 1. Various Virtual Rehabilitation therapeutic approaches: a) teaching by example [8] © Lawrence Erlbaum 2002. Reprinted by permission; b) video-game exercise simulation. © Rutgers University 2002. Reprinted by permission.

Finally, one can classify Virtual Rehabilitation according to the *proximity to the therapist* (or therapeutic team) assisting the patient. If the therapists are nearby, the therapy is local, such as in an outpatient clinic environment. However, if the therapist is remote, then therapy is administered through a Virtual Telerehabilitation approach. Telerehabilitation is a newer form of virtual rehabilitation than clinic-based therapy, and is less developed at this time.

## Benefits of Virtual Rehabilitation

Before discussing the benefits of Virtual Rehabilitation, let us first look at some of the characteristics of classical rehabilitation. One adjective comes to mind… "boring." Indeed, rehabilitation is by its nature repetitive, and repetition tends to "decouple" the mind, and reduce patient's motivation. Another characteristic is the predominance of simple mechanical devices with little or no computerized sensing. Thus there are no widespread online databases, and there are errors in interpreting evaluation data. Such errors are both positional and temporal, since the temporal granularity of manual data recording is low. Traditional rehabilitation is done one-to-one, meaning that one therapist (or sometimes several) is working with one patient. Thus costs are high, especially for demanding patients such as those with traumatic brain injury or spinal chord injury. For the portion of therapy that the patient is doing at home, there currently is no monitoring. This results in varying degrees of compliance with the prescribed exercise regimen, and a larger than necessary variability in treatment outcome. Finally, the distribution of therapists over the territory is uneven. They tend to gravitate towards urban areas, and away from rural or remote locations, where their practice is more difficult. More than 50 million Americans live in rural areas, however, only 10% of therapists practice there, according to a recent National Rural Health Association survey [9]. This situation forces patients to travel to mostly-urban clinics, with the resulting additional expenses and disruption in family life.

The advantages associated with the use of Virtual Rehabilitation are numerous. The same VR hardware can be used for various types of patients, as well as for various types of exercises done on those patients. For example, the same head-mounted display can be used for patients suffering from "Vietnam syndrome" (a form of post-traumatic stress disorder), as well as for children with attention deficits, or for post-stroke patients. Similarly, the same sensing glove can be used to train musculo-skeletal patients to squeeze "rubber balls," or to do a peg-board exercise. The rubber ball squeezing is a typical strengthening exercised prescribed after hand surgery, and corresponds with rehabilitation at the impairment level. The peg-board exercise, such as the one shown in Figure 2 [11], is a procedure done to improve hand-eye coordination (and possibly upper arm extension). It represents rehabilitation done at the (higher) functional level. Of course, there are no real peg-boards, or rubber balls, or any other equipment, except for the haptic glove. Thus a major advantage in all forms of Virtual Rehabilitation is *economy of scale*.

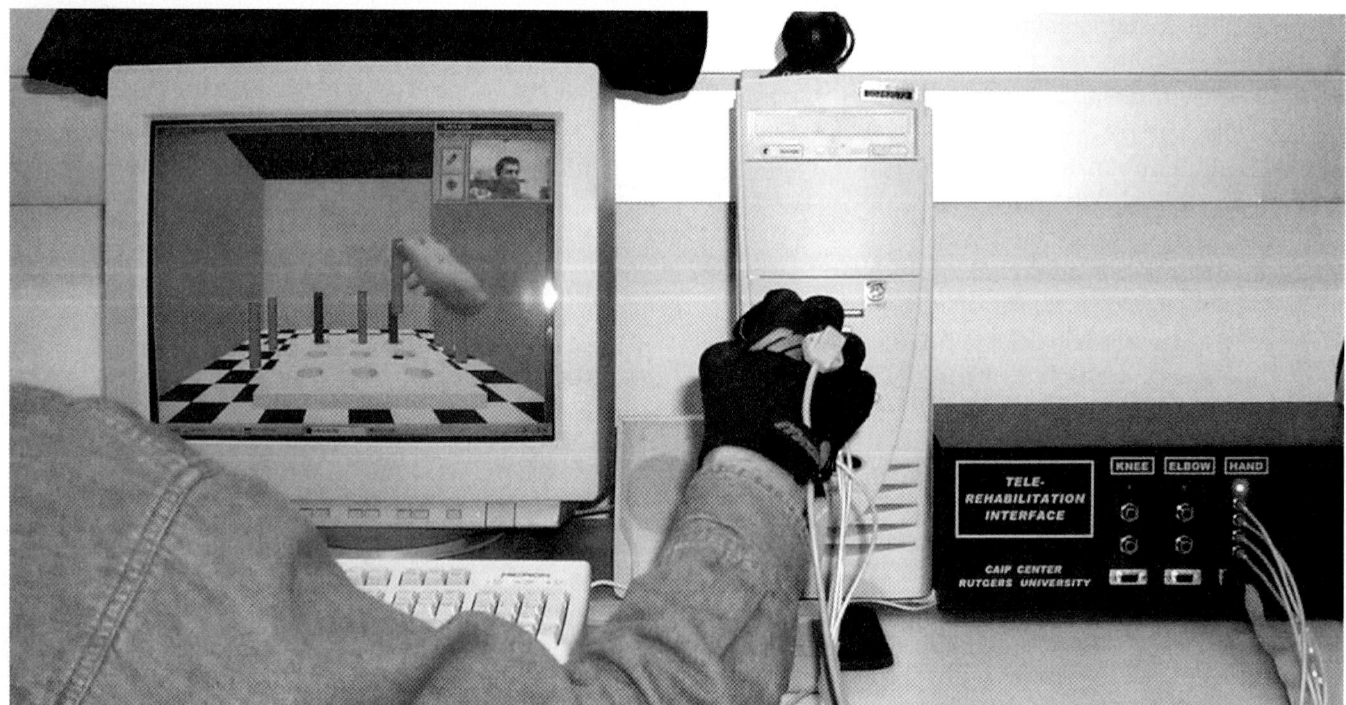


Fig. 2. The VR-based orthopedic rehabilitation using a haptic glove during a peg-board exercise. © IEEE 2000. Reprinted by permission.

Another advantage present in all forms of Virtual Rehabilitation is *interactivity* and *patient motivation*. This is especially true in video game-based therapeutic approaches, where the patient competes against the computer. By providing visual and auditory rewards, such as displaying gratifying messages in real time ("Great", "Very Good," etc.), patients are motivated to exercise. It has been even suggested that in the future patients may compete against each other in such rehabilitation games [5]. In other words they will get better while having fun!

Virtual Rehabilitation systems rely on computers to render and display the exercises, and on sensorized interfaces to mediate the patient's actions. As such data flows naturally to the host computer, at a frequency and resolution that are unmatched by traditional mechanical evaluation tools. The high temporal granularity of data, such as joint motion, or finger force output, is also important. One potential use of this intrinsic capability of Virtual Rehabilitation is to discern whether the patient is *"malingering."* This medical term describes patients that purposely do not exercise at their full capacity, for reasons of medical benefits, worker's compensation and such.

Thus patient data gathered during Virtual Rehabilitation is transparently stored in *online databases*, without the patient's or therapist's action. Access to this data can be done either through phone lines, or through the Internet. When the Internet is used, data can be uploaded through client-server communication, or through web access. If data is made available over the web, it needs to be password-protected, in order to preserve the patient's confidentiality. Once in a database, clinical measures can be viewed remotely, as shown in Figure 3. This represents the increase in a post-stroke patient's endurance during hand strengthening exercises over three weeks of VR-based therapy (August 13 to 30, 2001). The small bar graph to the left represents the baseline (the patient's initial capability before therapy). The data was sampled in Newark (New Jersey, USA), and accessed over the web, from the author's location 50 kilometers away.

Remote data access is one fundamental requirement of Telerehabilitation, where patients are remote from clinics and therapists. This represents a great benefit for rural patients, since they do not have to *travel* to urban clinics. Rural area therapy at home relies heavily on therapist assistants, who have less skill and experience than regular therapists. In that case Tele-consultation may provide expertise from specialists at tertiary care facilities, such as university hospitals, and thus improve quality of care and outcomes. Telerehabilitation is beneficial in *reducing healthcare costs* as well. For example, Buckley and colleagues at the Catholic University of America [4] report on a study of nursing management for stroke patients and their caregivers (usually spouses). They found that Tele-consultation visits averaged 20-25 minutes, compared to home care visits that took 30-60 minutes (plus another 60 minutes in travel time). Thus the cost of a nurse visit was reduced by more than half (from $75 to $30 for a Tele-consultation visit).

Another possible way in which costs will be reduced in the future is through multiplexed Telerehabilitation. This arrangement takes advantage of the intelligence available in the home PC, which can supplant the therapist some of the time. In this case a therapist will be able to monitor several patients exercising simultaneously at home, a departure from the one-to-one paradigm prevalent today. Telerehabilitation has also been found to improve compliance by musculo-skeletal patients exercising at home, as was recently reported in a study conducted by Eastman Kodak Company and Greenleaf Medical Systems [5].

The Virtual Rehabilitation advantages listed above are applicable across patient populations. There are however advantages which are specific to a

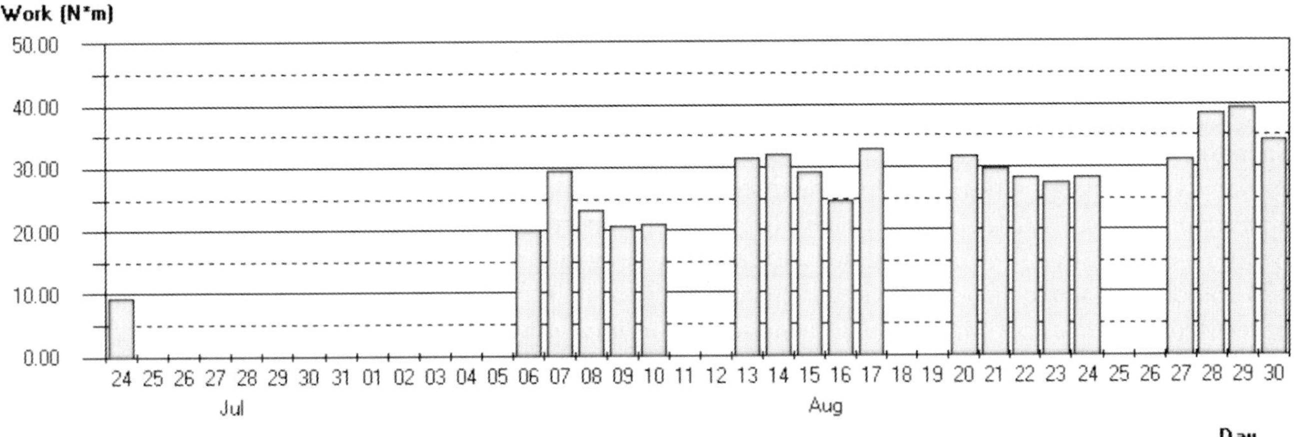



Fig. 3. Remote access of hand strengthening data obtained during VR-based rehabilitation of a post-stroke patient. © Rutgers University 2002. Reprinted by permission.

certain type of Virtual Rehabilitation. Patients with fear of flying, for example, are asked to take real flights with a therapist, as a way to desensitize them. Clearly, their privacy suffers, as sweating, tremor, and other manifestations of their illness are witnessed by passengers and crew. By contrast, Virtual Rehabilitation can be done in a therapist's office in complete privacy, as illustrated in Figure 4a [7]. Studies conducted at Georgia Institute of Technology and Emory Health Sciences [6] report that VR therapy was as efficacious as classical fear of flying therapy. A year after VR exposure 92% of patients maintained their gains and had flown on airplanes. Furthermore, the cost of therapy was reduced (cost of airline tickets, and therapist time).

Virtual Rehabilitation is particularly useful for those with post-traumatic stress syndrome, as found in Vietnam veterans. Again their privacy is maintained, as they are exposed to helicopter flights over hostile territory (see Figure 4b [7]). Taking patients to Vietnam is a more expensive and sometimes impractical solution. Exposure therapy in VR is also safer, as in the case of patients experiencing fear of spiders, or snakes. They can view these creatures in VR, without ever being poisoned.

## Challenges posed by Virtual Rehabilitation

For all its benefits, Virtual Rehabilitation does pose significant challenges for its widespread adoption. The first is *clinical acceptance*, which is conditioned on proven medical efficacy and on a proactive therapist response. Medical studies are underway, and not enough data exist to satisfy critics that VR-augmented, or VR-based rehabilitation, is viable. In all fairness it should be said that initial data from pilot studies is indeed

a)

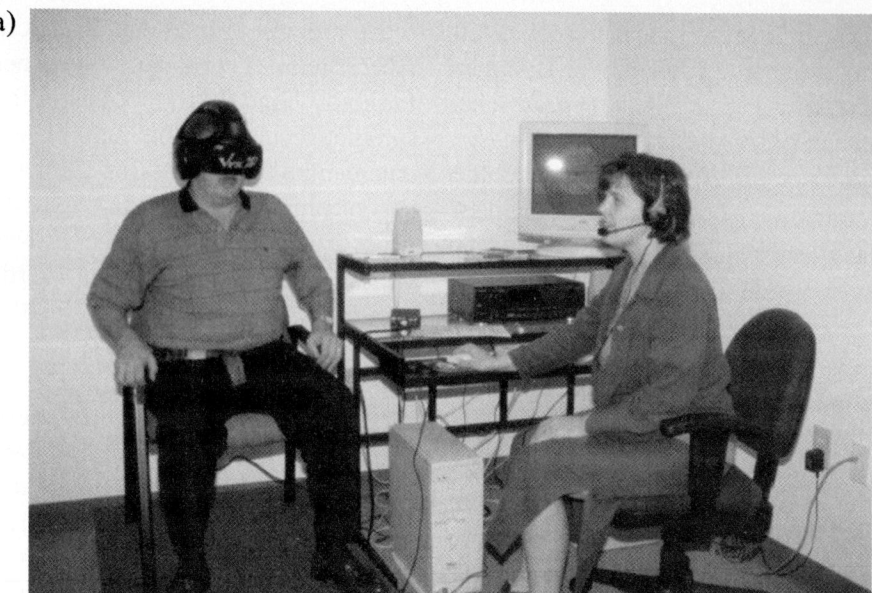

b)

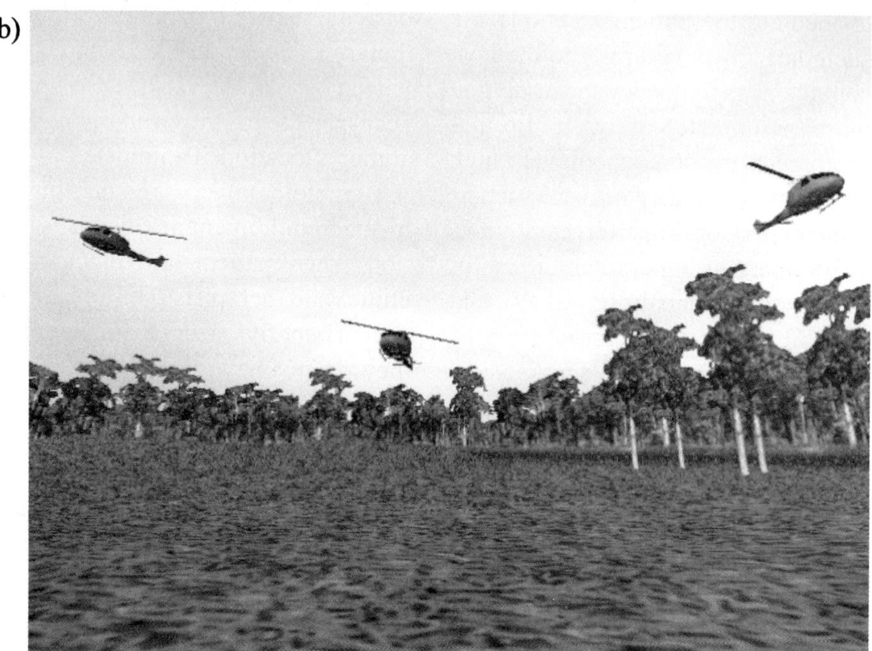

Fig. 4. Virtual Rehabilitation of patients with cognitive defficits: (a) office visit; (b) virtual scene used in desensitizing Vietnam vererans [7]. © Virtually Better 2000. Reprinted by permission.

encouraging, especially with respect to post-stroke chronic patients. VR by itself has been shown to improve them years after stroke, long after any classical therapy stopped [8,3].

The *therapist's attitude* towards the technology is another challenge. Certain unwise (and short-sighted) technologists have proclaimed that Virtual Rehabilitation will replace the therapists altogether with computers.

This misconception needs to be quickly rectified, lest our field is in danger. In truth Virtual Rehabilitation is a "force amplifier" for the therapist, allowing him to do more, and with more patients. The intricacies of computers, VR interfaces and networks is something therapists are not exposed to as part of their academic training, and resistance to such technology is widespread. This unfortunate *technology gap* is counterbalanced by a positive, accepting attitude from the patients and their caregivers. Faced with no alternative, the patients and their families clearly embrace Virtual Rehabilitation [4].

The *VR interfaces* currently in use are another challenge. They were not designed as medical equipment, which means they have difficulty being sterilized for repeated use by different patients. Furthermore, standard VR equipment cannot accommodate "special needs." One example is the lack of child-size equipment, which hampers VR-based assessment of children with attention deficit/hyperactivity syndrome [12]. Even adult-size equipment has shortcomings, for example patients that underwent hand surgery, or suffered a stroke, have difficulty donning sensing gloves, designed for normal anatomy. The commonly-recognized limited range of trackers, and the weight of haptic feedback equipment pose usability constraints, which reduce the naturalness of interaction, so important for cognitive patients.

*Equipment cost* has dropped significantly in recent years compared to the hundred of thousand of dollars that VR systems used to cost less than five years ago. Nevertheless, current prices are still prohibitive for health clinics, or for schools, and these institutions will be hesitant to invest in the absence of subsidies, or a vocal patient advocacy. Dhurjarty [5] suggests that game interfaces, such as the x-cube may be the answer. Of course, this assumes a more open programming environment than presently exists in the video-game industry.

Telerehabilitation has additional challenges relating to *inadequate (or absent) communication infrastructure*. The use of telephone lines does limit videoconferencing between therapist and the remote patient. Fortunately, certain forms of Telerehabilitation do not require constant supervision. Nevertheless, videoconferencing may be requested by patients when they have difficulty. If networks are used, then network traffic becomes the bottleneck, a problem that will eventually be solved by broadband, and widespread connections, some wireless.

Another important aspect of Telerehabilitation is *patient safety*. While patients exercise in VR, they are in danger of re-injury due either to large forces applied by robots or other feedback interfaces, due to cables and tethers, or due to over-exercising. Thus software "watch dog" programs need to be integrated at the patient's home to make sure he is not exercising at a higher level then prescribed, or for a longer duration than necessary.

Since Telerehabilitation is a newer form of therapy, it is unclear at this time how psychological factors will influence recovery. Certain patients may exercise less without direct therapist intervention, since they feel they get less attention than they deserve. Others will prefer less human contact, thus large-scale studies are needed to elucidate questions like: "Is Telerehabilitation as efficacious as Virtual Rehabilitation done at a clinic?" "Is it as good as classical rehabilitation, all else being equal?"

## Summary

This article reviewed the benefits brought by Virtual Rehabilitation use in various forms of therapy. A number of challenges exist at this time, and need to be addressed if Virtual Rehabilitation is to gain wide acceptance. Table 1 is a summary of our discussion. It is the belief of this author, based on years of related research, and on the review of pertinent literature, that Virtual Rehabilitation will overcome the current challenges. Of course, you the researcher will play a key role in the work that lies ahead. We wish you success!

## Acknowledgements

Research support for studies done by the author came from the National Science Foundation (BES-0201687), and from the New Jersey Commission on Science and Technology (R&D Excellence Grant).

Table 1. Virtual Rehabilitation benefits/challenges comparison © Rutgers University 2002

| Virtual Rehabilitation | Benefits of Virtual Rehab | Challenges posed by Virtual Rehab |
| --- | --- | --- |
| Neuro-muscular | Engaging/motivating<br>Economy of scale<br>Online data gathering<br>Fine time resolution<br>Impairment/Function<br>Malingering detection | Expensive equipment<br>Clinic and clinical acceptance<br>Technical expertise |
| Post-stroke | Engaging/motivating<br>Economy of scale<br>Repetitive/intensive<br>Adaptable to patient condition<br>Usable in chronic phase<br>Impairment/Function<br>Activities of daily living | Abnormal limb configuration<br>Applicable to upper functional population<br>Technical expertise<br>Clinical acceptance<br>Cognitive load |
| Cognitive | Economy of scale<br>Engaging/motivating<br>Increased privacy<br>Reduced costs<br>Increased safety<br>More realistic assessment | Lack of natural interfaces<br>Lack of child-size equipment<br>Large equipment cost (for schools)<br>Technical expertise |
| Tele-rehabilitation | Availability of therapists<br>Rehabilitation at home<br>Reduced therapist cost<br>Improved compliance<br>Reduced isolation<br>Remote database access | Equipment cost<br>Network bandwidth<br>Technical expertise<br>Safety at home<br>Sterilization for redeployment<br>Efficacy studies<br>Psychological factors |

## References

1. American Association of Orthopedic Surgeons. Broken Ankl; 2002. Also at orthoinfo.aaos.org.
2. American Stroke Association. Impact of Stroke; 2002. Also at www.strokeassociation.org.
3. Boian R, Sharma A, Han C, Burdea G, Merians A, Adamovich S, et al. Virtual Reality-Based Post-Stroke Hand Rehabilitation. Proceedings of Medicine Meets Virtual Reality 2002, Newport Beach CA, January 23-26 2002. IOS Press; 2002. p. 64-70.
4. Buckley K, Prandoni C, Tran B. Nursing Management and the Acceptance/Use of Telehealth Technologies by Caregivers of Stroke Patients in the Home Setting. Proceedings of State of the Science Conference on Telerehabilitation and Applications of Virtual Reality, Washington DC; October 2001. p. 35-8.
5. Dhurjaty S. Challenges of Tele-rehabilitation in the Home Environment. Proceedings of State of the Science Conference on Telerehabilitation and Applications of Virtual Reality, Washington DC; October 2001. p. 89-93.
6. Emory Health Sciences. Virtual Reality Therapy Proven Effective to Combat Fear of Flying. Press Release, December 18 2000. www.emory.edu.
7. Hodges L, Anderson P, Burdea G, Hoffman H, Rothbaum B. Treating Psychological and Physical Disorders with VR. IEEE Computer Graphics and Applications, November/December 2001: 25-33.
8. Holden M, Todorov E. Use of Virtual Environments in Motor Learning and Rehabilitation. In: Stanney K, editor. The Handbook of Virtual Environments Technology (HVET), Lawrence Erlbaum Associates, Inc.; 2002. p. 999-1026.
9. National Rural Health Association. Legislative and Regulatory Agenda. NRHA e-News, Washington DC 1999; 2(3). www.nrharural.org.
10. North M, North S, Coble J. Virtual Reality Therapy: An Effective Treatment for Psychological Disorders. In Stanney K, editor. The Handbook of Virtual Environments Technology (HVET). Lawrence Erlbaum Associates, Inc.; 2002. p. 1065-78.
11. Popescu V, Burdea G, Bouzit M, Girone M, Hentz V. Orthopedic Telerehabilitation with Virtual Force Feedback. IEEE Trans Inf Technol Biomed March 2000; 4(1):45-51.
12. Rizzo A, Schultheis M, Mateer C. Analysis of Assets for Virtual Reality Applications in Neuropsychology. Neuropsychological Rehabilitation (in press).



Address of the author:
Grigore Burdea, Ph.D.
CAIP Center, Rutgers University
96 Frelinghuysen Rd.
Piscataway NJ, 08854 USA
E-mail:    burdea@caip.rutgers.edu

# Research and Education Section

**J.E.C.M. Aarts, M. Berg, E. Huisman**

Institute of Health Policy and Management
Erasmus University Medical Center
Rotterdam, The Netherlands

# Research and Education

# *Health Information Management Education at the Institute of Health Policy and Management of the Erasmus University Medical Center*

**Abstract:** This paper presents a review of the philosophy and content of the Master course of Health Information Management that is being taught at the Institute of Health Policy and Management of the Erasmus University Medical Center in Rotterdam, the Netherlands. We present our experiences of teaching this master course, including its predecessor. Our work, both teaching and researching, can be characterized by the sociotechnical approach of health informatics, which means that we focus on the interrelation of technology and its social environment.

## Introduction

Within medical informatics, the recognition of the interplay of information technology and its social environment has become unchallenged. However, the understanding of this interplay is still problematic because its intrinsic complex nature and the fact that researchers and practitioners in medical informatics are not very familiar with the insights of the social sciences and the associated theoretical concepts.

The number of failed implementations of information systems in health care is large (1). The associated costs of destroyed capital and damaged reputations are high. The growing awareness that failures are not haphazard occasions but can be understood and acted upon led to one of us to conceive a postgraduate course for health care professionals who are involved in the design and implementation of information systems. A model

has been developed by Aarts, Peel and Wright to establish the contents of the course (2). The resulting master course, in which our department participated, was validated and established by the University of Surrey. Because of changing educational priorities, the University of Surrey decided not to continue the course after two intakes . This change of policy allowed us to take full responsibility for the course and to embed it in our research environment. The course was validated as an Erasmus University master course. We founded a new international network to ensure the European character of the course. Our international partners are Carelink in Sweden and CHIRAD in England. Also we reinforced collaboration with the Institute of Medical Informatics of the Erasmus Medical Center. The collaboration is described in a bit more detail below.

The master course links closely to our research on health information

systems in practice. Our institute might be seen as one of the first in the domain of medical informatics to address it in a more structured way.

Based on the same ideas, we have developed elective courses for students of health sciences and a ten day course for Dutch health care professionals and managers. These courses will not be discussed in this paper.

## Philosophy

The course contents are based on a model that summarizes how the introduction of information technology in different stages of change repeatedly interact with clinical work in its context of the health care system (3). Each stage has particular consequences for the knowledge, skills and behaviors that an experienced postgraduate must possess to interact effectively with clinical, managerial and informatics colleagues.

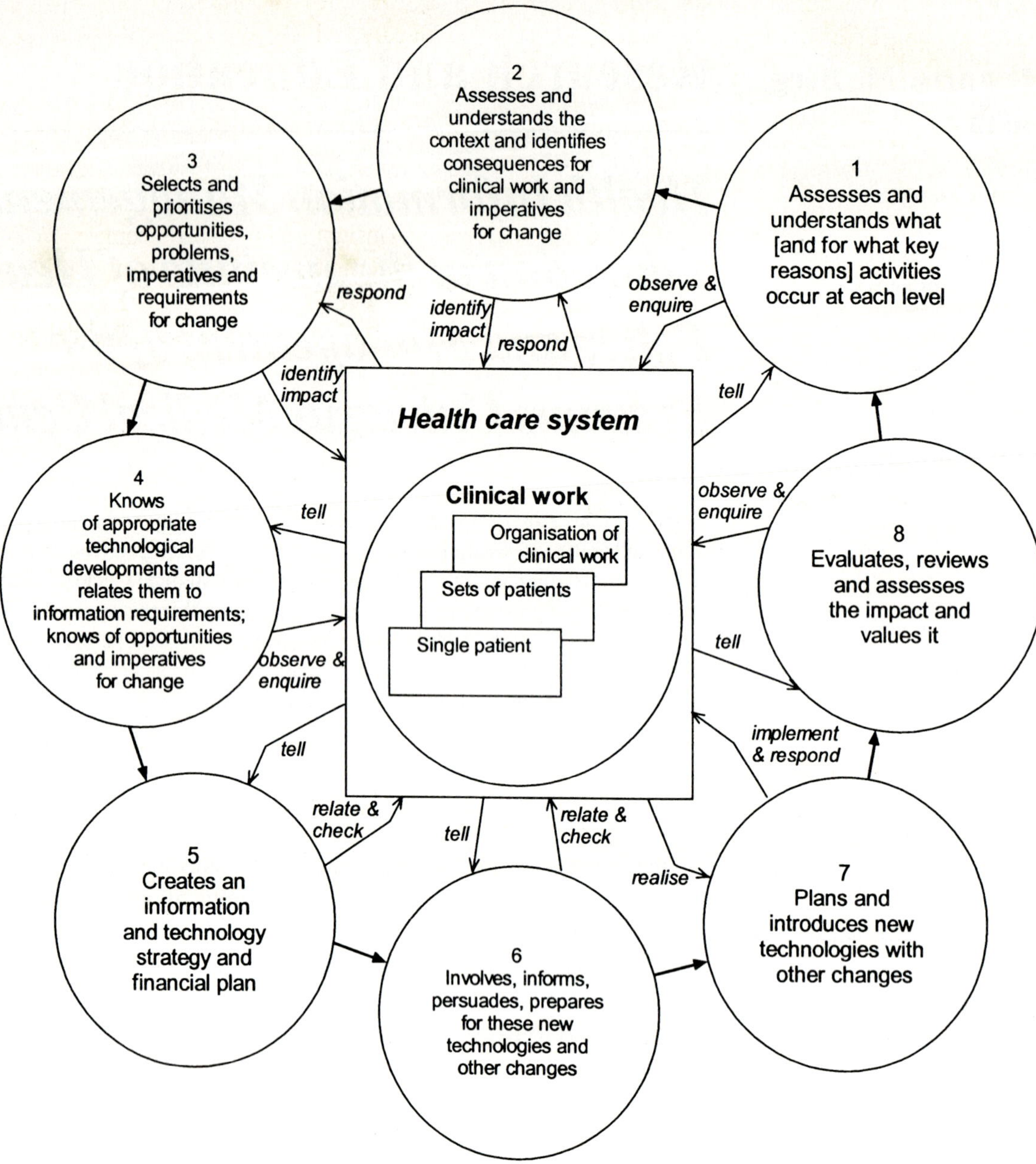



Fig. 1. Model of change and its stages.

The model is cyclic (see Figure 1), which means that managing such a change is a continuous process in health care. In reality, such a process rarely has a clear beginning or end and stages often overlap or iterate. The model might give the impression that the stages are linearly connected. This is not the case. For example, the stage of evaluation is important in each stage of design and implementation. It is vital that senior graduates possess the capacity to manage change in a fluid and demanding environment. Each stage and its interactions with clinical work translates into requirements involving knowledge, skills, attitudes and behaviors.

The stages have been translated into module contents which are described below.

As information technology consists of tools being used by, or at least affecting people, information systems cannot be studied without a focus on the interrelation of the technology and its social environment (4). Socio-technical approaches help to understand these relationships. These approaches have been adopted by our group in various research projects. The socio-technical approaches find their roots in the work of Mumford on information systems design, the Scandinavian tradition of strong worker involvement in the introduction of information technology in the workplace and studies in the field of science and technology studies where researchers recognize that the development of any technology cannot be separated from its social environment (see e.g. (5)). This thinking is a key element impacting the content and the teaching of the master course.

## Target audience

The master course is aimed at professionals in health care. We include clinicians (physicians, nurses and others) who are involved or take an interest in information technology, but also health care managers. We also welcome professionals of consultancy firms and health ICT companies. This mix of professionals can help to increase awareness for the specific problems of clinicians, and clinicians develop understanding for the managerial issues of health care and health care ICT in particular. The students are expected to stand back from their daily activities and reflect on it. Through this form of experiential learning we hope that the combination of reflection and acquiring new insight will provide the graduates with right skills and knowledge to introduce ICT successfully in health care practice. We therefore prefer that students have at least five years of professional experience in health care. The formal entrance qualification is a diploma of higher education in the relevant field (for example medicine, nursing or informatics).

## Program

The course is part-time and it is designed so that it can be completed within three years, taking into account a study load of twenty hours per week. The taught part consists of six modules upon the successful completion of a dissertation, the student is awarded the degree of Master of Health Information Management. We deliberately chose this title for the degree because we want to express the central role of the information function in health care. The technology, however important and influential, is supportive to that function.

The table below summarizes the structure and contents of the course.

| Module number | Module title | Study Points | Lead | Delivery location |
| --- | --- | --- | --- | --- |
| 1 | The health context | 4 study points | Institute of Health Policy and Management (iBMG) | Rotterdam |
| 2 | Informatics and the changing clinical and managerial environment | 4 study points | iBMG | Rotterdam |
| 3 | Medical informatics: concepts, technologies and infrastructures | 4 study points | Institute of Medical Informatics | Rotterdam |
| 4 | Integrated ICT strategies for the health care organization | 4 study points | Carelink | Sweden |
| 5 | Managing the transition | 4 study points | CHIRAD | UK |
| 6 | Evaluating the impact | 4 study points | iBMG | Rotterdam |
| - | Dissertation | 18 study points | iBMG | |

The student study load of each taught module is 160 hours of study including self study and the completion of study assignments. 40 hours of study is equivalent to 1 study point. Each module therefore yields 4 study points. The taught part of the master course totals 960 hours of study or 24 study points. The dissertation values 18 study points, thereby bringing the total study load of the master course to 1680 hours or 42 study points, which is a requisite to grant a masters degree. This would be equivalent to 70 ECTS points in the agreed system for accreditation of European higher education.

Below follows a summary of the student outcomes and contents of the six modules of the master course.

*1. The changing healthcare context*

The student understands the nature of health and health care, the formulation and realization of health policy, health care funding and the current issues for European health care systems, their commonality and impact.

*2. Informatics and the changing clinical and managerial practice*

The student appreciates how health care is delivered to the patient, the roles and professional practices of both clinicians and managers, the impact of the changes within the European context on these issues and their ramifications for health information management.

*3. Medical informatics: technologies and infrastructures*

The student knows about current developments and trends in health care information systems and technology infrastructures, for all forms of health care organizations, including their management, risks and effectiveness.

*4. Integrated strategies*

The student creates an integrated information and organizational strategy for the health care organization, and undertakes the requirements analysis, including the financial implications, necessary to implement an information and organizational strategy. This module combines stages 4 and 5 of the change model.

*5. Organizational development and managing the transition*

The student prepares and/or carries out the organizational development associated with the information and technology driven change within the organization; undertakes the innovative and effective procurement, implementation and change management of information, information systems and technologies and their associated organizational development and learning in the health care setting. This module covers stages 6 and 7 of the change model

*6. Evaluating the impact*

The student evaluates the efficiency and effectiveness of the information change management process and its associated information systems, its value to and impact on: the delivery of care; health outcomes; costs and resource usage; organizational impacts; benefits realized; and the management of the health care organization.

Research methods appropriate for information systems research are included in the course running throughout the modules in order to prepare the students for their dissertation work. The themes covered are research design, quantitative and qualitative methods, and evaluation approaches.

The Institute of Medical Informatics of the Erasmus University Medical Center takes responsibility for module 3. Modules 4 and 5 are respectively taught in Sweden and the United Kingdom. The responsible partners are Carelink, based in Stockholm, Sweden and CHIRAD in the United Kingdom. Carelink contributes to the development of a health information infrastructure in Sweden. CHIRAD is a IMIA recognized academic institute affiliated with King Alfred's College in Winchester.

We encourage students to take on a dissertation research project within their working environment. We think that the student can benefit from the close relationship between information and communication technology and the social environment that he or she experiences on a day-to-day basis. Of course, in such cases precautions should be taken in order to ensure that a dissertation will meet the academic standards of Erasmus University Rotterdam.

## Experiences

When we include the experiences gained through the University of Surrey, University of Manchester and Erasmus University collaboration we can summarize the following experiences.

The change model proved to be a sound basis for the program design and the contents of the course. It took about three years between conceiving the ideas and the start of the course in its first form at the University of Surrey. That time paid off, because the program design and contents also did not change dramatically in Rotterdam. However, it is important that the teaching of such a master course is strongly related to a strong research base. These conditions are definitely met at the Institute of Health Policy and Management.

Teaching staff are drawn from the participating institutes and partners. Apart from that we also invite external speakers who bring specific scientific or practical expertise not available in our research staff. We also try to enhance the European dimension by inviting people who bring the European overview of developments in health care and can place local issues in an international context.

The students come from different countries of Europe. Countries represented are Iceland, Ireland, United Kingdom, Sweden, the Netherlands, Luxemburg, Switzerland and Italy. With no exception, the students all combine learning with a busy working life. They represent the groups that we targeted on well. Among the 31 students, there are 14 belonging to the group of physicians and nurses and the rest are managers, and/or consultants with ICT-responsibility.

The course format suits the students well. For a module they travel to Rotterdam (or other places where the partners are located), spend a week following lectures and other educational activities and take home study assignments. They remain connected with us and their fellow students through the Internet. We have created a special web-based electronic learning environment for communication, document delivery, and where feasible, thematic discussion groups. We can monitor the progress of the student while he or she is taking part in the course work. It becomes more difficult when a student is doing the dissertation work alone and regular work may take precedence. We hope that through the Internet we can support the student to remain disciplined to finish the dissertation. Other help can come through peer support of the fellow students.

As it is often the case with postgraduate courses, students form their own networks for the exchange of experiences and ideas. They assume a critical but positive attitude towards the contents, the teaching and organization of the master course. A common denominator is their expectation that (invited) speakers relate the contents of their presentations to European developments.

## Conclusions

We believe that we established a unique master course both with regard to the contents and audience. The core of the master course is the intertwinement of information and communication technology and the social environment.

A deep understanding of this relationship is necessary for the successful design, implementation and evaluation of the information function in health care. The target audience is professionals in health care. We deliberately address their needs because through their experience they are often instrumental in or even responsible for introducing innovative information technology in health care practice. From the beginning we have put the course on a European level, because we are convinced that much common ground can be found despite local variations. Networking at a European level also provides the student with a unique learning experience and an international network that will last.

To our knowledge, there are no similar courses of this kind in Europe, or even in the world. Existing courses are focused at undergraduates or fresh graduates, or research graduates and offer mostly the broad theme of health informatics.

Embedding the course in a research environment allows for innovative insights to be shared among the students and the staff. As researchers we have been able to profit from the knowledge and experience of our students. Some students have already expressed their wish to pursue a doctorate in our institute and have shown to be prolific authors.

IMIA is setting up an accreditation system for health informatics courses (6). We support this initiative. We hope that IMIA will not only include pure health informatics courses, but also programs that address the close connection between information and technology, health care and its social environment.

We wish to acknowledge all the persons that have been involved in developing and delivering this master course. We would like to name specifically Vic Peel (formerly at the University of Manchester), Graham Wright (formerly at the University of Surrey, now CHIRAD), John Bryant (University of Surrey), Chris Atkinson (formerly University of Surrey, now Brunel University) and Mats Larson (Carelink).

## References

1. Berg M. Implementing information systems in health care organizations: myths and challenges. Int J Med Inf 2001;64(2-3):143-56.
2. Aarts JECM, Peel VJ, Wright G. Human and organisational issues in health care informatics: the conceptual basis for a higher educational programme. In: Mantas J, editor. Health telematics education. Amsterdam: IOS Press; 1997. p. 241-8.
3. Aarts J, Peel V, Wright G. Organizational issues in health informatics: a model approach. Int J Med Inf 1998;52:235-42.
4. Berg M, Aarts JECM, van der Lei J. ICT in heath care, sociotechnical approaches (editorial). Methods Inf Med 2003; forthcoming.
5. Bijker WE, Law J, editors. Shaping technology/building society, studies in technological change. Cambridge: The MIT Press; 1992.
6. Douglas JV, Hovenga EJ. Health and medical informatics competencies: call to participate in updating the IMIA recommendations. Methods Inf Med 2002;41:86-8.

Address of corresponding author:
Jos E.C.M. Aarts, MSc
Institute of Health Policy and Management
Erasmus University Medical Center
P.O. Box 1738
3000 DR Rotterdam
The Netherlands
E-mail: j.aarts@bmg.eur.nl

A. Geissbuhler, C. Lovis,
J. P. Vallée, S. Spahni,
R. Baud

Division of Medical Informatics
Geneva University Hospitals
Geneva, Switzerland

# Research and Education

## *A 2'200-bed laboratory: research and education in medical informatics at Geneva University Hospitals*

## Introduction

For more than three decades, the focus of medical informatics at Geneva University Hospitals has been the development of innovative, patient-centered computer-based tools to improve the quality and efficiency of healthcare delivery. Created under the visionary leadership of Professor Jean-Raoul Scherrer [1], the Division of Medical Informatics (Division d'Informatique Médicale, DIM) has always combined its service and research missions, leading to the development of influential real-world systems, such as the DIOGENE hospital information system [2,3], pioneering medical image management tools [4,5], and bio-informatics resources [6], as well as significant contributions to the fields of medical knowledge representation and natural language processing [7], image processing, federated health care records architectures, and e-health.

This paper presents the philosophy and scope of the research and education efforts of the Division of Medical Informatics at Geneva University Hospitals and School of Medicine.

## Geneva University Hospitals, a 2'200-bed laboratory

With the development of the DIOGENE hospital information system in the 70's, informatics made its way into the daily life of the collaborators of Geneva University Hospitals. Computing resources being limited, the idea at the time was to give priority to the applications for care-providers. Without terminals and 15 years before the advent of personal computers, the challenge was to create a convivial man-machine interface: a pool of phone operators who mediated the interactions between professionals and the mainframe computer, sending direct visual feedback through video cables, was an exemplary solution, the so-called "Geneva solution" [8], to an ergonomic, organizational and technical problem that can still be found in today's systems.

This example illustrates the key philosophy that has guided not only the service mission of the DIM, but also most of its research activity: innovative solutions for patient-centered, real-world problems. The emulation between these two missions, the proximity of researchers, informaticians and clinicians, and the cultural acceptance of innovative computer-based tools within the real-world care processes have enabled new synergies, development strategies, and production systems.

The importance of communication, collaboration and knowledge management within the hospital is now better understood, but the actual role of information and communication technologies in such complex organizations and processes need to be further studied. Ethnographic techniques, coupled with the analysis of usage logs and outcome measures, can be applied to this "laboratory" environment where actors can be finely observed, and, when necessary, randomized in prospective studies.

Today, Geneva University Hospitals (HUG) comprise a group of primary, secondary, and tertiary care facilities, employing 8'000 collaborators (including 1'300 physicians and 3'000 nurses), totaling 2'200 beds, 50'000 admissions, 70'000 emergency room visits, and 732'000 outpatient visits each year. Numbers reflect its level of computerization: there are 4'600 PCs, 500 physicians are equipped with institutionally-managed PDAs loaded with clinical information resources and dozens of wheel-mounted computers are used to provide point-of-care information through a wireless communication network. Digital information has been accumulated for decades, in the form of text, images, and encoded data. It is now available online within the computerized patient record and a clinical datawarehouse. The Picture Archiving and Communication System (PACS) handles 85 percent of all radiology images, which are available on all clinical workstations within the computerized patient record.

Based on a distributed component architecture [9], using HTTP/XML and DICOM as standards for inter-operability and a strong terminology management, the clinical information system can easily be extended to provide specific views or new business logic, while maintaining a globally coherent system. As interoperable components or applications can be shared over the internet, these extensions can be functional as well as geographical, leading to various telemedicine applications, ranging from sharing of knowledge components, to teleradiology and teleconsultations.

## The Division of Medical Informatics (DIM)

The DIM [10] is based in the Geneva University Hospital as a clinical service, and in the Geneva University School of Medicine as an academic division. This dual attachment facilitates the links between fundamental and applied research, and the transition between pre-graduate education and post-graduate or professional training.

The DIM consists of more than 50 collaborators who work in one or more of the four operational groups:

- the integrated patient record group: in charge of the design, development and deployment of the institution's clinical computer-based tools, including the computerized patient record, clinical data capture tools, and clinical decision support tools. Areas of research include: innovative human-machine interfaces, role-based information integration and presentation, and knowledge-coupling in clinical workflow,
- the digital imaging unit: in charge of the institution's image management system (PACS) and the support of clinicians for image analysis. Areas of research include the development of specific algorithms and tools for image analysis (segmentation, 3-D reconstruction, augmented reality), and, in connection with the radiology services, the development of new image acquisition techniques, in particular in the field of functional magnetic resonance imaging,
- the middleware group: in charge of the clinical information system's foundation components. Areas of research include open, component-based architectures, federated health-record systems, telemedicine infrastructures, and security in distributed systems,
- the natural language group: in charge of terminology management and the integration of operational natural language processing (NLP) tools in the clinical information system. Areas of research include innovative NLP techniques, clinical knowledge representation and engineering [11,12].

The DIM has established numerous academic collaborations that extend its research and education potential. These include:

- within Geneva University, the Faculty of Sciences and the Faculty of Literature, for the co-direction of doctoral students (computer

science, physics, mathematics, linguistics),
- other universities, and in particular the Swiss Polytechnical Schools in Lausanne (EPFL) and Zürich (ETHZ), with projects dealing with advanced image analysis and operational research for resource usage optimization,
- the Swiss Institute for Bio-informatics, whose director is also a member of the DIM,
- the European Nuclear Research Center (CERN), based in Geneva, with projects on medical imaging instrumentation, and others on grid- and super-computing.

---

## Current research activity

Current research activity at the DIM can be grouped in four mains areas:

- **techniques and tools for enabling the learning healthcare institution**: healthcare being fundamentally a knowledge business, there is a need for improving the ability of healthcare institutions to capture, manage, activate, and discover knowledge within the immense amount of information that is being produced by the care processes and by biomedical research. Tacit knowledge capture can be enhanced by various tools [13,14]. Knowledge representation techniques can improve the quality and reusability of knowledge bases. The combination of data mining with NLP techniques and image features extraction could lead to innovative "multidimensional" knowledge discovery applications. Links with bio-informatics open perspectives both for the integration of genomics and proteomics information in the clinical processes, and bioinformatics research can be helped by medical informatics tools such as ontology management tools and NLP techniques,

- **clinical information systems that make a difference**: with numerous different types of stakeholders involved in the process of care production, in a complex environment characterized by discontinuities and nomadism, the clinical information system must be able to adapt its human-machine interfaces to bring the appropriate information at the point of decision, in a form factor adapted to the needs of the user. Research topics include clinical decision-support systems, component- and agent-based open architectures, intelligent notification systems, workflow and resource usage optimization, and the evaluation of the cognitive and communication impact of information technology in clinical environments [15],
- **from medical image acquisition to augmented reality for clinicians**: the complete medical image production chain is a subject of research activities at the DIM. It starts with the optimization of medical image acquisition techniques [16], the storage, communication and integration of images in various clinical applications, automated feature extraction for diagnostic assistance, to the post-processing of images, automated segmentation [17], multi-modality co-registration, tridimensional reconstruction and use in augmented-reality tools for surgery,
- **medical information technologies as enablers for developing countries**: the potential of information and communication technologies to improve the health system of developing countries is real. Infrastructures that can survive rough environments must be designed, telemedicine applications that help distributing expertise, and medical contents that is adapted to the resources and culture of the country are current topics of research, through collaborations

with several Western Africa countries [18] and the deployment of a multilateral, south-south, network of tele-expertise and tele-teaching [19].

## Education

The DIM is involved in various educational activities. Medical students follow courses on medical information retrieval and critical appraisal of web-based information. In parallel, a web-based medical informatics course for medical students is being developed as part of the Swiss Virtual Campus [20]. This course will be used by all five Swiss medical schools starting in 2003.

At the post-graduate level, the DIM provides a biostatistics course for physicians, a medical imaging course for radiologists, and a short-course in medical informatics open to healthcare and informatics professionals [21]. Several doctoral students in computer science, physics or linguistics are hosted at the DIM and are co-directed with the Geneva University Faculty of Sciences of the Faculty of Literature.

Medical residents and post-graduate students interested in the field of medical informatics can spend a one- or two-year fellowship at the DIM. Physicians are usually encouraged to spend at least two years of clinical practice before joining the DIM, in order to develop clinical skills and a good understanding of the care production processes.

Medical informatics training is still in its infancy in Switzerland, but the need for trained professionals is pressing for the development of structured curricula. A master-level degree is being set up in collaboration with the DIM and the Geneva University Computer Science Department. It should be available in

2004 and followed by a PhD-level degree in 2005. It is also likely that the Federation of Swiss Physicians (FMH) will recognize medical informatics as a specialty within a few years.

## References


1. Geissbuhler A, Lovis C, Spahni S, Appel RD, et al. A Humanist's Legacy in Medical Informatics : Visions and Accomplishments of Professor Jean-Raoul Scherrer. Methods Inf Med 2002; 41:237-42.
2. Scherrer JR, Baud RH, Hochstrasser D, Ratib O. An integrated hospital information system in Geneva. MD Computing 1990 Mar-Apr;7(2):81-9.
3. Borst F, Appel R, Baud R, Ligier Y, Scherrer JR. Happy birthday DIOGENE: a hospital information system born 20 years ago. Int J Med Inf 1999 Jun;54(3):157-67.
4. Ratib O, Ligier Y, Hochstrasser D, Scherrer JR. Hospital Integrated Picture Archiving and Communication System (HIPACS) at the University Hospital of Geneva. In: Schneider R, Jost G, Dwyer III S, editors. Medical Imaging V: PACS design and Evaluation. vol. 1446. San-Jose: SPIE; 1991. p. 330-8.
5. Appel RD, Hochstrasser DF, Funk M, Vargas R, Pellegrini C, Muller AF, Scherrer J-R. The MELANIE project - From a Biopsy to Automatic Protein Map Interpretation by Computer. Electrophoresis 1991; 12:722-35.
6. Appel RD, Bairoch A, Hochstrasser DF. A new generation of information retrieval tools for biologists: the example of the expasy WWW server. Trends in Biochemical Sciences TiBS (222) 1994; 19(6):258-60.
7. Rassinoux AM, Miller RA, Baud RH, Scherrer JR. Modeling concepts in medicine for medical language understanding. Methods Inf Med 1998 Nov;37(4-5):361-72.
8. Coiera E. When Conversation Is Better Than Computation, J Am Med Inform Assoc 2000;7:277-86.
9. Geissbuhler A, Lovis C, Lamb A, Spahni S. Experience with an XML/http-based Federative Approach to Develop a Hospital-Wide Clinical Information System. Medinfo 2001;10:735-9.
10. http://www.dim.hcuge.ch. Accessed 02/9/20.
11. Baud RH, Lovis C, Ruch P, Rassinoux AM. A light knowledge model for linguistic applications. Proc AMIA Symp 2001;37-41
12. Ruch P, Baud R, Geissbuhler A, Rassinoux AM. Comparing General and Medical Texts for Information Retrieval Based on Natural Language Processing: An Inquiry

into Lexical Disambiguation. Medinfo 2001:261-5.

13. Tschopp M, Geissbuhler A. Institutional Clinical Knowledge Management using Web-enabled Processes and Palmtop Computers. Proc AMIA Symp. 2001. p.840.

14. http://www.genisis.ch/casimage. Accessed 02/9/13.

15. Tschopp M, Lovis C, Geissbuhler A. Understanding Usage Patterns of Handheld Computers in Clinical Practice. To appear in J Am Med Inform Assoc 2002.

16. Ivancevic MK, Zimine I, Lazeyras F, Foxall D, Vallée JP. FAST Sequences Optimization for Contrast Media Pharmacokinetic Quantification in Tissue. J Magn Reson Imaging 2001;14:771-8.

17. Bidaut LM, Vallée JP. Automated Registration of Dynamic MR Images for the Quantification of Myocardial Perfusion. J Magn Reson Imaging 2001;13:648-55.

18. http://www.keneya.org.ml. Accessed 02/9/13.

19. http://www.unige.ch/e-cours. Accessed 02/9/13.

20. http://www.swissvirtualcampus.ch Accessed 02/9/13.

21. http://www.unige.ch/formcont/AAdiplomant/infomed02.html. Accessed 02/9/13.

Address of the first author:
Prof. Antoine Geissbuhler, MD
Division of Medical Informatics
Hôpital Cantonal
24 rue Micheli-du-Crest
CH-1211 Genève 14
E-mail : antoine.geissbuhler@hcuge.ch

**Nicos Maglaveras,
C. Pappas**

Aristotle University, The Medical School
Lab of Medical Informatics
Thessaloniki, Macedonia
Greece

# Research and Education

# *Research and education directions in Medical Informatics at the Aristotle University of Thessaloniki*

**Abstract**: The field of Medical Informatics is one of the most active fields both in research and education at the Aristotle University of Thessaloniki. The nucleus of this scientific field at the Aristotle University resides in the Medical School and in particular in the Laboratory of Medical Informatics. Education programs exist in undergraduate, graduate and post-graduate levels, and are targeted towards medical students and doctors and information technology related students and professionals. Research projects cover a wide area of medical informatics including medical information processing and management, electronic health records design and implementation, medical decision support, biological systems simulation, telemedicine applications, integration and communication issues related to regional health information systems, and quality assessment of health services and systems. The description and brief presentation of the output of these educational and research directions shall be presented in this paper.

## Medical Informatics Education

### Undergraduate Courses and Education

Although Medical Informatics (MI) is a well established discipline in most European countries [1], in Greece for a long time only the Medical School at the Aristotle University through the Laboratory of Medical Informatics offered Medical Informatics courses since 1990 [2]. At the undergraduate level the Laboratory of Medical Informatics offers two courses entitled Medical Informatics I and Medical Informatics II. These courses are offered to the students of the medical and dental schools of the Aristotle University of Thessaloniki. Each of the two courses are semester courses and last for 13 weeks and 32 hours of lectures and laboratories. Medical Informatics I is a mandatory course for all medical and dental students whereas Medical Informatics II is an elective. Medical Informatics I is offered at the first semester while Medical Informatics II can be elected by students from the second semester and on.

The aim of the undergraduate courses in Medical Informatics is to make the medical students aware of the possibilities given by informatics and information technologies to the medical professionals as it regards the way the health services are practiced and delivered today and in the near future. The primary aim is to render the medical students good users of the IT solutions in health care. The students have to complete a number of applied projects, and as a reference, the Handbook of Medical Informatics is used [3]. The laboratories and projects are completed in the premises of the Laboratory of Medical Informatics, which is the INTERNET provider of the Medical School, being one of the main network nodes of the network of the Aristotle University of Thessaloniki. Currently more than 2000 active users are registered in the Medical School's node.

More specifically, the thematic areas covered by the two courses are the following:

*Medical Informatics I*

· Introduction to computer and telematics systems architecture
· Introduction to Boolean algebra and binary logic
· Programming essentials and logic diagrams

- Introduction to Windows environment, INTERNET and networking tools
- Basic tools for data management
- Introduction to WWW tools for searching and navigating
- Introduction to HTML and multimedia information acquisition and set-up for use in the WWW

*Medical Informatics II*

- Information Technologies (IT) for health in Greece and the European Union
- Principles of electronic health records
- Data entry mechanisms in electronic health records in diabetes and cardiology
- Principles and types of decision support systems
- Evaluation of medical decision support systems
- Telemedicine applications in the medical field

## Graduate Courses and Education

At the graduate level the Greek Ministry of Education launched in 1997 calls for the development of pilot graduate programs which would aid in bridging the technological and educational gap between Greece and the rest of the European Union (EU) countries. The call was under the umbrella of EPEAEK which was a joint initiative of Greece and the European Commission, (EC) for the development of educational activities in all levels of education. Especially in the context of higher education through EPEAEK it was the aim of the ministry to fund development of graduate programs with a unified approach in Greece, and to provide infrastructure such as digital libraries and technology for the development of graduate based research and development (R&D) activities. These programs were designed to lead to the acquisition of both Master and PhD degrees. The pilot phase for this initiative started in 1998, and was co-funded by the EC and the Greek State.

After the submission of proposals from the Greek Universities and following the selection process, the following programs linked to Medical Informatics and the Aristotle University were accepted for funding.

- The graduate program on Medical Informatics of the Aristotle University of Thessaloniki (PROMESIP) coordinated by the Medical School, with the collaboration of the Informatics School and the Department of Electrical & Computer Engineering of the Aristotle University.
- The graduate program on Medical Research Technology of the Medical School of the Aristotelian University of Thessaloniki (PROMESI).

The above mentioned programs started their pilot phase in 1998, and they awarded the first degrees (Masters) in the year 2000. PhD degrees are expected to be awarded from the year 2003 and on. It is important to stress here that the ministry of education favors the development of collaboration with international Medical Informatics related programs especially those belonging to European Universities, and thus suggests that the course material should be developed both in the Greek and English language.

In particular, as it concerns the program with acronym PROMESIP, this leads to the acquisition of two degrees, Master of Science (MSc) and Doctor of Philosophy (PhD). This program is an inter-departmental program involving the medical school, the department of electrical & computer engineering and the department of computer science. The degrees are awarded from the medical school which acts as the program coordinator. The students who participate have a degree in electrical & computer engineering, informatics, physics and mathematics. In this program, the Master lasts for two years (three semesters coursework and one for a thesis), and the PhD lasts for a minimum of two additional years. Coursework is offered in the following disciplines.

- Basics of Systems Physiology
- Basics of Systems Morphology and Anatomy
- Computer Networking
- Biomedical Signal Processing
- Biomedical Image Processing and Coding
- Applied Mathematics
- Electronic Health Record
- Medical Databases
- Simulation of nonlinear biological systems
- Telematics applications in medicine
- Medical Decision Support Systems
- Security aspects of health information systems
- Workshops and lectures of advanced topics in Medical Informatics

A full time student must take four courses per semester and in the fourth semester the student must prepare a thesis. Each semester, the student spends a minimum of 250 hours attending lectures and laboratories. Specialized workshops and lectures are also part of this program. The courses can also be attended by industry or hospital specialized personnel that needs quick access to advanced education for immediate applications in their working environment. The number of students registered annually in this program is in the order of 10.

The second graduate program available from the medical school of the Aristotle University addresses the issue of medical research methodology and technology bearing the acronym PROMESI. Medical students as well as students with degrees in biology, pharmacology or dentistry can participate in this program. This program aims to give the medical student the background needed on technology and MI related tools that shall be used for any research endeavor the student shall concentrate on. In this program, the Master lasts for two years (three semesters coursework and one for a thesis), and the PhD lasts for a minimum of two additional years. Coursework is offered in the following disciplines.

- Mathematics, especially calculus
- Biostatistics and principles of research methodology
- Medical Informatics and Biomedical Engineering
- Office automation and data management techniques
- Advanced physiology
- Systems morphology and anatomy
- Molecular biology
- Biological systems simulation and identification
- Medical technology and telematics applications
- Medical technology and sensors – instruments
- Workshops and lectures on advanced topics in Medical Research Technology

The coursework of PROMESI aims to provide the medical students with links to the basic sciences so that they can use them in their routine clinical practice or clinical research. The Master degree is concluded with the submission of a thesis, and lasts four semesters, just as is the case with PROMESIP. Each semester the student spends a minimum of 250 hours attending lectures and laboratories. Specialized workshops and lectures are also part of this program. The number of students registered in the PROMESI program on a yearly basis is in the order of 15.

The students who received a Master from both PROMESI and PROMESIP at a rate of 35% continued with their dissertation, whereas the rest are working in the industry, the informatics

education domain, in hospitals, and in applied research environments.

*Medical Informatics Research in the Aristotle University*

Research in the wider field of Medical Informatics and Information Technologies is going on since the early 90's in the Medical School through the Laboratory of Medical Informatics. A large number of research projects usually funded through the Greek Secretariat of Research and technology, the ministry of education, and the European Commission have been carried out covering different facets of Medical Informatics and IT in health. More specifically the following areas were primarily addressed over the past 12 years:

- Electronic health records
- Integration of IT platforms for health care telematics applications
- Medical data security and integrity
- Versatile medical data representation and interfacing
- Medical decision making
- Simulation and modeling of biological and clinical systems for aid in clinical research
- Telemedicine and pervasive computing applications in home care delivery for chronic disease patients
- Biomedical signal and image processing & interpretation

Research and development in the above mentioned areas have resulted in a number of publications, project deliverables and products. The list that follows summarizes the most important results of the research and development that took place in the Lab of Medical Informatics.

- New electronic health record systems were developed in the context of the I4C project where a multimedia electronic health record was developed for cardiac patients focusing on the continuity of care [4], and

in the DIABCARD-3 project where a chip card medical information system was developed for use in the routine treatment and management of diabetic patients [5].
- New information processing techniques were developed based on neural networks (NN) and spectrotemporal analysis. For example, real-time ischemia beat detection techniques based on neural networks and non-linear PCA were developed usable in ICU settings [6],[7]. QRS/PVC classification based on non-linear transformations and NN were also developed [8], and ECG spectrotemporal analysis for use in the clinical environment for evaluating the success of thrombolysis and for explaining atrial fibrillation mechanisms in patients who underwent CABG are other examples of the research efforts of the team in the Medical Informatics Laboratory, in collaboration with the clinical teams of the A' Cardiology Clinic in the AHEPA hospital [9].
- In the image processing domain, research concentrated on the processing of angiograms for the extraction of the coronary tree, and for the quantitative measurement of the geometric parameters of the arteries using primarily watersheds and region merging techniques [10], as well as in the analysis of 4-D MRI data from the heart concentrating on the left ventricular wall motion analysis using NN, deformable models and wavelet techniques [11].
- Research was also conducted in the development of versatile and user friendly interfaces especially related with the use of the electronic health records and the information processing modules [12].
- In the context of the IST project with acronym CHS (Citizen Health System), we developed a generic contact center, though which we

were able to deliver monitoring and prompting services to chronic disease patients such as congestive heart failure (CHF) and diabetic patients [13]. Clinical trials for the production of evidence based material regarding the feasibility of using such approaches in regional health delivery enhancing quality of care and quality of life are currently carried out.

· In the context of the IST project with acronym PANACEIA-ITV, the use of the iTV platform for the delivery of home care is addressed. In the context of this project research on the use of intelligent agents in regulating information and requests flow in a health provision environment based on the active service provision (ASP) model is very active at this moment [14].

· Finally simulation of important physiological phenomena in easy to use platforms for research and clinical purposes using applied mathematics is another important area of research. Such examples are models of the cardiac tissue simulating infarction, and studying reentrant mechanisms by simulating wave propagation in microscopic level [15],[16], as well as looking into problems related to the most accurate modeling of the dipole function at a cellular level and using this in the propagation velocity estimation as well as in the estimation of the electrode distance from the surviving myocardium for use in the ablation procedure and in detecting the correct activation instant from fractionated electrograms for use in implantable devices [17].

A number of dissertations were produced through the above mentioned activities, six of them are finished already and another five are under development, showing the close relation of applied research and projects that run on national and European levels.

## Discussion

At the Aristotle University and more specifically in the Laboratory of Medical Informatics, considerable work started in the previous years in Medical Informatics related areas. Analogous attempts have been made both in Europe [18] and the USA [19]-[21]. In the present paper the program for Medical Informatics in the Aristotle University of Thessaloniki was presented. Medical Informatics in the medical school of the Aristotelian University is offered both at the undergraduate and graduate levels, something that is unique in the Greek University system. The experience with the application of these programs are quite encouraging. Today more than 2000 users both students and faculty use the INTERNET and networking facilities offered by the Medical School's node of the Aristotelian University which is the Laboratory of Medical Informatics. It is also a fact that medical students, when they start learning MI just in time, for example during their freshman year, they can become extremely competent network managers and can engineer innovative solutions for the management of medical information that will be subsequently used to confront medical problems. Also, the strength and practice of the young medical students seems to affect the older generation too, by increasing awareness of the use of MI in everyday clinical practice, and thus creates the need for continuing education programs. This is also a reason why there is a high demand for graduate studies in the field of Medical Informatics and Medical Research Technology at the Aristotle University, since a number of medical and IT students realize that the future lies in the combination of scientific disciplines, and that the domain of health is one of those domains, where collaboration of multiple disciplines is a must for the development of successful systems and services.

## Acknowledgment

This work was supported in part by the EPEAEK projects PROMESI, PROMESIP and KEDIP of the Greek Ministry of Education and by the projects IST-1999-13352 with acronym CHS and IST-2001-33369 with acronym PANACEIA-ITV funded by the European Commission.

## References

1. Van Bemmel JH. Medical Informatics, Art or Science?, Methods Inf Med 1996;35:157-72.

2. Maglaveras N. Medical Informatics Education. In: Iakovidis I, Maglavera S, Trakatellis A. User Acceptance of Health Telematics Applications, Health Technology and Informatics Series. IOS Press; 1998;56:135-42.

3. Van Bemmel JH, Musen MA. Handbook of Medical Informatics. New York: Springer Verlag; 1997.

4. Van Bemmel JH, van Ginneken AM, Stam H, Assanelli D, MacFarlane PW, Maglaveras N, et al. Integration and Communication for the Continuity of Cardiac Care (I4C), J Electrocardiology 1998;31(supp):60-8.

5. Gogou G, Mavromatis A, Maglaveras N, Pappas C, Engelbrecht R. DIABCARD-CCMIS – A portable and scalable CPR for diabetes care. IEEE Trans Biomed Eng 2002;49(12) (in press).

6. Maglaveras N, Stamkopoulos T, Pappas C, Strintzis M. An adaptive back-propagation neural network for real-time ischemia episodes detection. Development and performance analysis using the European ST-T database. IEEE Trans Biomed Eng 1998;45(7):405-13.

7. Stamkopoulos T, Diamantaras KI, Maglaveras N, Strintzis M. ECG analysis using non-linear PCA neural networks for ischemia detection. IEEE Trans Signal Proc 1998;46(11):3058-67.

8. Maglaveras N, Stamkopoulos T, Diamantaras KI, Pappas C, Strintzis M. ECG pattern recognition and classification using non-linear transformations and neural networks: A review. Int J Med Inf 1998;52:191-208.

9. Maglaveras N, Chouvarda I, Dakos G, Vassilikos V, Mochlas S, Louridas G. Analysis of Atrial Fibrillation after CABG using Waveletes. Comput Cardiol, IEEE Comp Soc Press 2002 (in press).

10. Haris K, Efstratiadis SN, Maglaveras N, Pappas C, Gourassas J, Louridas G. Model-based morphological segmentation and

labeling of coronary angiograms. IEEE Trans Med Imaging 1999;18(10):1003-15.

11. Stalidis G, Maglaveras N, Efstratiadis S, Dimitriadis A, Pappas C. Model-Based Processing Scheme for Quantitative 4-D Cardiac MRI Analysis Version. IEEE Trans Inf Technol in Biomed 2002;6(1):59-72.

12. Maglaveras N, Chouvarda I, Koutkias V, Meletiadis S, Haris K, Balas EA. Information technology can enhance quality in regional health delivery. Methods Inf Med 2002;41(5) (in press).

13. Maglaveras N, Koutkias V, Chouvarda I, Goulis DG, Avramides A, Adamidis D, et al. Home Care Delivery through the Mobile Telecommunications Platform: The Citizen Health System (CHS) Perspective. Int J Med Inf 2002 (in press).

14. Koutkias V, Chouvarda I, Maglaveras N. Agent-based Monitoring and Alert Generation for a Home Care Telemedicine System. Proc AMIA Annual Conference; 2002.

15. Maglaveras N, de Bakker JMT, van Capelle FJL, Pappas C, Janse M. Activation delay in bifurcating strands of surviving myocardial tissue in healed infarction. A comparison between model and experiment. Am J Physiol 1995;269 (Heart Circ Physiol. 38):H1441-9.

16. Maglaveras N, van Capelle FJL, de Bakker JMT. Wave propagation simulation in normal and infarcted myocardium: Computational and modeling issues. Med Inform 1998;23(2):105-18.

17. Chouvarda I, Maglaveras N, de Bakker J, van Capelle FJL, Pappas C. Deconvolution and wavelet based methods for membrane current estimation from simulated fractionated electrograms. IEEE Trans Biomed Eng 2001;48(3):294-301.

18. Le Beux P, Burgum A, Jarno P, Siregar P. Medical Informatics Training and Research at Rennes University School of Medicine. In: van Bemmel JH, McCray AT. editors. 1998 IMIA Yearbook of Medical Informatics. Stuttgart: Schattauer; 1998. p.71-7.

19. Balas EA, Reid JC, Mitchell JA. Health Informatics training at the University of Missouri. In: van Bemmel JH, McCray AT, editors. 1997 IMIA Yearbook of Medical Informatics. Stuttgart: Schattauer; 1997. p.108-12.

20. Cimino JJ, Allen BA, Clayton PD. Medical Informatics training at the Columbia University and the Columbia-Presbyterian Medical Center. In: van Bemmel JH, McCray AT, editors. 1995 IMIA Yearbook of Medical Informatics. Stuttgart: Schattauer; 1995. p.125-9.

21. Shortliffe EH. Medical Informatics training at Stanford University School of Medicine. In: van Bemmel JH, McCray AT, editors. 1995 IMIA Yearbook of Medical Informatics. Stuttgart: Schattauer; 1995. p.105-9.

Address of the first author:
Nicos Maglaveras, PhD
Associate Professor
Aristotle University
The Medical School
Lab of Medical Informatics - Box 323
54124 Thessaloniki, Macedonia
Greece
E-mail:    nicmag@med.auth.gr

A. T. McCray

National Library of Medicine
Bethesda, Maryland
USA

# Research and Education

## *Informatics Research, Development, and Training at the Lister Hill National Center for Biomedical Communications*

The Lister Hill National Center for Biomedical Communications is a research and development division of the United States National Library of Medicine (NLM). The Center conducts and supports research, develops research tools and systems, and provides training opportunities to individuals at various stages of their careers. The Center has been in existence since 1968, when it was established by a joint resolution of the United States Congress, with the mandate to conduct research supporting the mission of the NLM. The Center's research programs are reviewed biannually by a Board of Scientific Counselors, an external advisory group of researchers from the informatics community. The most current information about Lister Hill Center research activities can be found at http://lhncbc.nlm.nih.gov/.

The Center's research staff are drawn from a variety of disciplines, including medicine, computer science, library and information science, linguistics, engineering, and education. Research projects are generally conducted by teams of individuals of varying backgrounds and often involve collaboration with other divisions of the NLM, other institutes at the National

Institutes of Health (NIH), and other academic partners. Center staff publish in the medical informatics, computer and information science, and engineering communities. (See [1-40] for a sample of recent publications by Center staff.) The Center is often visited by researchers from academic centers around the world, and our ongoing lecture series features presentations from many invited outside speakers.

Lister Hill Center research activities fall into several broad categories, and each of these is discussed in turn below. Our training program has grown significantly in the last few years and has brought many talented individuals to the Center to learn from and collaborate with our research staff. Our language and knowledge processing research involves basic research in medical language processing and medical knowledge representation, and image processing research involves the development of algorithms and methods to effectively process biomedical images of all types. We have developed and continue to support a number of information systems, all of which are informed by our basic research activities. In addition, Lister Hill Center staff are involved in a number of activities that define and support the

research infrastructure for next generation information systems.

## Training Opportunities at the Lister Hill Center

The Lister Hill Center provides training and mentorship for individuals at various stages in their careers. Fellowship programs may be as short as eight weeks or as long as one year, with possible renewal for a second year. Each fellow is matched with a mentor from the research staff who works closely with the fellow throughout the fellowship program. In all cases, fellows define a research project early in their stay and then give a mid-term progress report. At the end of the fellowship period, fellows prepare a final, often publishable, paper and make a formal presentation which is open to all interested members of the NLM and NIH community.

This past year, we provided training to 46 participants from 16 states and 9 countries. The participants included nine undergraduate students, 15 graduate or medical students, 15 postdoctoral or post-MD fellows, and seven visiting faculty scholars. Participants worked on projects in the areas of biomedical knowledge discovery, consumer health systems, history of medicine, image processing, information retrieval research, just-in-time systems, knowledge based research, natural language processing, ontology research, palm technology, semantic web research, text mining, distance education, and visualization.

We again offered the Clinical Elective in Medical Informatics for third and fourth year medical students in March and April, and we continue to participate in programs supporting minority students including the Hispanic Association of Colleges and Universities (HACU) and the National Association for Equal Opportunity in Higher Education (NAFEO) summer internship programs.

In the summer of 2001 we initiated the NLM Rotation Program. This program provides an opportunity for trainees in NLM supported Medical Informatics Training programs to spend eight weeks at the Lister Hill Center learning about our programs and collaborating with our research scientists. Trainees from any NLM sponsored training program are eligible. The rotation includes a series of lectures and the opportunity for trainees to work closely with established scientists conducting research at the Center. Trainees who participated in the summers of 2001 and 2002 were members of informatics programs at Columbia University, Duke University, Oregon Health and Science University, University of Pittsburgh, University of Minnesota, University of Missouri, and University of North Carolina.

Additional information about our training and visiting faculty programs is available at our web site (http://lhncbc.nlm.nih.gov/) under "Training Opportunities". Interested individuals will find descriptions of each of the training programs including specific application procedures.

# Language and Knowledge Processing

## Natural Language Processing Research

The Natural Language Systems research team investigates the contributions that natural language processing techniques can make to the task of mediating between the language of users and the language of online biomedical information resources. The successful integration of these techniques with other information retrieval strategies has the potential of contributing to the resolution of some of the most difficult problems underlying biomedical information management.

The focus of our natural language processing work is the development of SPECIALIST, an experimental natural language processing system for the biomedical domain. The SPECIALIST system includes several modules based on the major components of natural language: the lexicon, morphology, syntax, and semantics. The lexicon and morphological component are concerned with the structure of words and the rules of word formation. The syntactic component treats the constituent structure of phrases and sentences, while the semantic component seeks to extract biomedical content from text. All components of the SPECIALIST system rely heavily on the linguistic and domain knowledge in the Unified Medical Language System knowledge sources.

The Lexical Systems project builds and maintains the SPECIALIST lexicon, a large syntactic lexicon of medical and general English that is released annually with the UMLS Knowledge Sources. New lexical items are continually added using a lexicon-building tool, and the lexicon currently contains over 180,000 lexical items. Lexical access tools, including LVG, a set of algorithms for morphological variation in English, are also distributed

with the UMLS. Several additional modules have recently been completed and are now available independently as tools for a variety of natural language processing projects. These include a tokenizer, a lexical look-up utility, and a noun phrase extractor.

Innovative methods for providing more effective access to biomedical information depend on reliable representation of the knowledge contained in text. The Semantic Knowledge Representation project develops programs that extract usable semantic information from biomedical text by building on existing NLM resources, including the UMLS knowledge sources and the natural language processing tools provided by the SPECIALIST system. Two programs in particular, MetaMap and SemRep, are being developed, enhanced, and applied to a variety of problems in biomedical informatics. MetaMap maps noun phrases in free text to concepts in the UMLS Metathesaurus, while SemRep uses the UMLS Semantic Network to determine the relationships asserted between those concepts. Project resources are being applied in a variety of research initiatives aimed at identifying specific biomedical information in MEDLINE citations, including semantic predications asserting a treatment relationship between drugs and diseases. Several projects focus on molecular biology. One seeks to identify genes, gene products, and gene functions in abstracts and compares this information to that found in the Gene Ontology, and another supports comparison of protein function by identifying protein-protein interactions in text.

The Indexing Initiative project explores concept-based indexing methods. Project members have developed a system, Medical Text Indexer (MTI), that is being applied to automated and semi-automated indexing environments at the NLM.

We recently conducted experiments to evaluate the effectiveness of MTI terms for NLM indexers, and these recommendations are now available to all indexers. In addition, results of the MTI system have been assigned as keywords for collections of meetings abstracts in a fully automated mode. As part of the Indexing Initiative we have also conducted experiments using journal descriptors corresponding to biomedical specialties that are used to index journal titles. The goal of the work is to contribute to the reduction of ambiguity inherent in biomedical language. We have designed an experimental system that associates journal descriptors with words in titles and abstracts in a training set of about 435,000 MEDLINE records. The more words in the document co-occurring with a particular descriptor, the more likely it is that the document falls into that particular biomedical specialty.

## Unified Medical Language System

NLM regularly distributes a set of Unified Medical Language System (UMLS) knowledge sources to the research community. These include the Metathesaurus, Semantic Network and SPECIALIST lexicon. The Metathesaurus is a knowledge source representing multiple biomedical vocabularies organized as concepts in a common format. It thus provides a rich terminology resource in which terms and vocabularies are linked by meaning. (See Figure 1.)

Vocabularies proposed as standards by the Department of Health and Human Services in the rulemaking accompanying the Health Insurance Portability and Accountability Act (HIPAA) continue to be added and maintained in each release. The most recent release contains over two million names for almost 900,000 biomedical concepts in approximately 60 families of vocabularies or thesauri.

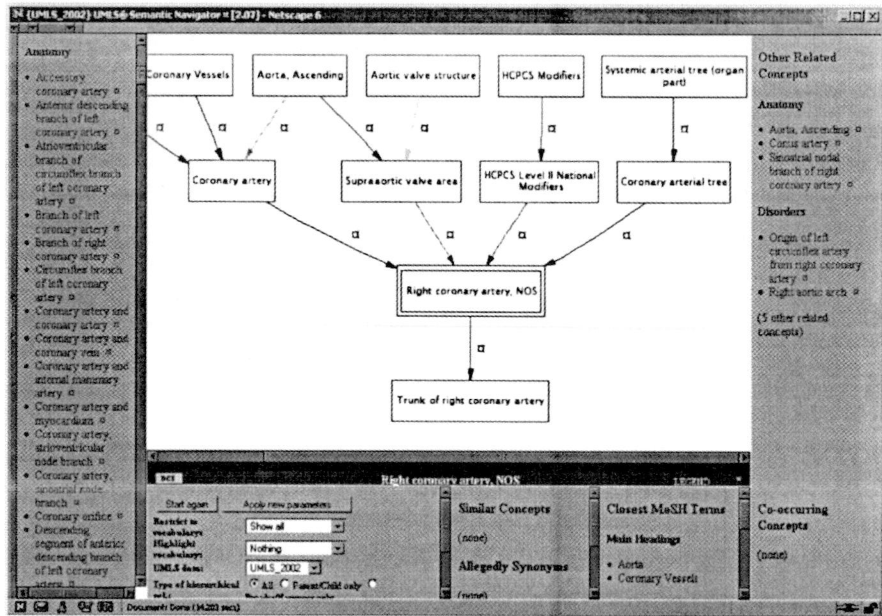

Fig. 1. The Semantic Navigator is a browser developed for visualizing and navigating biomedical concepts from the Unified Medical Language System. It displays the semantic space surrounding an arbitrary UMLS concept. Clicking on any concept dynamically generates a new display in which this concept becomes the center of the new semantic space. The concept entered above is "right coronary artery."

For a decade, the Metathesaurus had been released annually early in the year. Beginning with calendar year 2002, the Metathesaurus is being released quarterly. The systems and software used to create, manange, edit, and release the Metathesaurus are increasingly sophisticated, more automated, and better documented. This makes it possible to continue the schedule of more frequent releases and helps ensure the timely addition of content as required to keep the Metathesaurus current.

The UMLS Semantic Network provides a semantic framework for the Metathesaurus vocabularies. Each concept in the Metathesaurus is assigned to at least one semantic type, chosen from the set of 135 available types. There are semantic types for organisms, biologic and pathologic function, anatomy, chemicals and drugs, and concepts and ideas. More than 50 relationships bind the semantic types to each other. Thus, for example, a possible assertion might be "Disease or Syndrome" has_location "Ana-

tomical Structure". As we enhance the Metathesaurus with genomic terminology, we are also reviewing the Semantic Network for its coverage in this domain.

The UMLS data are made available over the Internet through the UMLS Knowledge Source Server, which provides direct access to each component of the UMLS. (See Figure 2.)

Using the Knowledge Source Server, users can request information about a particular concept in the Metathesaurus, including definitions, semantic types, and synonyms as well as other concepts that are related to the input term. The Knowledge Source Server also accommodates navigation in the Semantic Network, allowing users to investigate relationships among semantic types to retrieve a list of Metathesaurus concepts assigned to a particular semantic type. Finally, the data in the SPECIALIST lexicon are also made available, providing the user with the syntactic and morphologic information about each lexical item the lexicon contains.

The most recent release of the Knowledge Source Server incorporates several features designed to enhance performance by allowing faster access to UMLS data, providing flexibility through a rich API set, and facilitating scalability in handling ever-increasing user loads and constituent vocabularies. The redesigned architecture includes a web server implemented as a collection of Java servlets that provide quick and easy access to UMLS data. In addition to enhancements to the user interface, XML has been incorporated into the design of the Knowledge Source Server to provide flexibility in delivering data to users. In order to support the customization of UMLS terminologies for individual user needs, we are developing filters to help users select subsets of medical terms. Such tools will allow them to define terminologies relevant to their own domain and to tailor the UMLS data further for specialized needs.

While existing knowledge sources in the biomedical domain may be sufficient for information retrieval purposes, the organization of information in these resources is generally not suitable for reasoning. Automated inferencing requires the principled and consistent organization provided by ontologies. Our Medical Ontology Research project develops methods whereby ontologies can be acquired from existing resources and validated against other knowledge sources. Although the UMLS is used as the primary source of medical knowledge, OpenGALEN, CYC, and WordNet are being explored as well. Recent research has focused on two subdomains of biomedicine: anatomy and molecular biology. In one project, the representation of anatomical concepts in two ontologies, the Foundational Model of Anatomy and GALEN, were compared. In another project, we contributed to the integration of the Gene Ontology in the UMLS by studying the properties of this ontology.

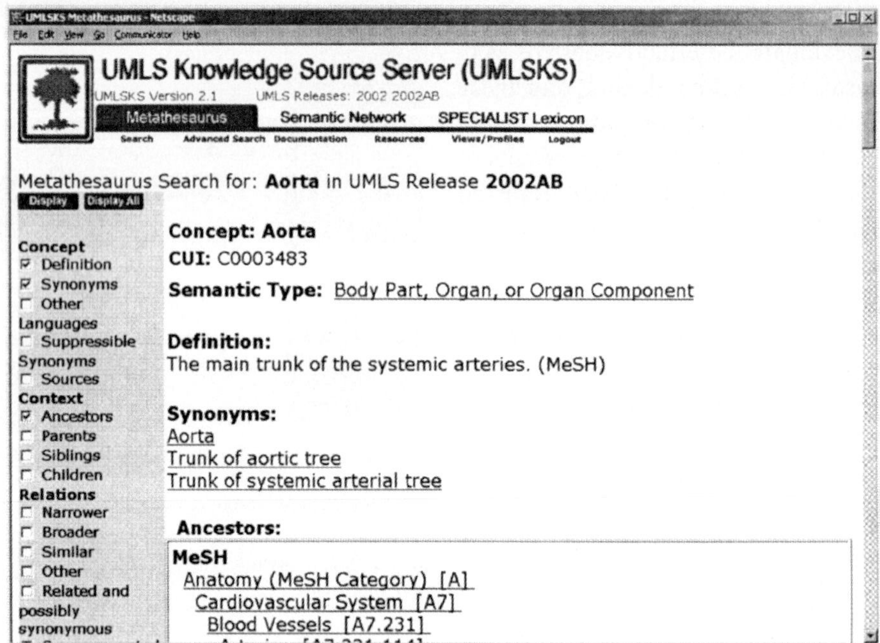

Fig. 2. The UMLS Knowledge Source Server is a tool for providing Internet access to the UMLS Knowledge Sources. Its purpose is to make UMLS data more accessible to users, and in particular to system developers. This represents a view of the UMLS concept "aorta."

## Image Processing

### Visible Human Project

The Visible Human project data sets are designed to serve as a common reference for the study of human anatomy, as a set of common public domain data for testing medical imaging algorithms, and as a test bed and model for the construction of image libraries that can be accessed through networks. The Visible Human data sets are distributed to licensees over the Internet at no cost. The data sets are being applied to a wide range of educational, diagnostic, treatment planning, virtual reality, artistic, mathematical, legal and industrial uses. We continue to maintain two databases to record information about Visible Human project use. The first, to log information about Visible Human Project license holders and record their plans for using the images, and the second, to record information about the applications that are being developed.

With research support from the NLM, the University of Colorado Health Science Center, Center for Human Simulation has developed a first version of a head and neck atlas titled "Functional Anatomy of the Visible Human: Version 1.0 The Head and Neck". The atlas, based on the Visible Human data set, is designed in educational modules covering the topics of mastication, deglutition, phonation, facial expression, extra-ocular motion, and hearing. QuickTime movies have been produced using live human subjects portraying the function of the regional anatomy described from a surface anatomy perspective. Tools include basic anatomic structure identification, a model builder, orthogonal plane browser, and links to the PubMed web site for automatic key word searches of the literature.

A Visible Human project inspired initiative, the Insight Toolkit, began beta testing last year. The toolkit makes available a variety of open source image processing algorithms for computing segmentation and registration on a variety of hardware platforms. Platforms currently supported are PCs running Visual C++, Sun Workstations running the GNU C++ compiler, SGI workstations, Linux based systems and Mac OS-X. This work is being conducted by a consortium of university and commercial entities.

Building on the earlier AnatLine system, the object-oriented database of Visible Human images indexed for the male thorax region, Lister Hill Center researchers created AnatQuest with the goal of providing widespread access to the Visible Human images. AnatQuest offers users thumbnails of the cross-section, sagittal and coronal images of the Visible Male, from which detailed (full-resolution) views are accessed. Low bandwidth connections are accommodated by a combination of adjustable viewing areas and image compression done on the fly as images are requested. Users may zoom and navigate through the images. (See Figure 3.)

## Medical Image Indexing and Retrieval

The Web-based Medical Information Retrieval System (WebMIRS) is an application that allows remote users to access x-ray and other data from two surveys conducted by the National Center for Health Statistics. These are the National Heath and Nutrition Examination Surveys (NHANES) II and III, carried out during the years 1976-1980 and 1988-1994, respectively. The project investigates fundamental questions that arise in the handling, organization, storage, access and transmission of very large x-ray images. WebMIRS allows a user to control a graphical user interface to construct a query for the data. A sample query might be equivalent to the English statements: "Find records for all individuals who reported chronic back pain. Return their age, sex, race, age when the pain began, and longest duration of pain. Also, return the record data required for statistical analysis

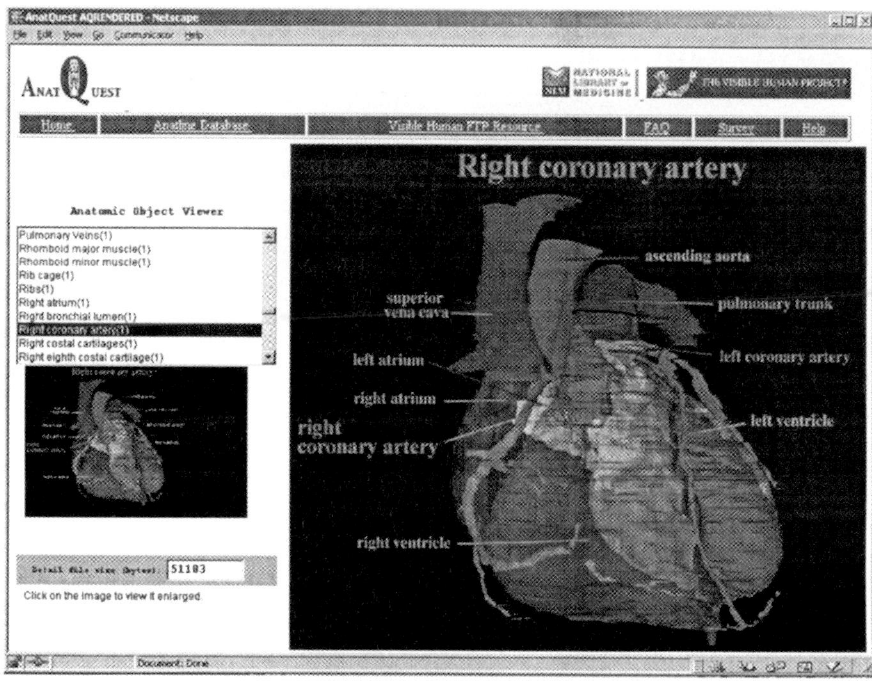



Fig. 3. AnatQuest is a web-based interface for viewing high resolution Visible Human anatomical images. The system provides viewers for rendered anatomical organs and the cut away slices of the body. AnatQuest allows browsing over images through an adjustable size viewing area, downloading portions of the 33-meg image slices to the browser as needed, thereby making it feasible to view the images

and display their x-ray images." WebMIRS allows the user to save the returned data to the local disk drive, where it may be analyzed with appropriate statistical tools.

The Content Based Image Retrieval project develops methods for effective extraction of biomedical information from digital images of the spine. This work has implications both for indexing of image data and for retrieval of those data. For example, for the NHANES II images, the only indexing data available is the collateral (alphanumeric) data collected in the questionnaires and examinations; no indexing information derived directly from the images is available, and the high cost of employing radiological experts to compile such data by physical viewing and interpreting each image makes it unlikely that such information will ever be acquired by purely manual means. These circumstances could be reversed if reliable, biomedically-validated soft-

ware could produce image interpretations automatically, or even semi-automatically. (See Figure 4.)

Computer-assisted image searching is a potential enabler of enhanced information extraction from a database that has already been indexed. The most popularized form of this type of search is "query by example" or a variant, "query by sketch". In query by example, the user inputs an image, perhaps by selecting from a set of choices provided by the system, or by providing a completely new image, and queries the database by asking, in effect, "Find records with images like this one", usually with respect to one or more characteristics of the example image, such as shape, histogram, or texture. In query by sketch, the input image is replaced by a sketch by the user, using drawing tools provided by the system. In either case, the system analyzes the input into component features, then searches the images in the database for those with similar features.

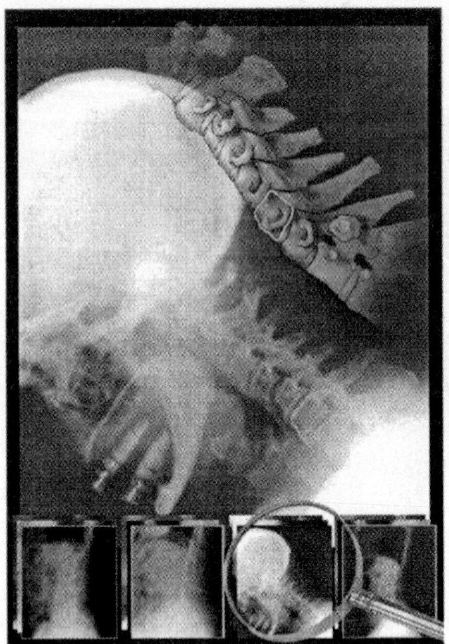

Fig. 4. Content-Based Image Retrieval of Biomedical Images comprises both indexing and retrieval. Indexing, the computer-assisted data reduction of images into mathematical features, may be subdivided into: segmentation, feature extraction, feature vector organization, and classification. Retrieving desired images from the databases comprises user query formulation, user query feature extraction, query search space strategy, and similarity matching method.

## Multimedia Research and Development

Our multimedia R&D efforts concentrate on the engineering of technical improvements applied to media issues such as image quality and resolution, color fidelity, transportability, storage, and visual information communication. In addition to the development by the staff of new methods and processes, the facilities and hardware infrastructure must reflect state-of-the-art standards in a very rapidly changing field. High definition video is a technology area being developed that represents the future for improved electronic image quality. Multimedia systems, scientific visualization and networked media are being pursued for the performance, educational, and economic advantages that they offer. Three dimensional computer graphics, animation techniques, and photorealistic rendering methods have changed the tools and products of the graphic artists in the Center. Digital video and image compression techniques are central to projects requiring storage of large images and rapid transmission.

One of our projects, the "Breath of Life Virtual Tour" was the centerpiece of the opening activities on World Asthma Day, and continued as part of program events on the CDC campus throughout that month. Another project, the "Movement Disorders" video database project is a collaborative project with the Yale University School of Medicine. This pilot effort established a digital video database of high quality, full-motion video clips of neurologically based movement disorders. The video database of patients with a variety of clinically diagnosed movement disorders, collected from the Yale University Movement Disorders Clinic underwent updated editing and compression to capitalize on advanced digitization and compression technology. "Expanding the Medical Universe", a new video shown daily in the NLM Visitors Center, is the first NLM video to be produced in the High Definition format. The new video also is presented in 'surround sound' and is delivered on a DVD which has both non-captioned and captioned versions.

## Information Systems

### Digital Library Research and Development

The Digital Library Research project involves all aspects of creating and disseminating digital collections, including standards, emerging technologies and formats, copyright and legal issues, effects on previously established processes, protection of original materials, and permanent archiving of digital surrogates. Research issues currently in focus are long-term preservation of digital archives, innovative methods for creating and accessing digital library collections, and the development of modular and open information environments. Investigations concerning interoperability among digital library systems, the role of well-structured metadata, and varying "points of view" on the same underlying data set are also being pursued.

The Profiles in Science web site makes the manuscript collections of prominent biomedical scientists available. The content of the database is created in collaboration with NLM's History of Medicine Division, which processes and stores the physical collections. The documents have been donated to NLM and contain published and unpublished materials, including books, journal volumes, pamphlets, diaries, letters, manuscripts, photographs, audio tapes and other audiovisual resources. (See Figure 5.)

Automatic data entry continues to be an active area of research and development in our digital library research program. MARS (Medical Article Records System) is a system that automates the production of MEDLINE records from biomedical journals. From bitmapped images of the first page of the articles, this system is designed to automatically extract the article title, author names, affiliations and the abstract. Our current research centers on the identification of rules for page segmentation, zone labeling, optical character recognition (OCR) error correction, and affiliation ranking. Operators enter fields (other than the ones automatically extracted), as well as perform text verification before the records are made available to indexers. The MARS system relies on image analysis and lexical analysis algorithms to correctly extract bibliographic data from images. These algorithms are based on rules constructed from features extracted from the layout geometry and OCR output.

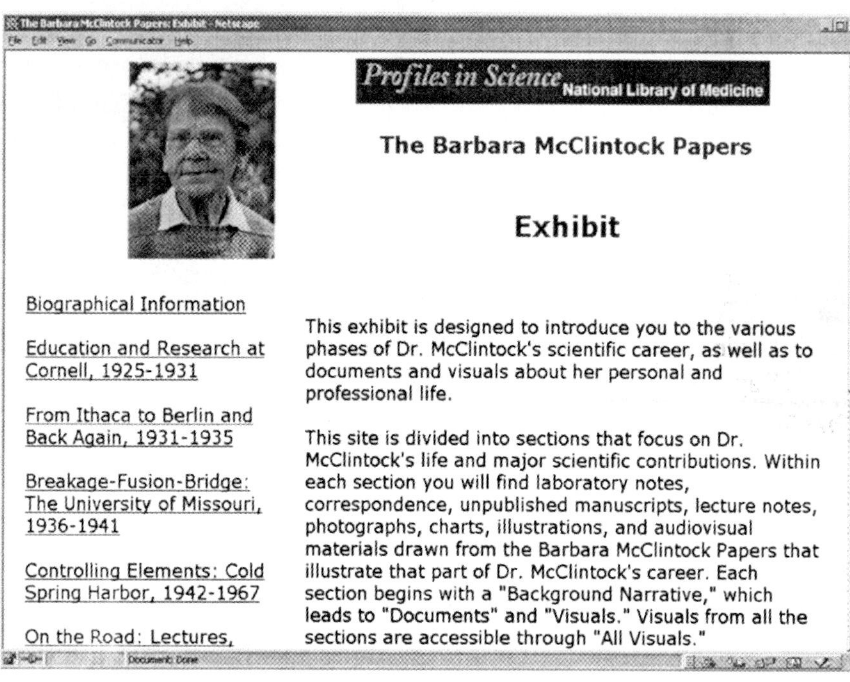



Fig. 5. Profiles in Science is a digital library site that makes the archival collections of prominent twentieth century biomedical scientists available to the public through modern digital technology. This is the introductory exhibit page for the Barbara McClintock collection.

The DocView project facilitates the delivery of library documents directly to the patron via the Internet in multiple ways. Once documents in bitmapped image form are received, the user may use DocView to retain them in electronic form, view the images, organize them into "folders" and "file cabinets", electronically bookmark selected pages, manipulate the images (zoom, pan, scroll), copy and paste images, and print them if desired. Users may receive document images either via Ariel FTP or Multipurpose Internet Mail Extensions protocols. DocMorph provides additional functionality for DocView users. DocMorph enables online users to convert files from one format to another for easier exchange or delivery.

## NLM Gateway

The National Library of Medicine offers an increasing number of Internet-based information resources, each with its own user interface. We have created the NLM Gateway to let users initiate searches in multiple retrieval systems from a single web interface.

The target audience for the new system is the Internet user who comes to NLM not knowing exactly what is available or how best to search for it. Results from the systems searched are presented in categories (for instance, journal article citations; books, serials and audiovisuals; consumer health information; meeting abstracts) rather than by database. The basic Gateway search interface is simple. It takes advantage of the capabilities of the retrieval systems it links to, for example, the advanced query parser and the "Related Articles" and "LinkOut" functions in MEDLINE/PubMed. Users may set preferences to adapt the interface to their needs, such as specifying which elements of a record they wish to see in the display of results.

## Consumer Health Informatics Research

Consumer Health Informatics research projects explore the needs, information seeking behavior, and cognitive strategies of health care consumers. The goal is to use medical informatics and information technolo-

gies to study ways to develop, organize, integrate, and deliver accessible health information to members of the public. We are currently conducting research that investigates readibility metrics and algorithms with the goal of providing health information to the public at all levels of health literacy.

ClinicalTrials.gov provides members of the public with comprehensive information about clinical trials. The site not only simplifies access to research protocols but also directs visitors to appropriate background information, such as health topics on MEDLINEplus and the biomedical literature on PubMed. (See Figure 6.)

Currently, ClinicalTrials.gov has thousands of protocol records sponsored by the Federal government, the pharmaceutical industry, and nonprofit organizations in tens of thousands of locations, mainly in the United States and Canada. We recently introduced several new search features in ClinicalTrials.gov to help users find relevant studies more easily. For example, "Search Within Results" enables users to narrow their search results with additional criteria and "TryIt" automatically suggests alternative queries when no studies are found. In addition, following the release of the Food and Drug Administration's "Guidance for Industry: Information Program on Clinical Trials for Serious or Life-Threatening Diseases and Conditions", ClinicalTrials.gov now regularly receives protocol information from pharmaceutical industry sponsors.

The Genetic Disease Home Reference is a new project that seeks to provide information about genes and diseases to members of the public. When completed, this resource will focus on diseases that are caused by single genes and, in turn, on the genes that cause these diseases. As knowledge of genetics expands, the interrelationships between genes and diseases will

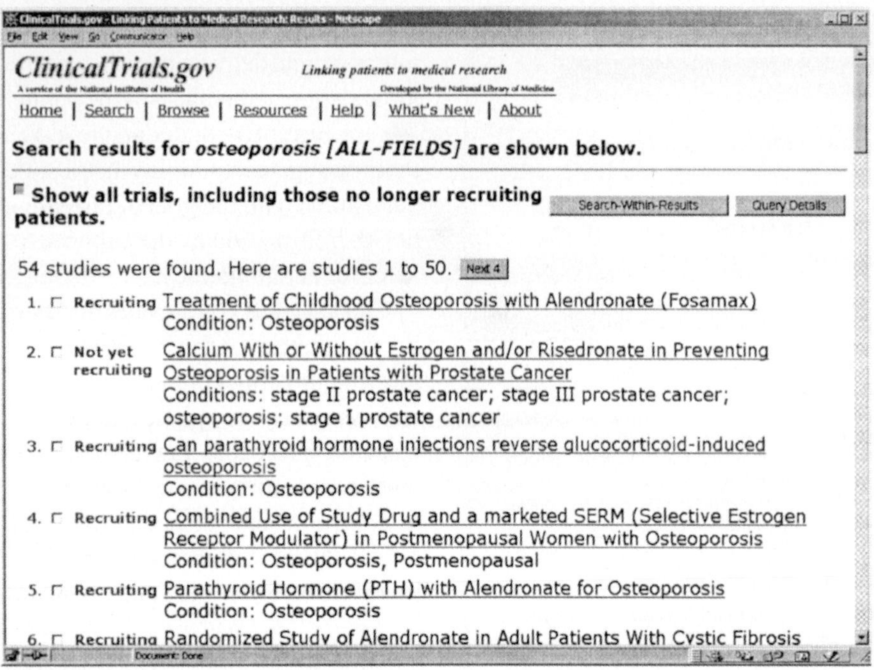

Fig. 6. ClinicalTrials.gov provides patients, family members, health care professionals, and members of the public easy access to information on clinical research studies for a wide range of diseases and conditions. Abstracts of the clinical study protocols include a summary of the purpose of the study, recruiting status, criteria for patient participation, location of the trial, and specific contact information. A list of trials for "osteoporosis" is shown above.

continue to unfold. Our goal is to provide a bridge between the clinical questions of the public and health professionals and the richness of data emanating from the Human Genome Project. Other resources will delve more deeply into the clinical aspects of the diseases and the details of the genes. This system is meant to serve as a guide into those other resources.

## Research Infrastructure and Support

### High Performance Computing and Communications

We are working to define and support Next Generation Internet (NGI) capabilities that will allow the NGI to be used routinely in health care, public health and health education, as well as biomedical, clinical and health services research. These capabilities include quality of service, security and medical data privacy, nomadic comput-ing, network management, and infra-structure technology as a means for collaboration. In 1998, NLM began a three-phase effort to support NGI capabilities in health care. The goal of the project is to gain a better under-standing of the impact of NGI on health care, health education, and health research in the areas of cost, quality, usability, efficacy, and security. Phase 1 was a planning effort, and Phase 2 supported the implementation of these plans within a limited geographic scope. Phase 3 was to be a test of scalability of applications to a national scope on public networks featuring quality of service. Such a network is, however, not available because of the rapid increase in available bandwidth and a decrease in the price of that bandwidth. In lieu of Phase 3, we began a new initiative in Scalable Information Infra-structure. The purpose of this initiative is to encourage development of health related applications of scalable, wire-less, geographic information systems, and identification technologies in a net-worked environment. The initiative focuses on situations that require or greatly benefit from the application of these technologies in health care, medical decision-making, public health, large-scale health emergencies, health education, and biomedical, clinical and health services research.

The Collaboratory for High Perform-ance Computing and Communication investigates innovative means for assisting health science institutions in their use of online distance learning technologies and explores advanced computer and network technologies for distance interactivity, including wireless technology and virtual reality research. We recently conducted a series of experiments combining wire-less and streaming video technology offsite to do live webcasts from NLM that originated at remote sites. Video encoding software on a laptop roaming the scientific poster session at the annual meeting of the American Medical Informatics Association (AMIA) sent the video stream through a wireless network installed onsite back to NLM for broadcast via the Collaboratory streaming server. We established a 802.11b wireless network at the AMIA NLM booth for the duration of the exhibits.

### System Security and Advanced Networks

Our research and development activities depend on advanced network capabilities as well as state of the art security systems. Lister Hill Center staff collaborate with other NLM divisions in the development of access controls and security classifications. A secure subnets working group last year developed a classification of NLM systems used to categorize different levels of required network access between each system and the Internet. The first phase of the secure subnets initiative has been implemented, with most desk-based systems placed on subnets that are not accessible from outside NLM. These systems can themselves access sites outside NLM, but transmissions originating outside of NLM cannot access them. The effect of this grouping has been to make these systems less vulnerable to external security attacks. A new network performance testing system generates live traffic for analyzing and tuning the performance of the NLM network. A very high capacity tape library system based on LTO tape technology is used for backups of the Center's computer systems. Most backup media are online at all times, available for restoration of older data and programs. Backup volumes are created in duplicate, with one set for offsite storage.

The Lister Hill Center is connected to two NGI networks, vBNS (very high speed Backbone Network Services) and Abilene, with connections to the Federal NGI network DREN, the Department of Defense Research Network. The Abilene network supports full IP (Internet Protocol) multicast. We use that mode to receive and transmit multicast voice and video sessions. We recently worked with the Uniformed Services University and its Medical Simulation Center in connecting to the Abilene network. Dark fiber was used to connect the institutions, and we arranged for connectivity to Abilene through the router at NLM. For a cross country test using large images, we conducted memory-to-memory tests between the Armed Forces Institute of Pathology in Maryland through NLM to the San Diego Supercomputing Center in California.

## Organizational Structure

The Lister Hill Center has five major components, each of which is listed below, together with its Branch or Office Chief. Many of our research activities involve collaboration not only across Lister Hill Center branches, but also across divisions of the NLM, the NIH, federal agencies, and university departments.

## Communications Engineering Branch (George Thoma, PhD)

The Communications Engineering Branch is engaged in applied research and development in image engineering and communications engineering motivated by NLM's mission-critical tasks such as document delivery, archiving, automated production of MEDLINE records, Internet access to biomedical multimedia databases, and imaging applications in support of medical educational packages employing digitized radiographic, anatomic, and other imagery. In addition to applied research, the branch also develops and maintains operational systems for production of bibliographic records for NLM's flagship database, MEDLINE. Research areas include: content-based image indexing and retrieval of biomedical images, document image analysis and understanding, image compression, image enhancement, image feature identification and extraction, image segmentation, image retrieval by "query by image content", image transmission and video conferencing over networks implemented via asynchronous transfer mode and satellite technologies, optical character recognition and man-machine interface design applied to automated data entry. The branch also maintains archives of large numbers of digitized spine x-rays and bit-mapped document images that are used for intramural and outside research purposes. The most current information about the Communications Engineering Branch can be found at http://lhncbc.nlm.nih.gov/ceb/.

## Cognitive Science Branch (Alexa T. McCray, PhD)

The Cognitive Science Branch conducts research and development in computer and information technologies.

Important research areas involve the investigation of a variety of techniques, including linguistic, statistical, and knowledge-based methods for improving access to biomedical information. Branch members actively participate in the Unified Medical Language System project and collaborate with other NLM research staff in the Indexing Initiative project, whose goal is to develop automated and semi-automated techniques for indexing the biomedical literature. The branch also conducts research in digital libraries and collaborates with NLM's History of Medicine Division on Profiles in Science, a project to digitize collections of prominent biomedical scientists. Several branch projects address the challenges involved in providing health information to consumers. ClinicalTrials.gov is a resource developed by the branch, and it affords an excellent testbed for conducting consumer health informatics research. The branch is currently developing a system designed to provide information about genes and diseases to the public. The most current information about the Cognitive Science Branch can be found at http://lhncbc.nlm.nih.gov/cgsb/

## Computer Science Branch (Lawrence C. Kingsland III, PhD)

The Computer Science Branch applies techniques of computer science and information science to problems in the representation, retrieval and manipulation of biomedical knowledge. Branch projects involve both basic and applied research in such areas as intelligent gateway systems for simultaneous searching in multiple databases, intelligent agent technology, knowledge management, the merging of thesauri and controlled vocabularies, data mining, and machine-assisted indexing for information classification and retrieval. Research issues include knowledge representation, knowledge base structure, knowledge acquisition, and the human-machine interface for complex systems. Important components of the research include embedded intelligence systems that combine local reasoning with access to large-scale online databanks. Computer Science Branch research staff include the teams that developed NLM's Gateway, Internet Grateful Med and HSTAT programs and the team that annually produces the UMLS Metathesaurus. Branch staff coordinate the NIH Clinical Elective in Medical Informatics for third and fourth year medical students. The most current information about the Computer Science Branch can be found at http://lhncbc.nlm.nih.gov/csb/.

## Audiovisual Program Development Branch (James Main)

The Audiovisual Program Development Branch supports the Lister Hill Center's research, development, and demonstration projects with high quality video, audio, imaging, and graphics materials. From initial project concept through project implementation and final evaluation, a variety of forms and formats of visuals are developed, and staff activities include content creation, editing, enhancement, transfer and display. Included in this effort is the production of a series of video modules, documenting the progress of Lister Hill Center research projects. Consultation and materials development are also provided by the branch for NLM's information programs. From applications of optical media technologies and teleconferencing to support for web design, the requirement for graphics, video, and audio materials has increased in quantity and diversified in format. Included within the branch is the Office of the Public Health Service Historian. This office provides information about the history of Federal efforts devoted to public health, preserves and interprets the history of PHS, and promotes historically oriented activities across the U.S. Department of Health and Human Services. The most current information about the Audiovisual Program Development Branch can be found at http://lhncbc.nlm.nih.gov/apdb/

## Office of High Performance Computing and Communications (Michael J. Ackerman, PhD)

The Office of High Performance Computing and Communications serves as the focal point for the NLM's High Performance Computing and Communications (HPCC) activities. It coordinates NLM's HPCC planning, research and development activities with federal, industrial, academic, and commercial organizations, and it collaborates with Lister Hill Center research branches and NLM Divisions in the development, operation, evaluation and demonstration of HPCC research programs and projects. In addition, it plans, coordinates, and administers the Inter-Agency HPCC research and development program. Office staff serve as NLM's liaison to scientific organizations at all levels of national, state and international government on planning and implementing research in HPCC. The major research activities of the office center around the Visible Human Project, NLM's Next Generation Internet Program, including telemedicine, the Collaboratory for High Performance Computing and Communications, and the 3D Informatics research program. The most current information about the Office of High Performance Computing and Communications can be found at http://lhncbc.nlm.nih.gov/ohpcc/.

## Conclusion

Lister Hill Center research and development is driven by the needs of an increasingly information based society. We work at the intersection of computer and information science and medicine, addressing the information problems faced by biomedical researchers, health care professionals, and, increasingly, members of the public. The health information needs of patients, families, and other members of the public bring new research challenges, especially as the complexity of biomedical knowledge continues to increase. We conduct basic and applied research to support open access to high quality biomedical information, and we develop information systems that are strongly informed by informatics principles and methods. As we look forward, we see a host of exciting research opportunities, and, through our training program, we continue to be committed to the development of the next generation of outstanding informatics researchers.

## Acknowledgments

I would like to thank all Lister Hill Center research staff for their contributions to the content of this report.

## References

1. Ackerman MJ, Banvard RA. Imaging outcomes from the National Library of Medicine's Visible Human Project. Comput Med Imaging Graph 2000; 24(3):125-6.
2. Aronson AR. Effective mapping of biomedical text to the UMLS Metathesaurus: The MetaMap program. Proc AMIA Symp. 2001; p. 17-21.
3. Aronson AR, Bodenreider O, Chang HF, Humphrey SM, Mork JG, Nelson SJ, et al. The NLM indexing initiative. Proc AMIA Symp. 2000; p. 17-21.
4. Bodenreider O, Rindflesch TC, Burgun A. Unsupervised corpus-based method for extending a biomedical terminology. Proceedings of the Workshop on Natural Language Processing in the Biomedical Domain, North American Chapter of the Association for Computational Linguistics. 2002; p. 53-60.
5. Bodenreider O. Experiences in visualizing and navigating biomedical ontologies and knowledge bases. Proceedings of the ISMB 2002 Bio-ontologies SIG meeting. 2002; p. 29-32.
6. Bodenreider O. Using UMLS semantics for classification purposes. Proc AMIA 2000; p. 86-90.
7. Burgun A, Bodenreider O. Aspects of the taxonomic relation in the biomedical domain. In: Welty C, Smith B, editors. Collected papers from the Second International

Conference on Formal Ontology in Information Systems. New York: ACM Press; 2001; p. 222-33.

8. Fan Y, Hwang K, Gill M, Huang HK. Some connectivity and security issues of NGI in medical imaging applications. Journal of High Speed Networks 2000; 9:3-13.

9. Ford G, Hauser SE, Le DX, Thoma GR. Pattern matching techniques for correcting low confidence OCR words in a known context. Proc SPIE, Document Recognition and Retrieval VIII. 2001. p. 241-9.

10. Hauser SE, Le DX, Thoma GR. Automated zone correction in bitmapped document images. Proc SPIE, Document Recognition and Retrieval VII. 2000. p. 248-58.

11. Humphrey SM, Rindflesch TC, Aronson AR. Automatic indexing by discipline and high-level categories: methodology and potential applications. In: Soergel D, et al. editors. Advances in classification research. Proceedings of the 11th ASIST SIG/CR Classification Research Workshop; 2001.

12. Kim J, Le DX, Thoma GR. Automated labeling in document images. Proc SPIE, Vol 4307, Document Recognition and Retrieval VIII; 2001. p. 111-22.

13. Le DX, Straughan SR, Thoma GR. Greek alphabet recognition technique for biomedical documents. Proc 6th World Multiconference on Systemics, Cybernetics and Informatics, Vol. III. ; 2002. p. 86-91.

14. Le DX, Tran LQ, Chow J, Kim J, Hauser SE, Moon CW, et al. Automated medical records citation records creation for web-based online journals. Proc 14th IEEE Symposium on Computer-Based Medical Systems; 2001. p. 315-20.

15. Locatis, C. Instructional design and technology in healthcare. In: Reiser R, Dempsey J, editors. Trends and Issues in Instructional Design and Technology, Upper Saddle River, New Jersey: Merrill/ Prentice-Hall; 2002. p. 225-38.

16. Long LR, Thoma GR. Identification and classification of spine vertebrae by automated methods. Proc SPIE Medical Imaging 2001: Image Processing; 2001. p. 1478-89.

17. Long LR, Thoma GR. Use of shape models to search digitized spine x-rays. Proc. IEEE Computer-Based Medical Systems; 2000. p. 255-60.

18. Long LR, Thoma GR. Landmarking and feature localization in spine x-rays. Journal of Electronic Imaging 2001; 10(4):939-56.

19. Lu CJ, Bangalore A, Tse T. Developing web browser recording tools using server-side programming technology. In: Proceedings of WebNet 2000, World conference on WWW and Internet. Association for the Advancement of Computing in Education; 2000. p. 372-7.

20. Marcelo AB, Fontelo PA. A pathology report metadata registry: Framework for semantic interoperability across disparate systems. Arch Pathol Lab Med 2001; 125(8):1014-15.

21. McCray AT, Gallagher ME. Principles for digital library development. Commun ACM 2001; 44(5):48-54.

22. McCray AT. Better access to information about clinical trials. Ann Intern Med 2000; 133(8):609-14.

23. McCray AT, Bodenreider O, Malley JD, Browne AC. Evaluating UMLS strings for natural language processing. Proc AMIA Symp; 2001 p. 448-52.

24. Nishinaga N, Tatsumi H, Gill M, Akashib A, Nogawa H, Reategui I. Trans-Pacific demonstration of Visible Human. Space Communications 2002; 17(4):303-11.

25. Parascandola, JA. From germs to genes: Trends in drug therapy, 1852-2002. Pharmacy in History 44; 2002. p. 3-11.

26. Parascandola J. The pharmaceutical sciences in America, 1852- 1902. J Am Pharm Assoc 2000; 40:733-5.

27. Pearson G, Moon CW. Bridging two biomedical journal databases with XML: A case study. Proc 14th IEEE Symposium on Computer-Based Medical Systems; 2001. p. 309-14.

28. Rindflesch TC, Tanabe L, Weinstein JN, Hunter L. EDGAR: extraction of drugs, genes and relations from the biomedical literature. Pacific Symposium on Bio-computing; 2000. p. 517-28.

29. Rindflesch TC, Rajan JV, Hunter L. Extracting molecular binding relationships from biomedical text. Proceedings of the 6th Applied Natural Language Processing Conference; 2000. p. 188-95.

30. Rodgers RPC, Sherwin Z. A management system for network-sharable locally installed software: Merging RPM and the depot scheme under Solaris. LISA XV: Proceedings of the Fifteenth Systems Administration Conference; 2001. p. 267-72.

31. Thoma GR, Ford G. Automated data entry system: performance issues. Proc SPIE Document Recognition and Retrieval IX.; 2002. p. 181-90.

32. Thoma GR, Ford G, Le DX, Li Z. Text verification in an automated system for the extraction of bibliographic data. Proc 5th International Workshop on Document Analysis Systems; 2002. p. 423-32.

33. Tran LQ, Moon CW, Le DX, Thoma GR. Web page downloading and classification. Proc 14th IEEE Symposium on Computer-Based Medical Systems; 2001. p. 321-6.

34. Walker FL, Thoma GR. A SOAP-enabled system for an online library service. Proc InfoToday 2002; 2002. p. 320-9.

35. Walker FL, Thoma GR. Web-based document image processing. Proc SPIE: Internet Imaging; 2000. p. 268-77.

36. Weeber M, Mork JG, Aronson AR. Developing a test collection for biomedical word sense disambiguation. Proc AMIA Symp; 2001. p. 746-50.

37. Xiaocheng L, Prettyman, M., Antonucci, R. System expansion and integration with agents in HSTAT. Proceedings of the World Multiconference on Systemics, Cybernetics, and Informatics; 2000.

38. Yoo TS, Morris J, Chen DT, Burgess J, Richardson AC. Template guided intervention: Interactive visualization and design for medical fused deposition models. Proceedings of the Workshop on Interactive Medical Image Visualization and Analysis; 2001. p. 45-8.

39. Yoo TS. Toward validation databases for medical imaging: Engineering a scientific rendezvous. Proceedings of VISIM Workshop on Information Retrieval; 2001. p. 7-10.

40. Zamora G, Sari-Sarraf H, Mitra S, Long R. Analysis of the feasibility of using active shape models for segmentation of gray scale images. Proceedings of SPIE Medical Imaging 2002: Image Processing; 2002. p. 1370-81.

Address of the author:
Alexa T. McCray
National Library of Medicine
8600 Rockville Pike
Bethesda, MD 20894
USA
Tel.:       +1 301 496 4441
Fax:        +1 301 435 3146
E-mail:     mccray@nlm.nih.gov

**H. Takeda**

Department of Medical Information
Science Osaka University Hospital
Osaka, Japan

# Research and Education

# *Introduction to the Department of Medical Information Science of Osaka University Hospital*

## Introduction

The department of Medical Information Science at Osaka University Hospital was established in 1986 and takes a double responsibility: research in medical informatics, and implementation, operation and maintenance of information systems in the hospital. The double function is a common characteristic in the Japanese department of medical informatics in national university hospitals.

The first professor (1986- 1997) and director was Michitoshi Inoue who is now the director of the Osaka National Hospital and the president of the Japanese Association of Medical Informatics. The second professor of the department is Hiroshi Takeda who has been the associate professor since 1986.

Research is conducted in both basic and applied medical informatics areas, ranging from the electronic patient record system, hospital information system, PACS system, clinical data warehouse, regional networks, telemedicine and remote consultation. Other topics include decision-support systems and check systems are also of concern. In 2000, the department also belonged to the Osaka University Graduate School of Medicine. In 2001,

Professor Hiroshi Takeda was appointed director of the department of Clinical Quality Management which is the first department for patient safety and clinical quality improvement in the Japanese national university hospitals.

## Research Activities

### 1. The Hospital Information System (HIS)

An integrated hospital information system called "HUMANE" (human oriented universal medical assessment system under network environment) was developed in 1993. There are two groups of application programs inside HUMANE: one is an interdepartmental or common application program including patient registration, an accounting and billing system, an order entry system (prescriptions, laboratory testing, radiological examinations, admission, operation, and meal service), disease name registration, a reporting system (laboratory test and radiological examination), reservation (re-visit, special examination), admission management, and a nursing care system; while the other is a department-specific application program including the pharmacy department, laboratory department,

radiological examination department, operational department and meal service department. The system architecture of the first generation was main-medium-micro frame link and featured a quick response time and a good man-machine interface by using GUI (Graphical User Interface). The hardware configuration was totally changed into a client-server system in 2000. The system has been developed with the Nippon Electric Company (NEC) since 1986. From the beginning, the physicians' direct order entry has been established in "HUMANE" and the database provides the basis for clinical data management in conjunction with the paper-based medical record that is totally integrated into one-patient-one-file in the central storage.

### 2. PACS system

In our hospital, image data of almost all modalities including CR, CT, MR, ultra-sound and RI are in PACS (Picture Archiving and Communication System). The Image data is sent through a Multi-image Terminal to a Multimedia Server with a jukebox type MO disk. A client PC can request the patient information as the reporting system of radiological examination by means of HIS-RIS (Radiological Information System)-PACS coupling.

Although there are some arguments against its costs, it does assist decision making of referring doctors in very short turn-around time.

### 3. The Electronic Patient Record (EPR) System

Due to the successful operation of the ordering and reporting system, an electronic patient record system of the Osaka University Hospital (EPROU) was deployed in January 2001. The system is also developed jointly with NEC. The EPROU features 1) physicians' direct structured data entry, 2) multi-modal output of registered clinical data and 3) dynamic problem oriented system.

Next, we are planning to transfer this structured data into a data warehouse and link it with speech recognition input with which may achieve other functional goals of an EPR, i.e. clinical decision support, access to knowledge resources, and improvement in the overall process of recording and retrieving clinical data.

### 4. Clinical Data Warehouse (CDW)

The nature of CDW as a source for analysis and rapid retrieval of data is tailor-made for EPR and provides a mechanism used to identify individuals at risk for target diseases and to identify costs and revenue opportunities. Thus, many hospitals are developing their data warehouses. We have finished implementing our data warehouse and installing "Business Objects" for data analysis this year and are now conducting the following research:

·   Methodology of deducing the regional morbidity from CDW;
·   Investigation and analysis of the occurrence frequency of drug side-effects;
·   Method of selecting specific data for diagnosis;
·   Predicting the prognosis of diabetes;
·   Evaluation of the effectiveness of risk reduction initiatives

·   Analysis of the costs affected by prescribing different types of hypo tensors.

### 5. Regional health care networks

For the sake of providing more efficient and effective health care to the patients and sharing the patients' information with other institutions, we have made our hospital system tightly connect in the regional health care institution networks. Last year, we contracted with the Ministry of Economics and Trade Industry in developing an introductory networked EPR system, which has been put in practice and is currently being evaluated. Further, with the progress of standardizations in medical informatics and the improved security environments, we are engaging to develop a digital radiological imaging and electronic prescription system among regional health care networks.

### 6. Telemedicine and remote consultation

Telemedicine is a cost-effective form of medical practice for rural area patients and a quick and easy method for primary care clinicians to get expert consultations via electronic access. We have successfully developed a high quality oriented teleconference system and remote Open MRI operation system with the function of sharing DICOM and 3-D images and the navigation of a remote operating process.

### 7. Decision-support and check system

The more developed the HIS decision-support function is, the more benefits can be seen by health care providers and patients. Currently when we conduct ordering, we can do some checking as well. For instance, we can check the overdoses, the repetitions, the contraindications, the drug-drug inter-effects, etc. In order to enforce this checking system, the well-estab-

lished knowledge base is inevitable.

Based on this incentive, we are also conducting research on selecting similar cases from CDW by using data mining technology.

### 8. Clinical quality management

In conjunction with the department of clinical quality management, the on-line incident report system has been developed and operated for two years by using the intranet of the HIS. The accumulated reports have been analyzed to prevent medical errors in the hospital. In order to respond to the implementation of the first Japanese DRG (diagnosis related group)/PPS (prospective payment system), which will be scheduled to start next April, the data gathering concerning clinical process, major diagnoses, major care procedures and their costs has started and is being entered into a database. Several studies will be conducted to measure the quantitative quality of health care in the very near future.

### 9. Health care standardization

As Prof. Takeda is a project leader of the work item: framework of emergency data sets in the working group 1 of ISO/TC215 (medical informatics), existing emergency data sets are collected world-wide and analyzed to make a framework that will position and map those data sets. Other standardization projects have been involved in this department to facilitate networked EPR systems in Japan.

---

### Staffs and students

For conducting studies and research, both the department of medical information science and clinical quality management have worked together. The greater department consists of three faculties (Prof. Hiroshi Takeda, Associate Prof. Yasushi Matsumura, and Assistant Prof. Kazue Nakajima) and three full-time staff (one registered

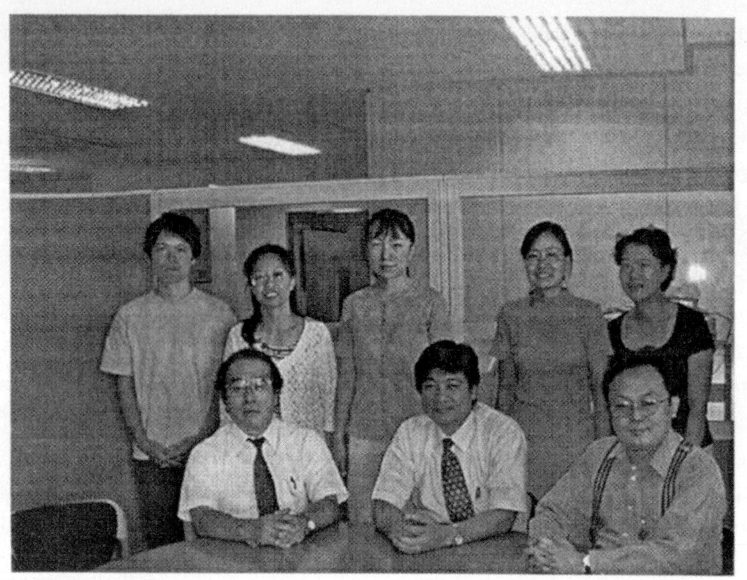

risk manager nurse, one registered health information administrator and one secretary). There are currently one post-doctoral fellow, two research fellows and seven graduate students. The maintenance of HIS is mainly provided by ten members in the administration office of the Osaka University Hospital.

Address of the author:
Professor Hiroshi Takeda, M.D., Ph.D.
Department of Medical Information Science
Osaka University hospital, 2-15
Yamada-Oka, Suita 565, Japan
E-mail: takeda@hp-info.med.osaka-u.ac.jp

**M.A. Musen**[1],
**J.H. van Bemmel**[2]

[1] Stanford Medical Informatics
Stanford University School of Medicine
Stanford, California, USA
[2] Institute of Medical Informatics,
Erasmus University Medical Center,
Rotterdam, The Netherlands

# Challenges in Medical Informatics

## *A Discipline Coming of Age*

Adolescence is a difficult time. Teenagers harbor doubts about themselves and about their relationship with others. They enter a period of deep introspection and begin to question their roots. They also begin to envision what it is that they truly want to become.

Medical informatics—after a prolonged period of development—is facing its own adolescence. During the past three to four decades, we have transitioned from a group of hospital-based technologists whose primary focus was the implementation of clinical information systems to a diverse community of scholars, clinicians, engineers, and pragmatists who often share common long-term objectives but who often have different agendas for achieving them. Today, academicians in medical informatics constitute a large group of scholars with their own professional societies, conferences, and journals—venues in which they happen to express quite heterogeneous scientific philosophies and goals. Although the emergence of organized elements of scholarship shows how far we have come, the variability in our scientific approach suggests that we are facing a period of continued development.

These are tough times in which to be an adolescent. Many health-care institutions are beginning to question the value of the investments that they have made in informatics. Some of our best scientists are leaving their university positions and many of our trainees seem ill prepared to take on academic jobs. Funding organizations are suddenly enraptured by the glamour of computational biology (which they confuse with bioinformatics), heightening the competition for limited resources. In these demanding times, workers in medical informatics do not have the luxury to act as teenagers and to brood about why the world may be treating them unfairly; they need to define their purpose clearly and to set achievable goals for the years ahead.

As we reported last year in these pages [1], a group of senior academicians in medical informatics convened in Madrid in March 2001 in conjunction with the meeting of the IMIA Board. The goal of the Madrid workshop was to define the challenges faced by medical informatics as an academic discipline and to suggest strategies to enhance the scholarly foundation of our field. Some of the position papers that were contributed to the Madrid

workshop appeared last year in a special issue of *Methods of Information in Medicine* [2]. Four of those papers are now reprinted in this edition of the *Yearbook*. These papers were selected because they provide a cross-section of opinions and are representative of all the contributions discussed at the workshop.

The papers point to the need for our community to define clearly what medical informatics is and why it is important. We cannot continue to characterize medical informatics in terms of other, more established disciplines. If we claim that medical informatics is a kind of "applied computer science," for example, then it remains unclear why medical informatics—at least academically—needs to exist apart from more traditional computer-science groups. If we claim that our field is simply an amalgam of other disciplines, such as computer science, biostatistics, health-services research, and cognitive science, then there is nothing that we can claim to be *our own*. Like teenagers struggling to understand what differentiates themselves from their parents, the participants at the Madrid workshop worked hard to characterize what are the unique elements of medical informatics that are distinct from those of the allied disciplines that contribute to our scientific enterprise.

Although it may seem obvious in retrospect, the universal conclusion from the Madrid workshop was that academic informatics is special because of its focus on information. Unlike computer science, for example, which typically places its emphasis on *computation*, our research community is dedicated to the study of *information* as a first-class object. It is modeling the data and knowledge required by our applications that requires unique skills, and where our academic research makes its distinguishing contribution. Ours is indeed the discipline that cares about the content. Our principal challenge in medical or health informatics is to understand better the structure of data, information, and knowledge, and to cast our scholarship in terms of appropriate models of these abstract entities.

Models of information, of course, lack cogency unless there are processes that operate on those models to perform useful tasks. Such tasks must be performed within complex social systems and must inform discerning and yet fallible human participants. Thus, it is impossible to consider information completely in isolation. Work in medical informatics is inherently interdisciplinary because of the need to draw on a large number of related fields that allow us to put the study of information into context. We are challenged to maintain our bridges to diverse, related fields such as cognitive science, image processing, and epidemiology, and to clarify the common foundation that we share with research in bioinformatics.

The participants at the Madrid workshop concluded their discussions articulating an urgent need to disseminate the perspective that informatics is both a science and an engineering discipline with a strong theoretical foundation. They saw a requirement to enhance our curricula to clarify the contributions of basic research in informatics—helping students to understand the underlying principles that transcend particular application domains and that provide coherency to our research programs. There also was a perception that professional societies, such as IMIA, must take the lead in educating both their members and funding bodies about the generalizable contributions of basic scholarship in informatics, and how a wide range of application areas—from health care to biology to other information-intensive activities—can benefit from academic research in informatics.

The papers reprinted in this edition of the *Yearbook* are a step toward the dissemination of the ideas discussed at the Madrid workshop. We hope that they will stimulate both continued introspection and a plan for action within our community as the field of medical informatics continues to come of age.

## References


1. Musen, MA and Van Bemmel, JH. Challenges for medical informatics as an academic discipline: workshop report. In: Haux R and Kulikowski C, editors. Yearbook of Medical Informatics 2002. Stuttgart: Schattauer; 2002. p. 194-7.
2. Musen, MA and Van Bemmel, JH. editors. Special issue on Challenges for Medical Informatics as an Academic Discpline. Methods Inf Med 2002; 41:1–63.



Address of the authors:
Mark A. Musen
Stanford Medical Informatics
Stanford University School of Medicine
251 Campus Drive, Room X-215
Stanford, CA 94305-5479
USA
E-mail:    Musen@SMI.Stanford.EDU

Jan H. van Bemmel
Institute of Medical Informatics
Erasmus University Medical Center
P.O. Box 1738
3000 DR Rotterdam
The Netherlands
E-mail:    vanbemmel@mi.fgg.eur.nl

# Medical Informatics as a Discipline at the Beginning of the 21$^{st}$ Century

J. L. Talmon, A. Hasman
Department of Medical Informatics, Maastricht University, Maastricht, The Netherlands

## Summary

*Objectives:* To analyse the present situation of the discipline medical informatics and to propose actions for change.

*Methods:* Evaluation of the current situation mainly based on anecdotal evidence.

*Results:* The difference between the scientific and the engineering aspects of medical informatics get blurred. Because of the requirements of European funding medical informatics focuses more on engineering than on science. Too many manuscripts are submitted that describe engineered artefacts without a scientific purpose. Some of the subjects (like security issues) that are studied in medical informatics are not considered important by medical faculties thus impeding support.

*Conclusions:* The methodological underpinnings of our research should be strengthened, impact studies should be more frequently performed; the quality of results reporting should be increased.

## Keywords

Medical informatics, methodology, impact studies, reporting quality

Methods Inf Med 2002; 41: 4–7

## Introduction

Medical informatics seems to be in a crisis. Most of our scientific journals have low citation rates. The founders and the second-generation researchers in Medical Informatics still reign the field; new talent is scarce. We have seen people moving from academia towards industry, and not necessarily toward the industry that delivers ICT (Information and Communication Technology) solutions for health care. The ICT industry is sceptical about the profitability of their market in health care. Apparently the need for information systems (be it hospital information systems or information systems for general practitioners) is not that large that hospitals or GPs are willing to pay a reasonable price for these systems. Physicians are complaining that the systems are not user friendly and focus more on registration than on supporting their daily work.

On the other hand, bio-informatics is flourishing. Risk capital is flowing into start-up companies in this domain. New departments are being created in many universities all over the world. We may ask ourselves why medical informatics is not profiting and what its position will be in the 21$^{st}$ century.

Before we further analyse the situation we would like to elaborate on what medical informatics entails. Medical informatics is the discipline concerned with the systematic processing of data, information and knowledge. The domain of medical informatics covers computational and informational aspects of processes and structures in medicine and healthcare. The aims of medical informatics are twofold: (i) to provide solutions for problems related to data, information and knowledge processing and (ii) to study the general principles of processing data, information and knowledge [1].

Hasman et al. [1] describe medical informatics as a modelling discipline. Medicine in general and health care in particular involve many kinds of processes (e. g. biological, communication, decision, educational, organizational or computational). It is the aim of medical informatics to design models for such processes in order to implement them in computer systems. This implies that the structure and the processes of the problem domain have to be methodically analysed, modelled, instantiated (with data or domain knowledge), and the corresponding algorithms and programs designed. How these models should be developed and how to determine their predictive strengths is the core business of medical informatics as a discipline. Making these models applicable for daily medical practice is the applied science/engineering side of medical informatics.

## Aspects of Medical Informatics

Medical informatics covers a broad domain. The processes that are studied are diverse in nature and may require different methodological approaches. When we study the Recommendations of the International Medical Informatics Association on Education in Health and Medical Informatics [2] not only does the extent become apparent, but also the broad range of professionals that are educated. The types of professionals range from physicians who use the acquired medical informatics knowledge to support research in their own medical discipline to professionals that can be hardly discriminated from professionals with a computer sciences background. This may give the impression that the field is fragmented, and that medical informatics does not have a clear theory.

The majority of the PhD studies performed in our department [3] is carried out in a combined effort with a medical discipline. This cooperation between medical informatics and a medical specialty is a consequence of the domain we are working in. The medical informatics researcher tries to develop methods or gain knowledge useful for the medical specialty, and at the same time tries to obtain more insight into the nature of data, information or knowledge processing. In these PhD studies, the medical informatics part focuses on, for example, the problem of how to represent knowledge so that a system can reason with this knowledge in order to solve a medical problem. Since the medical counterpart is usually interested in the quality of the output of the system, the study often also involves an evaluation element.

In research we try to extend the body of knowledge of medical informatics. Via education we try to train professionals by providing them with the necessary knowledge and skills so that they can develop information systems, be responsible for information delivery in e. g. the hospital, advise physicians, nurses, administrators etc. in decision making tasks, e. g. concerning the purchase of information systems, etc.

Medical informaticians as professionals work together with physicians and nurses and apply their medical informatics knowledge to solve a number of problems. Medical informaticians as researchers are modelling situations and trying to formalize these models so that they can be implemented in a program and be evaluated. They, also investigate whether the processes under consideration are found in other medical disciplines and if so they will study the general application of their developed methods.

Sometimes the difference between medical informatics as a profession and medical informatics as a science is blurred. This is for example apparent when manuscripts are submitted to scientific journals describing yet another system, without evidence of new design principles or new techniques. We do not say that systems should not be built. In research we have to build systems to prove the correctness of models or concepts. However, in research we should start with hypotheses and test these hypotheses by implementing the ideas into systems and evaluating them. Developing systems for practical use is important but usually cannot be considered as a scientific enterprise.

When we use tested models to build systems we are not so much interested in extending our knowledge, but more in the direct support of physicians and nurses.

We will discuss some of the applications of ICT in health care and argue why these have hardly contributed to the recognition of medical informatics as a scientific discipline. We are aware that we are making gross generalisations, and that exceptions exist. These exceptions, however, often deal with technological developments that have applicability beyond the medical domain.

# ICT Applications in Health Care

Hospital information systems are installed in nearly all hospitals in the developed countries. In their early days they supported the administrative processes in hospitals. In recent years there has been a move towards the support of clinical care. Although there are people that claim that health care cannot be compared with any other business, the administrative processes resemble those in other (service) industries. Therefore research in this area is not necessarily considered to be of relevance by medical faculties where the departments of medical informatics are located. For example, all issues related to security, authentication, etc. are not only relevant for the health care industry but also for many other industries, such as banking. Developing and implementing a HIS is seen as automating administrative processes. Developing integrated systems that support the chain of health care delivery from specialized clinics, via general hospitals and general practitioners to home nursing is more an organisational – if not political – problem rather than an ICT problem.

The medical community has rapidly adopted all kinds of medical imaging modalities. The modern imaging techniques such as CT, MRI, PET rely heavily on computational algorithms. Without computers, such imaging technologies would not exist. Medical imaging is seen as an important discipline in modern hospitals. Some consider it as a subdiscipline of medical informatics, but this view is not universally shared.

Bio-informatics is booming. Molecular biologists and genetics researchers embrace it. It covers a diverse domain, ranging from genetic sequencing, via analysis of mRNA microarrays to modelling of molecular structures e. g. proteins. Medical informaticians did not develop these techniques but computer scientists (efficient data base and search algorithms), (bio-) statisticians (clustering and classification algorithms) and mathematicians. It seems that medical informatics as a discipline has missed these developments and is now facing the rise of new research groups applying informatics to research in basic life sciences, and which are competing with medical informatics for scarce resources.

The fact that funds are directed to bio-informatics research has also to do with the fact that results in this area are believed to lead to applications that will change part of medicine. It is not bio-informatics itself but its close connection with the fields of genetics and proteomics that is important for the funding agencies. The results of medical informatics research are important but the expected financial benefits are estimated to be much lower.

The last two application domains have in common that without computers the work could not be done (or only with an enormous amount of effort). This is due to the large volume of data that has to be processed and managed to provide the information that is relevant for the user. There is an implicit necessity for computational techniques in these domains. In medical imaging and bio-informatics these techniques have a strong mathematical and physics foundation. As long as these computer systems assist the medical specialists or geneticists and do not stand in their way, these applications are accepted very rapidly.

In the early days of medical informatics, research concerning e. g. the processing of various types of biomedical signals and radiation dosage planning, belonged to the core of the field alongside early research on clinical decision making and (administrative) hospital information systems. When the price of computers plummeted the development of departmental information systems and patient data management systems, e. g. for ICUs and CCUs, became more common.

Due to rapid technological developments, the computer system and algorithm as such were no longer the subject of study, but instead their (possible) application in clinical practice became the focus. There was also a change in the focal point from computation towards an understanding of how humans process information and come to decisions with the objective to develop systems that can make close to expert decisions in difficult domains. These developments were in many cases not driven by a need from within the medical community, but by the technological opportunities and the interest of one or a few clinicians. This has led on the one hand to the creation of quite a body of knowledge about the possibilities and limitations of the use of ICT in health care. On the other hand, this body of knowledge has been rather local and has not been adopted on a larger scale. In addition, the medical community has remained rather sceptical with respect to decision support except for some specific applications such as reminders concerning e. g. drug-drug interactions or protocol adherence.

When we consider the three past EU funded research programmes on ICT in health care there has been a transition from exploring the technical possibilities (the exploratory phase of AIM [Advanced Informatics in Medicine]), via research and development (the AIM programme) towards the demonstration of the ICT technologies in health care (the TAP [Telematics Applications Programme]). These programs were successful to some degree. A few spin-off companies were created to market the results of the developmental work, but the more conceptual work has neither been widely published nor adopted. One could argue that this shift in focus has contributed to the view that medical informatics is more engineering than science or

even that it has sent out the message that research in medical informatics is no longer necessary.

If the shift in focus from research towards demonstration reflects the state of affairs in our domain, one has to face the question whether there is a solid basis for medical informatics to survive as a scientific discipline.

As editor and member of editorial boards of Medical Informatics journals, we noticed that many submissions are of low scientific quality. Many of the manuscripts describe applications that have been developed for the local situation. The clinical relevance is not always clear. Comparisons with the work of others are seldom made and if comparisons are made, there is little explanation provided when differences exist. Work as reported in the papers in our journals seldom extends the work of others. It seems that our domain suffers from the "Not-Invented-Here" syndrome. There are only a very few papers that contain a broader view of previously published methods or results.

# Hope for the Future?

In the above we have presented a rather negative view of how our community operates. There are, however, also activities that give hope for the future. When we can strengthen them, we might get the proper recognition in the medical community.

Firstly, we have to strengthen the scientific foundation of our discipline. Medical informatics contributes to the extension of medical knowledge and of knowledge about how health care can be delivered. This knowledge base is extending at such a rapid pace that physicians and nurses no longer have an overview of what has been published. To support the usage of this knowledge in daily care, it has to be represented in a usable way so that information systems can provide the physicians or nurses with relevant information when needed. How to model and represent this medical knowledge should be one of the (core) theories of our discipline. The theory should allow the representation of knowl-

edge such that it becomes usable for all kinds of purposes in various circumstances. Research should focus on what the general principles are for organizing ontologies such that they can be used and reused in all kinds of applications ranging from providing guideline-based medical care to clinical research.

To direct our research, we have to establish what the issues of concern are for the medical community and where our discipline can provide answers. In the past, our own interests have excessively driven our research. A prime example is the research on decision support systems. In the past, various research projects have developed (stand-alone) systems that could solve complex problems in a narrow domain. Such systems utilized the most advanced reasoning mechanisms and were of a technical beauty. Unfortunately, such systems were not very well integrated into the practice setting. Physicians or nurses had to remember for which situations the system was intended and in which of these situations their performance could be increased by using the system.

If we want to survive as a discipline, we have to address the issues that really count. Health care systems in many developed countries are changing. The NHS in the UK is reforming; the Clinton administration put health care on the political agenda in the USA; and also in the Netherlands, the roles of general practitioners and physicians in the health care system is changing. Also protocol/evidence based care is becoming more and more the standard. Hospitals are required to implement quality assurance programs to become accredited.

These changes in the organisation of health care systems as well as in the way medicine is practiced offer opportunities to our field to really contribute to these developments and to develop, implement and study solutions to the challenges that these reforms impose.

Taking decision support as an example again, understanding the context in which decisions are made and researching how the decision process may be restructured and supported by ICT to allow physicians and nurses to work and be accountable as professionals seems to be more promising.

Also the more fundamental problems of knowledge representation have to be addressed here. Theories are needed that describe how medical knowledge is structured and how it can be used in various contexts ranging from basic research to clinical practice.

Technical problems with respect to the ICT infrastructure are likely to be solved by industry, especially in countries where the government is promoting the electronic highway for health care use.

The role of standardisation committees like HL7 and CENTC251 can play a role here, but also the work of the OMG (Object Management Group) can bring forward solutions that do not only exist on paper, but that are actually implemented.

The role of academia could be to study how to best utilize such an infrastructure and to develop the technology for the applications that are needed to meet the requirements, which will be posed to the clinicians of the future. This requires that we add new tools to our toolbox and that we develop the methodologies to apply these tools appropriately. These tools can partly come from disciplines such as (cognitive) psychology, sociology and organisational sciences. A proper methodology will make it possible to compare results obtained in similar studies in different settings.

The quality of our research cannot be measured only with the standard used in medical research: the (double-blind) randomised clinical trial is not necessarily the gold standard. Qualitative methods are required as well.

The editorial boards of the relevant journals in our domain could play a role to strengthen the methodological foundation of our discipline. Clear guidelines should be developed as to what we expect from papers that can be considered as exemplary for our domain. Almost all major medical journals require a structured abstract. This is only possible when there exists a methodological framework for the research that is performed. The editors of our journals should develop similar guidelines. Medical journals are also discussing a further structuring of submitted papers, most notably the discussion section. We could improve the quality of our scientific reports by adopting similar guidelines across the board.

In our view, there is a need for a joint effort on three topics:

- The methodological underpinning of our work should be strengthened. This leads to an improved quality of our research. It will also support the mutual comparison of results from other similar studies.
- The study of the impact of ICT on health care delivery and health care organisations should have a more prominent place on our research agenda.
- The quality of the reporting of the results of our research should be improved.

The key aim is to improve our credibility among those who will utilize the results of our research. The second topic will allow us to better address the issues that are of relevance for health care organisations and health care providers.

# References


1. Hasman A, Haux R, Albert A. A systematic view on medical informatics. Comput Methods Programs Biomed 1996; 51: 131-9.
2. Recommendations of the International Medical Informatics Association (IMIA) on Education in Health and Medical Informatics. Methods Inf Med 2000; 39: 267-77.
3. Hasman A, Talmon JL. Education and Research at the Department of Medical Informatics Maastricht. In: van Bemmel JH, McCray AT, editors. IMIA Yearbook of Medical Informatics 2000. Patient-Centered Systems. Stuttgart, New York: Schattauer 2000; 100-6.



Correspondence to:
Arie Hasman or Jan Talmon
Department of Medical Informatics
Maastricht University
PO Box 616, 6200 MD Maastricht
The Netherlands
E-mail: {talmon,hasman}@mi.unimaas.nl

# Medical Informatics:
# Searching for Underlying Components

M. A. Musen
Stanford Medical Informatics, Stanford University School of Medicine, Stanford, California, USA

*"Yes, well, you may well ask,
what is my theory?"*
Anne Elk, in a skit by Monty Python, 1972

## Summary

*Objective:* To discuss unifying principles that can provide a theory for the diverse aspects of work in medical informatics. If medical informatics is to have academic credibility, it must articulate a clear theory that is distinct from that of computer science or of other related areas of study.

*Results:* The notions of reusable domain ontologies and problem-solving methods provide the foundation for current work on second-generation knowledge-based systems. These abstractions are also attractive for defining the core contributions of basic research in informatics. We can understand many central activities within informatics in terms defining, refining, applying, and evaluating domain ontologies and problem-solving methods.

*Conclusion:* Construing work in medical informatics in terms of actions involving ontologies and problem-solving methods may move us closer to a theoretical basis for our field.

## Keywords

Medical informatics, computing methodologies, artificial intelligence, academic training, professional training

Methods Inf Med 2002; 41: 12–9

## How do we Define our Field?

There is wide recognition that the management of medical information is central to the future of both health care and the world's health. Medical professional societies everywhere point to medical informatics as an essential element of medical practice. The word informatics increasingly is used as an adjective to sell the latest health-care technology. Vendors of clinical information systems hope to impress customers by claiming that their products are based on "informatics techniques" and "informatics methods". The recent report of the Institute of Medicine on the problem of medical errors specifically identified information technology as a large element of the required solution [1]. For the first time in its history, the American Society for Clinical Investigation – the major honor society for academic physician-scientists in the United States – now recognizes medical informatics as a specific area of investigation. With the concept of informatics finally entering the mainstream, one would think that these would be heady days for our research community. My problem, however, is that I am still sure not what "medical informatics" is.

The term *medical informatics* has become a universally applied term that, sadly, remains difficult to define. The latest edition of Shortliffe's textbook defines the discipline as, "a field of study concerned with the broad issues in the management and use of biomedical information, including medical computing and the study of the nature of medical information" [2]. Jan van Bemmel and I defined *informatics* as "the science that studies the use and processing of data, information, and knowledge", and *medical informatics* as "informatics applied to medicine, health care, and public health" [3]. Shortliffe's definition, by couching medical informatics in terms of unspecified "broad issues", leaves the dimensions of the discipline intentionally vague. This lack of specificity has the advantage of defining the field to be maximally inclusive. Van Bemmel and I, in using the word *science* to describe informatics, implicitly make strong claims as to the existence of an underlying theory and of an empirical methodology that can explore potentially defeasible hypotheses. As an academic, I very much want to believe that medical informatics is a science, or at least that it has scientific elements. It remains a challenge for our community, however, both to articulate the underlying theory of informatics and to embrace an empirical approach to validating hypotheses.

When most people talk about medical informatics, they speak not of theories or of methodologies, but simply of computer applications in medicine. Terms such as *clinical computing* permeate our culture. Descriptions that emphasize the computational aspects of our work are indeed much more understandable to most people than is the word *informatics* – which even my spell-checker insists is not a real word. The problem for our field – and the problem for more entrenched disciplines such as computer science – is that the emphasis on the role of the computer in defining our discipline is that we highlight the technology that facilitates our work, rather than put the focus squarely on the work itself. We don't call probability theory "dice science"; we don't call the study of literature "pencil science". We easily seem to be able to call medical informatics *medical computer science*, however.

## Medical Informatics and Computer Science

Our colleagues in traditional departments of computer science remain confused about the relationship between work in our community and that in their own. My own fellow faculty members at Stanford University have struggled to understand what motivates researchers in my group that might be different from what inspires workers in the Computer Science Department. My colleagues also wonder why the rather close relationship shared by medical informatics and computer science at Stanford does not seem to be replicated at many other universities.

Traditionally, workers in medical informatics have been somewhat estranged from their colleagues in computer science. They have worked in different faculties, often quite separated geographically. The two disciplines also have been quite separated intellectually, despite the fact that both are dependent, ultimately, on computational principles. The result is that the medical-informatics community as a whole has been extremely slow to build on the advances that have been achieved in computer science. In the 1970s, for example, the computer-science community was discovering structured programming and abstract data types; at the same time, the medical-informatics community, struggling to build time-shared applications that would execute within a minuscule memory space, was still discovering MUMPS. In the 1980s, when the computer-science community was turning to relational database technology and distributed architectures, our community still was promoting hierarchical databases and mainframe systems. In the 1990s, when the computer science community had come to grips with the significant limitations of rule-based architectures for building knowledge-based systems [4], the medical-informatics community was advocating the use of medical logic modules as the standard means for computer-based decision support. It is not that MUMPS and mainframe systems and medical logic modules did not make important contributions. Rather, the point is that, when the tradition-al computer-science community has made significant intellectual advances, the medical-informatics community often has trailed behind in its incorporation of these results. Our colleagues outside our community thus have not tended to view our work as advancing the science – or at least as advancing *their* science. The problem, of course, is that we in medical informatics have not done a very good job of articulating what our own science is.

It is significant, however, that there is substantial overlap in the goals of workers in medical informatics and those of researchers in the subset of the computer-science community concerned with the development of knowledge-based systems. My goal in this paper is to show how principles for building knowledge-based systems that began to be articulated by a large community of researchers in the 1990s are particularly germane to developing a theory for medical informatics. We are a long way from defining an overarching theory for our field, but these advances from the world of knowledge-based systems can offer our own research community a more solid theoretical footing – for purposes of communicating ideas both among ourselves and among our computer-science colleagues.

Although there are notable exceptions, workers in medical informatics tend not to present their work in a manner that would allow their computer-science colleagues to identify the generalizable results. It is often difficult for us to present our work detached of the contributions that we make specifically to biomedicine. Work in medical informatics, however, does lead to significant theoretical results – particularly when members of the medical-informatics community can elucidate the general principles and can stimulate their colleagues to build on them. A key question for our field, however, is whether medical informatics should be viewed as some admixture of generic computer science plus biomedicine. Current curricula in medical informatics suggest that much of what is traditionally taught as part of computer science is largely irrelevant to our own work. (Compiler design and computer architecture, for examples, are not at the core of what most of us define as informatics.) I believe that our goal as a discipline should be to communicate more effectively with the academic computer-science community, not to merge with it. I believe it would be wrong to construe current work in medical informatics simply as computer science with a biomedical bent. It also would be wrong to construe medical informatics as a form of software engineering that concentrates on the development of clinical computer systems.

## The Role of Building Artifacts

Many laboratories for medical informatics were created during the past four decades in response to pressing needs to assist clinical information management. Early information systems for health-care organizations frequently addressed administrative and financial concerns. Rarely did such systems provide assistance in the management of clinical data. As a result, academicians stepped in to fill a niche that industry at the time was refusing to address. The need to build information systems that could acquire, store, and communicate clinical data sparked the emergence of many of the great academic groups in medical informatics. Satisfying institutional requirements for clinical data management also provided the substrate for much of the seminal research in medical informatics.

Many academic groups still justify much of their existence on the basis of the support that they provide to their institutions in the area of clinical computing. Most of those groups argue that their service role leads them to generate more practical and more meaningful results than would be possible if the groups were to perform their research and development *in vitro*. There is no doubt that information systems such as HELP [5], COSTAR [6], and many others have provided tremendous substrates for research at the institutions that have developed them.

I have argued elsewhere that, despite the obvious advantages of having direct access to the information infrastructure of a health-care organization, a set of service commitments no longer necessarily enhances a laboratory's work in medical informatics [7]. Fundamentally, I believe that modern software systems have become much too large and much too complex to be designed, implemented, tested, and maintained by small groups of academicians who are supported on academic budgets. It simply is inconceivable to me that an academic unit without the discipline, procedures, and personnel resources of a commercial software-engineering organization could create and deploy a large-scale information system on the scale of HELP using today's programming conventions. It therefore seems dangerous to define medical informatics – at least in the academic sense – specifically in terms of the software artifacts that we can build for the clinical enterprise.

I recognize that many academic medical informatics groups consider their service role to their institutions as part of their *raison d'être*. I worry that this position ultimately will undermine the status of academic medical informatics in modern medical centers. Whereas once information-system vendors ignored the requirements of clinical data management, there now is no shortage of commercial systems that begin to address the clinical needs that sparked the growth of academic medical informatics a generation ago. There is considerable room for improvement in the capabilities of many commercial systems, but the market place is ensuring that the capabilities of clinical information systems are only getting better. Development of comprehensive electronic patient-record systems, for example, is a problem that industry is tackling with more resources (and, I believe, with more success) than is the case in any academic laboratory. Whereas once academic groups were needed to define basic structures such as HL-7 messages to assist in communication of clinical data among distributed systems and controlled medical terminologies to facilitate data entry and presentation, the expanding vendor community is now taking the lead in developing appropriate standards for data communication and management throughout the clinical enterprise. Historically, homegrown information systems, such as those at LDS Hospital [5] and Boston's Beth Israel Hospital

[8], have been the bedrock of academic work in medical informatics. Inexorably, however, those homegrown systems are being unplugged and replaced by commercial installations. Even when commercial systems lack many of the features available in academic software, health-care organizations are seeking the security of installing well tested and well maintained information systems that are backed by the technical support of large corporations that have large user communities. Even if their academic mission might benefit from a service commitment, opportunities for academic groups to characterize themselves in terms of responsibilities to the information infrastructure at their own institutions are simply disappearing. Just as many health-care organizations have had to redefine their missions and strategies in the wake of a changing economic climate, academic units in medical informatics are having to redefine themselves as their affiliated health-care organizations change. The time may soon be past when academic units in medical informatics can use the information systems of their associated clinical organizations as test beds for the development and evaluation of major software artifacts without careful negotiation with their associated clinical institutions.

The changing landscape of academic medical centers, at least in the United States, makes some of the broad issues of medical informatics to which Shortliffe [2] alludes no longer within the purview of most academic groups. As development and deployment of clinical information systems becomes squarely the province of industry, much of what used to be considered part of academic medical informatics suddenly has been taken away from university faculty. I will suggest, however, that our research contributions actually will be strengthened as we focus on the part of medical informatics that still remains solidly within the academic realm.

## The Beginnings of a Science

Investigators in any area of science require theories that can frame the interpretation

of observations and that can provide the basis for making advances in understanding. If medical informatics is to have credibility as an academic discipline, it is essential to identify its scientific foundations. We must articulate the basic theories, and explain how our individual contributions extend those theories. It is my belief that workers in medical informatics have difficulty explaining their academic enterprise to other faculty colleagues – and to one another – primarily because our community has not done a good job of articulating a set of fundamental assumptions. We are excellent at describing the surface behavior of our artifacts and quite good at measuring their success. We have a long way to go, however, in being able to explain why our artifacts are successful in terms of some underlying theory or set of basic principles.

We certainly can turn to principles of computer science to justify much of our systems' behavior. Theories of software engineering, of human-computer interaction, and of computational complexity certainly are essential to understanding and evaluating computer systems built for the clinical arena. When we define the theory of medical informatics only in terms of the theory of computer science, however, medical informatics loses any claim to being a scientific discipline in its own right. If we believe that the study of medical informatics itself contributes to a basic understanding of some aspect of the world that is intrinsically valuable, then it is imperative for us to articulate the theoretical underpinnings of medical informatics that are distinct from those of computer science – and from those of other fields, such as information theory, biostatistics, and health-services research.

Unfortunately, our discipline has had few philosophers with a penchant for suggesting underlying theories. Blois [9] made a landmark attempt at defining a theory of medical informatics in his monograph on the nature of medical information. Blois made the claim that medicine, as an area of human endeavor, is epistemologically unique. He argued that this uniqueness arises because clinical knowledge is dependent on understanding other knowledge that can be defined only at lower levels of abstraction

(e. g., that of organismal biology), which in turn can be understood only in terms of knowledge that needs to be defined at still lower levels of abstraction (e. g., that of biochemistry), and so on. Blois suggested that a vast hierarchy of informational levels creates a kind of complexity that is unknown outside of medicine. He justified medical informatics as an academic discipline on the basis of the singular need to model these different hierarchical levels when building information systems for use in clinical care.

Blois' hierarchy of information levels has compelling face validity. As a theory, however, it does little to explain our successes and failures in medical informatics. It is hard to think of a specific example of where a clinical information system may have failed expressly because it neglected to consider knowledge that exists at different hierarchical levels, or could not use knowledge at one level to reason about knowledge at another level. There are many compelling examples where systems have taken good advantage of reasoning at multiple levels of abstraction [10], but demonstration of this principle does mean that the hierarchical levels of knowledge described by Blois contribute to a fundamental theory of medical informatics.

Blois clearly was on to something, however. The principal contribution in Blois' work was the identification of *epistemology* as the core element of what makes medical informatics a cogent area for academic study. It was not the building of artifacts or the deployment of information technology in clinical settings per se that made medical informatics fitting for scientific inquiry. According to Blois, it was the elucidation of the underlying medical knowledge required to build such systems in the first place that demanded a theoretical foundation – a foundation that clearly remains the subject of active scholarly investigation.

Most work to develop epistemological models is no longer done by philosophers, but by workers in artificial intelligence who wish to build knowledge-based systems. The very essence of creating a knowledge-based system requires the construction of a model of human problem solving and the

representation of human knowledge in a computational form [11]. It is ironic that Blois himself had such doubts about the viability of much research in artificial intelligence [12]. Much of that doubt was in fact quite justified, given the overstated claims that were commonly made by many developers of expert systems at the time. In the years since Blois' death, however, there has been a revolution of thought among workers in the knowledge-based systems community regarding the modeling and representation of human knowledge. Many practitioners in traditional areas of computer science are not even aware that this transformation has taken place. For workers in medical informatics, it is particularly important to understand the foundational primitives for modeling human knowledge that now are commonly used to design and implement a wide range of intelligent computer systems.

# Ontologies and Problem Solving Methods

It is no coincidence that, from the beginnings of both disciplines, researchers in the area of artificial intelligence have contributed much to medical informatics. The earliest knowledge-based systems, such as INTERNIST-1 and MYCIN, stimulated workers such as Blois to think critically about medical epistemology and contributed substantially to our understanding of medical knowledge representation and automated reasoning [13]. Meanwhile, as the limitations of systems such as INTERNIST-1 and MYCIN became better understood, computer scientists were inspired to develop and evaluate new ways of representing and processing knowledge within computer systems. In the past decade, the emergence of *second-generation knowledge-based systems* has provided more explicit and more maintainable frameworks for encoding and applying clinical knowledge [4, 14].

Most workers in the artificial intelligence community now view intelligent computer systems as comprising the following four

essential conceptual components: (1) a *domain ontology*, which defines the primary concepts in the application area, and the relationships among those concepts [15]; (2) a knowledge base of detailed content knowledge, which consists of a set of propositions about the world cast in terms of the domain ontology; (3) a *problem-solving method*, which encodes an abstract, possibly domain-independent algorithm that can automate the task for which the intelligent system has been built [16]; and (4) a set of mappings, which defines how the concepts represented in the domain ontology and corresponding knowledge base satisfy the input–output requirements of the particular problem-solving method [17]. Although many knowledge-based systems still are implemented using traditional rule-based "shells", design methodologies such as CommonKADS [11] encourage developers to view the knowledge that such systems model in terms of these four kinds of conceptual building blocks. In Europe, CommonKADS has become the de facto standard for constructing intelligent systems in industry. Many software-engineering tools for building intelligent systems, such as Protégé-2000 [18], enforce the same perspective.

My own research during the past decade has followed that of the knowledge-based systems community, emphasizing how medical knowledge-based systems can be developed using these different components. For example, to build knowledge bases for the EON system for automation of guideline-based care [19], we begin with a domain ontology that characterizes the kinds of concepts that are found in typical clinical guidelines [20]. Developers instantiate that ontology to define the knowledge of particular clinical guidelines (e. g., a protocol for management of patients who have hypertension). EON includes discrete problem-solving methods that automate tasks such as (1) determining the correct therapy for a patient who is in a particular clinical situation and who is being treated according to a particular guideline or (2) reasoning about whether a particular patient might be eligible for treatment according to a given guideline. Like subroutines in a programming language, the problem-solving methods in EON have formal parameters that define the kinds of data on which the problem-solving methods operate. Each such parameter is mapped to a corresponding element of the domain ontology (e. g., the "plan" on which EON's therapy-determination problem-solving method operates maps to the concept of "guideline" in the domain ontology).

Ontologies and problem-solving methods potentially are highly reusable components [14]. They can be viewed as building blocks from which a variety of intelligent systems can be constructed by combining (and, when necessary, augmenting) appropriate components. In a sense, the particular ontology and problem-solving method that are used to automate a given task together define a *theory* for the knowledge required to solve that task. That theory is one that enumerates the domain concepts required for problem solving (the ontology) and the algorithm that must be applied to those domain concepts to achieve a solution (the problem-solving method).

The notion of viewing software as data structures and the algorithms that operate on those data structures is nothing new. The distinction between descriptions of data and specifications of procedures has been around since the early days of computer science [21]. What is new here is the view of the data descriptions – the ontology – as having central significance and an existence independent of particular algorithms. Ontologies thus become like database schemas in that they are separable and distinct from the set of algorithms that may operate on them. Unlike traditional database schemas, however, ontologies may express extremely complex relationships among the represented concepts – emphasizing a desire to capture a rich, reusable model of the domain, rather than to provide an efficient framework for storing data instances.

It is not an overstatement to claim that the theory for constructing any clinical information-processing system can be understood in terms of an ontology of the information being processed and the problem-solving methods that provide the procedures by which information processing takes place. In second-generation knowledge-based systems, the ontologies and the problem-solving methods are encoded as discrete pieces of software. When building conventional software systems, the ontologies and problem-solving methods often exist only as conceptual entities at design time, rather than as working pieces of code (although there is typically a direct relationship between a conceptual ontology and the hierarchy of classes used to build programs in object-oriented languages such as C++ or Java). If we can shift our focus so that we view the end product of our enterprise not as the construction of software, but instead as the development of ontologies and problem-solving methods, I believe that we will be closer to describing a foundation for the *science* of informatics. We will not have defined a complete theory by any means, but we will be able to suggest what the content of such a theory might need to address.

When Blois claimed that the essence of medical informatics lay in understanding the hierarchical nature of clinical knowledge, he was stating that elucidating the ontology of medicine was at the heart of the informatics enterprise. Although one can quibble as to whether the essential problem is in distinguishing the various layers of knowledge described in Blois' book, it is clear that a major contribution of medical informatics rests in the elucidation of the ontology needed to automate clinical tasks, as well as in the characterization of appropriate problem-solving methods that can drive the computation. If we can construe our academic discipline in terms of defining, using, and evaluating ontologies and problem-solving methods, we can move closer to articulating a theory that can allow us to present our work in terms of basic principles. Suddenly, the construction of a clinical information system is more than building a software artifact – it becomes the identification and validation of an appropriate ontology and problem-solving method for the task at hand. The notion of construing the development of a clinical information system in these terms entails more than simply applying new buzz words to a familiar software-engineering problem; by elucidating the ontology and the problem solving method, we can create a formal model of the clinical knowledge required to automate a given task, and have the potential to apply elements of that model systematically to the construction of future clinical systems.

There is a risk, however, in concentrating on these fundamental building blocks of informatics: Considerable, important work builds directly on the core elements of our discipline but itself has little to do with conceptual modeling using ontologies or problem-solving methods. Indeed, a strength of medical informatics is that it so readily can incorporate a wealth of perspectives within its interdisciplinary context. As we attempt to justify informatics as an academic enterprise in terms of its fundamental elements, it is important not to forget that basic research in our field contributes to a wide range of tools and practical applications that are worthy of study in their own right. In emphasizing basic principles, we should not diminish in any way the value of studying deployed systems. Rather, the goal simply is to clarify the elements of informatics that contribute to the basic science of our discipline and that may distinguish informatics from related areas of study.

# Toward a Scientific Basis for Medical Informatics

Casting work in medical informatics in terms of reusable ontologies and problem-solving methods gives us a helpful vocabulary for talking about the science of our discipline. Suddenly, research to create controlled clinical terminologies can be seen as work to construct new ontologies of medical descriptions that meet specific requirements [22]. Research on electronic patient record systems generally can be understood in terms of the ontologies needed to capture clinical information and to communicate that information effectively [23]. Development of improved algorithms for information retrieval, for image processing, or for signal analysis can be viewed as research to devise new problem-solving methods with enhanced performance characteristics. It may be simplistic to couch such diverse work in medical informatics in terms of these rather basic conceptual building blocks. The emphasis on underlying ontologies and problem-solving methods, however, provides a way of unifying the "broad issues" addressed by our discipline within a coherent framework.

It is clear that there are many elements of work in medical informatics that are not well captured by ontologies or problem-solving methods. Work to embed information systems within organizational structures and workflows, for example, seems outside of the computational elements that ontologies and problem-solving methods represent. There is no doubt that such efforts are essential to the successful deployment of clinical systems. At the same time, it is not clear what distinguishes workflow integration within clinical settings from similar activities that might be done in countless other industrial environments. The underlying theory of workflow integration is the same, whether one is deploying an information system in a hospital or a process-control system in a manufacturing plant. What is different in each case, of course, is the model of the relevant organization. Construction of that organizational model can be viewed as a problem in ontology development, and thus fits well within our framework.

One way to validate this emphasis on conceptual building blocks as fundamental to medical informatics is to identify the manner in which seminal work in our field contributes to our understanding of ontologies or problem-solving methods. There certainly is no consensus concerning what are the most significant accomplishments in medical informatics. There was considerable discussion of this topic, however, during September 2000 on the e-mail distribution list of the American College of Medical Informatics. Sittig [24] summarized the discussion, listing ten major achievements. Although there has been no attempt to ratify Sittig's synthesis, his list of "top ten accomplishments in biomedical informatics" is a convenient starting-off point for our own discussion. Let us consider each item on the list in turn.

**1. The entire MEDLARS and, more recently, MEDLINE database:** The primary scientific contribution of MEDLARS is one of ontology. U.S. governmental agencies such as the Social Security Administration had begun to create and manage enormous databases before the advent of MEDLARS and MEDLINE. Work on information retrieval had been ongoing for several decades before the National Library of Medicine provided online access to the biomedical literature. What had not been done before, however, was the construction of a rich, detailed ontology (the Medical Subject Headings; MeSH) for indexing the biomedical literature; of procedures for updating and maintaining the ontology (and the associated indexes) over time; and of problem-solving methods that could use the MeSH ontology to aid information retrieval.

**2. The Unified Medical Language System:** Construction of the UMLS and of each its incorporated controlled terminologies is a problem in ontology.

**3. The clinical decision support systems that work within large hospital information systems:** Building a decision support system is a problem in creating an appropriate domain ontology and of linking that ontology to an appropriate problem-solving method [14]. There has been considerable, important work to evaluate the effects of such decision-support systems on the behavior of health-care workers and on patient outcomes – but the theory that underlies such investigation seems to come more from the area of health-services research than it does from informatics.

**4. MUMPS:** As a programming language, MUMPS facilitated much seminal work in informatics. Construction of a programming language, however, fits more within the purview of computer science than it does informatics.

**5. Systems including QMR, DxPLAIN, MYCIN; software for individualizing dosage regimens of drugs:** Once again, ontologies and problem-solving methods are at the core of decision-support systems [14].

**6. Fully developed electronic medical record systems:** As emphasized by Kuhn and Giuse [23], the major contribution of patient record systems lies in the ontologies that allow practitioners to record clinical descriptions and to communicate those descriptions to their colleagues. There certainly are major software-engineering issues that developers of electronic medical record systems must address. The semantics of the underlying databases and of the user interfaces that capture clinical information in the first place, however, rely on extensive ontologies, development of which fits squarely within the province of informatics.

**7. The Visible Human project; the Digital Anatomist; the Slice of Life:** The construction of the data set of Visible Human images was not a problem in informatics; it was a problem in gross anatomy, specimen preparation, and photography. The development of the problem-solving methods to render three-dimensional reconstructions and other visualizations of the Visible Human images clearly constitutes important work in informatics, however. The Digital Anatomist project has explored significant problem-solving methods for rendering and presenting anatomical content, and now is moving into the development of the most comprehensive, machine-processable ontology of human structure in existence [25]. The Slice of Life project, while curating and distributing an enormous library of valuable anatomical images, does not seem to be addressing fundamental research questions in informatics.

**8. The HL-7 messaging standard:** The transmission of data packets on local-area networks is the stuff of electrical engineering. The description of what generic medical data look like and the development of a structure for their communication from one application to another is a problem in creating an appropriate ontology.

**9. Understanding the fundamental processes of medical diagnosis, therapy planning, reminder systems, uncertain reasoning (Bayesian belief nets, rule-based systems, neural networks), patients' information needs, problem-oriented and time-oriented records:** This item from Sittig's list lumps together a variety of major research results from different academic communities. Work in cognitive science to elucidate human-problem solving behavior clearly informs work in medical informatics, and leads to the development of computational problem-solving methods. Research in uncertain reasoning has at its core the elaboration of problem-solving methods. Understanding patients' information needs informs our ontologies. Construction of time-oriented and problem-oriented records is a problem in ontology development and evaluation.

**10. The human genome project's data:** The rapid sequencing of the human genome would not have been possible without the development of new problem-solving methods to assemble long stretches of nucleotide sequences by piecing together those of relatively short fragments. Problem-solving methods to determine homologies among base sequences are central to much current work in bioinformatics. At the same time, now that most of the genome is known, the bioinformatics community recognizes the importance of building ontologies that can help to structure this information and to relate specific genes to their physiological function [26].

# Informatics as an Academic Discipline

At Stanford, we now teach the course that introduces first-year graduate students to the principles of biomedical informatics in terms of the development and application of domain ontologies and problem-solving methods [27]. The course begins with a discussion of controlled terminologies, introduces basic principles of knowledge representation, and then segues into several lectures on ontology development and use – both for development of clinical applications and for work in bioinformatics. We then introduce the notion of abstract problem-solving methods. We discuss computational approaches to topics such as clinical diagnosis, therapy planning, sequence searching and alignment, and molecular structure determination in terms of problem-solving methods that can operate on ontologies. We find that this approach allows us to unify many otherwise diverse ideas in medical informatics. More important, our curriculum makes it

clear that there is considerable methodological overlap between clinical informatics and bioinformatics. In bioinformatics, the particular ontologies and problem-solving methods may be different from those in clinical informatics, but the fundamental problems of designing and using ontologies, and of selecting and refining problem-solving methods, clearly are the same.

In recent years, computational biology and bioinformatics have captured the imagination of the scientific community and of funding agencies. Many workers in clinical informatics have expressed concern that the application of informatics to problems related to genomics and biological-structure determination will soon eclipse long-established research paradigms to develop information technology for health-care settings and for medical education. It is my conviction that the boundary between biology and medicine will become more and more blurred as genetic information becomes increasingly relevant in the treatment of patients, and as the biological functions of more and more genes become known. Regardless, basic research on ontologies and problem-solving methods is required to advance both clinical informatics and bioinformatics. As we become better able to articulate a theory of *informatics* (undifferentiated with respect to application area), we should see profound cross-fertilization between our work in the clinical and basic-science arenas.

When we emphasize the role of domain-specific ontologies and generic problem-solving methods in building clinical systems, we highlight a way of viewing information technology that seems surprisingly untethered to health care. We begin to beg the question of what makes *medical* informatics different from informatics in general. Indeed, some European universities have departments of business informatics and social-science informatics, and one can imagine the study of information technology applied to a host of professional enterprises. My perspective is that informatics (without a modifier) is a basic science that concerns the computational modeling and application of human knowledge. Informatics involves the construction of ontologies that define the concepts relevant to differ-

ent aspects of human experience and the elucidation of problem-solving methods that can solve specific computational tasks. When the relevant ontologies are related to health and health care, we call the discipline *medical informatics;* when they are related to basic biology, we call the discipline *bioinformatics;* and so on. Because all subdisciplines within informatics rely on the same kinds of fundamental building blocks, basic advances in one branch of informatics will enhance all the others. At the same time, the historically fierce debates concerning whether our field should be called medical informatics or health informatics seem less important when our focus is on the unifying methodology. Basic research in clinical informatics, nursing informatics, and bioinformatics is pretty much the same thing.

There are important distinctions to be made, however. Each subdiscipline of informatics is unique because it needs to model its own set of professional activities and to define its own set of ontologies. Blois was correct: Medicine is complex and the ontology of medical knowledge is multilayered and multifaceted. Medical informatics deserves recognition as a specific discipline (distinct from other forms of informatics) because of the unusual intricacy of the ontologies that drive our systems. The practitioners of our craft need to understand not only the basic principles of informatics in general, but also the details of clinical practice that can make modeling the knowledge of health care such a thorny problem.

If there is a slogan that characterizes why informatics is different from computer science, it is "ours is the discipline that cares about the content". Although software engineers of all kinds certainly need to incorporate relevant domain knowledge into their program code, the conceptual modeling and computational representation of domain knowledge and data is the centerpiece of our discipline. Computer scientists always can work in tandem with application specialists to build useful software. Workers in informatics, however, play a role that is more than that of software engineer and more than that of domain informant: Informaticians are domain modelers who are primarily driven by a desire to get the content knowledge "right".

Computer scientists, particularly those who work in the area of knowledge-based systems, surely understand the importance of carefully modeling and applying content knowledge; they simply do not work at these tasks as a fulltime job. Although many academic computer scientists study questions concerning the representation and management of large-scale ontologies, the use of ontologies by particular problem solvers, and the computational performance of alternative algorithms for solving specific problems, such research questions are core to the science of informatics. Research in informatics certainly includes the study of more applied questions, such as those of system development, deployment, and evaluation [28]. Indeed, it often is only via systems-level evaluations that we can test the success of our basic models. If we are to claim that informatics is an academic discipline somehow distinct from computer science and information science, however, I believe that we need to highlight the conceptual modeling of content knowledge as the basic, fundamentally special element of our research agenda.

There is no doubt that the construction of the rich domain ontologies required for robust clinical systems is difficult and that many of the problem-solving methods required for many biomedical application systems represent significant computational challenges. It is precisely because the modeling work in biomedical informatics is so hard and requires so much innovation that our research has such high potential to be transferable to other areas outside of biomedicine that also require rich conceptual models. For our work to be generalizable, however, we must learn to couch our contributions in terms of primitives that transcend our particular application domain. The notions of domain-specific ontologies and of problem-solving methods are excellent initial candidates both to frame our research hypotheses and to communicate our results to other investigators.

**Acknowledgments**

Russ Altman, Patti Brennan, Milton Corn, Charles Friedman, and Michael Kahn provided extremely helpful comments on a previous draft of this manuscript. I only wish that I could have adequately reflected on all their good ideas in this paper.

# References


1. Kohn LT, Corrigan JM, Donaldson MS (eds.). To Err Is Human: Building a Safer Health System. Washington: National Academy Press 2000.
2. Shortliffe EH, Perreault LE, Wiederhold G, Fagan LM (eds.). Medical Informatics: Computer Applications in Health Care and Biomedicine, 2nd Edition. New York: Springer-Verlag 2001.
3. van Bemmel JH, Musen MA (eds.). Handbook of Medical Informatics. Heidelberg: Springer-Verlag 1997.
4. David J-M, Krivine J-P, Simmons R (eds.). Second Generation Expert Systems. Berlin: Springer-Verlag 1993.
5. Kuperman GJ, Gardner RM, Pryor TA. HELP: A Dynamic Hospital Information System. New York: Springer-Verlag 1991.
6. Barnett GO, Justice NS, Somand ME, Barclay Adams J, Waxman BD, Beaman PD, Parent MS, Van Deusen FR, Greelie JK. COSTAR system. Proceedings of the IEEE 1979; 67 (9): 1226-37.
7. Friedman CP (organizer and moderator), Frisse ME, Musen MA, Slack WV, Stead WW (participants). How should we organize to do informatics? Report of the ACMI debate at the 1997 AMIA Fall Symposium. J Am Med Inform Assoc 1998; 5: 293-304.
8. Safran C, Slack WV, Bleich HL. Role of computing in patient care in two hospitals. M.D. Computing 1989; 6 (3): 141-8.
9. Blois MS. Information and Medicine. Berkeley: The University of California Press 1984.
10. Patil RS, Szolovits P, Schwartz WB. Causal understanding of patient illness in medical diagnosis. In: Proceedings of the Seventh International Joint Conference on Artificial Intelligence. Vancouver, British Columbia, 1981; 893-9.
11. Schreiber AT, Akkermans JM, Anjewierden AA, De Hoog R, Shadbolt NR, Van de Velde W, Wielinga BJ. Knowledge Engineering and Management: The CommonKADS Methodology. Cambridge, MA: The MIT Press 2000.
12. Blois MS. Clinical judgment and computers. N Engl J Med 1980; 303 (4): 192-7.
13. Clancey WR, Shortliffe EH. Readings in Medical Artificial Intelligence: The First Decade. Reading, Massachusetts: Addison Wesley 1984.
14. Musen MA. Scalable software architectures for decision support. Methods Inf Med 1999; 38: 229-38.
15. Chandrasekaran B, Josephson, JR, Benjamins VR. What are ontologies, and why do we need them? IEEE Intelligent Systems 1999; 14 (1): 20-6.
16. Chadrasekaran B, Johnson TR, Smith JW. Task-structure analysis for knowledge modeling. Communications of the ACM 1992; 35 (9): 124-37.
17. Gennari JH, Tu SW, Rothenfluh TE, Musen MA. Mapping domains to methods in support of reuse. Int J Hum Comput Stud 1994; 41: 399-424.
18. Noy FN, Sintek M, Decker S, Crubézy M, Fergerson RW, Musen MA. Creating Semantic Web contents with Protégé-2000. IEEE Intelligent Systems 2001; 16 (2): 60-71.
19. Musen MA, Tu SW, Das AK, Shahar, Y. EON: A component – based approach to automation of protocol-directed therapy. J Am Med Inform Assoc 1996; 3: 367-88.
20. Musen MA. Domain ontologies in software engineering: Use of Protégé with the EON architecture. Methods Inf Med 1998; 37: 540-50.
21. Wirth N. Algorithms + Data Structures = Programs. Englewood Cliffs, New Jersey: Prentice-Hall 1976.
22. Musen MA, Wieckert KE, Miller ET, Campbell KE, Fagan LM. Development of a controlled medical terminology: Knowledge acquisition and knowledge representation. Methods Inf Med 1995; 34: 85-95.
23. Kuhn KA, Giuse DA. From hospital information systems to health information systems – problems, challenges, perspectives. Methods Inf Med 2001; 40: 275-87.
24. Sittig D. Top 10 accomplishments in biomedical informatics. Electronic mail posting to acmi-discussion@mail.amia.org, September 24, 2000.
25. Rosse CR, Mejino JL, Modayur BR, Jakobovits R, Hinshaw KP, Brinkley JF. Motivation and organizational principles for anatomical knowledge representation: The Digital Anatomist symbolic knowledge base. J Am Med Inform Assoc 1998; 5: 17-40.
26. The gene ontology consortium. Gene ontology: tool for the unification of biology. Nat Genet 2000; 1: 25-9.
27. Musen MA. Design and use of clinical ontologies: Curricular goals for the education of health-telematics professionals. In: User Acceptance of Health Telematics Applications: Education and Training in Health Telematics. Iakovidis I, Maglavera S, Trakatellis A (eds.). Amsterdam: IOS Press 2000; 40-7.
28. Friedman CP. Where's the science in medical informatics? J Am Med Inform Assoc 1995; 2: 65-7.



Correspondence to:
Mark A. Musen MD, PhD.
Stanford Medical Informatics
Stanford University School of Medicine
Stanford, California
94305-5479 USA
E-mail: musen@Stanford.EDU

# The Micro-Macro Spectrum of Medical Informatics Challenges: From Molecular Medicine to Transforming Health Care in a Globalizing Society

C. A. Kulikowski
Department of Computer Science, Rutgers University, New Jersey

## Summary

*Background:* Medical informatics has always encompassed a very broad spectrum of techniques for clinical and biomedical research, education and practice. There has been a concomitant variety of depth of specialization, ranging from the routine application of information processing methods to cutting-edge research on fundamental problems of computer-based systems and their relations to cognition and perception in biomedicine.

*Objectives:* Challenges for the field can be placed in perspective by considering the scale of each — from the highly detailed scientific problems in bioinformatics and emerging molecular medicine to the broad and complex social problems of introducing medical informatics into web-related global settings.

*Methods:* The scale of an informatics problem is not only determined by the inherent physical space in which it exists, but also by the conceptual complexity that it involves, reinforcing the need to investigate the semantic web within which medical informatics is defined.

*Results and Conclusion:* Bioinformatics, biomedical imaging and language understanding provide examples that anchor research and practice in biomedical informatics at the detailed, scientific end of the spectrum. Traditional concerns of medical informatics in the clinical arena make up the broad mid-range of the spectrum, while novel social interaction models of competition and cooperation will be needed to understand the implications of distributed health information technology for individual and societal change in an increasingly interconnected world.

## Keywords

Medical informatics, bioinformatics, biomedical imaging, languages, ontologies

Methods Inf Med 2002; 41: 20–4

## Introduction

Just as in human and machine vision the interpretation of a scene depends critically on the field of vision and the scale of what is being perceived [1], so our more abstract vision of the challenges facing medical informatics depends on where we focus within the broad spectrum of scales which our discipline spans – from the molecular to the societal. The challenges most amenable to scientific investigation tend to be at the micro (or more accurately nano) end of the spectrum, and they promise to revolutionize all aspects of medicine through our increasing understanding of the molecular basis of disease [2]. The most refractory problems are at the other, societal end of the spectrum, where individual and group behaviors are beginning to be studied in terms of collaborative and cooperative processes [3], that must be better understood if the impact of informatics on human health is itself to be better understood.

Figure 1 illustrates one way in which we can conceptualize the scales along which some of the challenges for medical informatics present themselves. In the first scale (a) we show medical information systems, around which most traditional medical informatics has focused, spanning the range from individual to hospital practice, and thereby defining the emphasis of our field to date. The challenge for medical informatics at the micro end of the spectrum is to support more patient-centered, or consumer health, as is now beginning to happen, and to prepare for much deeper involve-

ment with molecular medicine as this field develops. At the macro end of the practice scale, greater overlap with public health and involvement with global health initiatives can be anticipated as medical informatics methods are applied to new challenges, such as identifying disease-resistant organisms and the environmental and social conditions that make them thrive.

In (b) we illustrate how the academic discipline of medical informatics is positioned along a micro-macro scale of discipline content, ranging from the molecular/cellular environments of genomics and proteomics, to the large-scale human populations studied in environmental health and epidemiology. A major challenge for medical informatics is to uncover principles of information and knowledge organization and application that span this wide range of health-related disciplines, while developing specific systems that best suit the radically different problems that arise at the different levels of scale.

We now consider a number of specific challenges and opportunities that face medical informatics in terms of where they appear on the micro-macro spectrum.

## The Bioinformatics and Medical Imaging Challenges

Bioinformatics, genomics, proteomics, and pharmacogenetics have become the most promising directions for achieving break-

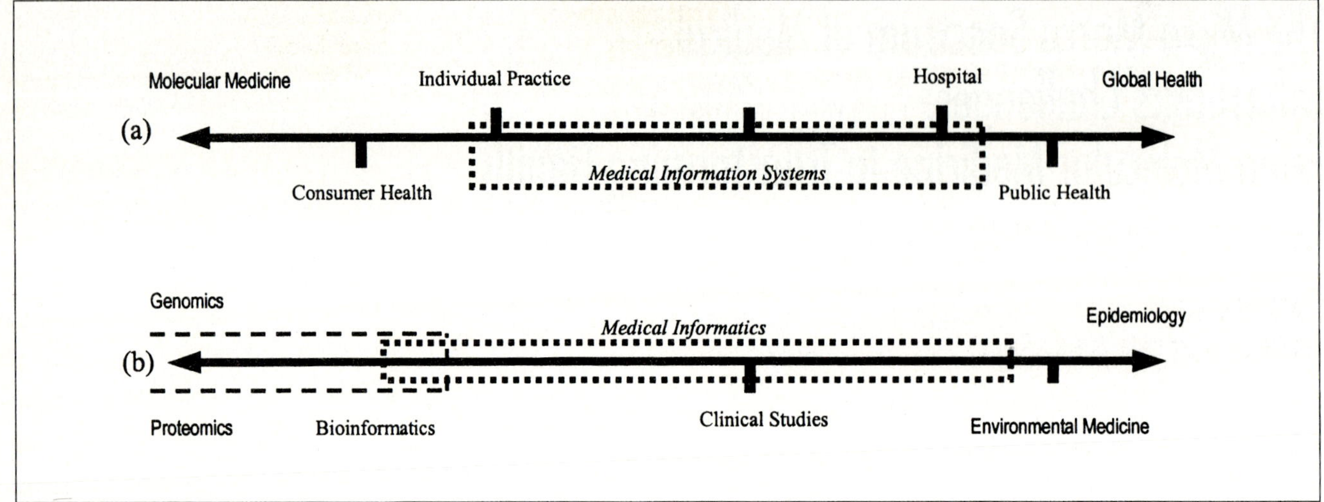



**Fig. 1**   Micro-to-Macro Scales of Medical Informatics: (a) Focus of traditional medical information systems at the clinical mid-range of the scale of medical practice; (b) Range of medical informatics as a discipline overlapping with bioinformatics at the micro-level, and environmental medicine/.epidemiolgy at the macro-level.

throughs in 21st century medicine [4]. It is ironic that bioinformatics, which had early connections to medical informatics, is now among the leading fields of research, while the broader discipline frequently finds it hard to define a focus, or share in the novelty of bioinformatics [5]. This follows a somewhat similar path to what has happened historically to medical informatics in relation to medical computer-based imaging. Thirty years ago, most computational medical imaging research involved general methods of pattern recognition, feature extraction and segmentation, and fit easily within medical informatics in its early stage of development. By the mid 1980's, however, highly specialized techniques of tomographic imaging had spawned an independent field of medical image analysis which depended so much on exploiting the biophysics and bioengineering of the medical imaging devices to obtain the best segmentations and analyses, that a wide professional gap grew between most imaging and informatics research. It is to the credit of the Visible Human Project [6] that this gap has begun to be narrowed in recent years, by focusing on the creation of a unique set of multimodal reference images. By making the correlation of CT and MR with cryogenic tissue images pos-

sible for the first time, the Visible Human has brought medical informatics in designing image databases, visual information retrieval strategies, and annotation of images with existing and extended medical nomenclatures and vocabularies to the fore [7]. New symbolic and image-oriented ontologies for characterizing structural biological entities [8] are being developed from the molecular level to the whole body level. Graphical modeling and simulation, fundamental problems of multimodal, knowledge-based [9] and 3-D color segmentation [10] and registration [11] of large, frequently dynamic image datasets of elastic, biological tissues have become the subject of investigation [12].

Development of a similar pattern of shared research interests would be highly desirable vis-a-vis bioinformatics, and this presents a major challenge for our discipline. Progress along these lines will depend very much on medical informatics researchers getting involved in the next stage of bioinformatics: the development of multilevel knowledge representations at the cellular, tissue, organ, and whole-body levels. Developing specialized digital atlases [7, 13] of different aspects of human biology is an excellent area where medical informatics can confront problems of

language and ontology construction, and intelligent image annotation linked to schematic medical illustrations. This in turn raises interesting issues of diagrammatic, visual reasoning.

At the molecular end of the spectrum, the challenge is to answer the informatics questions surrounding the proliferating studies of gene expression, gene finding, and comparative genomics, all of which are in the process of being connected to metabolic and regulatory pathway databases and models [14]. Fundamental work is beginning in detecting or diagnosing potential conflicts between data and models using metadata [15]. Finding the right integrative cellular and tissue models is a challenge in the modeling of complex biological systems which medical informaticians rarely handle alone. Collaboration with bioengineers, biophysicists, biochemists and molecular biologists is essential for any effective project in this field. Yet informatics has an important role to play in introducing models of decision analysis, experimental design, and knowledge representation systems that will enable not only routine information handling, but also the exploration of semi-automated methods of hypothesis formation, evaluation, and testing over multi-level biological systems [16]. Characterizing and making accessible information from studies of human biological variability, the design and evaluation of biological reference sets and their relation to more aggregative physiological and population models also present important challenges and opportunities for medical informatics.

# Informatics Transforming Health Care in a Globalizing Society

At the other end of the scale of challenges for medical informatics we find many traditional directions of our field, which allied with rapidly advancing information technology, promise to transform health care practices worldwide. The web and other shared information mechanisms (wireless, satellite, smart cards, etc.) provide an increasingly economical means for expediting and distributing more equitable quality health care in developed economies – if societal priorities prove enabling rather than constraining. For developing countries the challenge is considerably greater. Many regions of the world are becoming increasingly socially disrupted, less well off and have weaker health care systems, and are loosing their more educated and well-informed members of society to migration. The role of medical informatics is secondary to social and environmental action in handling the dire health problems involved. However, since a lack of information and knowledge frequently compounds problems of conflict, famine, and disruption, it is not out of the question that medical informatics could have some positive effect. Creating factual databases, simulation models, and information dissemination strategies might, with the right sway on public opinion around the world, have some influence on policy-makers who could try harder to alleviate the suffering of the people affected. Epidemiological models have much to offer, but there is need to go beyond the interpretive to better understand how human competition

and cooperation interact in the increasingly realistic game-theory models [17], and how different objectives and value choices affect our rational decision models. How such models can be extended to include more realistic aspects of human cognition and perception, all are fair play for medical informatics. There are preliminary approaches to consider the social and organizational factors that influence the applicability and probable effectiveness of health informatics in a variety of settings [18].

Within the developed world with its various schemes for health insurance and financing, a concern of medical informatics has been to consider standardized medical records and identification for individuals, such as a smart-card based system [19]. However, given the complexities that have been repeatedly noted in designing standardized electronic medical records [20], progress is much slower than anticipated. Many problems involve societal and economic constraints, but there are many challenging informatics problems in producing such a record: standards of medical vocabulary and nomenclature for describing findings, conditions, and therapies, and translations across medical nomenclatures and systems nationally and internationally. The Unified Medical Language System (UMLS) has made great progress in providing a common set of linkages between existing nomenclatures and various health specialty terminologies [21, 22]. Progress on standard data interchange formats are also encouraging [23], but much more needs to be done.

In consumer medicine, developing health care information retrieval strategies that maximize the amount of peer-reviewed, edited, evaluated and validated results for answering specific queries by patients, their families, and advocates, as well as different sets of providers, is becoming a major issue for people navigating the web in search of answers to their health problems [24, 25]. Providing accurate equitably distributed medical information to patients for self-help and for referral to the right health professionals represents a related set of challenges [26]. Professional societies have always borne the brunt of assessing and editing knowledge content within their

specialties. Medical informatics might take a more forceful role in asking how its practitioners can help other medical specialties cope with the novel problems of information competition and filtering at the large scales demanded by the web. Scientific "clearing-houses" or "knowledge-cooperatives" can be experimented with to explore how consensus panels can be made more efficient and disseminate their results in more timely ways than is traditional.

All the above will require more research on medical languages and sub-languages: unified vs. distributed, evolutionary vs. standardized, local and national variants of medical terminology, vocabulary, nomenclature, and rules of usage. While the Unified Medical Language System (UMLS) [21] has made a great start in these directions, it is clear that new ontologies for software engineering [27] that will also help structure medical knowledge and its application in specific health care contexts are becoming very necessary [28]. A challenge is to envision the digital medical libraries of the future in terms of how information is dispersed and aggregated, filtered and customized for personal and group use [29]. The functions and responsibilities of intelligent human and machine librarians and agents (bots) at different levels needs to be better understood, and related to various representations of information and knowledge. The processes of screening/editing and validating medical information (content, presentation, and sources) require considerable further investigation into its societal as well as technological dimensions [30].

# Challenges for Medical Guidelines and Reasoning

The centrality of medical guidelines in managed care has resulted in the development of numerous approaches to making guidelines computationally available. A standard syntax has been proposed to make them more interoperable [31]. For helping advance the science of medical informatics, a critical element is to get the semantics of medical guidelines right. This involves understanding better what is the basis of consensus reasoning, its evidence base, its customization to the individual patient, and the handling of exceptions. All these require considerable work in connecting guidelines to more formal medical decision and action models, and supporting them by patient simulations, both qualitative and quantitative.

Investigation into the nature of valid arguments in medical guidelines, and how they are supported by different types of evidence and experience (ranging from meta-analysis, decision models and case-based analysis) sets the task of standardizing the basis for guideline development and application [32]. Large scale longitudinal studies are essential to the data for such evidence models. Understanding better how to apply methods of stratification and aggregation in spatio-temporal databases and develop appropriate probabilistic models for medical events and management [33] will be critical in ensuring confidence in automated or semi-automated guideline systems [34]. Today's basic one-size-fits-all data mining systems need to evolve into more sophisticated data-and-knowledge exploration environments. These will need to go beyond the detection of simple logical and numeric patterns in data, and find visual and temporal constraints [35] that connect to hypotheses of underlying structural and functional components of health and disease. How to develop useful representations of knowledge (ontologies) [36] that support human and machine learning over massive datasets of such structured objects and processes is a major challenge for medical informatics. We can also expect that cognitive science approaches which support deeper understanding of the perceptual and cognitive bases of health care behavior will be as important as the information technology itself [37].

# Challenges for Medical Informatics Technology and Engineering

The technological and engineering aspects of building working informatics systems continues to define the pragmatic challenges in our field. Informatics issues in software engineering arise as we must integrate large numbers of signals from increasingly sophisticated medical sensors and images, often remotely. Telemedicine [38] for critical health care problems that have well-engineered human interfaces and are easy to use under conditions of high stress or emergency, such as during strokes or heart attacks, present an important set of challenges in going beyond current, platform independent software towards highly reliable and secure medical plug-and-play devices.

A different yet related set of challenges arises from the increased proportion of the population of developed countries that are living into old age, with its many long-term chronic health problems. The development of medical and nursing web-ware that can be made uniquely personal yet ubiquitously shareable is a major challenge to our field. Besides the connection to various monitoring, prosthetic and health support technologies, our information systems must deal with an increasing need for patient (or consumer) level education in accessing the myriad of health related resources on the web. This can be increasingly envisaged as being carried out through info-bots or intelligent negotiating agents that can assist them in the management of health care problems. Rapid connection to laboratories for the analysis of biochemical and physiological tests that can be performed in the home presents yet another challenge in technological and information management, as well as many cost-effectiveness challenges.

In developed countries the proportion of the aging population that remains mobile and in good health continues to grow. This leads to opportunities for medical informatics in addressing the more complex issues of gerontological risks involved in active sports-travel-lifestyle interactions (such as choices in nutrition, exercise, and medication modalities in different environments).

Also at the societal level, serious ethical and legal issues arise when developing information systems that support markets in human organs, tissues, and reproductive materials. The trans-national capabilities of the web have already highlighted these problems in several cases.

For medical informatics, the problems of privacy and confidentiality of medical information is a central concern which is being addressed technologically, but which has complex policy implications in pitting individual patients against third party payers in market-based systems like the USA [39]. As information about genotypes and their relation to phenotype and disease (SNP consortium and genetic network research) increase the predictive power of lifetime individual risks for disease, the sensitivity of this information becomes critical in its effects on employment, and access to rationed care. Medical informatics can play an important role in developing methodologies for modeling the health care implications of such social choices.

The challenges of disseminating research widely and fairly, while protecting intellectual property of medical informatics researchers are emphasized by the current rapid changes in the technologies, practices, and economics of publishing. There is need for more web-based publication and flexible access mechanisms that are responsive to professional and consumer needs while maintaining a viable economic base.

In summary, the socio-technological opportunities and challenges facing medical informatics have grown considerably over the past decade with the development of the world wide web, the ubiquity of inexpensive distributed computing, and a multitude of new biological and medical tests and knowledge. As in the past [40] we continue to face definitional and organizational challenges in channeling and focusing our energies so that the medical informatics community can pursue these opportunities most productively.

# References


1. Koenderink JJ. The structure of images. Biol Cybern 1984; 50: 363-70.
2. Altman R. The interactions between clinical informatics and bioinformatics. JAMIA 2000; 7: 439-43.
3. Simon H. A mechanism for social selection and successful altruism. Science 1990; 250: 1665-9.
4. Parrish D, Liebman M, Miller P, Altman R. Bioinformatics and molecular medicine applicability and future impact on healthcare informatics, AMIA 2000 Annual Symposium, Los Angeles, CA.
5. Talmon JL, Hasman A. Medical informatics at the beginning of the 21st century, Methods Inf Med 2002; 41: 4-7.
6. Ackerman MJ, Spitzer VM, Scherzinger AL, Whitlock DG. The Visible Human Data Set: An image resource for anatomical visualization. Medinfo 8 1995; 1195-8.
7. Brinkley JF, Bradley SW, Sundsten JW, Rosse C. The Digital Anatomist information system and its use in the generation and delivery of web-based anatomy atlases. Comp Biomed Res 1997: 472-503.
8. Rosse C, Mejino JL, Modayur BR, et al. Motivation and organizational principles for the Digital Anatomist Symbolic Knowledge-base: an approach towards standards in anatomical knowledge representation. JAMIA 1998; 5: 17-40.
9. Kulikowski CA, Gong L, Mezrich RS. Knowledge-based medical image analysis and representation for integrating content definition with the radiological report, Methods Inf Med 1995; 34: 96-103.
10. Imielinska C, Metaxas D, Udupa J. Hybrid Segmentation of the Visible Human data, Proc. Third Visible Human Project Conference, National Library of Medicine, NIH, Bethesda, MD, 2000: 41-4.
11. Schiemann T, Tiede U, Hohne KH. Segmentation of the Visible Human for high quality volume-based visualization. Med Image Anal 1996; 1: 263-70.
12. Udupa JK, Herman GT, eds. 3D Imaging in Medicine (2nd Ed) CRC Press, Boca Raton, FL, 2001.
13. Toga AW. Three Dimensional Neuroimaging. New York: Raven Press 1990.
14. Karp PD. Pathway Databases: A Case Study in Computational Symbolic Theories. Science 2001; 293: 2040-4.
15. Chen RO, Altman RB. Automated diagnosis of data-model conflicts using metadata. JAMIA 1999; 6: 374-92.
16. Karp PD. Design methods for scientific hypothesis formation and their application to molecular biology. Machine Learning 1993; 12: 89-116.
17. Ridley M. The Origins of Virtue: Human instincts and the evolution of coorperation. London; Penguin Books 1996.
18. Kaplan B, Brennan PF, Dowling AF, et al. Towards an informatics research agenda: Key people and organizational issues. JAMIA 2001; 8: 235-41.
19. Takahashi T. Current status of the world health card system. Yearbook of Medical Informatics 98; 1998: 103-7.
20. Institute of Medicine, Committee on Improving the Patient Record. The Computer-based patient record: An essential technology for health care. Washington, DC; National Academy Press 1997.
21. Lindberg DAB, Humphreys BL, McCray AT. The Unified Medical Language System, Methods Inf Med 1993; 32: 281-91.
22. McCray AT. Conceptual complexity in biomedical terminologies: The UMLS approach, in Classification and Knowledge Organization. Berlin, Springer Verlag 1997: 475-89.
23. Wang C, Ohe K. A CORBA-based object framework with patient identification, translation and dynamic linking. Methods for exchanging patient data. Methods Inf Med 1999; 38: 56-65.
24. Wyatt JC. Commentary: measuring quality and impact of the World Wide Web. BMJ 1997; 314: 1879-81.
25. Jadad AR, Gagliardi A. Rating health information on the Internet: navigating to knowledge or to Babel? JAMA 1998; 279: 611-4.
26. Morris TA, Guard JR, Marine SA. Approaching equity in consumer health information delivery, JAMIA 1997; 4: 6-13.
27. Musen MA. Domain ontologies in software engineering: Use of Protégé with the EON architecture. Methods Inf Med 1998; 37: 540-50.
28. Joubert M, Fieschi M, Robert J-J, et al. UMLS-based conceptual queries to biomedical information databases. JAMIA 1998; 5: 52-61.
29. Li Y-C. Towards a medical information collective: trends in the development of digital libraries in medicine. IMIA Yearbook 2001: 77-82.
30. Brown JS, Duguid P. The Social Life of Information., Boston, MA. Harvard Business School Press 2000.
31. Ohno-Machado L, Gennari JH, Murphy SN, et al. The GuideLine interchange format: A model for representing guidelines. JAMIA 1998; 5: 357-72.
32. Miller PL. Domain-constrained generation of clinical condition sets to help test computer-based clinical guidelines, JAMIA 2001; 8: 131-45.
33. Sonnenberg FA. Decision analysis in disease management. Disease Management and Clinical Outcomes 1997; 1: 20-34.
34. Hagerty CG, Pickens D, Kulikowski CA, Sonnenberg FA. HGML: A hypertext guideline markup language, Proc. AMIA Fall Symposium 2000.
35. Shahar Y, Musen MA. Knowledge-based temporal abstraction in clinical domains. Artif Intelligence in Medicine 1996; 8: 267-98.
36. Maedche A, Staab S. Ontology learning for the semantic web, IEEE Intelligent Syst. 2001, March/April: 72-9.
37. Golland P, Kokinis R, Halle M, et al. Anatomy Browser: A novel approach to visualization and integration of medical information. Comput Aided Surg 1999; 4: 129-43.
38. Bashshur R. (ed.). Telemedicine: Theory and Practice; CC Thomas Publications 1997.
39. Halamka JD, Szolovits P, Rind D, Safran C. A WWW implementation of national recommendations for protecting electronic health information. JAMIA 1997; 4: 458-64.
40. van Bemmel JH. Medical informatics, Art or science? Methods Inf Med 1996; 35: 157-72.



Correspondence to:
Dr. Casimir A. Kulikowski
Department of Computer Science
Rutgers University
Hill Center, Busch Campus
Piscataway, New Jersey 08855
USA
E-mail: kulikows@cs.rutgers.edu

# Challenges in Medical Informatics: Perspectives of an International Medical Informatics Organization

K. C. Lun
School of Biological Sciences, Nanyang Technological University, Singapore

## Summary

*Objective:* As an international organization with the missions to promote informatics in health care and biomedical research, advance international cooperation, stimulate research, development and education, and disseminate and exchange information, the International Medical Informatics Association (IMIA) must be constantly cognizant of new developments in medical informatics and address the challenges to the discipline. From an international organization standpoint, it perceives three major challenges viz. the Identity, Organizational and Leadership challenges.

*Method:* This paper attempts to identify and discuss these challenges and to offer ways to overcome them through the activities of an international organization for medical informatics.

*Results and Conclusion:* From an international organization standpoint, IMIA can help overcome these organizational challenges by ensuring strong leadership throughout its echelon, actively promoting its goals and objectives worldwide through its national and institutional members as well as its regional groups and encouraging strategic partnerships between its many Working Groups and Special Interest Group on Nursing with other international organizations and industry to further promote the awareness and the perception of the relevance of medical informatics to health and medicine by the international community.

## Keywords

Identity challenge, organizational challenge, leadership challenge, medical informatics organization, international organization

Methods Inf Med 2002; 41: 60–3

## 1. Introduction

The International Medical Informatics Organization (IMIA – http://www.imia.org) was founded in 1967 as a Technical Committee (TC4) of the International Federation of Information Processing (IFIP – http://www.ifip.or.at). It became a formal organization in 1979 with the following goals and objectives:

- promotion of informatics in health care and biomedical research
- advancement of international cooperation
- stimulation of research, development and education
- dissemination and exchange of information

Today, IMIA is a global organization that has a national membership of some 50 member countries together with 12 corporate and 13 academic institutional members. To further promote its activities worldwide, IMIA has also established three regional groups viz. the European Federation of Medical Informatics (EFMI), the Asia Pacific Association for Medical Informatics (APAMI) and the IMIA-Latin American and Carribean group (IMIA-LAC). There are ongoing efforts to establish a regional group for North America and also for Africa. MEDINFO, the triennial World Congress of Medical Informatics, is a major IMIA scientific activity that began with the first MEDINFO in Stockholm in 1974. MEDINFO 2001, the 10th World Congress, was recently held in London from 2-5 September. San Francisco will be the host city for MEDINFO 2004.

As a major international organization promoting and supporting medical informatics, IMIA has to be constantly cognizant of new developments in medical informatics and address the challenges to the discipline.

From an international organization standpoint, the three major challenges confronting medical informatics today are:

- The Identity Challenge
- The Organizational Challenge
- The Leadership Challenge

## 2. The Identity Challenge

### 2.1 Medical Informatics: A Diffused Science ?

In many parts of the world, medical informatics is still perceived as a diffused science, a tool for the health and medical sciences rather than a science in its own right. This is because medical informatics education, research and development straddle many health and medical disciplines and specialists in those disciplines view medical informatics as "a means to an end". Such a view of medical informatics is probably the underlying reason why many medical schools, particularly those in the developing world, find it difficult to justify setting up an academic department of medical informatics. For example, among Asian countries, Japan is undoubtedly the leading nation in developing and promoting medical informatics. That country has far more medical informatics departments in universities than any other country in the region. Yet, most medical informatics departments in Japanese universities have largely evolved from a service function to support data, information and image processing in the delivery of patient care in university teaching hospitals than from recognition of an academic function to teach and train medical informatics specialists [1]. Even in North America and Europe, many universities have yet to establish academic departments of medical informatics and of those that have done so, medical informatics degree courses are usually offered at graduate level. As further evidence of its diffusion, variants of the discipline are commonly found within the fields of biomedical engineering, biomedical informatics and also classical methodological fields of computer science, nursing, statistics and engineering. The same view can be perceived by an analysis of journals publishing papers that are relevant to the fields of medical informatics. As an example, papers reproduced in the 2001 Yearbook of Medical Informatics originally appeared in journals as diverse as IEEE Transactions on Biomedical Engineering, American Journal of Roentgenology, Computers and Biomedical Research and Journal of Advanced Nursing [2].

## 2.2 Pervasiveness of IT: A Challenge to Medical Informatics

When medical informatics started to develop in the early '60s, mainly out of a necessity to use IT to process large volumes of data in the hospital setting, it was all encompassing [3,4]. The use of IT in medicine was novel at that time and the state-of-the-art of computing and software tools then necessitated the creation of medical informatics specialists to teach clinicians and other health and medical professionals how these tools could be applied in hospital and clinical settings.

Today, the state-of-the-art allows a clinician to effectively use these tools to create applications for himself in his own field. Hence a radiologist now has powerful imaging tools to assist him in doing a better job. A clinician has powerful database tools that can even allow him to store clinical information on his Personal Digital Assistant (PDA) for decision-making. The biomedical scientist can blast his way through to an array of sequence databases for the analysis of genomic data. With the increasing level of computer literacy among these health and medical professionals, coupled with the pervasive proliferation of powerful yet user-friendly IT tools, the need to consult and work with medical informatics specialists has often been overlooked. The pervasiveness of IT has also resulted in medical informatics awareness and applications transcending many levels of activities within a healthcare setting, from people supporting administrative processes to hospital information processing, decision support, nursing, radiology and laboratories. As a result, the medical informatics demands within a health care setting have become increasingly very specialized and focused. Today, you cannot practice radiology without the informatics influence of PACS and DICOM. But many radiologists have neither heard of IMIA nor attended MEDINFOs. They present their informatics projects at their own professional conferences, such as the US Academy of Radiologists whose annual conference has participants outnumbering those attending a MEDINFO.

One of the latest challenges to medical informatics comes from the discipline of bioinformatics. To the medical informatics purist, bioinformatics is a subset of medical informatics. Many bioinformatics practitioners, however, view their newly emerging field as complementary to medical informatics. The medical informatics community must be cognizant of the growing emergence of bioinformatics and the life sciences that have started to bring winds of change to the global economy. As many of the tools in medical informatics can be deployed to handle the massive data that are being generated by genomic and proteomic research, it will be strategic for practitioners of medical informatics to explore synergy with their bioinformatics colleagues to jointly address the many research and development issues and opportunities in the life sciences in the coming years [5,6].

# 3. The Organizational Challenge

The current position of IMIA comprises some 50 national member societies and a smaller number of corresponding and institutional members. Compared to the membership of 189 countries in the United Nations, IMIA is still very far from being a truly international organization. Some may say that this is not an equitable comparison as there are still many countries in the world that have not embraced information technology, let alone medical informatics. But if we look at IMIA statistics over the past several years, the numbers of national member societies as well as institutional membership and affiliations with international organizations have not grown significantly over the last several years.

IMIA could do more to actively promote itself as an international body. Many international organizations, research institutions, pharmaceutical companies and companies in healthcare-related industries have not heard of IMIA. It has to build "bridges" to connect to these organizations. The recognition of medical informatics as a scientific discipline depends very much on the promotion of its awareness and the perception by the international community of its relevance to health and medicine. Much of this recognition can be achieved through the activities of IMIA as an international organization.

# 4. The Leadership Challenge

The Organizational Challenge in turn depends on meeting the Leadership Challenge, for the success of the work of an international organization depends on the leadership and commitment of the individuals that lead the organization. To play out its international role, an international organization like IMIA must reach out to all corners of the world. To achieve this effort, it requires leaders not just on its Executive Board but also passionate leaders and champions in countries in which medical informatics is practised or promoted. A case in point is Africa. Apart from South Africa, there is no other country in that vast continent that is a member society of IMIA. For several years now, IMIA has been trying to promote medical informatics in Africa by supporting the HELINA conference, which held its inaugural conference in Nigeria in 1993 [7]. There is general expectation within the IMIA leadership that HELINA can be the catalyst for the formation of its fourth regional group after EFMI, IMIA-LAC and APAMI. The IMIA leadership is therefore supportive of HELINA and the efforts to see it grow. Currently the HELINA leadership largely comes from individuals outside Africa. Therefore, it is imperative that champions of the medical informatics cause must be identified within Africa to rise up to the leadership challenge for the continent.

## 5. Meeting the Challenges

One of our best resources that IMIA has is its Working Groups and Special Interest Group in Nursing Informatics (Table 1). Many of these groups have already attracted the participation of experts and enthusiastic practitioners in various fields of medical and nursing informatics. To meet future challenges in medical informatics, IMIA, as an international organization, should leverage on the expert resources of its WGs and SIG so that these groups can better assist the organization to reach out to individuals, groups, organizations and countries in the promotion of IMIA's aims and missions.

IMIA Working Groups and its SIG can positively contribute in the following ways:
- Raise awareness of their fields among countries that are beginning to adopt information technology in health and medicine
- Build bridges to foster liaisons with other professional organizations working in related fields
- Actively promote smart international partnerships with industries, organizations and institutions
- Serve as expert resource panels which industries, educational institutions and research organizations could tap

**Table 1**  IMIA Working Groups and Special Interest Group

| Working Group | Topic |
|---|---|
| Special Interest Group 1 | Nursing |
| WG1 | Health and Medical Informatics Education |
| WG2 | Consumer Health Informatics |
| WG3 | Intelligent Data Analysis and Data Mining |
| WG4 | Data Protection in Health Information Systems |
| WG5 | Primary Health Care Informatics |
| WG6 | Medical Concept Representation |
| WG7 | Biomedical Pattern Recognition |
| WG8 | Mental Health Informatics |
| WG9 | Health Informatics for Development |
| WG10 | HIS and Health Profession Workstations |
| WG11 | Dental Informatics |
| WG13 | Organization and Dental Issues |
| WG15 | Tech Assessment & Quality Developn in Hlth Info |
| WG16 | Standards in Health Care Informatics |
| WG17 | Computerized Patient Records |
| WG18 | Telematics in Healthcare |

For objectives, activities and contact details of each WG or SIG, please visit: http://www.imia.org and link to information on *Working Groups*

The following are some examples of how IMIA WGs and SIG can rise up to the challenges of medical informatics:
- Currently, there are several international and regional groups already actively promoting telehealth activities. IMIA Working Group 18 on Telematics in Healthcare could establish links with these organizations. One of these is the International Society for Telemedicine (http://www.isft.org) which organizes an international meeting every year. It could also be very useful for WG18 to linkup with APAN, the Asia Pacific Advanced Networking group whose members are involved with high-speed, advanced network projects like NGI, Internet2, Abilene, and Dante (http://www.apan.org).
- Working Group 5 on Primary Health Care Informatics could establish liaison with WONCA, the World Federation of Family Physicians (http://www.globalfamilydoctor.com) in promoting primary care informatics among general practitioners and family physicians.
- Working Group I on Health and Medical Informatics Education could build bridges with the many international education agencies and groups promoting distance learning such as the Global University System.

The IMIA WG1 recommendations on 'Education in Health and Medical Informatics' [8] and the Group's current efforts to promote a 'Virtual University for Medical Informatics' are steps in the right direction. However, one swallow does not a summer make. Our other WGs and SIGs have similar resources to form committees of experts to come up with recommendations on data protection and security, on standards and on minimum data sets.

Should medical informatics be driven by academia? One common comment on the MEDINFOs that IMIA hosts triennially is that many of the sessions are too academic and do not generally appeal to the medical informatics user communities e.g. the hospital CIOs and industry. Therefore, one of the challenges for IMIA is to dispel the notion that it is does 'ivory tower' medical informatics. Increasingly the working conferences hosted by IMIA Working Groups, especially those in collaboration with industries, are helping to correct that misconception. In future, IMIA would do well in encouraging its Working Groups to organize conferences with greater focus on industry solutions and to attract greater industry participation.

Some concern has also been expressed over medical informatics academics leaving for the private sector. The IMIA Executive Board has a balance of individuals who are either in academia or industry. Out of the 10 board members, 4 are in industry. Some of those in industry were former academics who now run successful industry startups. The emergence of the new world economy and the strong emphasis that many universities place on entrepreneurship are driving many of medical informatics academics towards the direction of the private sector. Good R&D in medical informatics can equally come from the private sector. That concern has been expressed is indeed surprising.

## References


1. Lun KC, Kaihara S. Hospital Information Systems in Japan. Methods Inf Med 1986; 5: 4-14.
2. Haux R, Kulikowski C (eds. ). IMIA Yearbook of Medical Informatics 2001: Digital Libraries and Medicine. Stuttgart: Schattauer 2001.
3. Priest SL. Managing Hospital Information Systems. Aspen Publication; 1982.
4. van Bemmel JH, Musen MA, editors. Handbook of Medical Informatics. Heidelberg: Springer 1997.
5. Luscombe NM, Greenbaum D, Gerstein M. What is bioinformatics? An introduction and overview. In: Haux R, Kulikowski C (eds). IMIA Yearbook of Medical Informatics 2001. Digital Libraries and Medicine. Stuttgart: Schattauer 2001; 83-99.
6. Lun KC. Inaugural address of the IMIA President at MEDINFO 2001. British Journal of Healthcare Computing and Information Management (to be published).
7. Mandil SH, Korpela M, Forster D, Moidu K, Byass P, editors. Health Informatics in Africa – HELINA 93. First international conference on health informatics in Africa, Nigeria, Excerpta Medica 1993; 19-23.
8. Recommendations of the International Medical Informatics Association (IMIA) on Education in Health and Medical Informatics. Methods Inf Med 2000; 39: 267-77.



**Correspondence to:**
Dr. K. C. Lun
Professor and Vice Dean
School of Biological Sciences
Nanyang Technological University
1 Nanyang Walk, Block 5 Level 3
Singapore 637616
E-mail: kclun@ntu.edu.sg

# *Special Section:*

**T. Bürkle**

Department of Medical Informatics
and Biomathematics
University of Münster
Münster, Germany

# Synopsis

# *Quality of Healthcare: The Role of Informatics*

## Introduction

From the very beginning, the promoters of computer use in medicine emphasized the potential of medical computing to improve medical care. Early adopters such as Pipberger et al [1], who introduced data processing methods for electrocardiogram analysis rigorously examined how well the computer would perform and compared its abilities with those of the best experts in the field. The fathers of the early hospital information system HELP at LDS hospital built a system centered around decision rules [3] and noted that the system helped to reduce severe adverse drug events from 41 in 1990 to 12 in 1991 [4]. In 1992 they performed a controlled study to find out that the system had prevented 982 patients from staying on average 1.94 days longer in hospital due to an adverse drug event. They calculated that LDS hospital thus would save more than one million dollars in treatment costs in a single year. McDonald continued such work and evaluated the Regenstrief Medical record in another controlled study to show that physicians would react to 51 percent of adverse events in patient condition such as elevated blood pressure or required liver enzyme controls when the computer generated an alert compared to only 22 percent when no alert was given [5]. Other studies such as the influencing work of deDombal et al [6], who showed that the computer might even perform better than physicians in diagnosing acute abdominal pain were discussed controversially. Transfer of the results to other institutions proved difficult and despite favorable evaluation results, the system was not well received in different environments.

Today there are more controlled trials [7,8,9] and even systematic reviews [8,9] which let us believe with some confidence that, in medical computing, we have tools to improve process quality in medical care. The analysis of Johnston et al in 1994 [8] concludes that there is strong evidence that several computer applications will improve the treatment process. This is shown for computer assisted drug dosing as well as preventive care reminders (e.g. to give required vaccinations or perform scheduled screening procedures) and for protocol or guideline based alerts (e.g. in hypertensive care, diabetes care etc). Two years later Balas et al [9] confirm in a meta-analysis based on nearly 100 randomized clinical trials that reminder functions will improve physician performance and that computer assisted drug dosage surveillance may outperform the physician. They note that interactive patient education or instruction programs will also be successful. Other applications such as computer assisted diagnosing or simple access to computerized medical records however did not show significant influence on patient care in this analysis.

We do have some evidence that not only the quality of the treatment process but also patient outcome may be influenced positively when computer functions are employed. Some of this evidence is rather weak as in [10], when the computerized reminder seemed to reduce the frequency of urinary incontinence in elder persons, some is stronger, e.g. in [11]. There, White et al. examined the influence of a computerized decision support system on patients receiving warfarin and found a reduced length of stay.

Under these circumstances it is enlightening to read the work of Bates et al [12] in this section who take up the conclusions of the November 1999 report of the Institute of Medicine: *To Err is human: Building a Safer*

*Health System* [13]. The IOM report estimates that an incredible number of more than a million injuries and between 44.000 and nearly 100.000 deaths per year alone in the US are actually attributable to medical errors. Clearly, information technology has a potential to prevent some of those medical errors. But Bates et al., besides citing many positive effects of medical computing, tempt us also with the demanding question of what errors are caused by the use of information technology. Quite simply, the information system might be faulty. But there is also another inherent source of errors: As systems become more reliable, we tend to rely on them. But what, if the system just misses to send an alert in a certain condition and we rely solely upon the system abilities? In this case the system is not "faulty", it has just (like humans) overlooked some facts. Bates and his colleagues cite the survey of the institute for safe medical practice (ISMP) [14] that performed a field test in 1998 to prescribe deadly drug doses within several different computerized pharmacy prescription systems. Fatally it turned out that the majority of those computer systems failed to detect those life threatening situations and did not generate an alert. Clearly physicians and pharmacists must double check such prescriptions and should detect the dosing error. But their attention might diminish in view of an otherwise effective computerized prescription system. Bates et al consequently propose a set of recommendations to ensure safe and valuable clinical decision support. Those recommendations center not only on reinforced use of clinical information systems e.g. in order entry and computerized prescribing in order to detect and prevent human error, but simultaneously the authors recommend to put the new technology itself rigorously under test in order to assure that it works correctly and does not induce new errors. The latter has been emphasized by other authors before: "*Clinicians would be unwise to use any system unless it has been shown to be safe and effective*" [15].

This implies continuous measurement of quality. Consequently, the other papers in this section deal extensively with the evaluation of information technology regarding value and effectiveness. The three papers of Vasallo et al [16], van't Riet et al. [17] and Roine et al [18] demonstrate the difficulties one faces in the attempt to assess information technology splendidly. The three evaluation studies range from a simple descriptive case study which demonstrates positive effects of a telemedicine link between the UK and a developing country [16] on to a qualitative evaluation of a patient information system for children with amblyopia and their parents [17] and to a sophisticated review study of controlled studies on the effects of telemedicine [18].

The topic of system evaluation has been discussed extensively in medical informatics [see e.g. 19-23]. Several authors have promoted the idea to use not only descriptive evaluation (the system is evaluated as is) but to concentrate on formative evaluation as well (evaluation results influence system layout and design directly in order to lead to an improved and accepted system) [21,22,23]. Evaluation strategies have been presented for various situations and topics [21,22]. Problems of evaluation have been discussed and methods to overcome them have been described [21,22,23]. For brief recapitulation we may just cite a few conclusions from those papers:

·  Goals of the evaluation must be clearly stated [21,22]
·  The evaluation object is complex [23]
·  The evaluation environment is complex [23]
·  There is no generic solution for evaluation. Different evaluation goals demand different evaluation strategies [22]
·  Full control of environmental factors is not possible in all evaluations [22]
·  High quality studies rely on a mix of multiple evaluation methods [21,22]
·  High evaluation quality may impose a high workload and evaluation costs [22]
·  Information systems induce a change process which must be understood [21]
·  Consequently study design must be adapted to capture changes over time [21]
·  Evaluation builds on user interaction which must be understood [21,23]

The paper by Vasallo and colleagues [19] describes a case study which is used to evaluate the benefit of a telemedicine link for a rehabilitation center in a developing country. All 27 telemedicine referrals made during a 12 month study period are qualitatively assessed regarding the benefit for the patient and the referring institution. The authors cite cost effectiveness of the telemedicine link as the goal for their evaluation. Their evaluation does not control environmental effects, but mainly restricts to a comparison between costs of equipment and perceived benefits. The merits of this study are clearly a proof of feasibility for the use of high tech telemedicine equipment under adverse circumstances and a proof of user acceptance at least during study period. To show both is very appropriate in an area where either new technology is implemented or proven technology is transferred to a different environment which is the case in this example. The proof of cost effectiveness, a cited goal of the authors, however is rather weak. The authors do not only totally omit the expense in time and money for the physicians in the UK who deal with the referrals beside their normal clinical activity, obviously without extra payment. Nor do the authors really compare a situation with telemedicine link with a situation where another effort of comparable size is undertaken to improve patient care at the referring institution. Nevertheless, we should not overemphasize these weak points. The study is a valuable formative evaluation in a setting where modern technology is used for the first time under adverse situations to improve patient care. It demonstrates practical feasibility of the underlying approach and good user acceptance at least during the study period. On a case by case base, positive effects for individual patients and the referring institution itself are shown. We may conclude that a telemedicine approach such as this one may be a feasible and potentially even cost effective approach to improve quality of health care in a developing country. Clearly further studies of improved design are needed to confirm the latter.

Van't Riet et al. [17] face a different situation. They are asked to perform an external evaluation study for an existing patient information system. In principle they have the choice to either perform a descriptive evaluation of the system or to use a formative approach. Typically, in this situation where the evaluation object is a completed system, most evaluators would decide in favour of a descriptive evaluation. Then proven evaluation tools such as controlled trials, approved questionnaire designs etc. could be used. However, van't Riet and colleagues decided differently. In order to define evaluation criteria and to come to grips with the patient information system they started with a qualitative assessment as a pilot study instead. A small group of 14 families with 15 children affected by amblyopia were included in a study design which relied on direct observations, virtual observations of computer based chatting and semi-structured open-ended interviews. The researchers noted that actual use of the information system was weak and from their study results concluded that there was a misfit between the content and functionality of the information system and the needs and capacities of the target group. Besides, several specific flares such as inappropriate operation times of the chat room and inappropriate assumptions which were programmed into the information system could be pinpointed. Van't Riet et al. conclude that the system is not addressing the users' needs at all. As those results came somewhat late to influence system design (which would be the goal of a typical formative evaluation study), they led to the discontinuation of the examined information system, thus preventing unnecessary further expenditure. Obviously, in this case the information system did not influence the quality of healthcare, but we hope with the authors that succeeding projects will build on the evaluation results, thus leading to improved patient information.

When we think about descriptive evaluation of procedures and applications in healthcare we should refer to methodologies developed in the context of evidence based medicine [24,25]. Sacket [24] defines evidence-based medicine as

> "The central demand to link best individual clinical knowledge with best available external, scientific evidence to achieve optimal patient care."

Scientific evidence in this context relies on preferably exact knowledge. Applications in medical informatics, if influencing patient health directly, must at least demonstrate that they do not harm the patient [12,15]. More rigorous evaluation of clinical software may become a must in the future, when within new regulations software programs are considered to be medical devices [26]. In an ascending hierarchy improved scientific evidence originates when higher levels of the following study designs are achieved:

I. *At least one systematic review based upon methodically sound RCT's (randomized controlled trials)*
II. *At least one methodically sound RCT of sufficient size*
III. *Methodically sound non randomized or non prospective controlled trials*
IV. *More than one methodically sound non experimental trial*
V. *Gold standard, experts opinion, descriptive studies*

In this hierarchy the review of Roine and colleagues [18] adapts the highest level of scientific evidence in order to assess potential effects and cost effectiveness of telemedicine applications. In a comprehensive literature search the authors include 50 out of 1124 studies on telemedicine applications for a systematic review. They reject non-controlled studies and feasibility studies as well as studies giving insufficient outcome data. However, within those 50 selected papers they could pinpoint only six RCTs whereas the other included studies varied between non-randomized controlled studies, cohort studies, case control studies and descriptive studies. Due to different evaluation goals within the 50 studies as well as different study designs, Roine et al refrain correctly from a meta analysis and restrict their review to a description of the study results, grouped into the areas of telemedicine in medical consultation, telemedicine in patient monitoring, teleradiology and telemedicine in various clinical areas. The researchers conclude that the data about effectiveness and cost-efficiency in telemedicine derived from the 50 examined studies is still poor. They find evidence for the effectiveness of telemedicine applications in the areas teleradiology, teleneurosurgery, telepsychiatry, transmission of electrocardiographic images and electronic referrals between primary and secondary healthcare providers. Regarding cost-efficiency, the researchers quote "economic analyses suggest that teleradiology, especially transmission of CT images, can be cost saving". Their final suggestion: "Based on current scientific evidence, only a few telemedicine applications can be recommended for broader use".

What can we learn from this review? It is a well known fact that even systematic reviews of RCT's, albeit on the highest evidence level, cannot deliver good evidence if the underlying RCT's have poor quality or insufficient data. When looking at the highly structured review studies of the Cochrane Collaboration [27] on medical treatment of patients, we find many which recommend that further large-sample controlled trials are needed in order to come to a final conclusion regarding scientific evidence pro or contra a certain treatment strategy (see e.g. [28]). Based on only six RCT's on telemedicine applications one would be very lucky to gain clear evidence about effectiveness and cost-efficiency of such applications. The review of Roine and colleagues does give us hints that we may improve quality of healthcare effectively using telemedicine applications and should encourage to continue research and evaluation in this area towards a stage where we may be able to find clear evidence, thereby advancing such applications beyond the current pilot project phase.

Within this section *Quality of Healthcare: The role of Informatics* we have seen four different papers.
- A strong recommendation to make extensive use of information technology to avoid human error, paired with the urgent suggestion to improve this technology and to assess its effects on patient safety [12].

- A descriptive case study for the use of a known technology in a new area presenting a positive picture of feasibility, but clearly asking for further methodically sound evaluation studies to confirm effectiveness and cost-efficiency [16]

- A formative evaluation of an application which does not meet the needs of its projected users [17].

- A review study on a modern information technology which indicates positive effects without being able to demonstrate conclusive evidence that the new technology is superior to other methods [18].

From these and many other cited sources [4-11,28] a picture emerges. If we consider medical informatics as a young field, which it clearly still is compared to other medical fields, we find many indicators and increasing evidence that information technology will and must play an important role in improving the quality of healthcare now and in the future. When de Dombal et al [6] evaluated a decision support system in 1971, they were still among the first to do such work and no one would have recommended to use such systems everywhere at that time. Today instead, some areas of information processing are made mandatory in medicine, for example the use of computerized physician order entry systems in Californian hospitals [29]. We notice that there is a change in argumentation: In the future we may find ourselves in a situation where we do not need to demonstrate why we used information technology, but instead we may be asked why we did not use this technology. Thanks e.g. to Pipbergers work [1] the computerized ECG machine which delivers an automated assessment of the ECG stripe is a fact today. Hardly anyone would argue with the machine regarding QRS time span and signs of ventricular

blockage in its printed assessment. This does not mean that we may refrain from further checks and just accept the use of information technology. The more we use such technology in areas which directly affect patient care, the more rigorously we must perform evaluations and prevent technology from becoming harmful. Information technology implies a change process [21]. This renders evaluation difficult in many cases and requires continuing effort [21-23]. We must adapt our methods to the evaluation object and we will not always be able to measure effects with RCTs or review studies. Examples of other methods can be found in this section [17] and in literature (e.g. [22,23]). It will certainly be interesting to see more studies emerge which demonstrate that no harm is done by an information technology which then is commonplace.

## References


1. Pipberger HV, Arms RJ, Stallmann FW. Automated Screening of normal and abnormal electrocardiograms by means of a digital computer. Proc Soc Exp Biol Med 1961;106:130-2.
2. Warner HR, Olmsted CM, Ritherford BD. HELP, a program for medical decision making. Comp Biomed Res 1972;5:65-74.
3. Evans RS, Pestotnik SL, Classen DC, Horn SD, Bass SP, Burke JP. Preventing adverse drug events in hospitalized patients. Ann Pharmacother 1994;28:523-7.
4. Evans RS, Pestotnik SL, Gardner RM. Evaluating the impact of computer-based drug monitoring on the quality and cost of drug therapy. In: Prokosch HU, Dudeck J, editors. Hospital information systems: Design and development characteristics; Impact and future architectures. Elsevier; 1995. p. 201-20.
5. McDonald CJ. Protocol-based computer reminders, the quality of care and the non-perfectability of man. N Engl J Med 1976;295:1351-5.
6. De Dombal FT, Leaper Dj, Staniland JR, McCann AP, Horrocks JC. Computer – aided diagnosis of acute abdominal pain. BMJ 1972;2:9-13.
7. Adlassnig KP, Horak W. Development and retrospective evaluation of HEPAXPERT-I: a routinely-used expert system for interpretive analysis of hepatitis

A and B serologic findings. Artif Intell Med 1995;7:1-24.

8. Johnston ME, Langton KB, Haynes RB, Mathieu A. Effects of computer-based clinical decision support systems on clinician performance and patient outcome. Ann Intern Med 1994;120:135-42.

9. Balas EA, Austin SM, Mitchel JA, Ewigmann BG, Bopp KD, Brown GD. The clinical value of computerized information services. A review of 98 randomized clinical trials. Arch Fam Med 1996;5:271-8.

10. Petrucci K, Petrucci P, Canfield K, McCormick KA, Kjerulff K, Parks P. Evaluation of UNIS: Urological Nursing Information System. Proceedings Fifteenth Annual Symposium on Computer Applications in Healthcare SCAMC;1992:43-7.

11. White RH, Hong R, Venook AP, Daschbach MM, Murray W, Mungall DR, et al. Initiation of warfarin therapy: comparison of physician dosing with computer assisted dosing. J Gen Intern Med 1989;2:141-8.

12. Bates DW, Cohen M, Leape LL, Overhage M, Shabot MM, Sheridan T. Reducing the frequency of errors in medicine using information Technology. J Am Med Inform Assoc 2001;8:299-308.

13. Kohn LT, Corrigan JM, Donaldson MS, editors. To Err is Human: Building a Safer Health System. Washington DC: National Academic Press, 1999.

14. Institute for Safe Medication Practices. Over-reliance on computer systems may place patients at great risk. ISMP Medication Safety Alert , Feb 10, 1999. Huntingdon Valley, Pa.: ISMP; 1999.

15. Van Bemmel JH, Musen MA, editors. Handbook of Medical Informatics, Heidelberg: Springer; 1997.

16. Vasallo DJ, Hoque F, Farquharson R, Patterson V, Swinfen P, Swinfen R. An evaluation of the first years's experience with a low-cost telemedicine link in Bangladesh. J Telemed Telecare 2001;7:125-38.

17. van't Riet A, Berg M, Hiddema F, Sol K. Meeting patients' needs with patient information systems: potential benefits of qualitative research methods. Int J Med Inf 2001;64:1-14.

18. Roine R, Ohinmaa A, Hailey D. Assessing telemedicine: a systematic review of the literature. Can Med Assoc J 2001;165(6): 765-71.

19. Ohmann C, Boy O, Eich HP. Arbeitskreis Evaluation im MEDWIS-Programm. Leitfaden zur Evaluierung von wissensbasierten Systemen. Informatik, Biometrie und Epidemiologie in Medizin und Biologie 1998;29:77-83.

20. Ohmann C, Boy O, Yang Q. A systematic approach to the assessment of user satisfaction with health care systems: constructs, models and instruments. Stud Health Technol Inform 1997; 43 Pt B:781-5.

21. Kaplan B. Addressing Organizational Issues into the Evaluation of Medical Systems. J Am Med Inform Assoc 1997;4:94-101.

22. Bürkle T, Ammenwerth E, Prokosch HU, Dudeck J. Evaluation of clinical Information Systems - What can be evaluated and what cannot ? J Eval Clin Pract. 2001 Nov;7(4):373-85.

23. Ammenwerth E, Kaiser F, Bürkle T, Gräber S, Herrmann G, Wilhelmy I. Evaluation of User Acceptance of Data Management Systems in Hospitals - Feasibility and Usability. In: Brown A, Remenyi D, editors. Proceedings of the 9th European Conference on Information Technology Evaluation (ECITE) 2002, Paris. Reading: MCIL; 2002. p. 31-8.

24. Sackett DL, Richardson WS, Rosenberg W, Haynes RB. Evidence Based Medicine – How to practice and teach EBM. Churchill Livingstone; 1997.

25. Perleth M, Antes G. Evidenz-basierte Medizin. München: MMV Medizin Verlag; 1998.

26]. Miller R, Gardner R. Recommendations for responsible monitoring and regulation of clinical software systems. J Am Med Inform Assoc 1997;4:442-57.

27. The Cochrane Library, http://www.cochrane.org

28. Walton RT, Harvey E, Dovey S, Freemantle N. Computerised advice on drug dosage to improve prescribing practice (Cochrane Review). In: The Cochrane Library, Issue 3/2002. Oxford: Update Software.

29. California Senate Bill No. 1875. Chapter 816, Statutes of 2000. (http://www.mederrors.com/pdf/SB1875.pdf)

Address of the author:
Dr. Thomas Bürkle
Department of Medical Informatics and Biomathematics
University of Münster
Domagkstrasse 9
D-48129 Münster, Germany
E-mail: Thomas.Buerkle@mednet.uni-muenster.de

# Reducing the Frequency of Errors in Medicine Using Information Technology

DAVID W. BATES, MD, MSC, MICHAEL COHEN, MS, RPH,
LUCIAN L. LEAPE, MD, J. MARC OVERHAGE, MD, PHD,
M. MICHAEL SHABOT, MD, THOMAS SHERIDAN, SCD

**Abstract** **Background:** Increasing data suggest that error in medicine is frequent and results in substantial harm. The recent Institute of Medicine report (LT Kohn, JM Corrigan, MS Donaldson, eds: *To Err Is Human: Building a Safer Health System.* Washington, DC: National Academy Press, 1999) described the magnitude of the problem, and the public interest in this issue, which was already large, has grown.

**Goal:** The goal of this white paper is to describe how the frequency and consequences of errors in medical care can be reduced (although in some instances they are potentiated) by the use of information technology in the provision of care, and to make general and specific recommendations regarding error reduction through the use of information technology.

**Results:** General recommendations are to implement clinical decision support judiciously; to consider consequent actions when designing systems; to test existing systems to ensure they actually catch errors that injure patients; to promote adoption of standards for data and systems; to develop systems that communicate with each other; to use systems in new ways; to measure and prevent adverse consequences; to make existing quality structures meaningful; and to improve regulation and remove disincentives for vendors to provide clinical decision support. Specific recommendations are to implement provider order entry systems, especially computerized prescribing; to implement bar-coding for medications, blood, devices, and patients; and to utilize modern electronic systems to communicate key pieces of asynchronous data such as markedly abnormal laboratory values.

**Conclusions:** Appropriate increases in the use of information technology in health care— especially the introduction of clinical decision support and better linkages in and among systems, resulting in process simplification—could result in substantial improvement in patient safety.

■ **J Am Med Inform Assoc.** 2001;8:299–308.

Affiliations of the authors: Harvard Medical School, Boston, Massachusetts (DWB); Institute for Safe Medication Practices, Huntingdon Valley, Pennsylvania (MC); Harvard School of Public Health, Boston (LLL); Indiana University of Medicine, Indianapolis, Indiana (JMO); University of California–Los Angeles School of Medicine, Los Angeles, California (MMS); Massachusetts Institute of Technology, Cambridge, Massachusetts (TS).

This work is based on discussions at the AMIA 2000 Spring Congress; May 23–25, 2000; Boston, Massachusetts.

Correspondence and reprints: David W. Bates, MD, MSc, Division of General Medicine and Primary Care, Brigham and Women's Hospital, 75 Francis Street, Boston, MA 02115; e-mail: <dbates@partners.org>.

Received for publication: 10/09/00; accepted for publication: 3/16/01.

Our goal in this manuscript is to describe how information technology can be used to reduce the frequency and consequences of errors in health care. We begin by discussing the Institute of Medicine report and the evidence that errors and iatrogenic injury are a problem in medicine, and also briefly mention the issue of inefficiency. We then define our scope of discussion (in particular, what we are considering an error) and then discuss the theory of error as it applies to information technology, and the importance of systems improvement. We then discuss the effects of clinical decision support, and errors generated by information technology. That is followed by management issues, the value proposition, barriers, and recent developments on the national front. We conclude by making a number of evidence-based general and specific recommendations regarding the use of information technology for error prevention in health care.

## The Institute of Medicine Report and Iatrogenesis

Errors in medicine are frequent, as they are in all domains in life. While most errors have little potential for harm, some do result in injury, and the cumulative consequences of error in medicine are huge.

When the Institute of Medicine (IOM) released its report *To Err is Human: Building a Safer Health System* in November 1999,[1] the public response surprised most people in the health care community. Although the report's estimates of more than a million injuries and nearly 100,000 deaths attributable to medical errors annually were based on figures from a study published in 1991, they were news to many. The mortality figures in particular have been a matter of some public debate[2,3] although most agree that whatever the number of deaths is, it is too high.

The report galvanized an enormous reaction from both government and health care representatives. Within two weeks, Congress began hearings and the President ordered a government-wide feasibility study, followed in February by a directive to governmental agencies to implement the IOM recommendations. During this time, professional societies and health care organizations have begun to re-assess their efforts in patient safety.

The IOM report made four major points—the extent of harm that results from medical errors is great; errors result from system failures, not people failures; achieving acceptable levels of patient safety will require major systems changes; and a concerted national effort is needed to improve patient safety. The national effort

recommended by the IOM involves all stakeholders—professionals, health care organizations, regulators, professional societies, and purchasers. Health care organizations are called on to work with their professionals to implement known safe practices and set up meaningful safety programs in their institutions, including blame-free reporting and analysis of serious errors. External organizations—regulators, professional societies, and purchasers—are called on to help establish standards and best practice for safety and to hold health care organizations accountable for implementing them.

Some of the best available data on the epidemiology of medical injury come from the Harvard Medical Practice Study.[4] In that study, drug complications were the most common adverse event (19 percent), followed by wound infections (14 percent) and technical complications (13 percent). Nearly half the events were associated with an operation. Most work on prevention to date has focused on adverse drug events and wound infections. Compared with the data on inpatients, relatively few data on errors and injuries outside the hospital are available, although errors in follow-up[5] and diagnosis are probably especially important in non-hospital settings.

While the IOM report and Harvard Medical Practice Study deal primarily with injuries associated with errors in health care, the costs of inefficiencies related to errors that do not result in injury are also great. One example is the effort associated with "missed dose" medication errors, when a medication dose is not available for a nurse to administer and a delay of at least two hours occurs or the dose is not given at all.[6] Nurses spend a great deal of time tracking down such medications. Although such costs are harder to assess than the costs of injuries, they may be even greater.

## Scope of Discussion

In this paper, we are discussing only clear-cut errors in medical care and not suboptimal practice (such as failure to follow a guideline). Clearly, this is not a dichotomous distinction, and some examples may be helpful. We would consider a sponge left in the patient after surgery an error, whereas an inappropriate indication for surgery would be suboptimal practice. We would consider it an error if no postoperative anticoagulation were used in patients in whom its benefit has clearly been demonstrated (for example, patients who have just had hip surgery). However, we would not consider it an error if a physician failed to follow a pneumonia guideline and prescribed a commonly used but suboptimal antibiotic, even though adherence to such guidelines will almost certainly improve outcomes. Although we believe that information technology can play a major role in both domains, we are not addressing suboptimal practice in this discussion.

## Theory of Error

Although human error in health care systems has only recently received great attention, human factors engineering has been concerned with error for several decades. Following the accident at Three Mile Island in the late 1970s, the nuclear power industry was particularly interested in human error as part of human factors concerns, and has produced a number of reports on the subject.[7] The U.S. commercial aviation sector is also very interested in human error at present, because of massive overhaul of the air traffic control network. A few excellent books on human error generally are available.[8–10]

While it is easy and common to blame operators for accidents, investigation often indicates that an operator "erred" because the system was poorly designed. Testimony of an operator of the Three Mile Island nuclear power plant in a 1979 Congressional hearing[11] makes the point, " If you go beyond what the designers think might happen, then the indications are insufficient, and they may lead you to make the wrong inferences. ...[H]ardly any of the measurements that we have are direct indications of what is going on in the system."

The consensus among man–machine system engineers is that we should be designing our control rooms, cockpits, intensive care units, and operating rooms so that they are more "transparent"—that is, so that the operator can more easily "see through" the displays to the actual working system, or "what is going on." Situational awareness is the term used in the aviation sector. Often the operator is locked into the dilemma of selecting and slavishly following one or another written procedure, each based on an anticipated causality. The operator may not be sure what procedure, if any, fits the current not-yet-understood situation.

Machines can also produce errors. It is commonly appreciated that humans and machines are rather different and that the combination of both thus has greater potential reliability than either alone. However, it is not commonly understood how best to make this synthesis. Humans are erratic, and err in surprising and unexpected ways. Yet they are also resourceful and inventive, and they can recover from both their own and the equipment's errors in creative ways. In comparison, machines are more dependable, which means they are dependably stupid when a minor behavior change would prevent a failure in a neighboring component from propagating. The intelligent machine can be made to adjust to an identified variable whose importance and relation to other variables are sufficiently well understood. The intelligent human operator still has usefulness, however, for he or she can respond to what at the design stage may be termed an "unknown unknown" (a variable which was never anticipated, so that there was never any basis for equations to predict it or computers and software to control it).

Finally, we seek to reduce the undesirable consequences of error, not error itself. Senders and Moray[10] provide some relevant comments that relate to information technology: "The less often errors occur, the less likely we are to expect them, and the more we come to believe that they cannot happen... . It is something of a paradox that the more errors we make, the better we will be able to deal with them." They comment further that, "eliminating errors locally may not improve a system and might cause worse errors elsewhere."

A medical example relating to these issues comes from the work of Macklis et al. in radiation therapy[12]; this group has used and evaluated the safety record of a record-and-verify linear accelerator system that double-checks radiation treatments. This system has an error rate of only 0.18 percent, with all detected errors being of low severity. However, 15 percent of the errors that did occur related to use of the system, primarily because when an error in the checking system occurred, the human operators assumed the machine "had to be right," even in the face of important conflicting data. Thus, the Macklis group expressed concern that over-reliance on the system could result in an accident. This example illustrates why it will be vital to measure to determine how systems changes affect the overall rate of not only errors but accidents.

## Systems Improvement and Error Prevention

Although the traditional approach in medicine has been to identify the persons making the errors and punish them in some way, it has become increasingly clear that it is more productive to focus on the systems by which care is provided.[13] If these systems could be set up in ways that would both make errors less likely and catch those that do occur, safety might be substantially improved.

A system analysis of a large series of serious medication errors (those that either might have or did cause harm)[13] identified 16 major types of system failures associated with these errors. Of these system failures, all of the top eight could have been addressed by better medical information.

Currently, the clinical systems in routine use in health care in the United States leave a great deal to be desired. The health care industry spends less on information technology than do most other information-intensive industries; in part as a result, the dream of system integration been realized in few organizations. For example, laboratory systems do not communicate directly with pharmacy systems. Even within medication systems, electronic links between parts of the system—prescribing, dispensing, and administering—typically do not exist today. Nonetheless, real and difficult issues are present in the implementation of information technology in health care, and simply writing a large check does not mean that an organization will necessarily get an outstanding information system, as many organizations have learned to their chagrin.

Evaluation is also an important issue. Data on the effects of information technology on error and adverse event rates are remarkably sparse, and many more such studies are needed. Although such evaluations are challenging, tools to assess the frequency of errors and adverse events in a number of domains are now available.[14–19] Errors are much more frequent than actual adverse events (for medication errors, for example, the ratio in one study[6] was 100:1). As a result, it is attractive from the sample size perspective to track error rates, although it is important to recognize that errors vary substantially in their likelihood of causing injury.[20]

## Clinical Decision Support

While many errors can be detected and corrected by use of human knowledge and inspection, these represent weak error reduction strategies. In 1995, Leape et al.[13] demonstrated that almost half of all medication errors were intimately linked with insufficient information about the patient and drug. Similarly, when people are asked to detect errors by inspection, they routinely miss many.[21]

It has recently been demonstrated that computerized physician order entry systems that incorporate clinical decision support can substantially reduce medication error rates as well as improve the quality and efficiency of medication use. In 1998, Bates et al.[20] found

in a controlled trial that computerized physician order entry systems resulted in a 55 percent reduction in serious medication errors. In another time series study,[22] this group found an 83 percent reduction in the overall medication error rate, and a 64 percent reduction even with a simple system. Evans et al.[23] have also demonstrated that clinical decision support can result in major improvements in rates of antibiotic-associated adverse drug events and can decrease costs. Classen et al.[24] have also demonstrated in a series of studies that nosocomial infection rates can be reduced using decision support.

Another class of clinical decision support is computerized alerting systems, which can notify physicians about problems that occur asynchronously. A growing body of evidence suggests that such systems may decrease error rates and improve therapy, thereby improving outcomes, including survival, the length of time patients spend in dangerous conditions, hospital length of stay, and costs.[25–27] While an increasing number of clinical information systems contain data worthy of generating an alert message, delivering the message to caregivers in a timely way has been problematic. For example, Kuperman et al.[28] documented significant delays in treatment even when critical laboratory results were phoned to caregivers. Computer-generated terminal messages, e-mail, and even flashing lights on hospital wards

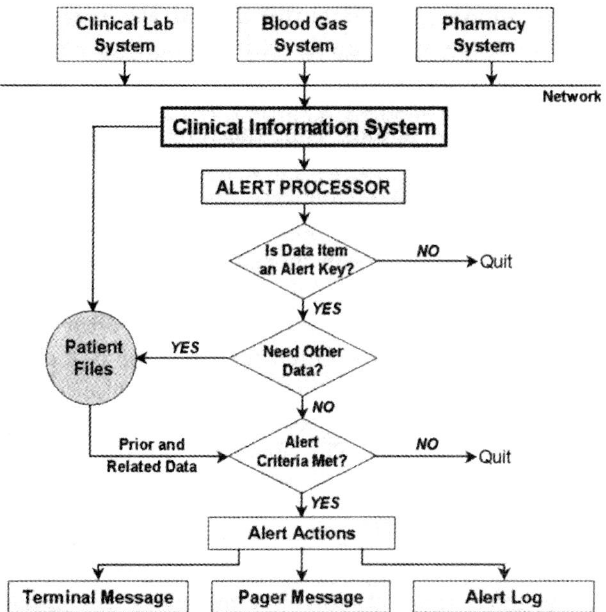


**Figure 1** Alert detection system. Three major forms of critical event detection occur—critical laboratory alerts, physiologic "exception condition" alerts, and medication alerts.

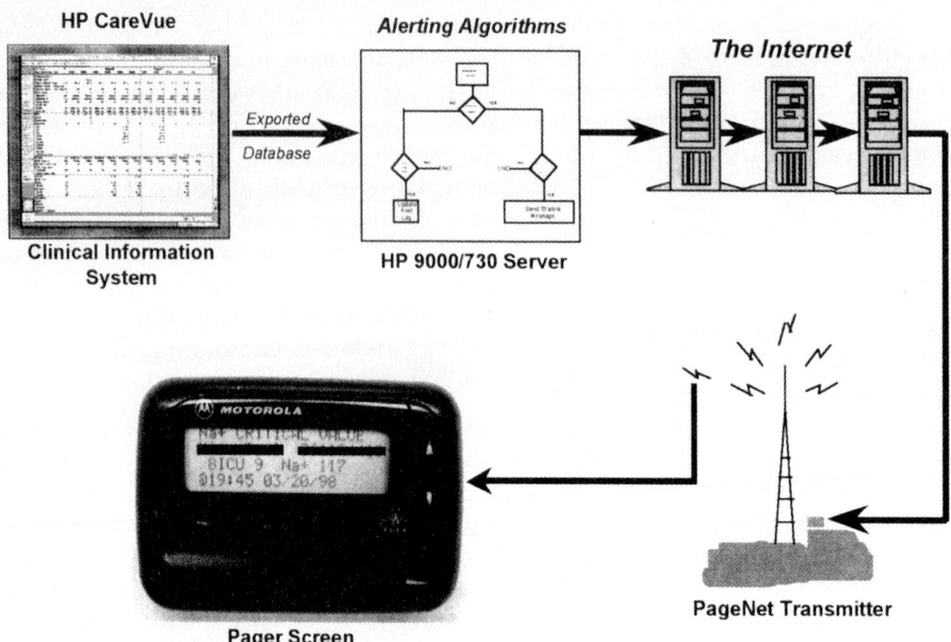


**Figure 2** Wireless alerting system. In the Cedars-Sinai system, alerts are initially detected by the clinical system, then sent to a server, then via the Internet, then sent over a PageNet transmitter to a two-way wireless device.

have been tried.[29–32] A new system, which transmits real-time alert messages to clinicians carrying alphanumeric pagers or cell phones, promises to eliminate the delivery problem.[33,34] It is now possible to integrate laboratory, medication, and physiologic data alerts into a comprehensive real-time wireless alerting system.

Shabot et al.[33,34] have developed such a comprehensive system for patients in intensive care units. A software system detect alerts and then sends them to caregivers. The alert detection system monitors data flowing into a clinical information system. The detector contains a rules engine to determine when alerts have occurred.

For some kinds of alert detection, prior or related data are needed. When the necessary data have been collected, alerting algorithms are executed and a decision is made as to whether an alert has occurred (Figure 1). The three major forms of critical event detection are critical laboratory alerts, physiologic "exception condition" alerts, and medication alerts. When an alert condition is detected, an application formats a message and transmits it to the alphanumeric pagers of various recipients, on the basis of a table of recipients by message type, patient service type, and call schedule. The message is sent as an e-mail to the coded PIN (personal identification number) of individual caregivers' pagers or cell phones. The message then appears on the device's screen and

includes appropriate patient identification information (Figure 2).

Alerts are a crucial part of a clinical decision support system,[35] and their value has been demonstrated in controlled trials.[27,35] In one study, Rind et al.[27] alerted physicians via e-mail to increases in serum creatinine in patients receiving nephrotoxic medications or renally excreted drugs. Rind et al. reported that when e-mail alerts were delivered, medications were adjusted or discontinued an average of 21.6 hours earlier than when no e-mail alerts were delivered. In another study, Kuperman et al.[35] found that when clinicians were paged about "panic" laboratory values, time to therapy decreased 11 percent and mean time to resolution of an abnormality was 29 percent shorter.

As more and different kinds of clinical data become available electronically, the ability to perform more sophisticated alerts and other types of decision support will grow. For example, medication-related, laboratory, physiologic data can be combined to create a variety of automated alerts. (Table 1 shows a sample of those currently included in the system used at Cedars-Sinai Medical Center, Los Angeles, California.) Furthermore, computerization offers many tools for decision support, but because of space limitations we have discussed only some of these; Among the others are algorithms, guidelines, order sets, trend monitors, and co-sign forcers. Most sophisticated systems include an array of these tools.

*Table 1* ■

## Sample of Wireless Alerts Currently in Use at Cedars-Sinai Medical Center, Los Angeles, California

Laboratory alerts:
  Chemistries:
    Sodium
    Potassium
    Chloride
    Calcium
  Hematology:
    Hemoglobin
    Hematocrit
    White blood cell count
    Prothrombin time
    Partial thromboplastin time
  Arterial blood gas:
    pH
    $PO_2$
    $PCO_2$
  Laboratory trend alerts:
    Hematocrit
    Sodium
  Drug levels:
    Phenytoin
    Theophylline
    Phenobarbital
    Quinidine
    Lidocaine
    Procainamide
    NAPA (N-acetyl-procainamide)
    Digoxin
    Thiocyanate
    Gentamicin
    Tobramycin
  Cardiac enzymes:
    Troponin I

Exception alerts:
  $FiO_2 > 60\%$ for > 4 hours
  PEEP (positive end-respiratory pressure) > 15 cm $H_2O$
  Systolic BP < 80 mm Hg and no pulmonary artery catheter
  Systolic BP < 80 mm Hg and pulmonary wedge pressure
    < 10 mm Hg
  Pulmonary wedge pressure > 22 mm Hg
  Urine output < 0.3 cc/kg/hour and patient not admitted in
    chronic renal failure
  Ventricular tachycardia
  Ventricular fibrillation
  Code Blue
  Re-admission to intensive care unit < 48 hours after discharge

Medication dose alerts:
  Gentamicin ≥ 200 mg
  Tobramycin ≥ 200 mg
  Vancomycin ≥ 1,500 mg
  Phenytoin ≥ 1,000 mg
  Digoxin ≥ 0.5 mg
  Heparin flush ≥ 500 units
  Heparin injection ≥ 5000 units
  Enoxaparin ≥ 30 mg
  Epogen (epoetin alfa) ≥ 20,000 units

Medication–physiology alerts:
  Alert if urine output is low (< 0.3 cc/kg/hour for 3 hours) and the
  patient is receiving gentamicin, tobramycin, vancomycin, penicillin,
  ampicillin, Augmentin (amoxicillin/clavulanic acid), piperacillin,
  Zosyn (piperacillin/tazobactam), oxacillin, Primaxin (imipenem/
  cilastatin), or Unasyn (ampicillin/sulbactam).

Medication–laboratory data trend alerts:
  Alert if serum creatinine level increases by > 0.5 mg/dL in
  24 hours and the patient is receiving any of the following drugs:
  gentamicin, tobramycin, amikacin, vancomycin, amphotericin,
  digoxin, procainamide, Prograf (tacrolimus), cyclosporin, or ganciclovir.

## Errors Generated By Information Technology

Although information technology can help reduce error and accident rates, it can also cause errors. For example, if two medications that are spelled similarly are displayed next to each other, substitution errors can occur. Also, clinicians may write an order in the wrong patient's record.

In particular, early adopters of vendor-developed order entry have reported significant barriers to successful implementation, new sources of error, and major infrastructure changes that have been necessary to accommodate the technology. The order entry process with many computerized physician order entry systems currently on the market is error-prone and time-consuming. As a result, prescribers may bypass the order entry process totally and encourage nurses, pharmacists, or unit secretaries to enter written or verbal drug orders. Also, most computerized physi-

cian order entry systems are separate from the pharmacy system, which requires double entry of all orders. This may result in electronic/computer-generated medication administration records (MARs) that are derived from the order entry system database, not the pharmacy database, which can result in discrepancies and extra work for nurses and pharmacists.

Furthermore, many computerized physician order entry systems lack even basic screening capabilities to alert practitioners to unsafe orders relating to overly high doses, allergies, and drug–drug interactions. While visiting hospitals in 1998, representatives of the Institute for Safe Medication Practices (ISMP) tested pharmacy computers and were alarmed to discover that many failed to detect unsafe drug orders. Subsequently, ISMP asked directors of pharmacy in U.S. hospitals to perform a nationwide field test to assess the capability of their systems to intercept common or serious prescribing errors.[36] To participate, pharmacists set up a test patient in their computer system, then entered actual physician prescription errors that had actually led to a patient's death or serious injury during 1998 (Table 2). Only a small number of even fatal errors were detected by current detection methods.

These anecdotal data suggest that current systems may be inadequate and that simply implementing the current off-the-shelf vendor products may not have the same effect on medication errors that has been reported in research studies. Improvement of vendor-based systems and evaluation of their effects is crucial, since these are the systems that will be implemented industry-wide.

## Management Issues

A major problem in creating the will to reduce errors has been that administrators have not been aware of the magnitude of problem. For example, one survey showed that, while 92 percent of hospital CEOs reported that they were knowledgeable about the frequency of medication errors in their facility, only 8 percent said they had more than 20 per month, when in fact all probably had more than this.[37] Probably in part as a result, the Advisory Board Company found that reducing clinical error and adverse events ranked 133rd when CEOs were asked to rank items on a priority list.[38] A number of efforts are currently under way to increase the visibility of the issue. For example, a video about this issue, which was developed by the American Hospital Association and the Institute for Healthcare Improvement, has been sent to all hospital CEOs in the United States, and a number of indicators suggest that such efforts may be working.

## The Value Proposition

For information technology to be implemented, it must be clear that the return on investment is sufficient, and far too few data are available regarding this in health care. Furthermore, there are many horror stories of huge investments in information technology that have come to naught.

Positive examples relate to computer order entry. At one large academic hospital, the savings were estimated to be $5 million to $10 million annually on a $500 million budget.[39] Another community hospital predicts even larger savings, with expected annual savings of $21 million to $26 million, representing about a tenth of its budget.[40] In addition, in a randomized controlled trial, order entry was found to

*Table 2* ■

Percentage of Pharmacy Computer Systems That Failed to Provide Unsafe Order Alerts*

| Order | Unsafe Order Not Detected | Can Override Without Note |
|---|---|---|
| Cephradine oral suspension IV | 61 | 36 |
| Ketorolac 60 mg IV (patient allergic to aspirin) | 12 | 64 |
| Vincristine 3 mg IV x 1 dose (2-year-old) | 62 | 56 |
| Colchicine 10 mg IV for 1 dose (adult) | 66 | 55 |
| Cisplatin 204 mg IV x 1 dose (26-kg child) | 63 | 62 |

* All these orders are unsafe and have resulted in at least one fatality in the United States. However, most pharmacy systems did not detect them, and even among those that did, a large percentage allowed an override without a note. Data reprinted, with permission, from ISMP Medication Safety Alert! Feb 10, 1999.[36] Copyright © Institute for Safe Medication Practices.

result in a 12.7 percent decrease in total charges and a 0.9 day decrease in length of stay.[41] Even without full computerization of ordering, substantial savings can be realized: data from LDS Hospital[23] demonstrated that a program that assisted with antibiotic management resulted in a fivefold decrease in the frequency of excess drug dosages and a tenfold decrease in antibiotic-susceptibility mismatches, with substantially lower total costs and lengths of stay.

## Barriers

Despite these demonstrated benefits, only a handful of organizations have successfully implemented clinical decision support systems. A number of barriers have prevented implementation. Among these are the tendency of health care organizations to invest in administrative rather than clinical systems; the issue of "silo accounting," so that benefits that accrue across a system do not show up in one budget and thus do not get credit; the current financial crisis in health care, which has been exacerbated by the Balanced Budget Amendment and has made it very hard for hospitals to invest; the lack, at many sites, of leaders in information technology; and the lack of expertise in implementing systems.

One of the greatest barriers to providing outstanding decision support, however, has been the need for an extensive electronic medical record system infrastructure. Although much of the data required to implement significant clinical decision support is already available in electronic form at many institutions, the data are either not accessible or cannot be brought together to be used in clinical decision support because of format and interface issues. Existing and evolving standards for exchange of information (HL7) and coding of this data are simplifying this task. Correct and consistent identification of patients, doctors, and locations is another area in which standards are needed. Approaches to choosing which information should be coded and how to record a mixture of structured coded information and unstructured text are still immature.

Some organizations have moved ahead with adopting such standards on their own, and this can have great benefits. For example, a technology architecture guide was developed at Cedars-Sinai Medical Center to help ensure that its internal systems and databases operate in a coherent manner. This has allowed them to develop what they call their "Web viewing system," which allows clinicians to see nearly all results on an Internet platform. Many health care organizations are hamstrung, because they have implemented so many different technologies and databases that information stays in silos.

A second major hurdle is choosing the appropriate rules or guidelines to implement. Many organizations have not developed processes for developing and implementing consensus choices in their physician groups. Once the focus has been determined, the organization must determine exactly what should be done about the selected problem. Regulatory and legal issues have also prevented vendors from providing this type of content. Finally, despite good precedents for delivering feedback to clinicians for simple decision support, changing provider behavior for more complex aspects of care remains challenging.

## The National Picture

A national commitment to safer health care is developing. Although it is too soon to determine how it will "play out" (the initial fixation on mandatory reporting has been an unwelcome diversion, for example), it seems clear that many stakeholders have a real interest in improving safety. Doctors and other professionals are in the interesting position of being expected to be both leaders in this movement and the recipients of its attention. Already a national coalition involving many of the leading purchasers, the Leapfrog Group, which includes such companies as General Motors and General Electric, have announced their intention to provide incentives to hospitals and other health care organizations to imple-

ment safe practices.[42] One of the first of these practices will be the implementation of computerized physician order entry systems. Similarly, a recent Medicare Patient Advisory Commission report suggested that that the Health Care Financing Administration consider providing financial incentives to hospitals that adopt physician order entry systems.[43] The Agency for Healthcare Research and Quality has received $50 million in funding to support error reduction research, including information technology–related strategies. California recently passed a law mandating that non-rural hospitals implement computerized physician order entry or another application like it by 2005.[44] Clearly, many look to automation to play a major role in the redesign of our systems.

## Recommendations

Recommendations for using information technology to reduce errors fall into two categories—general suggestions that are relevant across domains, and very specific recommendations. It is important to recognize that these lists are not exhaustive, but they do contain many of the most important and best-documented precepts. Although many of these relate to the medication domain, this is because the best current evidence is available for this area; we anticipate that information technology will eventually be shown to be important for error reduction across a wide variety of domains, and some evidence is already available for blood products, for example.[45,46] The strength of these recommendations is based on a standard set of criteria for levels of evidence.[47] For therapy and prevention, evidence level 1a represents multiple randomized trials, level 1b is an individual randomized trial, level 4 is case series, and level 5 represents expert opinion.

### General Recommendations

- Implement clinical decision support judiciously (evidence level 1a). Clinical decision support can clearly improve care,[48] but it must be used in ways that help users, and the false-positive rate of active suggestions should not be overly high. Such decision support should be usable by physicians.

- Consider consequent actions when designing systems (evidence level 1b). Many times, one action implies another, and systems that prompt regarding this can dramatically decrease the likelihood of errors of omission.[49]

- Test existing systems to ensure that they actually catch errors that injure patients (evidence level 5).

The match between the errors that systems detect and the actual frequency of important errors is often suboptimal.

- Promote adoption of standards for data and systems (evidence level 5). Adoption of standards is critical if we are to realize the potential of information technology for error prevention. Standards for constructs such as drugs and allergies are especially important.

- Develop systems that communicate with each other (evidence level 5). One of the greatest barriers to providing clinicians with meaningful information has been the inability of systems, such as medication and laboratory systems, to readily exchange data. Such communication should be seamless. Adopting enterprise database standards can vastly simplify this issue.

- Use systems in new ways (evidence level 5). Electronic records will soon facilitate new, sophisticated prevention approaches, such as risk factor profiling and pharmacogenomics, in which a patient's medications are profiled against their genetic makeup.

- Measure and prevent adverse consequences (evidence level 5). Information technology in general and clinical decision support in particular can certainly have perverse and opposite consequences; continuous monitoring is essential.[50] However, such monitoring has often not been carried out. It should also be routine to measure how often recommendations are presented and how often suggestions are accepted and to have some measures of downstream outcomes.

- Make existing quality structures meaningful (evidence level 5). Quality measurement and improvement groups are often suboptimally effective. Increasing the use of computerization should make it dramatically easier to measure quality continually. Such information must then be used to make ongoing changes.

- Improve regulation and remove disincentives for vendors to provide clinical decision support (evidence level 5). The regulation relating to information technology is hopelessly outdated and is currently being revised to address such issues as privacy in the electronic world.[51] One issue that relates to error in particular is that vendors, with some cause, fear being sued if they provide action-oriented clinical decision support. Thus, the support either is not provided or is watered down. This problem must be addressed.

## Specific Recommendations

- Implement provider order entry systems, especially computerizing prescribing (evidence level 1b). Provider order entry has been shown to reduce the serious medication error rate by 55 percent.[20]

- Implement bar-coding for, for example, medications, blood, devices, and patients (evidence level 4). In other industries, bar-coding has dramatically reduced error rates. Although fewer data are available for this recommendation in medicine, it is likely that bar-coding will have a major impact.[52]

- Use modern electronic systems to communicate key pieces of asynchronous data (evidence level 1b). Timely communication of markedly abnormal laboratory tests can decrease time to therapy and the time patients spend in life-threatening conditions.

Our hope is that these recommendations will be useful for a variety of audiences. Error in health care is a pressing problem, which is best addressed by changing our systems of care—most of which involve information technology. Although information technology is not a panacea for this problem, which is highly complex and will demand the attention of many, it can play a key role. The informatics community should make it a high priority to assess the effects of information technology on patient safety.

*References* ■


1. Kohn LT, Corrigan JM, Donaldson MS (eds). To Err Is Human: Building a Safer Health System. Washington, DC: National Academy Press, 1999.
2. McDonald CJ, Weiner M, Hui SL. Deaths due to medical errors are exaggerated in Institute of Medicine report. JAMA. 2000;284:93–5.
3. Leape LL. Institute of Medicine medical error figures are not exaggerated [comment]. JAMA. 2000;284:95–7.
4. Leape LL, Brennan TA, Laird NM, et al. The nature of adverse events in hospitalized patients: results from the Harvard Medical Practice Study II. N Engl J Med. 1991;324:377–84.
5. Gurwitz JH, Field T, Avorn J, et al. Incidence and preventability of adverse drug events in nursing homes. Am J Med. 2000;109:87–94.
6. Bates DW, Boyle DL, Vander Vliet MB, Schneider J, Leape LL. Relationship between medication errors and adverse drug events. J Gen Intern Med. 1995;10:199–205.
7. Rasmussen J. Human errors: a taxonomy for describing human malfunction in industrial installations. J Occup Accid. 1982;4:311–35.
8. Reason J. Human Error. Cambridge, UK: Cambridge University Press, 1990.
9. Norman DA. The Design of Everyday Things. New York: Basic Books, 1988.
10. Senders J, Moray N. Human Error: Cause, Prediction and Reduction. Mahwah, NJ: Lawrence Erlbaum, 1991.
11. Testimony of the Three Mile Island Operators. United States

President's Commission on the Accident at Three Mile Island, vol 1. Washington, DC: U.S. Government Printing Office, 1979:138.

12. Macklis RM, Meier T, Weinhous MS. Error rates in clinical radiotherapy. J Clin Oncol. 1998;16:551–6.

13. Leape LL, Bates DW, Cullen DJ, et al. Systems analysis of adverse drug events. ADE Prevention Study Group. JAMA. 1995;274(1):35–43.

14. Brennan TA, Leape LL, Laird N, et al. Incidence of adverse events and negligence in hospitalized patients: results from the Harvard Medical Practice Study I. N Engl J Med. 1991;324:370–6.

15. Barker KN, Allan EL. Research on drug-use-system errors. Am J Health Syst Pharm. 1995;52:400–3.

16. Classen DC, Pestotnik SL, Evans RS, Burke JP. Computerized surveillance of adverse drug events in hospital patients. JAMA. 1991;266:2847–51.

17. Jha AK, Kuperman GJ, Teich JM, et al. Identifying adverse drug events: development of a computer-based monitor and comparison to chart review and stimulated voluntary report. J Am Med Inform Assoc. 1998;5(3):305–14.

18. Gandhi TK, Seger DL, Bates DW. Identifying drug safety issues—from research to practice. Int J Qual Health Care 2000;12:69–76.

19. Karson AS, Bates DW. Screening for adverse events. J Eval Clin Pract. 1999;5:23–32.

20. Bates DW, Leape LL, Cullen DJ, et al. Effect of computerized physician order entry and a team intervention on prevention of serious medication errors. JAMA. 1998;280(15):1311–6.

21. Bates DW, Cullen D, Laird N, et al. Incidence of adverse drug events and potential adverse drug events: implications for prevention. JAMA. 1995;274:29–34.

22. Bates DW, Miller EB, Cullen DJ, et al. Patient risk factors for adverse drug events in hospitalized patients. Arch Intern Med. 1999;159:2553–660.

23. Evans RS, Pestotnik SL, Classen DC, et al. A computer-assisted management program for antibiotics and other anti-infective agents. N Engl J Med. 1998;338:232–8.

24. Classen DC, Evans RS, Pestotnik SL, et al. The timing of prophylactic administration of antibiotics and the risk of surgical-wound infection. N Engl J Med 1992;326:281–6.

25. Tate K, Gardner RM, Scherting K. Nurses, pagers and patient specific criteria: three keys to improved critical value reporting. Proc Annu Symp Comput Appl Med Care. 1995;19:164–8.

26. Tate K, Gardner RM, Weaver LK. A computerized laboratory alerting system. MD Comput. 1990;7:296–301.

27. Rind D, Safran C, Phillips RS, et al. Effect of computer-based alerts on the treatment and outcomes of hospitalized patients. Arch Intern Med. 1994;154:1511–7.

28. Kuperman G, Boyle D, Jha AK, et al. How promptly are inpatients treated for critical laboratory results? J Am Med Inform Assoc. 1998;5:112–9.

29. Bradshaw K. Computerized alerting system warns of life-threatening events. Proc Annu Symp Comput Appl Med Care. 1986;10:403.

30. Bradshaw K. Development of a computerized laboratory alerting system. Comput Biomed Res. 1989;22:575–87.

31. Shabot M, LoBue M, Leyerle B. Inferencing strategies for automated alerts on critically abnormal laboratory and blood gas data. Proc Annu Symp Comput Appl Med Care. 1989;13:54–7.

32. Shabot M, LoBue M, Leyerle B. Decision support alerts for clinical laboratory and blood gas data. Int J Clin Monit Comput. 1990;7:27–31.

33. Shabot M, LoBue M. Real-time wireless decision support alerts on a palmtop PDA. Proc Annu Symp Comput Appl Med Care. 1995;19:174–7.

34. Shabot M, LoBue M, Chen J. Wireless clinical alerts for critical medication, laboratory and physiologic data. Proceedings of the 33rd Hawaii International Conference on System Sciences (HICSS); Jan 4–7, 2000; Maui, Hawaii [CD-ROM]. Washington, DC: IEEE Computer Society, 2000.

35. Kuperman G, Sittig DF, Shabot M, Teich J. Clinical decision support for hospital and critical care. J HIMSS. 1999;13:81–96.

36. Institute for Safe Medication Practices. Over-reliance on computer systems may place patients at great risk. ISMP Medication Safety Alert, Feb 10, 1999. Huntingdon Valley, Pa.: ISMP, 1999.

37. Bruskin Goldring Research. A Study of Medication Errors and Specimen Collection Errors. Commissioned by BD (Becton-Dickinson) and College of American Pathologists. Feb 1999. Available at http://www.bd.com/bdid/whats_new/survey.html. Accessed Mar 12, 2001.

38. The Advisory Board Company. Prescription for change: toward a higher standard in medication management. Washington, DC: ABC, 1999.

39. Glaser J, Teich JM, Kuperman G. Impact of information events on medical care. Proceedings of the 1996 HIMSS Annual Conference. Chicago, Ill.: Healthcare Information and Management Systems Society, 1996:1–9.

40. Sarasota Memorial Hospital documents millions in expected cost savings, reduced LOS through use of Eclipsys' Sunrise Clinical Manager [press release]. Delray Beach, Fla.: Eclipsys Corporation; Oct 11, 1999. Available at: http://www.eclipsys.com. Accessed Nov 8, 2000.

41. Tierney WM, Miller ME, Overhage JM, McDonald CJ. Physician inpatient order writing on microcomputer workstations: effects on resource utilization. JAMA. 1993;269:379–83.

42. Fischman J. Industry Preaches Safety in Pittsburgh. U.S. News and World Report. Jul 17, 2000.

43. Medicare Payment Advisory Commission. Report to the Congress: Selected Medicare Issues, Jun 1999. Available at: http://www.medpac.gov/html/body_june_report.html. Accessed Mar 12, 2001.

44. California Senate Bill No. 1875. Chapter 816, Statutes of 2000.

45. Lau FY, Wong R, Chui CH, Ng E, Cheng G. Improvement in transfusion safety using a specially designed transfusion wristband. Transfus Med.2000;10(2):121–4.

46. Blood-error reporting system tracks medical mistakes [press release]. Dallas, Tex: The University of Texas Southwestern Medical Center at Dallas; Nov 22, 1999. Available at http://irweb.swmed.edu/newspub. Accessed Mar 12, 2001.

47. Centre for Evidence-based Medicine. Levels of evidence and grades of recommendation; Sep 8, 2000. Available at: http://cebm.jr2.ox.ac.uk/docs/levels.html. Accessed Mar 12, 2001.

48. Haynes RB, Hayward RS, Lomas J. Bridges between health care research evidence and clinical practice. J Am Med Inform Assoc. 1995;2:342–50.

49. Overhage JM, Tierney WM, Zhou X, McDonald CJ. A randomized trial of "corollary orders" to prevent errors of omission. J Am Med Inform Assoc. 1997;4:364–75.

50. Miller R, Gardner RM. Summary recommendations for responsible monitoring and regulation of clinical software systems. Ann Intern Med. 1997;127:842–5.

51. Gostin LO, Lazzarini Z, Neslund VS, Osterholm MT. The public health information infrastructure: a national review of the law on health information privacy. JAMA.1996;275:1921–7.

52. Bates DW. Using information technology to reduce rates of medication errors in hospitals. BMJ. 2000;320:788–91.

# Guided Medication Dosing for Inpatients With Renal Insufficiency


Glenn M. Chertow, MD, MPH

Joshua Lee, MD

Gilad J. Kuperman, MD

Elisabeth Burdick

Jan Horsky

Diane L. Seger

Rita Lee

Aparna Mekala

Jean Song

Anthony L. Komaroff, MD

David W. Bates, MD, MSc



**Context** Usual drug-prescribing practices may not consider the effects of renal insufficiency on the disposition of certain drugs. Decision aids may help optimize prescribing behavior and reduce medical error.

**Objective** To determine if a system application for adjusting drug dose and frequency in patients with renal insufficiency, when merged with a computerized order entry system, improves drug prescribing and patient outcomes.

**Design, Setting, and Patients** Four consecutive 2-month intervals consisting of control (usual computerized order entry) alternating with intervention (computerized order entry plus decision support system), conducted in September 1997–April 1998 with outcomes assessed among a consecutive sample of 17 828 adults admitted to an urban tertiary care teaching hospital.

**Intervention** Real-time computerized decision support system for prescribing drugs in patients with renal insufficiency. During intervention periods, the adjusted dose list, default dose amount, and default frequency were displayed to the order-entry user and a notation was provided that adjustments had been made based on renal insufficiency. During control periods, these recommended adjustments were not revealed to the order-entry user, and the unadjusted parameters were displayed.

**Main Outcome Measures** Rates of appropriate prescription by dose and frequency, length of stay, hospital and pharmacy costs, and changes in renal function, compared among patients with renal insufficiency who were hospitalized during the intervention vs control periods.

**Results** A total of 7490 patients were found to have some degree of renal insufficiency. In this group, 97 151 orders were written on renally cleared or nephrotoxic medications, of which 14 440 (15%) had at least 1 dosing parameter modified by the computer based on renal function. The fraction of prescriptions deemed appropriate during the intervention vs control periods by dose was 67% vs 54% ($P<.001$) and by frequency was 59% vs 35% ($P<.001$). Mean (SD) length of stay was 4.3 (4.5) days vs 4.5 (4.8) days in the intervention vs control periods, respectively ($P=.009$). There were no significant differences in estimated hospital and pharmacy costs or in the proportion of patients who experienced a decline in renal function during hospitalization.

**Conclusions** Guided medication dosing for inpatients with renal insufficiency appears to result in improved dose and frequency choices. This intervention demonstrates a way in which computer-based decision support systems can improve care.

*JAMA. 2001;286:2839-2844*          www.jama.com


RENAL INSUFFICIENCY IS RELAtively common among hospitalized patients, and is associated with an increase in hospitalization-related morbidity and mortality.[1-4] Persons with acute and chronic renal insufficiency are hospitalized with increased frequency compared with those nonaffected, due to renal disease per se, and to the effects of renal insufficiency on other medical conditions, including congestive heart failure and chronic liver disease.[5,6] Practitioners caring for these patients are faced with the challenges of managing the complex interplay between renal insufficiency and other organ system disease, and of altering diagnostic studies (eg, angiography) and therapeutics to avoid further renal injury. With regard to renal insufficiency and pharmacotherapeutics, the majority of clinicians' attention has been directed at avoiding nephrotoxic drugs in patients at risk for worsening renal failure; comparatively little attention has been paid to the disposition of drugs, nephrotoxic and non-nephrotoxic, in patients with renal in-

**See also Patient Page.**

sufficiency. In prescribing drugs for patients with renal insufficiency, most practitioners rely on their clinical experience or the advice of consultant physicians or pharmacists to guide dosing regimens. Since few clinicians are expert in this area, and medication orders can rarely be delayed until consultation is obtained, the capacity to provide information on drug disposition in real


**Author Affiliations:** Division of General Internal Medicine (Drs J. Lee, Komaroff, and Bates and Mss Burdick, Horsky, and Seger), and Renal Division, Department of Medicine, Brigham and Women's Hospital, Harvard Medical School (Dr Chertow), Department of Information Systems, Partners HealthCare System (Dr Kuperman and Mss R. Lee, Mekala, and Song) Boston, Mass. Dr Chertow is now with the Division of Nephrology, Department of Medicine, University of California, San Francisco.
**Financial Disclosures are listed at the end of this article.**
**Corresponding Author and Reprints:** Glenn M. Chertow, MD, MPH, Department of Medicine Research, UCSF Laurel Heights, 3333 California St, Suite 430, San Francisco, CA 94118 (e-mail: chertowg@medicine.ucsf.edu).

time might be of great value to the practicing clinician and the patient.

The problem of error in medicine has been found to be important and costly.[7] Adverse drug events (ADEs) are common and often associated with errors.[8] Even basic computerization of physician ordering with relatively little decision support was associated with a 55% decrease in serious medication errors, and an 84% decrease in near misses or potential ADEs in 1 study by our group.[9] However, only a 17% decrease was seen in preventable ADEs. The study suggested that computerized advice regarding the dosing of drugs in the setting of renal insufficiency might be among the most potent additional preventive strategies.[10]

Thus, we hypothesized that the incorporation of guided dosing algorithms for inpatients with renal insufficiency into an existing computer order entry system would result in a larger proportion of appropriate dose and frequency orders, and would be associated with shorter lengths of stay (LOS), lower costs, and a lower frequency of worsening renal function.

## METHODS
### Study Setting

The study was carried out at Brigham and Women's Hospital, a 720-bed urban tertiary care academic medical center in Boston, Mass. The Brigham Integrated Computing System (BICS) provides administrative and clinical computing services at BWH. All inpatient orders are entered into BICS, including orders for medications, laboratory and radiology studies, and for nursing interventions. The BICS order entry application provides the physician with a range of possible dose amounts for that medication (dose list) along with 1 dose that is highlighted as the default or recommended dose amount (FIGURE 1A). The clinician is also offered a highlighted frequency as the recommended dosing interval (Figure 1B). The clinician can also hit an additional key to see the data used for calculation of creatinine clearance. Nearly all laboratory, radiology, and pathology results, admission vital signs (including weight), and demographic information can be accessed.

The BICS system had for some years contained an on-line, noninteractive version that could be accessed separately from the order entry system. In an attempt to enhance the impact of this application within the BICS, its internal logic was integrated with the computerized laboratory results reporting system, and was incorporated into the order entry system. Based on information already in the reporting system, the new application first determined whether a patient had renal insufficiency, defined as an estimated creatinine clearance of less than 80 mL/min (1.34 mL/s), by the Cockroft-Gault equation.[11] Next, based on the real-time calculation of the estimated creatinine clearance and the drug being prescribed, the application would modify the above-described dose list, default dose amount, and default frequency (dosing interval) in the BICS (FIGURE 2).

### Knowledge Base

After reviewing the relevant literature, an expert panel including a nephrologist, a pharmacist, and a general internist con-

**Figure 1.** Screen Displays of Brigham Integrated Computing System's New Application for Dose List and Frequency

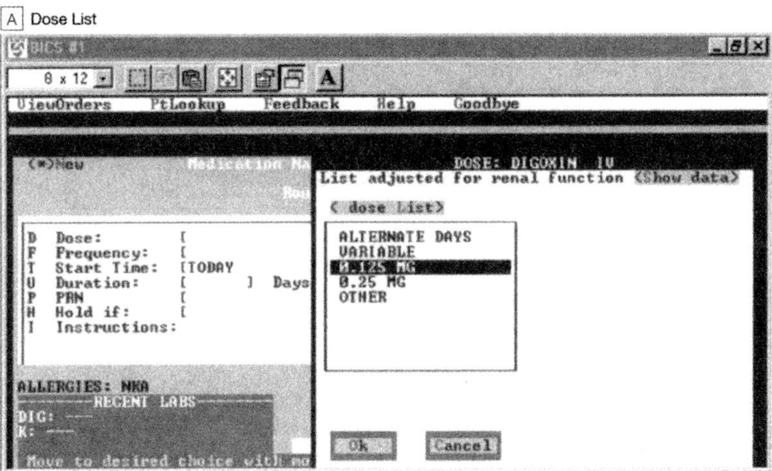

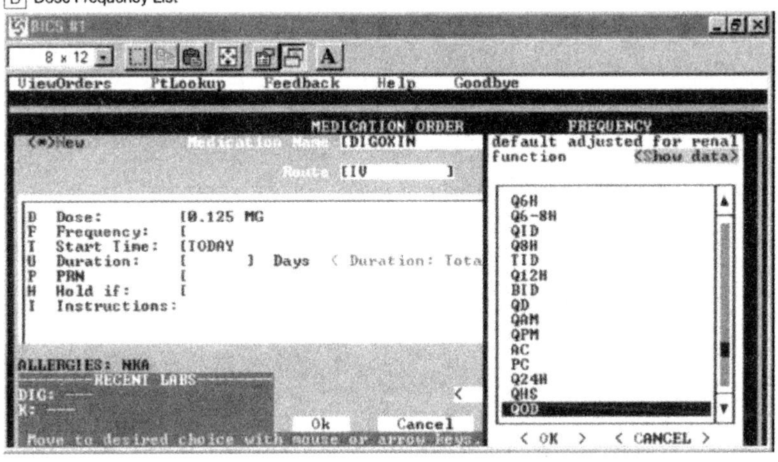

The dose and dose frequency lists in which defaults were chosen by the system were based on a simulated patient's estimated creatinine clearance.

vened to review all medications in the hospital's drug formulary and selected those medications that were renally cleared and/or nephrotoxic. New dosing suggestions were generated in a subset of approximately 500 medications (approximately 2500 in total). To smooth dose recommendations, renal insufficiency was divided into 3 categories: mild (estimated creatinine clearance, 50-80 mL/min [0.84-1.34 mL/s]), moderate (estimated creatinine clearance, 16-49 mL/min [0.27-0.82 mL/s]), and advanced (estimated creatinine clearance, ≤15 mL/min [≤0.25 mL/s]). The expert panel then determined optimal adjustments in dose list, default dose amount, and default frequency for each of the medications in the application in each of the renal insufficiency categories. The nonfixed variables in the estimated creatinine clearance calculation (ie, weight, serum creatinine) were the weight entered by the nurse or physician into the BICS database on admission. The latest serum creatinine level was entered by the laboratory and updated regularly during the hospital stay.

### Patient Population

All persons admitted to the medical, surgical (including subspecialty surgical services), neurology, and obstetrics and gynecology services between September 1997 and April 1998, whose admission and discharge were within the boundaries of 4 consecutive 2-month periods were included in the study. Admission periods did not overlap.

### Intervention and Evaluation

When renal insufficiency was detected and any medication was ordered, the application potentially modified 1 or more of the dose list, default dose amount, and default frequency. To test the effect of this application, an intervention trial was designed. The study periods consisted of 4 alternating 8-week blocks of intervention and control subperiods. Throughout the intervention and control periods, the application was active, determining whether the dose list, default dose amount, and default frequency needed adjustments. During the

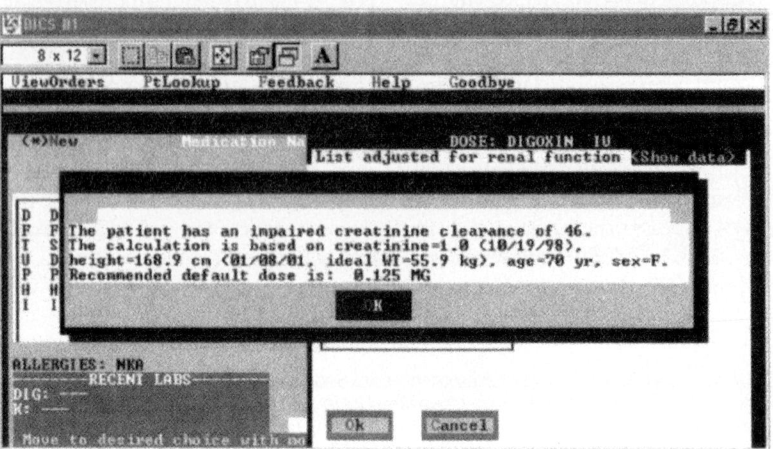

**Figure 2.** Screen Display of Brigham Integrated Computing System's New Application for Actual Calculation



Screen that appears when clinician requests drug in which the dose or frequency may be modified for renal function.

intervention periods, the adjusted dose list, default dose amount, and default frequency were displayed to the order-entry user and a notation was provided that adjustments had been made based on renal insufficiency. During the control periods, these recommended adjustments were not revealed to the order-entry user, and the unadjusted parameters were instead displayed.

A log was kept of all instances in which an application medication was ordered and the application adjusted the dose list, default dose amount, and/or default frequency. A log was also kept of the order finally made by the ordering physician. A selection was considered appropriate if the dose amount or frequency interval did not exceed the parameters set forth by the expert panel.

If use of a particular medication was considered potentially harmful, the application would provide feedback to the ordering clinician, accompanied by a recommendation for a suitable substitute when appropriate. For instance, if meperidine hydrochloride were prescribed for a patient with an estimated creatinine clearance of less than 15 mL/min (<0.25 mL/s), a warning regarding its potential for promoting seizures would be issued, with a suggestion that an alternative narcotic analgesic be prescribed. The clinician could then either accept or override such a recommendation.

### Patient Outcomes

Patient outcomes were determined during discrete admissions. Length of stay was recorded in days. Hospital and pharmacy costs were estimated from billed charges and institution-specific charge-to-cost ratios.

### Statistical Analysis

Continuous data were presented as mean (SD) or median (interquartile range), and compared with the $t$ test or Wilcoxon rank-sum test, as appropriate. Categorical data were presented as proportions and compared using the $\chi^2$ test. Multivariable linear regression analysis was used to compare LOS and costs (both log-transformed) in the intervention and control periods. Age, sex, and diagnosis related group (DRG) weight[12] were used as covariates in these analyses. In addition, we evaluated (using multiplicative interaction terms) whether the effect of the application intervention differed by age, sex, or DRG weight. To determine whether the exclusion of patients whose admission extended across study periods exerted any meaningful effects on the analyses of

**Table 1.** Catalog of Application Suggestions

| | | No. of Orders | |
|---|---|---|---|
| Type of Intervention | Total No. of Orders | Control Period (Alteration Not Revealed) | Intervention Period (Alteration Revealed) |
| All types | 97 151 | 58 160 | 38 399 |
| **Total** | **14 440** | **8950** | **5490** |
| Dosing alteration only | 3490 | 2136 | 1354 |
| Frequency alteration only | 4787 | 2986 | 1801 |
| Dosing and frequency alteration | 6163 | 3828 | 2335 |
| Warnings | 253 | 0 | 253 |
| Substitute medication | 27 | 0 | 27 |

LOS, costs, and renal function, we repeated the analyses without these exclusions. Each patient was assigned to the group (intervention or control) based on the day of admission. All reported $P$ values were based on 2-tailed tests of statistical significance. Analyses were conducted using SAS statistical software (SAS Institute Inc, Cary, NC).

## RESULTS
### Patients

There were 19 982 admissions that either began or ended during the 8-month study period; we focused on the 17 828 that were wholly contained within a study subperiod. There were 7887 (39.5%) admissions wholly contained in the 2 intervention periods and 9941 (49.7%) admissions wholly contained in the 2 control periods (corresponding to 58 912 and 70 821 patient-days, respectively). There were 2154 (10.8%) admissions that straddled a study-period boundary and were excluded. In-hospital mortality rates were 1.8% and 1.9% (intervention vs control, $P = .61$). Mean (SD) age (52.5 [18.4] years vs 52.5 [18.3] years; $P = .95$) and sex (61.4% vs 61.8% female; $P = .78$) were not significantly different across periods. The mean DRG weight was higher during the control periods (2.3 vs 2.1 in intervention periods; $P = .004$). The majority of patients (11 896 [60.1%]) had estimated creatinine clearance values greater than 80 mL/min ($>1.34$ mL/s). One in 4 patients (4927 [24.9%]) had mild renal insufficiency. Fifteen percent had moderate (2563 [12.9%]) or advanced (414 [2.1%]) renal insufficiency. The mean estimated creatinine

clearance at admission was higher during the intervention periods (90.9 vs 84.7 mL/min [1.52 vs 1.41 mL/s] in control periods; $P < .001$).

### Drug Orders

There were a total of 2 278 723 orders during the study period, 773 113 of which were medication orders and 108 537 of which were orders for nephrotoxic and/or renally cleared medications. We excluded 11 386 orders because of missing dose amount (3794 [33.3%]) or frequency interval (5102 [44.8%]), or because of an uninterpretable estimated creatinine clearance value (3696 [32.5%]), usually indicating an aberrant weight measurement, and for a variety of other less common reasons (2588 [22.7%]). These exclusions left 97 151 orders for analysis (orders could be excluded for $>1$ reason).

Of the 97 151 analyzable orders, the application generated a suggestion for the clinician in 14 440 (15%). **TABLE 1** shows a detailed array of these suggestions. **TABLE 2** shows the proportion of orders deemed appropriate, stratified by whether the the application's suggestion was dose-related, frequency-related, or both. In the intervention vs control periods, the frequency of appropriate orders was 51% vs 30% for all relevant orders, 67% vs 54% for orders involving dose changes, and 59% vs 35% for orders involving frequency changes, respectively ($P < .001$ for all comparisons).

### LOS, Costs, and Renal Function

**TABLE 3** shows unadjusted LOS and costs (hospital and pharmacy) during

the intervention and control periods. The rightward half of the table shows the effect of including the 2154 hospitalizations that overlapped. Hospitalizations were categorized as intervention or control based on conditions on the day of admission.

The adjusted mean LOS (adjusted for age, sex, and DRG weight) remained significantly shorter during the intervention period, both when overlapping admissions were included ($P = .002$) and when they were excluded ($P < .001$). The effect of the application on LOS was attenuated at higher DRG weights ($P < .001$). In contrast, there were no significant differences in adjusted mean total or pharmacy costs between intervention and control periods.

A 10-mL/min (0.17-mL/s) decrement in estimated creatinine clearance from admission to discharge was considered to be of clinical significance. The percentage of patients whose estimated creatinine clearance declined by more than 10 mL/min (0.17 mL/s) was 11.8% and 11.5% (intervention vs control, $P = .43$). The mean (SD) changes in estimated creatinine clearance were 1.9 (0.2) mL/min (0.03 [0.003] mL/s) and 2.3 (0.2) mL/min (0.04 [0.003] mL/s) during the corresponding periods ($P = .18$).

## COMMENT

We were successful in designing and implementing a computer order entry-based application that provided real-time drug prescription decision support to physicians. Compared with control periods during which information was readily available on-line but not incorporated into the order-entry process, the application intervention led to a statistically significant and clinically meaningful increase in the proportion of prescriptions considered appropriate for inpatients with renal insufficiency.

The large improvements in appropriateness of dosing and frequency were probably realized in part because the application is largely transparent to the clinician. Its key characteristics are that it remembers a huge amount of data essentially impossible for clinicians to master (and keep updated), and it makes it easy to do the right thing. Nonetheless, despite the overall improved appropriateness of dosing, 49% of orders for the application's drugs were still inappropriate in the intervention group. Some physicians may have been reluctant to reduce drug dosages, particularly among more critically ill patients. Others may have simply disregarded the advice in favor of their own established practice patterns. Future studies with this application and similar applications should investigate the reason(s) for accepting or rejecting on-line advice regarding medication ordering, and it might be worthwhile to consider stronger suggestions in specific situations.

A number of other studies have evaluated the impact of decision support on dosing of medications for patients with renal insufficiency. For example, Rind et al[13] developed an application that alerted physicians caring for inpatients when there was an increase in the patient's serum creatinine concentration. An alert was triggered by a 0.5 mg/dL (44.2 μmol/L) increase in serum creatinine if the patient was prescribed a potentially nephrotoxic medication (eg, aminoglycoside), and a 50% increase in serum creatinine, to at least 2.0 mg/dL (176.8 μmol/L), if prescribed a medication that was renally excreted (eg, digoxin). The alert was delivered by e-mail to physicians who had accessed computer-based information on the affected patient in the 3 days preceding and following the increase in serum creatinine. The intervention resulted in a significant decrease in the frequency of more severe renal dysfunction, although fewer than half of the recipients (44%) found the alerts helpful and 28% found them "annoying." It is also noteworthy that Rind et al excluded patients on all services other than medicine, and all patients with preexisting moderate or severe renal insufficiency (serum creatinine >3.0 mg/dL [265.2 μmol/L]).

In another important study, one in a series evaluating the influence of computerized decision support, investigators at LDS Hospital in Salt Lake City, Utah, incorporated renal function assessment into an application that assisted physicians in prescribing antibiotics in an intensive care unit.[14] These authors found that the use of their program decreased the frequency of inappropriate antimicrobial prescriptions (ie, orders for drugs to which patients had reported allergies, antibiotic susceptibility mismatches, and excessive drug dosages), and ADEs. Among patients who received recommended regimens, there was a significant decrease in LOS and drug and total hospital costs. More recently, Nightingale et al[15] implemented a program in the renal unit of a British teaching hospital. Clinicians cancelled more than half of their orders when they were warned that the drug dosage they had requested was excessive. In the Nightingale et al study, there were no formal comparisons made between presystem and postsystem implementation periods with regard to appropriateness of orders, costs, complications, or hospital LOS.

The application used here differs from prior applications in that it is generalized to all hospitalized patients, provides suggestions for a wide range of drugs, and does so in real time. Feedback is most likely to be successful if it is delivered in real time, and in close temporal proximity to the decisions being made.[9] As noted earlier, while we found that computerized physician order entry reduced the frequency of serious medication errors, it had a bigger impact on errors that did not actually cause injury compared with those that did injure patients.[9] We believe—although this needs to be validated—that part of the reason for the larger impact on potential ADEs than actual ADEs was that the systems evaluated did not include sophisticated decision support, such as that pro-

**Table 2.** Rates of Appropriate and Inappropriate Orders in Intervention vs Control Periods*

| | All Orders With Dose or Frequency Alteration | | | Dose Alteration | | | Frequency Alteration | | |
|---|---|---|---|---|---|---|---|---|---|
| | Intervention | Control | P Value‡ | Intervention | Control | P Value‡ | Intervention | Control | P Value‡ |
| Inappropriate† | 2714 (49) | 6298 (70) | <.001 | 1211 (33) | 2743 (46) | <.001 | 1689 (41) | 4456 (65) | <.001 |
| Appropriate | 2776 (51) | 2652 (30) | | 2478 (67) | 3221 (54) | | 2447 (59) | 2358 (35) | |
| **Total** | **5490** | **8950** | | **3689** | **5964** | | **4136** | **6814** | |

*Values expressed as number (percentage).
†Defined as an excessive dose (higher than recommended) or frequency (more frequent than recommended).
‡$\chi^2$ Test of proportions.

**Table 3.** Unadjusted Length of Stay and Costs in Intervention and Control Periods*

| | Without Overlapping Admissions† | | | With Overlapping Admissions† | | |
|---|---|---|---|---|---|---|
| | Intervention | Control | P Value | Intervention | Control | P Value |
| Length of stay, mean (SD), d‡ | 4.3 (4.5) | 4.5 (4.8) | .009 | 5.3 (7.1) | 5.4 (7.4) | .05 |
| Total costs, $ | 4881 (2974-9383) | 4968 (3035-9590) | .52 | 5211 (3093-10 497) | 5282 (3156-10 570) | .51 |
| Pharmacy costs, $ | 168 (77-417) | 166 (79-416) | .64 | 185 (82-497) | 179 (83-479) | .45 |

*Values presented as median (interquartile range) unless otherwise indicated.
†An overlapping admission is defined as an admission spanning across intervention and control periods. For the purpose of the comparison, the admission was assigned to the group (intervention vs control) active on the first admission day.
‡Median (interquartile range) for intervention and control is 3 (2-6), although Wilcoxon rank-sum tests are significant due to differences in distribution.

vided by the application described here. With widespread application of sophisticated decision support, major reductions in ADE frequency as well as improvements in efficiency should be possible.

It is unclear why LOS was reduced by the new application's activity. Typically, LOS is a downstream indicator of quality of care. Because of resource constraints, we were unable to evaluate the more subtle effects of the application. For example, avoidance of overdosing of selected drugs in elderly patients may have led to fewer central nervous system or gastrointestinal tract adverse effects or other complications. Alternatively, LOS may have been reduced by other severity factors, which were not adjusted for by age, sex, and DRG weights.

The application had no effect on costs, but an effect may have been present but obscured since all patients were included in the cost analyses. In other words, restricting the analytic population to individuals prescribed selected nephrotoxic or renally cleared medications might have allowed us to show a difference. Regardless, the application itself is inexpensive to implement within the context of an order-entry system, in contrast to other prescription–quality-improvement programs, which generally have significant labor costs and require ongoing expenditure or the effect wanes.

Our study has several limitations. First, the intervention and control periods were not entirely analogous, since the number of admissions and the hospital census were higher during the control periods. The higher census may have prompted shorter LOS (in an effort to open beds), potentially decreasing the relative effect of the application on LOS. Second, the calculation of creatinine clearance by the Cockcroft-Gault formula may not accurately reflect renal function under nonsteady-state conditions (ie, with increasing or decreasing serum creatinine concentrations). In other words, the Cockcroft-Gault formula may overestimate renal function when the serum creatinine is increasing, and underestimate renal function when the serum creatinine is decreas-

ing. However, this misclassification should have affected individuals equally during the intervention and control periods, and would tend to diminish the effect of any intervention toward the null. Third, we did not consider the degree to which individual orders differed from those considered optimal by the application's definitions. In other words, we would have expected that dose-list modification by the application would have led to a larger fraction of near-miss orders during intervention periods, but due to the immense number of orders and resource constraints, these were not calculated. Fourth, the program did not send notices (pages or e-mails) to clinicians as soon as it had evidence of worsening renal function, as did that of Rind et al,[13] but only alerted the clinician at the next occasion when the clinician was ordering a medication. Finally, since the intervention was tested at a teaching hospital where house officers write the majority of medication orders, the results may not be generalizable to other, nonteaching hospital settings.

In summary, a computer order entry-based application to guide medication dose and frequency choices for inpatients with renal insufficiency was tested and resulted in a significant improvement in the appropriateness of drug prescription. Provision of real-time advice in drug prescription may prove to be among the most useful applications of medical informatics technology. Such applications may provide clinicians "a better cockpit" and results in enhanced safety and increased efficiency at minimal cost, with little intrusion into practice.

**Author Contributions:** *Study concept and design:* Chertow, Kuperman, Komaroff, Bates.
*Acquisition of data:* J. Lee, Kuperman, Burdick, Horsky, Seger, R. Lee, Mekala, Song.
*Analysis and interpretation of data:* Chertow, J. Lee, Kuperman, Burdick, Horsky, Mekala, Komaroff, Bates.
*Drafting of the manuscript:* Chertow, J. Lee, Kuperman, Bates.
*Critical revision of the manuscript for important intellectual content:* Chertow, J. Lee, Kuperman, Burdick, Horsky, Seger, R. Lee, Mekala, Song, Komaroff, Bates.
*Statistical expertise:* Chertow, Burdick, Horsky, Bates.
*Administrative, technical, or material support:* Kuperman, Burdick, Seger, R. Lee, Mekala, Song, Komaroff, Bates.
*Study supervision:* Chertow, Kuperman, Komaroff, Bates.
**Financial Disclosures:** Dr Bates is a consultant and serves on the advisory board for McKesson Med-Management, a company that assists hospitals in preventing adverse drug events. He has received honoraria for speaking from Automated Healthcare, which makes robots that dispense medications. He is on the clinical advisory board for Becton Dickinson, which develops drug delievery systems, and the advisory board for Zynx, which develops evidence-based algorithms. He is a consultant for Alaris, which makes intravenous drug delivery systems.
Dr Bates also has received honoraria for speaking from the Eclipsys Corp, which has licensed the rights to the Brigham and Women's Hospital Clinical Information System for possible commercial development. Dr Bates is also a coinventor on patent No. 6029138 held by Brigham and Women's Hospital on the use of decision support software for medical management, licensed to the Medicalis Corp. He holds a minority equity position in the privately held company Medicalis, which develops Web-based decision support for radiology test ordering, and serves as a consultant to Medicalis.
**Previous Presentation:** Presented in abstract form at 31st Annual Meeting of the American Society of Nephrology, Philadelphia, Pa, October 25-28, 1998.

**REFERENCES**

1. Hou SH, Bushinsky DA, Wish JB, et al. Hospital-acquired renal insufficiency: a prospective study. *Am J Med.* 1983;74:243-248.
2. Levy EM, Viscoli CM, Horwitz RI. The effect of acute renal failure on mortality: a cohort analysis. *JAMA.* 1996;275:1489-1494.
3. Nolan CR, Anderson RJ. Hospital-acquired acute renal failure. *J Am Soc Nephrol.* 1998;9:710-718.
4. Obialo CI, Okonofua EC, Tayade AS, Riley LJ. Epidemiology of de novo acute renal failure in hospitalized African Americans. *Arch Intern Med.* 2000;160:1309-1313.
5. Wang R, Mouliswar M, Denman S, Kleban M. Mortality of the institutionalized old-old hospitalized with congestive heart failure. *Arch Intern Med.* 1998;158:2464-2468.
6. Dries DL, Exner DV, Domanski MJ, et al. The prognostic implications of renal insufficiency in asymptomatic and symptomatic patients with left ventricular systolic dysfunction. *J Am Coll Cardiol.* 2000;35:681-689.
7. Leape LL. Institute of Medicine medical error figures are not exaggerated. *JAMA.* 2000;284:95-97.
8. Bates DW, Cullen DJ, Laird N, et al. Incidence of adverse drug events and potential adverse drug events. *JAMA.* 1995;274:29-34.
9. Bates DW, Leape LL, Cullen DJ, et al. Effect of computerized physician order entry and a team intervention on prevention of serious medication errors. *JAMA.* 1998;280:1311-1316.
10. Jha AK, Kuperman GJ, Teich JM, et al. Identifying adverse drug events. *J Am Med Inform Assoc.* 1998;5:305-314.
11. Cockcroft DW, Gault MH. Prediction of creatinine clearance from serum creatinine. *Nephron.* 1976;16:31-41.
12. Edwards N, Honemann D, Burley D, Navarro M. Refinement of the Medicare diagnosis-related groups to incorporate a measure of severity. *Health Care Financ Rev.* 1994;16:45-64.
13. Rind DM, Safran C, Phillips RS, et al. Effect of computer-based alerts on the treatment and outcomes of hospitalized patients. *Arch Intern Med.* 1994;154:1511-1517.
14. Evans RS, Pestotnik SL, Classen DC, et al. A computer-assisted management program for antibiotics and other antiinfective agents. *N Engl J Med.* 1998;338:232-238.
15. Nightingale PG, Adu D, Richards NT, Peters M. Implementation of rules based computerised bedside prescribing and administration: intervention study. *BMJ.* 2000;320:750-753.

# Assessing telemedicine: a systematic review of the literature

**Risto Roine,* Arto Ohinmaa,† David Hailey‡**


Abstract

**Background:** To clarify the current status of telemedicine, we carried out a systematic review of the literature. We identified controlled assessment studies of telemedicine that reported patient outcomes, administrative changes or economic assessments and assessed the quality of that literature.

**Methods:** We carried out a systematic electronic search for articles published from 1966 to early 2000 using the MEDLINE (1966–April 2000), HEALTHSTAR (1975–January 2000), EMBASE (1988–February 2000) and CINALH (1982–January 2000) databases. In addition, the HSTAT database (Health Services/Technology Assessment Text, US National Library of Medicine), the Database of Abstracts of Reviews of Effectiveness (DARE, NHS Centre for Reviews and Dissemination, United Kingdom), the NHS Economic Evaluation Database and the Cochrane Controlled Trials Register were searched. We consulted experts in the field and did a manual search of the reference lists of review articles.

**Results:** A total of 1124 studies were identified. Based on a review of the abstracts, 133 full-text articles were obtained for closer inspection. Of these, 50 were deemed to represent assessment studies fulfilling the inclusion criteria of the review. Thirty-four of the articles assessed at least some clinical outcomes; the remaining 16 were mainly economic analyses. Most of the available literature referred only to pilot projects and short-term outcomes, and most of the studies were of low quality. Relatively convincing evidence of effectiveness was found only for teleradiology, teleneurosurgery, telepsychiatry, transmission of echocardiographic images, and the use of electronic referrals enabling email consultations and video conferencing between primary and secondary health care providers. Economic analyses suggested that teleradiology, especially transmission of CT images, can be cost-saving.

**Interpretation:** Evidence regarding the effectiveness or cost-effectiveness of telemedicine is still limited. Based on current scientific evidence, only a few telemedicine applications can be recommended for broader use.



*Research*

*Recherche*

**From the *Finnish Office for Health Care Technology Assessment, Helsinki, Finland; the †Department of Economics, Health Services Research Unit, University of Oulu, Oulu, Finland; and the ‡Alberta Heritage Foundation for Medical Research, Edmonton, Alta.**

*This article has been peer reviewed.*


Telemedicine is the use of information and communications technology to provide health care services to individuals who are some distance from the health care provider. Rather than being a single technology, telemedicine is part of a wider process or chain of care. It has been assumed that telemedicine can improve this chain and thus enhance the quality and efficiency of health care. Telemedicine is also expected to increase the fairness and equality of the distribution of services, because the accessibility of health services, especially in remote areas, can be improved. Although the use of older approaches (telephone, fax) is commonplace, telemedicine applications increasingly use the latest innovations in computer and network technologies and other equipment.

Before adoption into routine use, any new technology has to be proved to be superior to the approach that it is intended to replace, that is, it has to be more effective or more cost-effective than the alternative(s). Telemedicine is no exception to this rule. There is growing acceptance that telemedicine systems require assessment and the ongoing collection of relevant data for administrative purposes before they can be considered for routine use on a large scale. Furthermore, assessment of telemedicine applications is needed to assist purchasing and planning decisions and also to monitor and modify the use of the technology when it is in place.[1]

Ideally, assessment should provide a broad description of telemedicine that covers technical, clinical, economic, ethical, legal and organizational issues. In practice, assessments have been constrained by the availability of data, the timing of policy and administrative decisions, a shortage of evaluators and inertia within health care systems. Earlier reviews[2–7] have indicated that assessment studies dealing with telemedicine are scarce. In a 1997 review of telemedicine applications,[8] only one cost-effectiveness study could be identified. Since then several other economic studies have been published, but there is still a great need for high-quality evaluation.

In this paper, we examine the evidence for the effectiveness and economic efficiency of telemedicine in order to clarify the current status of the technology. The review is intended to help decision-makers who are under commercial or public pressure to establish telemedicine services, by providing an objective view of what is known at present about the effectiveness and cost-effectiveness of telemedicine.

## Methods

Computerized literature searches were performed using the MEDLINE (1966–April 2000), HEALTHSTAR (1975–January 2000), EMBASE (1988–February 2000) and CINALH (1982–January 2000) databases and the search strategy described in Table 1. In addition, the HSTAT database (Health Services/Technology Assessment Text, US National Library of Medicine), the Database of Abstracts of Reviews of Effectiveness (DARE, NHS Centre for Reviews and Dissemination, United Kingdom), the NHS Economic Evaluation Database and the Cochrane Controlled Trials Register were searched using the search term "telemedicine." Some articles were also identified by reading reference lists of published review articles and by consulting experts in the field of telemedicine.

Inclusion criteria were the following: articles had to consider, in a scientifically valid manner, the outcomes of a form of telemedicine in terms of administrative changes, patient outcomes or economic assessment. In addition, studies were required to include a comparison between a telemedicine application and a conventional alternative. Criteria for scientific validity were that the nontelemedicine alternative was related to the same application and health system as the telemedicine project and that sufficient data were included to permit comparison of the outcomes of the telemedicine and nontelemedicine alternatives.

The exclusion criteria required the rejection of articles that were limited to describing the feasibility or technical evaluation of a certain system, and to the rejection of noncontrolled studies. Articles that were duplicates of the same authors' other published studies were also excluded; the most representative of the studies was included for further consideration.

Initial screening of the articles that were identified was based on their abstracts. All abstracts were read independently by at least 2 of the authors, who recorded their opinions. The selection of the relevant articles was based on the information obtained from those abstracts, which gave some expectation that inclusion criteria would be met, and was agreed upon in consensus meetings among the reviewers. Full-text articles that were obtained for closer inspection were again evaluated independently by 2 of the authors who, in a consensus meeting, made the final decision on whether or not an article should be included in the final review. Abstracts and full-length papers were examined by the same criteria.

The strength of the evidence in each of the studies included, other than those concerned only with economic analysis, was judged according to the classification system drawn up by Jovell and Navarro-Rubio,[9] in which study design is specified as one of 9 levels in descending order of strength (Table 2). Each level is further qualified by conditions of scientific rigour for the study.

Each selected article was described using the strength of evidence according to the 9-level classification, the objectives of the study, approach, setting and subjects, type of economic analysis, and the results and conclusions of the authors. Original descriptions by the authors were mainly used, although in some cases they appeared to be misleading.

## Results

The use of this approach enabled us to identify 1124 articles dealing with telemedicine. One hundred and thirty-three full-text articles were obtained for closer inspection. Of these, 50 were deemed to fulfill the inclusion criteria of the review and are listed and briefly described in Tables 3–6.[10–59] Fourteen of the studies considered the application of telemedicine to medical consultation of various types, and 7 dealt with patient monitoring or counselling. A further 13 were concerned with teleradiology, and the remainder with emergency department care, psychiatry, dermatology, cardiology, ophthalmology and pathology.

Thirty-four of the articles assessed at least some clinical outcomes; the remaining 16 were mainly economic analyses. Some kind of economic analysis was included in 30 (60%) of the studies. In terms of study design, the quality of the clinical studies ranged in most cases from fair to poor. Ac-

**Table 1: Search strategy**

| | |
|---|---|
| 1. | exp telemedicine/ |
| 2. | telemedicine [TW] NOT 1 |
| 3. | telepsychiatry [TW] NOT 1 |
| 4. | teleradiology [TW] NOT 1 |
| 5. | teleconsult$ [TW] NOT 1 |
| 6. | OR 1–5 |
| 7. | assess$ [TW] AND 6 |
| 8. | evaluat$ [TW] AND 6 |
| 9. | validat$ [TW] AND 6 |
| 10. | feasib$ [TW] AND 6 |
| 11. | pilot [TW] AND 6 |
| 12. | OR 7–11 |
| 13. | OR 6–12 |

Note: TW = text word, $ = wild card.

**Table 2: Classification of study design**

| | |
|---|---|
| 1. | Meta-analyses of randomized controlled trials |
| 2. | Large-sample randomized controlled trials |
| 3. | Small-sample randomized controlled trials |
| 4. | Nonrandomized controlled prospective studies |
| 5. | Nonrandomized controlled retrospective trials |
| 6. | Cohort studies |
| 7. | Case–control studies |
| 8. | Noncontrolled clinical series, descriptive studies, consensus methods |
| 9. | Anecdotes or case reports |

Note: Information derived from Jovell and Navarro-Rubio.

cording to the Jovell and Navarro-Rubio classification,[9] 6 were randomized controlled trials (RCTs), corresponding to levels 2 or 3, 4 were level 4 or 5, 13 level 6, 6 level 7 and 5 level 8. Conditions of scientific rigour varied considerably. In many papers, procedures for the selection of patients and for the reading and interpretation of clinical findings were not adequately described. The outcome measures used were sometimes vaguely defined or clinically not very relevant.

Although RCTs provide the strongest study design, the strength of the evidence obtained will also be dependent on the quality of the study. The 6 papers that were located that described RCTs provide an illustration of the variation in study quality and reported outcomes. Two of the larger RCTs[29,52] were well described in terms of the randomization and subsequent procedures. The first of these, which considered automated telephone calls and management of diabetes, showed improvement in glycemic control and other benefits through the use of a telemedicine approach. However, no effect on health-related quality of life (HRQOL) was demonstrated. The second, which considered real-time teledermatology, indicated that there was no significant clinical difference from conventional consultations. A linked economic analysis indicated that teledermatology was not cost-effective under the conditions of the trial.

A further report of a large RCT[28] had a more limited description of randomization but showed that telelemedicine using a telephone-based system improved compliance with medication and led to a significant decrease in blood pressure.

Of the papers about smaller RCTs, that by Brennan and colleagues[45] appeared to have been well performed; the authors found that clinical outcomes were similar for telemedicine and for the alternative approach in an emergency department setting. Another paper, which described a pilot project for a larger RCT, indicated time savings for patients as a result of video consultations, but no significant difference in HRQOL between groups.[17] This study appeared to be more limited in quality, with substantial dropping out of patients and possibly insensitive outcome measures. The third small RCT found no significant difference between tele–exercise monitoring and a hospital-based program.[24] The power of the study was low, and further investigations would be needed to assess this application.

The nonrandomized clinical studies also varied in their quality, as judged by the descriptions in the articles, and in their outcomes. Some would have provided useful indications to decision-makers in the health systems concerned. For example, the study by Trippi and colleagues[44] showed that 72% of patients scheduled for hospital admission had normal results in dobutamine stress tele-echocardiography and could, therefore, be discharged instead of being admitted to hospital. Giovas and colleagues[46] reported that pre-hospital diagnosis by electrocardiography, using a telemedicine

## Table 3: Telemedicine applications to medical consultations

| Application studied* | Effect size or outcome |
|---|---|
| Patient consultations in a general medical clinic[10] | NSD in outcome measures among TV, hands-free telephone, face-to-face consultations |
| Interactive cable TV in pediatric primary care[11] | Cost of consultation via TV two-thirds that of a physician providing direct care |
| Telemedicine in a prison system[12] | 95% of telemedicine consultations saved trips to clinics, at 30% of cost of transportation |
| Telemedicine for HIV-positive prison inmates[13] | Increased access to care, cost savings in transportation and care delivery |
| Clinical decision-making for patients with urolithiasis[14] | Recommendation in 37.5% of initial consultations altered after telemedicine consultation |
| General hospital consultations, electronic referral; video conferencing for outpatient services[15,16] | Direct outpatient costs of internal medicine 20% lower with electronic referrals. Outpatient visits reduced by 67% |
| Video consultation, GP referral for hospital consultation[17] [RCT] | No difference in patient well-being; time to visit surgery 20% of conventional consultations |
| Consultations for ENT problems, primary care centre and university clinic[18] | Cheapest options were patient travel for < 56 patients per year, teleconsultation for > 56 and < 325 patients per year, visiting specialist at > 325 patients per year |
| Video-conferencing system, medical centre, remote primary site[19] | System saved about US$102 per hour |
| Teleoncology for patients in a medically underserved area[20] | Costs per patient US$149, US$897, US$812 for conventional, outreach and telemedicine clinics |
| Web site pro forma to aid management plans in rheumatology clinic[21] | No changes in tests requested in 62% of cases; suggested treatment remained same in 74% |
| Outpatient care via telemedicine[22] | Break-even point 1449 consultations per year |
| Prison telemedicine program[23] | Break-even point 1575 consultations per year |

Note: NSD = no significant difference, GP = general practitioner, ENT = ear, nose and throat, RCT = study was a randomized controlled trial.
*A fuller description of the studies referred to in the table is available from the authors.

link to the ambulance, took place 25 minutes before hospital diagnosis for a control group. Other studies indicated important clinical benefits through avoiding the unnecessary transfer of patients. For example, Goh and colleagues[37] reported that the use of teleradiology in the management of neurosurgical patients reduced both numbers of transfers and adverse events during transfer and also increased the number of therapeutic measures before transfer was undertaken.

In most of the studies, effectiveness was defined in clinical terms. Only 2 studies[17,29] included standardized HRQOL measures. No studies employed quality-adjusted life-year (QALY) calculations. Given the diversity of the studies in terms of design, topics covered, populations and health care settings, calculation of a notional average for effect size was not feasible. Indications of effect sizes for some of the studies are given in Tables 3–6.

### Table 4: Telemedicine applications to patient monitoring and counselling

| Application studied* | Effect size or outcome |
|---|---|
| Home exercise program, telephonic exercise monitoring[24] [RCT] | NSD between groups before or after training |
| Self-monitoring, dietetic education in diabetes management[25] | Dietetic knowledge and some biologic parameters improved. No significant decrease in HbA1c |
| Transtelephonic arrhythmia monitoring[26] | Appeared more effective than ambulatory ECG |
| Electronic information system (telephone), diabetes management[27] | Diabetes-related crisis fell 3-fold. HbA1c fell 1.0%–1.3% |
| Automated telephone patient monitoring, counselling in hypertension management[28][RCT] | 50% improvement in adherence to medication. Greater decrease in diastolic BP (5.2 v. 0.8 mm Hg) |
| Automated telephone disease management, self-care education in management of diabetes[29,30] [RCT] | Follow-up HbA1c levels 0.3% lower, better glycemic control, fewer symptoms. No difference in measures of anxiety and HRQOL |

Note: HRQOL = health-related quality of life.
*A fuller description of the studies referred to in the table is available from the authors.

### Table 5: Telemedicine applications to radiology

| Application studied* | Effect size or outcome |
|---|---|
| Regional neuroradiology department, 6 referring hospitals[31] | Significant change in management in 81% of cases |
| Image transmission in management of neurosurgical emergencies[32] | Significantly reduced interhospital transfer of patients |
| Teleradiologic case conference system for oncologists[33] | Changes in treatment planning and outcomes equivalent to in-person sessions |
| Rural radiology services: teleradiology, examinations at remote and host sites[34] | The teleradiology option did not seem to be cost-saving |
| Teleneuroradiology, district hospital and neurosurgical centre[35] | Images transferred in only 25% of cases; with this usage, cost of avoided patient transfer was high (French Fr 10 800) |
| Teleradiology network for neurologic surgery[36] | Of 100 patients, 33 did not require transportation; savings of US$502 638 |
| Teleradiology in management of neurosurgical patients[37] | Unnecessary transfers reduced (21%), more therapeutic measures before transfer (27% v. 20%), adverse events during transfer reduced (8% v. 32%) |
| Teleradiology in the context of neurosurgical emergencies[38] | 16%–50% of unnecessary patient transfers avoided |
| Comparison of teleradiology with a visiting radiologist service[39] | Break-even point was 1576 patients per year. With an equipment lifetime of 4 years rather than 6 years, threshold value was 2320 patients per year |
| Primary MRI interpretation of examinations generated at distant sites[40] | At 2000 cases per year, cost US$470 per case using teleradiology, US$544 using film and courier |
| Teleradiology system in 3 scenarios[41] | Teleconferencing within the hospital or with an external PC broke even at 1817 and 528 consultations per year |
| Emergency CT service provided to a remote hospital by teleradiology[42] | Cost per examination by teleradiology DM 372, films by taxi for reporting DM 156, patient to nearest central hospital DM 524 by road or DM 4667 by helicopter |
| Conversion of videotape review network to one based on telemedicine[43] | Net monthly savings in nonfixed costs US$7405–US$8585 |

*A fuller description of the studies referred to in the table is available from the authors.

Few comprehensive economic analyses were included in the articles. The analyses mainly measured direct medical costs, although some kind of estimation of transportation costs was included in 25 studies. Indirect costs were assessed in 4 studies,[22,34,53,59] incremental cost analysis was performed in one[18] and cost-effectiveness ratios were also calculated in one.[28] Discounting of costs was included in 7 studies,[18,20,22,34,39,52,58] and 14 included some kind of sensitivity analysis or break-even analysis of the study results.

Most of the economic analyses were variants of cost analysis. Cost–benefit analysis was said to have been carried out in 3 studies.[13,41,52] However, these were methodologically more like cost-analysis studies, because the benefits were estimated as savings (mainly the cost of travel) compared with the conventional alternative.

Demonstrated savings in costs of transportation varied considerably among the different health care situations described in the papers, from a 40% reduction to no savings as a result of telemedicine. Three of 4 studies of the transmission of diagnostic images indicated that telemedicine was more costly than the cheapest alternative.[42,54,59]

Economic analyses have mostly shown that teleradiology, especially transmission of CT images, can be cost-saving, although one of the studies, which was of good quality, did not find this to be the case.[34] An important contribution to the discussion about the cost-effectiveness of teleradiology is the study by Bergmo,[39] which explicitly provides a measure of the workload that has to be exceeded in order to achieve cost savings by using teleradiology (break-even analysis). A similar study, also undertaken by Bergmo, has

**Table 6: Telemedicine applications to other services**

| Application studied* | Effect size or outcome |
| --- | --- |
| **Emergency department** | |
| Dobutamine stress tele-echocardiography (DSTE)[44] | 72% of patients scheduled for hospital admission because of cardiac risk factors discharged after normal DSTE results |
| Emergency department telemedicine[45] [RCT] | Equal to face-to-face consultations in terms of return visits within 72 hours, additional care |
| ECG transmission from an ambulance[46] | Pre-hospital ECG diagnosis took place 25 minutes before in-hospital diagnosis |
| **Psychiatry** | |
| Videoconferencing in rural psychiatric services[47] | Break-even point 396 consultations per year |
| Telepsychiatry for remote communities[48] | 40% reduction in patient transfers. Savings A$85 380 in first year, A$112 790 in subsequent years |
| **Dermatology** | |
| Store-and-forward teledermatology, in care of nursing home residents[49] | Correct treatment plan seen in 70%, 87% and 90% of the patients given history alone, image alone, and both |
| Real-time teledermatology consultations, low-cost equipment[50] | Management plan the same in 64% of cases, suboptimum in 8%, inappropriate in 9%, unable to recommend in 20% |
| Simple teledermatology system, management of rural patients[51] | Teledermatology increased the number of referrals for specialist evaluation |
| Real-time teledermatology[52] [RCT] | No major differences in clinical outcomes or reattendance rates. Net societal cost £132.10 for teledermatology, £48.73 for conventional consultation |
| **Cardiology** | |
| Transmission of echocardiographic images[53] | 31% cost savings; unnecessary patient transfer avoided in 23% of cases |
| Telemedicine use in NICU[54] | Cost per test US$33 higher with telemedicine; NSS 5.4-day reduction in length of stay |
| Transmission of echocardiograms[55] | Little evidence of reduction in the use of respiratory therapy |
| Pediatric cardiography[56] | NSD in rates of use of additional studies. Missed diagnosis in 10% of cases |
| **Ophthalmology** | |
| Teleophthalmology for patients presenting in emergency department[57] | 400% reduction in referrals for urgent assessment, 37% reduction in nonurgent referrals |
| Examination of patients with glaucoma[58] | At 300 consultations per year, costs of telemedicine and visits equal except for US$55 savings per visit in travel costs |
| **Pathology** | |
| Processing of histopathology specimens[59] | Cost of telepathology 15% more than courier, 18% less than on-site pathology at a small centre |

Note: NICU = neonatal intensive care unit, NSS = not statistically significant.
*A fuller description of the studies referred to in the table is available from the authors.

shown that specialist consultations in the field of otorhinolaryngology can be performed in a cost-saving way when the workload exceeds a certain number of patients.[18]

Pilot projects in telepsychiatry, the provision of orthopedic and dermatology services via telemedicine and the evaluation of the costs and benefits of a prison telemedicine program used a similar approach.[22,23,47] Such studies that give a clear number needed to treat by the telemedicine option are helpful for decision-makers when faced with the question of whether or not to start a new telemedicine service. Teledermatology, with short distances (26 km) between sites, appeared not to be cost-saving in one study.[52]

The quality of the economic analysis in the papers was relatively low, with a few exceptions. The papers by Bergmo,[18,39] Agha and colleagues,[59] Stensland and colleagues,[22] Halvorsen and colleagues[34] and Wootton and colleagues[52] provide examples of better-quality economic studies. The costs included varied significantly among studies, so that comparison of the cost estimates may not be feasible in many cases. There were also several economic studies that did not give detailed information about the empirical background of the costs or benefits, or both, included in the calculations. These studies were excluded from the review. For example, we excluded a teleradiology cost–benefit analysis,[60] because the theoretically good economic model did not make use of the empirical cost and benefit estimations made at specific sites by the study group.

## Interpretation

The review shows that there are still few data on the effectiveness and cost-effectiveness of telemedicine. Of the more than 1000 articles surveyed, most were reports about the feasibility of various applications, and only a few of the studies reported a controlled comparison of a telemedicine application with conventional means of providing services.

The review indicates that, at the moment, the most convincing published evidence regarding the effectiveness of telemedicine deals with teleradiology, teleneurosurgery (transmission of CT images before patient transfer), telepsychiatry, transmission of echocardiographic images, and the use of electronic referrals enabling email consultations and video conferencing between primary and secondary health care providers. However, even for these applications, most of the available literature refers only to pilot projects and short-term outcomes, and in many cases the efficacy of the application was being considered, rather than its effectiveness. Promising results have been obtained for the transmission of electrocardiograms and teledermatology. For other applications, scientific data concerning the effectiveness of telemedicine remain limited.

There are still few cost-effectiveness studies of telemedicine. A systematic comparison of the costs and more work on the effects of the alternatives should be done in the future. Although the term "cost-effectiveness" was frequently used in the studies, the effectiveness (and sometimes costs) were assumed to be established for telemedicine without any scientific evidence. As a result, decision-makers must be cautious regarding the degree to which they can apply the results of such assessments to their own circumstances. Assessments of telemedicine have so far been on stronger ground when considering the effects of the technology on the time-related consequences of health care services and on organizational issues.

Five years ago, an editorial in the *Lancet* stated that "although much is claimed, the economic benefits of telemedicine have yet to be proved."[61] Although a limited number of telemedicine applications have up to now been shown to be effective and cost-effective in specific settings, that original conclusion still remains valid for most of the suggested ways in which to use telemedicine. Although a number of detailed studies are in progress in several countries, the assessment literature has yet to address aspects of telemedicine applications as they move into routine use, or their longer-term impact on health status, costs and organization. Other dimensions will also require consideration when formulating approaches to further economic analysis. These will include the sustainability of a telemedicine service, decisions about equipment and telecommunications, impact on the overall use of health program resources and measurement of outcomes.[62]

We conclude that further assessment studies in the field of telemedicine are still clearly needed. Decision-makers who are under public and commercial pressure to start new telemedicine services should link the implementation of new and, in many instances, costly technology to realistic development of a business case and subsequent data collection and analysis. Guidance for performing such an assessment can be found easily in a number of frameworks formulated by various authors.[1,8,63–67]

*Competing interests:* None declared.

*Contributors:* Drs. Roine and Ohinmaa selected and reviewed the retrieved abstracts and papers. Dr. Hailey assisted in checking papers and in preparing the classification of selected studies. The text of the manuscript was prepared collaboratively by all 3 authors.

*Acknowledgements:* The help of Ms. Leigh-Ann Topfer, Institute of Health Economics, Edmonton, Alta., in undertaking the literature searches is gratefully acknowledged. An earlier version of this systematic review (covering literature until November 1998) has been published as part of a joint report by the Finnish Office for Health Care Technology Assessment and the Alberta Heritage Foundation for Medical Research in August 1999.

## References

1. Hailey D, Jacobs P. *Assessment of telehealth applications.* Edmonton (Alta): Alberta Heritage Foundation for Medical Research; 1997.
2. Grigsby J, Kaehny M, Sandberg EJ, Schlenker RE, Shaughnessy PW. Effects and effectiveness of telemedicine. *Health Care Financ Rev* 1995;17:115-31.
3. Baer L, Elford R, Cukor P. Telepsychiatry at forty: What have we learned? *Harv Rev Psychiatry* 1997;5:7-17.
4. Wootton R. Telemedicine: a cautious welcome. *BMJ* 1996;313:1375-7.
5. Taylor P. A survey of research in telemedicine. 2: Telemedicine services. *J Telemed Telecare* 1998;4:63-71.
6. Wootton R. Telemedicine: the current state of the art. *Minim Invasive Ther Allied Technol* 1997;5/6:393-403.
7. Allen A. A review of cost effectiveness research. *Telemed Today* 1998;6:10-2,14-5.
8. McDonald I, Hill S, Daly J, Crowe B. *Evaluating telemedicine in Victoria: a generic framework.* Melbourne (Australia): Centre for the Study of Clinical Practice, St. Vincent's Hospital; 1997.

9. Jovell AJ, Navarro-Rubio MD. Evaluation de la evidencia cientifica. *Med Clin (Barc)* 1995;105:740-3.

10. Conrath DW, Dunn EV, Bloor WG, Tranquada B. A clinical evaluation of four alternative telemedicine systems. *Behav Sci* 1977;22:12-21.

11. Muller C, Marshall CL, Krasner M, Cunningham N, Wallerstein E, Thomstad B. Cost factors in urban telemedicine. *Med Care* 1977;15:251-9.

12. Brecht RM, Gray CL, Peterson C, Youngblood B. The University of Texas Medical Branch — Texas Department of Criminal Justice Telemedicine Project: findings from the first year of operation. *Telemed J* 1996;2:25-35.

13. McCue MJ, Mazmanian PE, Hampton C, Marks TK, Fisher E, Parpart F, et al. The case of Powhatan Correctional Center/Virginia Department of Corrections and Virginia Commonwealth University/Medical College of Virginia. *Telemed J* 1997;3(1):11-7.

14. Hayes WS, Tohme WG, Komo D, Dai H, Persad SG, Benavides A, et al. A telemedicine consultative service for the evaluation of patients with urolithiasis. *Urology* 1998;51:39-43.

15. Harno KSR. Telemedicine in managing demand for secondary-care services. *J Telemed Telecare* 1999;5:189-92.

16. Harno K, Arajärvi E, Paavola T, Carlson C, Viikinkoski P, Böckerman M, et al. *Assessment of an electronic referral and teleconsultation system between secondary and primary health care.* Helsinki (Finland): FinOHTA; 1999. Report no.: 10.

17. Harrison R, Clayton W, Wallace P. Virtual outreach: a telemedicine pilot study using a cluster-randomized controlled design. *J Telemed Telecare* 1999;5:126-30.

18. Bergmo TS. An economic analysis of teleconsultation in otorhinolaryngology. *J Telemed Telecare* 1997;3:194-9.

19. Crump WJ, Tessen RJ. Communication in integrated practice networks: using interactive video technology to build the medical office without walls. *Tex Med* 1997;93:70-4.

20. Doolittle GC, Williams A, Harmon A, Allen A, Boysen CD, Wittman C, et al. A cost measurement study for a tele-oncology practice. *J Telemed Telecare* 1998;4:84-8.

21. Pal B, Laing H, Estrach C. A cyberclinic in rheumatology. *J R Coll Physicians Lond* 1999;33:161-2.

22. Stensland J, Speedie SM, Ideker M, House J, Thompson T. The relative cost of outpatient telemedicine services. *Telemed J* 1999;5:245-56.

23. Zollo S, Kienzle M, Loeffelholz P, Sebille S. Telemedicine to Iowa's correctional facilities: initial clinical experience and assessment of program costs. *Telemed J* 1999;5:291-301.

24. Sparks KE, Shaw DK, Eddy D, Hanigosky P, Vantrese J. Alternatives for cardiac rehabilitation patients unable to return to a hospital-based program. *Heart Lung* 1993;22:298-303.

25. Turnin MC, Bolzonella-Pene C, Dumoulin S, Cerf I, Charpentier G, Sandre-Banon D, et al. Evaluation multicentrique du systeme telematique Nutri-Expert aupres de patients diabetiques. *Diabetes Metab* 1995;21:26-33.

26. Wu J, Kessler DK, Chakko S, Kessler KM. A cost-effectiveness strategy for transtelephonic arrhythmia monitoring. *Am J Cardiol* 1995;75:184-5.

27. Albisser AM, Harris RI, Sakkal S, Parson ID, Chao SC. Diabetes intervention in the information age. *Med Inf* 1996;21:297-316.

28. Friedman RH, Kazis LE, Jette A, Smith MB, Stollerman J, Torgerson J, et al. A telecommunications system for monitoring and counseling patients with hypertension. Impact on medication adherence and blood pressure control. *Am J Hypertens* 1996;9(4 Pt1):285-92.

29. Piette JD, Weinberger M, McPhee SJ. The effect of automated calls with telephone nurse follow-up on patient-centered outcomes of diabetes care. *Med Care* 2000;38:218-30.

30. Piette JD, Weinberger M, McPhee SJ, Mah CA, Kraemer FB, Crapo LM. Do automated calls with nurse follow-up improve self-care and glycemic control among vulnerable patients with diabetes? *Am J Med* 2000;108:20-7.

31. Spencer JA, Dobson D, Hoare M, Molyneux AJ, Anslow PL. The use of a computerized image transfer system linking a regional neuroradiology centre to its district hospitals. *Clin Radiol* 1991;44:342-4.

32. Eljamel MS, Nixon T. The use of a computer-based image link system to assist inter-hospital referrals. *Br J Neurosurg* 1992;6:559-62.

33. Teslow TN, Gilbert RA, Grant WH III, Woo SY, Butler EB, Liem JH. A teleradiology case conference system. *J Telemed Telecare* 1995;1:95-9.

34. Halvorsen PA, Kristiansen IS. Radiology services for remote communities: cost minimisation study of telemedicine. *BMJ* 1996;312:1333-6.

35. Fery-Lemonnier E, Brayda E, Charpentier E, Couturon I, Fay A, Souag A. *Transmission interhospitaliere d'images radiologiques pour la prise en charge des urgences neurochirurgicales. Resultats de l'evaluation.* Paris: Comité d'Evaluation et de Diffusion des Innovations Technologiques (CEDIT); 1996.

36. Bailes JE, Poole CC, Hutchison W, Maroon JC, Fukushima T. Utilization and cost savings of a wide-area computer network for neurosurgical consultation. *Telemed J* 1997;3:135-9.

37. Goh KYC, Lam CK, Poon WS. The impact of teleradiology on the inter-hospital transfer of neurosurgical patients. *Br J Neurosurg* 1997;11:52-6.

38. Heautot JF, Gibaud B, Catroux B, Thoreux PH, Cordonnier E, Scarabin JM, et al. Influence of the teleradiology technology (N-ISDN and ATM) on the inter-hospital management of neurosurgical patients. *Med Inform Internet Med* 1999;24:121-34.

39. Bergmo TS. An economic analysis of teleradiology versus a visiting radiologist service. *J Telemed Telecare* 1996;2:136-42.

40. Davis MC. Teleradiology in rural imaging centres. *J Telemed Telecare* 1997;3:146-53.

41. Lehmann KJ, Walz M, Bolte R, Georgi M, Schinkmann M, Busch C. Einsatzmöglichkeiten des KAMEDIN-Teleradiologiesystems unter besonderer Berücksichtung einer Wirtschaftlichkeitsanalyse. *Radiologe* 1997;37:278-84.

42. Stoeger A, Strohmayr W, Giacomuzzi SM, Dessl A, Buchberger W, Jaschke W. A cost analysis of an emergency computerized tomography teleradiology system. *J Telemed Telecare* 1997;3:35-9.

43. Malone FD, Athanassiou A, Craigo SD, Simpson LL, D'Alton ME. Cost issues surrounding the use of computerized telemedicine for obstetric ultrasonography. *Ultrasound Obstet Gynecol* 1998;12:120-4.

44. Trippi JA, Lee KS, Kopp G, Nelson DR, Yee KG, Cordell WH. Dobutamine stress tele-echocardiography for evaluation of emergency department patients with chest pain. *J Am Coll Cardiol* 1997;30:627-32.

45. Brennan JA, Kealy JA, Gerardi LH, Shih R, Allegra J, Sannipoli L, et al. Telemedicine in the emergency department: a randomized controlled trial. *J Telemed Telecare* 1999;5:18-22.

46. Giovas P, Papadoyannis D, Thomakos D, Papazachos G, Rallidis M, Soulis D, et al. Transmission of electrocardiograms from a moving ambulance. *J Telemed Telecare* 1998;4(Suppl 1):5-7.

47. Doze S, Simpson J, Hailey D, Jacobs P. Evaluation of a telepsychiatry pilot project. *J Telemed Telecare* 1999;5:38-46.

48. Trott P, Blignault I. Cost evaluation of a telepsychiatry service in northern Queensland. *J Telemed Telecare* 1998;4(Suppl 1):66-68.

49. Zelickson BD, Homan L. Teledermatology in the nursing home. *Arch Dermatol* 1997;133:171-4.

50. Loane MA, Corbett R, Bloomer SE, Eedy DJ, Gore HE, Mathews C, et al. Diagnostic accuracy and clinical management by realtime teledermatology. Results from the Northern Ireland arms of the UK Multicentre Teledermatology Trial. *J Telemed Telecare* 1998;4:95-100.

51. Perednia DA, Wallace J, Morrisey M, Bartlett M, Marchionda L, Gibson A, et al. The effect of a teledermatology program on rural referral patterns to dermatologists and the management of skin diseases. *Medinfo* 1998;9(Pt 1):290-3.

52. Wootton R, Bloomer SE, Corbett R, Eedy DJ, Hicks N, Lotery HE, et al. Multicentre randomised control trial comparing real time teledermatology with conventional outpatient dermatological care: societal cost-benefit analysis. *BMJ* 2000;320:1252-6.

53. Finley JP, Sharratt GP, Nanton MA, Chen RP, Bryan P, Wolstenholme J, et al. Paediatric echocardiography by telemedicine — nine years' experience. *J Telemed Telecare* 1997;3:200-4.

54. Rendina MC, Downs SM, Carasco N, Loonsk J, Bose CL. Effect of telemedicine on health outcomes in 87 infants requiring neonatal intensive care. *Telemed J* 1998;4:345-51.

55. Rendina MC, Bose CL, Gallaher KJ, Long WA, Ciszek TA, Baush CM, et al. The effect of a neonatal telecardiology system on respiratory therapy in very low birthweight infants. *Medinfo* 1998;9(Pt 1):298-301.

56. McConnell ME, Steed RD, Tichenor JM, Hannon DW. Interactive teleradiology for evaluation of heart murmurs in children. *Telemed J* 1999;5:157-61.

57. Blackwell NAM, Kelly GJ, Lenton LM. Telemedicine ophthalmology consultation in remote Queensland. *Med J Aust* 1997;167:583-6.

58. Tuulonen A, Ohinmaa A, Alanko HI, Hyytinen P, Juutinen A, Toppinen E. The application of teleophthalmology in examining patients with glaucoma: a pilot study. *J Glaucoma* 1999;8:367-73.

59. Agha Z, Weinstein RS, Dunn BE. Cost minimization analysis of telepathology. *Am J Clin Pathol* 1999;112:470-8.

60. Heckermann D, Wetekam V, Hundt W, Reiser M. Nutzwert-und Wirtschaftlichkeitsanalyse verschiedener Teleradiologieszenarien. *Radiologe* 1997;37:285-93.

61. Telemedicine: Fad or future? *Lancet* 1995;345:73-4.

62. Hailey D, Jennett P. The evolution of economic evaluation of telemedicine applications. *G7/8 SP4 Workshop — towards a framework for evaluation of telemedicine;* 1999 Feb 19-20; Melbourne (Australia). Melbourne: Australian Department of Health and Aged Care; updated 1999 July 5. Available: http://partners.health.gov.au/index.htm (accessed 2001 Aug 20).

63. Perednia DA. Telemedicine system evaluation, transaction models, and multicentered research. *J AHIMA* 1996;67:60-3

64. Institute of Medicine. Committee on evaluating clinical applications of telemedicine. In: Field MF, editor. *Telemedicine: a guide to assessing telecommunications in health.* Washington: National Academy Press; 1996.

65. McIntosh E, Cairns J. A framework for the economic evaluation of telemedicine. *J Telemed Telecare* 1997;3:132-9.

66. Ohinmaa A, Reponen J, Working Group. *A model for the assessment of telemedicine and a plan for testing the model within five specialities.* Helsinki (Finland): National Research and Development Centre for Welfare & Health (STAKES); 1997. FinOHTA report no.: 5.

67. Sisk JE, Sanders JH. A proposed framework for economic evaluation of telemedicine. *Telemed J* 1998;4:31-7.

**Correspondence to:** Dr. David Hailey, Alberta Heritage Foundation for Medical Research, Suite 1500, 10104 – 103 Avenue, Edmonton AB T5J 4A7; fax 780 429 3509; dhailey@interact.net.au

# Meeting patients' needs with patient information systems: potential benefits of qualitative research methods

Annemarie van 't Riet [a], Marc Berg [a,*], Frans Hiddema [b], Kees Sol [b]

[a] *Institute of Health Policy and Management, Erasmus University Rotterdam, L4-117, P.O. Box 1738, 3000 DR Rotterdam, The Netherlands*
[b] *Eye Hospital Rotterdam, P.O. Box 70030, 3000 LM Rotterdam, The Netherlands*

Received 9 January 2001; accepted 4 July 2001

## Abstract

This article reports on our pilot evaluation of an electronic patient information system for children with amblyopia and their parents. The aim was to investigate whether the information system would be able to improve the quality of care, as indicated by an improvement in the effectiveness and efficiency of care, and in an increase in patient satisfaction. In the pilot evaluation, we used qualitative research methods, exploring the impact of the information system on children and their parents, with the aim to find suitable indicators for a potential further, quantitative study. Yet we found that the system was little used and had marginal effects on the quality of care for children with amblyopia and their parents. It appeared that the main problem underlying this patient information system was that the needs of those people who actually would be using the system had never really been investigated. The designers had built their assumptions about these needs into the system. These appeared to be mistaken at so many levels that the system could not become a success. As a result of this pilot evaluation, the patient information project was thoroughly transformed. This study makes clear that a thorough exploration of user needs before building the system, using qualitative research methods, may be crucial because it can prevent mismatches and maximizes the chance that the eventual information system meets its most important aim: to enhance patient empowerment and improve the quality of care. © 2001 Elsevier Science Ireland Ltd. All rights reserved.

*Keywords:* Electronic patient information system; Amblyopia; Pilot evaluation; Quality of care; Qualitative research methods

## 1. Introduction

Adequate patient information is important for the quality of care: it is one of the key indicators of patient satisfaction and it improves the effectiveness and efficiency of care giving [1]. The traditional means of disseminating patient information is the face-to-face explanation of the caregiver to the patient during the consultation. More extensive, background information can be given through paper-based flyers and, more re-

---

* Corresponding author.
*E-mail address:* m.berg@bmg.eur.nl (M. Berg).

cently, videos. The problem with these media, however, is that they address the 'average' patient, and deliver a uni-directional flow of information in a pre-fixed sequence. Electronic patient information systems, on the other hand, can use more interactive ways of informing patients, and may thus be better geared towards the needs and capacities of individual patients. In addition, electronic patient information systems can establish virtual meeting groups for patients, discussion lists, or occasions for (public or private) electronic interchanges between patients and experts. Through these means, such systems may enhance social support systems, may support patient decision making and planning [2], enhance the patient's trust in the caregiver and increase compliance [3].

Patient information systems are increasingly popular, but there are not many documented success stories about patient information systems (see for a concise review [4]). A core issue for such systems is their 'usability', which includes the extent to which the system takes the actual user's needs and capacities into account (ibid.). This issue might seem obvious, but failing to meet users' needs has been a recurrent failure factor in the wider field of information system development [5–7], and is often caused by paying too little attention to these needs in the early, design phase of the system [8–11]. For the success of patient information systems, the necessity to address the projected users' needs is especially vital.

This article reports on our pilot evaluation of an electronic patient information system for children with amblyopia and their parents. Building upon the work of Forsythe and others, we will argue that qualitative research methods, as we used in our evaluation, can be of help in meeting patients' needs with patient information systems.

## 2. Background

In amblyopia, normal vision in one eye fails to develop because of a difference in vision between the two eyes in early life. Amblyopia can only develop in very young children and the treatment has to start as early as possible, but in any case before the child has reached the age of 6 years. Treatment usually involves patching the unaffected eye to stimulate the use of the amblyopic eye. To improve the quality of care for children with amblyopia and their parents the Rotterdam Eye Hospital has developed an interactive, electronic patient information system directed at both the children and the adults [12].

The Rotterdam Eye Hospital is the only freestanding hospital in the Netherlands that is specifically oriented towards eye afflictions. More than 125 000 patients a year visit the hospital and there are approximately 9500 operations each year. At the moment that the Internet was becoming a frequently used medium in the Netherlands, the Eye Hospital wanted to find out if using this medium for giving patient information could help improve the quality of care. They chose children with amblyopia and their parents as a target-group, because amblyopia is a frequently occurring eye-problem (in the Netherlands amblyopia affects one of every 40 children) and because children and their parents were considered to be a population that were more commonly using computers than older people. [Had another frequent affliction been chosen (such as, e.g. glaucoma), the target population would have been unlikely to be very computer-oriented].

The Rotterdam Eye Hospital developed the patient information system for children with amblyopia and their parents together with the Dutch Digital Hospital[1]. The Dutch

[1] www.ziekenhuis.nl

Digital Hospital is an organization that develops information technology-based communication and information tools, focused on patients and healthcare employees, for the whole hospital sector. They assisted the Eye Hospital primarily with the technical aspects of building the system components.

The system consisted of a CD-ROM and an Internet site. The basic material on the CD-ROM had been developed a few years earlier by the Rotterdam Eye Hospital, together with other CD-ROMs directed at other eye-afflictions. The amblyopia CD-ROM contained information on the Rotterdam Eye Hospital, on amblyopia, on the investigations done to establish the diagnosis of amblyopia, on possible results of these tests, on causes, consequences and treatment methods of amblyopia, and on possible complications. The information was presented by an orthoptist, an ophthalmologist and a child health center physician in brief video fragments. Other fragments showed amblyopic children and parents speaking about their experiences. In addition, the CD-ROM featured a cartoon about Paul, a boy with amblyopia, who wears glasses and an eye patch. At school the other kids make fun of him, until the teacher tells them to make a pair of glasses from paper. Paul's pair of glasses turns out to be the most beautiful.

The Internet site, specifically developed for this project by the Dutch Digital Hospital, consisted of four parts: a Chatbox, a Question and Answers section, a Newsletter and Games. The Chatbox afforded virtual contact with fellow sufferers, supervised by an orthoptist or ophthalmologist. During the pilot evaluation phase, the Chatbox was open for use 1 night a week, during 1 h (see also Section 4.3). In the Question and Answer section patients could ask questions to one another. The Newsletter was a general information bulletin of the Rotterdam Eye Hospital, featuring medical news items on eye treatments and so forth. The Games, which were not especially designed for this project, consisted of coloring pictures, simple computer games and jokes for children. In the design of both the Internet site and the CD-ROM, images and voice recordings were used so as to make them accessible for children.

## 3. Methods

### 3.1. Research approach

To find out whether this electronic information system for patient information giving would improve the quality of care, the Eye Hospital wanted a scientific evaluation of the system. Their initial idea was that a controlled study would have to be done to proof the increased effectiveness, efficiency and patient satisfaction that this system would bring. Some 200 patients would constitute a control group, who would receive the common information that is given to patients with amblyopia (like paper-based flyers and videotapes). The experimental group—also some 200 patients—would use the electronic information system. The Eye Hospital asked the Institute of Health Policy and Management from the Erasmus University Rotterdam to perform this evaluation. The researchers of the Erasmus University, however, doubted whether the proposed evaluation design was suitable for this situation. It was not clear as yet what kind of effects could be expected from the system. Also it was still a question what kind of impacts would be interesting and valuable to explore in the quantitative study. It was still even unclear whether such a larger evaluation would be feasible at all. Because of all these unanswered questions we decided to do a small qualitative pilot evaluation first.

Qualitative research is primarily inductive and explorative in its procedures; it is therefore perfectly suited in situations such as these, where the *nature* of the impacts are to be investigated, and where the question *why*, and on which dimensions, the patient information system would be (un)successful is of paramount importance [13–16]. The research consisted primarily of in-depth interviews with users of the patient information system. These interview data were complemented with an in-depth exploration of the functionality of the patient information system, observation of orthoptist's and ophthalmologist's consultations, observation of the system in the actual setting of use (i.e. the patient's home), and virtual observation of chat sessions. All data gathering activities were performed by Annemarie van't Riet.

During some days the orthoptists that participated in the project were asking the patients that were visiting them to join the project. If they did, they received the CD-ROM from their orthoptist. The first 17 families who joined the project were also asked whether they would want to join the evaluation of the project. Of the 17 families, 14 families did so. Three families did not want to join the evaluation because of a lack of interest or a lack of time. One of the families had two children with amblyopia, so in all 15 children joined the evaluation. The age of the parents who joined the evaluation was between 29 and 60 years old; their mean age was 35 years. The age of the children was between 2 and 9 years old, mean age 4.9 years. Most of the parents were highly educated; in nine out of 14 families at least one of the parents had a college degree. Only two of the 15 patients were 'new' patients (defined as being in treatment for less than 3 months) at the moment of joining the project. The other patients had been in treatment by the orthoptist between 4 and 89 months (mean:

24.3 months) at the moment that they joined the project.

We first did some observations of orthoptist's and ophthalmologist's consultations. This primarily served to make us familiar with the treatment setting of amblyopia. It taught us how patients and caregivers deal with amblyopia and it showed us what kind of questions patients ask during a consultation and what kind of information is given by the caregivers. During the in-depth exploration of the functionality of the patient information system we worked with the system as if we were a patient looking for information. We did this to find out how the system was set up, how it works in practice and to get a feel for what kind of information the system gives. Virtual observations of chat sessions were also data sources. These showed us how many people joined the chat sessions, how long they stayed in the chat box, what kind of questions they asked, to whom they preferred to talk and what type of discussions ensued. We wrote down our observations in a notebook, and from every chat session we could print out the dialogues.

As a result of these three brief investigations, we were more familiar with the context in which the information system would operate. We subsequently undertook in-depth interviews with one or both parents of the 14 families. We had planned to ask the children themselves some questions too, but soon it appeared that almost all of them were too young or too shy to answer our questions. So parents informed us about the experience of their child with amblyopia and what their child had done with the project and how he or she liked it. The interviews were semi-structured and open-ended, which means that, although there was a topic list, the respondents were able to tell their own story about their experience with amblyopia and the information system. Topics were for example the respondent's experience with amblyopia, information collection about amblyopia, contact with the ophthalmologist and orthoptist, the reason of joining the project, computer experience, opinion about the CD-ROM and about the internet components, potential benefits from the patient information system and the overall opinion about the project. The interviews were all tape-recorded and transcribed. Finally, we also undertook observation of the system in the actual setting of use (i.e. the patient's home). This made clear how patients actually worked with the system, which parts of the system they used and how they liked it. A written report was made from every observation. As a result of these different research methods there were three different types of textual documents to analyze (observation notes, interview texts, and print outs from the chat sessions). All these documents were coded, and the codes were subsequently clustered per topic. The initial coding categories and topics were partly derived from our original interest in the different potential impacts of the patient information system (see also Section 3.2), but also emerged from the observations and interviews themselves. In addition, the analysis of the empirical material was crucial in the iterative refinement and categorization of the codes [13,14].

## 3.2. Operationalization of research questions

The aim of our qualitative pilot evaluation, then, was to find out which effects could be expected from the system, which effects would be interesting and valuable to explore in a quantitative study, and how these effects could be measured. The starting question of the Eye Hospital had been to investigate whether this information system would improve the quality of delivered care—as measured by the effectiveness and efficiency of the system, and the patients' satisfaction in using it.

These three key aspects, often used as the core dimensions of the quality of care [17], are by themselves rather indefinite terms, requiring operationalization. The aspects 'effectiveness' and 'efficiency' were each made operational by selecting indicators that were expected to be affected by the introduction of the system. These indicators covered different dimensions of these key aspects (for the selected indicators per key aspect see Figs. 1–3). Some of the indicators were drawn from documents stating the Eye Hospital's own expectations about the system [12,18]; other indicators were added by the researchers on the basis of our initial experiences with the system (through the initial observations). The kind of indicators we selected are common in evaluation studies of patient information systems [1,19–21].

- use of the system  (patients/parents would use the system)
- trust in caregivers  (trust in caregivers would increase)
- support network  (informal support networks would emerge or grow)
- patient's anxiety  (patient's/parents' anxiety would be reduced)
- coping ability  (patient's/parents' ability to cope would be increased)
- compliance  (patient's/parents' compliance would be increased)
- outcome of the treatment  (better vision would be achieved)
- quality of life  (patient's/parents' quality of life would increase)

Fig. 1. Selected indicators of the effectiveness of the patient information system, and the expectation of the impact of the system on the indicator.

- costs for gathering information   (parents costs for gathering information would be reduced)
- amount of consultations   (the amount of consultations per patient would be reduced)
- length of waiting lists   (the Eye Hospital's waiting lists would be reduced)

Fig. 2. Selected indicators of efficiency of the patient information system, and the expectation of the impact of the system on the indicator.

The 'effectiveness' of an intervention in the medical care process is ideally measured in terms of whether it achieves a better clinical outcome for the patient, and a higher quality of life. Yet in the case of this research, these indicators were deemed to be very ambitious. A patient information system is not an ordinary 'treatment' intervention; it may very well be beneficial to the patient without directly impacting on the outcome of the treatment to which it is geared. It may, for example, help to reduce anxiety, or help build trust in the caregivers. So we added other indicators, and we listed them in the order of increasing ambition: the further the indicator in the list, the more ambitious the goals to be achieved by the system. Both that the system is 'used' and that the system improves 'quality of life', for example, are indicators of 'effectiveness'—yet the former indicator is a much less ambitious goal than the latter (see Fig. 1).

A similar hierarchy of indicators was created for the aspect of 'efficiency': although the Eye Hospital ultimately hoped to reduce waiting lists through the utilization of this system, it was also deemed to be important to study some more realizable efficiency gains (see Fig. 2). Again, these lists of indicators and their mutual relations emerged iteratively by drawing upon the Eye Hospital's starting documents and our initial experiences with the system and its contexts of use. The hierarchies we describe are certainly not absolute, nor are the lists themselves intended to be complete nor mutually exclusive. Their main purpose was to function as a heuristic starting point for the interview's topic list, and for the analysis of the data obtained.

The satisfaction of patients with the patient information system finally, was investigated by several different features of the system (see Fig. 3). These features were not listed in increasing ambition, because here there is no question of more or less ambitious indicators; they all are different, equally important features of the system.

## 4. Results

### 4.1. Effectiveness

The actual *use of the system* by the patients was disappointing. Most families only checked the CD-ROM once or twice. Afterwards, they never used the CD-ROM again. From the Internet site, only the Chatbox part was really used, but just by half of the 14 respondents. The only reason to use the Chatbox was to ask questions to the orthoptist or the ophthalmologist. No chatting between users evolved. As a result, a *support network* did not emerge or grow through use of the system.

Almost all of the respondents, on the other hand, stated that the system had a positive influence on the *trust* they had in their caregivers. These respondents felt that the very existence of the system showed that caregivers took amblyopia seriously, that there were many professionals working on it and that these professionals would be easily accessible when they would need them. The system, however, did not reduce the children's and parents' *anxiety*. The reason for this was not primarily that the patient information system was not used much—although this in itself made a high impact on the emotional well-being of patients and their parents unlikely. The principal reason of a lack of impact was that the amblyopia problem did not create much anxiety in the children and parents in the first place. Our respondents stated that they did feel a bit frightened when the diagnosis amblyopia was made: they were uncertain about the consequences of this diagnosis, and worried about the impact of it on their child. Yet this did not last long, and a state of anxiety did not develop. All respondents indicated that they soon realized that amblyopia is not a severe illness, that it is a temporary affliction, and that it can be treated well if they follow the instructions from the orthoptist. Where there is no patient's anxiety, a patient information system cannot reduce it. Similar conclusions can be made with regards to the system's effect on the *coping ability* of patients and their parents. Because most children do not really suffer from their affliction at all (see also Section 3.2), there is not much to cope with in the first place.

Three of the 14 respondents said that the information system made it easier to follow the instructions from the orthoptist, and some respondents stated that the information system would make it possible to better prepare oneself for consultations with the caregivers. Most respondents, however, stated that the system did not have an effect on their *compliance* at all. These respondents stated that they already followed the instructions from the orthoptist strictly. Further-more, most parents also indicated that the system would not be able to stimulate children's patching, because children cannot do much with the system and because it is too difficult for them to relate the information the system gives to their own treatment. The parents stated that if they were motivated to patch the eye well, their children were in a short time also well motivated. The information, therefore, should be primarily directed at the parents rather than at the child.

With regards to the indicators *treatment outcome* and *quality of life*, finally, it can be safely deduced that the impact of the system was negligible. The system was hardly used and compliance with treatment was already high. In addition, most parents indicated that amblyopia could not be said to reduce the quality of life in the first place.

## 4.2. Efficiency

The information system did not seem to decrease the *costs for gathering information* by patients. If anything, the opposite was true. Most respondents had never before gathered information themselves outside the context of the consultations with their caregivers and the flyers and booklets they obtained from them. All the costs they made in using this information system (for instance, the patients were supposed to buy the CD-ROM and had to access the Internet from their homes), therefore, were additional costs.

The system could lead to a reduction in the *amount of consultations per patient* in two ways: a patient's condition could improve

- interactive, electronic nature of information system
- accessibility of system
- user-friendliness of system
- fit between content and functionality of system and needs and capacities of target group

Fig. 3. Patient satisfaction: the features of the patient information system investigated.

faster through better compliance, or the number of consultations that center on the providing of information could be reduced. The first route, it has become clear, could not emerge. The second route also appeared to be very unlikely, because most parents and orthoptists who were enrolled in the pilot evaluation indicated that consultations were rarely requested just to ask questions. On the other hand, the fact that parents used the Chatbox to consult their caregivers could have led to a reduction in the number of telephonic consultations. Since the Chatbox was not often used, this potential effect did not actually occur.

*Waiting lists*, finally, could also be reduced through a reduction in the number of consultations. This did not occur, however. In addition, waiting lists could also be reduced when the number of consultations would not decrease, but the duration of these consultations would reduce. We did not actually measure consultation lengths in this study, but we conjecture that this hope is problematic, because it might equally be possible that more informed patients lead to even *longer* consultations rather than shorter ones. For some people, all this additional information might lead to information overload [22] and even to extreme anxiety [23]. In addition to being an unwanted effect in and by itself, these 'side effects' of supplying more information may by itself increase physicians' workloads [24].

### 4.3. Patient satisfaction: the lack of fit between the system and the user's needs

The respondents appreciated the *interactive, electronic nature* of the patient information system (computer, CD-ROM and Internet). They preferred these media to other possible media. If, for instance, they had to choose between a book, a videotape or a CD-ROM, they would opt for the last one.

Contrary to an information leaflet, the *accessibility* of a CD-ROM and Internet-based information system is dependent on the availability of a computer, a CD-ROM player and Internet access. Although current Internet and PC utilization rates are still increasing, at the moment we started this research still a large part of the Dutch population would not be able to access this system. At the end of 1999 one-third of Dutch households, for example, did not have a computer and two-thirds of the households did not have access to the Internet [25]. Because the participants of the pilot evaluation did have a computer, CD-ROM player and Internet access (otherwise they would not have been participants in the pilot), they all rated the *accessibility* of the information system as good.

In general the respondents were satisfied with the *user-friendliness* of the information system when it came to the adult users, although most of the parents complained about the structure of the content on the CD-ROM and the Internet site. Considering the user-friendliness for children, however, the respondents were not satisfied at all. For most children in our evaluation sample, both the content of the information and the operation of the CD-ROM and the Internet site were much too difficult.

The respondents, finally, were not satisfied at all about the *fit between the content and functionality of system and the needs and capacities of target group*. During the analysis of the data, this lack of fit appeared to be the main problematic feature of the system, explaining much of the low impact on the effectiveness and efficiency indicators. First of all, the children themselves, a core target group, could do almost nothing with the system, because the system seemed to be designed for an age group that was older than the average age of the children who actually constitute the target group. Parents estimated that 7 years would be the minimal age for a child to do something meaningful with the system (i.e. to use the system in such a way that it would affect the child in any of the ways hoped for by the designers of the system). However, the Eye Hospital's orthoptists stated that the majority of children are diagnosed with amblyopia, and have to start patching the eye, at the age of approximately 2–4. And such children are too young to be able to talk about their eye and their treatment or to be interested in it:

> For him it's just 'oh the patch has to be stuck on my eye, well, just do it'. And anyway... he doesn't ask questions of course. A 4-year-old just accepts such things (respondent K).

When the children reach the age at which they can really use the system, they are often already 'experienced eye patchers' that no longer need an information system such as this:

> It is well done for the older kids. But when the kids get older, the frequency of the patching decreases. And then you're so familiar with it, that you don't need something like this anymore (respondent F).

Second, several more specific features of the system were criticized by the parents as being poorly adapted to their needs. The Chatbox, for example, was operational only between 19:00 and 20:00 h, 1 night a week. That is a very poor choice, because this time slot is exactly 'rush hour' in Dutch households with young children, who are then be-

ing fed, bathed, and put to bed. As another example, parents felt it was very unpractical that they could only ask their questions to their caregivers once a week. They do not need real-time on-line contact with these professionals: they would rather like to be able to put their questions on a discussion list that can be accessed whenever they please.

Thirdly, parents indicated that they have only a minimal need for an information system such as this. A child with amblyopia is not thought to be afflicted with a serious condition, nor is it seen to have much impact on daily life. Furthermore, most parents report no difficulties with the treatment of amblyopia. Children usually get used to wearing the patch rather fast, and then they become rapidly indifferent to it. In addition, amblyopia is so frequent that most parents reported no awkward reactions from their environments. A patched eye is not something 'strange': most children were never teased. One of the basic assumptions built into the information system, however, is that having a patched eye is something you suffer from, that sets you apart (like in the cartoon of Paul), that pains parents, and that therefore requires support both for the child and his/her parents. Parents, however, argue that they do not need the support or the contacts a (virtual) parents' network could bring:

> Chatting only for amblyopia, I think that's exaggerated. Who would need a Chatbox only because your child has to wear an eye patch? I don't want to be rude, but for me that's really overdone. Normally I never think about that eye; I trust the doctors, I do what they say, my son doesn't need to be anaesthetized, it doesn't hurt, it doesn't cost anything, it's just no big deal. So why not just leave it like it is? If it would be a severe illness, I would really appreciate to chat and visit a virtual support group and

so on. In such a situation—of course. But only for wearing that patch... there are so many more pressing issues (respondent D).

In addition, the system attempts to joke about amblyopia, and attempts to transform the child's negative self-perception of in a positive feeling of 'being special'. The project, for example, is called 'Land of Squint' (Land van Loens), in which the child will enter and experience 'adventures', and the main logo is a pirate with a patched eye. Yet as the children did not have much negative emotions about their patched eye, the system failed the opportunity to tap into the child's actual experiences. A few parents actually objected against the fact that the information system portrayed their child as 'being special'. They were eager to emphasize that their kid was *normal*, nothing special at all:

For him it's normal and I want to prevent that he's going to think that it's something special (respondent D).


Those parents that did appreciate the attempt to make their child with amblyopia feel special in a pleasant way, stated that this could be achieved much easier with different means. Printing the pirate on the patch itself, for example, was said to be a much more feasible and practical way to make patching pleasant for children rather than an elaborate patient information system.

That the parents did not experience a need for this information system was also related to the fact that amblyopia is an affliction that is rather easy to understand, with a simple treatment that has no real complications and rarely poses difficulties. Likewise, the treatment methods have been the same for many years, and because the affliction is rather

common, most people have friends or relatives who they can turn to for information. In addition on an emotional level, the system would also seem to be superfluous at the cognitive level.


## 5. Discussion and conclusion


I think that the designers have been thinking too much from their own point of view. With the best intentions. But the people who worked on it haven't really put themselves in the position of the people who get the information, the parents. That's what I think I'm seeing in this system (respondent J).

I still know what I first thought when I heard about the system: 'it's nice that they made this, but is all this necessary for amblyopia?' (respondent J)


This interactive electronic information system, then, was little used and had marginal effects on the quality of care for children with amblyopia and their parents. These disappointing conclusions are mainly due to the lack of fit between the content and functionality of the system and the needs and capacities of the target group. Most important here is the observation that amblyopia does not generate a large need for information in the first place. Most parents actually feel that an elaborate patient information system for this affliction overshoots its aims.

One caveat that must be made at this point is that most of the parents who joined the pilot evaluation were highly educated. Maybe the system would have been more 'effective' (as indicated by the indicators) if there had been a larger portion of less educated people using the system. We might assume that less educated people would be more in need to 'be informed', less compliant, and/or less able to cope than well-educated people, for example. If these assumptions were true, having mainly well-educated people in your sample reduces the potential of the system to be 'effective'. Yet it is an ironic fact that it is exactly amongst this less educated group that the problem of having access to a computer with a CD-ROM and Internet access would be the most acute [25].

Another caveat we must make at this point is that almost all respondents were already rather experienced eye-patchers at the time they started using the information system. Maybe somewhat better results could have been obtained if the group had primarily consisted of newly diagnosed amblyopia patients and their parents. These patients and parents might be more anxious, more in need of information and peer support. Yet the respondents stated that even new patients would not get much support or essential information from the system. The experience with the system of the two newly diagnosed patients who joined the evaluation also showed this. The system does not target the children appropriately, and the explanations and comfort that the orthoptist, friends and relatives can offer are deemed to be sufficient.

When an information system is not used much by the target group and when the expected effects are not reached, designers often blame the users for being lazy, or for being afraid of change or technological innovations [26]. Indeed, after the results of the pilot evaluation were known, the designers sometimes centered the discussion on the fact whether parents were competent enough to surf the Internet and operate the CD-ROM. Yet the unexamined assumptions of the designers themselves might be much more important in explaining the failure of information systems [27]—as it was the case in the patient information system studied here. When building an information system, designers cannot but start out with what they know and/or take for granted about the prospected users and their worlds. Designers often take for granted that the perspective with which they look at the system and would use the system, is also the perspective of the actual users of the system. These assumptions affect both the kind of information given and the way in which it is given [8,28]. If these assumptions remain unexamined, as they often are, many wrong assumptions may end up being built into the system, resulting in a mismatch between the system and its potential users (ibid.).

This is exactly what happened in the project we studied here: the designers of the system built their assumptions about the needs and capacities of the target group into the system. Parents and children were seen to be anxious, to have compliance and coping problems, to be in emotional and cognitive need for information, to be eagerly looking for support networks and real-time virtual contacts, etc. All these assumptions turned out to be wrong, explaining to a large extent the minimal impact of this system. Before the project had started many of these assumptions seemed quite reasonable (about parents and children being anxious, for example). Other assumptions seem to have been due to the project being focused too much on its technical feasibility rather than on its social usability (such as the chat-sessions being open only one, very unpractical, hour a week). That many of the built-in assumptions were in fact wrong only became evident during our evaluation.

If the qualitative pilot evaluation had not been done and we had started immediately with the quantitative evaluation, it would have been likely that we would have stuck to the explanation that the lack of results were due to problems of access to the technology, to a lack of 'traffic' on the Internet site, or to parents not being used enough to these technologies. Thanks to our qualitative pilot evaluation, however, we learned more than only the extent of the expected effects. We also found the underlying causes for the limited impact of the system. From the interviews it became clear that the users were all relatively highly educated, and that computer experience was not a limiting factor. We found out that the main problem underlying this patient information system, in fact, was that the needs of those people who actually would be using the system had never really been investigated. The designers had built in their own assumptions about these needs in the system, which appeared to be mistaken at too many levels for the system to become a success. A thorough exploration of user needs before building the system, using qualitative research methods, like we did in our pilot evaluation, could have prevented this mismatch.

With hindsight, it is obvious that we should have undertaken our study *before* the patient information system was developed, or in the early stages of its development. In that case, our findings could have informed the design, resulting in a much improved fit between system and users.

Because qualitative research methods can grasp the contexts of use of a (future) information system, and the meanings that (future) users attach to the situations in which they find themselves, they are very useful in designing and evaluating electronic information systems [11,27,29,30]. Such a development process implies involving the target group early on in the design of the information system, and creating a rich base of interview and observation data. Qualitative research methods can elucidate what the assumptions of the designers and of the potential users are exactly, and how they may be different. They can help elucidate whether prospected users really need information and/or support, what information or support they need, from whom they want it, and in which way the information or support could be presented and created.

As mismatched assumptions and other potential user-problems can be spotted early, the system can be optimized and fine-tuned from the first beginning, which will make the final patient information system more usable and suitable for the target group. Not doing this introduces a crucial flaw in the design. This can be very problematic, since these flaws can remain hidden until the system is actually introduced in the field. It is only then that the system will meet the problem of user acceptance, and that it will be discovered that fatal mistakes were made during the designing process [31]. At that moment, these mistakes are much more costly to repair (since the assumptions might be quite basic to the set-up of the system), and much resources may have been spent on implementing and evaluating a system that, wholly or partially, *cannot* work.

In addition, running into the problem of user acceptance might produce exactly the opposite effect of what is aimed for: it may irritate users and reduce their motivation and/or trust in those care-givers that have given them unfit information-resources. The most important advantage of using qualitative research methods in developing information systems, then, is not only to minimize the chance of costly failures, but also to maximize the chance that the eventual information system may meet its most important aim: to enhance patient empowerment and improve the quality of care.

In our situation, as a result of the qualitative pilot evaluation, the Eye Hospital has discontinued the Land of Squint project. They have thus not wasted their time and money on a large scale evaluation, and on continuing a project that cannot work. With the information gathered through this evaluation, the Eye Hospital is currently targeting a much broader group of eye patients directly through the Internet, for the time being mainly through general information and individualized question and answer facilities. This study prevents them from making the same faults again in their following projects and it enables them to use the insights discussed here to help make their following projects more successful.

# References


[1] J.S. Silva, A.J. Zawilski, The health care professional's workstation: Its functional components and user impact, in: M.J. Ball, M.F. Collen (Eds.), Aspects of the Computer-based Patient Record, Springer, New York, 1992, pp. 103–123.

[2] P. Brennan, I. Strombom, Improving health care by understanding patient preferences: The role of computer technology, JAMIA 5 (1998) 257–262.

[3] P. Tang, C. Newcomb, Informing patients: A guide for providing patient health information, JAMIA 5 (1998) 563–570.

[4] P.F. Brennan, Y.S. Kuang, K. Volrathongchai, Patient-centered information systems, in: J.H.v Bemmel, A.T. McCray (Eds.), Yearbook of Medical Informatics 2000: Patient Centered Systems, Schattauer, Stuttgart, 2000, pp. 79–86.

[5] K.C. Laudon, J.P. Laudon, Management Information Systems. New Approaches to Organization and Technology, 5 ed., Macmillan, New York, 1998.

[6] M.E. Collen, A History of Medical Informatics in the United States, 1950 to 1990, American Medical Informatics Association, 1995.

[7] C. Sauer, Why Information Systems Fail: A Case Study Approach, Alfred Waller, Henley-on-Thames, 1993.

[8] D.E. Forsythe, Using ethnography in the design of an explanation system, Expert Systems Appl. 8 (1995) 403–417.

[9] J. Greenbaum, M. Kyng (Eds.), Design at Work: Cooperative Design for Computer Systems, Lawrence Erlbaum Associates, Hillsdale, NJ, 1991.

[10] G. Button (Ed.), Technology in Working Order. Studies of Work, Interaction, and Technology, Routledge, London, 1993.

[11] B. Kaplan, Objectification and negotiation in interpreting clinical images: implications for computer-based patient records, AI Med. 7 (1995) 439–454.

[12] U.F. Hiddema, Improving health care quality by innovative use of CD-ROM and Internet for patient education and support in mother language (Dutch); Concept Project Plan, 1999.

[13] M.P. Hammersley, P. Atkinson, Ethnography: Principles and Practice, Routledge, London, 1989.

[14] A.L. Strauss, Qualitative Analysis for Social Scientists, Cambridge University Press, Cambridge, 1987.

[15] B. Kaplan, J.A. Maxwell, Qualitative research methods for evaluating computer information systems, in: J.G. Anderson, C.E. Aydin, S.J. Jay (Eds.), Evaluating Health Care Information Systems, Sage, Thousand Oaks, CA, 1993, pp. 45–69.

[16] C.P. Friedman, J.C. Wyatt (Eds.), Evaluation Methods in Medical Informatics, Springer, New York, 1997.

[17] N. Klazinga, Quality Management of Medical Specialist Care in the Netherlands. An Explorative Study of its Nature and Development, Belvédère, Overveen, 1997.

[18] U.F. Hiddema, Improving quality through better patient education: a case study by Francis Hiddema, MD. International Forum Meeting May 3–5 1998, The Ritz Carlton Hotel, Arlington, VA, 1998.

[19] H. Jimison, A. Adler, M. Coye, Health care providers and purchasers and evaluation of interactive health communication applications, Am. J. Prev. Med. 16 (1999) 16–22.

[20] J. Henderson, J. Noell, T. Reeves, T. Robinson, V. Strecher, Developers and evaluation of interactive health communication applications. The Science Panel on Interactive Communications and Health, Am. J. Prev. Med. 16 (1999) 30–34.

[21] D. Gustafson, R. Hawkins, E. Boberg, Impact of a patient-centered, computer-based health information/support system, Am. J. Prev. Med. 16 (1999) 1–9.

[22] G. Eysenbach, T.L. Diepgen, Labeling and filtering of medical information on the Internet, Methods Inf. Med. 38 (1999) 80–88.

[23] J. Gregory, J.E. Mattison, C. Linde, Naming notes: Transitions from free text to structured entry, Meth. Inf. Med. 34 (1995) 57–67.

[24] C. Appleby, Net gain or net loss? Healthcare consumers become Internet savvy, Trustee 52 (2) (1999) 20–23.

[25] H. Schmeets, Vooral hoogopgeleiden hebben toegang tot digitale wereld, Index-CBS 1999 (1999) 7.

[26] D.E. Forsythe, Blaming the user in medical informatics: the cultural nature of scientific practice, Knowledge Soc.: Anthropol. Sci. Technol. 9 (1992) 95–111.

[27] D.E. Forsythe, M.S. Brostoff, B.G. Buchanan, Information exchange and the problem of perspective: what should an explanation system explain? In 16th Symposium on Computer Applications in Medical Care, 1993.

[28] T. Winograd (Ed.), Bringing Design to Software, ACM Press, New York, 1996.

[29] M. Berg, Patient care information systems and healthcare work: A sociotechnical approach, Int. J. Med. Inf. 55 (1999) 87–101.

[30] J. Bardram, M. Sølvkjær, Computer supported cooperative work in clinical practice, in: J. Brender, J.P. Christensen, J.R. Scherrer, P. McNair (Eds.), Medical Informatics Europe'96, IOS Press, Amsterdam, 1996, pp. 853–857.

[31] M.L. Markus, S. Axline, D. Petrie, C. Tanis, Learning from adopters' experiences with ERP: Success and problems, J. Inf. Technol. 5 (2000) 245–265.

# D J Vassallo*, F Hoque[†], M Farquharson Roberts[‡], V Patterson[§], P Swinfen** and R Swinfen**

*Royal Hospital Haslar and 33 Field Hospital, Gosport, UK; [†]Centre for the Rehabilitation of the Paralysed, Dhaka, Bangladesh; [‡]Royal Hospital Haslar, Gosport, UK; [§]Royal Group of Hospitals, Belfast, UK; **The Swinfen Charitable Trust, Canterbury, UK

## Summary

In July 1999, the Swinfen Charitable Trust in the UK established a telemedicine link in Bangladesh, between the Centre for the Rehabilitation of the Paralysed (CRP) in Dhaka and medical consultants abroad. This low-cost telemedicine system used a digital camera to capture still images, which were then transmitted by email. During the first 12 months, 27 telemedicine referrals were made. The following specialties were consulted: neurology (44%), orthopaedics (40%), rheumatology (8%), nephrology (4%) and paediatrics (4%). Initial email replies were received at the CRP within a day of referral in 70% of cases and within thee days in 100%, which shows that store-and-forward telemedicine can be both fast and reliable. Telemedicine consultation was complete within three days in 14 cases (52%) and within three weeks in 24 cases (89%). Referral was judged to be beneficial in 24 cases (89%), the benefits including establishment of the diagnosis, the provision of reassurance to the patient and referring doctor, and a change of management. Four patients (15% of the total) and their families were spared the considerable expense and unnecessary stress of travelling abroad for a second opinion, and the savings from this alone outweighed the set-up and running costs in Bangladesh. The latter are limited to an email account with an Internet service provider and the local-rate telephone call charges from the CRP. This successful telemedicine system is a model for further telemedicine projects in the developing world.

## Introduction

Telemedicine is a process in which expert medical advice from afar is provided using telecommunications technology. The system chosen depends primarily on the needs of the user, but must also take account of the available finances and technical resources. This is particularly relevant in the developing world.

Telemedicine based on store-and-forward email techniques has become increasingly affordable in the last few years with the advent of high-quality yet inexpensive still digital cameras and easy access to the Internet[1].

Accepted 25 December 2000

Correspondence: Lt Col David J Vassallo RAMC, Defence Medical Services Telemedicine Unit, Royal Hospital Haslar, Gosport, Hants PO12 2AA, UK (Fax: +44 2392 762 960; Email: DJVassallo@aol.com)

Many civilian and military organizations in the industrialized world now have experience of telemedicine. The United States military medical services have been developing and using telemedicine systems in support of their forces overseas since the early 1990s[2–4]. Their initial focus was on the use of realtime videoconferencing links, but emphasis is now shifting towards the use of email with still images, which is cheaper and simpler[5]. This is partly as a result of British military experience with this method.

In January 1998, the British Defence Medical Services (DMS) set up their first telemedicine link, between a field hospital in Bosnia and specialists at the Royal Hospital Haslar in the UK[6]. The DMS system relied on the transmission of still images attached to email messages containing clinical information. The success of this simple and cheap system led to its rapid adoption by other British military medical units worldwide[7–9]. These features also make it suitable for telemedicine projects in the developing world.

## Centre for the Rehabilitation of the Paralysed

The Centre for the Rehabilitation of the Paralysed (CRP) is a 100-bed hospital at Savar, near Dhaka, in Bangladesh. The CRP has grown from humble beginnings in 1979 to become one of the best management and rehabilitation centres for patients with spinal cord injuries in South Asia (Fig 1). It is the only such centre in the whole of Bangladesh (whose population is in excess of 120 million) and the majority of its patients are extremely poor. The CRP provides services for disabled people in a hospital setting and in the community[10]. It is fully accredited by the government of Bangladesh. The CRP clinical staff consists of one full-time consultant orthopaedic surgeon, one resident medical officer and two medical officers. There are three visiting neurosurgeons and one visiting urologist. There are 20 physiotherapy staff, 12 occupational therapy staff and 23 nursing staff, in addition to administrative and domestic staff.

## The Swinfen Charitable Trust

The Swinfen Charitable Trust (SCT) was set up in the UK in 1998 with the aim of assisting poor, sick and disabled people in the developing world[11]. The Trust's policy is to do this by helping to establish telemedicine links between hospitals in the developing world and specialists who generously give free advice by email. The simple telemedicine protocols used are modelled on those of the DMS system[1,6–8] (see below).

## The CRP telemedicine link

In November 1998, Olympus UK donated two digital cameras (C-1400XL, Olympus) and accessories, two tripods and a laptop computer to the SCT in order to

establish a telemedicine link at the CRP. Two SCT administrators delivered this equipment to the CRP in July 1999. They trained a small team of local staff in its use and how to send email referrals, and provided them with an initial list of specialists and their email addresses. Most of the staff had no previous experience of using computers.

## Equipment and software

### The CRP

To be suitable for telemedicine, a digital camera has to produce images of sufficient resolution for a clinician to give a confident second opinion on the images and clinical details alone. The Olympus C-1400XL digital camera (known as the D620L in the USA) fulfilled this requirement. It was the highest-resolution digital camera available commercially until mid-1999. It is still widely used by the DMS (although it is now being superseded by the Olympus C-2500). Two Olympus C-1400XL digital cameras, two 6 V AC power adaptors, two sets of rechargeable batteries and rechargers, and two tripods were procured for the CRP (thus allowing some redundancy to prevent disruption of the telemedicine service should any single component fail).

A laptop computer was used (ThinkPad 365XD, IBM) with a standard modem (19.2 kbit/s).

The digital camera was supplied with basic image manipulation software (C-W95, Olympus). This was used to import, display, crop, compress and store images in the laptop. No other image software was required at the CRP.

The CRP took out an email subscription with Bangla-net Dhaka. An ordinary telephone line (not an ISDN line) was used at the CRP for the connection.

### The SCT

Individual specialists and the staff at the SCT used a variety of laptop or desktop computers, choosing their own communication and image manipulation software. It was not usually necessary to enhance images on receipt.

## Telemedicine protocols

### Image capture at the CRP

The camera was usually used on a tripod to photograph clinical images or electrocardiograms; 'macro mode' was used for close-ups. For radiographs or magnetic resonance or computerized tomography images, the camera was used in self-timer mode, on a tripod, in a darkened room, with the radiographs or scans illuminated by a viewing box, at a distance of 40 cm

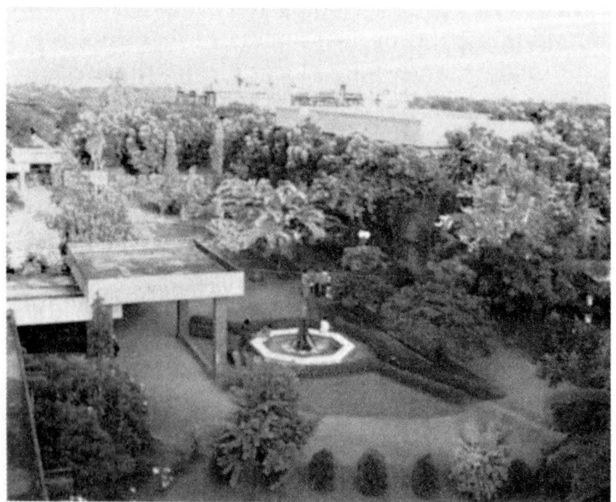

**Fig 1** Centre for the Rehabilitation of the Paralysed, Bangladesh.

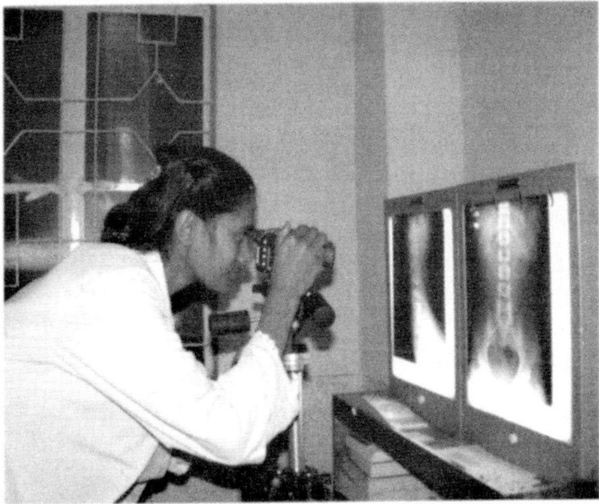

**Fig 2** Digital camera in use at the CRP by Shamsun Nahar Begum, the operating theatre nurse.

from the camera (Fig 2). Images were taken in 'high-quality mode' (1280 × 1024 pixels) for maximum definition. The images were then downloaded into the computer using a Fuji floppy path adaptor (this method was faster than using the serial adaptor cable provided with the camera). The images were automatically compressed as JPEG images (Joint Photographic Experts Group algorithm) and cropped as necessary. This resulted in file sizes of 30–200 kByte, depending on whether the image was saved in 256-level greyscale (for radiographs) or 24-bit colour format.

The images were then attached to an email containing the necessary clinical information and appropriate subject header (as described below).

### Patient confidentiality

Patient confidentiality was ensured by the use of a sequential number for each patient (e.g. CRP 001 was the first referral) and the avoidance of any mention of details that could identify the patient. There was therefore no need for encryption software. The patient's consent was obtained beforehand for telemedicine referral.

### Email subject header

The subject header for each referral was written in the following format: *Tmed xxxx CRP nnn.*

(1) *Tmed* identified the email as a telemedicine referral;
(2) *xxxx* identified the specialty whose opinion was being sought, such as neuro for neurology, orth for orthopaedics, rheum for rheumatology, xray for radiology and so on;

(3) *CRP* identified the referring site;
(4) *nnn* was the sequential patient number.

Thus Tmed orth CRP 007 identified the seventh telemedicine referral from the CRP, requesting an orthopaedic opinion.

### Email transmission

Each email referral was sent to a specialist's own email address and copied (for coordination and evaluation) to two further SCT addresses. The specialists' replies were sent to the CRP and also copied to the SCT. The SCT thereby built up a central database of all referrals and replies. The SCT administrator or a deputy logged onto the Internet to check for email referrals three or four times a day throughout the evaluation period, including at weekends, and occasionally telephoned consultants to notify them of the more urgent referrals. The SCT also sought the aid of different specialists as required to cover for absences on leave, or if a referral to a new specialty was required.

## Methods

The evaluation period lasted from the date of the first telemedicine referral from the CRP on 19 July 1999 to the completion of the first telemedicine referral for July 2000, the study ending on 20 July 2000. All email referrals, replies and follow-up email messages were copied to the SCT (as described above, or after a reminder in the few early instances where either the CRP or the specialist inadvertently omitted to send copies). At the end of the study period the email traffic was analysed to determine the specialties involved, speed of initial reply, time to completion of each consultation, number of email messages for each referral, number of images and size of files, and the frequency of referrals. Only email messages directly relating to patient management were included in the evaluation. Email copies were excluded.

The neurologist graded the difficulty of his consultations as 'difficult' or 'straightforward'. The lead clinician at the CRP documented what benefits accrued to the patient or to the referring doctor as a result of telemedicine. Clinical staff at the CRP evaluated the outcomes of telemedicine interventions in relation to the likely outcome if a telemedicine service had been unavailable. The set-up and ongoing costs of the telemedicine service were compared with the potential or actual savings to assess the cost-effectiveness of the link.

**Table 1** Telemedicine referrals from the CRP during the study period

| Patient | Specialty | No. of email messages | First reply | Completion | Diagnosis | Telemedicine result | Benefit |
|---|---|---|---|---|---|---|---|
| CRP 001 | Orthopaedics | 4 | < 1 day | < 1 week | Tetraplegia (see Appendix) | Management endorsed | Flight avoided |
| CRP 002 | Orthopaedics | 5 | < 1 day | < 1 day | Paraplegia | Pain management refined | Travel avoided |
| CRP 003 | Orthopaedics | 6 | < 3 days | < 3 days | Pathological fracture | Local management endorsed | Reassurance |
| CRP 004 | Orthopaedics | 4 | < 3 days | < 3 days | Vertebral tumour | Local management endorsed | Reassurance |
| CRP 005 | Orthopaedics | 9 | < 3 days | < 3 weeks | Tuberculosis, cord compression | Local management refined | Reassurance |
| CRP 006 | Neurology | 7 | < 1 day | < 3 weeks | Neuropathy (see Appendix) | Differential diagnosis clarified | Flight avoided |
| CRP 007 | Rheumatology | 4 | < 1 day | < 2 weeks | Juvenile chronic rheumatoid arthritis | New management plan | Management changed |
| CRP 008 | Orthopaedics | 15 | < 1 day | < 3 months | Paraplegia, cause? | Diagnosis established | Reassurance |
| CRP 009 | Neurology | 10 | < 1 day | < 7 months | Chronic inflammatory demyelinating peripheral neuropathy (see Appendix) | Diagnosis established | Management changed |
| CRP 010 | Medicine | 3 | < 1 day | < 1 day (died) | Tetraplegia, renal failure | n/a | No benefit |
| CRP 011 | Orthopaedics | 5 | < 3 days | < 1 week | Leg injury (see Appendix) | Management options clarified | Reassurance |
| CRP 012 | Rheumatology | 2 | < 3 days | < 3 days | Rheumatic fever | Management plan clarified | Reassurance |
| CRP 013 | Neurology | 4 | < 3 days | < 3 weeks | Stroke | Management plan clarified | Management changed |
| CRP 014 | Neurology | 6 | < 1 day | < 3 weeks | Abnormal posture | Differential diagnosis clarified | No benefit to patient |
| CRP 015 | Orthopaedics | 3 | < 1 day | < 1 day | Paraplegia | Local management endorsed | Reassurance |
| CRP 016 | Orthopaedics | 4 | < 1 day | < 3 days | Congenital hip dislocation (see Appendix) | Management plan clarified | Surgery avoided |
| CRP 017 | Neurology | 5 | < 1 day | < 3 weeks | Early-onset dementia | Diagnosis established | Reassurance |
| CRP 018 | Neurology | 4 | < 1 day | < 3 days | Parkinson's disease | Management plan clarified | Management changed |
| CRP 019 | Neurology | 2 | < 3 days | < 3 days | Stroke | Management plan clarified | Reassurance |
| CRP 020 | Neurology | 2 | < 1 day | < 1 day | Cerebral palsy, spasms | Management plan clarified | Management changed |
| CRP 021 | Neurology | 13 | < 1 day | < 3 months | Neurological deterioration | Differential diagnosis, management options | No benefit to patient |
| CRP 022 | Paediatrics | 7 | < 3 days | < 3 weeks | Osteogenesis imperfecta | Management plan clarified | Travel avoided |
| CRP 023 | Neurology | 3 | < 1 day | < 3 days | Stroke | Management plan clarified | Management changed |
| CRP 024 | Neurology | 2 | < 1 day | < 1 day | Depression | Management plan clarified | Management changed |
| CRP 025 | Orthopaedics | 2 | < 1 day | < 1 day | Ankylosing spondylitis | Management plan clarified | Surgery avoided |
| CRP 026 | Neurology | 4 | < 1 day | < 3 weeks | Neurological deterioration | Differential diagnosis clarified | Reassurance |
| CRP 027 | Orthopaedics | 2 | < 1 day | < 1 day | Ankylosing spondylitis (see Appendix) | Management plan clarified | Surgery avoided |

# Results

Twenty-seven telemedicine referrals were sent during the first 12 months (Table 1), relating to both inpatients and outpatients. Twenty-three referral messages (85%) contained images, the number ranging from one to seven, apart from one referral containing 13 images. Apart from this one referral, the total file size was always less than 500 kByte. The file transfer times (i.e. the length of time it took to send the email with attachments from the PC to the ISP) were less than 2 min. There was no loss of definition in transmitted images.

Five different specialties were consulted (Table 1). Rheumatology referrals were sent to a British rheumatologist working at the Patan Hospital in Nepal, which illustrates the feasibility of referrals between two developing countries.

The frequency of referrals gradually increased, reaching a maximum of six in two separate months.

Twice as many referrals were sent on a Monday than on any other day of the week. The Bangladeshi weekend starts on Thursday afternoon, with Friday being the main holiday. Saturday and Sunday are normal working days, and the pattern of referrals reflected this. There was a tendency for a slight delay before reply to Sunday referrals, probably because Sunday is a holiday in the UK and there is a 5 h time difference between the UK and Bangladesh. Paradoxically, the one Sunday referral that received a reply on the same day was sent on Boxing Day (26 December 1999), a public holiday in the UK. The day of referral did not otherwise affect the time before a reply was received.

Initial email replies were received at the CRP within a day of referral in 70% of referrals and within three days in 100% (Table 1).

The number of email messages per referral ranged from two (in the most straightforward cases, i.e. a referral and a reply) to 15 (in a combined orthopaedic and neurological case), the mean being five email messages per referral. There was no significant difference between specialties in the number of email messages per referral (Table 1).

Telemedicine consultation was completed within one day in seven cases overall (26%), within three days in 14 cases (52%), within a week in 16 cases (59%) and within three weeks in 24 cases (89%). Of the remaining three cases, two were completed within three months and in the last, a complicated neurological case, the correspondence lasted seven months. The time to completion of the telemedicine consultation was significantly longer for neurology referrals than for orthopaedic referrals. Thus the respective figures for completion within one day were two out of 12 neurology cases (17%) and four out of 11 orthopaedic cases (36%). For completion within three days the figures were five out of 12 neurology cases (42%) and seven out of 11 orthopaedic cases (64%), and at one week the figures were still five out of 12 for neurology (42%) but nine out of 11 for orthopaedics (82%). By three weeks after initial referral most consultations were finished, with 10 out of 12 neurology cases (83%) and 10 out of 11 orthopaedic cases (91%) being completed.

Notwithstanding the difference between specialties, this short time overall compares very favourably with standard (non-telemedicine) outpatient referrals (even between hospital specialists) within the UK, especially for orthopaedics and neurology.

Of the 12 neurological referrals, eight were graded as 'difficult' and four as 'straightforward'. The cases therefore represented a highly selected and difficult patient population. The UK neurologist considered this method of email consultation to be sufficient in the four straightforward cases but stated that he would have preferred video-consultation to email in the other eight. Nonetheless, the CRP staff perceived benefit to the patient and/or to the referring clinician in six of the eight complicated neurological cases.

Telemedicine referral was judged by the CRP staff to be beneficial to the patient in 24 cases (89%), the three exceptions being a patient who died very shortly after referral (CRP 010), one who probably had a psychiatric disorder (CRP 014) and one with a rapidly progressive complex neurological condition (CRP 021). The benefits included establishment of the diagnosis, reassurance to the patient and referring doctor, and a change of management. These results do not take into account the considerable educational benefits to the referring doctor and his colleagues at the CRP — and indeed to the specialists — even in those few cases where no benefit accrued to the patient.

Four patients (15% of the total referred) and their families were spared the considerable expense and unnecessary stress of travelling abroad for a second opinion. They had expressed the intention of travelling before the telemedicine referral, but changed their minds on receipt of the replies.

The cost to the patients for the telemedicine service was a nominal Tk1000 ($18 — Tk1 is $0.018, EU0.020), paid to the CRP to partially defray the cost of the email subscription. This fee was waived for two patients.

## Discussion

There has been little practical experience with telemedicine of a direct clinical kind in the developing world, which contains 80% of the world's population. In the 45 poorest countries, it is estimated that only 50% of the population has access to health services[12]. Arguably, it is those same countries that stand to gain most from a simple and cheap telemedicine system, on the principle that it could improve access to health-care and specialists, and enhance research and the education of local health-care workers[13]. However, the fundamental assumption — that telemedicine in a developing country is cost-effective — can be proved only by carrying out pilot projects[14]. The potential for telemedicine to play a useful role in the developing world has been the focus of attention for several years[15–21]. The dearth of formal evaluations of the cost-effectiveness of telemedicine projects and the almost complete lack of evaluations of the outcomes of telemedicine interventions have unfortunately militated against the wider use of telemedicine[21]. The

International Telecommunication Union has reviewed the telemedicine experience of various countries and published its recommendations for the development of telemedicine services in developing countries[17,18]. A major recommendation was that developing countries should undertake pilot projects in order to identify the most cost-effective telemedicine solutions, especially for the provision of health-care to people living in remote and rural areas.

It has been suggested[14] that the logical steps to determine the place of telemedicine in the developing world would include:

(1) identifying potential telemedicine projects;
(2) establishing one or more pilot projects in order both to demonstrate technical feasibility and to measure the benefits to the health-care system;
(3) calculating the cost of large-scale deployment.

Various concerns have been raised regarding the use of telemedicine in the developing world[14]. The following questions are pertinent:

(1) Can health workers do anything on the basis of the advice they receive?
(2) Is telemedicine an appropriate use of resources?
(3) Can the difficult organizational and administrative problems be overcome in a developing country? (In telemedicine projects in the industrialized world it has been shown that success depends on much more than the delivery of the right equipment to the user.)
(4) Are neurological consultations based on still images and store-and-forward email effective? (It has been shown that this specialty can safely be carried out using video-consultation[22,23].)

In addition, there are particular logistical concerns in attempting to set up a telemedicine project in the developing world[24]. These include:

(1) delivering the equipment;
(2) doing the initial user training;
(3) supporting the project afterwards.

These questions can be answered only on the basis of experience with telemedicine in the developing world[14].

The establishment of the CRP telemedicine link followed the logical strategy outlined above and sought to determine whether telemedicine in the developing world could be cost-effective and therefore whether it ought to be more widely employed.

## Identification of a suitable site for a telemedicine project

The CRP is situated in one of the 45 poorest countries of the world and cares for the poorest of the poor. It has a well deserved reputation as a centre for the management and rehabilitation of patients with spinal cord injuries throughout South Asia and yet is handicapped by a lack of specialists in various disciplines. It originally sought advice from the SCT and others about a suitable telemedicine system that would enhance the care it could offer its patients. The Bangladesh Ministry of Health gave its approval to the CRP for telemedicine advice to be sought from overseas.

## Choice of telemedicine system

The simplicity and effectiveness of telemedicine based on pictures taken with a digital camera and email had been established by the DMS. This system was deemed to be potentially suitable for the CRP. The equipment requirements were modest and in the event the costs were met through donations.

## Evaluation

The results of the first year of the pilot project at the CRP show the technical feasibility of telemedicine based on a digital camera and email in a developing country and show measurable benefits to the patients at the referring institution. The fact that initial replies were received within one day in 70% of referrals and within three days in 100% of referrals demonstrated that store-and-forward telemedicine could be both fast and reliable. Follow-up email messages were equally prompt, resulting in completion of the consultation within three days in 14 cases (52%) and within three weeks in 24 cases (89%). Such results are not often obtained, even for non-telemedicine referrals, within the UK.

## Cost of large-scale deployment

The essential elements of the system used at the CRP were a digital camera, computer and email link, one or more coordinators, and a network of specialists. How best to scale up the system to encompass a large number of referring sites — and therefore what the costs of large-scale deployment would be — is a current topic for research.

## Can health workers do anything on the basis of the advice they receive?

Our evaluation shows that the telemedicine advice received is useful, so long as common sense is applied and so long as specialists can be relied upon to reply promptly, with consistently high-quality advice and a choice of management options. The referring doctor then chooses the best option in the circumstances. This worked well in the present study. Specialists soon realized what was feasible locally and tailored their advice accordingly. This is illustrated in the case reports (see Appendix), especially CRP 011, a very difficult case where amputation would probably have been the best surgical option, but parental influence overrode this, so further advice was modified accordingly.

It is essential that specialists always reply promptly to referrals. Only thus will they materially influence patient management and maintain the confidence and trust of the referring doctor. The CRP experience shows that the quality of service (i.e. response time, quality of consultation and the expertise of the consultants) is important in sustaining such a telemedicine link.

## Is telemedicine an appropriate use of resources?

In considering the introduction of low-cost telemedicine for the developing world, this question might be better phrased as 'Is telemedicine the most effective use of resources?' and 'What would have happened if telemedicine had not been available?' Can it be shown, for instance, that the funds produce a greater health gain when spent on telemedicine rather than on conventional public health measures? These questions can now be answered on the basis of the CRP's experience.

The main aim of the CRP telemedicine project was to provide access to specialist consultation for the patients at the CRP, often very poor people, at little or no cost. A secondary consideration was to prevent unnecessary and expensive travel for treatment to another country. Both aims were achieved. In four cases, a personal outlay of Tk1000 each saved the patients and respective families the considerable cost of travelling abroad for a second opinion (Table 1). The ongoing costs to the CRP were low, mainly consisting of the email account with an Internet service provider and the cost of local-rate telephone calls. The cost to the CRP for the email account and all telephone bills for the period of the evaluation was about Tk20,000.

Staff at the CRP were asked specifically to evaluate what would have happened if telemedicine had not been available in their assessment of the appropriateness of the use of resources. The results were as follows:

(1) Four patients (15% of the total) would have travelled abroad for a second opinion. Two of them, including a tetraplegic patient, would have travelled, with at least one relative each, by air to the UK and two would have travelled overland to India, accompanied by two relatives each. The expenses saved in these four instances more than made up for the set-up and maintenance costs of the telemedicine project. The costs of travel and treatment abroad would have been fully borne by the patients and families concerned. Instead, this money was available for their care at home in Bangladesh. Both the CRP staff and the patients were delighted with this outcome.

(2) Seven patients (26%) whose management was changed as a result of telemedicine would have suffered longer and might well have undergone inappropriate treatment.

(3) Three patients would not have received a firm diagnosis and would probably have undergone inappropriate investigation and management, and unnecessary stress.

(4) Three patients might have undergone possibly deleterious or unnecessary surgery.

(5) Three patients would have been referred to another hospital in Dhaka for investigation and further management, at significant cost to the patients. One of these, CRP 010, underwent telemedicine referral almost in extremis (without it interfering with his clinical care) and he died shortly afterwards, during transfer to another hospital.

(6) The referring clinician would have missed out on the educational aspects of professional consultation, possibly to the detriment of future patients (see below).

The question about appropriate use of resources has to be placed in the context of the CRP's specialist work, the costs involved in setting up and maintaining a telemedicine link, and the benefits accruing to the staff and patients. In this project, the equipment was donated to the CRP; the SCT transported it, carried out the training, made two subsequent visits (see below) and provided the connection to overseas specialists, who gave their advice free of charge. There was therefore almost no cost to the CRP. The potential outlay for equipment would otherwise have been in the region of £2500 (£1 is $1.49, EU1.57) (for two cameras, accessories, tripods and a laptop computer). The potential outlay for travel (including the follow-up visits) would have been at least £4000 (for two persons and three return journeys each, with economy-class return flight to the UK from Dhaka costing £650 per person).

The main impingement on local resources at the CRP was on personnel, but their work in the local telemedicine team was performed without detriment to other duties. Analysis showed that it took 90–120 min from the time the CRP clinician requested the help of his telemedicine team with a new referral to the time the email message was sent. The steps and the time involved were:

(1) to obtain patient's consent and contact address form, 10 min;
(2) to compose an email message containing the relevant clinical information, 30–60 min, depending upon the specialty, with non-orthopaedic referrals taking longer (it should be noted that referrals were not being composed in the clinician's native language and that the email was typed by another person, not a clinician, who was also unfamiliar with the English language);
(3) to photograph a radiograph or computerized tomography or magnetic resonance scan, 20 min;
(4) to download images to the computer, 10 min;
(5) to attach the relevant images to the email message, 10 min
(6) to perform a final check and send the referral, 10 min.

On the basis of the results of the referrals, the CRP staff judged this to be time and effort well spent.

Our results show that the minimal expenditure incurred by the CRP in using the telemedicine link significantly improved the service it could provide. The CRP already had ready access to medical supplies, clean drinking water and proper sanitation, so this was not an issue. The CRP management and clinical staff could not identify any alternative health measure locally where such a small expenditure would have had as great or as lasting an effect on patient care, and they were in no doubt that the introduction of telemedicine had been both appropriate and a most effective health measure.

## Teleneurology

Can the specialist consulted give appropriate advice on the basis of the transmitted information? This question is particularly pertinent to neurology[22,23,25]. In the industrialized world, teleneurology has concentrated on realtime high-quality video-links, mainly using transmission at 384 kbit/s via ISDN lines because this is what is required to transmit a neurological examination accurately. It had been assumed that store-and-forward techniques would not be sufficient to enable accurate diagnosis and therefore management recommendations to be made. Our results suggest that this may not always be the case. While the neurologist felt that video-consultation would have given him more diagnostic confidence, he was still prepared to provide a reasoned differential diagnosis and suggest further management on the basis of the excellent

clinical history and examination findings recorded by an experienced orthopaedic surgeon. The clinical images themselves were less important. What is particularly interesting is that the perceptions of usefulness were so different between the neurologist, who was not happy that he had always made the diagnosis correctly, and the referring doctor, who thought that the neurologist's advice was extremely useful in 10 of the 12 cases. Store-and-forward techniques are not just less expensive to set up than a video-link but also much easier to use, since they do not require the referring doctor and the consultant to be dealing with the patient's problem at the same time. Moreover, a video-link is particularly difficult to organize where there is a substantial difference in time zones between the two sites. Our results indicate that store-and-forward telemedicine for neurology would be of substantial potential benefit to the developing world, where neurologists are scarce. Consequently this technique merits further study.

## The logistics of setting up telemedicine

Can the organizational and administrative problems of setting up a telemedicine service be overcome in a developing country? There were different organizational and administrative issues at each end (the UK and Bangladesh) of this telemedicine link, some of which were unique to it, but others which are generally applicable (see below). There were no insurmountable technical, administrative or logistical problems.

### *Delivering the equipment*

Before importing the digital cameras and accessories into Bangladesh, a number of bureaucratic formalities had to be completed. These were done with the aid of the Bangladesh High Commission in London, but still took some months. Two SCT administrators transported the equipment by Emirate Airlines to Dhaka in early July 1999. All went well until they reached Dhaka Airport, where the customs officers initially refused to let the equipment through, despite all the relevant forms having been completed in both Bengali and English. However, obduracy finally paid off and the equipment was allowed through to the CRP.

### *Initial user training*

At the CRP, four personnel were selected for involvement in telemedicine. The same two SCT administrators who had delivered the equipment collaborated with the local team leader in training these staff. They concentrated on teaching them how to use the camera to take the best possible images, and how to compose email messages to ensure that correct subject headers were used and that referrals were sent to appropriate addresses. Local staff quickly grasped the basics of the system and the unfamiliar technology, even though they were learning through the medium of English, when their native language was Bengali. There were inevitably some amusing incidents during the teaching sessions, with everything said having to be translated into Bengali.

The CRP team leader was a clinician, who was responsible for initiating all telemedicine referrals. Other team members were responsible for taking and downloading photographs, and for the composition and transmission of email messages.

## Supporting the network

At the UK end, an SCT administrator or deputy checked the email three or four times a day and followed the progress of each referral, occasionally prompting replies by email or by telephone calls to relevant specialists. New specialists were enrolled as required through personal contacts. The SCT also sent two administrators to visit the CRP on two occasions to monitor its progress during the evaluation period, to encourage local staff, to help in further training and to participate in telemedicine workshops. These two visits (in October 1999 and April 2000) were followed by a significant surge in telemedicine referrals as local staff regained confidence in their skills. Both visits were considered crucial in this regard. The second visit resulted in a sustained level of activity, with the project gaining a momentum of its own. A drop in referrals in May 2000 was due to the referring clinician going abroad on a postgraduate course, and the number of referrals picked up after his return.

At each end of the link, a particular concern was how best to keep track of email messages and images relating to particular referrals, especially as email traffic increased and involved more specialists in different locations. For this reason, the SCT began to assess the free telemedicine software system specially developed for the DMS Telemedicine Unit at the Royal Hospital Haslar for use with the telemedicine protocols described above[26].

## Additional benefits of telemedicine

The educational aspects have already been alluded to. For example, two weeks after telemedicine advice was given for better pain management in a patient with cerebral palsy and painful muscle spasms (CRP 020), a similar outpatient presented to the CRP. This new patient was managed successfully according to the same treatment regime, without the need for further consultation.

Two telemedicine workshops were also held during the year, and these generated considerable interest among local Bangladeshi medical consultants, politicians, non-governmental organizations, other interested persons and the local press[27].

The CRP is now developing itself as a centre for telemedicine within Bangladesh, a welcome offshoot of this project. Digital photographs are also being used in teaching local personnel, and the Haslar Hospital library's Website[28] is being used by CRP staff as a portal to medical sites on the Internet. A Web-based presentation on the work of the CRP has been prepared with the aid of the supplied digital cameras and has been published on the 'Good Medicine in Bad Places' Website[10].

## Satellite telephones

An Inmarsat-A satellite telephone was donated to the SCT by Nera Satellite Services to provide an emergency backup at the CRP in the event of conventional telephone lines breaking down, which would be most likely during the monsoon season. The satellite telephone was delivered to the CRP by the SCT in July 1999. In practice, the telephone line at the CRP broke down only twice during the study period and these interruptions were overcome by using another line. The satellite telephone itself, on the few occasions it was tried, ran up a prohibitively large telephone bill, so its use was discontinued. On the basis of this experience we hesitate to recommend satellite telephones for telemedicine links in the developing world, primarily because of the cost of the calls.

## Unique aspects

The present work has provided invaluable experience in how to set up a successful telemedicine project in the developing world. It has also shown that the most pressing concerns about such projects (the logistical aspects of delivering the equipment, doing the initial user training and supporting the network afterwards) can be overcome by the use of simple yet effective equipment, straightforward protocols and dedicated personnel.

This telemedicine project is also unique in that it was established under the aegis of a new telemedicine charity[11]. This charity donated and transported the relevant equipment to a centre already equipped with email, it helped train local staff and it has continued to support the local staff and supervise the progress of the project. It aims to help establish further telemedicine projects in the developing world[29].

## Conclusions

Other health workers have independently confirmed the usefulness of digital cameras and email for telemedicine in the developing world[30,31]. The low-cost telemedicine project described in this article is one of very few clinical projects in the developing world. Evaluation of the project has proven that telemedicine in a developing country is cost-effective. It is simple and can readily be emulated.

Its example is already being followed in similar pilot projects set up by the SCT in two other countries: Nepal (at Patan Hospital) and in the Solomon Islands (Gizo Hospital in Gizo, and Helena Goldie Hospital in New Georgia, Western Province)[32]. The LAMB Hospital, also in Bangladesh, followed suit in late 2000. The CRP digital camera and email telemedicine link is a model for further telemedicine projects in the developing world. In the words of one of the CRP telemedicine team:

> Telemedicine has provided us with tremendous support for our patient management at CRP and in Bangladesh. If this service had not been available, some of our patients would have definitely suffered longer from their disease process and money would have been wasted travelling overseas. Telemedicine has lessened the suffering of our patients, given them assurance too and provided teaching for our consultant.

*Acknowledgements:*   We thank Chris Bowen, Digital Division Manager of Olympus UK, for the donation of two Olympus C-1400XL cameras and accessories, and a laptop computer to the SCT for use at the CRP. We also thank Bob Chewter, Nera Satellite Services, for donating a satellite telephone to the SCT as backup at the CRP. Emirate Airlines kindly waived all excess baggage charges for the transport of the telemedicine equipment. We are particularly grateful to Professor Richard Wootton, who has a special interest in telemedicine for the developing world, for his advice and help in establishing the telemedicine link to Bangladesh. We also thank the other specialists who have provided telemedicine advice and help with this project, and those who have offered to help but not yet been called upon. In particular, we thank Dr Lorraine Graham at Patan Hospital, Nepal, and Mr Stephen Wood (of World Orthopaedic Concern — see http://www.boa.ac.uk), Mr John Beavis (of the Leonard Cheshire Centre for Post-Conflict Recovery), Lieutenant Colonel John Bowen RAMC and Surgeon Commander Chris Kershaw RN, as well as Surgeon Commander Peter Buxton RN and Wing Commander John Kilbey RAF at the DMS Telemedicine Unit. We also thank Shamsun Nahar Begum, Deb Dulal Chakraborty and Ahadullah of the telemedicine team at the CRP.

## References

1 Vassallo DJ. Digital camera telemedicine for British and NATO forces — a simple solution with civilian and humanitarian applications. *Journal of Telemedicine and Telecare* 2000;**6** (suppl. 1):197

2 Zajtchuk R, Sullivan GR. Battlefield trauma care: focus on advanced technology. *Military Medicine* 1995;**160**:1–7

3 Calcagni DE, Clyburn CA, Tomkins G, *et al.* Operation Joint Endeavor in Bosnia: telemedicine systems and case reports. *Telemedicine Journal* 1996;**2**:211–24

4 Zajtchuk R, Gilbert GR. Telemedicine: a new dimension in the practice of medicine. *Disease-a-Month* 1999;**45**(6):197–262

5 Vidmar DA. The history of teledermatology in the Department of Defense. *Dermatology Clinics* 1999;**17**:113–24

6 Vassallo DJ, Buxton PJ, Kilbey JH, Trasler M. The first telemedicine link for the British Forces. *Journal of the Royal Army Medical Corps* 1998;**144**:125–30

7 Scerri GV, Vassallo DJ. Initial plastic surgery experience with the first telemedicine link for the British Forces. *British Journal of Plastic Surgery* 1999;**52**:294–8

8 Vassallo DJ. Twelve months' experience with telemedicine for the British armed forces. *Journal of Telemedicine and Telecare* 1999;**5** (suppl. 1):117–18

9 See http://www.emergency-medical.com/case01_01.htm

10 See http://www.emergency-medical.com/case06_01.htm

11 The Swinfen Charitable Trust. Registered charity no. 1077879 (see http://www.coh.uq.edu.au/swinfen), c/o Dene House, Wingham, Canterbury CT3 1NU, UK (email: swinfen@dene73.freeserve.co.uk)

12 UNDP. *Human Development Report 1996.* New York: Oxford University Press, 1996

13 Mitka M. Developing countries find telemedicine forges links to more care and research. *Journal of the American Medical Association* 1998;**280**:1295–6

14 Wootton R. The possible use of telemedicine in developing countries. *Journal of Telemedicine and Telecare* 1997;**3**:23–6

15 Wright D, Androuchko L. Telemedicine and developing countries. *Journal of Telemedicine and Telecare* 1996;**2**:63–70

16 Wright D. Telemedicine delivery to developing countries. *Journal of Telemedicine and Telecare* 1997;**3** (suppl. 1):76–8

17 Wright D. The International Telecommunication Union's report on Telemedicine and Developing Countries. *Journal of Telemedicine and Telecare* 1998;**4** (suppl. 1):75–9

18 Wright D. Telemedicine and developing countries. A report of study group 2 of the ITU Development Sector. *Journal of Telemedicine and Telecare* 1998;**4** (suppl. 2):1–87

19 Adeyinka MB. Fundamentals of modern telemedicine in Africa. *Methods of Information in Medicine* 1997;**36**:95–8

20 Darkwa O. An exploratory survey of the applications of telemedicine in Ghana. *Journal of Telemedicine and Telecare* 2000;**6**:177–83

21 Hakansson S, Gavelin C. What do we *really* know about the cost-effectiveness of telemedicine? *Journal of Telemedicine and Telecare* 2000;**6** (suppl. 1):133–6

22 Craig JJ, McConville JP, Patterson VH, Wootton R. Neurological examination is possible using telemedicine. *Journal of Telemedicine and Telecare* 1999;**5**:177–81

23 Craig J, Patterson V, Russell C, Wootton R. Interactive videoconsultation is a feasible method for neurological inpatient assessment. *European Journal of Neurology* 2000;**7**:699–702

24 R Wootton, personal communication

25 Craig J, Chua R, Wootton R, Patterson V. A pilot study of telemedicine for new neurological outpatient referrals. *Journal of Telemedicine and Telecare* 2000;**6**:225–8

26 See http://www.bktelemed.com

27  Swinfen P. Telemedicine service. *The Independent* (Bangladesh), 9 May 2000

28  See http://www.medical-bookmarks.org.uk

29  See http://www.coh/uq.edu.au/swinfen/

30  Corr P, Couper I, Beningfield SJ, Marss M. A simple telemedicine system using a digital camera. *Journal of Telemedicine and Telecare* 2000;**6**:233–6

31  Fraser HS, McGrath SD. Information technology and telemedicine in sub-Saharan Africa. *British Medical Journal* 2000;**321**:465–6

32  Vassallo DJ. Telemedicine kept simple. *Images in Paediatric Cardiology* 2000;**3**:1–14. Also available on line at http://www.magnet.mt/health/impaedcard/issue/issue3/vassallod/vassallod.htm#top, or go to http://www.medical-bookmarks.org.uk then click on Telecommunication (including Telemedicine) and go to electronic journal article 'Telemedicine kept simple'

# Appendix. Case reports

## Patient CRP 001 (orthopaedic)

### *Referral*

I would be most grateful if you would look at this email and its attachments. This patient is a complete tetraplegic, neurological level C5. A male aged 18 years. His tetraplegia developed following a road traffic accident in December 1998. He is now rehabilitated in a wheelchair, suffering frequent attacks of vertigo, probably due to postural hypotension. He has bladder and bowel incontinence, and is using a clean intermittent rubber catheter. This patient's relatives are convinced that he needs further treatment, and they are thinking seriously of travelling to the UK with him, in order to obtain it. We therefore need an opinion as to whether he has any chance of improvement if he should undergo further treatment, by surgery or any other means. Attached are two cropped magnetic resonance images.

### *Reply (same day)*

The replying consultant endorsed the local management regime, and advised that useful neurological recovery was highly unlikely and that the only benefit obtainable by travel overseas would be for aid in occupational therapy. The patient and his family were persuaded that the local doctor's management was appropriate and that they would gain little from overseas travel. They were therefore spared the expense of overseas travel. The patient's quality of life improved slightly afterwards.

### *Result (four emails total)*

There were significant cost savings to patient and family.

## Patient CRP 006 (neurological)

### *Referral*

A 38-year-old man attended the CRP outpatient department with gradual weakness in his upper limbs for the last one and a half years. For the last couple of months he has noticed wasting in the right arm and hand. He has also noticed weakness of the left upper limb. For the last seven years he has been suffering from sexual dysfunction (loss of desire, delayed erection and rapid loss of erection). His attending physician on that visit detected that he had some weakness in the left side of his face. Functionally he is unable to perform fine hand functions such as buttoning his clothes and eating with his right hand. Now he has tremor (coarse) in both hands and is unable to extend the fingers of his right hand. Gradually all the motor symptoms are progressing but his sensory function remains normal. . . . The neurophysiological studies reveal chronic active denervation confined to both upper limbs. . . .

### *Initial reply*

Thanks for the case history which is really difficult! I'm going to discuss the magnetic resonance images with a neuroradiologist colleague but meanwhile answers to the following questions (if they're available) would help. . . .

### *Further reply after supply of answers*

This is extremely difficult! As part of the Royal College of Physicians Membership Examination there are tests called 'grey cases' which are easy compared with this. I will run through my thought processes. First this appears to be a problem with the lower motor neurone system because. . . . I don't think I've been much help to you and I'm still concerned we haven't got a perfect diagnostic fit. This has reinforced my prejudice that teleneurology is best dealt with by realtime ISDN-6 connections (but I realize that this is not always possible!) . . . I look forward to future challenges which I hope will be easier!

### *Result (seven emails total)*

The neurologist's differential diagnosis and expected outcome of the likeliest two diseases (differing mainly in their rate of progression) were thoroughly explained to the patient by the CRP physician. The patient had initially reacted by suggesting that he would travel abroad to try to ascertain the exact diagnosis, but on reflection he decided against this. He accepted that, as there was no effective treatment in either case, he would gain little by doing so.

### Patient CRP 009 (Boxing Day referral) (neurological)

#### Initial referral (when patient was confined to a wheelchair)

A 48-year-old lady, non-diabetic, normotensive, right-handed housewife. Presented with the following complaints: (1) Gradual weakness of both lower limbs since nine months ago. (2) Pain in both calves nine months ago. . . . On examination. Lower limb: All the tendon jerks are absent, muscle tone reduced, muscle power grade III proximal and grade II in distal group of muscles. . . . Disease process [Fig 3] is slowly progressive. . . .

#### Initial reply

This lady seems to have a motor peripheral neuropathy. The likely cause is chronic inflammatory demyelinating peripheral neuropathy (CIDP). If you have access to nerve conduction velocities these should be slow. Your investigations seem to have excluded myeloma and also diabetes; the other condition that needs to be excluded is lead poisoning. CIDP should respond well to steroids — prednisolone 60 mg daily is what I would use. . . .

#### Further email

Following your advice, I started prednisolone . . . after one month of the course I found she was improving.

#### Result (10 emails)

The diagnosis was established, the management changed and the patient fully recovered, walking unaided.

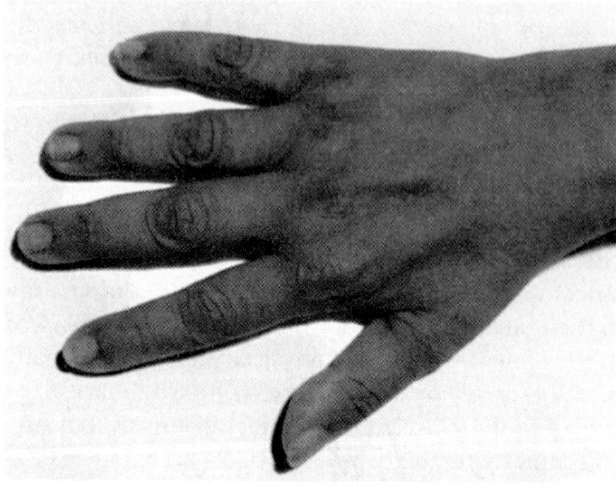

**Fig 3** Wasting of intrinsic hand muscles in CRP 009.

### Patient CRP 011 (orthopaedic)

#### Referral

A young man, 20 years old, had a road traffic accident two months ago and had a closed comminuted fracture of the left tibia and fibula. He was initially treated at the district hospital conservatively and developed compartment syndrome. Four days after the accident he was referred to me. On examination, the left foot was found to have loss of sensation and motor function on dorsum of the foot and anterior compartment of the leg. We immediately did a fasciotomy but after seven days we found necrosis of the anterior and lateral compartment muscles. Finally we performed debridement of the necrotic tissue and subsequently good granulation tissue has formed and the fibula has healed well. However, the fracture area of the shaft of tibia was exposed and had become necrotic; this we removed [Figs 4, 5]. Now the flexor muscle of the leg and foot has normal power. The patient is very much interested

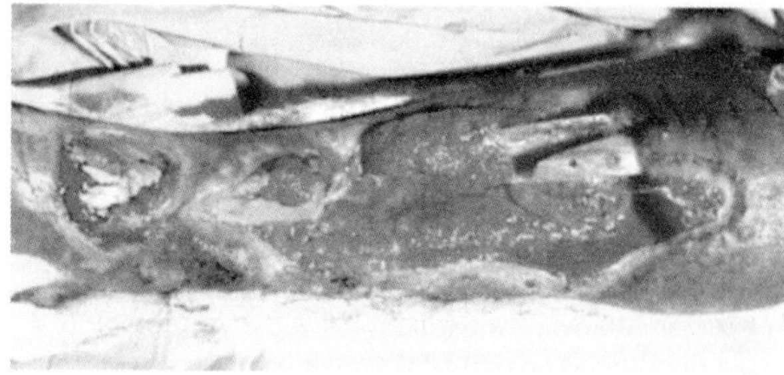

**Fig 4** Extensive leg wound of CRP 011 (after excision of necrotic tibial shaft and necrotic muscles).

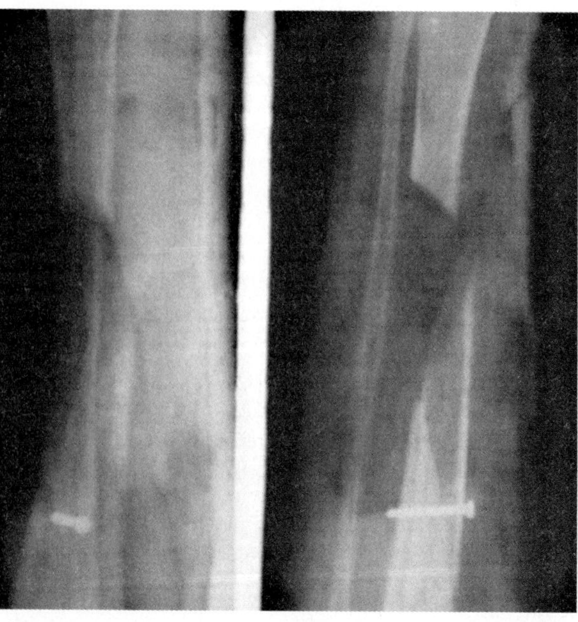

**Fig 5** Radiographs of CRP 011 after excision of necrotic tibial shaft.

in saving his leg. I need your opinion at present as to what should be the line of treatment.

## Initial reply

This is a dreadful case. This would be an appallingly difficult case even in a major trauma unit; I do not envy you. To save the leg, the first essential is skin cover. The extent of the defect is such that only a free flap, probably latissimus dorsi, is the only way to get cover. To deal with the bone defect, there are two options. First an external fixator at anatomical length and once there is good skin cover do an Ilizarov-type bone transport, from proximal to distal. The alternative is to trim the bone ends at the time of the free flap, externally fix and oppose the bone ends and then distract as it starts to unite — risky, but it might work. However, if that were one of my sons (three) I would recommend a below-knee amputation. Otherwise, it's going to be multiple procedures, prolonged period under care, and a far from guaranteed result. Looking at the pictures, you should be able to get a long posterior flap of good skin, so it should be a reasonable stump. Sorry to be so nihilistic, but I think it would be for the best.

## Reply from CRP

Thank you for your detailed explanation. I explained the possibility of amputation but the parents of the patient do not accept this owing to social prejudice. They want to keep the leg even if it is totally inactive. I have removed all the necrotic bone; now the wound is infection free and a good granulation tissue has formed with a big area of bone loss from the tibia. I am planning for skin grafting very soon. After skin grafting I will send you a picture and X-ray of the foot.

## Further reply from UK

If amputation is not an option, there is one rather old and forgotten technique you might consider. The Papineau method for treating infected non-unions was very good at filling in bony defects, even with poor skin cover. If you put on an external fixator to hold anatomical position and to allow the limb to be supported clear of the bed, pack the defect with fine autogenous bone graft, and leave open, and then a continual gentle irrigation with saline over a period of weeks. If you wish, I could dig out some references, though it might take a few days.

## Follow-up after five months

, . . the leg wound is now healed except a tiny point anteriorly lower end of tibia. He is walking with axillary crutch and AFO. He needs bone grafting for an area of 1 cm in the shaft of the tibia.

## Result (five emails)

The management options were clarified and modified according to local circumstances, and moral support was provided for the referring clinician.

# Patient CRP 016 (orthopaedic)

## Referral

A four-year-old boy presented to me at the CRP outpatient department with the complaints of huge swelling of both thighs, shortening of both thighs and unable to walk without support. The boy is quite normal in his other functions and system. He looks very short for his age: height is 70 cm and the diameter of each mid-thigh is 28 cm. It seems that both thighs are short in comparison to his legs and trunk. I did not find any other abnormalities in the boy or any other congenital anomalies in his family. I attach X-rays of both femurs and pictures of his thighs [Figs 6, 7].

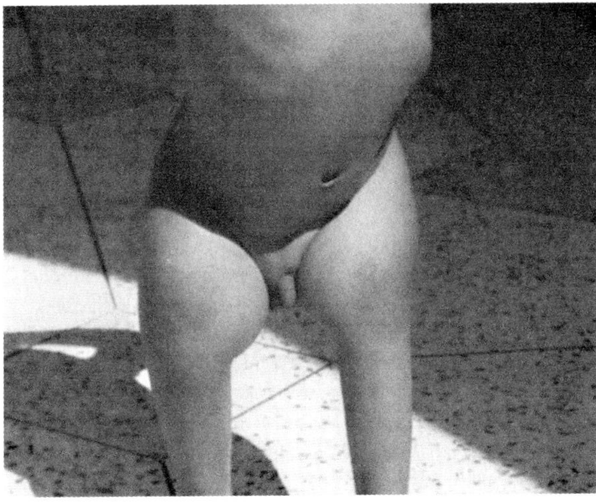

**Fig 6** CRP 016 — neglected congenital dislocation of both hips.

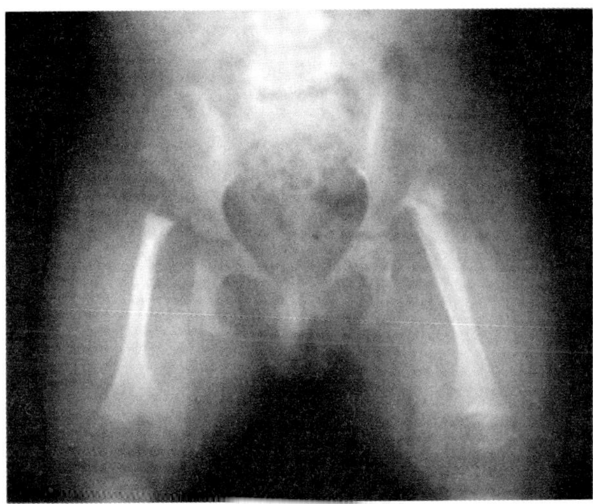

**Fig 7** Radiographs of CRP 016.

### Reply (same day)

I think it is possible he has bilateral congenital dislocation of the hip. That said, on the basis of the photos it is a very severe case. The Canadian experience suggests that leaving them is probably best with late presenters.

### Further reply (next day)

I showed these films in Edinburgh today [at an orthopaedic meeting]. No real consensus, but the absence of the femoral head epiphysis was noted . . . with the acetabular deficiency, I don't feel you have much prospect of getting an anatomical hip joint. My feeling is leave alone for fear of making it worse.

### Result (four emails)

The diagnosis was established, the management plan clarified and no surgery undertaken.

## Patient CRP 027 (orthopaedic)

A 22-year-old boy attended the CRP outpatient department with severe stiffness of both hips and knees. He is unable to bend his spine forward and chest expansion is only 0.5 cm. His blood ESR 106 mm in the first hour (Westergreen). Plain X-ray of both hips shows complete fusion and both knees are dislocated, deformed and have lost contour of the articular surfaces [Figs 8, 9]. His upper limbs and hand functions are normal but both legs have severe disuse atrophy with equinus deformity of both ankles. He is a case of ankylosing spondylitis and now he is pain free and receiving active physiotherapy and NSAID (ibuprofen). At this stage, what could I do for his mobility? What kind of surgery of hips and knees would be helpful for his mobility? Would you please give me a management plan for this patient?

### Reply (same day)

Firstly, let me say that with a chest expansion of only 0.5 cm any surgical intervention would be fraught with danger. As he is pain free his ankylosing spondylitis is largely burnt out although I note his high ESR. I think the most important thing is to strengthen his upper limbs and shoulder girdle so that he can transfer from his wheelchair unaided. If he is able to sit reasonably comfortably I would not recommend any surgical interference. In view of the

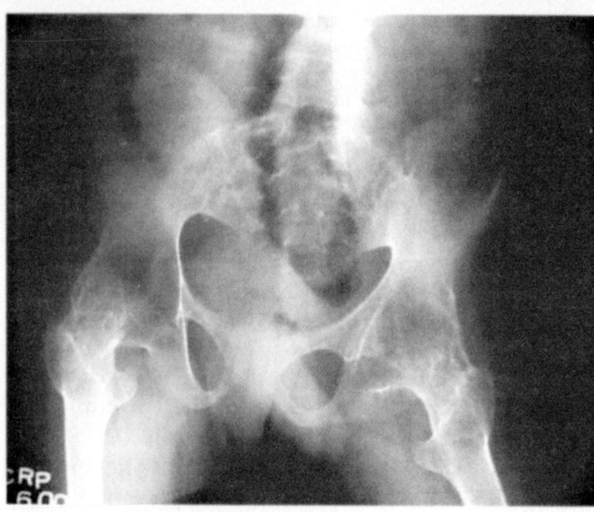

**Fig 8** Pelvic radiographs of CRP 027 (ankylosing spondylitis).

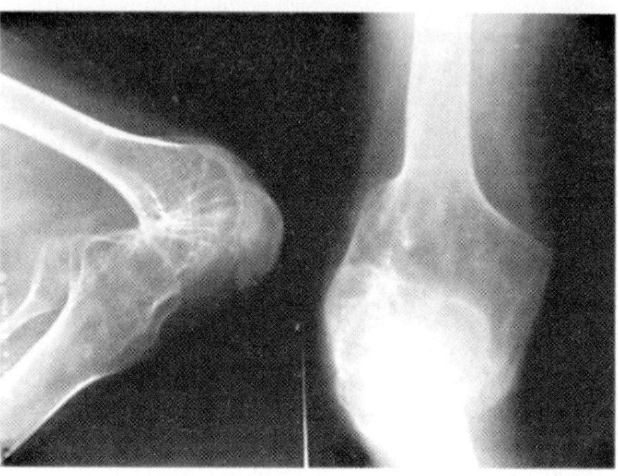

**Fig 9** Knee radiographs of CRP 027.

general state of his lower limbs I feel any surgery to provide mobility of his ankylosed joints would be doomed to failure. I know that people argue that spinal anaesthetics do not interfere with breathing but that is not my experience here. The respiratory effects are just as severe and surgery is to be avoided unless absolutely necessary.

### Result (two emails)

The management plan was clarified and surgery was avoided on the basis of the advice received.

# Section 1:

<table>
<tr><td valign="top" width="35%">

## Health and Clinical Management

<br><br><br><br><br><br><br><br>

*Reprinted by kind permission of:*
*Blackwell Science Ltd. (307)*
*Elsevier Science (322), Sage*
*Publications, Inc. (336), Schattauer*
*GmbH (296,318)*

</td><td valign="top">



</td></tr>
</table>

**Ling Zhu**

Beijing Lianshi Technology Co. Ltd.
Beijing, PR China

# Synopsis

# *Health and Clinical Management*

The Healthcare industry is certainly one of the most information intensive industries. Medical information and clinical data are growing at close to explosive rates each day. Processing medical information and clinic data has become increasingly difficult in medical and clinic management. Computer-assisted information management systems have been used to provide an effective mechanism to present the relevant information/knowledge that is essential in the decision-making processes in Healthcare.

The papers selected for this section address the issues of information applications in health care, especially in clinical management.

The paper by Chakravarty et al. presents a pattern specification language (CAPSUL) to support both acquiring knowledge about patterns from domain experts and searching for these patterns in clinical data sets.

Patterns, as standard solutions to repeating problems, have become increasingly important in formulating the problem-solving processes in many areas of information technology. Some major research focuses with regard to patterns is how to capture patterns as well as how to describe them.

In many medical domains, care providers and clinical researchers need to specify and detect recurring trends, not only at the level of time-stamped data, but also at higher levels of data abstraction. As a result, the detection of repeating patterns in time-oriented clinical data often becomes an important component of the analysis of a large set of clinical data. The pattern specification language (CAPSUL) presented in the selected paper is used as a critical component in a data analysis system. CAPSUL defines a set of expressive constraints upon temporal entities that already exist in the knowledge case. Using a graphical knowledge acquisition tool, expert physicians can specify pattern queries using a variety of temporal and value constraints. CAPSUL provides an expressive language in which one-time only and repeating patterns of intervals can be described. The CAPSUL language is designed both for the task of knowledge acquisition as well as data interpretation, which is very significant to build knowledge-based intelligent medical and clinical information systems.

The paper describes CAPSUL in details as a language to capture the repeating patterns. Many examples are discussed to display the expressive power of the language, its flexibility as well as its limitations. The article also discussed CAPSUL as a knowledge acquisition tool to obtain the domain expertise from experienced expert physicians.

The intensive care unit (ICU) is an environment with abundant data. Each second, a patient data set is produced by online monitoring systems. Clinical data is collected manually at various time intervals. A computer-based patient date management system (PDMS) stores data that has been collected online or entered manually within a specified time frame. Even if these electronic patient records are complete and correct, they are difficult to analyze because they contain so much data. The paper by Horn et al. describes a graphic tool, VIE-VISU, a graphic visualization system, as an aid to comprehending and analyzing a large amount of data.

Graphic representation offers a wide variety of methods to support data integration. Which method is chosen depends mainly on what information is to be displayed for clear comprehension. The article discusses the domain of neonatal intensive care in which recognizing changes of neonatal status over time is critical. As an example, the article describes the 24 hours display of VIE-VISU by using metaphor graphical objects that represent circulatory data, respiratory data and fluid balance.

The nurse change of shift report occurs on most hospital wards everyday. Little study and research, however, has been done upon examining how changing the style and information content of the shift report may affect an individual's ability to process information on her/his duty. The paper by Dowding presents a study that suggests that how individuals structure their knowledge, is an important consideration when examining how they process information.

The nurse change of shift report provides information about patients in the ward or unit to those nurses who are beginning their shift. Often information is provided verbally. The aim of this experimental study was to explore the possible ways that information is processed during the change of shift report on an acute medical and surgical ward in order to provide evidence with which to explore the relevance of the change of shift report to nursing practice. Various assumptions are made about the importance of the information communicated during the shift report. The information which nurses receive during the report is perceived to subsequently enable them to plan and to give care effectively and efficiently to patients. Specific research studies that have examined the nature of the nursing shift report have concentrated too much on the information content of the communication. Those studies have concluded that the verbal communication at the change of shift can be characterized by being retrospective and task orientated, focusing on actions that the nurse has carried out and the medical treatment the patients have received. Despite those assumptions, no research currently

appears to exist to support the claims which have been made. There have been attempts to replace the verbal shift report with written communication, however, these studies have not examined the effect this has had on patient care. There is also no apparent information regarding its usefulness depending on the skill or expertise of the nurses involved in the communication.

It appears from the previously discussed literature that the purpose of the verbal change of shift report is assumed to be to communicate information from one nurse to another nurse(s), and that through this communication, the nurse receiving the report will be able to plan care effectively for his/her patients. Therefore, it could be suggested that the nurse receiving the report has to "process" the information he/she receives in some way. As the theory of information processing suggested, human beings have limited capacities for processing information. And there are only a small number of studies that have examined how nurses process information to form plans of care and make decisions regarding patient care.

The paper discusses the result of an experimental study where report style (retrospective vs. prospective) and schema information (schema consistent vs. schema inconsistent) were compared in a factorial design. A sample of 48 registered nurses from acute medical and acute surgical wards were randomly allocated to one of the four experimental conditions. Outcome measures included the amount of information that subjects accurately recorded and recalled from the shift report, together with their ability to plan patient care. The results of the study indicated that the type of report has a significant effect on an individual's ability to plan patient care, and the type of information content has an

effect on their ability to accurately record and recall the information they heard.

The paper discusses the insufficiency of the current theories of knowledge organization which fail to address how knowledge categories may be linked together, or how new information is accumulated into existing knowledge structures. As an alternative explanation for how knowledge may be organized in the long-term memory, the article describes a schema theory which is regarded as more complicated net-works of represented information, using common themes or situations as a way of organizing knowledge. A number of examples of different types of schema have been given in the article.

This study, however, was based on a fabricated shift report situation and therefore the results need to be treated with some caution. The results of this study did indicate that verbal communication at the change of shift may not be the most effective way of communicating information about patients to enable patient care to be planned effectively. Further research needs to be carried out into the exact role that the change of shift report plays within the context of patient care. Further research also needs to be carried out examining how nursing knowledge affects how information is processed in patient care situations.

Chemotherapy has been regarded as an important component of childhood cancer treatment. Because of the intensity of the therapy, an error in calculating the dosage of the cytostatic drug would have severe consequences. The paper by Knaup et al. presents a computer-aided therapy planning system in pediatric oncology (CATIPO) that aims at reducing errors and saving time during the development of a therapy plan.

CATIPO is actually a knowledge-based expert planning system that aims at determining the adequate therapy for individual patients by determining a complete chemotherapy cycle in advance. It consists of three system components 1) CATIPO-kam, a knowledge acquisition module that formulates the therapy protocol guidelines; 2) CAPITO-dss, a decision-making module that is able to process the formulated protocol guidelines and produce a patient-specific therapy plan; and 3) a knowledge base.

One of the major tasks in CATIPO is to identify, model and formulate the general knowledge of the protocols. Such knowledge is formally represented which allows for use of the implicit knowledge for various patients and for various trials. Part of this process of identifying, modeling and formulating knowledge is the analysis of the explicit knowledge that is acquired by the knowledge acquisition tool, CATIPO-kam. Such knowledge consists of 1) drugs, which are to be used in the chemotherapy cycle; 2) solutions containing an active agent; 3) infusion, which is composed of drugs and solutions; 4) sequential order of drug applications; and 5) inclusion criteria, which takes patients' variables or conditions into account for planning the chemotherapy cycle. All of the formulated knowledge will be used by CAPITO-dss, a decision making tool, to generate a patient-specific therapy plan that adheres to the definition of a therapy protocol.

The paper also discusses some other systems supporting the protocol-guided therapy in oncology and compares them with CAPITO.

In medicine, business, and other domains, people tend to assume that more information cannot hurt. Underlying this assumption is the belief that people have clear and stable preferences that can only be refined by becoming informed. Research in psychology, on the other hand, suggests that individuals' preferences are often unclear and tend to be constructed during the process of making a decision. Psychological research has discovered systematic inconsistencies that stem from individuals' imperfect ability to distinguish relevant from redundant information. One weakness is the tendency to pursue no instrumental information that may be relevant but ought not to alter the decision. In this vein, people sometimes pursue more information than necessary and, once they receive it, tend to see it as crucial for the decision.

The paper by Redelmeier et al. presents a study that investigated whether clinicians also show a tendency to pursue and potentially misapply non-instrumental medical information.

The study tested whether clinicians make different decisions if they pursue information than if they receive the same information from the start. The study was carried out on three participating groups of clinicians: dialysis nurses, practicing urologists and academic physicians with medical scenarios formulated in 1 of 2 versions. And the result of the study indicates that the pursuit of information can increase its salience and cause clinicians to assign more importance to the information than establish that such an awareness of this cognitive bias may lead to improved decision making in difficult medical situations.

The survey that the study was based upon adapted methods developed by psychologists for evaluating how decisions are prone to systematic errors. One scenario with the two different versions was given in the survey, and each version was formulated with different descriptions of information on the scenario. The survey aimed at providing evidence of whether or not clinicians are prone to make different decisions when they pursue information than when they are given the information all at once.

The study suggests that one factor influencing clinicians' decisions is their own behavior. Using scenarios, the article shows how the pursuit of information can lead nurses and doctors to weigh information more heavily than if the information were available at once. As a result, the paper suggested physicians to consider the relevance of missing information before it is pursued. In situations where a piece of information is non-instrumental but is hard to forgo, physicians might be well served by constraining themselves to a pre-specified course of action. For situations in which missing information has been sought without a clear pre-specified plan, the physician may want to consult with a colleague who can review the data easily without biases related to an involved search.

Address of the author:
Dr. Ling Zhu
Beijing Lianshi Technology Co. Ltd.
4/F, Building 7, No.28 Yuhua Road
Area B, Beijing Airport Industrial Zone
101300 Beijing, PR China
or:
Dr. Ling Zhu
China Medical Informatics Association
No.17, Zhengjue Jiadao, Xinjiekou
Xicheng District,
100035 Beijing, PR China
E-mail:  lzhu_md@yahoo.com

# Acquisition and Analysis of Repeating Patterns in Time-oriented Clinical Data

S. Chakravarty, Y. Shahar
Stanford Medical Informatics, Stanford University, California, USA

## Summary

*Objectives:* (1) Creation of an expressive language for specification of temporal patterns in clinical domains, (2) Development of a graphical knowledge-acquisition tool allowing expert physicians to define meaningful domain-specific patterns, (3) Implementation of an interpreter capable of detecting such patterns in clinical databases, and (4) Evaluation of the tools in the domains of diabetes and oncology.

*Methods:* We describe a constraint-based language, named CAPSUL, for specification of temporal patterns. We implemented a knowledge-acquisition tool and a temporal-pattern interpreter within Résumé, a larger temporal-abstraction architecture. We evaluated the knowledge-acquisition process with the help of domain experts. In collaboration with the Rush Presbyterian/St. Luke's Medical Center, we analyzed data of bone-marrow transplantation patients. The expert compared the detected patterns to a manual inspection of the data, with the help of an experimental information-visualization tool we are developing in a related project.

*Results:* The CAPSUL language was expressive enough during the knowledge-acquisition process to capture almost all of the patterns that the experts found useful. The patterns detected in the data by the pattern interpreter were all verified as correct. Completeness (whether all correct patterns were found) was difficult to assess, due to the size of the database.

*Conclusions:* The CAPSUL language enables medical experts to express temporal patterns involving multiple levels of abstraction of clinical data. The ability to reuse both domain-patterns and abstract constraints seems highly useful. The Résumé interpreter, augmented by the CAPSUL semantics, finds the complex patterns within a clinical time-oriented database in a sound fashion.

## Keywords

Temporal Reasoning, Pattern Matching, Temporal Abstraction, Periodicity

Methods Inf Med 2001; 40: 410–20

## 1. Introduction

The detection of repeating patterns in time-oriented clinical data is often an important component of the analysis of large data sets. In many medical domains, from diabetes to oncology, care providers and clinical researchers need to specify and detect recurring trends, not only at the level of time-stamped data, but also at higher levels of data abstraction. For example, an oncologist is often interested in monitoring trends in a patient's systemic toxicity as measured by the level of anemia (from moderate to severe) and the level of fever. The concepts of anemia and fever must be derived from a patient data set that contains only individual test values indicating the level of hemoglobin or temperature at a certain time point. To support the detection of repeating patterns, an intelligent medical data analysis system must first recognize a higher level, clinically meaningful concept, such as anemia from raw level hemoglobin values. Second, the system must combine individual data points into larger intervals, such as systemic toxicity. Finally, the system must detect trends in repeating intervals of systemic toxicity. Fig. 1 shows these levels of data analysis.

In order to accomplish the task of pattern abstraction, our data analysis system needs the following components: a language for expressing the sort of patterns that we want to detect, a knowledge base to define the abstract concepts relative to the domain, a knowledge acquisition tool that domain experts can use to modify and maintain the knowledge base, a patient database that can be mapped to the format expected by the interpreter, and an interpreter to derive the abstractions from the data set. Together, these components comprise a temporal abstraction system. The computational tool of this system is the Résumé system (1). The Résumé system uses the **knowledge-based temporal-abstraction (KBTA)** method (2) to derive high level concepts, or *abstractions*, from raw level data. Each derived abstraction must be associated with a *context*, since the definitions of these abstractions can change depending on the context in which the data were acquired (3). Using a knowledge base of domain-specific contexts, parameters, events, patterns, and a database of time-stamped raw-level data, the Résumé interpreter derives a set of abstractions that can then be visualized and summarized for a user. The knowledge base not only contains the definitions of the concepts, but also the properties of these concepts (such as persistence) that are necessary for deriving them from raw data.

To acquire and detect knowledge about patterns, Résumé uses the **Constraint-Based Pattern Specification Language (CAPSUL)** both to acquire knowledge about patterns from domain experts and to search for these patterns in a data set. CAPSUL defines a set of expressive constraints upon temporal entities that already exist within the Résumé temporal ontology. Using a graphical knowledge acquisition (KA) tool, whose frames mirror the syntax of CAPSUL, expert physicians can specify pattern queries using a variety of temporal and value constraints. These patterns are then combined with the rest of the Résumé temporal ontology and can be derived from a data set by the Résumé interpreter, which includes the CAPSUL language interpreter. The output of the Résumé interpreter is a set of interval-based abstractions (including pattern abstractions) that are directly useful to applications, such as a therapy planner (EON) (4), or that can be displayed and explored using a visualization

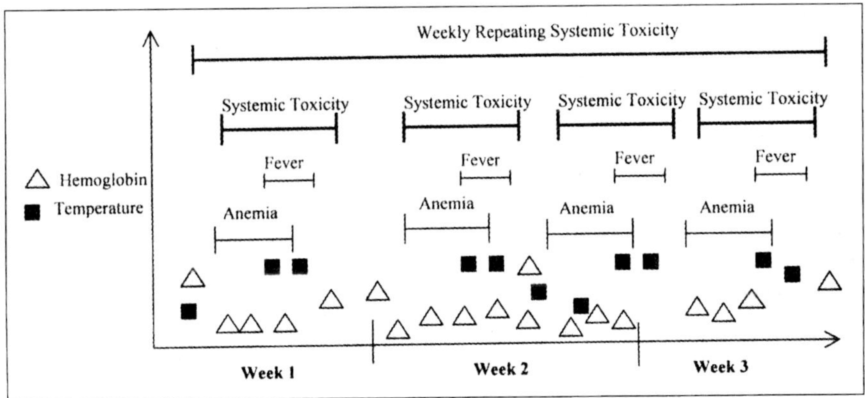


**Fig. 1** The levels of temporal data abstraction. The lowest level of this graph shows raw data indicating the results of hemoglobin tests and temperature measurements. These data points are combined into intervals of the higher level concepts of *Fever* and *Anemia*. These intervals can then be combined into an overall interval of repeating *Systemic Toxicity*. A physician examining this patient record can immediately see that the patient has frequent periods of systemic toxicity.

tool, such as the Knowledge-Based Abstraction Visualization and Exploration (KNAVE) system (5).

In this paper, we first describe the CAPSUL language briefly, providing examples of the types of patterns we can specify and detect. Second, we discuss the knowledge acquisition process, including our success in having domain experts use our KA tool. Third, we will provide results of a recent evaluation of our pattern detection system using data sets in the domains of oncology and diabetes and an expert in each domain. Fourth, we briefly survey related work in the representation of repeating patterns. The results of our evaluation indicate that CAPSUL can capture most useful patterns in which experts are interested, that our KA tool is usable by domain experts with the help of a knowledge engineer, and that the Résumé interpreter can correctly derive patterns when they exist in a data set.

# 2. Language

CAPSUL provides an expressive, yet simple, language in which one-time only ("linear") and repeating ("periodic") patterns of intervals can be described. The CAPSUL language is designed for the twin tasks of knowledge acquisition and data interpretation. At a high level, CAPSUL is

a template for a pattern. Users can fill in this template with a variety of temporal objects and constraints to form a pattern specification. This pattern template is not specific to Résumé. Moreover, it can be used to specify and detect temporal patterns in any domain. To better understand CAPSUL, we examined three key distinctions that structure the syntax of the language.

## 2.1 Description of the Language

CAPSUL distinguishes between *what repeats* (the *single repeating component* of the pattern) from *how it repeats* (the *global repeating-pattern constraints* of the pattern). The repeating pattern components are temporal entities that have previously been defined in the temporal ontology. They may be patterns, events, parameters, or contexts. Each repeating pattern is defined by exactly one repeating component. So, the content of what is to repeat must be expressed as a single abstraction. For example, a component can be a parameter-component such as *Anemia*, where anemia has been defined in the Résumé knowledge base. The constraints define everything about the temporal and value relations between the components. Both the components and the constraints of the pattern are specified in disjunctive normal form. In other words, the user can define more than one set of components or constraints, each of which

comprises a valid definition of the pattern. The separation of components and constraints has important implications for the semantics of CAPSUL patterns: this distinction separates the CAPSUL language from other pattern languages that define repeating patterns as intersections of non-convex intervals (6).

CAPSUL distinguishes between linear and repeating patterns. Linear patterns consist of a set (of one or more) *linear pattern components* that occurs exactly once, such as the linear sequence of high glucose followed by an insulin injection (note, in this example, the first linear component is a parameter, while the second is an event). Meanwhile, repeating patterns consist of exactly one *repeating component* that repeats over time, such as daily glucose measurements. Either type of pattern can be used as a component of its own or of the other type of pattern.

CAPSUL distinguishes three different levels of constraints: local, global, and repeating. All constraints are defined as ranges to enhance flexibility. Local constraints apply to a single interval. They define the duration and value of the interval, as well as the relevant time period in which the interval might occur. For example, an *Anemia*-component could have a local value constraint of *severe* (where a "severe" value of anemia has been defined in the Résumé knowledge base), and a local duration constraint of 3-5 days. Similarly, the relevant time period of a pattern component, including the anemia-component, might be defined as the first midnight following the administration of a drug that might cause the anemia. Global constraints define the temporal and value relations between two components of a linear pattern. For example, a gap between two intervals is a global constraint that defines the temporal distance between any two (of four) endpoints of the intervals (begin-begin, begin-end, end-begin, end-end). Gaps can be qualitative (using Allen's algebra [7]) or quantitative (using numerical values). Furthermore, gaps can be specified using calendaric or absolute units. An *absolute* day is twenty-four hours, even if those twenty-four hours occur from 4 p.m. to 4 a.m. By contrast, a *calendaric* day requires that the twenty-four hours occur from midnight to the next midnight. Finally, CAPSUL allows a limited number of statistical constraints that can be applied to intervals of a linear pattern. A statistical constraint applies to the mean, variance, minimum, or maximum value of a parameter-component. An example of the use of a statistical constraint is: 2 weeks of blood glucose values where the average value of the first week is less than the average value of the second week.

Repeating-pattern constraints define the temporal and value relations between successive intervals of a repeating pattern. Gap and value constraints of this sort, once defined, apply to every successive pair of intervals of the pattern; users cannot specify a different gap or value relation for each pair of intervals of the pattern. Recall, however, that these gap and value relations can be specified as a disjunction of constraints that applies to every pair of successive intervals. Repeating-pattern constraints can also apply to the entire set of intervals that comprise the pattern. For example, the cardinality of the set, the duration of the pattern, or the relevant time period in which the pattern must occur are all examples of repeating-pattern constraints that apply to a whole set of intervals rather than a pair of successive intervals. Furthermore, repeating-pattern constraints can define sub-patterns, or *clusters*, of intervals within the larger pattern over which a set of sub-constraints applies (e.g., an overall pattern of monthly episodes of *Anemia* must contain at least one month in which there are 2 episodes of *Anemia*, both severe). A more complete description of these constraints can be found in Chakravarty and Shahar (8). A complete BNF syntax is included in the appendix to this paper. We now present two examples to better understand the semantics of the CAPSUL constraints.

## 2.2 Examples

A patient who has undergone a bone-marrow transplant (BMT) receives frequent platelet transfusions until the patient's body recovers and starts to produce platelets on its own again. The context of this pattern is BMT, since it applies only to pa-

tients who have had a bone-marrow transplant. The half-life of a platelet transfusion is defined as the time it takes for the platelet level to decrease to one half of the level that was measured immediately post-transfusion. Thus, each platelet transfusion has an associated half life. A physician who is monitoring such a patient wants to know if these successive platelet half lives are increasing or decreasing over time (in order to see how well the patient is adjusting to the transfused platelets). In this pattern, the repeating component is the half life of a single transfusion. The cardinality is 3-5 intervals (to ensure that the trend is not random) and the repeating temporal constraint between intervals is decreasing inter-interval gaps. Each *Platelet-half-life* is itself a linear pattern that consists of a platelet transfusion, the immediate post-transfusion platelet level (the *High* level), and the later *Low* platelet level. These levels, in turn, are abstractions of raw platelet counts. Also, the linear pattern imposes certain local constraints on their values (e.g., one is at least *High*, and the other is *Low* or *Very_Low*) and global temporal constraint on the relation between them (e.g., the high value interval is *before* the low value inter-

val; both are *after* the transfusion event, etc.). This pattern can be parsed using CAPSUL as in Fig. 2.

The design of the CAPSUL syntax includes several limitations that prevent CAPSUL from expressing every possible repeating pattern. CAPSUL cannot handle repeating patterns for which the content of what repeats cannot be expressed as a single repeating component. Consider the following example from diabetes: suppose we want to compare how the average weekend glucose, as monitored by a diabetic patient, compares to the level of glycated hemoglobin, which is measured every other month and provides a more reliable measure of blood glucose. The pattern we are interested in consists of high average glucose on weekends, 3 times a month, for at least 6 months of the year. Additionally, the pattern contains an episode of glycated hemoglobin during every other month in which the weekend glucose is high. Either of these patterns can be expressed using CAPSUL. However, the combination of weekend glucose measurements and bimonthly glycated hemoglobin measurements cannot be expressed as a single CAPSUL pattern, since it consists of two independently repeating

**Repeating Pattern:** *Declining Platelet Half Life*
    **Context**: BMT
    **Repeating Component**: Platelet Half Life
    **Constraints**:
        **Cardinality**: 3-5 repetitions
        **Temporal Envelope**: 5 weeks
        **Value Constraint between successive intervals**: Less-than-or-equal

**Linear Pattern:** *Platelet Half Life*
    **Context**: BMT
    **Linear Components**:
        **Event Component**: Transfusion-Component
          **Abstracted from**: Platelet Transfusion
        **Parameter Component**: High-Platelet-State
          **Abstracted from**: Platelet-State
          **Local Constraints**: value HIGH
        **Parameter Component**: Low-Platelet-State
          **Abstracted from**: Platelet-State
          **Local Constraints**: value LOW
    **Global Constraints**:
        **Quantitative Gap Constraint**: High-Platelet-State <= 1 hour AFTER Transfusion-Component
        **Qualitative Gap Constraint**: Low-Platelet-State AFTER High-Platelet-State
    **Output Value of Pattern**:
        **Duration Function**: [(Start of Low-Platelet-State) – (Start of High-Platelet-State)]/2

**Fig. 2** A partial parsing of the pattern "Declining Platelet Half Life" in the CAPSUL syntax. The repeating component slot of the repeating pattern points to an instance of a linear pattern, namely, the "Platelet Half Life" pattern. Note that the repeating pattern and linear pattern exist as instantiated temporal objects of their respective classes in the knowledge base. These patterns have pointers to other temporal objects in the knowledge base, such as "Platelet State" and "Platelet Transfusion".

components that repeat at different frequencies. A repeating component cannot consist of both a high average weekend glucose and a glycated hemoglobin interval, since for most episodes of *High-Weekend-Glucose* there is no corresponding *Glycated Hemoglobin* measurement. We call this example the *Weekend-Glucose-and-Glycated Hemoglobin* pattern.

For this pattern, the best we can do using CAPSUL is to create two patterns, one consisting of a year in which the average weekend glucose constraints are satisfied, and a second pattern consisting of repeating glycated hemoglobin measurements for 1 year. We can combine these two repeating patterns into a single linear pattern in which the two separate components overlap, but we cannot constrain the individual episodes of high glycated hemoglobin to occur during every other month in which the average weekend glucose is high.

## 2.3 Expressivity

Examples such as the previous one, which cannot be expressed in CAPSUL, lead us to ask: what set of patterns can be expressed using CAPSUL? There are three noteworthy design decisions that effect the expressivity of CAPSUL.

CAPSUL patterns are represented as single components that repeat over time. In this regard, CAPSUL patterns differ from intersections of nonconvex intervals (6). If we considered any intersection of nonconvex intervals as a pattern, the previous *Weekend-Glucose-and-Glycated Hemoglobin* pattern example could be expressed. The reason being that we could check if the two nonconvex intervals were aligned so that the glycated hemoglobin values occurred at the same time as every other month of high weekend glucose. CAPSUL patterns represent a subset of such patterns; CAPSUL patterns are those in which a one-to-one correspondence between convex sub-intervals of the two (or more) nonconvex intervals exists. In such cases, the convex subintervals can be paired up exactly, where each pair represents one component of a repeating pattern.

CAPSUL pattern constraints are specified as relationships between consecutive intervals. The user may specify exactly one set of constraints to define this relationship. The same set of constraints (or disjunction of constraints) must hold between each pair of consecutive intervals. In other words, the user may not specify a different set of constraints for each pair of intervals that comprise the pattern. This limitation implies, for example, that CAPSUL cannot represent patterns in which the gaps between intervals follow a Fibonacci sequence.

CAPSUL also cannot handle patterns that require "non-linear" constraints. By non-linear, we mean the evaluation of the constraint over a given set of intervals requires a non-linear algorithm with respect to the number of intervals in the set. In other words, constraints must be evaluated by comparing pairs of single repeating components rather than considering the entire set of such repeating components at once. All of the constraints in the CAPSUL syntax can be evaluated linearly for a set of elements. The CAPSUL interpreter can step down the set of (temporally ordered) intervals and evaluate the constraints in one pass. For example, the gap constraint defines one relation (which may be a disjunction of relations) to be evaluated for each consecutive pair of intervals. Once the constraint has been evaluated for a pair of intervals, the interpreter never revisits the intervals to evaluate this constraint. Thus the running time of the constraint-satisfaction, given a set of $m$ sorted elements, is $O(m)$. This is called the linearity characteristic of CAPSUL constraints. Also, the CAPSUL constraints were designed specifically to maintain this characteristic. These design properties of the language help define a CAPSUL pattern more precisely.

# 3. Knowledge Acquisition

To complete the temporal abstraction task, Résumé requires a domain-specific knowledge base of concepts related to the domain. The four types of concepts in a Résumé knowledge base are parameters (e.g., *glucose*), contexts (e.g., *diabetes*), events (e.g., *platelet transfusion*), and patterns (e.g., *Platelet-Half-Life*). The interface to the Résumé knowledge base is a graphical tool through which domain experts can create, modify, visualize, and maintain the Résumé knowledge base. This graphical tool was created using the Protégé tool set (4). It can be used to create knowledge acquisition (KA) tools in any domain. The Résumé KA tool we are currently using has been designed for the medical domain. The Résumé knowledge base, as visualized in the KA tool, is organized in an IS-A class hierarchy. The top-level view of the Résumé KA tool contains frames for the definitions of the four knowledge classes. Each entity in the ontology can be viewed and edited in a separate window with slots allowing the user to specify the various parameters, event, and pattern values. The window slots containing pattern definitions closely follow the CAPSUL syntax. A domain expert uses this KA tool to create and modify an ontology of terms and concepts that applies to his/her specific domain, such as diabetes. In order to maintain knowledge specific to different medical domains, we have created a separate knowledge base for each of our domain areas.

## 3.1 Example

As an example for entering knowledge using the Resume KA tool, consider the following CAPSUL pattern. The pattern monitors how well the glucose level can be controlled by a patient. The relevant context in this case is diabetes. The *Recurring Weekend Glucose Monitoring* repeating pattern consists of low or very low morning glucose and high evening glucose (with at least one insulin injection in-between), occurring during the weekend, for 5-7 weekends during the summer. Most diabetic patients record insulin administrations and blood glucose values on a daily basis. In this case, the repeating component is a linear pattern called *Weekend Glucose Monitoring* that consists of three linear components: *Low-Morning-Glucose, High-Evening-Glucose,* and *Insulin-Injection.* To define the repeating-pattern constraints associated with this pattern, we must first define a calendar-specific term, *Summer*, which itself is a repeating temporal interval. The repeating pattern contains a cardinality constraint (5-7 repetitions) and a period-constraint that specifies that the relevant scope of the pattern is Summer. Further, the *Recurring Weekend Glucose Monitoring* pattern contains a cluster constraint that requires at least two consecutive so-called *Highly Variable Weekends* in which the value of the single repeating component is Very_Low. For this cluster, we must also define a repeating calendar interval of *Weekend*, just as we defined Summer.

To enter the *Recurring Weekend Glucose Monitoring* pattern in the Resume KA tool, the domain expert first uses the KA tool to abstract the concept of *Glucose-State* from individual glucose counts. The user maps numeric ranges of glucose values to symbolic terms. (e.g., for a diabetic patient, a glucose count below 88 corresponds to an abstraction of *Low* Glucose-State). Building upon this abstraction, the user defines more complicated abstractions, that depend on the level of Glucose-state. An important feature of any Protégé KA tool is that any entity of the ontology, once defined, is reusable in any other part of the ontology. However, currently, the system does not warn users when they modify definitions of entities that are referenced elsewhere in the ontology. The new parameter, Glucose-State, can now be used in the definitions of other entities in the ontology.

The second step in the definition of our example, as shown in the screen shot depicted in Fig. 3, is to define the linear pattern called *Weekend Glucose Monitoring*. The domain expert uses the Glucose-State abstraction in the definition of two of the three components of this linear pattern: *Low-Morning-Glucose* (the patient's Glucose-State has a value of *Low* in the morning), *High-Evening-Glucose*, and *Insulin-Injection* (classified in the Resume ontology as the event of giving oneself insulin). By selecting any of the three components listed in the "Linear Components" frame and clicking "Edit", a new window, containing slots for local level constraints, appears. This allows the user to define local constraints on any of these components. The

other major frame of interest in this figure is the "Constraints" frame. Here, the user defines global constraints. These specify that the interval of Low-Morning-Glucose must precede the Insulin-Injection, which must precede the interval of High-Evening-Glucose. Given these constraints, which define the temporal ordering of the components, the linear sequence of components, which defines the Weekend Glucose Monitoring pattern, can be defined.

As the third and final step of using the KA tool to define this example pattern, Figs. 4 and 5 show the knowledge acquisition screens of the constraints associated with the *Recurring Weekend Glucose Monitoring* repeating pattern. Once the user specifies that the repeating component of this pattern is the Weekend Glucose Monitoring linear pattern, as defined above, the pattern's repeating-pattern constraints can be defined, which are a cardinality constraint, a period constraint (which defines the relevant time period of the pattern), and a cluster constraint. The cluster con-

straint specifies that, within the pattern, there must exist 2-5 consecutive weekends for which the value of the repeating component is *Very_Low*. The graphical specification of this cluster constraint is shown in Fig. 4. One of the constraints on this sub-pattern is a gap constraint of 7 days, shown in Fig. 5. This gap constraint requires that the weekends of the sub-pattern must be consecutive.

To facilitate the knowledge acquisition process, the knowledge base ontology differs slightly from the knowledge base used by the Résumé interpreter. The filtering process, which converts the knowledge base, as defined by the user, into the knowledge base to be interpreted by Résumé, handles small, but important, tasks, such as adding back pointers between temporal objects. (This is necessary so that each temporal object points to both what it is abstracted from as well as what it is abstracted into). The filter also restructures the class hierarchy to eliminate intermediate classes, which are useful for knowledge acquisition,

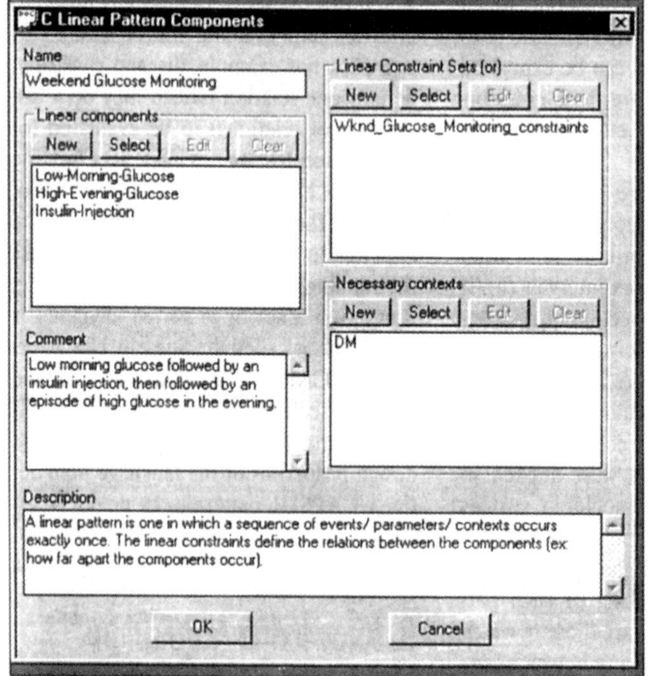



**Fig. 3**  A linear pattern definition. The window defines the linear pattern "Weekend Glucose Monitoring". The frame "linear components" contains pointers to the three linear components of this pattern. The "constraints" window contains pointers to the constraints associated with these linear components. Note that all temporal objects, including constraints, exist as separate entities in the knowledge base; the user can reference a constraint or component that is used in another pattern definition by clicking the "select" button and choosing a pointer to a previously-defined component or constraint.

but are inefficient for the detection process. For example, when acquiring knowledge, it is useful to store each type of constraint as a separate class (so that each constraint can be named and reused by other patterns), so the KA tool has separate classes for each type of constraint. However, the abstraction process can be much faster if all constraints are bundled with the appropriate pattern. In this way, the Résumé knowledge base does not store constraints as separate objects from the pattern objects.

## 3.2 KA Evaluation

To test the knowledge acquisition process, as well as the usability of the CAPSUL language, we have worked with two domain experts with moderate computer experience to create knowledge bases for two medical domains, diabetes and oncology. The domain experts have already shown their capability for independent use of the KA tool without the repeating pattern frames (9). Our domain experts tried to use the enhanced KA tool with the help of a knowledge engineer. The process has proven very useful both for domain experts, as well as knowledge engineers. Also, the users pointed out the features and bugs of our KA process. As a domain, diabetes lends itself to specifying complex patterns of parameters, such as glucose, that are measured on a daily basis. These are of particular interest to physicians as weekly and monthly trends. For this, the calendar-based constraints of CAPSUL have proven very useful for specifying patterns, such as repeating states of high Glucose on consecutive weekends for a period of at least two months.

For the bone marrow transplant (BMT) knowledge base, our domain expert worked with us to create a knowledge base consisting of over 70 parameters typically of interest when a patient has received a bone-marrow transplant, such as White Blood Cell count, Total Bilirubin, and Platelet Count. We began by selecting the 70 most useful parameters often measured for BMT patients from a group of 550 such parameters. We categorized the chosen parameters into eight classes: hematological, drug levels, electrolytes, infection, metabolic, pancreatic, renal, and respiratory. For each parameter, we not only defined the concept and its range, but also, mapped the numerical values of the parameters, as encountered in a database, into symbolic values, such as *Platelet-State*, as described earlier.

The next phase of the knowledge acquisition was to elicit useful patterns in the domain. We defined a total of 10 patterns that were of interest to the oncologist. Due to space limitations, we cannot include the full specifications of all 10 patterns. We realized during this process that the CAPSUL patterns in the oncology domain were of a different nature than those in the diabetes domain. We learned that many of the most useful patterns were not concepts that we would usually classify as patterns, but that are easily represented in CAPSUL patterns. The *Platelet Half Life* pattern described earlier is an example of this. Although physicians usually think of the half life of a platelet transfusion as a single measurement rather than a pattern, the most appropriate CAPSUL representation of this measurement is a linear pattern as shown in Fig. 2. In practice, most of our pattern specifications consisted of linear patterns and their corresponding repeating pattern, where the repeating pattern is a simple extension of the linear one. For example, after defining the linear pattern for the half life of transfused platelets, it was

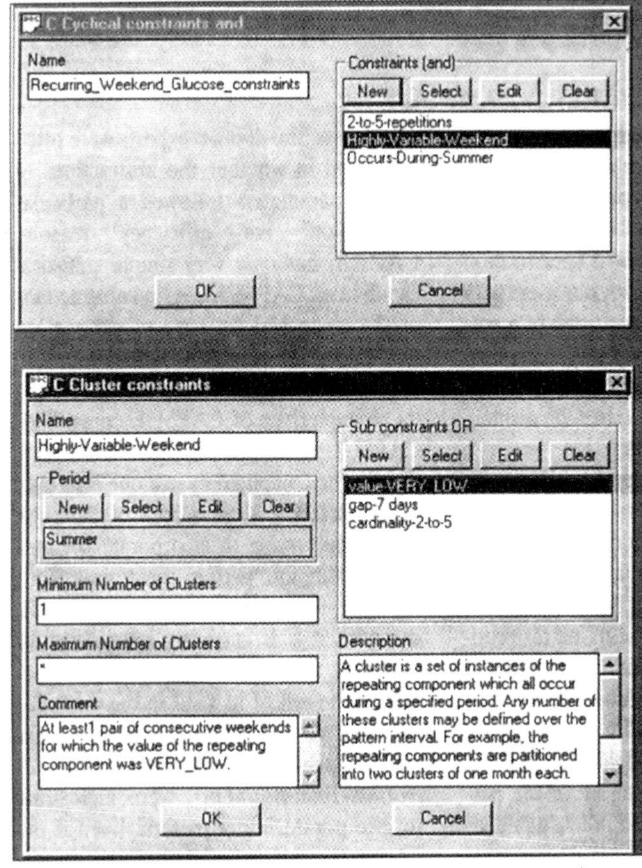

**Fig. 4**   Definition of repeating-pattern constraints. The top window shows the definition of the set of repeating-pattern constraints associated with the pattern Recurring-Weekend-Glucose-Monitoring. The set contains a cardinality constraint, a period constraint, and a cluster constraint. The period, or relevant scope, of the pattern is Summer (where Summer is a repeating time interval, defined elsewhere in the knowledge base). The bottom window shows the specification of a cluster constraint. The sub-pattern consists of at least one pair of consecutive weekends during which the value of the repeating component was VERY_LOW. The 7 day gap constraint ensures that the intervals are consecutive, while the cardinality constraint ensures that there are at least 2 such weekends in the cluster. The definition of the 7-day gap constraint is shown in Figure 6.

natural for the oncologist to inquire whether these half lives decrease over time. For this, we defined the repeating pattern "Declining Platelet Half Life" to see if the values of the platelet half life patterns repeated over time, and if so, if the values decreased steadily over time, as shown in Fig. 2.

In the BMT ontology, we also defined a pattern that describes the simultaneous toxicity levels of several organ systems. The pattern *Multiple-Organ-Toxicity* consists of overlapping intervals of Renal, Liver, and Myelotoxicity levels. Toxicity levels for each organ are characterized by different parameters: Renal toxicity is measured by Creatinine, Liver toxicity is governed by Total Bilirubin and Alkaline Phosphatase, and Myelotoxicity is defined by White Blood Cell count and Platelet-State. Thus the pattern of *Multiple-Organ-Toxicity* summarizes the values of 5 different raw level data elements, which would be very difficult for a person to try to find by hand in a patient data file. We also defined a pattern, called *Time to T-Bili Recovery*, to measure the time required for the total Bilirubin parameter to recover to a normal level after a bone marrow transplantation. For this, we defined a linear pattern consisting of a BMT followed by a sustained period of normal Total Bilirubin; the value of the parameter was the gap between these components. We defined similar time-to-recovery patterns of several parameters of interest, such as White Blood Cells and Platelets. Additionally, we classified the intervals of abnormality for the Total Bilirubin and SGPT parameters as overlapping or disjoint. The last two patterns looked for intervals in which the Total Bilirubin and Creatinine levels fluctuated within the normal range after recovery.

The users, who tested the KA tool, liked several features of the graphical tool. The Windows/NT design of the windows allows for intuitive browsing and filling of the slots in the various windows and frames. The users could quickly find the windows for the objects they wanted to modify. Within windows, the users were almost always able to quickly understand the meanings of different slots. For simple parameter definitions, the users were able to use the tool

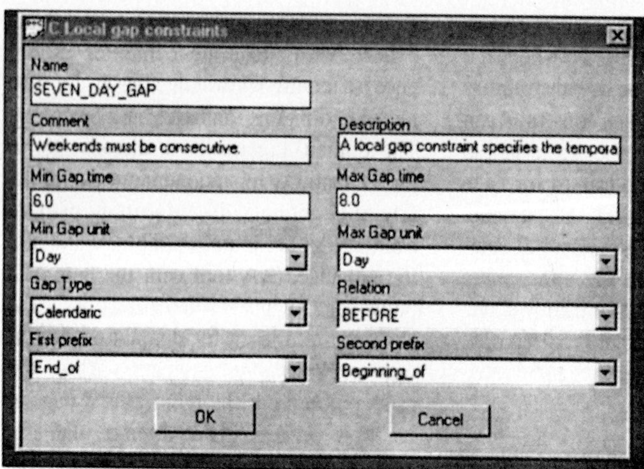


**Fig. 5** Definition of a gap constraint. This constraint, which is part of the Highly-Variable-Weekend sub-pattern, specifies that all weekends that are part of the sub-pattern must be 6-8 days apart. We use a gap measured in days rather than weeks to enhance flexibility. Since the periodic components are already required to occur during a weekend, this gap constraint is enough to ensure that the sub-pattern will consist of consecutive weekends. The gap type is calendaric, meaning that the gap must be measured using calendar days. Note that there is no slot in this window to specify which pair of Weekend-Glucose-Monitoring components this constraint applies to; once any repeating-pattern constraint is specified, that constraint applies to every consecutive pair of intervals of the pattern.

without assistance to modify existing definitions of ranges or symbolic values. Although the users found pattern specification a bit more complex, the disjunctive normal form of the pattern specification was surprisingly intuitive for our users with little explanation. The structuring of a pattern definition in an AND-OR tree made sense to them. Also. they were able to describe their patterns in terms of disjunctions of sets of constraints.

With regard to the expressive power of our pattern specification language, we found that CAPSUL could specify almost all of the patterns in which our users expressed interest. We had more success in using more expressive repeating-pattern constraints in the diabetes domain. In that domain, we could successfully input 6 out of the 8 patterns suggested by the expert. In the BMT domain, although we had a bit more trouble in expressing all of the patterns of interest, we gained the valuable insight of recognizing and expressing concepts that we do not normally think of as a series of repeating events, such as the *Platelet Half Life* example from Section 2.

Two primary types of patterns were determined that CAPSUL could not express, but in which our domain experts were interested. The first area is that of statistical constraints. The domain experts were often interested in whether the abstractions of certain parameters followed a particular distribution. For efficiency reasons, CAPSUL has only very simple statistical capabilities: CAPSUL can find abstractions of the mean and variance of parameters, but CAPSUL cannot fit distributions to sets of data. This goes along with the linearity characteristic of CAPSUL constraints: CAPSUL is limited to those constraints that can be computed by just one pass over a data set. The second area of difficulty arose when trying to incorporate the idea of ordinality into pattern constraints. Since the derivation of abstractions occurs in random order, it is currently impossible for CAPSUL to specify that a certain component is the $n$th of its kind in the data. For the *Time To T-Bili Recovery* pattern, constraints, such as "find the first occurrence of *Normal-Total-Bilirubin*", were impossible to incorporate into a pattern. Even if the interpreter were to find and sort all instances of Normal-Total-Bilirubin at every step of the abstraction process, there would be no way to verify that an earlier interval of Normal-Total-Bilirubin would not be found later in the data set. We intend to enhance the computational framework somewhat to enable constraints such as "First occurrence". Most of the other difficulties encountered by the users can be solved with a more extensive help file, or tutorial, that explains the meanings of the slots in a more intuitive way for users with moderate computer experience. One commonly encountered problem was dealing both with the number of windows required, as well as the number of slots per window. Because of the large number of slots associated with patterns, our users often required the assistance of a knowledge engineer to input patterns into the KA tool.

Overall, however, the domain experts were quite satisfied with the ability of CAPSUL to express complicated patterns useful in the analysis of patient records. Furthermore, all patterns that could be expressed theoretically in CAPSUL, were successfully entered into the knowledge base via the graphical KA tool, demonstrating the ability of the current Résumé/ CAPSUL KA tool to support entry of CAPSUL expressions.

# 4. Implementation

The pattern-matching module of Résumé is currently implemented as a rule-based system in the CLIPS expert system shell. Each abstraction is associated with a rule that governs how it is derived from data points and a set of constraints. The left hand side of such a rule is a translation of a CAPSUL repeating pattern specification, including its repeating component and all repeating-pattern constraints. The right hand side of the rule consists of commands that generate an instance of the repeating pattern, including the appropriate start and end times, value, and contexts. Recall that once generated, a Résumé abstraction is added to a general pool of instances upon which further abstractions may be derived. This allows the inputs to a repeating pattern to consist not only of raw level data, but also of high level abstractions (such as linear patterns) that have already been generated.

Résumé uses the specifications of repeating patterns filtered from the knowledge base to generate rules, which check for these patterns in the database. When a repeating pattern rule fires, the resulting instance that is created contains the name of the pattern, the start and end times of the pattern (in real time points, in the same units as the database), and the value of the pattern, as defined in the knowledge base. The Résumé interpreter outputs these instances of repeating patterns along with the all the other abstractions that it has derived from the data set. The running time of the Résumé interpreter varies between 1 to 12 hours, depending on the size of the knowledge base and the amount of data.

For the purpose of pattern detection, we have found that a more goal-directed approach works much more efficiently than allowing Résumé to derive a full set of abstractions on an entire data set. If we are interested in asking a query about a particular pattern, then we can run Résumé as follows: First we extract all the data points that are used in the definition of the pattern in question from the data set. We then run Résumé using just the pattern definition as a knowledge base (and its related lower level abstractions) and the relevant data. For the *Platelet Half Life* pattern example, we would extract (using a linear-time search procedure) all of the data points of *Platelet transfusion* and *Platelet count* from the data. The abridged knowledge base consists of the rules for the abstractions of *Platelet-state* and *Platelet Half Life*. When run in this fashion, the time required to detect a pattern in data is at most a few minutes, compared to several hours if Résumé is run in the more comprehensive way.

# 5. Data Analysis

In collaboration with the Rush Presbyterian/St. Luke's Medical Center, we have evaluated the pattern-matching Résumé interpreter in the oncology domain by analyzing data sets from patients who have received bone marrow transplants. We obtained an extensive database from the Rush Bone Marrow Transplantation (BMT) Center that contained full records of over 100 patients. Each patient was hospitalized between 2 months and 3 years.

During the course of treatment, the patients had daily tests taken for a subset of some 550 laboratory parameters. In addition, the data contained the various blood transfusions that the patients received during their hospitalization. Overall, each patient data set contains several thousand test values, including the date(s) of transplant operation(s) and basic biographical information. The data was recorded during the period 1993-1996 using a Paradox (DOS-based) database. First, we converted this database into a Microsoft Access database; from this format we converted it into a text-based format that could be read in by the Résumé interpreter.

After creating the BMT knowledge base (including parameters, events, linear and repeating patterns) as described in Section 3.2, we moved on to the actual derivation of these abstractions in the patient data files. With help from our domain expert, we then selected the full records of ten patients. For 4 of these patients, we used the Résumé interpreter, combined with the BMT knowledge base, to derive a full set of abstractions for these patients. These abstractions included 3 types of higher-level parameters (states, gradients, and rates), as well as the 10 patterns discussed above. On average, the output of Résumé was about five times the size of the input; each element of raw data was used in the derivation of about 4 higher-level abstraction intervals. The average running time for these files was 5 hours. We also used the goal-directed approach, described in Section 4, to search for these patterns in the other 6 patient data files. When run using the goal-directed approach, the running time was reduced to about 5 minutes. The results of the analysis are shown in Fig. 6.

With over 3000 output intervals, our domain experts could not hope to examine all of the text output of Résumé. Instead, the output intervals were entered into an online visualization tool, a derivation of KNAVE (5). In this way, both the raw level data, as well as the abstracted intervals could be explored. After visualizing the output, we went through several iterations of modifying the pattern specifications, rerunning Résumé, then looking at the output again. As the pattern specifications be came more precise, several instances of them were found in the data; however, missing data points often served as a hindrance to the detection of patterns. For example, although each patient received between 10 and 20 platelet transfusions, we often found only a few (or no) instances of the Platelet Half Life patterns, since the measurement of a platelet count was often not recorded soon enough after the transfusion to be considered an accurate measure of the post-transfusion platelet count. In other cases, we often had to make the constraints of a pattern more flexible by widening the range of a gap constraint, or adding another term to a conjunction of constraints, in order for the pattern to be found in the data.

Through this process of evaluation, we addressed two questions. First, how much time can we save by analyzing the patient data sets using Résumé, and second, what insights can Résumé provide that are impossible to discover without the use of such a tool? With regard to the first question, the sheer size of the data set made it difficult to analyze the patient data without the help of some computer software. By reformatting and creating charts of small, selected parts of the data set, the expert could identify trends in the values of individual, raw-level parameters. Within just a couple of hours, the expert was able to reformat the data and plot it using a spreadsheet package. Thus, for the task of looking only at individual raw data values and identifying extrema, using a regular spreadsheet program may actually be easier than using Résumé. Résumé is most useful when trying to identify trends not only in raw data, but in higher level abstractions, and when trying to identify trends in more than one parameter at once. Many interesting patterns that involve more than one parameter are very time-consuming to find by hand. For example, consider the earlier example of *Liver-toxicity*, a high level concept that is derived from the states of Alkaline Phosphatase and Total Bilirubin. When both of these parameters are high at the same time, Résumé can derive the abstraction of *Liver-toxicity*. To find this pattern in the patient data record by hand, the expert must (mentally or using a spreadsheet) align the graphs for

|  | Patient 1 | Patient 2 | Patient 3 | Patient 4 |
|---|---|---|---|---|
| Number of data points | 3061 | 2437 | 1449 | 3834 |
| Time period of recorded data | 14 months | 35 months | 19 months | 9 months |
| Number of outputed abstractions | 5207 | 3781 | 6217 | 10659 |
| Total Pattern Intervals found: | 16 | 17 | 6 | 23 |
| Platelet Half Life | 5 | 10 | 0 | 14 |
| Declining Platelet Half Life | 1 | 2 | 0 | 3 |
| Total Bilirubin recovery time | 1 | 1 | 1 | 1 |
| White Blood Cell recovery time | 1 | 1 | 1 | 1 |
| Platelet recovery time | 1 | 1 | 1 | 1 |
| Bilirubin-SGPT abnormalities | 1 | 1 | 1 | 1 |
| Total Bilirubin fluctuations | 1 | 0 | 1 | 0 |
| Creatinine fluctuations | 2 | 1 | 0 | 1 |
| Multi-organ toxicity | 2 | 0 | 1 | 1 |
| Repeating Multi-Organ Toxicity | 1 | 0 | 0 | 0 |

**Fig. 6** Results of data analysis. We analyzed 10 full patient records with the Résumé interpreter using 10 pattern specifications relevant to the bone marrow transplantation domain. Results are reported above for six representative patients; two of these data sets were run in the goal-directed mode. On average, Résumé outputs 4 times as many abstractions as inputed data points. By visualizing the raw data points along with the outputed abstractions, we concluded that the Résumé interpreter correctly finds linear and repeating patterns when they exist in the data.

Total Bilirubin and Alkaline Phosphatase and see if, and when, they both are high at the same time. For tasks such as these, the Résumé interpreter can greatly speed up the time required to analyze data.

In other cases, Résumé not only speeds up data analysis, but also makes the detection of patterns possible, that could not be found at all by looking at raw level data only. Patterns that involve trends in one or more parameter over years, for example, or those that require more complex intermediate levels of abstraction (that cannot be easily derived mentally) are made tractable by Résumé. For example, consider the pattern of a quickly changing glucose level at least once a week for more than half of the weekends in a year. Such a pattern is useful to both patient and physician, to identify lifestyle patterns that cause rapid changes in glucose level. Such a pattern could have

important implications for a patient's diabetes control. To find this pattern by hand, an analyst would first have to plot the glucose levels, derive the *Glucose-state* values, then count the weekends in which the value of *Glucose-state* changed sharply (either decreasing or increasing). He would then determine if this occurred more than 26 times within any given 12 month period in the database. For practical purposes, it is impossible for a physician to detect such a pattern, making a system like Résumé necessary.

# 6. Related Work

Most work in the area of temporal reasoning, involving interval-based representations of time, refers to Allen (7), who defined an interval algebra of 13 basic binary temporal relations for convex time intervals. These temporal relations are the basis for the qualitative temporal relations allowed in CAPSUL. Ladkin (6) developed a taxonomy of binary relations between non-convex intervals. In that work, Ladkin also showed that the number of relations between unions of nonconvex intervals is at least exponential in the number of convex subintervals, a result that proved useful to us. Rather than allowing any possible union of nonconvex intervals, CAPSUL allows only those unions in which the convex subintervals can be matched one-to-one.

In another work, Ladkin (10) dealt with the representation of calendar-based time. He developed a formal representation of repeating intervals, such as *Mondays,* that we referred to when incorporating repeating events into our framework. In a paper dealing with the representation of events in calendar time, Clifford and Rao (11) identified different types of elements in their temporal universe, all of which could be represented in different time units. Unlike us, they did not allow the problematic use of weeks as a time unit, since weeks can overlap with months and years and, therefore, do not fit into the natural subset chain of <seconds, minutes, hours, days, months, years>.

Several people have proposed frameworks similar to ours, defining repeating events. Cukierman and Delgrande (12) studied calendar-based repeating temporal objects. In this language, a series of $n$ repeats is represented as follows: $<r_1, g_1, r_2, g_2, ..., r_n, g_n>$, where $r$ refers to a repeat (an instance of the repeating event) and $g$ refers to a gap. An important component of the Cukierman language is the pattern of gaps $<g_1, g_2, ..., g_n>$, which allows each gap to be the same, to be different, or to be defined probabilistically. More recently, Cukierman and Delgrande (5) introduced a revised framework for representing repetition with the notion of a *time loop.* Such a loop is made up of a cycle (or a repeat), as well as the relations between cycles. Furthermore, this loop may be "flattened" to form a "closed-view representation" of the sequence of instances that constitutes the loop's semantics. Thus, all re-

peats can be represented in only a single cycle. In this way, the object that repeats does *not* vary with time. In the Cukierman-Delgrande language, loops are represented in closed time: a pattern, Math class on Monday and English class on Tuesday, is represented as the convex interval <Math before English> that repeats weekly. Representing this same pattern in Ladkin's language involves correlating the two nonconvex intervals <Math on Monday> and <English on Tuesday>. Cukierman's representation was useful to us: CAPSUL operates entirely under this closed-view scheme.

The temporal-repetition language presented by Terenziani (14) contains many important distinctions that we used in our language. For example, Terenziani introduces a distinction between a *time frame* (which can be seen as a relevant time period in which the entire pattern occurs) and a *period* (which could be a specific Monday on which one instance of the pattern occurs) which we use as well. Furthermore, Terenziani's constraint-based language distinguishes local and global constraints (where *local* constraints are applied to instances of the repeating event, and *global* constraints apply to the overall pattern) and between qualitative and quantitative constraints.

Morris and Khatib (15) have discussed a set of temporal constraints in detail. In their representation, gaps can be specified either by a fixed length or by a probability distribution. They also discussed the idea that there is a set of possible constraints, but that only a subset is necessary to completely specify a repeating event. More recently, Morris and Khatib (16) have developed the matrix of binary relations to represent the temporal relations between every pair of nonconvex intervals in a pattern. This matrix idea helped us to think about the advantages and limitations of allowing only one relationship to be specified for all the pairs of consecutive intervals.

# 7. Conclusion

In this paper, we have shown the ability of the Résumé system to detect repeating

trends in time-oriented medical data. The pattern matching module of Résumé – consisting of a temporal pattern specification language (CAPSUL), a KA tool, and an interpreter – provides an invaluable tool for efficiently summarizing large data sets. The CAPSUL language that we have designed allows a domain expert to express complicated patterns involving multiple levels of parameter abstractions in the data set. The graphical KA tool allows the user to enter such patterns into the Résumé knowledge base, the Résumé interpreter then finds these patterns in the data sets. We are currently conducting an evaluation of the usability of the KA tool, as well as the performance of the Résumé interpreter. Our initial results indicate that experts with moderate computer experience are able to use the KA tool with help from a knowledge engineer, and that the Résumé interpreter can correctly derive abstractions that would otherwise be unattainable to data analysts.

In the future, we plan to expand our ongoing evaluation of the diabetes domain, as well as to study the performance of the interpreter on more and larger data sets. We also plan to work more on the theoretical aspects of CAPSUL, including the formulation of the exact limitations and expressive powers of the language. Finally, we plan to extend the statistical capabilities of the CAPSUL constraints and explore the possibilities for more dynamic means of pattern specification and detection. Once the Résumé system has been tested and evaluated, it can be combined with visualization tools, such as KNAVE, to provide a new level of clinical data analysis.

**Acknowledgments**
We would like to thank Dr. Herbert Kaizer and Dr. Lawrence Basso, our domain experts in oncology and diabetes, respectively. Furthermore, we thank the Rush Presbyterian/St. Luke's Medical Center, which, through Dr. Kaizer, allowed us to use collected patient data. Mr. Arthur Menaker assisted us in expanding and maintaining the Résumé system. Mr. Eddie Schwalb facilitated the data analysis with an online visualization tool similar to KNAVE. This work has been supported by the grants 5R01-LM05708 and 5R29-LM06245 from the National Library of Medicine (NLM) and LM-06806 from the National Institutes of Health.

## Appendix. BNF syntax for CAPSUL

**pattern:** <linear pattern> | <repeating pattern>
**linear pattern:** <name> <disjunctive-linear-component-set>[+] <value> <output context> <necessary context>
**repeating pattern:** <name> <disjunctive-periodic-component-set>[+] <value> <output context> <necessary context>

**disjunctive-periodic-component-set:** <pattern-component> <disjunctive-periodic-constraint-set>
**disjunctive-periodic-constraint-set:** <name> <conjunctive-periodic-constraint-set>[+]
**conjunctive-periodic-constraint-set:** <name> <periodic-constraint>[+]
**periodic-constraint:** <cardinality-constraint> | <value-constraint> | <global-gap-constraint> | <local-gap-constraint> | <cluster-constraint>
**cardinality-constraint:** <minimum-number-of-repetitions> <maximum-number-of-repetitions>
**value-constraint:** <minimum-difference-between-instances> <maximum-difference> | <qualitative-value-relation>
**global-gap-constraint:** <qualitative-temporal-relation>
**local-gap-constraint:** <minimum-time-difference> <maximum-time-difference> <gap-type> <qualitative-temporal-relation>
**cluster-constraint:** <period> <minimum-number-of-clusters> <maximum-number-of-clusters> <disjunctive-sub-constraint-set>[+]
**disjunctive-sub-constraint-set:** <conjunctive-periodic-constraint-set>[+]

**disjunctive-linear-component-set:** <pattern-component>[+] <disjunctive-linear-constraint-set>[+]
**disjunctive-linear-constraint-set:** <conjunctive-linear-constraint-set>[+]
**conjunctive-linear-constraint-set:** <linear-constraint>[+]
**linear-constraint:** <gap-constraint> | <interval-constraint> | <period-constraint> | <value-constraint>
**gap-constraint:** <first-point> <second-point> <minimum-time-difference> <maximum-time-difference> <gap type>
**interval-constraint:** <first-interval> <second-interval> <qualitative-temporal-relation>
**period-constraint:** <period>
**linear-value-constraint:** <first-interval> <second-interval> <value-constraint>

**qualitative-temporal-relation:** <before> | <after> | <starts> | <ends> | <within> | <meets> | <overlaps> | <equal>
**qualitative-value-relation:** <greater-than> | <less-than> | <greater-than-or-equal> | <less-than-or-equal> | <equal>
**period:** <time-period> | <repeating-interval>
**time-period:** <name> <period-type> <minimum-amount-of-time> <maximum-amount-of-time>
**repeating-interval:** <name> <hour-start> <hour-end> <week-start> <week-end> <year-start> <year-end> <minute-start> <minute-end> <day-start> <day-end> <month-start> <month-end> <global-start-time> <global-end-time>

**pattern-component:** <proposition> <local-constraint>[+]
**proposition:** <linear-pattern > | <repeating-pattern> | <parameter> | <context> | <event>
**local-constraint:** <duration> | <value> | <earliest-starting-time> | <latest-starting-time> | <earliest-ending-time> | <latest-ending-time>
**value:** <true> | <function> | <mapping-function>

# References

1. Shahar Y, Musen M. Knowledge-based temporal abstraction in clinical domains. Artif Intell Med 1996; 8 (3): 267-98.
2. Shahar Y. A framework for knowledge-based temporal abstraction. Artificial Intelligence 1997; 90 (1-2): 79-133.
3. Shahar Y. Dynamic Temporal Interpretation Contexts for temporal abstraction. Annals of Mathematics and Artificial Intelligence 1998; 22 (1-2): 159-92.
4. Musen MA, Tu SW, Das AK, Shahar Y. EON: A component-based approach to automation of protocol-directed therapy. JAMA 1996; 3 (6): 367-88.
5. Shahar Y, Cheng C. Intelligent Visualization and Exploration of Time-Oriented Clinical Data. In press for Topics in Health Information Management (THIM) 1999.
6. Ladkin P. Time representation: A taxonomy of interval relations. In: Proceedings of the AAAI-86, 1986; 360-6.
7. Allen J. Towards a general theory of action and time. Artificial Intelligence 1984; 23 (2): 123-54.
8. Chakravarty S, Shahar Y. A constraint-based specification of periodic patterns in time-oriented data. In: Proceedings of the International Workshop on Temporal Representation and Reasoning (Time)-99. IEEE Press 1999; 29-40.
9. Shahar Y, Chen H, Stites DP, Basso L, Kaizer H, Wilson DM, Musen MA. Semiautomated Acquisition of Clinical Temporal-abstraction Knowledge. In press for Journal of the American Medical Informatics Association (JAMIA) 6 (6) 99.
10. Ladkin P. Primitives and Units for Time Specification. In: Proceedings of the AAAI-86, 1996; 354-9.
11. Clifford J, Rao A. A simple, general structure for temporal domains. Temporal Aspects in Information Systems, IFIP 1988; 17-28.
12. Cukierman D, Delgrande J. Characterizing Temporal Repetition. In: Proceedings of the International Workshop on Temporal Reasoning and Representation (TIME)-96, IEEE Press 1996; 80-7.
13. Cukierman D, Delgrande J. Towards a formal characterization of temporal repetition with closed time. In: Proceedings of the International Workshop on Temporal Reasoning and Representation (TIME)-98. IEEE Press 1998; 140-7.
14. Terenziani, P. Qualitative and Quantitative Temporal Constraints About Numerically Quantified Periodic Events. In: Proceedings of the International Workshop on Temporal Reasoning and Representation (TIME)-97, IEEE Press 1997; 94-101.
15. Morris R, Khatib L. Quantitative Structural Temporal Constraints on Repeating Events. In: Proceedings of the International Workshop on Temporal Reasoning and Representation (TIME)-98, IEEE Press 1998; 74-9.
16. Morris R, Khatib L. Periodic and Repeating Events. Florida Institute of Technology 1996; 1-17.
17. Khatib L. Reasoning with Non-convex Time Intervals. PhD. Thesis. Florida Institute of Technology 1994.

**Correspondence to:**
Yuval Shabar, MD, Ph.D,
Department of Information Systems Engineering
Ben-Gurion University of the Negev
Beer-Sheva 84105
Israel
E-mail: yshabar@bgumail.bgu.ac.il

# Examining the effects that manipulating information given in the change of shift report has on nurses' care planning ability

Dawn Dowding PhD BSc RGN

*Senior Research Fellow, Nursing Research Initiative for Scotland, Nursing and Midwifery Building, University of Stirling, Stirling, UK*

Submitted for publication 9 September 1999
Accepted for publication 27 October 2000

Correspondence:
*Dawn Dowding,*
*Senior Research Fellow,*
*NRIS,*
*Nursing and Midwifery Building,*
*University of Stirling,*
*Stirling FK9 4LA,*
*UK.*
*E-mail: dwl1@stir.ac.uk*

DOWDING D. (2001) *Journal of Advanced Nursing* 33(6), 836–846

**Examining the effects that manipulating information given in the change of shift report has on nurses' care planning ability**

**Aim of the study.** To investigate the effect that manipulating the style and content of the nurse change of shift report had on an individual's ability to plan patient care.

**Background.** The nurse change of shift report occurs on most hospital wards at least two if not three times a day. However, little research exists examining how changing the style and information content of the shift report may affect an individual's ability to process the information they hear. It is suggested that how individuals structure their knowledge, in the form of schema, is an important consideration when examining how they process information.

**Design.** This was an experimental study where two independent variables, report style (retrospective vs. prospective) and schema information (schema consistent vs. schema inconsistent) were compared in a factorial design. A convenience sample of 48 registered nurses from acute medical and acute surgical wards were randomly allocated to one of the four experimental conditions. Outcome measures included the amount of information that subjects accurately recorded and recalled from the shift report, together with their ability to plan patient care.

**Results.** Results indicated that the type of report had a significant effect on an individual's ability to plan patient care, and type of information content on their ability to accurately record and recall the information they heard.

**Conclusions.** The implications of the results, both for schema theory as an explanation of nursing knowledge, and for the type of report which should be used in acute medical and acute surgical wards are discussed, together with the implications of the study for further research.

**Keywords:** shift report, schema theory, nursing knowledge, information processing, experimental methods

## Introduction

The nurse change of shift report provides information about patients in the ward or unit to those nurses who are beginning their shift. Often verbal in nature, it has been discussed by individuals from a variety of countries (Kihlgren *et al.* 1992, Luikkonen 1993, McKenna & Walsh 1997, Lamond 1998) implying that it may be important to nursing practice across cultures. However, most of the literature that discusses the change of shift report does so at an anecdotal level, with many assumptions being made concerning its purpose, without adequate research evidence to support these claims. The aim of this experimental study was to explore the possible way that information is processed during the change of shift report in acute medical and surgical wards in order to provide evidence with which to explore the relevance of the change of shift report to nursing practice.

## Background literature

### Research into the nursing shift report

Relevant literature considering the nature of the change of shift report was identified using electronic databases (Cinahl, Medline, Bids ISI; key words included 'handover(s)', 'shift report(s)', 'oral communication'), by hand searching relevant journals and following up references from lists provided in published material. This provided 49 articles or reports, of which 19 were reports of research carried out into the shift report. The research considers the role of the shift report as a ritual (Ekman & Segesten 1995), patient reactions to bedside reports (Cahill 1998), evaluates alternative forms of report to that of verbal communication (Wallum 1995, Kennedy 1999) and examines the content of the shift report (Georgopoulos & Sana 1971, Norberg & Asplund 1987, Kihlgren *et al.* 1992, Luikkonen 1993). The remaining articles are anecdotal in nature, either describing how communication of information during the shift report had been changed (Mosher & Bontomasi 1996), or suggesting what information should be contained in the shift report (Kilpack & Dobson-Brassard 1987).

Various assumptions are made about the importance of the information communicated during the shift report. The information which nurses receive during the report is perceived to enable them subsequently to plan and to give care effectively and efficiently to the patients whom they look after (Clair & Trussell 1969, Glen 1988), contributing both to the quality and continuity of the care that patients receive (Georgopoulos & Sana 1971, Kilpack & Dobson-Brassard 1987, Kihlgren *et al.* 1992). The context within which the shift report operates (in terms of how it relates to initial patient assessments and the written care plan) has not been considered. However, the assumption in the literature appears to be that without the information communicated during the shift report, an individual nurse's ability to assess the status of a patient and plan care for them at the beginning of a shift would be compromised.

Specific research studies that have examined the nature of the nursing shift report have concentrated on the information content of the communication. They have identified that certain types of information appear to be communicated consistently during the verbal report, including information regarding patients' communication, moving, elimination, medication and medical treatment (Georgopoulos & Sana 1971, Norberg & Asplund 1987, Kihlgren *et al.* 1992,

Luikkonen 1993) and summary statements about the individual patient's condition such as 'feeling well' (Kihlgren *et al.* 1992, Luikkonen 1993) or 'self caring' (Lamond 1998). The patient's name, age and diagnosis also seem to be reported consistently, often in a specific order at the beginning of the communication (Sherlock 1995, Lamond 1998). They have also criticized the verbal shift report for failing to provide information regarding the patient's psychological state and their social situation (Kihlgren *et al.* 1992, Luikkonen 1993).

These studies have concluded that the verbal communication at the change of shift can be characterized by being retrospective and task orientated, focusing on actions that the nurse has carried out and the medical treatment the patient has received (McMahon 1990, Kihlgren *et al.* 1992, Luikkonen 1993). In the anecdotal literature discussing the nature of the shift report in the context of patient centred care, it has been suggested that both the location of the verbal report and the content should be altered (from office to patient bedside and from a medical to a patient focus) (Rowe & Perry 1984, Ward 1988, McMahon 1990, McKenna & Walsh 1997, Watkins 1997). More specifically, it has been suggested that the content of the report should be altered to focus on the patient's needs and problems, together with their nursing solutions, and move away from discussing a patient's medical care and treatment (McMahon 1990, Kihlgren *et al.* 1992, Luikkonen 1993). The implicit assumption made by authors suggesting this change is that by altering the shift report in this way so that it is more prospective in nature, a nurse's ability to plan care for patients will be facilitated.

Despite these assumptions no research currently appears to exist to support the claims made. There have been attempts to replace the verbal shift report with written communications or a 'silent report' (where patient documents are reviewed) (Wallum 1995, Kennedy 1999), however, these studies have not examined the effect this has had on patient care. There is also no apparent information regarding its usefulness depending on the skill or expertize of the nurses involved in the communication. The research study presented here aims to explore the effect that giving different types of information to nurses during a shift report may have on their ability to plan care, in order to provide some evidence with which to explore the assumptions surrounding the verbal change of shift report.

### Information processing and the shift report

It appears from the literature previously discussed that the purpose of the verbal change of shift report is assumed to be to communicate information from one nurse to another nurse(s), and that from this communication the nurse receiving the report will be able to plan care effectively for his/her patients. Therefore, it could be suggested that the nurse receiving the report has to 'process' the information he/she receives in some way.

The theory of information processing (Newell & Simon 1972) suggests that human beings have limited capacities for processing information. Factors that need to be taken into account when considering how information is processed include:
• the inputs or information identified as being relevant for the task at hand;
• how this information is subsequently processed in the human brain (including the influence knowledge has on processing);
• the output of the process (what judgements, decisions or plans the individual has made).
In nursing there are a small number of studies that have examined how nurses process information to form plans of care and make decisions regarding patient care (Corcoran 1986a, Tanner *et al.* 1987). They have suggested that nurses use a hypothetico-deductive approach to information processing, where information cues are used to form possible hypotheses regarding the patient's state or condition. These hypotheses are then 'tested' against available information until the most appropriate hypothesis for that patient has been identified. Decisions are then taken on the basis of this hypothesis (Tanner *et al.* 1987). Many of these studies have found that nurses' ability to process information accurately increases with expertize in an area (Corcoran 1986b, Tanner *et al.* 1987, Greenwood & King 1995).

Other studies have suggested that nurses, like other humans, use a number of reasoning 'short cuts' or heuristics to help them process large amounts of information, such as representativeness (used to judge the probability that certain signs and symptoms are indicative of a clinical condition previously encountered) and availability (instances of a similar condition which are easily recalled) (Cioffi & Markham 1997). Both of these heuristics rely on an individual having existing knowledge about previous cases to draw on.

All of these findings also suggest that the individual's knowledge has an important effect on how information is processed. Research into expertize in particular has suggested that how an individual's knowledge is organized within their long-term memory is the key influence on their ability to process information (Norman *et al.* 1985, Grant & Marsden 1988, Parrino & Mitchell 1989).

How knowledge is structured appears to be a key influence on how information is processed. For situations such as that of the nursing shift report, where a large amount of information could potentially be processed, it is therefore important to consider the effect of an individual's knowledge structure or organization on the output of the situation (in this case planning care).

*Theories of knowledge organization*
A considerable body of literature exists examining possible ways in which knowledge may be organized in memory, in order to facilitate information processing. Many of the studies have suggested that information is 'chunked' or classified, so that items which are similar are categorized together in 'concepts' (Smith & Medin 1981). Within these overarching concepts are 'categories' of information, objects or items of information that are equivalent in some way (Rosch 1978). By classifying information in this way it is suggested that individuals are able to access all the knowledge they have about an entity (Ross & Spalding 1994) and can use it to make inferences about unobservable characteristics, to predict future events and to understand the cause of events (Lingle *et al.* 1984, Ross & Spalding 1994). For example, Crow and Spicer (1995) suggested that district nurses might categorize the patients they look after by criteria based on a patient's severity of illness (whether they are acutely or chronically ill). This categorization may then allow the nurse to predict what might happen to the patient, infer certain things about them, and perhaps therefore plan patient care effectively.

The structure of such categories has been suggested to be 'probabilistic' in nature, with members of a concept category varying in their 'typicality' or 'goodness of fit' within a category. The more typical a member of a category is, the more attributes it has in common with other members of the category and the fewer attributes with members of another category (Rosch 1978). This has implications for how information cues may be processed in order to provide 'accurate' judgements. In medicine, Cantor *et al.* (1980) found that the more prototypical a patient was with respect to a psychiatric diagnosis category, the more likely they were to be diagnosed accurately. However, theories of knowledge organization based on the idea of classification have been criticized for failing to address how knowledge categories may be linked together, or how new information is accumulated into existing knowledge structures (Ross & Spalding 1994).

Schema theory offers an alternative explanation for how knowledge may be organized in the long-term memory and deals with some of the criticisms of theories of categorization. In contrast to 'categories' of knowledge, schema are considered to be more complicated networks of represented information, which have categories as their variables (Wyer & Gordon 1984), using common themes or situations as a way of organizing knowledge. Examples of different types of schema have been given, such as scene schema, which represent what one would expect to see when looking at or entering a scene (e.g. hospital ward – beds, curtains, nurses, IV infusions, etc.) and event schema which represent sequences of events (e.g. what I do when I give a patient an injection, Mandler 1979).

Marshall (1995) suggests that schema contain four different types of knowledge:

*Identification knowledge:* The characteristics which lead to the initial recognition of a situation, event or experience through the simultaneous processing of a number of features from that situation, event or experience.

*Elaboration knowledge:* This type of knowledge consists of elaboration about the main features of the event or situation around which the schema has developed, and may use specific examples from experience. Elaboration knowledge identifies an appropriate schema, and then interprets the details of the current situation in order to fit it into the template.

*Planning knowledge:* This is used to make plans, create expectations and set up goals and sub goals, in order to guide the individual's actions.

*Execution knowledge:* The choice and order of operation of execution knowledge is determined by the planning knowledge.

Together, identification and elaboration knowledge allow the individual to create a tentative framework about a situation and test it (the process of categorization). However, planning knowledge is needed in order to make inferences and to determine actions once identification and elaboration have occurred (Marshall 1995). In unfamiliar situations the individual will not possess well-formed schema, so they will access several schema in order to find the best match for that situation (Marshall 1993) which may lead to mistakes being made.

Narayan and Corcoran-Perry (1997) have identified similar types of knowledge to that described by Marshall (1995) when studying nursing practice. They suggest that a situation contains 'triggering cues' (identification knowledge) that activate relevant concepts in the memory, accessing domain concept information (elaboration knowledge). Subsequently 'intermediate' conclusions are drawn which indicate what needs to be performed before action can be taken (planning knowledge). Lamond (1998) examined possible knowledge organization in nursing through the use of card sorts and interviews with registered nurses. This study found that knowledge appeared to be organized in categories based

around the patient's medical diagnosis and acuity, with information details for 'typical' members of the category that contained both elaboration and planning knowledge (characteristics of the patient, plus what the nurse would do for them in a particular situation). Similarly, Grobe *et al.* (1991) have found that nurses' perceptions of patient problems and necessary interventions were inextricably linked and Benner *et al.* (1996) have found evidence that nurses have knowledge of patients which allows them to predict the care patients need and generate expectations concerning patients' recovery. All of these studies suggest that planning knowledge is an integral part of the way individual nursing knowledge may be organized, and they lend support to schema theory.

## The study

### Rationale

As has been highlighted in the literature reviewed, it is suggested that nurses receiving information from the shift report need to process it in some way. This processing can be considered within the framework of information processing theory (Newell & Simon 1972) together with schema theory (Figure 1). A possible scenario could therefore be that a nurse has knowledge about patients organized as schema. They receive information regarding patients they will be caring for during a shift report, which contains information that allows them to identify an appropriate schema (forceful feature information in Figure 1). They use identification knowledge to recognize an appropriate schema for these patients. They then use elaboration knowledge to access this schema knowledge (which gives them access to information which may allow them to predict what could happen to the patient(s)), exemplified by the 'process' in Figure 1. Through accessing this schema they also have planning knowledge, which allows them to develop plans of care for the patient. Once plans have

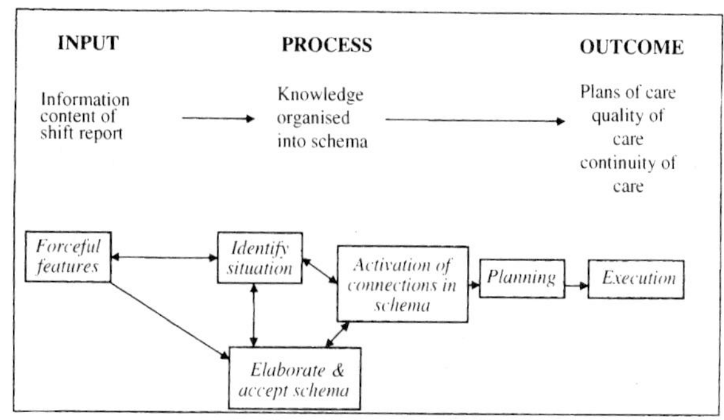



**Figure 1** How information processing and schema theory can be applied to the shift report situation (Lamond 1998).

been developed, then care is given and outcomes achieved (such as continuity of care and quality care), again identified in the outcomes of information processing in Figure 1. If, however, the shift report contains information that does not allow an individual nurse to access appropriate identification knowledge, they may be unable to access other schema information and this may affect the outcomes of the process such as their ability to plan patient care.

The literature on shift reports makes various assumptions regarding their purpose and the types of information that should be contained within them, without adequately testing the effect that this may have on patient care. Schema theory offers a potential framework within which one can consider the effect providing different types of information in a shift report may have on an individual's ability to plan patient care. This study therefore was designed, using an experimental approach, to test some of the assumptions apparent in the literature regarding the shift report and also to test whether nurses' knowledge could be organized in schema. The two specific research questions were:

- Does altering the structure of the shift report (retrospective and task orientated, or prospective and patient focused) affect a nurse's ability to access appropriate knowledge and plan patient care?
- Does altering the information content of the shift report (schema consistent or schema inconsistent) affect a nurse's ability to access appropriate knowledge and plan patient care?

## Study design

### Method

In order to have control over the information that subjects in this study received and ensure that the structure was consistent across conditions, an experimental methodology was employed. If 'real life' shift reports had been used it would not have been possible to compare subjects across groups, and would have also raised issues regarding patient confidentiality.

A factorial design with two independent variables was utilized. The two variables were shift report structure (retrospective and task orientated vs. prospective and patient centred) and type of schema information (schema consistent vs. schema inconsistent). This study design gave four subject groups (Table 1). Dependent variables included the amount of information subjects accurately recorded about the patients during the shift report, the amount of information subjects accurately recalled after the shift report, and the quality of the plan of care they were able to construct.

**Table 1** The four subject groups within the experimental condition

| Handover structure | Schema consistency | |
| --- | --- | --- |
| | Consistent patients | Inconsistent patients |
| Retrospective | A | B |
| Prospective | C | D |

### Experimental materials

Separate shift report scenarios were constructed for each experimental condition and for medical and surgical subjects, giving a total of eight different shift report situations. The shift reports consisted of information regarding five patients with varying medical diagnoses/surgical conditions and severity of illness. The patient descriptions were based on information gained from the research into schema content carried out by Lamond (1998). Examples of retrospective and prospective reports, together with schema consistent and inconsistent information, can be seen in Table 2.

### Outcome measures

The amount of information accurately recorded and recalled by subjects was measured using a checklist. All the information features included in the shift report were listed and the percentages of the total amount of information the subject accurately recorded/recalled calculated. In order to assess the quality of the plans of care the subjects produced, an expert panel was asked to construct plans of care for each patient in each condition. The expert panel consisted of four expert clinicians, two medical and two surgical, who had been qualified between 10 and 14 years and were currently working as specialists in acute medical and acute surgical environments. The plans they constructed were considered to be the 'gold standard'. Each item they mentioned in the plan of care for each patient was placed on a checklist. If the subject mentioned these items they scored 2 points and every item they mentioned that they would do which was not mentioned in the expert plan, given 1 point. The plan scores awarded to each subject gave an indication of how like the expert plan the subject's plan was and an overall score. For the purpose of the experiment it was decided that a high score indicated a more complete plan of care and a lower score a less complete plan of care. The total possible plan score varied slightly according to the condition, however, those individuals who had plans similar to those produced by the experts produced higher plan scores.

### Reliability and validity

In order to ensure that the calculations for the dependent variables were reliable, interrater reliability measures were

**Table 2** Examples of schema consistent and schema inconsistent information, together with retrospective and prospective reports, used within the experimental conditions

| Schema consistent information | Schema inconsistent information |
|---|---|
| Aged 70 | Aged 70 |
| Lady | Lady |
| Exacerbation of COPD | Exacerbation of COPD |
| Admitted yesterday | Admitted yesterday |
| Chest Infection | Chest Infection |
| Breathing worse | Breathing worse |
| Very breathless | Not breathless |
| On continuous 28% oxygen | Not on oxygen |
| Four hourly nebulisers | Four hourly nebulisers |
| Pre- and post-peak flows | Pre- and post-peak flows |
| Peak flows unrecordable | Peak flows measuring 400–500 |
| Four hourly observations | Four hourly observations |
| Observations are fine | Observations are fine |
| Oxygen saturations being measured | Oxygen saturations being measured |
| Oxygen saturations 85% | Oxygen saturations 85% |
| On steroids | On steroids |
| Steroids have been increased | Steroids have not been increased |
| On IV antibiotics | Not on IV antibiotics |
| Antibiotics have been given | Has an IV infusion |
| Has an IV infusion | IV infusion running over 8 hours |
| IV infusion running over 8 hours | IV infusion is due at 16:00 hours |
| IV infusion is due at 16:00 hours | Eating all her food without problems |
| Not eating very much | Looks quite pink |
| Looks grey | Didn't need assistance with washing and dressing |
| Needed a lot of assistance with washing and dressing | Managing to mobilize around the ward quite well |
| Not walking very far | Hasn't been referred to a physiotherapist |
| Has been referred to a physiotherapist | Seems fine |
| Quite anxious | Not anxious |
| Needs a lot of reassurance | |

Retrospective report

In bed 1 is X, a 70-year-old lady with exacerbation of her COPD who was admitted yesterday. She has a chest infection which has made her breathing worse. She's very breathless, on continuous 28% oxygen and four hourly nebulisers. She's on pre- and post-peak flows, which are unrecordable, and four hourly observations, which are fine, her oxygen saturations are around 85%. Her steroids have been increased, and she's on IV antibiotics, which have been given today. She's got an IV infusion running eight hourly, which is due at 16:00 hours, and she's not really eaten very much this morning. She looks quite grey. She needed a lot of assistance with washing and dressing this morning, and isn't really managing to walk very far. She's been referred to the physiotherapist. She's quite anxious and needs quite a lot of reassurance

Prospective report

In bed 1 is X, a 70-year-old lady admitted yesterday. Her main problem is breathlessness, and she's for continuous 28% oxygen and four hourly nebulisers. She's also for pre- and post-peak flows, which at present are unrecordable and oxygen saturations, which at present are around 85%. Her next main problem is nutrition, she isn't really eating very much, so we need to try and encourage her. She's also on an IV infusion, running eight hourly, which is due at 16:00 hours this afternoon. She has a problem with mobility and caring for her own hygiene, she needs assistance with washing and dressing, and help to mobilize around the ward. At present she isn't walking very far. She has also been referred to the physiotherapist. Her final problem is anxiety, she is very anxious about her health and needs to have quite a lot of reassurance

calculated. A separate coder was trained by the researcher to use the checklists for accurate recording and recall of information and plan scores. A sample of 10% of the experimental responses was then independently scored and interrater reliabilities calculated utilizing Cohen's κ coefficient (Cohen 1960). These results indicated high reliability for the dependent measures (Table 3) (Landis & Koch 1977).

**Table 3** Reliability calculations for experimental outcome measures

| Measure | Agreement (%) | κ |
|---|---|---|
| Information recorded | 88·2 | 0·76 |
| Information recalled | 93·1 | 0·84 |
| Plan score | 93 | 0·86 |

To increase the validity of the experiment, it was designed to simulate an actual shift report situation, with only the variables being tested in the experiment varying. Subjects from surgical wards were given a shift report for surgical patients and subjects from medical wards a shift report for medical patients. The expert panel was used to assess the validity of the content of the reports, ensuring that the information given was clinically correct and consistent across experimental conditions. Subject evaluations of the shift reports indicated that in general they were representative of reports that they would normally hear.

### Subjects

The convenience sample consisted of 48 registered nurses working in general medical and general surgical wards from two district hospitals located in central Scotland. They were randomly allocated to one of the four experimental conditions, giving a total of 12 subjects in each experimental condition. Specific characteristics of each subject group can be seen in Table 4.

### Ethical issues

The appropriate committee at each hospital gave ethical approval for the study. Permission to access staff from

**Table 4** Details of sample characteristics for each subject group

| | Experimental condition | | | |
|---|---|---|---|---|
| | A | B | C | D |
| **Age (years)** | | | | |
| Mean | 30·7 | 29·7 | 31·6 | 28 |
| Range | 23–51 | 21–40 | 22–50 | 20–45 |
| **Grade (frequency)** | | | | |
| C | 2 | 0 | 1 | 0 |
| D | 5 | 8 | 3 | 10 |
| E | 5 | 2 | 6 | 2 |
| F | 0 | 1 | 0 | 0 |
| G | 0 | 1 | 2 | 0 |
| **Length of time qualified (years)** | | | | |
| Mean | 5·8 | 7 | 6·1 | 5·3 |
| Range | 9 months–16 years | 6 months–16 years | 6 months–16 years | 1–24 years |

Grades indicate level of seniority of the nurse, with C the lowest level and G the highest.

relevant wards was given by managers, before both verbal and written information regarding the study was given to all potential subjects who worked in the appropriate specialist areas. Only those individuals who indicated their willingness to take part in the study were approached, and only once it was apparent that they clearly understood the nature of the study and consented to take part, did the study begin.

### Procedure

Subjects were randomly allocated to an experimental condition and were played an audiotape of the appropriate shift report. During this report they were encouraged to take notes if they normally did so and wished to. Once the report was complete, subjects were asked to count backwards from 100 to 1 whilst their notes were removed (preventing rehearsal in the short-term memory, meaning that all information subsequently recalled should be schema knowledge retrieved from long-term memory).

After subjects had finished counting they were asked to write down as much information as they could remember within a time limit of 5 minutes. They were then asked to write down what care they would plan to give the patients if they were looking after them for the afternoon, this time with a time limit of 10 minutes.

### Data analysis

Data were analysed using SPSS version 9 for Windows (SPSS Inc., Chicago), and two-way analysis of variance. Before the analysis was carried out the data were checked for normality using the Shapiro Wilks test (Norusis 1993), which was nonsignificant, indicating that the hypothesis that the data were normally distributed could be accepted (i.e. all the data were normally distributed). Analysis of variance allows comparison of variation between different factors in the experimental design, as well as considering interactions between the two variables. The *F*-test examines whether or not the data suggest equivalent populations, through examining the variation in means (Everitt 1995).

## Results

### General findings

In order to confirm that subjects' speciality and expertize did not confound the experimental results, significant differences in the samples (medical vs. surgical, nonexpert vs. expert) were detected by comparing them using an independent samples *t*-test. Experts were defined as subjects at grades E and above (in the English grading system this represented nurses with considerable experience at staff nurse level, together with ward managers), nonexperts grade D and below (this represented nurses with less experience at staff nurse level and enrolled nurses). The results of this analysis for all of the outcome measures indicated that there were no significant differences between medical and surgical subjects ($P > 0.05$), and no significant difference according to subject expertize ($P > 0.05$). Therefore, for the remaining analyses subjects were grouped according to their experimental condition.

Overall, subjects accurately recorded a mean of 45.2% of the total information given during the shift report (range 10.6–76.3%), accurately recalled a mean of 27% of the total information given (range 8.4–50%) with a mean plan score of 33.5 (range 3–78).

*Effect of type of shift report*
The effect the type of shift report had on subjects' ability to accurately record and recall information, together with their plan score, was examined using two-way analysis of variance (Table 5). Type of shift report appeared to have little effect on the amount of information subjects accurately recorded and recalled ($P > 0.05$). However, it did appear to have a significant effect on their ability to plan care ($P < 0.01$), with those subjects who heard a retrospective report having a higher mean plan score than those who heard a prospective report (40.1 vs. 26.9).

*The effect of schema consistent and schema inconsistent information*
The effect that the different types of information content (schema consistent or schema inconsistent) had on subjects' ability to accurately record and recall information, together with their plan score, was also examined using two-way analysis of variance (Table 6). Type of information had a significant effect on the information accurately recorded ($P < 0.01$) and recalled ($P < 0.05$) by subjects, but no effect on their ability to plan care ($P > 0.05$). Subjects who heard schema consistent information were more likely to record and recall information more accurately than those subjects who had heard schema inconsistent information.

*Interaction between shift report type and schema information*
Two-way analysis of variance was carried out to examine any interactions between shift report type and schema information (Table 7). This analysis indicated no significant interactions between the two independent variables for the amount of

**Table 5** Results for analysis of variance for effect of shift report type on outcome measures. Bold text indicates significant results

| | Mean | | | | | |
| | Retrospective | Prospective | d.f. | F | Significant | Power |
|---|---|---|---|---|---|---|
| Accurately recorded (%) | 42.8 | 47.4 | 1.40 | 1.6 | P = 0.2 | 0.2 |
| Accurately recalled (%) | 26.9 | 27.1 | 1.44 | 0.008 | P = 0.9 | 0.04 |
| Total plan score (max 114) | **40.1** | **26.9** | **1.44** | **10.6** | **P = 0.002**** | **0.9** |

**$P < 0.01$.

**Table 6** Results for analysis of variance for effect of schema information on outcome measures. Bold text indicates significant results

| | Mean | | | | | |
| | Consistent | Inconsistent | d.f. | F | Significant | Power |
|---|---|---|---|---|---|---|
| Accurately recorded (%) | **50.7** | **38.5** | **1.40** | **11.6** | **P = 0.002**** | **0.9** |
| Accurately recalled (%) | **29.8** | **24.1** | **1.44** | **4.5** | **P = 0.04*** | **0.5** |
| Total plan score (max 114) | 35.4 | 31.7 | 1.44 | 0.8 | P = 0.4 | 0.2 |

*$P < 0.05$; **$P < 0.01$.

**Table 7** Results for analysis of variance for the interaction between schema information and shift report type. Bold text indicates significant results

| | Mean (experimental condition) | | | | | | | |
| | A | B | C | D | d.f. | F | Significant | Power |
|---|---|---|---|---|---|---|---|---|
| Accurately recorded (%) | 46 | 38.5 | 55.5 | 38.6 | 1.40 | 1.6 | P = 0.2 | 0.2 |
| Accurately recalled (%) | **25.5** | **28.2** | **34.2** | **20.1** | **1.44** | **9.8** | **P = 0.003**** | **0.9** |
| Total plan score (max 114) | 41.6 | 38.7 | 29.2 | 24.7 | 1.44 | 0.03 | P = 0.8 | 0.04 |

**$P < 0.01$.

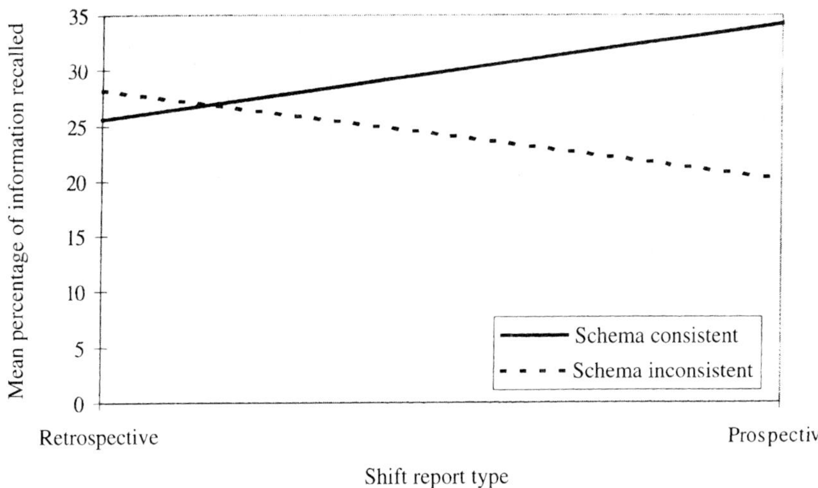



**Figure 2** The interaction effect between shift report and schema information for amount of information subjects accurately recalled.

information accurately recorded and plan scores ($P > 0.05$). However, it did show a significant effect for the amount of information subjects accurately recalled ($P < 0.01$).

Figure 2 seems to indicate that subjects were able to recall more information accurately when they heard a prospective shift report and schema consistent patient information (mean 34·2% accurately recalled), and least accurately when they heard a prospective report with schema inconsistent information (mean 20·1% accurately recalled). When they heard a retrospective report, regardless of the type of schema information, they appeared to recall approximately the same amount of information (means 25·5% and 28·2% accurately recalled).

## DISCUSSION

The first research question considered whether altering the structure of the shift report (from retrospective and task orientated to prospective and patient focused) would affect a nurse's ability to access appropriate knowledge and plan patient care. The results of the study indicate that shift reports that are 'retrospective' in nature may be more appropriate for the effective communication of information to enable individuals to plan care (indicated by the higher plan scores in this experimental condition). This is in contrast to the literature, which suggests that a prospective report is more effective (McMahon 1990, Kihlgren *et al.* 1992, Luikkonen 1993). However, the overall ability of any subject accurately to recall information they heard during the report was limited (mean 27% accurately recalled). This could indicate that verbal communication is perhaps not an effective way of communicating such vital information, and indeed there are some authors who have suggested alternative means of giving a shift report (Baldwin & McGinnis 1994,

Prouse 1995, McKenna & Walsh 1997, Kennedy 1999). It could be argued that this result might be an artefact of the experiment. However, when examining the notes made by nurses, on average less than half of the information presented in the reports was accurately recorded (45·2%). This suggests that over 50% of the information communicated during the report could be considered to be 'unimportant'. Examination of the notes and information recalled in the experiment indicated a pattern which could support schema knowledge structure (further examination of this data is outside the remit of this study, and readers are referred to Lamond 1998 for more information). Although this study offers some insight into how changing the way information is given during a shift report may affect the assumed outcomes of report, a large amount of research into the area still needs to be carried out.

The second research question considered whether altering the information content of the shift report, to contain either schema consistent or schema inconsistent information, would affect a nurse's ability to access appropriate knowledge and plan care. Schema theory suggests that schema consistent information should be recalled more accurately, as access to schema knowledge allows connection to a large amount of additional information (Abelson 1981). In this respect the higher accurate recall of information in the schema consistent experimental conditions gives support to nursing knowledge being organized in schema. However, the low level of recall of information overall in the experiment, together with the lack of effect of subject expertize on the outcome measure, could suggest that in this instance schema knowledge has not been accessed (or that knowledge may not be organized in schema at all). One would perhaps expect experts (with more a richer and more organized knowledge schema) to accurately recall more information than less expert practitioners, and that overall the amount of information recalled would be higher if schema were being utilized fully.

The complex nature of the results of the interaction between the report structure and schema information type could suggest that a shift report structuring information giving around patients' needs and problems facilitates access to appropriate knowledge schema when the information is schema consistent, but prohibits it when the information is schema inconsistent. The lack of ability to plan care (indicated by lower plan scores) in the prospective shift report condition also suggests that this type of report may inhibit access to appropriate planning knowledge. Again, further research is needed to examine the complex relationship between the information given and how it may be processed.

### Study limitations

This study was based on a fabricated shift report situation and therefore the results need to be treated with some caution, despite the attempts made to ensure that the materials used during the experiment were as realistic as possible. Because the reports were on audiotape they consisted of a one-way communication. Many of the subjects indicated that in a 'normal' shift report they would be able to ask questions in order to clarify information that was communicated during the report. The study also considered only a small subset of the types of patients subjects would normally look after and, as the information was constructed on a fictional basis, they had no experience of nursing the patients. Also, the reports given in the experimental conditions for schema inconsistent information may not have been as believable as those for schema consistent information, which again may have affected the results slightly. The plan scores were a crude measure of what care subjects thought the patients might need, based on the limited information available to them. In a normal situation they would be able to look at patient documentation and discuss care plans with the patient before finally deciding on what actions to take. The plan scores did not take into account actions that might be detrimental to the patient (i.e. there was no indication of the appropriateness of care), and would not give an indication of individuals' actual planning behaviour.

### Conclusions

This study attempted to study a particular aspect of nursing practice using a controlled experimental situation. Because of this, many of the results need to be treated with caution and further research into the role and effectiveness of the shift report needs to be carried out in a more naturalistic environment. The results of this study did indicate that verbal communication at the change of shift may not be the most effective way of communicating information about patients to enable patient care to be planned effectively. Further research needs to be carried out into the exact role that the change of shift report plays within the patient care context (i.e. how does it link in with the use of patient documentation and patient assessment), and the effect that subjects 'knowing the patient' has on their information needs. It could be that the shift report is not the 'vital' method of communication that is intimated in much of the nursing press. Further research also needs to be carried out examining how nursing knowledge (including the way it may be structured) affects how information is processed in patient care situations. In order to ensure that nursing practice is based on evidence, the whole area of the nursing shift report, the assumptions made about it, and the effect it has on patient care need to be examined more closely.

### Acknowledgements

I would like to thank Prof. Rosemary Crow and Dr Jonathon Chase for their help and support during this project. I would also like to thank those individuals who helped with the expert panel, and all the nurses who volunteered to take part in this study. A final thank goes to Dr Anne Scott, for her assistance with the interrater reliability coding.

### References

Abelson R.P. (1981) Psychological status of the script concept. *American Psychologist* 36, 715–729.

Baldwin L. & McGinnis C. (1994) A computer-generated shift report. *Nursing Management* 25, 61–64.

Benner P., Tanner C. & Chelsa C. (1996) *Expertise in Nursing Practice. Caring, Clinical Judgement and Ethics.* Springer, New York.

Cahill J. (1998) Patients' perceptions of bedside handovers. *Journal of Clinical Nursing* 7, 351–359.

Cantor N., Smith E., French R. & Mezzich J. (1980) Psychiatric diagnosis as prototype categorisation. *Journal of Abnormal Psychology* 89, 181–193.

Cioffi J. & Markham R. (1997) Clinical decision-making by midwives: managing case complexity. *Journal of Advanced Nursing* 25, 265–272.

Clair L.L. & Trussell P.M. (1969) The change of shift report: study shows weaknesses and how it can be improved. *Hospitals* 43, 91–95.

Cohen J. (1960) A coefficient of agreement for nominal scales. *Educational and Psychological Measurement* 20, 37–46.

Corcoran S.A. (1986a) Task complexity and nursing expertise as factors in decision making. *Nursing Research* 35, 107–112.

Corcoran S.A. (1986b) Planning by expert and novice nurses in cases of varying complexity. *Research in Nursing and Health* 9, 155–162.

Crow R. & Spicer J. (1995) Categorisation of the patient's medical condition – an analysis of nursing judgement. *International Journal of Nursing Studies* 32, 413–422.

Ekman I. & Segesten K. (1995) Deputed power of medical control: the hidden message in the ritual of oral shift reports. *Journal of Advanced Nursing* 22, 1006–1011.

Everitt B.S. (1995) Analysis of variance designs. In *Psychological Research Methods and Statistics* (Colman A.M. ed.), Longman, Essex, pp. 18–34.

Georgopoulos B.S. & Sana J.M. (1971) Clinical nurse specialization. *American Journal of Nursing* 71, 538–545.

Glen J. (1988) What's in a report? *Nursing Standard* 2, 28.

Grant J. & Marsden P. (1988) Primary knowledge, medical education and consultant expertise. *Medical Education* 22, 173–179.

Greenwood J. & King M. (1995) Some surprising similarities in the clinical reasoning of 'expert' and 'novice' orthopaedic nurses: report of a study using verbal protocols and protocol analyses. *Journal of Advanced Nursing* 22, 907–913.

Grobe S.J., Drew J.A. & Fonteyn M.E. (1991) A descriptive analysis of experienced nurses' clinical reasoning during a planning task. *Research in Nursing and Health* 14, 305–324.

Kennedy J. (1999) An evaluation of non-verbal handover. *Professional Nurse* 14, 391–394.

Kihlgren M., Lindsten I.G., Norberg A. & Karlsson I. (1992) The content of the oral daily reports at a long-term ward before and after staff training in integrity promoting care. *Scandinavian Journal of Caring Science* 6, 105–112.

Kilpack V. & Dobson-Brassard S. (1987) Intershift report: oral communication using the nursing process. *Journal of Neuroscience Nursing* 19, 266–270.

Lamond D. (1998) *Information Processing and Handover: An Investigation.* PhD Thesis. University of Surrey, Surrey.

Landis J.R. & Koch G.G. (1977) The measurement of observer agreement for categorical data. *Biometrics* 33, 159–174.

Lingle J.H., Altom M.W. & Medin D.L. (1984) Of cabbages and kings: assessing the extendibility of natural object categories to social things. In *Handbook of Social Cognition*, vol. 1. (Wyer R.S. & Srull T.K. eds), Lawrence Erlbaum Associates, New Jersey, pp. 71–117.

Luikkonen A. (1993) The content of nurses' oral shift reports in homes for elderly people. *Journal of Advanced Nursing* 18, 1095–1100.

Mandler J.M. (1979) Categorical and schematic organization in memory. In *Memory Organization and Structure* (Puff C.R. ed.), Academic Press, New York, pp. 259–299.

Marshall S.P. (1993) Assessing schema knowledge. In *Test Theory for a New Generation of Tests* (Frederikson N., Mislevy R.J. & Bejar I.I. eds), Lawrence Erlbaum Associates, New Jersey, pp. 155–180.

Marshall S.P. (1995) *Schemas in Problem Solving.* Cambridge University Press, New York.

McKenna L. & Walsh K. (1997) Changing handover practices: one private hospital's experiences. *International Journal of Nursing Practice* 3, 128–132.

McMahon R. (1990) What are we saying? *Nursing Times* 86, 38–40.

Mosher C. & Bontomasi R. (1996) How to improve your shift report. *American Journal of Nursing* 96, 32–34.

Narayan S.M. & Corcoran-Perry S. (1997) Line of reasoning as a representation of nurses' clinical decision making. *Research in Nursing and Health* 20, 353–364.

Newell A. & Simon H.A. (1972) *Human Problem Solving.* Prentice-Hall, New Jersey.

Norberg A. & Asplund K. (1987) Patterns of speech. *Nursing Times* 83, 64–66.

Norman G.R., Tugwell P., Feightner J.W., Muzzin L.J. & Jacoby L.L. (1985) Knowledge and clinical problem-solving. *Medical Education* 19, 344–356.

Norusis M.J. & SPSS Inc. (1993) *SPSS for Windows Base System Users Guide Release 6.0.* SPSS Inc., Chicago.

Parrino T.A. & Mitchell R. (1989) Diagnosis as skill: a clinical perspective. *Perspectives in Biology and Medicine* 33, 18–44.

Prouse M. (1995) A study of the use of tape-recorded handovers. *Nursing Times* 91, 40–41.

Rosch E. (1978) Principles of categorization. In *Cognition and Categorisation* (Rosch E. & Lloyd B.B. eds), Lawrence Erlbaum Associates, Hillsdale, New Jersey, pp. 27–48.

Ross B.H. & Spalding T.L. (1994) Concepts and categories. In *Thinking and Problem Solving. Handbook of Perception and Cognition,* 2nd edn (Sternberg R.J. ed.), Academic Press, San Diego, pp. 119–149.

Rowe M.A. & Perry A. (1984) Don't sit down nurse – it's time for report! *Nursing Times* June 27, 42–43.

Sherlock C. (1995) The patient handover: a study of its form, function and efficiency. *Nursing Standard* 9, 33–36.

Smith E.R. & Medin D.L. (1981) *Categories and Concepts.* Harvard University Press, Cambridge, MA.

Tanner C.A., Padrick K.P., Westfall U.E. & Putzer D.J. (1987) Diagnostic reasoning strategies of nurses and nursing students. *Nursing Research* 36, 358–363.

Wallum R. (1995) Using care plans to replace the handover. *Nursing Standard* 9, 24–26.

Ward K. (1988) Not just the patient in bed 3. *Nursing Times* 84, 39–40.

Watkins S. (1997) Introducing bedside handover reports. *Professional Nurse* 12, 270–273.

Wyer R.S. & Gordon S.E. (1984) The cognitive representation of social information. In *Handbook of Social Cognition*, vol. 2 (Wyer R.S. & Srull T.K. eds), Lawrence Erlbaum Associates, New Jersey, pp. 73–150.

# Support for Fast Comprehension of ICU Data: Visualization using Metaphor Graphics


W. Horn[1], C. Popow[2], L. Unterasinger[2]
[1]Department of Medical Cybernetics and Artificial Intelligence, University of Vienna, and Austrian Research Institute for Artificial Intelligence, Vienna
[2]NICU, Division of Neonatology, Department of Pediatrics, University of Vienna, Austria



## Summary

*Objectives:* The time-oriented analysis of electronic patient records on (neonatal) intensive care units is a tedious and time-consuming task. Graphic data visualization should make it easier for physicians to assess the overall situation of a patient and to recognize essential changes over time.

*Methods:* Metaphor graphics are used to sketch the most relevant parameters for characterizing a patient's situation. By repetition of the graphic object in 24 frames the situation of the ICU patient is presented in one display, usually summarizing the last 24 h.

*Results:* VIE-VISU is a data visualization system which uses multiples to present the change in the patient's status over time in graphic form. Each multiple is a highly structured metaphor graphic object. Each object visualizes important ICU parameters from circulation, ventilation, and fluid balance.

*Conclusion:* The design using multiples promotes a focus on stability and change. A stable patient is recognizable at first sight, continuous improvement or worsening condition are easy to analyze, drastic changes in the patient's situation get the viewers attention immediately.

## Keywords

Computer Graphics, Data Display, Intensive Care

Methods Inf Med 2001; 40: 421–4


## 1. Introduction

The intensive care unit (ICU) is a data rich environment. Each second, a patient data set is produced by online monitoring. Moreover, clinical data (patient's state, lab values, diagnoses, medication, as well as other therapeutic and nursing actions) are collected manually at various time intervals. A computer-based patient data management system (PDMS) stores data that has been collected online or entered manually within a specified time frame.

Even if these electronic patient records are complete and correct, they are difficult to analyze because they contain so much data. The amount of data stored in electronic form outperforms the amount of data available in paper records by far. This should serve an important function: the investigation of problems in great detail. However, the overall assessment of the patient's situation becomes more difficult. Physicians face the difficult task of selecting relevant information from the vast amounts of available data.

The monitoring devices of a modern ICU are usually optimized to support instantaneous problem recognition. Usually, only a limited amount of past data can be reviewed on the monitor itself. Sophisticated PDMS, such as HP's CareVue 9000, allow complete review of the data over the entire period of a patient's stay on the ICU.

Most of the data are presented in the form of a spreadsheet. A few parameters can also be displayed as X-Y plots. This kind of display makes it easy to find the value of a specific parameter at a specific time. It is more difficult to extract a summary of a patient's condition at a specific time point. Finding the essential change(s) in a patient's state over a given time interval is even more complicated.

There are several reasons why spreadsheet tables and X-Y plots are difficult to use:

- Too many parameters are displayed to be easily comprehended by humans.
- Usually, no comprehensive indicator for value ranges (normal, critical, or out of range) exists. This would require a conceptual understanding of value ranges. Moreover, in medicine, parameter ranges are context dependent: What is *normal* often depends on the patient's actual situation, i.e., on several other parameters.
- X-Y plots give the impression of a linear development of parameters between the tics shown. This is often misleading.
- The shown data have to be representative of the period of time they cover. A PDMS with time-stamped data usually shows the data value received at a fixed time point. No provisions are made to present the value most representative of a given time interval. This creates a severe problem when the time interval covered by one data point is increased. Usually this happens by decreasing the resolution of the time axis in the display. Depending on the starting time of the time axis of the display, quite different data values may be shown if the PDMS merely picks out the values stored at the time of the axis tics.

Representation graphic tools are an aid to comprehending and analyzing data (1). We

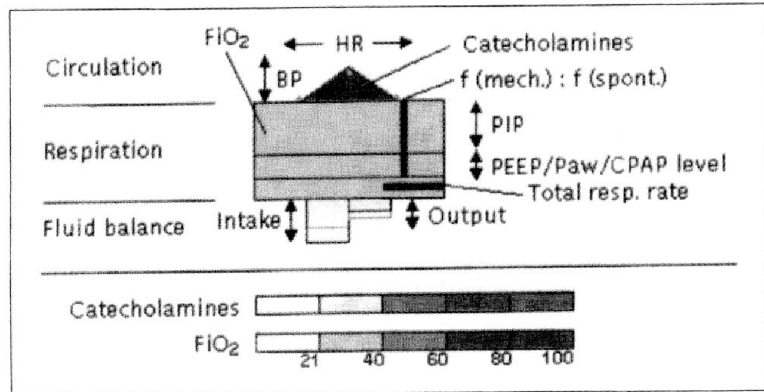

**Fig. 1**
The metaphor graphic object

have developed a graphic visualization system, VIE-VISU, which uses metaphor graphics. In the following section, we present the design of the graphical objects and the display. A discussion of the design and its usability is given in Section 3.

# 2. Using Metaphor Graphics to Visualize ICU Data

Graphic representation offers a wide variety of methods to support humans in easily integrating data (1-4). Which method is chosen depends mainly on what information you would like to display, to ease comprehension. In our domain, neonatal intensive care, we would like to be able to recognize changes in neonatal status over time. The most relevant parameters for such a view are circulatory, respiratory, and fluid balance data.

Small multiples present a good way to represent changes over time (2). They resemble the frames of a movie: the same graphical object changes its shape and color from frame to frame. The time intervals between frames are fixed, as is the basic design of the frame. The fixed design focuses attention on the data shifts over time.

Volume rectangles were used as a metaphor graphic by Cole and Stewart (5) to represent respiratory data. Breath rates and breath volumes are sketched by the size and volume of rectangles. Rectangles do not offer sufficient degrees of freedom for our problem. Our first goal was to combine the following parameters into one metaphor object:

- Circulatory data:
  - mean blood pressure ($BP$)
  - heart rate ($HR$), and
  - a catecholamine index ($CI$). The index gives the summarized (and weighted) administration of dopamine, dobutamine, epinephrine, and norepinephrine
- Respiratory data:
  - spontaneous breathing frequency ($f_{spont}$)
  - oxygen saturation measured by pulsoximetry ($S_PO_2$)
  - fraction of inspired oxygen concentration ($FiO_2$)
  - type of ventilation: none, continuous positive airway pressure (CPAP), high frequency ventilation (HFOV), or intermittent positive pressure/ mandatory ventilation (IPPV/IMV). Depending on the type of ventilation
  - *CPAP level* for CPAP ventilation
  - mean airway pressure ($Paw$) and
  - pressure amplitude of the oscillator ($\Delta P$) for HFOV
  - peak inspiratory pressure ($PIP$),
  - positive end-expiratory pressure ($PEEP$), and
  - mechanical ventilatory rate ($f$) for conventional mechanical ventilation
- Fluid balance:
  - total fluid intake, and
  - total urinary output.

It took several design steps to find a metaphor graphic able to include most of these parameters in a way which is easy to comprehend. It is quite clear, such a graphic object must be rather complex.

For our first design, we used a very simple object: a circle with twelve sectors. Each sector represents one parameter. A "normal" circle represents the normal situation, i.e. all parameters are normal. The sectors grow, or shrink, in corre-

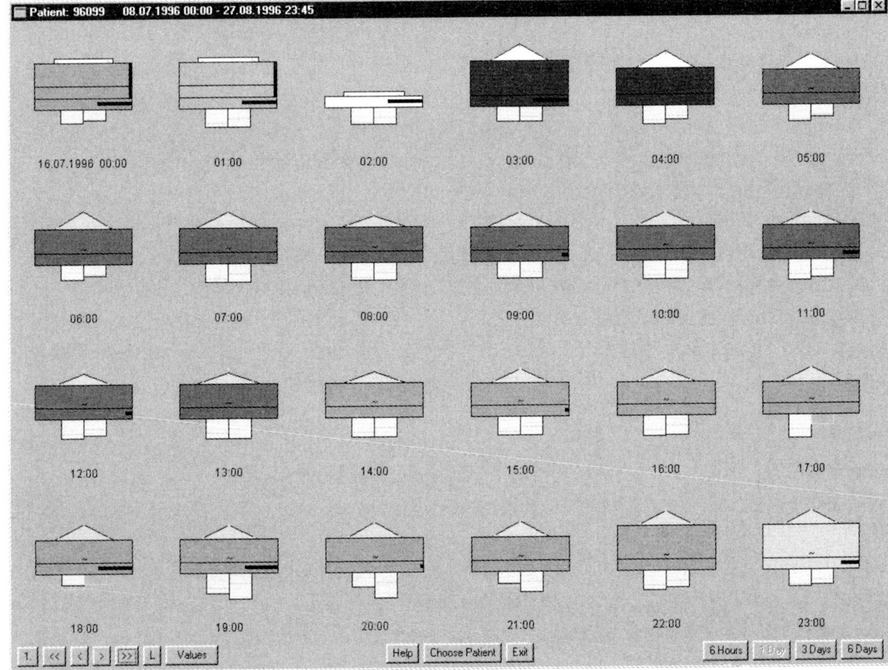

**Fig. 2**   The 24 hours display of VIE-VISU

spondence to the deviation from the normal value.

The first use gave us a clear impression of the major flaws of this design: there is no overall impression of how the patient's situation "looks". The bad experience with a uniform object forced us to try a completely different approach, using a highly structured object.

## 2.1 A Structured Metaphor Graphic Object

A highly structured object has the advantage of allowing easy identification of several parameters. The object we designed is explained in Fig. 1.

The actual value of a parameter is either depicted by the size of an object, or by its color. The larger a value, the larger the object, or the darker the color. Heart rate is the only parameter which varies in size horizontally (size of the top triangle). Blood pressure, *PIP, PEEP, Paw*, fluid intake, and urinary output vary the size of the drawn object vertically. The total respiratory rate is given by a slider, which increases from right to left. The relation between the mechanical ventilatory rate and the spontaneous breathing rate is depicted by a vertical slider, which moves to the left the higher the spontaneous respiratory rate. $FiO_2$ is represented by the color of the respiration block. The higher the $FiO_2$ concentration, supplied by the ventilator, or by the incubator, the darker the blue of the respiration block. The color of the triangle changes in intensities of red when increasing amounts of catecholamines are applied. $S_pO_2$ and $\Delta P$ are not displayed.

The graphic object forms the basis for recognition of change over time. By repetition of the object in 24 frames ($6 \times 4$), the situation of the ICU patient during the past 24 hours, is presented in one display. Each multiple shows the situation of a specific hour. The multiples should enable physicians to focus on repetition and change. A sample display is shown in Fig. 2.

The display draws attention to the change from IPPV ventilation (at 01:00) to HFOV ventilation (at 03:00; data are missing at 02:00). HFOV ventilation begins with a high $FiO_2$ supply, which decreases over time. Simultaneously, *Paw* settings decrease over time until 22:00. At this time, *Paw* is again high. The circulation is quite good. Fluid balance shows a considerable increase in output most of the time.

A comprehensive view over 24 h supports focus on continuity and surprise. It is easy to recognize a stable patient. Continuous improvement is made transparent. Attention is directed toward critical situations in patient care: the change from IPPV to HFOV and the increase in *Paw* at 22:00, in our example. With respect to our initial goal, namely to ease the comprehension of essential changes in patient status over time, the display fulfills its task.

## 3. Discussion

Multiples directly depict comparison. They are well-suited to reveal repetition and change, enabling the user to see patterns and surprise. A first evaluation of VIE-VISU was conducted by two expert neonatologists, using data from 167 neonatal ICU patients. This evaluation has shown, the 24 metaphor graphic objects are able to focus the attention of physicians toward critical situations in patient care. A very fast understanding of the situation is supported. This is consistent with results stemming from a human performance evaluation of respiratory data recognition (6).

However, the quality of the metaphor is of essential importance to recognition. Cole and Stewart (5) used volume rectangles to represent two ventilatory parameters: breathing/ventilation rate and tidal volume. Width and height of the rectangles are modified in accordance to these two parameters. The size of the rectangle represents metaphor of the minute breathing volume of the patient.

Our first design used a circle with sectors to represent our manifold parameters (see [7]). Physicians did not find this useful in practice. Uniform objects do not seem adequate for helping to analyze the complex situation of a patient, which is represented by a set of *different* parameters. In contrast, a quite similar design, Aberdeen polygons, is reported to be quite useful (8). However, an Aberdeen polygon shows the deviation from normal values for a set of physiological parameters. For our task, a norm circle is inappropriate. It is confusing: some parameters may be lower, or higher, compared to normal (e.g., *BP,HR*). Other values are never below normal (e.g., $FiO_2$ is never less than 21%), and others have a normal value of zero (e.g., *PIP*). As a result, some sectors never shrink and the display is biased. With a uniform object it is hard to learn which parameter is located in each sector. It forces attention on the sectors, instead of on the change between frames. The highly structured object we have used in our second design avoids such problems. It further supports the ability to learn and orientate, due to the different shapes and colors within one object.

Highly structured objects have one disadvantage: there is very limited space for each of the different parameters. This makes it nearly impossible to recognize subtle changes of a parameter's value. Inappropriate scales effectively hide the essentials (4). We tried to avoid such hiding effects by carefully setting scales. In addition, we marked expected (normal) values with green dots and lines. This makes it easy to recognize deviations from the expected values. An evaluation study should provide us with details about the accuracy a viewer is able to achieve. We cannot expect great precision in recognizing slight modifications of individual parameters (the values displayed should serve this task), but we expect high accuracy in recognizing essential changes.

A different, and quite problematic, question is about the representative value of a parameter over a certain time interval. This becomes significant if the resolution of the time axis of the display is less than the time resolution of the data collection process. We use the median value of all data values within the time interval as the representative value. This is somewhat consistent with data collection methods of the PDMS, averaging data received every five seconds. However, it is quite questionable. It loses extreme values which may be of specific importance to patient care. However, in practice, extreme values are very often artifacts. Data validation (9) offers only very limited methods to recognize such artifacts should the data density be low and the data has been already averaged by the PDMS preprocessing. The VIE-VISU server is confronted with such a situation. Therefore, it serves the median value over an interval, instead of the most severe value within that interval, which may be more interesting. Temporal data abstraction (10, 11) provides an alternative. However, it usually looks for an abstract symbolic characterization of a parameter over time. Associated visualization tools for temporal clinical data (12, 13) try to find appropriate visual representations to display an (abstracted) medical event. In contrast, VIE-VISU's data server must find a numeric value which represents all values of the parameter within a fixed time period at regular intervals.

The design of graphic displays for ICU data comprehension must look for easy learnability, high accuracy, and increased comprehension speed. We are preparing a clinical study to examine the usefulness of VIE-VISU, both for expert neonatologists and novice physicians. The results should provide us with detailed insight about the three criteria: learnability, accuracy, and speed.

# 4. Conclusion

VIE-VISU is a visualization system for data collected on intensive care units. The change in the patient's status over time is depicted by 24 multiples. Each multiple is a highly structured metaphor graphics object. Each object visualizes important parameters, such as circulation, ventilation, and fluid balance. A display presents a metaphor graphics summary on a time scale of six hours to six days, depending on the users' choice.

Fast comprehension and easy analysis of changes in a patient's situation by physicians was the primary goal of VIE-VISU. The design using multiples promotes focus on stability and change. A stable patient can be recognized at first sight, continuous improvement, or worsening condition, is easy to analyze. Drastic changes in the patient's situation gains the viewers attention immediately. In summary, VIE-VISU provides access to the complex without complicating the simple.

Metaphor graphics are quoted for easy learnability, long remembering periods, and good decision support, if the task is finding patterns in a mass of data. A clinical study, now in its early stage, should justify these claims for VIE-VISU.

**Acknowledgments**
The first version of VIE-VISU was implemented by Barbara Riepl, as part of her master's thesis. Major parts of the current Java code were implemented by Christoph Stocker.
We greatly appreciate the support given to the Austrian Research Institute of Artificial Intelligence (ÖFAI) by the Austrian Federal Ministry of Education, Science and Culture.

# References

1. Tufte ER. Visual Explanations. Cheshire CT: Graphics Press 1997.
2. Tufte ER. The Visual Display of Quantitative Information. Cheshire CT: Graphics Press 1983.
3. Tufte ER. Envisioning Information. Cheshire CT: Graphics Press 1990.
4. Wainer H. Visual Revelations: Graphic Tales of Fate and Deception from Napoleon Bonaparte to Ross Perot. New York: Copernicus/Springer 1997.
5. Cole WG, Stewart JG. Metaphor graphics to support integrated decision making with respiratory data. Int J Clin Monit Comput 1993; 10: 91-100.
6. Cole WG, Stewart JG. Human performance evaluation of a metaphor graphic display for respiratory data. Methods Inf Med 1994; 33: 390-6.
7. Horn W, Popow C, Unterasinger L. Metaphor graphics to visualize ICU data over time. In: Bellazzi R, Zupan B, eds. ECAI-98 Workshop on Intelligent Data Analysis in Medicine and Pharmacology (IDAMAP-98), Brighton, UK 1998; 76-81.
8. Green CA, Logie RH, Gilhooly KJ, Ross DG, Ronald A. Aberdeen polygons: computer displays of physiological profiles for intensive care. Ergonomics 1996; 39: 412-28.
9. Horn W, Miksch S, Egghart G, Popow C, Paky F. Effective data validation of high-frequency data: time-point-, time-interval-, and trend-based methods. Comp Biol Med 1997; 27: 389-409.
10. Shahar Y. A framework for knowledge-based temporal abstraction. Artif Intell 1997; 90: 79-133.
11. Combi C, Chittaro L. Abstraction on clinical data sequences: an object-oriented data model and a query language based on the event calculus. Artif Intell Med 1999; 17: 271-301.
12. Shahar Y, Cheng C. Model-based visualization of temporal abstractions. Fifth International Workshop on Temporal Representation and Reasoning (TIME'98), Sanibel Island, Florida 1998; 11-20.
13. Combi C, Portoni L, Pinciroli F. Visualizing temporal clinical data on the WWW. In: Artificial Intelligence in Medicine. Horn W, et al., eds. Berlin: Springer 1999; 301-10.

Correspondence to:
Prof. Werner Horn
Department of Medical Cybernetics
and Artificial Intelligence
University of Vienna
Freyung 6, A-1010 Vienna
Austria
E-mail: werner@ai.univie.ac.at

# Efficiency and safety of chemotherapy plans for children: CATIPO—a nationwide approach

Petra Knaup[a,*], Timm Wiedemann[a], Andreas Bachert[b], Ursula Creutzig[c], Reinhold Haux[a], Freimut Schilling[d]

[a]*Department of Medical Informatics, University of Heidelberg, Institute for Medical Biometry and Informatics, Im Neuenheimer Feld 400, D-69210 Heidelberg, Germany*
[b]*HMS GmbH, Schillerstr. 4-8, D-69115 Heidelberg, Germany*
[c]*Gesellschaft für Pädiatrische Onkologie und Hämatologie, Thea-Bähnisch-Weg 12, D-30657 Hannover, Germany*
[d]*Olga Hospital Stuttgart, Child and Adolescent Medicine, Pediatrics 5 (Oncology/Hematology, Immunology), Bismarckstr. 8, D-70176 Stuttgart, Germany*

Received 20 June 2001; received in revised form 24 September 2001; accepted 10 October 2001

## Abstract

Chemotherapy is an important component of childhood cancer treatment. Due to the intensity of this therapy, an error in calculating the dosage of the cytostatic drugs would have severe consequences. Therefore, a computer-aided therapy planning system in pediatric oncology (CATIPO) was introduced into routine use in approximately 20 clinics across Germany. The system consists of a knowledge acquisition module for acquiring knowledge about chemotherapy protocols and a decision support module for producing a patient-specific therapy plan. The main benefits of the system are the reduction of errors and saving time during the development of a particular therapy plan. CATIPO's success is based on the enormous demand for this kind of decision support and its development in tight cooperation with future users. © 2002 Elsevier Science B.V. All rights reserved.

*Keywords:* Therapy planning; Decision support; Pediatric oncology; Chemotherapy

## 1. Introduction

### 1.1. Subject and relevance

The treatment of childhood cancer in Germany has improved continuously over the last decades. According to a report by the German Childhood Cancer Registry [12], the

---

*Corresponding author. Present address: Adolph-Kolping-Str. 48, D-61118 Bad Vilbel, Germany.
Tel.: +49-6101-85818; fax: +49-6221-564997.
*E-mail address:* petra_knaup@med.uni-heidelberg.de (P. Knaup).

recurrence-free survival rate has increased to an average around 70%. This average varies depending on the particular diagnosis: the 5-year survival rate is approximately 38% for acute non-lymphatic leukemia and around 97% for retinoblastoma. It is assumed that nationwide multi-center trials have contributed considerably to this success. For each of the 18 most common diagnoses of childhood cancer, trial centers have been established to produce therapy protocols for respective treatment. In Germany, approximately 90% of the children with cancer are treated according to these protocols. Research in multi-center trials currently focuses primarily on the survival rate, as well as on minimizing the side effects of the intense treatment.

*1.2. Problems and motivation*

Chemotherapy is the core treatment in the most cases of childhood cancer. Cytostatic drug dosage depends on age, height and weight of the patients. Therefore, the therapy protocol guidelines must be adjusted for each patient. These calculations are time-consuming and complex (cf. [19]). An error could have severe consequences for the child [7]. If the dosage is too low, the tumor will be attacked insufficiently and therefore, the child will not be cured. Should, however, the dosage be too high, the side effects will harm the child to a non-justifiable extent. Due to these problems, the Department of Medical Informatics of the University of Heidelberg, in cooperation with the German Society of Pediatric Oncology and Hematology (GPOH), has developed the application system computer-aided therapy planning in pediatric oncology (CATIPO) [1]. CATIPO is currently in routine use in approximately 20 pediatric cancer clinics across Germany. Considering that 70% of the childhood cancer patients are treated in 30 hospitals, this number is rather high [12].

*1.3. Aim of this paper*

The aim of this paper is to discuss the effectiveness of using computer-aided chemotherapy planning in a number of German cancer clinics and to share our experiences with the reader. We will begin by introducing the application system in further detail.


## 2. Introduction of CATIPO

Clinically, CATIPO aims at determining the adequate therapy for an individual patient according to the guidelines of the respective protocol. Most often, CATIPO determines a complete chemotherapy cycle in advance. Such a cycle can last for several weeks, or even months. This is an important difference to comparable systems in adult oncology, in which daily decisions must often be supported. Additionally, the eligibility of a patient for a trial is not a relevant problem for computer-aided decision support in this field.

CATIPO consists of two main modules: the knowledge acquisition module (CATIPO-kam), helps to formalize the therapy protocol guidelines of the trial centers, independent of a particular patient. The decision-support module (CATIPO-dss), is able to process

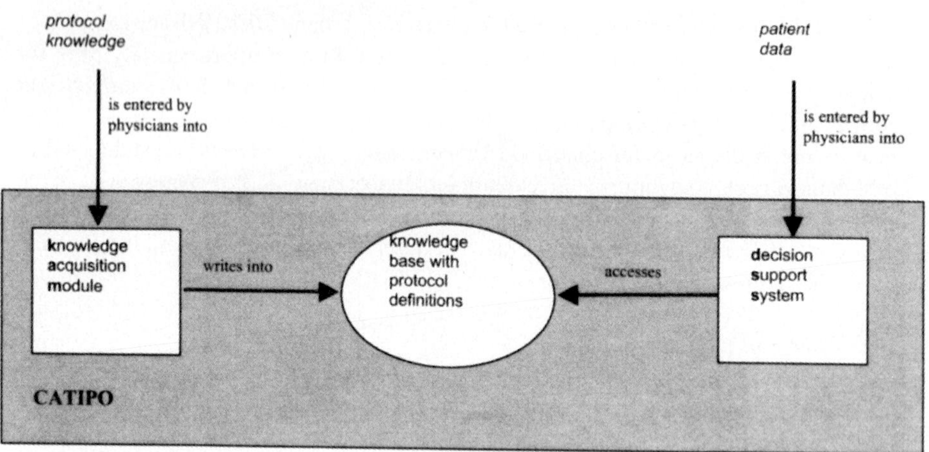



Fig. 1. Basic architecture of CATIPO. The physician specifies protocol-specific knowledge with the help of the CATIPO-kam. The knowledge is also accessed by the decision support tool, which produces patient-specific therapy plans. For this purpose, the CATIPO-dss needs certain data about the patient.

formalized guidelines, to ask for patient data, and to produce a patient-specific therapy plan. Fig. 1 shows the basic architecture of CATIPO.

CATIPO has been in routine use since 1993. An easy to use DOS-interface was implemented at that time to lead the users through all necessary steps.

### 2.1. Knowledge acquisition: defining therapy protocols

The GPOH began the first clinical trials during the end of the 1970s. Since different chairmen have been responsible for establishing the trials that followed, structure, layout, and conventions of the various trial protocols differ considerably. Thus, the first task in developing CATIPO was to identify, model and specify the general knowledge implicitly inherent in the protocols of the GPOH trials. The formal representation of this knowledge in CATIPO allows use of the implicit knowledge for various patients and for various clinical trials. Part of this modeling process was the analysis of the explicit knowledge that must be entered into the knowledge acquisition tool, CATIPO-kam, by the clinicians. The most important entities of explicit knowledge are:

- *Drugs*: All drugs used in the chemotherapy cycle must be formally defined, e.g. standardized information about the unit, type of administration, calculation mode, maximum dosage, rounding precision, tolerated deviation of calculated doses.
- *Solutions containing an active agent*: For infusion drugs, the concentration of the active agents contained in the solution must be declared.
- *Infusions*: Each infusion can be composed of drugs and solutions that have been defined beforehand. The addition of hydration fluid can occur in four ways. Examples are: according to the patient's body surface, or by fixed volume. Additionally, volume and speed of the infusion are defined. Fig. 2 presents an example of how the components of an infusion are defined.

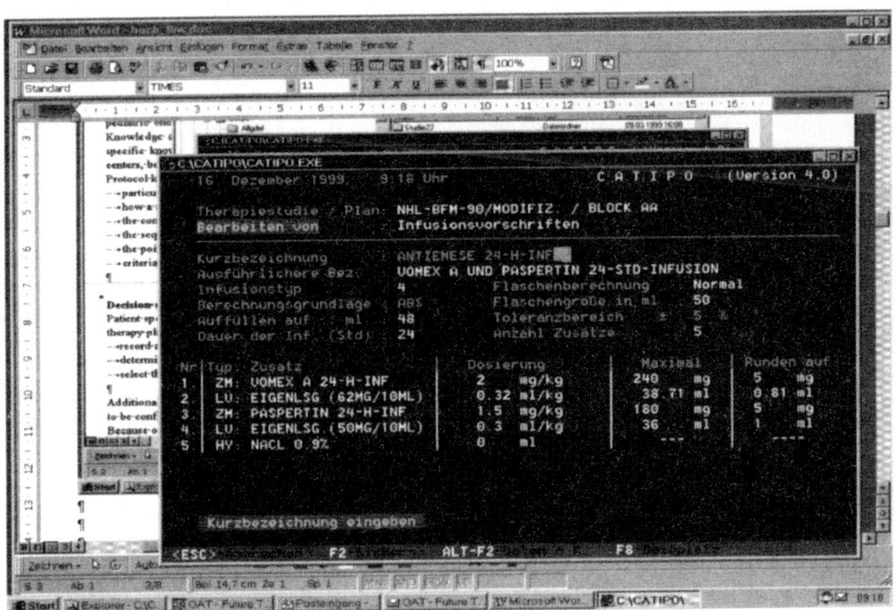

Fig. 2. Definition of the components of an infusion using the (CATIPO-kam). The upper part of the figure shows the name of the trial, function of the screen, name of the infusion and several parameters pertaining to the make-up of the infusion (volume, duration, number of components, etc.). In the lower part of the figure, all components of the infusion are declared formally: name, dosage per unit of weight, maximum dosage and necessary precision.

- *Sequential order of drug applications*: The entities mentioned above can be arranged to form the course of a chemotherapy cycle. Drugs and infusions can be administered at various points in time, which are defined relative to the beginning of the chemotherapy cycle. The formal definition of the therapy plan can be enhanced by passages of free text, e.g. to remind the nursing staff of necessary measures, or to explain certain administrations.
- *Inclusion criteria*: Patient variables, or conditions, necessary for starting the chemotherapy cycle can be described informally.

Following a detailed examination of the modeling results, we determined that the explicit knowledge could be stored efficiently in relational database tables. Algorithms could represent the general course of calculating a particular therapy plan of a patient. This includes, e.g. implicit knowledge about handling rounding precisions and tolerated limits, should a physician decide to reduce the dosage indicated in the protocol. The most important parameters in calculating patient-specific dosages are body surface (calculated using weight and height), age and weight. Rules for checking the plausibility of these parameters have been implemented to warn the user whether a particular combination of parameters is outside the normal range.

Knowledge acquisition with CATIPO-kam takes place in the participating hospitals. The physicians enter the explicit knowledge. Unfortunately, this process cannot take place in the trial centers, because each hospital has its own conventions, e.g. concerning drug usage or solutions.

### 2.2. Decision support: achieving patient-specific therapy

Patient-specific data must be entered into CATIPO's decision support module, CATIPO-dss, to generate a patient-specific therapy plan that adheres to the definition of a therapy protocol. The treating physician must:

- record the age, height, weight and gender of the patient;
- determine the starting point of the chemotherapy cycle;
- select the therapy protocol and chemotherapy cycle according to which the patient is to be treated.

In addition, the criteria necessary for including a patient in a selected chemotherapy cycle must be confirmed.

Because of toxic reactions to previous radio- or chemotherapy, the physician may decide that the complete dosage, as proposed by the therapy protocol, should not be administered to the child. In this case, the physician has the opportunity to reduce the dosage of all or certain drugs. If, during the administration of a chemotherapy cycle, the physician decides that the remaining doses of this cycle should be reduced, the physician can calculate a new therapy plan. The new plan then begins on the respective day of the current cycle using a reduced dosage.

The generated therapy plan can be printed as a structured document. It contains all drug administrations of a single chemotherapy cycle in chronological order, the cytostatic drugs as well as any supportive medication. All administrations of a particular therapy day within a cycle can be regarded as a unit. The printed therapy plan is used as an organizational and documentation aid on most wards. The schedule is used for ordering drugs from the dispensary and for making final preparations on the ward. In addition, it may happen that a drug is not given exactly at the calculated time, or there may be slight variations in the dosage. In this case, the modifications are recorded in the therapy plan. Otherwise, each administration is signed by the responsible person and given as calculated. Finally, this document is stored in the patient record. Fig. 3 shows a typical example of a therapy plan being used in clinical routine.

## 3. Discussion—lessons learned

### 3.1. Brief comparison with other available approaches

Several information systems supporting protocol-guided therapy in oncology have been introduced and their benefits evaluated during the last two decades (e.g. [4–7,18,22]). Most of the systems are designed for use in adult cancer treatment. These systems usually offer decision support based on earlier treatment responses and changes in vital parameters or laboratory findings (cf. [2,6,9,20]), and help select patients eligible for a certain protocol or medication.

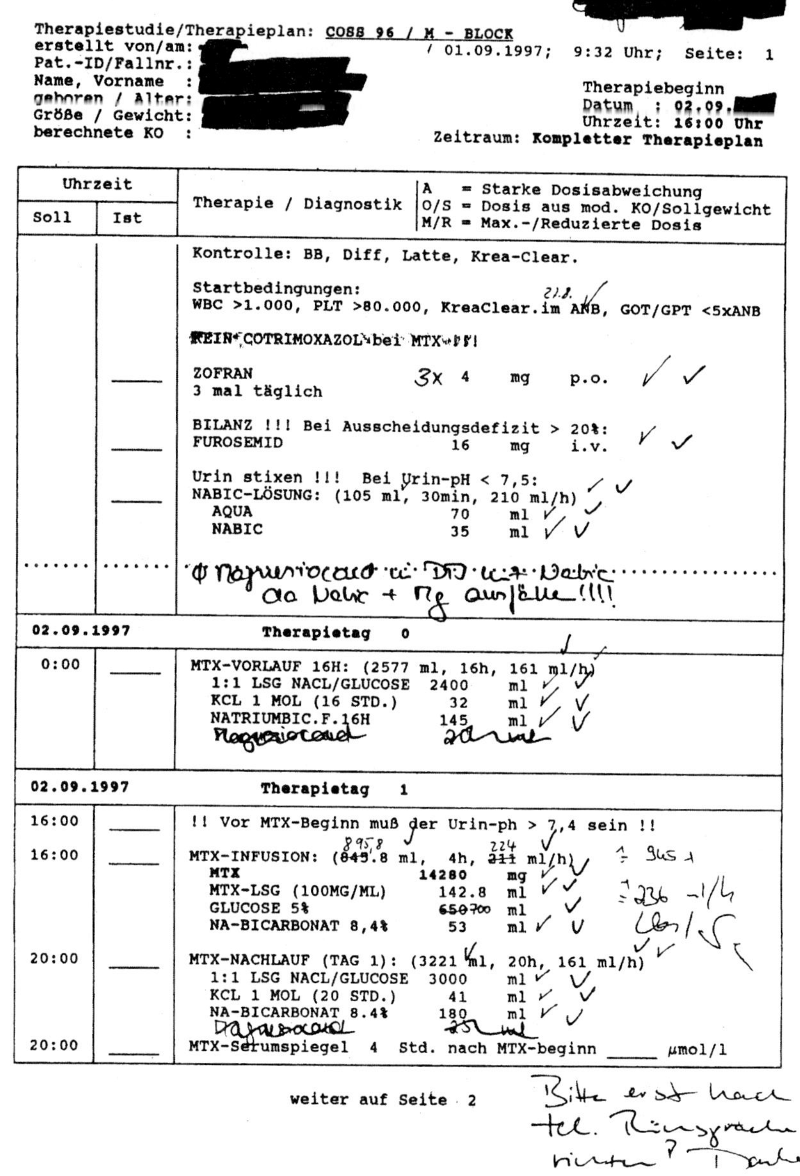



| Uhrzeit | | Therapie / Diagnostik | A = Starke Dosisabweichung |
| Soll | Ist | | O/S = Dosis aus mod. KO/Sollgewicht |
| --- | --- | --- | --- |
| | | | M/R = Max.-/Reduzierte Dosis |



| 02.09.1997 | | Therapietag  0 | |
| --- | --- | --- | --- |



| 02.09.1997 | | Therapietag  1 | |
| --- | --- | --- | --- |



weiter auf Seite  2

Fig. 3. Example of a therapy plan printed by CATIPO-dss and used for documentation purposes. The part above the big rectangle shows the official name of the trial, its date and time, and the demographic patient data. The left column contains the time at which a new dose is administered. The upper part, not associated to certain time periods, contains general remarks important to the chemotherapy cycle. The handwritten notes document whether a calculated administration took place.

These problems are not relevant to pediatric oncology in Germany. In most cases, an adequate protocol can be assigned unambiguously, because just one nationwide protocol exists for each of the most common diagnoses. Furthermore, the treating physician is not solely responsible for making this decision, he is supported by the German Childhood Cancer Registry [11] and the respective trial centers.

Additionally, children, in contrast to adults, can tolerate higher doses of chemotherapy rather well. Therefore, the proposed chemotherapy cycle can often be applied as calculated in advance. Daily decisions regarding therapeutic actions normally pertain only to supportive medication, or slight dosage reductions.

Another reason why most of the available systems are not applicable for widespread use in pediatric oncology in Germany is the need for flexible and easy to use knowledge acquisition tools dedicated to processing the GPOH protocols. The physicians of the treating clinics must enter the protocol-specific knowledge. Most of the 18 multi-center trials last about 5 years; so, three to five new protocols are delivered every year.

THEMPO is a well-directed system aimed at meeting the needs of pediatric oncology [15]. Beside presenting and calculating therapy plans, it allows the representation of causal, temporal and other clinical contexts [14]. However, THEMPO has been developed in a NEXTSTEP environment and therefore, is not yet applicable for widespread use in clinics across Germany.

The basic idea underlying the development of CATIPO during early 1990s was to obtain an application system dedicated to the needs of pediatric oncology in Germany relative quickly, and to immediately make it available for routine clinical use. Therefore, we did not fall back on more sophisticated approaches, such as [13,16]. While the system was validated by routine clinical use, direct feedback led to several improved versions.

### 3.2. *What effort is involved in adapting CATIPO for use in a particular hospital?*

CATIPO itself can be used quite easily in any pediatric oncology hospital. It is available on request by GPOH (Gesellschaft für Pädiatrische Onkologie und Hämatologie) and is delivered by the developers of the system. In principle, it can be used immediately without any adaptations. Nevertheless, certain parameters can be adapted, making it as comfortable to use as possible for each clinic:

- global definition of drugs and solutions can be adopted for various protocols;
- parameters for printing the therapy plan (layout);
- parameters for printing labels (e.g. for the dispensary).

No special qualification is needed to adapt the system, since the user is guided through the adaptation of these and other parameters. CATIPO is delivered with a standard setting of these parameters.

Of course, one must be aware of the fact that no patient-specific therapy plan can be calculated before the guidelines of a protocol have been implemented with the knowledge acquisition module. Because of the mentioned hospital-specific conventions, CATIPO is delivered without any protocol knowledge. A physician who knows the protocol for each relevant chemotherapy cycle quite well should enter this knowledge. In the beginning, it will take the physician about an hour to define a new cycle. In the course of time, the definition process will become much faster, since global definitions of drugs and solutions can be made and used for various chemotherapy cycles, even in different protocols.

### 3.3. What are the benefits of using CATIPO for planning chemotherapy in cases of childhood cancer?

CATIPO's main task is to support physicians in developing patient-specific protocol-guided therapy plans for childhood cancer patients. Due to the complexity and scope of multi-center trial therapy protocols (cf. [18]), CATIPO can help avoid mistakes, which could have severe consequences. CATIPO has been in routine use now for several years. All cytostatic drug dosages used in pediatric oncology are calculated at least twice. This ensures that experienced physicians have double-checked all calculations made by CATIPO using conventional calculation forms. Due to these checks, a high quality could be shown for CATIPO calculations over the years. Obviously, the prerequisite for a high quality therapy plan is a correctly defined therapy protocol using CATIPO-kam.

Helping to avoid mistakes is not CATIPO's only benefit. Moreover, it can also reduce the effort required for developing protocol-guided therapy plans, because upon definition, each chemotherapy cycle can be used for several patients.

CATIPO provides additional tasks for supporting routine clinical processes. First, the calculated therapy plans can be printed and used for administrative and documentation purposes. After the medical staff has recorded the application of the calculated doses on the printed sheets, they are filed in the patient record. Additionally, CATIPO prints labels and forms for ordering drugs from the dispensary.

As stated earlier, the basic idea underlying CATIPO was to provide, and gain experience in using, a simple and easy to use computer-aided decision support system. Therefore, one of CATIPO's main tasks is to produce a chemotherapy plan that fulfills the criteria of a therapy protocol. It is not yet possible to use CATIPO for computer-aided documentation. It may happen, e.g. that the physician decides to change the calculated dosage due to toxic reactions by the child. In this case, it is not possible to record and store the actually administered application electronically using CATIPO. Currently, CATIPO can calculate only a single chemotherapy cycle. It is neither able to give an overview of the complete and overall chemotherapy received by a patient, nor to include received radiotherapy and surgery.

The integration of decision support systems into hospital information systems is often mentioned as an important aspect to avoid multiple data entry [3,8,17]. In the case of CATIPO, the amount of data to be entered after a protocol has been defined is rather low. Therefore, the physicians have not yet regarded the lack of integration as a shortcoming of the system.

### 3.4. How well is CATIPO accepted by the users?

In order to evaluate the number of hospitals and physicians actually using CATIPO, to assess user acceptance, user satisfaction and problems in using CATIPO, two surveys were conducted in 1993 and 1995. Standardized questionnaires were sent to all hospitals that had requested to install the program.

### 3.4.1. Survey results 1993

Out of 31 hospitals, 21 responded. Sixteen hospitals used CATIPO to routinely calculate individual therapy plans. Seven hospitals reported severe problems in using CATIPO; nevertheless, five of them were using it. The problems that arose involved either CATIPO itself (four hospitals), the connected printers (two hospitals), or the definition of protocol knowledge (four hospitals).

Despite the mentioned problems, 19 out of 21 hospitals considered CATIPO an adequate tool for calculating patient-specific therapy plans. Two hospitals did not answer this question.

Out of 21 hospitals, 18 confirmed that routine use of CATIPO is changing the clinical tasks of physicians, as well as of the nursing staff. Fifteen hospitals regarded these changes as tolerable or minor, while three reported major changes in clinical tasks.

The time needed to define protocol knowledge and calculate individual plans—compared to the conventional procedure—is considered higher (three hospitals), only initially higher (four hospitals), identical (five hospitals) or lower (nine hospitals). Four hospitals reported that the acceptance of the patient-specific therapy plan generated by CATIPO was lower than that of the plans used before.

Reasons mentioned for not using CATIPO in clinical routine were:

- insufficient hardware resources (three hospitals);
- time too limited for training (three hospitals);
- disapproval among nursing staff (two hospitals).

### 3.4.2. Survey results 1995

Out of 46 hospitals, 22 responded. Sixteen of these hospitals routinely used CATIPO to calculate individual therapy plans. While one hospital reported severe problems in using CATIPO, twelve reported minor, and four no problems. The problems that arose either involved CATIPO itself (six hospitals), the connected printers (one hospital), or the definition of protocol knowledge (ten hospitals).

The number of therapy protocols defined using CATIPO ranges from 4 to 29, with a mean of 12. The number of chemotherapy cycles of these protocols range from 9 to 133, with a mean of 56. At certain times, about 16–20 GPOH clinical trials were active.

The hospitals not routinely using CATIPO mentioned the following reasons:

- the task of preparing the cytostatic drugs had been transferred to the dispensary, which uses its own forms;
- the hospital was using an electronic medication system, which they had developed and were afraid of replacing a system they were already familiar with;
- the hospital had only a few patients for each clinical trial, so the effort of defining the protocol knowledge appeared too high.

### 3.4.3. Discussion of the results

The 16 responding hospitals of the 1993 survey, which mentioned routine use of documentation system for pediatric oncology (DOSPO), are not identical with those hospitals responding in the 1995 survey. Thus, it can be concluded that about 20 German hospitals have routine experience with CATIPO. The lack of sufficient hardware resources was a severe problem for several years, but is no longer an obstacle today.

The nursing staff disapproved of the computer-generated therapy plans only in few cases. The 1993 survey made obvious that the introduction of computer-based application systems changes clinical tasks. This problem is often underestimated. Comprehensive situation analyses should be conducted in advance, and the concerned staff should be involved in the development and introduction process as early as possible.

A severe and, still remaining, problem is the limited time available to the involved staff. The time for training and becoming acquainted with a new application system is an obstacle, even if timesaving is expected by using the application system in the long run. Another time problem, not reported in either survey, but often reported to us in discussions with potential users, is that some clinicians regard the process of knowledge acquisition as too time-consuming. Whether this time is invested highly depends on the user's motivation and attitude, and obviously, is worthwhile only if a minimum amount of patients can be expected for a trial in a particular hospital.

All severe problems mentioned in the surveys were discussed with the users and resulted in new versions of the system (up to version 4.0).

Another severe problem we have observed during the years of CATIPO usage is the need of a contact person within each hospital, who is experienced in using CATIPO, and who holds the position over a certain length of time. In most hospitals, only one or two physicians are familiar with CATIPO. If these individuals leave the ward, e.g. due to career or rotation reasons, the danger arises that CATIPO is no longer used if experiences are not transferred to another physician in time.

### 3.5. Further factors for CATIPO's success

The most important aspect of CATIPO's success is that the demand for such a computer-aided therapy planning system came from physicians working in pediatric oncology clinics. A real necessity for a decision support of this kind existed. CATIPO was developed in close cooperation with its future users and therefore, is adapted well to their requirements. The limitations of the system are accepted well by the users, because they enable easy application and use of the system.

Another important factor is that by using CATIPO, the physician does not feel the system is explicitly suggesting decisions. CATIPO merely supports physicians with calculations based on formally represented knowledge of therapy protocols. The physician is very well aware that he is responsible for the final decision. This can be shown with the help of an example: CATIPO is able to reduce the dosage of cytostatic drugs in comparison to those proposed by the protocol. However, the decision that the cytostatic drugs should be reduced is left to the physician. To date, the users have not asked for additional decision support of this kind. They want to fall back on their own experience and knowledge, or that of the trial centers. Trial centers offer telephone support in critical cases, based on the latest data of the current trial. It is also very important that possible side effects of the treatment are immediately reported to the trial centers.

Currently, maintenance of the knowledge base is left to the hospital physicians. It is up to them to keep the definitions of chemotherapy cycles up to date, especially if a new version of a therapy protocol is released. Often, a new cycle differs only slightly from its previous version. In this case, the physician can copy and modify the old one, instead of completely redefining it. Of course, the quality of the knowledge depends strongly on the processes and attitudes of the various hospitals. An important factor for quality is the availability of a core ward staff not only able to handle CATIPO very well, but also to maintain the quality of the formalized protocols over several years. Unfortunately, this is not always the case. Due to educational reasons, physicians sometimes change wards as often as every 6 months.

CATIPO is a specialized system for a medical area with a limited number of patients. As demanded by Horn [10], it is embedded in daily clinical patient care activities, it enables the application of clinical standards to guarantee a high quality of care, and the results are tailored to meet the needs of individual patients. The fact that CATIPO represents knowledge highly relevant to routine patient care activities constitutes its success, not the complexity and scope of knowledge representation. Relevance and adequacy of the represented knowledge could be gained by carefully analyzing the clinical tasks and the general knowledge inherent in the GPOH protocols. The printed therapy plans are used directly as instructions by nursing and medical staff, as documentation sheets for drug administration, and as documents to be filed in the medical record.

Routine use of DOSPO has led to several versions and a validated system. During recent years, no complaints about errors in the calculation process were reported, provided that clinicians had correctly defined the protocol knowledge.


## 4. Perspectives of CATIPO

CATIPO currently offers basic decision support functions within pediatric oncology. A further benefit for patient care and research can be assumed by additional knowledge-based functions, although the physicians have not yet explicitly demanded them. For example, the protocol definition could be enhanced by knowledge of clinical actions other than drug administrations. During the production of a patient-specific therapy plans, reminders could be given, e.g. if a laboratory examination must be ordered, diagnostic material must be sent to reference institutions, or a report on toxic reactions must be transmitted to the trial center.

The more patient data that can be taken into account, the more effective knowledge-based functions can be. Currently, CATIPO's functions are integrated into a computer-aided clinical DOSPO [21], making a considerable amount of patient data available for decision support. This offers new perspectives for supporting the routine work of physicians. Among others, with DOSPO the physician is able to:

- store the actually applied therapy in comparison to the calculated therapy for further patient care provision;
- generate therapy reports for filing in the conventional patient record;
- present an overview of the complete and overall chemotherapy received by a patient, which means that therapy planning is no longer restricted to a single chemotherapy cycle;
- automatically add important therapy items to a medical report or discharge letter;
- electronically transmit research data to the trial centers.

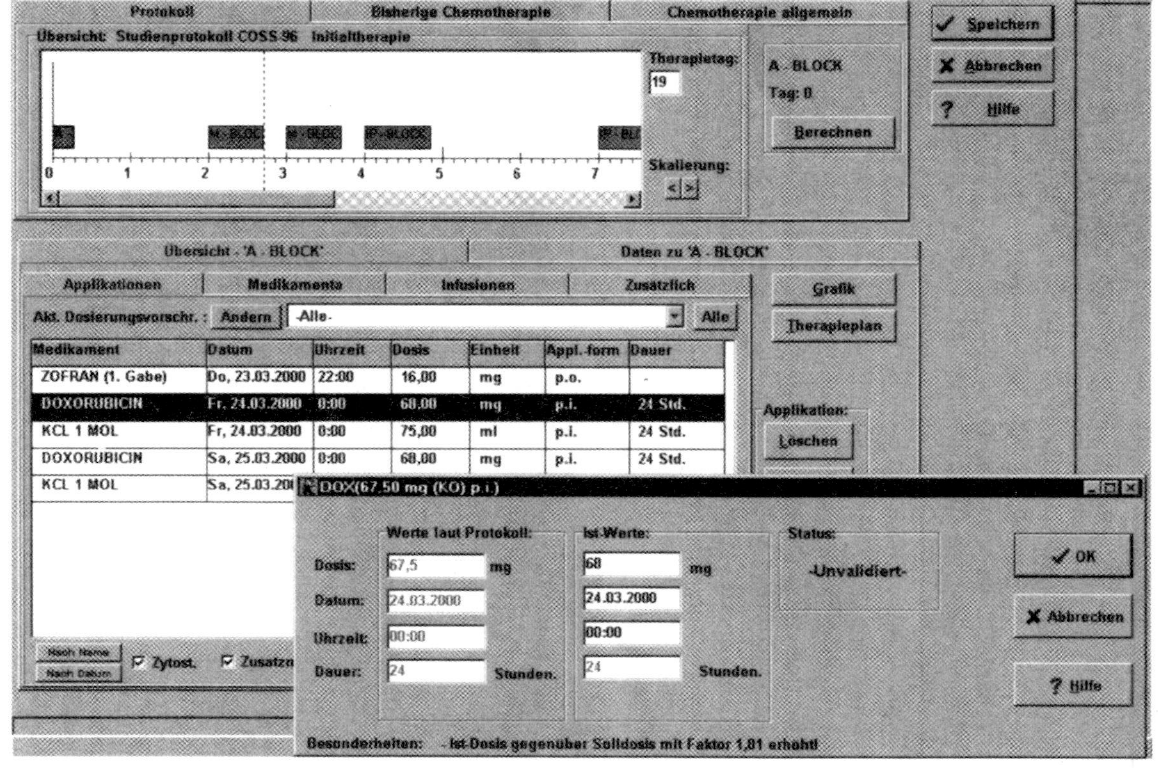



Fig. 4. Integration of CATIPO-dss functions into pediatric oncology and hematology documentation. The diagram seen in the upper part of the screen shows the various chemotherapy cycles of the chosen therapy arm. The table contains the chemotherapy drug administrations that have been calculated for a particular patient (name, date, time, dosage, type of administration and duration). The little window in front of the screen appears when a single administration is double clicked, in this case, doxorubicin. The left column shows the calculated parameters (dosage, date, time and duration). In the right column, the treating physician can document whether it was necessary to deviate from the generated calculations.

Within the framework for integrating therapy planning into the documentation system, the knowledge acquisition tool has been enhanced by the possibility to define sequences of chemotherapy cycles and to arrange them as a therapy arm of a protocol. Additional knowledge has been integrated about how therapy protocols can be composed of various therapy arms by stratification and randomization. Fig. 4 shows an example of this enhanced function.

We plan to evaluate the benefits and other consequences arising in connection with the integration of therapy planning into a comprehensive documentation system.

## Acknowledgements

The development of CATIPO was funded by the German Leukemia Research Aid and took place in tight cooperation with members of the 'Applied Informatics' work group of the German Society for Pediatric Oncology and Hematology (GPOH). The authors wish to acknowledge Margret Baugh and Sebastian Garde for their assistance in the preparation of this paper.

## References

[1] Bachert A, Classen C-F. Wissensbasierte Chemotherapieplanung in der pädiatrischen Onkologie: Ein Beispiel zur Therapieunterstützung. In: Buchholz W, Haux R, editors. Informationsverarbeitung in den Universitätsklinika Baden-Württembergs. Heidelberg: Hörning, 1995. p. 117–24.

[2] Bornhauser M, Schmidt M, Ehninger U, von Keller J, Schuler U, Ehninger G. Computer-based quality control in high-dose chemotherapy and bone marrow transplantation. Bone Marrow Transplant 1998;21:505–9.

[3] Brigl B, Ringleb P, Steiner T, Knaup P, Hacke W, Haux R. An integrated approach for a knowledge-based clinical workstation: architecture and experience. Meth Inform Med 1998;37:16–25.

[4] Enterline JP, Lenhard R, Blum B. A clinical information system for oncology. New York: Springer, 1989.

[5] Friedman RB, Entine SM, Carbone PP. Experience with an automated cancer protocol surveillance system. Am J Clin Oncol 1983;6:583–92.

[6] Gaglio S, Ruggiero C, Spinelli G, Bonadonna G, Valagussa P, Nicolini C. BREASTCAN: an expert system for postoperative breast cancer therapy. Comp Biomed Res 1986;19:445–61.

[7] Hammond P, Harris AL, Das SK, Wyatt JC. Safety and decision support in oncology. Meth Inform Med 1994;33:371–81.

[8] Haug PG, Gardner RM, Tate KE, Evans RS, East TD, Kuperman G et al. Decision support in medicine: examples from the HELP system. Comp Biomed Res 1994;27:396–418.

[9] Hickam DH, Shortliffe EH, Bischoff MB, Scott AC, Jacobs CD. The treatment advice of a computer-based cancer chemotherapy protocol advisor. Ann Internal Med 1985;103:928–36.

[10] Horn W. AI in medicine on its way from knowledge-intensive to data-intensive systems. Artif Intel Med 2001;23:5–12.

[11] Kaatsch P, Haaf G, Michaelis J. Childhood malignancies in Germany—methods and results of a nationwide registry. Eur J Cancer 1995;31A:993–9.

[12] Kaatsch P, Kaletsch U, Michaelis J. Annual Report 1997. German Childhood Cancer Registry, Institute for Medical Statistics and Documentation, University of Mainz, Germany, 1998.

[13] Leaning MS, Ng KEH, Cramp DG. Decision support for patient management in oncology. Med Informat 1992;17:35–46.

[14] Müller R, Thews O, Rohrbach C, Sergl M, Pommerening K. A graph–grammar approach to represent causal, temporal and other contexts in an oncological patient record. Meth Inform Med 1996;35:127–41.

[15]  Müller R, Sergl M, Nauerth U, Schoppe D, Pommerening K, Dittrich HM. THEMPO: a knowledge-based system for therapy planning in pediatric oncology. Comp Biol Med 1997;27:177–200.

[16]  Musen MA, Tu SW, Das AK, Shahar Y. EON: a component-based approach to automation of protocol-directed therapy. J Am Med Informat Assoc 1996;3:367–88.

[17]  Shortliffe EH. The adolescence of AI in medicine: will the field come of age in the 90s? Artif Intel Med 1993;5:93–106.

[18]  Soula G, Puccia J, Fieschi D, Bernard J-L, Le Boeuf C, Fieschi M. Impact of the TOP-FORUM hypermedia system in a pediatric oncology care unit. In: Cesnik B, McCray AT, Scherrer JR, editors. MedInfo'98, Proceeding of 9th World Congress on Medical Informatics. Amsterdam: IOS Press, 1998. p. 809–13.

[19]  Teich JM, Schmiz JL, O'Connell EM, Fanikos J, Marks PW, Shulman LN. An information system to improve the safety and efficiency of chemotherapy ordering. In: Cimino JJ, editor. Beyond the superhighway: exploiting the Internet with medical informatics. Proceedings of the 1996 AMIA Annual Fall Symposium, Washington. Philadelphia: Hanley&Belfus, 1996. p. 498–502.

[20]  Tu SW, Kahn MG, Musen MA, Ferguson JC, Shortliffe EH, Fagan LM. Episodic skeletal-plan refinement based on temporal data. Commun ACM 1989;32:1439–55.

[21]  Wiedemann T, Knaup P, Bachert A, Creutzig U, Haux R, Schilling F. Computer-aided documentation and therapy planning in pediatric oncology. In: Cesnik B, McCray AT, Scherrer J-R, editors. MedInfo'98, Proceedings of the Ninth World Congress on Medical Informatics. Amsterdam: IOS Press, 1998. p. 1306–9.

[22]  Wirtschafter D, Carpenter JT, Mesel E. A consultant–extender system for breast cancer adjuvant chemotherapy. Ann Internal Med 1979;90:396–401.

# The Beguiling Pursuit of More Information

*Donald A. Redelmeier, MD, MSc, Eldar Shafir, PhD, Prince S. Aujla, BSc*

**Background.** *The authors tested whether clinicians make different decisions if they pursue information than if they receive the same information from the start.* **Methods.** *Three groups of clinicians participated (N = 1206): dialysis nurses (n = 171), practicing urologists (n = 461), and academic physicians (n = 574). Surveys were sent to each group containing medical scenarios formulated in 1 of 2 versions. The simple version of each scenario presented a choice between 2 options. The search version presented the same choice but only after some information had been missing and subsequently obtained. The 2 versions otherwise contained identical data and were randomly assigned.* **Results.** *In one scenario involving a personal choice about kidney donation, more dialysis nurses were willing to donate when they first decided to be tested for compatibility and were found suitable than when they knew they were suitable from the start (65% vs. 44%, P = 0.007). Similar discrepancies were found in decisions made by practicing urologists concerning surgery for a patient with prostate cancer and in decisions of academic physicians considering emergency management for a patient with acute chest pain.* **Conclusions.** *The pursuit of information can increase its salience and cause clinicians to assign more importance to the information than if the same information was immediately available. An awareness of this cognitive bias may lead to improved decision making in difficult medical situations.* **Key words:** *uncertainty, reasoning, judgment, rationality.* **(Med Decis Making 2001;21:376-381)**

**M**edical schools have traditionally trained physicians to follow an exhaustive approach when collecting data. A common recommendation, for example, is to "conduct a complete history and a thorough physical examination."[1] This adage implies that more information—particularly if available at little cost—is always good. This adage is further reinforced by professional standards that recommend knowing all that you can, especially if it is easily knowable.[2] The strategy of collecting large amounts of information is often appropriate because of the complexity of medical disorders, the possibility that a patient may have multiple concurrent diseases, and the reality that a single neglected disorder could lead to irreparable harm.[3]

Two common arguments justify a more conservative approach to collecting information. The 1st concerns the economic pressure to limit procedures that are not cost-effective.[4] For example, guidelines recommend against performing a cerebral angiogram on otherwise healthy adults with headaches because the high costs of testing greatly exceed the small chances of finding a treatable disorder.[5] The 2nd argument for a conservative approach is respect for patient autonomy.[6] For example, patients may refuse a cerebral angiogram because of the invasiveness of the procedure.[7] Neither of these 2 arguments is compelling for information that is available from history, examination, or simple test.

Other arguments call for restraint even toward data that are easy to obtain. The data occasionally represent false-positive or false-negative results and mandate some insight about baseline probabilities.[8] Obtaining the data can be associated with significant opportunity costs for patients; for example, an ultrasound of the abdomen is an inappropriate test for a patient with an acute gastrointestinal bleed because time spent in radiology represents time unavailable for monitoring vital signs, securing blood transfusions, or receiving other

Received 16 January 2001 from the Department of Medicine, University of Toronto, Ontario, Canada (DAR, PSA); Department of Psychology and the Woodrow Wilson School of Public Affairs, Princeton University, Princeton, New Jersey (ES); and Clinical Epidemiology and Trauma Programs, Sunnybrook and Women's College Health Sciences Centre, Toronto, Ontario, Canada (DAR). Revision accepted for publication 30 April 2001.

Address correspondence and reprint requests to Donald A. Redelmeier, Sunnybrook Hospital, G-151, 2075 Bayview Avenue, Toronto, Ontario, Canada M4N 3M5; telephone: (416) 480-6999; fax: (416) 480-6048; e-mail: dar@ices.on.ca.

treatments.[9] Finally, data can sometimes disengage the doctor-patient relationship so that clinicians (and sometimes patients) focus primarily on numbers and neglect other profound aspects of the situation.[10,11]

We propose that the preceding arguments overlook other adverse effects that arise from weaknesses in human reasoning. In particular, psychological research has discovered systematic inconsistencies that stem from individuals' imperfect ability to distinguish relevant from redundant information.[12–15] One weakness is the tendency to pursue noninstrumental information— information that may be relevant but ought not to alter the decision.[16,17] In this vein, people sometimes pursue more information than necessary and, once they receive it, tend to see it as crucial for the decision.[18] In this study, we investigate whether clinicians also show a tendency to pursue and potentially misapply noninstrumental medical information.

## METHODS

We adapted methods developed by psychologists for evaluating how decisions are prone to systematic errors.[18] In one experiment, university students ($n = 539$) were given a scenario involving applications to their university. By random assignment, one-half received the following simple version, which provided the information directly:

> Imagine that you are on the admissions committee. You are reviewing the file of an applicant who plays varsity soccer, has supportive letters of recommendation, and is editor of the school newspaper. The applicant has a combined SAT score of 1250 and a high school average grade of B. Do you decide to accept or to reject the applicant?

The other respondents evaluated the same applicant but in a different version that involved a possible search for one piece of missing information:

> Imagine that you are on the admissions committee. You are reviewing the file of an applicant who plays varsity soccer, has supportive letters of recommendation, and is editor of the school newspaper. The applicant has a combined SAT score of 1250 but 2 differing reports about high school average grade. The guidance counselor's report indicates a B, whereas the school office report indicates an A. The school has notified you that the records are being checked, and that you will be informed within a few days which grade is correct. Do you decide to accept the applicant, to reject the applicant, or to wait for further clarification from the applicant's school before deciding?

> If you chose to wait for further clarification, answer the following:
> The school informs you that the applicant's high school average is a B. Do you decide to accept or to reject the applicant?

Results in the simple version showed that most respondents accepted the applicant when they knew the grade was a B. Naturally, most would also have accepted the applicant had the grade been A. Thus, the uncertainty between an A and a B was noninstrumental for this decision for most respondents. Nonetheless, in the 2nd version the respondents faced uncertainty about the grade being A or B, and most chose to pursue that information. These respondents then received the same information as in the simple version; namely, a grade of B. However, the pursuit of the information altered subsequent choices. Once they found that the grade was a B and not an A, most rejected the applicant. As a result, fewer respondents overall accepted the applicant in the search version compared to the simple version (46% vs. 57%, $P = 0.020$).

In the present study, we investigated whether clinicians are also prone to make different decisions when they pursue information than when they are given the information all at once. To do so, we asked clinicians to consider a hypothetical written scenario that described a medical situation. The scenario was formulated in 1 of 2 versions. The simple version of the scenario had the information immediately available. The search version presented the same medical situation but left a piece of information missing and available through a plausible search (such as simply waiting or conducting a test). Those who chose to search in this version then obtained the same information that was available in the simple version, thus rendering the 2 versions comparable.[19]

The basic design of each survey was a randomized comparison trial in which clinicians' management decisions were compared across the 2 versions of the same scenario. By random assignment, one-half of the clinicians received the simple version and one-half received the search version. Participants remained blinded to the intervention (and, indeed, unaware of the possibility of an alternative version). Our main hypothesis was that having pursued a piece of information, clinicians tend to focus on the obtained information, thereby leading to different decisions than if the same information had been available from the start. The study was approved by the Research Ethics Board of Sunnybrook and Women's College Health Sciences Centre

**Table 1**  Summary of Results

| Group | Option | Simple Version | | | Search Version | | | | |
| | | | | | Search Forgone | | Search Pursued | | |
| | | Accept | Reject | (% accept) | Accept | Reject | Accept | Reject | (% accept)[a] |
| Dialysis nurses | Donate kidney | 38 | 48 | 44 | 0 | 26 | 55 | 4 | 65 |
| Practicing urologists | Recommend surgery | 97 | 136 | 42 | 49 | 46 | 10 | 123 | 26 |
| Academic physicians | Continue flight | 32 | 268 | 11 | 6 | 208 | 51 | 9 | 21 |

a. Percentage who accept combining both search forgone and search pursued responses.

## RESULTS

### Dialysis Nurses

The 1st survey involved nurses affiliated with kidney dialysis centers in Toronto. All individuals ($n = 211$) were sent a 1-page survey and offered a lucky draw of $50 for participation. In total, 171 surveys were returned, representing a response rate of 81%. By random assignment, one-half received the following simple version of the scenario:

> Suppose that a 68-year-old relative of yours needed a kidney as a result of renal failure. Suppose that you were a suitable match. Would you donate?

The other nurses received the search version of the scenario, which contained the same data but involved a possible search for information:

> Suppose that a 68-year-old relative of yours needed a kidney as a result of renal failure. Suppose that it was not known whether you were a suitable match. You could be tested to determine whether you are suitable. Would you choose to be tested?

> If you indicated a willingness to be tested, please answer the following:
> Suppose that you had undergone the test and that the test showed that you were a suitable match. Would you donate?

A minority of nurses in the simple version chose to donate a kidney (44%). This notwithstanding, a majority of nurses in the search version were willing to be tested for compatibility (69%). A willingness to be tested presumably arises because the donation decision is not trivial for anyone, is tempting to postpone, and can be avoided by a negative test result. However, once they underwent testing and were found (as in the simple version) to be compatible, most nurses who searched were willing to donate (93%). As a consequence, more overall were willing to donate in the search version than in the simple version (65% vs. 44%, $P = 0.007$). The discrepancy was found for both those who replied early and those who replied late (before and after median reply time).

### Practicing Urologists

The 2nd survey involved practicing urologists affiliated with the American Urologic Association. A sample of English-speaking individuals ($n = 1076$) were surveyed and offered a lucky draw of $5000 for participation. In total, 461 completed surveys were returned, representing a response rate of 43%. By random assignment, one-half received the following simple version of the scenario:

> N.F. is a 69-year-old man with stage T1C prostate cancer. His prostate-specific antigen level is marginally elevated at 7.0 ng/ml, and biopsy reveals Gleason 6 cancer. Review of systems is otherwise remarkable only for shortness of breath on exertion (2 flights of stairs). Otherwise, he is in good health. A medical consultation documents chronic emphysema with moderate obstruction (FEV1 of 1000 ml, equivalent to 40% predicted). In this situation, would you recommend surgery or radiation therapy?

The other urologists received the search version of the scenario, which contained the same data but involved a possible search for a piece of missing information:

> N.F. is a 69-year-old man with stage T1C prostate cancer. His prostate-specific antigen level is marginally elevated at 7.0 ng/ml, and biopsy reveals Gleason 6 cancer. Review of systems is otherwise remarkable only for shortness of breath on exertion (2 flights of stairs). Otherwise, he is in good health. In this situation, would you recommend surgery, recommend radiation therapy, or obtain a medical consultation before deciding?

If you decided to obtain a medical consultation, consider the following:
A medical consultation documents chronic emphysema with moderate obstruction (FEV1 of 1000 ml, equivalent to 40% predicted). In this situation, would you recommend surgery or radiation therapy?

In the simple version, many of the urologists (42%) chose to operate. Yet, in the search version, somewhat more (58%) chose to obtain a medical consultation, presumably because the data might help in patient care. However, having obtained the consultation and learned the extent of emphysema (identical to that in the simple version), most who obtained the consultation recommended against surgery (92%). As a consequence, fewer urologists were willing to operate in the search version than in the simple version (26% vs. 42%, $P = 0.001$). The discrepancy was found for both those who replied early and those who replied late (before and after median reply time). Note that unlike the nurse scenario, medical consultation is not mandatory before surgery.

## Academic Physicians

The 3rd survey involved academic physicians whose addresses were obtained from the Internet. A sample of physicians in the United States and Canada ($n = 1596$) were surveyed by e-mail and given no incentive for participation. In total, 574 completed surveys were returned, representing a response rate of 36%. By random assignment, one-half received the following simple version of the scenario:

> You are traveling on an airplane and respond to the appeal "Is there a doctor on board?" Apparently, a 60-year-old male passenger experienced 15 to 20 minutes of "crushing" chest pain during takeoff (now resolved). Past medical history is unremarkable. The patient looks sick. The heart rate is about 80. The first-aid kit has a blood pressure cuff. You obtain a systolic pressure of 120 (cabin too noisy for auscultation). In this situation, would you recommend that the pilot land the airplane for medical reasons or would you recommend that the pilot continue the flight as scheduled?

The other physicians received the search version of the scenario, which contained the same data but involved a possible search for information:

> You are traveling on an airplane and respond to the appeal "Is there a doctor on board?" Apparently, a 60-year-old male passenger experienced 15 to 20 minutes of "crushing" chest pain during takeoff (now resolved). Past medical history is unremarkable. The patient looks sick. The heart rate is about 80. The first-aid kit does not have a blood pressure cuff, but the flight attendant knows there is one in a second kit elsewhere in the plane. Would you recommend that the pilot land the airplane for medical reasons, recommend that the pilot continue the flight as scheduled, or ask for the blood pressure cuff before making a decision?

If you chose to have the blood pressure cuff, answer the following:
You obtain a systolic pressure of 120 (cabin too noisy for auscultation). In this situation, would you recommend that the pilot land the airplane for medical reasons or would you recommend that the pilot continue the flight as scheduled?

Few physicians in the simple version recommended continuing the flight (11%). In contrast, a substantial number in the search version asked for the blood pressure cuff (22%), presumably because baseline data could be valuable if the patient's condition changed. Once having obtained the relatively favorable blood pressure results (which were the same as in the simple version), most of the physicians who asked for the blood pressure cuff recommended continuing the flight (85%). Consequently, more physicians recommended continuing the flight in the search version than in the simple version (21% vs. 11%, $P = 0.001$). The discrepancy was found for both those who replied early and those who replied late to the survey (before and after median reply time). Note again that measuring blood pressure is not mandatory for the decision.

## DISCUSSION

In medicine, business, and other domains, people tend to assume that more information cannot hurt. Underlying this assumption is the belief that people have clear and stable preferences that can only be refined by becoming informed.[20] Research in psychology, on the other hand, suggests that individuals' preferences are often unclear and tend to be constructed during the process of making a decision.[21–23] As a result, preferences can be significantly altered by subtleties in context.[24,25] Like the fuzzy boundary between education and advertising, it is hard to tell when clarification ends and distortion begins. Individuals' priorities can be malleable, so that minor changes in circumstances can sometimes alter individuals' preferences and lead to discrepant decisions.

**Table 2**   Summary of Recommendations

| Recommendation | Violation | Example of Error |
| --- | --- | --- |
| Consider whether missing information is relevant | Seek all available data from history and exam | Rectal exam in a patient who is having an acute aortic dissection |
| Make a plan in advance of data becoming available | Forestall planning until after data are collected | Ignoring the patient's history when acting on unexpected lab test results |
| Check with colleagues who can review data impartially | Disregard new views after gathering the data | Dismissing colleague's idea because you have "known the patient longer" |

The present study suggests that one factor influencing clinicians' decisions is their own behavior. Using scenarios, we show how the pursuit of information can lead nurses and doctors to weigh information more heavily than if the information were available at once. The findings cannot be attributed to thoughtless or deceptive responses, which work against the observed pattern. The findings are consistent with past studies of decisions—with both hypothetical and real pay-offs—involving consumer purchases, mortgage applications, and difficult negotiations.[16,26–29] A number of forces may be relevant, such as the influence of cognitive dissonance or sunk costs, although we feel the most germane notion is self-perception.[30–32] That is, clinicians infer from the pursuit that the data are crucial. This, we argue, has medical care implications (Table 2).

First, we urge physicians to consider the relevance of missing information before it is pursued. Good physicians collect a lot of information. Yet, in some cases missing information may be irrelevant and at other times it may be worth acquiring only for reasons outside the current choice (e.g., for research).[33] In cases where the information is not instrumental to the decision at hand, this reality needs to be appreciated and the pursuit of data adjusted accordingly.[16] Determining relevance is not easy, but after a search one may shift perspective and feel obliged to act. Although a warning against pursuing noninstrumental information may sound banal, the data suggest that such predispositions can emerge when facing difficult decisions.

Second, in situations where a piece of information is noninstrumental but is hard to forgo, physicians might be well served by constraining themselves to a prespecified course of action. That is, physicians should consider making a contingency plan for when the data become available. Doing so encourages people to think through the uncertainty and identify the features that truly ought to matter. In contrast, delaying deliberation until the information is available risks focusing undue attention on the one piece of information. In many situations, moreover, foresight and advanced planning are essential for allowing time for patients and families to contribute to the decision. Finding ways to teach people to think through uncertainty is a priority for future research.

Third, for situations in which missing information has been sought without a clear prespecified plan, the physician may want to consult with a colleague who can review the data easily without biases related to an involved search. Although it is hard to simulate how influential the pursued information would have been had it been known all along, a colleague might provide a fresh perspective that is free of the investments made during a difficult or long search. This technique is analogous to review boards who evaluate transplant candidates after each patient has been fully evaluated by his or her own physician. Colleagues who are presented with all the data at one time often see things differently than the physician who obtains the same data through gradual struggle.

A limitation of our research is the low survey response rate, yet this weakness is unlikely to explain our findings. Our research design tests for discrepancies between 2 versions of the same scenario. It avoids inferences about overall choice, and the discrepancies cannot be explained by a willingness to respond. In addition, past studies have found discrepancies regardless of whether response rates were high or low; indeed, the largest discrepancy we observed was in the sample with the highest response rate. Moreover, the observed patterns would still be statistically significant in each case even if all nonresponders were to give identical replies (either positive or negative). Finally, real-world situations may be much more intense and involved than the gentle delays induced through survey research.

One interesting feature of our scenarios is that reasonable people could disagree on which decision is correct. Yet, the discrepancies between the simple and search versions are disturbing. Although more research is needed, we think that choices made following a search have added reasons for worry. One reason is that information can be pursued along different search paths, which may shift priorities in different directions and result in divergent decisions. The simple version, in contrast, is a single perspective that is consistent for all decision makers. In addition, undue searching has the markings of a "self-erasing error."[34] That is, people might initially "err" by pursuing noninstrumental information but then proceed to make choices that endow the information with instrumental value, thereby "erasing" the error. At no point will the decision maker recognize having made a mistake.

Dr. Redelmeier was supported by a career scientist award from the Ontario Ministry of Health, the de Souza Chair in Trauma at the University of Toronto, and a grant from the Physicians' Services Incorporated Foundation. Mr. Aujla was supported by a Medical Research Council scholarship.

## REFERENCES


1. Bates B. A Guide to the Physical Examination and History Taking. 6th ed. Philadelphia: JB Lippincott Company; 1995.

2. Eisenberg JM. Doctors' Decisions and the Cost of Medical Care: The Reasons for Doctors' Practice Patterns and How to Change Them. Ann Arbor (MI): Health Administration Press; 1986.

3. Redelmeier DA, Tan SH, Booth GL. The treatment of unrelated disorders in patients with chronic medical diseases. N Engl J Med. 1998;338:1516–20.

4. Ubel PA, Goold S. Recognizing bedside rationing: clear cases and tough calls. Ann Intern Med. 1997;126:74–80.

5. Pryse-Phillips WE, Dodick DW, Edmeads JG, et al. Guidelines for the diagnosis and management of migraine in clinical practice. Can Med Assoc J. 1997;156:1273–87.

6. Asch DA, Hershey JC. Why some health policies don't make sense at the bedside. Ann Intern Med. 1995;122:846–50.

7. Kassirer JP. Adding insult to injury: usurping patients' prerogatives. N Engl J Med. 1983;308:898–901.

8. Sox HC, Blatt MA, Higgins MC. Medical Decision Making. Stoneham (MA): Butterworths; 1988.

9. Goitein M. Waiting patiently. N Engl J Med. 1990;323:604–8.

10. Ong LM, de Haes JC, Hoos AM, Lammes FB. Doctor-patient communication: a review of the literature. Soc Sci Med. 1995;40:903–18.

11. Cook DJ. Health professional decision-making in the ICU: a review of the evidence. New Horizons. 1997;5:15–9.

12. Simon H. Models of Man: Social and Rational. New York: Wiley Company; 1959.

13. Tversky A, Kahneman D. Judgment under uncertainty: heuristics and biases. Science. 1974;185:1124–31.

14. Nisbett RE, Ross L. Human Inference: Strategies and Shortcoming of Social Judgment. Englewood Cliffs (NJ): Prentice Hall; 1980.

15. Green LA, Yates JF. Influence of pseudodiagnostic information on the evaluation of ischemic heart disease. Ann Emerg Med. 1995;25:451–7.

16. Tversky A, Shafir E. The disjunction effect in choice under uncertainty. Psychol Sci. 1992;3:305–9.

17. Baron J, Beattie J, Hershey JC. Heuristics and biases in diagnostic reasoning II: congruence, information, and certainty. Organizational Behav Hum Perform. 1988;42:88–110.

18. Bastardi A, Shafir E. On the pursuit and misuse of useless information. J Personality Social Psychol. 1998;75:19–32.

19. Grice HP. Logic and conversation. In: Cole P, Morgan JL, editors. Syntax and Semantics, 3: Speech Acts. New York: Academic Press; 1975. p. 41–58.

20. Kassirer JP. Our stubborn quest for diagnostic certainty: a cause of excessive testing. N Engl J Med. 1989;320:1489–91.

21. Slovic P. The construction of preference. Am Psychol. 1995;50:364–71.

22. Slovic P, Lichtenstein S. Preference reversals: a broader perspective. Am Econ Rev. 1983;73:596–605.

23. Shafir E, Tversky A. Decision making. In Smith EE, Osherson DN, editors. An Invitation to Cognitive Science (vol 3). 2nd ed. Boston: MIT Press; 1995. p. 77–100.

24. Ubel PA. How stable are people's preferences for giving priority to severely ill patients? Soc Sci Med. 1999;49:895–903.

25. Shafir E, Simonson I, Tversky A. Reason-based choice. Cognition. 1993;49:11–36.

26. Festinger L. A Theory of Cognitive Dissonance. Evanston (IL): Row & Peterson; 1957.

27. Kachelmeier SJ, Shehata M. Examining risk preferences under high monetary incentives: experimental evidence from the People's Republic of China. Am Econ Rev. 1992;82:1120–41.

28. Camerer C, Babcock L, Loewenstein G, Thaler R. Labor supply of New York City cab drivers: one day at a time. Q J Econ. 1997;112:407–41.

29. Bastardi A, Shafir E. Nonconsequential reasoning and its consequences. Curr Direc Psychol Sci. 2000;9:216–9.

30. Arkes HR, Blumer C. The psychology of sunk cost. Organizational Behav Hum Perform. 1985;35:129–40.

31. Aronson E. The theory of cognitive dissonance: a current perspective. In: Berkowitz L, editor. Cognitive Theories in Social Psychology. New York: Academic Press; 1978.

32. Bem DJ. Self-perception theory. In: Berkowitz L, editor. Cognitive Theories in Social Psychology. New York: Academic Press; 1978.

33. Asch DA, Patton JP, Hershey JC. Knowing for the sake of knowing: the value of prognostic information. Med Decis Making. 1990;10:47–57.

34. Sherman SJ. On the self-erasing nature of errors of prediction. J Personality Social Psychol. 1980;2:211–21.

# *Section 2:*

<table>
<tr><td valign="top">

**Patient Records**

<br><br><br><br><br><br><br><br>



</td><td valign="top">



</td></tr>
</table>

**J. van der Lei**

Department of Medical Informatics
Erasmus MC - University Medical
Center Rotterdam
The Netherlands

# Synopsis

## *The changing scenery of patient records*

Looking at the papers selected for inclusion in the Yearbook Medical Informatics 2003, one is confronted with the changing scenery provided by research and development of patient records. These changes include new perspectives on the role of the patient him/herself as custodian of the medical record, and research from the social sciences underscoring that technology is often not the limiting factor in getting the electronic record implemented and accepted. Other papers in this section show that some topics remain in the forefront of research: how can we support coding and how do we deal with multilingual environments.

In their paper "Personal Health Records: Evaluation of Functionality and Utility", Kim and Johnson examine the Web sites that provide personal health records for patients. In most western countries we have delegated the role of custodian of the medical record to the medical community. In line with the increased emphasis on patient empowerment and involvement, it seems only logical that patients are also given an active role in managing their own medical record. Provide patients with the opportunity to create on a website their own, personal records; they can subsequently grant access to the care provider. The idea is simple and appealing.

In other parts of the world, it would be considered strange if a medical community would hold on to the medical record. In India, as was pointed out by one of our students who came from there, it is common that the patients carry their own paper medical record with them. When the patients visit a physician, they hand over their record to the physician who adds notes to that record and returns it. I recall the Indian student asking me what is new about this idea of a personal medical record on the Web – my response, for lack of better, was "the technology".

In their study, Kim and Johnson test the claims made by the providers of websites for personal health records. The design of the study is compellingly simple. First, take stock of the claims made by the providers of the Web sites in their promotional material. Second, take a concrete example (albeit in this case a fairly complicated example). Finally, see if it works. The results are sobering. The promises and claims of the industry are not met. One might be tempted to respond with a sarcastic statement such as "Only fools believe the claims and promises of the software industry". That, however, would do injustice to this study. Certainly, the websites examined in this study showed many shortcomings. That, in my mind, is not the essence of the paper. For me, the paper posed a question I had never asked myself before: Given the same set of medical data, what is the difference between patient entry and physician entry? Or, in the words of the authors: "Of principal concern is the fact that the entire process of data entry assumes that individuals can accurately categorize and prioritise their own medical information." This thought-provoking paper deserves reading. It supplied me with the question I should have asked our Indian student: In your hometown, who writes on the patient-held paper record, the patient or the physician?

In their paper "Adoption of Smart Cards in the Medical Sector: The Canadian Experience", Aubert and Hamel report an evaluation study that examines the factors influencing the adoption of smart cards in the medical sector. Using methodology from the social sciences, they examine the introduction of smart cards in the complex and interwoven setting of the health-care delivery system. Their conclusions will not surprise the experienced researcher in medical informatics: technology is not the limiting factor, the system must be of direct benefit to the user, and the system is beneficial only if the information on the card is complete.

The paper underscores that the implementation of smart cards (or, for that reason, patient records) is no longer limited by the technology. Poor technology will kill a project. Good technology, however, does not guarantee success. Even better technology will still not guarantee success. In order to better understand the success or failures of our systems, medical informatics will have to collaborate with the social sciences. Although the methodology employed by the social sciences may be foreign to many researchers in medical informatics, we stand to gain from the collaboration.

The paper also illustrates the danger of separate communities addressing the same issue. In the past years, several initiatives have attempted to introduce cards with varying degrees of success. Aubert and Hamel do not make a single reference to these initiatives. Moreover, in the discussion section, the natural place to discuss how this work relates to the work of others, the authors do not discuss related work in medical informatics – the discussion is a summary of their findings without any attempt to relate their findings to the work of others.

In their paper "Evaluation of a Method that Supports Pathology Report Coding", Hasman, de Bruijn and Arends revisited a classical theme: The accuracy of coding by physicians. One of the purposes of electronic record is to use the data in those records not only for patient care but also for other purposes, such as research or management. Understanding the accuracy of the codes found in records is of paramount importance. The paper, as many other papers, documents the struggle researchers have to identify a "silver standard" because a gold standard, the truth, is not available. The silver standard is, for lack of better, based on agreement between experts. In this study, the authors conclude that the system, when judged against the silver standard provided by pathologists, does not function optimal. At first glance, their results are disappointing. The authors, however, report a second finding: despite the limitations of the system, the agreement among pathologists increased when the system was used during coding. This intriguing conclusion begs further research into how the system influenced the coding-process of the pathologists. Given the role of coded data when using medical records for a wide variety of purposes, increasing agreement is important. The paper shows that even if a system codes sub-optimally, its usage improves the quality of coding by physicians (that is, under the assumption that agreement is an indicator of quality).

The final paper in this section is entitled "Building a Controlled Health Vocabulary in Japanese" by Liu and Satomura. In the scientific community, English is the lingua franca. The most widely used coding systems and controlled vocabularies are in English. Countries that rely on other languages often use translations of these English coding systems. Liu and Satomura built a standard clinical vocabulary for the Japanese language. The authors report that Japanese medical terms mainly come from western medicine. Their use of SNOMED, therefore, is not surprising. Building controlled vocabularies is a daunting task. Having to build a controlled vocabulary and at the same time having to incorporate work done in a total different language adds layers of complexity. The paper provides the reader with a flavour of the many issues that need to be addressed in that context.

Address of the author:
Johan van der Lei, M.D., Ph.D.
Department of Medical Informatics
Erasmus MC - University Medical Center Rotterdam
PO Box 1738
NL-3000 DR Rotterdam
The Netherlands
Tel:       +31 10 408 7050
Fax:       +31 10 408 9447
E-mail:    vanderlei@mi.fgg.eur.nl

# Adoption of smart cards in the medical sector: the Canadian experience

Benoit A. Aubert[a,b,*], Geneviève Hamel[b,1]

[a] *Ecole des HEC, Service des Technologies de l'information, 3000 Chemin de la Cote Ste-Catherine, Montréal, Canada H3T 2A7*
[b] *CIRANO, 2020 University, 25th floor, Montréal, Canada H3A 2A5*

## Abstract

This research evaluates the factors influencing the adoption of smart cards in the medical sector (a smart card has a micro-processor containing information about the patient: identification, emergency data (allergies, blood type, etc.), vaccination, drugs used, and the general medical record). This research was conducted after a pilot study designed to evaluate the use of such smart cards. Two hundred and ninety-nine professionals, along with 7248 clients, used the smart card for a year. The targeted population included mostly elderly people, infants, and pregnant women (the most intensive users of health care services). Following this pilot study, two surveys were conducted, together with numerous interviews, to assess the factors influencing adoption of the technology. A general picture emerged, indicating that although the new card is well-perceived by individuals, tangible benefits must be available to motivate professionals and clients to adopt the technology. Results show that the fundamental dimension that needs to be assessed before massive diffusion is the relative advantage to the professional. The system must provide a direct benefit to its user. The relative advantage of the system for the professional is directly linked to the obligation for the client to use the card. The system is beneficial for the professional only if the information on the card is complete. Technical adequacy is a necessary but not sufficient condition for adoption. © 2001 Elsevier Science Ltd. All rights reserved.

## Introduction

A smart card is a card with micro-processor containing information. It is the size of a regular credit card. In the medical sector, it contains information about the patient: identification, emergency data (allergies, blood type, etc.), vaccination, drugs used, and the general medical record. Therefore, the card becomes an electronic medical record for the patient. For two years, a smart card has been tested by 7248 clients of the health care system in Canada. These cards (known as "*Health Cards*" in the project) enable doctors, pharmacists,

nurses and ambulance workers to share information more easily. The card is very easy to use. When interacting with a health care professional, the client produces his card. The professional inserts it into the computer and has access to the information stored in the card. Depending on the type of professional (doctor, nurse, pharmacist, etc.) some areas may not be accessible, or accessible in a read-only mode (no modification allowed). It is important to note that the system stores the information solely on the card (not on the computer or a server). Therefore, if a patient, voluntarily or not, omits to use the card for a period, the information will be missing on the card until a professional enters it (patients have a read-only access to the information). These entries are very easy to make. They rely on codes and abbreviations professionals have been using already. The smart card reduces delays for taking charge of a patient and improves caregiver-patient communication since it provides information

---

*Correspondence address: Ecole des HEC, Service des Technologies de l'information, 3000 Chemin de la cote ste-Catherine, Monteral, Canada H3T 2A7.

*E-mail address:* aubertb@cirano.umontreal.ca (B.A. Aubert).

[1] Also at Royal Bank of Canada.

that was not readily available before (because it was only stored in another hospital or clinic for example). This smart card was also linked to an expert system that detected potential drug interactions. The system was expected to reduce costs because all exams, results and prescriptions would be filed and professionals would not have to redo work already performed by a colleague. Before using the smart card, professionals had no access to files kept in another establishment. This was a pilot study meant to evaluate the potential of smart cards.

For such a system to be useful, massive adoption is required. However, the confidentiality of medical records is currently guaranteed by law, and so the use of the card cannot be made mandatory. Even if the value of the Health Card is recognised by everyone in the health system, there has to be some individual advantage to motivate adoption. This has to be true for professionals and clients. Usage is conditional on adoption by both groups. The study described in this paper looks at the critical factors that would lead to adoption of the system.

In the research, certain adoption factors were reviewed and tested. Two surveys were conducted, together with numerous interviews, to assess the factors. A general picture emerged, indicating that although the new card is well-perceived by individuals, tangible benefits must be available to motivate professionals and clients to adopt the technology.

## Theoretical framework

Rogers (1962) defined innovation as *"an idea perceived as new by the individual"*. For an organization, an innovation can be any product, input, process, service or technology perceived as new by the adopting organization (Moore, 1994). Its success can be measured by assessing its benefits, both financial and of other types. The adoption process has previously been studied from a variety of standpoints. Langley and Truax (1994) identified three types of model for innovation adoption: sequential, political, and serendipitous.

Sequential models consider innovation adoption as a sequence of steps that the adopter must go through. The most widely used and referenced sequential model is Rogers'. The steps defined by Rogers are: *Awareness, Interest, Evaluation, Trial,* and *Adoption.* The advantages of sequential models include their user-friendliness and their relative explanatory power to explain the adoption process. However, their linearity and simplicity have been subject to criticism by the proponents of the political and serendipitous models.

Political models integrate the role of power into innovation adoption. They consider that adoption is influenced by negotiation, political tactics and promotion, often by champions (Dean, 1987). These cham-

pions usually have personal characteristics that are valued by the users of the technology, giving them influence over the final users. However, the political models do not consider economic imperatives in the adoption of technological innovation.

Serendipitous models suggest that innovations will be adopted easily when organizational routines are compatible with the innovation, and when the innovation itself is considered within the natural conduct of the activities. The models indicate that some environments are more favourable to technological innovation because of their natural openness to innovation. Langley and Truax (1994) also identify a number of serendiptitious events that facilitate the adoption of innovation, including the hiring of new employees or the desire to imitate a competitor (who had adopted new technology already). In this approach, inertia is an impediment to technological adoption.

In fact, any of these three models, if taken separately, would offer a fragmented view of the factors affecting the adoption of new technology. When integrated, however, they provide a much more interesting perspective of the phenomenon. The potential user of any given innovation will doubtlessly assess the possible benefits and losses, before going through the various steps described in the sequential model. Along the way, he or she will be subjected to pressure by individuals inside and outside the organization (political influence). Moreover, the evaluation itself (the potential user's perception of the innovation) will be biased by the culture and the attitude of the user's organization toward technology (serendipitous model). The adoption process is therefore complex, non-linear, and subject to very different influences. This research draws on all three models, incorporating insights from each to provide a more complete view of all the factors influencing adoption.

### Adoption factors for technological innovations

This section presents the factors that influence the adoption process. A review of the relevant literature shows that most authors refer first to the factors mentioned by Rogers (1962) and then complete them with others (Frambach, 1993; Herbig & Day, 1992; Moore & Benbasat, 1991; Ramiller, 1994; Tornatzky & Klein, 1982). These additional factors are taken from the various perspectives mentioned in the previous section. The factors and their corresponding hypotheses are presented in Table 1.

### Adoption factors linked to the technical system

This group of factors encompasses all the characteristics of the technical system that influence the individual adoption process. It is linked to how the system is designed, perceived and used in the final user environment.

Table 1
Factors influencing adoption

| Variable | Description | Anticipated effect hypothesised |
|---|---|---|
| Compatibility | Quality of an innovation that fits easily into the values, culture and routine of an individual | Increase probability of adoption |
| Ease of use | Perception of the ease with which the innovation can be made usable (or integrated) in daily tasks. | Increase probability of adoption |
| Image | Perception of the prestige and value attributed to the use of the innovation | Increase probability of adoption |
| Information | Perception of the availability, quality and value of the information produced by the innovation. | Increase probability of adoption |
| Involvement | Mechanisms through which an individual feels part of the development, design, or implementation process of an innovation. | Increase probability of adoption |
| Mandatoriness | Use of the card conditional to the payment of the services | Increase probability of adoption |
| Membership | Sense of belonging to the professional association (promoting the adoption) | Increase probability of adoption |
| Perceived usefulness | Perception of the innovation's utility in the individual's routine | Increase probability of adoption |
| Quality of the support | Perception of accessibility, rapidity, and how the support is provided. | Increase probability of adoption |
| Relative advantage | The level to which an innovation is perceived as superior to the technology it is replacing. | Increase probability of adoption |
| Satisfaction | Evaluation of the fulfilment of the individual's expectations after a tryout of an innovation. | Increase probability of adoption |
| Triability | Opportunity to try the innovation before adopting it. | Increase probability of adoption |
| Visibility | Visibility of the innovation, the people using it, and the results. | Increase probability of adoption |
| Voluntariness | Individual perception of the freedom (no pressure) to adopt an innovation | Increase probability of adoption |

The first factor in this group is system complexity, referring to the difficulty inherent in understanding and using the innovation. The more users think the innovation is difficult to integrate into their daily practices, the slower its adoption will be. This factor was refined by Moore and Benbasat (1991) who referred to it as "ease of use" when adapting it to the context of information technology, and by Seddon and Kiew (1994) in a study of the user-friendliness of interfaces.

Pitt and Watson (1994) assessed the impact of information systems support on adoption. This factor is linked more directly to information technology innovation. It is usually measured with three indicators: accessibility of support, the time lapse between the request for support and the delivery, and how support is provided (attitude of support staff).

The adoption process can also be facilitated if the technical system proposed is visible in the organization (Moore & Benbasat, 1991). In this particular study, visibility did not play a discriminating role since the technology was highly visible for all respondents. PCs were used by the health care professionals with the clients. As this element was controlled, it was not measured. Another factor not assessed was the triability of the system, which is said to facilitate adoption (Rogers, 1962). Because the pilot study was in reality a tryout of the system, this factor was also controlled and will not be investigated further.

The last factor is the information produced by the new technology (Herbig & Day, 1992; Seddon & Kiew, 1994). It is assessed on the basis of three criteria: availability, quality, and value. Information must be provided in sufficient quantity, in a simple and precise manner. It is assessed according to its relevance for the user and according to the ease with which it can be obtained.

*Adoption factors related to individuals*
The perceived relative advantage is the first factor related to the individual. It refers to the extent to which the innovation is perceived as superior to the technology it is replacing. An innovation is more likely to be welcomed by an individual when it is perceived as bringing advantages (Hebert & Benbasat, 1994).

Rogers (1962) also discussed the compatibility of the innovation with the values, culture and practices of individuals. An innovation that fits well with individual norms is much more likely to be adopted. The compatibility of the innovation lowers the probability that the potential adopter will be rejected by the social group. This is linked to the notion of social approbation (Tornatzky & Klein, 1982). If adoption creates positive recognition within a social group, it may facilitate the adoption process. Adoption may also be facilitated if the use of the innovation improves the image of the user (Moore & Benbasat, 1991). Prestige and other valued attributes linked to the use of the innovation are directly related to the adoption rate.

User involvement in the design and implementation of new technology also influences adoption (Seddon & Kiew, 1994). User involvement helps in identifying key requirements and improving design, thus increasing the probability of adoption. In this study, the technology was developed without the participation of users, therefore impeding the potential influence of user involvement.

Another individual factor is voluntariness (Moore & Benbasat, 1991). It can be defined as the absence of pressure forcing individuals to use an innovation against their will. Innovations introduced on a voluntary basis are adopted more easily by individuals, and forcing adoption can increase resistance to change. The last factor identified in the literature is satisfaction after tryout. Individuals have expectations about innovations, and disappointment can impede adoption (Seddon & Kiew, 1994). Gagliardi and Compeau (1995) observed that adopters with lower (more realistic) expectations tended to adopt the innovation more easily. High expectations often resulted in rejection of the technology after a trial period.

*Technological innovation adoption in the medical sector*

The medical sector encompasses all the services offered by medical and paramedical personnel. It includes services related to the physical and psychological well-being of individuals, and services given by employees with different skills in the medical and paramedical sector. This definition supposes the notion of a direct relationship between the client and the supplier of the services, as was mentioned in the preceding section. This relationship is extremely important in the medical sector because the service offered by a health professional to a client is based on the confidence existing between the two parties. Innovations should therefore not threaten this personalized relationship (Harris, 1990). The most important thing to remember in the service sector is its main peculiarity: clients and employees of a service organization usually have a direct relationship. Therefore, a new technology introduced in the work routine of a service sector employee is much more visible (for the client) than a new technology implemented in a production organization. Moreover, in many instances the client will be required to adopt and use the innovation (ATM machines are an excellent example of this).

Although some research was conducted in the service sector (Herbig & Day, 1992), it is interesting to note that none of the authors studied the influence that one group (e.g. the clients) might have on the other (e.g. the employees). It may well be, especially in the medical service industry, that the adoption of an innovation by one group might influence its adoption by the other.

*Types of innovation*

The scientific literature refers to two types of innovation in the medical sector. The first, clinical innovation, includes elements such as new apparatus, vaccines, drugs, and tools that directly improve the clients' health. The second type, organizational innovation, improves the method of dispensing and distributing services. Both types seek to improve service quality, increase productivity or reduce costs. It is important to note that these two categories are not always mutually exclusive, but innovations are usually oriented toward one of the two types (Anderson & Jay, 1984).

The Health Card is an innovation of the second type. Its introduction modifies the way health professionals organize their work. This implies that the service given to the client will also be modified, to an extent that has yet to be determined. Implementation of the innovation must address both adoption processes, while preserving the relationship of trust between the client and the health professional.

*Actors in the medical sector*

In this project, four groups shared the task of providing services to clients: doctors (MDs and specialists), pharmacists, nurses, and ambulance personnel. All these groups are represented by one or more professional association(s) or union(s). They work in a regulated environment, where most strategic decisions are taken by government agencies. Financial resources are limited and work habits and privileges are well established among the various groups. Such a context might prevent the introduction of an innovation. Even if the client demanded the innovation, it would need approval from government agencies, the various professional associations, and the practitioners themselves before being implemented. These groups would assess the consequent modifications to their practices, their relative power and their hierarchical position before recommending adoption.

Adoption by all groups is pivotal to the success of the innovation's diffusion. If one group resists the introduction of a technology, the success of the project would be threatened. The notion of critical mass, *the point at which enough individuals have adopted an interactive innovation to cause the perceived cost–benefit of adoption to change from negative to positive so that the innovation's rate of adoption becomes self-sustaining* (Rogers, 1991; p. 245), applies in the Health Card project. The number of individuals adopting the innovation must attain a certain level if users are to benefit from the technology. If the Health Card is to realize its full potential, it is crucial that all the groups should decide to adopt it. This is the only way to maximize information transfer between practitioners. This unique characteristic arising from adoption by many different groups forced the developers of the innovation to recognize the distinctive characteristics of the various groups and to adapt both the innovation and the diffusion process.

These considerations lead to the introduction of two new factors. The first will be labelled "membership", referring to the extent to which the practitioners have a strong sense of belonging to their professional association (all associations had approved the project, encouraging their members to adopt the technology). The other is linked to the client. Since clients are refunded by the public medical insurance system, it would be possible to make use of the smart card mandatory for free service. This possibility was tested in the model. All the factors are summarized in Table 1.


**Methodology**

*The smart card project*

The small card project was undertaken by a research team from Laval University, in Quebec City. It was financed by a government agency and approved by all professional associations. All those facts were public and known by the health care professionals (it was advertised in bulletins and other publications from the various professional associations). The professionals were given training before the beginning of the experimentation. All the required equipment (PCs equipped with a card reader and appropriate security devices) was given to them and installed by a technician. Information stored on the cards could only be read with this special equipment. The actual use of the card always remained voluntary. The survey data were collected after one year of use.

In the pilot study, all participation, both from the professionals and the clients, was voluntary. In all cases, publicity was made in various associations, in local newspapers, and directly by distributing flyers to the households. The professionals were also contacted directly by a member of their profession. The participation among the professionals was extremely good. A total of 332 professionals were targeted to enrol in the study and 90% of them did (299/322). Specifically, 73% of the physicians agreed to participate (90), and all the pharmacists (54), the nurses (at the hospital and in the clinics) (111) and the ambulance workers (44) enrolled in the study. The professionals were to use the card for all their interactions with clients having such a card and agreeing to use it (since the whole experiment remained on a voluntary basis). Data on actual use of the card were recorded for three periods of four months each. The utilisation profile (intensive, average, or low) was stable for individual professionals throughout the three periods (all correlations are significant at the $p < 0.01$ level).

The clients were in two different cities. In the smallest one, all the population was invited to participate. Seventy-two percent of the population agreed to do so (1317 persons). In the second city (population of approximately 50,000 persons), three groups were targeted: pregnant women (303 participants, 19.8% of the corresponding population), infants from 0 to 18 months (953 participants, 36.3% of the corresponding population), and finally elderly people aged 60 and over (4675 participants, 41.4 % of the corresponding population). Overall, 7248 persons participated in the pilot study, representing 42% of the targeted population. This high participation rate reduces the risk that the sample was unrepresentative of the overall targeted population. No information was collected from non-respondents.

The current research was conducted to measure the outcome of the pilot site and to evaluate the appropriateness of wider use of smart cards. The literature review presented led to the identification of adoption factors for technological innovations in a medical service context. These factors had been studied in previous research (in other sectors) and measures therefore already existed. They were simply identified and adapted to the context of this study. A survey of the pilot site along with numerous interviews was used to pinpoint the critical elements related to adoption of the smart card during the pilot project. A second survey and another series of interviews were conducted to obtain the opinions of populations that had not experienced the technology (selected to ensure representativeness). Their aim was to identify the expectations of potential adopters.

*Sample description*

The research was conducted in four separate groups. Two of the groups actually tested the Health Card in the pilot study. One was composed of health professionals who had more than a year's experience with the smart card system, and the other of health service clients in the pilot region. The other two groups had never used the card. One was composed of health care practitioners, and the other of health care clients, both outside the pilot region.

*Population inside the pilot area*

Questionnaires were sent to all the health care professionals participating in the pilot study and still active in the area ($n = 287$). A reminder was send two weeks later. The response rate was excellent (66.4%) especially compared to other studies (Aubert, Rivard, & Patry, 1996). Table 2 presents the response rates for each sub-group.

For the clients of the health care system, a random list of telephone numbers was drawn up and interviews were conducted, selecting numbers from the list at random

Table 2
Response rates for each sub-group

|  | Doctors | Pharmacists | Nurses | Ambulance workers |
|---|---|---|---|---|
| Pilot study | 69.7% | 74.5% | 69.2% | 47.8% |
| Potential users | 22.7% | 26.4% | 29.9% | — |

until 300 interviews were completed. This number largely surpasses the number required for analysis.

*Population outside of the pilot area*

The respondents outside of the pilot area were carefully selected to ensure that they were representative of the overall population. This task was facilitated by the professional associations of the health care professionals. They randomly selected a sample ($n = 2000$) from their entire population (excluding those inside the pilot study area) and questionnaires were mailed to those respondents. Questionnaires were distributed to 750 doctors, 500 pharmacists, and 750 nurses. Questionnaires were sent without prior contact with the respondents. A total of 526 completed questionnaires were returned, for a response rate of 26.3% (see Table 2 for a detailed breakdown of response rates). Since all active professionals have to be listed in their respective association repertory, a random sample drawn from this repertory should be representative of the population. For the clients, three regions were selected for the interviews: one urban (3 million inhabitants in the metropolitan area), one rural, and a last one described as a mid-sized city (350,000 inhabitants). This variety ensured that the interviews would provide a valid picture of the Canadian population's opinions (from the results, all three sub-samples provided similar responses).

For clients outside the pilot study area, a series of face-to-face interviews (123) was conducted in three regions outside the pilot study area.

*Measures*

The research methodology was adapted to the characteristics of each group. For the professionals, a survey was used. Health care professionals are an educated population, familiar with questionnaires and similar methods of evaluation, and the questionnaire format was therefore appropriate. The clients, on the other hand, were interviewed. They were often elderly, and tended to be less educated than the health care professionals. A questionnaire would therefore have been inappropriate. Clients who had participated in the pilot study were interviewed by telephone. Those in other regions who had not participated in the study were interviewed in person. This enabled the interviewers to explain the basics of the Health Card before conducting the interview.

*Health care professionals*

As mentioned, a survey was carried out among the health care professionals. The measures identified in the literature review on adoption factors were collated and combined. Available instruments from all the authors cited were compiled to obtain as extensive a list of items as possible to measure the variables under study. All the instruments used Likert scales (note: A Likert scale is a statement (the question) followed by a series (usually five or seven) of ordered choices (the possible answers), each one described in words). It is important to note that three factors were not investigated at all: involvement, trialability, and visibility. As mentioned in the literature review, because of the project design, these factors could not vary from one respondent to another. They were therefore not able to provide information on the reasons for the different opinions of individual clients concerning adoption.

All items were adapted to the context of the study. This was done using a group of health care and information technology specialists. Each question was analysed and discussed to ensure that it was unambiguous and suited to the context. The questionnaire was pretested with two doctors (MDs), two pharmacists, two nurses and two ambulance workers, all from the target population. The pretests helped clarify some questions and eliminate others for which information would not be available.

Potential users were defined as health care professionals not participating in the pilot study. They were located in different regions of the country outside the pilot study area. The committee that designed the original questionnaire adapted a new one for this group. The new version was as similar as possible to the original, so that meaningful comparisons could be made. However, some questions were removed because professionals who had not used the system could not answer them. Each question was reassessed to ensure that it could be understood by someone who had not been involved in the pilot study. The final questionnaire was pretested with members of the target sample.

Health care professionals outside the pilot site were generally well informed about the experiment. The various professional associations regularly circulated information about the goals of the project and the functionalities of the system. This prior knowledge of the system enabled respondents to form an opinion. The only group that had not received information was the ambulance workers. They were therefore excluded from the sample because they did not have the information required to answer the questionnaire meaningfully.

*Clients of the health care system*

A significant portion of the target population in the pilot study was composed of elderly people, who are the most intensive users of health care services. However, unlike the health professionals, they are not familiar with questionnaires and Likert scales. For this reason, telephone interviews were preferred. A standardized interview procedure was developed. Questions were simple and there were only three possible choices of answer — one positive, one neutral and one negative — to simplify the process as far as possible. Pretests were carried out and improvements made to both the format and the wording of the questions.

As mentioned earlier, face-to-face interviews were conducted for clients outside the pilot area. The first part of the interview consisted in providing interviewees with information about the Health Card and its use. Once they were sufficiently informed, they were asked about their intention to adopt the card or not. The overall interview protocol, including the information section, was highly standardized to ensure that comparisons would be meaningful.

The responses obtained were not standardized because respondents expressed their opinions freely. Each response was coded by three different people trained for the project. Thirty interview transcripts were used to establish a uniform codification scheme on which all three coders agreed. The coders then coded all the remaining transcripts (93). Coding was compared across coders for each transcript and any discrepancies were identified, discussed and resolved. This method provided a high level of reliability and increased confidence in the results, which are presented in the section. Results of interviews of the clients outside the client area.

*Statistical Procedures*

Data collected were evaluated first by assessing means for each variable to have an indication of the overall perceptions. To ensure that each variable (the factors or the dependent variable (adoption) was consistently measured by the indicators used, Cronbach's alpha (Nunally, 1978) and individual item reliability as evaluated with PLS were computed. To indicate that significant variance is shared between each item and the construct, the loadings should be higher than 0.5 (Aubert et al., 1996). In this research, items that did not share enough variance with their respective constructs were removed from the scales. Correlation between variables was also assessed.

The data from the questionnaire were analysed using partial least squares (PLS). PLS enables the evaluation of a causal model. In this research, many factors are expected to influence adoption. Each factor, as well as the independent variable, is measured by several indicators (questionnaire items). For example, adoption is evaluated by three items in the questionnaire. From these indicators, PLS computes latent variables and evaluates the links between the factors and the independent variable. PLS computes a regression coefficient for each relationship specified in the causal model. Special cases of PLS models overlap well-known models like first principal components or first canonical correlation (Wold, 1984; Stoica & Söderström, 1998). PLS analyses models as wholes rather than evaluating each relationship separately (Fornell & Larcker, 1981). Instead of simply aggregating measurement error in a residual error term, PLS simultaneously evaluates both the measurement model and the theoretical model, and adjust the relationships between the variables accordingly.

In this study, PLS was appropriate considering the size of the model (see Fig. 1). It enabled us to obtain meaningful results from the number of responses obtained. The rule of thumb for determining the smallest sample size required to perform PLS analysis is that the sample must comprise ten times the number of items present in the largest construct (or the number of links

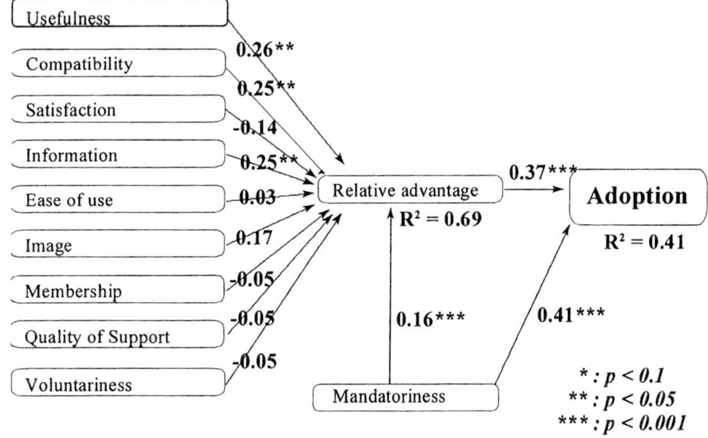


Fig. 1. Diffusion model for the professionnels in the pilot study.

to one variable) (Gopal, Bostrom, & Chin, 1992–1993). In this study, there were nine independent variables linked to a dependant variable. Consequently, a sample of at least 90 questionnaires was needed. This requirement was exceeded.

The models evaluated were built using information from two sources. The first one was the literature review. Anticipated relationships were identified and taken into account. This would have led to a simple model where all factors would have influenced directly the adoption. Discussion with the research team members and interviews with professionals involved in the study provided a second source of information and enabled the refinement of the models. All the factors do not affect the adoption process in the same way. Some appeared to be antecedents of others. These discussions led to the model presented in the result section.

## Results

Results from the four groups are presented. First the results of the survey of professionals using the Health Card in the pilot study are reported, followed by the survey results of the professionals outside the pilot region. Coming after are the results of the interviews with the clients using the Health Card, followed by the ones of the interviews with the clients outside the pilot region.

### Results of the survey of professionals using the Health Card

This section briefly presents the results obtained with the health care professionals who used the smart card system in the pilot study. The first part is a general description of the observed situation. It shows the general perceptions with regard to the factors related to technology adoption.

In the second part, the links between the variables are analysed. The model suggests that some variables influence others. Since the theoretical model does not identify the factors that should have the greatest influence on the adoption decision, it will be interesting to see which are really critical in the adoption process.

The dependent variables were the adoption of the Health Card and its utilization by health care professionals. The adoption of the Health Card, with an average score of 4.02 (5 being the maximum value), received widespread support among respondents, who favoured the extension of the project to other regions and to a larger subset of the overall population. They also wanted to continue to use the Health Card after the pilot study. When the results were broken down by type of professional, no significant difference emerged

$(F_{3,140} = 1.2; \ p = 0.31)$. The results are presented in Fig. 3, at the end of this section.

### The adoption factors

The independent variables encompass all the factors influencing the decision to adopt an innovation or not. The results show that the Health Card system ranked high on *ease of use* (4.22). *Quality of support* was almost as high (4.00), indicating that professionals requiring support during the pilot study received it diligently and efficiently. This suggests that use of the system was not restricted by technical factors.

The factors that received a favourable score include those related to the use of the Health Card. *Voluntariness* obtained a score of 3.85, indicating that the respondents did not feel they were under undue pressure to use the system. An interesting paradox is the score obtained for the factor *mandatoriness*. Although utilisation of the card was on a voluntary basis, the respondents from the professional group indicated that it would be more useful if clients were required to use the system (3.75).

*Quality of the information* was favourably evaluated (3.63), indicating that the information provided by the system was relevant, in a useful format and satisfied the needs of users. The system itself was evaluated as moderately useful (3.50) (*usefulness* measures the fundamental contribution of the system, its relevance). Similarly, the *relative advantage* linked to the use of the system received a moderate score (3.14). Respondents indicated that the system improved communications between professionals and made them slightly more efficient. As mentioned in the literature review, an innovation must be compatible with the environment in which it is introduced. *Compatibility* obtained a score of 3.36, indicating that the system was fairly compatible with the work habits of the health care professionals and with the vision these professionals had of their relationship with their clients. The last factor to receive a favourable evaluation was *satisfaction of expectations* (3.12), indicating that the system met the expectations of the respondent professionals.

Two factors received an unfavourable evaluation: *membership* (2.83) and *image* (2.55). This underlines the fact that use of this type of information technology in the provision of medical services does not seem to improve the image of the health care professional, and that professional use of the system is not really influenced by the official position taken by the professional association.

### Links among variables

Observation of the values obtained for each of the variables is interesting, but the main interest of the study lies in the analysis of the links between the variables. These links, and a model assessed using PLS, are discussed in the following section (All the links discussed are significant at the $p < 0.01$ level. The correlation matrices are given in the appendix).

Although there was a strong emphasis in the pilot study on the voluntary aspect of use of the Heath Card, the factor most strongly correlated with *adoption* was *mandatoriness* (of use of the card by clients) ($r = 0.53$). Health care professionals are only inclined to adopt the Health Card if it is compulsory for clients. One explanation is the significant and positive link between *mandatoriness* and *relative advantage* ($r = 0.34$). This means that the advantage of using the system is greater when the client is required to use the card. The mandatory nature of the card would ensure that all relevant information about the client is on the card. If use of the card is elective, the professional can never be sure that the information is complete and reliable. The relative advantage of using the card is therefore reduced.

As expected, the link between *relative advantage* and *adoption* was also significant and positive ($r = 0.49$). For health care professionals to adopt a smart card system, there must be a perceived advantage. The factor *relative advantage* had the largest number of significant links with other factors. It had a strong link with *compatibility* ($r = 0.72$), *image* ($r = 0.43$), *ease of use* ($r = 0.37$), and *quality of support* ($r = 0.22$). These links suggest that all the factors (compatibility, image, ease of use and quality) are important in obtaining an advantage from using the Health Card.

*Compatibility* was also linked to adoption ($r = 0.42$). This suggests that the technology must not disturb the environment, values and work habits of the professionals. The link between *satisfaction of expectations* and *adoption* was also significant and positive ($r = 0.37$), as was that with *usefulness* of the system ($r = 0.38$) and the *information* factor ($r = 0.35$).

Surprisingly, four elements identified in the literature review as influencing the adoption of an innovation were not found to be significant in this study. These were the correlations between diffusion and voluntariness, image, quality of support and ease of use, which did not meet the criterion of $p \leqslant 0.05$.

*Discussion*

To obtain a holistic view of the relationships, a PLS analysis was done. Numerous discussions between the health care professionals and the project team led us to expect a strong link between *relative advantage* and *adoption*. This factor is a key component in the adoption process. The others factors were considered important but were viewed more as prerequisite for the creation of an advantage. This configuration of the adoption model suggests that *relative advantage* acts as a moderating variable in the adoption process. It underlines the importance, for successful implementation of an innovation, of a tangible advantage to the adopter. Other

factors can be seen as sine qua non conditions for the creation of such an advantage, factors required for the creation of the advantage but not sufficient to justify the adoption. The variance explained for the factor *relative advantage* is excellent (0.69). For *adoption*, the variance explained is very good (0.41).

The dual role of the factor *mandatoriness* is apparent in the model. Mandatoriness has a significant effect on the relative advantage perceived by health care professionals and significantly increases the diffusion potential. Mandatory use of the Health Card by clients provides a guarantee that the information on the card is reliable and complete. Elective use of the card means that the professional must ask questions to ensure that no information is missing (the same procedure as when no card is used). This increases the time required for consultations and eliminates most of the advantages for the practitioner.

*Factual data on usage*

Throughout the project, *utilization* by doctors and pharmacists was automatically recorded by the system. The data are therefore unbiased by perceptions. They were compared and analyzed with the information gathered in the questionnaire. The data represent actual utilization of the Health Card by health care professionals, and might therefore be considered more representative of the intention to adopt the technology or not. However, it is possible that the factual data are potentially biased by a Hawthorne[2] effect and that the results cannot be extrapolated. Notwithstanding these considerations, the analysis of factual data, in association with perceptions and intentions, gives a fuller picture of what actually took place in the pilot study.

*Ease of use* was the first factor with a positive link to *utilization* ($r = 0.38$). Logically, the easier the system, the more the user will be inclined to use it. As was observed with *adoption*, *utilization* varies in the same direction as *compatibility* ($r = 0.36$). *Quality of support* was the third factor with a positive relationship to *utilization* ($r = 0.36$). This suggests that utilization of the Health Card by professionals was linked to their evaluation of the support they received. *Utilization* was also correlated with *voluntariness* ($r = 0.32$; *p*), suggesting that freedom to use the system had a positive influence on actual usage. There was also a positive correlation between *information* and *utilization* ($r = 0.28$). The professionals

---

[2] Hawthorne studies showed the bias on the results introduced by the simple fact that people participating in an experiment knew they were in such an experiement and modified their behavior because of this. For more information, see Roethlisberger, F.J., & Dickson, W.J. (1939). *Management and the worker: An account of a research program conducted by the Western Electric Company, Hawthorne works.* Chicago: Harvard University Press.

having the most intensive utilization profile were those who assessed the quality of the information provided by the system more positively. Two explanations are possible here. First, the system was used more intensively by the professionals for whom the information was more relevant. Second, by using the system frequently, intensive users obtained more benefit from it and were able to extract information that was more relevant to their work.

A PLS model similar to the one presented in Fig. 1 was tested, replacing *adoption* by *utilization*. The variance explained is marginal (0.03) and the links between relative advantage and utilization and between mandatoriness and utilisation are not significant. Interestingly, we also tested the link between the *utilization* and the opinion about *diffusion* and this link was not significant. This reinforces the idea that the use of the system was really perceived as a trial, with little implication on future obligation to adopt of not the system.

*Survey results for professionals not involved in the pilot study (potential users)*

This section presents the results of the survey carried out to assess the opinions of health care professionals not involved in the pilot study. Since these respondents had no hand-on experience with the system, they could not assess some of the factors. The items related to these factors were therefore removed from the questionnaire (namely: *usefulness, satisfaction, information, involvement, quality of the support, and ease of use of the system*). The results, included in Fig. 3 show which factors were considered as most important in the decision to adopt the innovation or not.

The innovation was generally well perceived by respondents. The value of 4.52 (on a scale of 1–5) reflects a very favourable opinion of the Health Card. This measure evaluated both the intention of respondents to adopt the system and their perception as to whether or not their colleagues would do so.

*Relationships among variables*

Three factors strongly influenced adoption: mandatory use of the card by clients, the relative advantage for the professional and the compatibility of the innovation with current practices. These three elements all obtained values close to four. Image and membership were not considered important by respondents. These results are consistent with those obtained from pilot study participants (correlations were all significant at the $p<0.01$ level).

Four factors exhibited a significant and positive relationship with *adoption* (see the appendix). The highest correlation coefficient was obtained for the relationship between *adoption* and *relative advantage*

($r = 0.54$). This result is very similar to that obtained with the pilot study group. The more advantages health care professionals anticipate from the use of the Health Card, the more interested they are in adopting it. There is also a strong correlation between *relative advantage* and *compatibility* ($r = 0.58$).

*Compatibility* also exhibited a significant and positive relationship with *adoption* ($r = 0.44$). As was the case at the pilot site, the mandatory factor exhibited a significant relationship. The major difference with the pilot study was the voluntariness factor. It seems that if use of the smart card by clients is totally voluntary, it will not be adopted by practitioners. In this sense, the potential user group was more consistent in its answers than the pilot study participants. Their perception of *mandatoriness* is in line with the results of the *voluntariness* factor. If clients are required to use the card, the professionals will have to use it too.

These links are apparent when observed in a PLS model similar to the one built for the pilot study. The effects are strong and the links are significant. The variance explained is very good. *Relative advantage* and *mandatoriness* are key factors in the decision to adopt an innovation such as the Health Card. *Relative advantage* is determined by the compatibility of the innovation, the image associated with the adoption, and the mandatory character of the innovation. These results are similar to those obtained in the pilot study and indicate that this study was probably highly representative of what could happen in a larger scale implementation of the innovation (Fig. 2).

*Results of the interviews with clients in the pilot area*

The results presented in this section were gathered through interviews conducted with health care system clients who participated in the pilot study. Three hundred people expressed their opinions on various aspect of the Health Card after using it for two years.

It should be remembered that the scales used in the interviews were simplified, three-point scales, with 1 representing a positive evaluation, 2 a neutral evaluation, and 3 a negative evaluation of the factors. The involvement factor was coded on a two-point scale, with 1 indicating that the respondent felt involved in the development process and 2 that he or she did not feel involved. Finally, the questions about quality of the support were omitted from most of the analysis process because only 14 respondents answered them. It seems that almost none of the participants required support during the two-year pilot study. The results are included in Fig. 3.

The score obtained for the variable *adoption* (1.24) indicates a marked positive attitude toward the Health Card, suggesting that respondents would continue to use it after the end of the trial period. Most of the

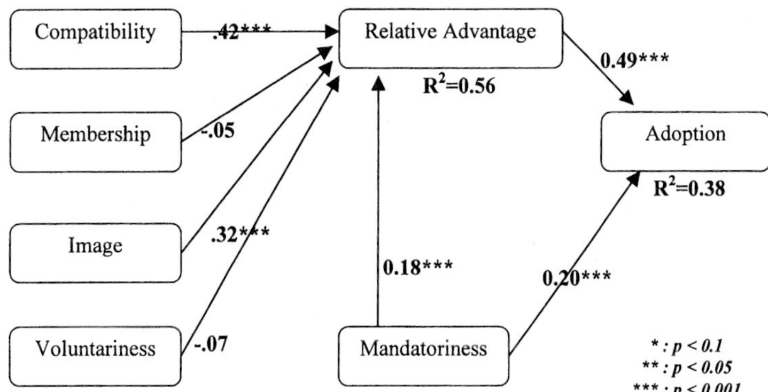



Fig. 2. Adoption model — professionals outside the pilot study.

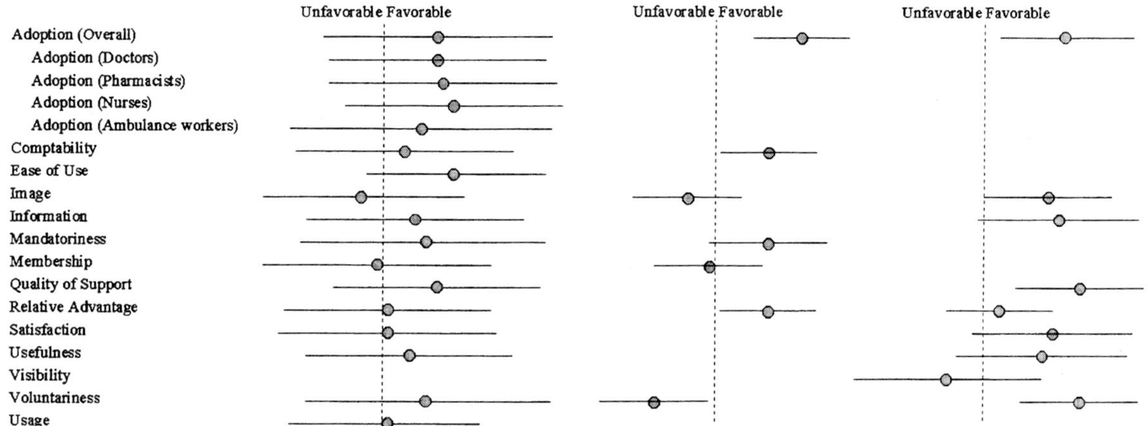



Fig. 3. Survey results (professionals using the card, potential users, clients).

independent variables were positively evaluated. The most positive result was obtained for *voluntariness*. Almost all participants said they were not pressured to use the card. They felt that every time they used it, they did so of their own free will. The information on the card also seemed to satisfy the population. More than one-third of respondents had looked at the information on their card (with the help of a health care professional, they could examine it on-screen or ask for a print-out) and found it clear and easy to read. On the other hand, almost two-thirds of the clients did not ask to see the information on their card. The interviews showed that these people did not appropriate their medical records and perceived the information as being the property of the health care professional treating them. The score obtained for the *usefulness* factor confirms this. Responses were between positive and neutral (1.44). Most respondents felt the card was useful for the professionals, but that the information was of little interest to them.

*Satisfaction of expectations* was fair (1.36). This suggests that most participants felt their expectations were met. Some clients said they expected the card to be used more intensively by the professionals. In some cases, when the patients consulted a professional more than once for the same reason, no additional information needed to be recorded. In some of these cases, the patients were disappointed.

The last factor to receive a positive evaluation was *image*. Most respondents said the fact that they were using the card was viewed favourably by their peers and by health care professionals. Many participants were also proud to have participated in a pilot study. As mentioned previously, this may have introduced a Hawthorne effect. Most clients did not see any direct *advantage* in using the Health Card (1.86). They did not think using the card gave access to better services, nor to more information about their own health records. They perceived the information as being useful mainly to health professionals.

*Links among variables*

The first observation to emerge from the analysis is the weakness of the links between the independent variables and the adoption variable. The factors presenting the strongest correlations were quality of information, image and usefulness. However, none of these correlations was over 0.24, which is relatively low.

Analysis of the results suggests that quality of *information* is linked significantly to the decision to adopt the Health Card. The people who evaluated the information more positively had a greater incentive to adopt the card. One explanation of this is probably the fact that the more clients are able to visualize the information provided by the system, the more lilely they are to understand its role and utility, and thus the more inclined they are to adopt it.

The second significant correlation was between *image* and *adoption* ($r = 0.23$). The intention of the clients to adopt the Health Card or not depended on the positive opinion of the other people associated with its use. The participants knew they were participating in a pilot study, and there was some "hype" around the project. It is possible that their positive image was due mostly to this factor. In the case of large-scale diffusion, the clients would not have the impression of participating in a unique project, which might affect their willingness to adopt the technology.

Finally, *usefulness* was the last factor to have a significant relationship with *adoption* ($r = 0.21$; $p = 0.033$). The interpretation of this result is analogous with that of quality of information.

The other factors did not have meaningful links with the decision to adopt the innovation or not. Respondents said they found it difficult to evaluate a technology that, in their opinion, was mainly of concern to health care professionals. This poses a problem in the case of a possible large-scale diffusion. Since clients do not think the innovation will provide them with an advantage, this might adversely affect their intention to use it on a permanent basis. Efforts should therefore be made to explain the advantages of using the Health Card — faster treatment, prevention of dangerous drug interactions, etc.

*Results of interviews of the clients outside the pilot area*

To see how the Health Card would be received if its use were extended to other regions, 123 personal interviews were conducted to assess the opinion of the general population. The interview transcripts suggest that the population as a whole is in favour of the innovation.

The reasons most often mentioned for adopting the card are shown in Table 3.

Table 3
Opinions given during interviews population outside the pilot area

| Opinion mentioned | | | % of respondents |
|---|---|---|---|
| I would adopt the Health Card if it was offered to me | | | 92 |
| Reason mentioned | Number of people mentioning the reason | % | |
| Security/Emergency use | 34 | 27.4 | |
| Access to information for the professional | 31 | 25.2 | |
| Usefulness | 20 | 16.3 | |
| Communication with the professional | 9 | 7.3 | |
| Rapidity of the consultation | 6 | 4.9 | |
| The Health Card should be merged with the insurance card (used to pay for the services) | | | 89 |
| I would like to know what the professional writes on my card | | | 89 |
| I would give the pharmacist access to my medical file | | | 84 |
| I would like to see the information on the computer during a consultation | | | 81 |
| The Health Card would lead to a better service for the client | | | 78 |
| The use of the Health Card would be well perceived by my peers | | | 73 |
| I would like to have access to the information on my card | | | 72 |
| I would obtain better information from the health care specialists | | | 71 |
| The Health Card should be well received by health care professionals | | | 68 |
| I would pay to have a Health Card | | | 67 |
| The Health Card should be mandatory for everyone | | | 59 |
| The Health Card would enable me to obtain more explanations about my health | | | 58 |
| The Health Card should improve my relationship with the nurses | | | 50 |
| The Health Card should improve my relationship with the doctors | | | 50 |
| The Health Card should improve my relationship with the pharmacists | | | 47 |
| The professionals should ask for the Health Card (instead of waiting for client to show it) | | | 27 |

Among the people interviewed, 93% said they were willing to adopt the Health Card if its use was generalized to other regions. Sixty-seven percent even said they were willing to pay for the innovation.

A high proportion of respondents were in favour of combining the Health Card with the insurance card used to pay for medical services. This did not always mean they were in favour of making the Health Card mandatory. Only 59% said the voluntary element should be abandoned.

With respect to the possible impacts of the Smart Card, 78% of respondents said the smart card would improve the service received from health care professionals. Among the items mentioned to explain this perception were the fact that the professionals would have more information on their health profile (49.6%) and that the duration of consultations would be reduced (13.8%).

Most respondents wanted to retain some form of control over the use of the card. They wanted to know what was written on the card (89%) and to see the information (81%). This is surprising when these results are compared with those obtained in the pilot study. Seventy-two percent of respondents said they wanted access to the information stored in their card.

A total of 64% thought it was the responsibility of the patient to give the card to the professional. Only 27% thought the professional should ask for the card. When questioned about access to the information, 84% of respondents said it would be acceptable for pharmacists to have access to medical records, and 71% said nurses should have access.


## Discussion

The study provides interesting results on many aspects. First, the role played by the classical adoption factors was investigated and the critical nature of some of these factors revealed. Second, the complexity linked to an innovation for which two distinct (but interacting) groups had to adopt the technology was brought to light. Finally, the most important finding is probably the critical role of the relative advantage provided to the adopter. This is particularly important for an innovation that is socially desirable.

The study results suggest that the adoption factors mentioned in the literature play very different roles in the adoption process. Some appear to be critical. Some others are necessary for the adoption, but not sufficient. In this research, the relative advantage provided by the innovation was the key element identified from the data collected. It was the most influential factor motivating an individual to adopt the technology. The technical factors did not have direct influence on the adoption decision. They were all evaluated as good by the users of

the Health Card. A poor evaluation might be sufficient to reject the adoption, but a positive one does not guarantee adoption. This situation is consistent with a frequently observed pattern for information technology: the system must be user-friendly and well-supported to be adopted, but will not be adopted simply because it is easy to use and well-supported. Technical adequacy is a necessary but not sufficient condition for adoption.

The study also illustrated the particular complexity of an innovation that requires the adoption by two different groups. In this case, the Health Card needs to be adopted by both the practitioners and the clients in order for the innovation to be used. The clients did not see any significant advantage in using the Health Card. Among the professionals, the advantage perceived was viewed as moderate. Interviews revealed that the system was perceived as being of use to the professionals, and there was no appropriation of the technology by the clients. It seems that clients will used the system if the professionals decide to adopt it, but they will not lead the diffusion process. This fact emphasises the need to provide perceptible benefits to the professionals in order to motivate them to adopt the innovation.

The perceived advantage was much higher (3.99 instead of 3.14) among the professionals who had not been part of the pilot study. This result indicates that expectations may be high regarding the smart card and that a trial of the card might be deceptive for the professionals. Such a deception might impede the adoption of the innovation. All these elements raise the question of the potential of smart cards in the medical sectors, as well as the tangible benefits associated with information sharing among professionals.

Another important finding made during this study is the caution that must be taken when extrapolating the results of a pilot study, considered as a trial by the potential adopters. Agreeing to participate in a pilot study requires a much lower commitment than actually adopting a technology for good. In this study, actual use of the smart card system differed significantly from the intention to adopt. It was not influenced by the same factors and the comparative advantage, critical in the decision to adopt the technology, did not influence its use during the trial period. This underlines the importance of carefully measuring the intentions of the potential adopters after a pilot study.

Finally, the study unveiled an important aspect of adoption of innovations that are socially desirable. In this case, the idea of sharing the information among all health care professionals is appealing. Evaluation of the technical factors indicates that the technology works. A social planner would probably evaluate that, on a global perspective, this technology is beneficial and should be adopted. However, to ensure adoption, the results show that some of the social benefits must be captured by the adopters. In this case, the health care practitioners indicated that the technology must bring them benefits for adoption to occur. This finding is clearly aligned with an underlying postulate of the various adoption theories, assuming that adoption is mainly an individual decision based on individual evaluation. This aspect poses a special challenge when diffusing innovations for which multiple-group adoption is required. It implies that a distribution mechanism must be established to ensure that each group obtain a portion of the overall innovation benefits. This mechanism may be difficult to devise and costly to implement, however, it remains critical to permit the adoption of the innovation.

### Limitations and avenues for future research

The most important limitation of this study is the fact that it was conducted as a pilot study. Although the number of participants was high (299 professionals and 7248 clients), all the persons involved knew that it was carried in a pilot setting and that adoption of the technology in the pilot study was not a commitment for definitive adoption. Curiosity regarding the technology and peer pressure could also have increased temporary adoption. These considerations might explain why the analysis of the factual data on usage did not mirror intentions regarding adoption.

Another limitation of the study pertains to the research strategy used. The questionnaires sent to the professionals were extensively validated and tested. However, for investigating the client population, we could not use such measures. A majority of the respondents were elderly people and the research team evaluated that questionnaires would not be appropriate to survey their opinions. For this reason, interviews were conducted. Although interview procedures, coding, and analysis were standardised, it is possible, because of the direct interaction, that some respondents did not reveal some negative opinions. Social desirability might have prevented the expression of such opinions.

A next step in evaluating the potential of a smart cad would be to conduct another study in a different (larger) setting. It would be interesting to verify the use of the smart card in a very large city, where clients might be less inclined to visit systematically the same practitioners and more prone to use less personalised services in larger clinics. It is logical to expect that it would be in such context that the benefits of the card would be maximised. Such an experiment would unfortunately involve much larger costs, since a very large number of professionals would need to be equipped with the technology. It might not be justifiable to conduct such study without a very strong probability to implement the technology permanently afterward.

Another interesting element would be to verify if the effect of mandatoriness on the relative advantage and the intention to adopt is as important as unveiled in this study. Linking the use of the system to the payment system (from the public insurance agency and the insurance companies) would undoubtedly motivate the professionals to use the system. We could measure the realised benefits of the system afterward. However, such an obligation would be very difficult to justify and might be considered unethical. Nevertheless, any subsequent project should include a more formal assessment of the realised benefits.

This study unveiled many interesting aspects linked to the use of a smart card. Advantages exist but each party needs to find a relative gain when adopting the technology. New developments, for example web based systems, might improve the innovation and provide the same benefits at a smaller cost. Such possibilities should be investigated. However, special care should be taken in planning any new venture to address the issues related to the relative advantage perceived by the professionals.

### Appendix

Correlation matrices (see Table 4–6).

### Acknowledgements

The authors wish to thank Jean-Paul Fortin and his team at Laval University for their precious contribution. This project was financed by the RAMQ.

### References

Anderson, J. G., & Jay, S. J. (1984). The diffusion of computer applications in medical settings. *Medical Information Science, 9*, 251–254.

Aubert, B. A., Rivard, S., & Patry, M. (1996). Development of Measures to Assess Transactional Characteristics of IS Operations. *Omega International Journal of Management Science, 24*(6), 661–680.

Dean, J. (1987). *Deciding to innovate: How firms justify advanced technology*, (p. 165). Cambridge, MA, Ballinger.

Frambach, R. T. (1993). An integrated model of organizational adoption and diffusion of innovations. *European Journal of Marketing, 27*(5), 2241.

Fornell, C., & Larcker, D. (1981). Evaluating structural equation models with unobservable variables and measurement error. *Journal of Marketing Research, 18*, 39–50.

Gagliardi, P., & Compeau, D. (1995) The effects of group presentations on intentions to adopt smart card technology: A diffusion of innovations approach. *ASAC Proceedings,* Windsor (pp. 20–32).

Table 4
Correlation among variables – professionals inside the pilot area

| Correlation | Adoption | Usage | Ease of use | Quality of support | Voluntariness | Mandatoriness | Information | Usefulness | Compatibility | Relative advantage | Satisfaction | Membership |
|---|---|---|---|---|---|---|---|---|---|---|---|---|
| ** : $p<0.001$ | | | | | | | | | | | | |
| *: $p<0.05$ | | | | | | | | | | | | |
| Adoption | 1.00 | | | | | | | | | | | |
| Usage | −0.04 | 1.00 | | | | | | | | | | |
| Ease of use | 0.15 | 0.38** | 1.00 | | | | | | | | | |
| Quality of support | 0.13 | 0.36** | 0.32** | 1.00 | | | | | | | | |
| Voluntariness | 0.15 | 0.33* | 0.26* | 0.10 | 1.00 | | | | | | | |
| Mandatoriness | 0.53** | −0.10 | 0.06 | 0.10 | 0.11 | 1.00 | | | | | | |
| Information | 0.35** | 0.28* | 0.24* | 0.38** | 0.10 | 0.16 | 1.00 | | | | | |
| Usefulness | 0.38** | 0.16 | 0.39** | 0.15 | 0.11 | 0.27* | 0.40** | 1.00 | | | | |
| Compatibility | 0.42** | 0.36** | 0.44** | 0.32** | 0.23* | 0.20* | 0.49** | 0.59** | 1.00 | | | |
| Relative Advantage | 0.49** | 0.04 | 0.35** | 0.22* | 0.11 | 0.34** | 0.58** | 0.67** | 0.67** | 1.00 | | |
| Satisfaction | 0.40** | 0.06 | 0.31** | 0.22* | 0.10 | 0.20* | 0.52** | 0.48** | 0.53** | 0.60** | 1.00 | |
| Membership | 0.25 | 0.11 | −0.01 | 0.04 | 0.43** | 0.28* | 0.09 | 0.32* | 0.33** | 0.26* | 0.22* | 1.00 |
| Image | 0.14 | −0.06 | 0.10 | 0.05 | 0.16 | 0.25* | 0.20* | 0.34** | 0.30** | 0.43** | 0.24* | 0.39** |

Table 5

Correlation between variables — professionals Outside of the Pilot Study

| Correlation<br>** : $p<0.001$<br>* : $p<0.05$ | Adoption | Voluntariness | Mandatoriness | Compatibility | Relative Advantage | Membership |
|---|---|---|---|---|---|---|
| Adoption | 1.00 | | | | | |
| Voluntariness | 0.52** | 1.00 | | | | |
| Mandatoriness | 0.44** | 0.27**. | 1.00 | | | |
| Compatibility | 0.44** | 0.047** | 0.54** | 1.00 | | |
| Relative advantage | 0.54** | 0.54** | 0.48** | 0.58** | 1.00 | |
| Membership | −0.03 | 0.01 | 0.01 | 0.01 | 0.00 | 1.00 |
| Image | 0.21** | 0.29** | 0.36** | 0.21** | 0.42** | 0.22** |

Table 6

Correlation between variables — clients inside the pilot area

| Correlation<br>** : $p<0.001$<br>* : $p<0.05$ | Image | Advantage | Information | Usefulness | Satisfaction | Voluntariness |
|---|---|---|---|---|---|---|
| Advantage | 0.25** | 1.00 | | | | |
| Information | 0.07 | −0.06 | 1.00 | | | |
| Usefulness | 0.26* | 0.26* | −0.03 | 1.00 | | |
| Satisfaction | 0.46** | 0.15* | −0.03 | 0.26* | 1.00 | |
| Voluntariness | −0.03 | −0.07 | 0.20* | −0.09 | −0.02 | 1.00 |
| Adoption | 0.23** | 0.15* | 0.24* | 0.21* | 0.16* | 0.05 |

Gopal, A., Bostrom, R., & Chin, W. (1992–1993). Applying Adaptive Structuration Theory to Investigate the Process of Group Support Systems Use. *Journal of Management Information System, 9* (3), 45–69.

Harris, B. L. (1990). Becoming deprofessionalized: One aspect of the staff nurse's perspective on computer–mediated nursing care plans. *Advances in Nursing Science, 13*(2), 6374.

Hebert, M., & Benbasat, I. (1994). Adopting information technology in hospitals: The relationship between attitudes/ expectations and behavior. *Hospital & Health Services Administration, 39*(3), 369383.

Herbig, P. A., & Day, R. L. (1992). Customer acceptance: The key to successful introductions of innovations. *Marketing Intelligence Planning, 10*(1), 4–15.

Langley, A., & Truax, J. (1994). A process study of new technology adoption in smaller manufacturing firms. *Journal of Management Studies, 31*(5), 619–652.

Moore, S. (1994). Understanding innovation in social service delivery systems. *Health Marketing Quarterly, 11*(4), 61–74.

Moore, G. C., & Benbasat, I. (1991). Development of an instrument to measure the perceptions of adopting an information technology innovation. *Information Systems Research, 2*(3), 192–222.

Nunnally, J. (1978). *Psychometric theory.* New York: McGraw-Hill.

Pitt, L., & Watson, R. (1994). Longitudinal measurement of service quality in information systems: A case study. *ICIS,* Vancouver (pp. 419–428).

Ramiller, N. C. (1994). Perceived compatibility of information technology innovations among secondary adopters: Toward a reassessment. *Journal of Engineering and Technology Management, 11,* 1–23.

Rogers, E. M. (1962). *Diffusion of innovations.* New York: The Free Press.

Rogers, E.M. (1991). *The Critical mass in the diffusion of interactive technologies in organizations.* Harvard Business Research Colloquium, Publishing Division, Harvard Business School, Boston (p. 245).

Seddon, P., & Kiew, M. (1994). A partial test and development of the DeLone and McLean model of IS success. *ICIS,* Vancouver (pp. 99–110).

Stoica, P., & Söderström, T. (1998). Partial least squares: A first order analysis. *Scandinavian Journal of Statistics, 25,* 17–24.

Tornatzky, L., & Klein, K. (1982). Innovation characteristics and innovation adoption–implementation: A meta-analysis of findings. *IEEE Transactions on Engineering Management, FM-29*(1), 28–45.

Wold, H. (1984). In Johnson, & Kotz (Eds.), *Partial least squares regression, encyclopædia of statistical science,* Vol. 6 (pp. 581–591) New York:Wiley.

# Evaluation of a Method that Supports Pathology Report Coding

A. Hasman, L. M. de Bruijn, J. W. Arends
Department of Medical Informatics, University of Maastricht, The Netherlands
Department of Pathology, Academic Hospital Maastricht, Maastricht, The Netherlands.

## Summary

*Objectives:* The paper focuses on the problem of adequately coding pathology reports using SNOMED. Both the agreement between pathologists in coding and the quality of a system that supports pathologists in coding pathology reports were evaluated.

*Methods:* Six sets of three pathologists each received a different set of 40 pathology reports. Five different SNOMED code lines accompanied each pathology report. Three pathologists evaluated the correctness of each of these code lines. Kappa values and values for the reliability coefficients were determined to gain insight in the variance observed when coding pathology reports. The system that is evaluated compares a newly entered report, represented as a multi-dimensional word vector, with reports in a library, represented in the same way. The reports in the library are already coded. The system presents the code lines belonging to the five library reports most similar to the newly entered one to the pathologist in this way supporting the pathologist in determining the correct codes. A high similarity between two reports is indicated by a large value of the inproduct of the vector of the newly entered report and the vector of a report in the library.

*Results:* Agreement between pathologists in coding was fair (average kappa of 0.44). The reliability coefficient varied from 0.81 to 0.89 for the six sets of pathology reports. The system gave correct suggestions in 50% of the reports. In another 30% it was helpful for the pathologists.

*Conclusions:* On the basis of the level of the reliability coefficients it could be concluded that three pathologists are indeed sufficient for obtaining a gold standard for evaluating the system. The method used for comparing reports is not strong enough to allow fully automatic coding. It could be shown that the system induces a more uniform coding by pathologists. An evaluation of the incorrect suggestions of the system indicates that the performance of the system can still be improved.

## Keywords

Coding, reliability, inter-observer variation, computer system evaluation, pathology

Method Inform Med 2001; 40: 293–7

## 1. Introduction

Clinical pathology is a diagnostic service – tissue or cell samples are examined by the pathology department on order of an attending physician. The result of the examination is reported and included in the patient record. In the Netherlands, pathologists not only record the diagnostic findings, but additionally summarize them in a so-called diagnosis line at the end of the report. The terms used in the diagnosis line are taken from a restricted vocabulary. Excerpts of all pathology examinations (including the diagnosis line) are sent to the PALGA foundation (Dutch Network and National Database for Pathology) where, after several checks have been performed, they are stored in a database. In 1996, the database contained approx. 20,000,000 excerpts and showed an annual increase of approx. 2,000,000. The database is queried for patient data nearly 1,800,000 times per year.

The pathologists have adopted and still use SNOMED II to formally represent their findings. Terms for all appropriate axes are to be recorded by the pathologists. Minimally, however, the topology axis should be coded. In this context, the word 'coding' refers to the recording of the appropriate terms contained in the vocabulary, not the proper SNOMED codes. Based on the terms generated by the pathologists, the translation to SNOMED codes is performed by PALGA.

Coding requires deciding which of the formal terms best represent the situation since the terms are not always concordant. Coding is also a generalization and hence demands deciding which level of detail is appropriate. Good coding leads to a correct, complete and concise summary of the report. The according literature makes it clear that manual coding is not error-free and is subject to the personal preferences of the coders [1].

When the pathologists use terms in the diagnosis lines that are not present in the restricted vocabulary, PALGA returns the reports for correction. This occurs relatively often and leads to additional work for the pathologist. Also, the quality of the content of the diagnosis lines appears to vary [2].

To improve this situation, we have developed a system that supports the pathologist in coding an examination. In this way, reports with a better coding quality are obtained. The system is described in the next section.

The performance of the method used by the system was determined by presenting pathology reports to the system and then comparing the suggested diagnosis lines with those actually given by pathologists. As stated earlier, the diagnosis lines given by pathologists are not totally reliable. Therefore, although the method suggested correct codes in 87.5% of the cases, the actual performance of the system was not clear. This was due to the lack of a gold standard.

In this contribution, we describe how we have determined a gold standard and how we have evaluated the system using this gold standard. As a side effect, we also obtained quantitative insight in the coding variability of pathologists.

We will describe the system in the next section. Following this description, we will present the method of evaluation, the material and the experts. The results will be presented and discussed in the last section of this paper.

# 2. Description of the System

The pathologist enters a report into the system. The system then suggests five diagnosis lines for this report. The suggestions stem from the diagnosis lines of the five most similar reports found by the system. The system selected these five reports from a collection of 7500 manually coded reports (containing approx. 20,000 different words all together). Following his own judgment, the user selects an appropriate diagnosis line, if available, for the current report.

The system works as follows: First it creates a multi-dimensional vector of the report text that has just entered the system. Each word represents a dimension. In case a word is absent, the value of the corresponding dimension is zero, otherwise it is equal to a weight factor. The weight factor of each word is determined so that it favors words occurring more often in certain reports, but rarely occur in the remaining collection of reports [3, 4]. The collection's report texts (not including the diagnosis lines) are also represented by multi-dimensional vectors. The vector of the current report is compared to the vector of each report in the collection. Each comparison is based on the inner product of both vectors. The larger the inner product, the more similar these reports are (in a statistical sense). The diagnosis lines corresponding to the five most similar reports are presented to the user.

In an experiment based on 30 reports, agreement among four pathologists using the system increased by 10% as compared to their agreement when coding manually.

The system was also evaluated on a larger scale. For this purpose, the system was changed: the user interface of the system was replaced by a module that randomly selected a report from the collection. According to the process described above, the similarity between each of the reports remaining in the collection and the randomly selected report was determined. The report showing the highest statistical similarity (as obtained via the inner product) was then selected. Our aim was to prove that a high statistical similarity

implies a high semantic similarity. To achieve this, the semantic similarity between the randomly selected report and its statistically most similar report was determined by comparing the contents of the diagnosis line accompanying each report. This procedure was repeated 1000 times. We found that the randomly selected report was also semantically similar to the statistically most similar report in 65.2% of the trials. 87.5% of the trials contained at least one semantically similar report when the five statistically most similar reports were selected during each of the 1000 trials [5, 6].

The quality of the method was tested by using the terms contained in the diagnosis lines as the gold standard. However, since the diagnosis lines may contain errors or may be incomplete, a better gold standard was needed to evaluate the system.

# 3. Methods and Material

## 3.1 Evaluation Method

A gold standard can be obtained by having a panel of pathologists code a large number of reports. This approach, however, is very time consuming and, in our setting, can not be carried out on a large scale. Therefore, as mentioned in the section above, a possibility was to conduct a small scale study with four pathologists, each composing diagnosis lines for 30 reports. However, this study would not suffice to create a gold standard.

Alternatively, we presented a set of 40 reports to each member of a panel of pathologists. Every report included five diagnosis lines which were suggested by the system. The experts were instructed to rate the adequacy of each diagnosis line on a three-point scale:

++ the diagnosis line is correct or can be
    made correct with a slight intervention
+/– the diagnosis line is partially correct
–/– the diagnosis line is incorrect

In this way, each pathologist rated 200 diagnosis lines and each diagnosis line was

rated by three different pathologists. The pathologists did not know which diagnosis line was initially from the report. In fact, in most of the cases, the initial diagnosis line was not present.

The agreement between pairs of pathologists as well as the kappa value between them were determined. While the mentioned agreement can be expressed as the number of diagnosis lines to which two raters gave the same rating divided by 200 (the total number of diagnosis lines assessed), the kappa value measures the agreement beyond chance between the raters. Landis and Koch [7] have characterized kappa value ranges for interpretation purposes: Values larger than 0.75 usually represent excellent agreement, values below 0.4 represent poor agreement, and values between 0.4 and 0.75 represent the range spanning fair to good agreement.

The performance of the system was determined by calculating the percentage of reports for which the majority of the pathologists rated at least one of the diagnosis lines as being correct. The majority decision made by the three pathologists regarding each diagnosis line was taken as the gold standard.

To determine whether the majority decision is an appropriate reference, the reliability coefficient (Cronbach's alpha) was calculated. Reliability is a measure for the reproducibility of the classification (in this case, obtained via the majority decision). The larger the number of raters, the better the reliability: individual opinions are averaged out this way. Literature states that a reliability of 0.7 is adequate if a standard is used to estimate the performance of a system [8, 9].

To determine the causes of incorrect diagnosis lines, the reports that proved to be difficult (the corresponding diagnosis lines were rated +/– or –/–) were studied more closely.

## 3.2 Material

The collection of reports was acquired from two laboratories: the pathology laboratory of the Academic Hospital Maastricht, Maastricht, Netherlands, supplied 5000 reports and the laboratory of the Elkerliek Hospital in Helmond, Netherlands, provided 2500 reports. In both cases, the reports were unfiltered productions of histology examinations covering a period of approx. three months.

From this collection, 240 reports were selected. These 240 reports were divided into six sets of 40 reports: three sets from each of the two laboratories. The sets were compiled as follows: starting from a number of random points in the chronologically sorted report text file, each report was included in the set until the set contained enough reports.

It was verified that this batch was a representative sample of the total collection. The reports contained texts on:

skin tissue (85)
- naevus (17)
- verruca (11)
- basal cell carcinoma (9)
- multiple samples with different diagnoses (6)
- dermatitis (5)
- other (37)

intestinal tissue (57)
- stomach (26)
  - helicobacter pylori (10)
  - gastritis/slightly abnormal (15)
  - adenocarcinoma (1)
- appendix (4)
- colon and sigmoid (21)
  - inflammation (13)
  - other (8)
- other (6)

gynecological tissue (19)
- cervix/corpus (12)
- uterus (3)
- other (4)

mammary tissue (11)
bone (9)
vasa deferentia (6)
other (53)

For each experimental report, the ten most similar reports were retrieved by the method from the remainder of the site's collection (4999 and 2499 reports respectively). From the ten diagnosis lines ordered according to the similarity score, the first five were selected such that this set contained no duplicates. The order of the five diagnosis lines was then randomized for presentation to the pathologist. By using this procedure, we were sure that some of the diagnosis lines would be quite similar. In this way, the pathologist would not be confronted with a majority of clearly incorrect diagnosis lines. Moreover, because of the selection procedure, most of the presented diagnosis lines showed some overlap with the diagnosis line of the report under scrutiny.

## 3.3 Experts

Experts were invited by mail to participate in the experiment until 18 experts could be recruited. The response rate was approx. 65%.

15 pathologists and 3 residents from 15 different hospitals were finally recruited to participate in the experiment. Their average working experience was 16 years (standard deviation 9.9 years), 8 of the participants possessed over 23 years of experience. The experts participated on a voluntary basis.

# 4. Results

## 4.1 Agreement among Raters

Table 1 presents the ratings of the three participating experts. The 1200 diagnosis lines were judged by 18 pathologists. There were six sets of 200 diagnosis lines whereby each set was rated by another group of three pathologists. In Table 1, we have abstracted the fact that each set had different raters. We have identified the raters as experts 1, 2 and 3, independent of the set of diagnosis lines. This abstraction serves presentation purposes only. The calculations are based on the fact that there are six sets of 200 diagnosis lines each having a unique set of judges.

The first two columns of this table present the coding combinations given by two of the experts. The third column indicates how many of the 1200 diagnosis lines were given each coding combination. The last four columns indicate which codes were given by the third rater for each of the coding combinations of his two colleagues. Each of these columns represent a possible rating by this expert. For sake of simplicity, the codes 1, 2 and 3 were used to denote ++, +/- and -/- respectively. For example, the fourth row in Table 1 indicates that two of the experts were in agreement regarding 117 diagnosis lines, both giving code 1. Expert 3, however, did not provide a rating twice (missing), agreed with his colleagues 81 times (code 1), gave code 2 a total of 31 times and code 3 three times.

One rating was missing in 6% of the diagnosis lines and all three experts gave the same rating in 54% of the diagnosis lines. The majority of these cases concerned the rating 'incorrect diagnosis line'. In 8% of the diagnosis lines, one expert rated ++ whereas another rated the same line as -/-.

When measured between pairs of experts, an average agreement of 0.70 (range between 0.6 and 0.8) was obtained. The average kappa value was 0.44 (range 0.299-0.667).

In 63 reports, one of the suggested diagnosis lines was exactly equal to the diagnosis line originally given to that report. These diagnosis lines were unanimously seen as correct by the experts in only 29 cases. Two of the experts rated the diagnosis lines as correct in 13 cases. The original classification of the remaining 21 cases were rated +/- or -/- by two or more of the experts.

In the experiment in which the system was used to compose diagnosis lines (see the section 2, Description of the system), the agreement between four pathologists on 30 reports was 0.77 (standard deviation 0.15).

The reliability coefficient varied from 0.81 to 0.89 for the six sets (when not taking the diagnosis lines containing missing values into account). Since one set of cases contained most of the missing values (caused by one expert) the reliability coefficient for this set was 0.71 instead of 0.81. Considering these missing values as a separate category, the reliability coefficients of the other sets hardly changed.

**Table 1**  The two left-hand columns indicate the rating combinations given by two of the experts. (1 = ++, 2 = +/–, 3 = –/–). The third column indicates the total number of diagnosis lines which received the ratings presented in the previous two columns of the same row. The four remaining columns show the total number of cases divided according to the ratings given by the third expert.

| Expert Ratings | | Number of diagnosis lines | Ratings given by Expert 3 | | | |
|---|---|---|---|---|---|---|
| Expert 1 | Expert 2 | | Missing | 1 | 2 | 3 |
| Missing | 2 | 2 | | 1 | | 1 |
| Missing | 3 | 10 | | 1 | | 9 |
| 1 | Missing | 1 | | | 1 | |
| 1 | 1 | 117 | 2 | 81 | 31 | 3 |
| 1 | 2 | 67 | 3 | 26 | 31 | 7 |
| 1 | 3 | 25 | | 5 | 12 | 8 |
| 2 | 1 | 54 | | 31 | 20 | 3 |
| 2 | 2 | 81 | 1 | 19 | 46 | 15 |
| 2 | 3 | 83 | 5 | 4 | 27 | 47 |
| 3 | Missing | 6 | | | 4 | 2 |
| 3 | 1 | 22 | 1 | 15 | 4 | 2 |
| 3 | 2 | 113 | 3 | 16 | 29 | 65 |
| 3 | 3 | 619 | 35 | 13 | 54 | 517 |

## 4.2 Performance of the System

The system suggested diagnosis lines for 121 reports of which at least one of the five obtained a majority rating ++. The system suggested at least one diagnosis line that was rated +/– for 71 reports. For the remaining 48 reports, the system suggested only incorrect diagnosis lines. Therefore, the system was accurate in 50% of the reports and helpful in another 30%. In 20% of the cases, the system was not helpful.

When comparing two reports, the use of the highest similarity measure value is based on the following assumption: the higher the similarity measure, the higher the semantic similarity. Indeed, we observed that the higher the textual similarity of two reports, the higher the probability that experts rate the adequacy of the corresponding diagnosis line as ++. However, there were a number of cases showing high textual similarity in which the diagnosis line still received a low rating. These cases appeared to be what we call multiple reports. These reports describe an examination of sections stemming from two or more different locations: typical combinations are stomach + colon, stomach + esophagus, appendix + gall bladder and endometrium + endocervix. In 42 cases, the report described a multiple section. In 16 instances, one of the diagnosis lines was rated ++, in 9 instances the best diagnosis line was rated +/– and in 17 instances all diagnosis lines were rated –/–.

For another 42 reports used in the experiment, it was determined that none of the cases in the report collection were really suitable and therefore a relatively small text similarity was obtained (average value 0.53). For diagnosis lines rated ++, a similarity value of over 0.8 was usually obtained.

Finally, a problem occurred in skin reports. For 25 reports used in the experiment, the reports describing skin tissue was correctly classified. However, the location of the skin was incorrect, thus leading to a – rating.

## 5. Discussion

### 5.1 Agreement among Pathologists

Average agreement among the experts was 'fair' (an average kappa value of 0.44). This indicates that coding is indeed error-prone or subject to personal interpretation. That experts do not always agree becomes apparent in the observation that in 94 cases one expert gave a ++ rating and another a –/– rating for the same diagnosis line. Also supporting this conclusion is the fact that the experts agreed with the diagnosis lines originally assigned to the reports in only 42 of 63 cases (67%). It emphasizes the need for decision support during the coding process.

It may be objected that the rating procedure is not natural to the pathologists. Had they directly coded the reports, they may have reached a higher agreement. However, we could not corroborate this objection. We determined the agreement between the earlier mentioned four pathologists by manually coding each of the 30 reports. An average agreement of 0.77 was found. This result does not differ statistically from the result of our panel.

## 5.2 Performance of the System

Clearly, the performance of the system is not optimal. One of the reasons being that the diagnosis lines of the reports from the collection were coded manually. From this study, we now know that the accuracy of these diagnosis lines is near the order of 70%. The performance of the system will increase once we begin using a collection of reports with diagnosis lines that have been validated.

Another reason why the system is not optimal, is the presence of multiple reports. To cope with this problem, the findings concerning the different locations should be reported and coded separately.

The errors observed with skin reports can be corrected easily since the location is always mentioned in another part of the report and can be copied to the diagnosis line.

Also, the collection of reports apparently does not contain enough cases. This explains why no counterpart could be found for 42 reports. This situation can be improved by uniformly distributing the different case types. Since our base was formed by the unfiltered reports produced within a period of three months, some case types were underrepresented while others appeared more frequently. This situation can, of course, be changed easily.

We could prove that the agreement among pathologists improved by 10% with support of the system as compared to manual coding.

## 5.3  Evaluation of the Method

The method described earlier in this contribution [5, 6] is capable of making good or partially good suggestions in approximately 80% of the reports. In 50% of the cases, the suggestions were good. Literature describes that methods based on syntactic or semantic analyses of texts perform successfully in 54% to 71% of the cases [10–12]. The material used in these studies consisted of short pieces of text and was restricted to limited domains: discharge summaries and head cancer reports. Our method, applied to a wide range of full pathology reports, performed errorless in a lower percentage of cases. This observation implies that the method is not strong enough for fully automatic coding. When used by pathologists, it leads to more uniform coding. Therefore the method appears worthwhile to support the pathologists in their coding process. The method could also be used as a first step to be followed by another method. We have shown that the method can provide correct suggestions in 50% of the cases. These suggestions can be recognized because they have a high statistical similarity (over 0.75). Croft [13] advocates the design of hybrid systems in which statistical and knowledge-based elements promise more effective systems.

In conclusion, we can state that we have found a considerable variance in the quality of coding. The overall agreement between coders was nearly 70%. We have evaluated a statistical method that provides good or partially good coding suggestions in 80% of the cases and provides a basis on which pathologists can code their reports more uniformly. An evaluation of the incorrect suggestions made by the system indicates that the performance of the system can still be improved.

## References


1. Hall PA, Lemoine NR. Comparison of manual data coding errors in two hospitals. J Clin Path 1986; 39: 622-6.
2. Wilhelm WW, Nap M. From data to concept management in health care reports. Is there a need for it? Int J Biomed Comp 1996; 42: 103-9.
3. Sparck Jones K. Index term weighting. Information storage and retrieval 1973; 9: 619-33.
4. Hersch WR. Information Retrieval – a health care perspective. New York, Springer Verlag 1996.
5. de Bruijn LM, Hasman A, Arends JW. Automatic SNOMED classification – a corpus-based method. Comp Meth Prog Biomed 1997; 54: 115-22.
6. de Bruijn LM, Hasman A, Arends JW. Automatic coding of diagnostic reports. Method Inform Med 1998; 17: 260-5.
7. Landis JR, Koch GG. The measurement of observer agreement for categorical data. Biometrics 1979; 33: 159-74.
8. Friedman CP, Wyatt JC. Evaluation methods in medical informatics. New York: Springer, 1997.
9. Hripcsak G, Kuperman GJ, Friedman C, Heitjan DF. A reliability study for evaluating information extraction from radiology reports. JAMIA 1999; 6: 143-50.
10. Sager N, Bross ID, Story G, Bastedo P, Marsh E, Shedd D. Automatic encoding of clinical narrative. Comput Biol Med 1982; 12: 43-56.
11. Brigl B, Mieth M, Haux R, Gluck E. The LBI method for automated indexing of diagnoses using SNOMED. Part 2: Evaluation. Int J Biomed Comput 1995; 38: 101-8.
12. Spyns P, De Moor G. A Dutch medical language Processor. Int J Biomed Comput, 1996; 41: 181-205.
13. Croft WB. Knowledge-based and statistical approaches to text retrieval. IEEE Expert 1993, 8-12.



Correspondence to:
Prof. Dr. Arie Hasman
Department of Medical Informatics
University of Limburg
P.O. Box 616, NL-6200 MD Maastricht
The Netherlands
E-mail: hasman@mi.unimaas.nl

# Personal Health Records:

## Evaluation of Functionality and Utility

MATTHEW I. KIM, MD, KEVIN B. JOHNSON, MD

**Abstract** **Objectives:** Web-based applications have been developed that allow patients to enter their own information into secure personal health records. These applications are being promoted as a means of providing patients and providers with universal access to updated medical information. The authors evaluated the functionality and utility of a selection of personal health records.

**Design:** A targeted search strategy was used to identify eleven Web sites promoting different personal health records. Specific criteria related to the entry and display of data elements were developed to evaluate the functionality of each PHR. Information abstracted from an actual case was used to create a series of representative PHRs. Output generated for review was evaluated to assess the accuracy and completeness of clinical information related to the diagnosis and treatment of specific disorders.

**Results:** The PHRs selected for review employed data entry methods that limited the range and content of patient-entered information related to medical history, medications, laboratory tests, diagnostic studies, and immunizations. Representative PHRs created with information abstracted from an actual case displayed varying amounts of information at basic and comprehensive levels of representation.

**Conclusions:** Currently available PHRs demonstrate limited functionality. The data entry, validation, and information display methods they employ may limit their utility as representations of medical information.

Affiliation of the authors: Johns Hopkins University School of Medicine, Baltimore, Maryland.

Correspondence and reprints: Matthew I. Kim, MD, Division of Endocrinology and Metabolism, Johns Hopkins University School of Medicine; 1830 East Monument Street, Suite 333, Baltimore, MD, 21287-0003; e-mail: <mkima@mail.jhmi.edu>.

Consumer advocates have raised concerns about the extent to which decentralization of health care has led to the dispersal of personal medical information.[1-3] Recognizing that increased mobility and managed care restrictions may drive patients to seek care from different providers, some advocates have recommended that patients adopt a proactive stance toward collecting and organizing their own medical

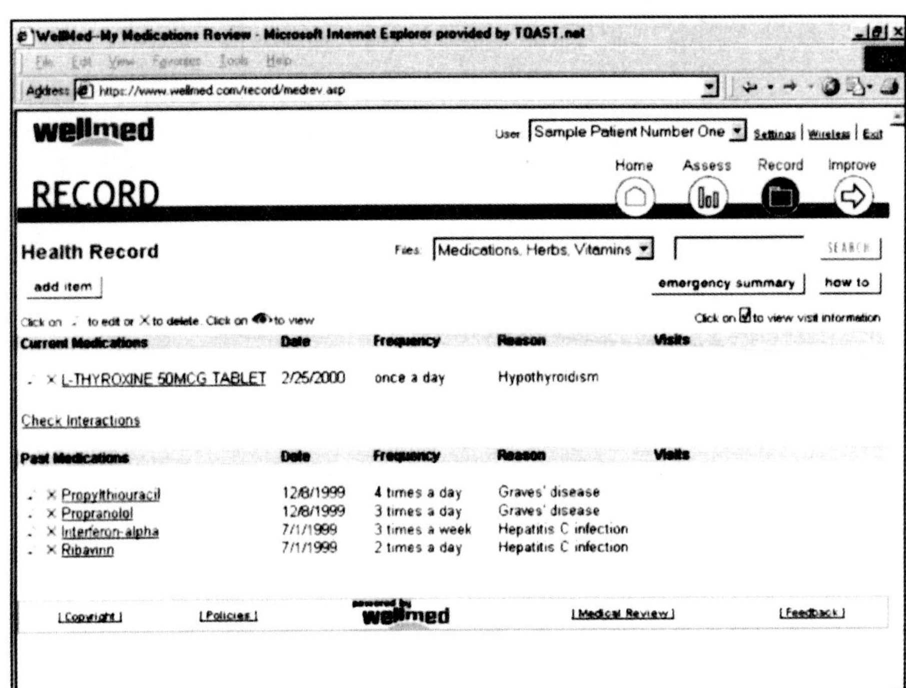

**Figure 1** WellMed Personal Health Record screen displaying current and past medication information

information.[4,5] Until recently, efforts directed at providing patients with approaches to this task have promoted document organization systems and specialized software applications. Document organization systems provide patients with templates and binders to store copies of medical records.[6] Software applications allow patients to enter information abstracted from medical records into files stored on personal computers.[7]

Recently, a number of Web-based applications have been developed as resources to provide patients with secure access to personal medical information.[8–10] Configured along the lines of standard provider-entered records, these personal health records (PHRs) allow patients to directly enter information about their own diagnoses, medications, laboratory tests, diagnostic studies, and immunizations. Host sites use this information to generate records that can be displayed for review or transmitted to authorized receivers (Figure 1).

Versions of these records are being promoted by a number of different consumer health care Web sites. Although a few have been set up by nonprofit organizations, most have been developed as commercial ventures. While initial revenue models were based on sales of advertising, current business strategies aim to use PHRs to provide laboratory, prescription, and billing information to designated providers.[11] One prominent commercial site recently reported enrollment of 10,000 active users based in the United States.[12]

Most PHRs in current use are designed to serve as static repositories for personal medical information. Advertisements depict hypothetical situations in which access to a centralized record might help patients relate accurate histories during clinical encounters, check for drug interactions when filling new prescriptions, or avoid unnecessary duplication of laboratory tests and diagnostic studies.[13] Promotional materials place a particular emphasis on the potential use of PHRs in emergency situations.[14] In circumstances in which a patient might be incapacitated or unable to provide a history, providers could access an updated PHR to obtain critical information about allergies, medications, and diagnoses.[15] A few PHRs are being promoted as resources to guide self-monitoring and disease management.[16,17]

To date, there have not been any studies evaluating the accuracy or utility of medical records generated using patient-entered information.[12] One pilot study focused on evaluating the performance of a Web-based application designed to collect verifiable patient-entered information detailing family health histories.[18] A few studies have evaluated the utility of patient-held summaries of institutional records, documenting significant improvements in levels of compliance with monitoring protocols and immunization schedules.[19–22] A number of recent initiatives have focused on the development of resources targeted to provide patients with direct online access to their own institutional records.[23–25] One recent study reviewed a selection of PHRs with a specific focus on features that might affect their utility as resources for critical care, noting significant problems with provisions for emergency access and storage of digitized images.[26]

In an effort to carry out an assessment of these untested resources, we adopted a systematic approach to evaluate the functionality and clinical utility of a selection of currently available PHRs.

## Methods

Our assessment was carried out in three phases. The first phase focused on the identification and selection of candidate PHRs. The second phase focused on the development of criteria related to the entry and dis-

*Table 1* ■

Personal Health Records

| Web Site | Record | URL |
| --- | --- | --- |
| Dr. I-Net | My Medical Record | www.aboutmyhealth.com |
| HealthCompass | Lifelong Health Record | www.healthcompassnet.com |
| MedicalEdge | Medical Registry | www.medicaledge.com |
| MedicalRecord.com | Your Medical Record | www.medicalrecord.com |
| MedicData | MedicData | www.medicdata.com |
| Medscape AboutMyHealth | Personal Health Record | www.aboutmyhealth.com |
| myhealthnotes.com | Personal Health Manager | www.myhealthnotes.com |
| PersonalMD | My Medical Records | www.personalmd.com |
| TheDailyApple | Health Records | www.thedailyapple.com |
| VistaLink | Health Profile | www.vistalink.com |
| WebMD | My Health Record | www.webmd.com |
| WellMed | Health Record | www.wellmed.com |

play of data elements that would need to be met for PHRs to serve as adequate representations of information. These criteria were used to evaluate the functionality and utility of a selected group of PHRs during the third phase of our assessment.

### Identification and Selection of Candidate Personal Health Records

We performed a search to identify sites promoting PHRs. Entered search terms included combinations of the words "patient," "own," "online," "personal," "health," "medical," and "record." We explored identified sites in detail, following links from articles, specialty guides, commercial sites, and personal Web pages to locate sites providing access to PHRs. We identified 19 independent sites promoting different versions of PHRs. We excluded four of these sites from consideration because of their narrow focus on specific diseases. We excluded two additional sites because of their connections to disease management programs. We also excluded a site that provided access to a hospital information system. Twelve remaining sites were selected for review (Table 1). During the course of our evaluation, we opted to exclude one of these sites because of recurrent problems encountered while trying to establish and maintain access.

### Development of Criteria

We identified five prospective functions of PHRs, based on our survey of aggregate claims appearing in advertising and promotional materials (Table 2). To establish a basis for systematic evaluation, we identified specific criteria that would need to be met for a given PHR to perform each of these functions. Given the lack of professional oversight in the creation of PHRs, most of these criteria outlined requirements for accurate entry of information and verification of reported test and study results. Other criteria outlined requirements for the provision of different routes of access, links to consumer health care information, functions to process and interpret information, and functions to provide secure communication between patients and providers. We identified specific data elements that would need to be included in a PHR to fulfill each of these requirements.

### Evaluation of Functionality and Utility

Our evaluation of the functionality of each PHR focused on testing different routes of access while documenting and characterizing representations of specific data elements in each category of required information (Table 3). To evaluate the functionality of each

*Table 2* ■

Criteria for Evaluation of Functionality

| Function | Requirements |
|---|---|
| Providing Web-based access to personal medical information | ■ Secure password-protected patient access<br>■ Capacity to provide authorized provider access<br>■ Capacity to provide directed emergency access |
| Providing an organized summary of personal medical information for presentation to health care providers | ■ Accurate entry of past and current medical conditions, including information about diagnosis and treatment<br>■ Accurate entry of past and current medications, including information about indication, dose, frequency, and duration<br>■ Verification of laboratory test results<br>■ Verification of diagnostic study results<br>■ Verification of immunizations, including information about dates and sequences |
| Serving as a portal to patient-specific consumer-level health care information | ■ Accurate entry of medical conditions<br>■ Accurate entry of medications<br>■ Capacity to provide links to consumer health care information |
| Providing interpretive information about laboratory test and diagnostic study results | ■ Accurate entry of medical conditions<br>■ Accurate entry of medications<br>■ Verification of laboratory test results<br>■ Verification of diagnostic study results<br>■ Capacity to interpret laboratory test and diagnostic study results |
| Serving as a database of information for patient-specific self-monitoring and disease management | ■ Accurate entry of medical conditions<br>■ Accurate entry of medications<br>■ Verification of monitoring study results<br>■ Capacity to interpret monitoring study results<br>■ Capacity to provide evaluation and treatment recommendations<br>■ Capacity to provide secure communication between patients and providers |

site, we generated representative PHRs using a standard profile of information. We identified six categories of required information that fell under general headings of personal information, medical history, medications, laboratory tests, diagnostic studies, and immunizations. We entered requested information without any truncation or omission, documenting the data-entry methods used to enter each type of information. Completed PHRs were printed for review. If a summary version was available for electronic transmission, it was relayed and printed for review.

To evaluate the clinical utility of the PHRs selected for review, we used objective information abstracted from an actual test case to generate a series of representative PHRs. We reviewed the output of each PHR to document the extent to which it accurately and completely presented diagnostic and therapeutic information.

The case selected for this purpose represented a patient seen in consultation for a thyroid condition. The initial referral had been prompted by identification of possible hyperthyroidism ascribed to Graves' disease. Subsequent evaluation revealed an extensive history incorporating a prior diagnosis of hepatitis C infection, immunization against hepatitis A and hepatitis B, treatment with ribavirin and interferon-alpha, development of autoimmune thyroiditis precipitated by interferon-alpha, and eventual progression to a state of persistent hypothyroidism.[27,28]

This case presented a number of considerations that would test the limits of any representation of medical information. Each diagnosis represented a chronic condition requiring specific treatment with an oral or subcutaneously injected medication. Clinical evaluation was based on a range of laboratory tests and radiographic studies used to establish diagnoses and monitor treatments. Specific indices reflected a transition from a hyperfunctioning condition to a hypofunctioning condition, prompting a change in diagnosis with alteration of therapy. Treatment of one of the conditions included specific immunizations, one of which was administered as a series of injections.

Outpatient chart records related to this case covered a span of 19 months. After reviewing these records, we abstracted relevant data elements from clinic notes and test reports to generate a standard profile

*Table 3* ◼

Functionality of Personal Health Records

| Web Site* | 1 | 2 | 3 | 4 | 5 | 6 | 7 | 8 | 9 | 10 | 11 |
|---|---|---|---|---|---|---|---|---|---|---|---|
| **Access:** | | | | | | | | | | | |
| Password-protected patient access | X | X | X | X | X | X | X | X | X | X | X |
| Authorized provider access | | | X | X | | X | | | X | | |
| Directed emergency access | X | | X | | X | X | X | | X | | |
| **Medical conditions:** | | | | | | | | | | | |
| Verification | | | | | | | | | | X | |
| Distinction between past and current | X | | | | | | X | | | | X |
| Diagnosis | X | | | X | X | | X | X | X | X | X |
| Treatment | | | | | X | | | X | X | X | X |
| Links | X | | | | | | | | | | |
| **Medications:** | | | | | | | | | | | |
| Verification | | | | | | | | | | | |
| Distinction between past and current | X | | | | | | X | | | X | X |
| Indication | X | | | | | | | | | X | X |
| Dose | X | | X | X | X | | X | X | X | X | |
| Frequency | | | X | X | X | X | X | | | X | |
| Duration | X | | X | | X | | X | | X | | |
| Links | X | | | | | | | | | | |
| **Laboratory tests:** | | | | | | | | | | | |
| Verification | | X | | | X | X | X | | | | |
| Results | X | X | X | X | X | X | X | X | | X | |
| Interpretation | | | | | | | X | | | | |
| Links | X | | | | | | X | | | | |
| **Diagnostic tests:** | | | | | | | | | | | |
| Verification | | | | | X | X | | | | | |
| Results | X | | X | X | X | X | | | | X | |
| Interpretation | | | | | | | | | | | |
| Links | X | | | | | | | | | | |
| **Immunizations:** | | | | | | | | | | | |
| Verification | | | | | | | | | | | |
| Results | X | X | X | X | X | X | X | X | | | X |
| Interpretation | | | | | X | | X | | | | X |
| Links | X | | | | | | | | | | |

*De-identified from listing in Table 1.

of information. This information was entered along with a profile of anonymous personal information to generate a series of representative PHRs. In the course of entering medical history information, we elected to use the term "Graves' disease" in place of "autoimmune thyroiditis," since Graves' disease was more likely to appear on pick lists of diagnoses. The PHRs that were generated were checked for accuracy before completed versions were printed for review.

Our evaluation of the utility of each PHR focused on a stratified assessment of output presented for display from a clinical perspective. In an effort to establish rigorous criteria for evaluation, we opted to review this output from the standpoint of different providers who might be presented with a PHR as a summary of a patient's medical history. To provide a balanced view with regard to different levels of complexity, we elected to evaluate each PHR at two distinct levels of representation.

At a basic level, we reviewed the output of each PHR to see if it provided the minimum amount of information a primary care provider would need to manage a simple problem based on the results of objective laboratory tests. Our evaluation at this level focused on the identification of essential data elements related to the diagnosis and treatment of persistent hypothyroidism (Table 4). At a more comprehensive level, we reviewed the output of each PHR to see whether it provided the minimum amount of information a consulting subspecialist would need to accurately trace the course of events contributing to a complete clinical history. Our evaluation at this level

*Table 4* ■

## Clinical Utility of Personal Health Records

| Web Site* | 1 | 2 | 3 | 4 | 5 | 6 | 7 | 8 | 9 | 10 | 11 |
|---|---|---|---|---|---|---|---|---|---|---|---|
| **Basic level:** | | | | | | | | | | | |
| Diagnostic elevated TSH and low T4 | X | | X | | X | | X | | | X | |
| Decline in TSH indicating response to therapy | X | | X | | X | | | | | X | |
| Current levothyroxine dose | X | | * | X | † | X | X | X | X | X | |
| **Comprehensive level:** | | | | | | | | | | | |
| Diagnosis of hepatitis C infection | | | | | | | | | | | |
| Elevated transaminases | X | | X | | X | | X | | | X | |
| Hepatitis C antibodies | X | | X | | X | | X | | | X | |
| Treatment with interferon-alpha | | | | | | | | | | | |
| Liver biopsy results | X | | X | X | | | X | | | X | |
| Interferon-alpha regimen | X | | X | X | † | | | X | X | | |
| Hepatitis A immunization | X | † | X | X | X | X | X | X | | | |
| Hepatitis B immunization | ‡ | † | ‡ | X | X | ‡ | X | ‡ | | | |
| Diagnosis of interferon-alpha-associated autoimmune thyroiditis | | | | | | | | | | | |
| Suppressed TSH, elevated T4 | X | | X | | X | | X | | | X | |
| Thyroid scan results | X | | X | X | | | X | | | X | |
| Timing relative to treatment | | | X | | | | | | | | |

* Unable to specify dose of levothyroxine in micrograms or fractions of milligrams.
† Unable to display entered information
‡ Unable to specify series.

focused on the identification of essential data elements related to the diagnosis of hepatitis C infection, subsequent treatment with interferon-alpha, and the emergence of complications associated with the development of autoimmune thyroiditis (Table 4). To set reasonable limits, we excluded additional tests that might be indicated to eliminate different causes of hepatitis. We also excluded quantitative hepatitis C RNA results that might be used to guide the treatment of hepatitis C infection, as documented values were not available at the time the PHRs were generated.[29]

## Results

### Functionality

#### Access

Each of the 11 sites displayed explicitly stated privacy and security policies at the point of registration. Each site provided password-protected access to entered information, with one requiring entry of an additional identification phrase. Four sites provided authorized physicians with password-protected access to viewable summaries of entered information.

Seven sites provided emergency access to patients' information. Three of these sites allowed patients to create a wallet card listing a URL along with an identification phrase. In an emergency situation in which a patient might be incapacitated or unable to relate a history, providers would be able to use the information on this card to access a viewable summary of a patient's PHR. Two sites allowed patients to transmit a printable summary of a PHR to a designated fax number, although neither elaborated a mechanism that would enable providers to receive this information if a patient were completely incapacitated.

#### Personal Information

Each site allowed patients to enter personal contact information that typically included a current home address, home phone number, work phone number, cellular phone number, fax number, and e-mail address. Each site also allowed patients to enter information for an individual designated as a primary emergency contact, with seven sites allowing patients to enter information for a secondary emergency contact.

Each site allowed patients to enter contact information for a designated primary physician, with nine sites allowing patients to enter contact information for other physicians. Ten sites allowed patients to enter insurance coverage information.

## Medical History

Each site used a different method to guide patients through the process of entering information related to medical conditions. Eight sites directed patients to select conditions from categorized lists. These lists varied widely in content and organization. Most included examples of nonspecific symptoms, general systemic disorders, and specific etiologic diagnoses. In most cases, entry was limited to simple identification, although there were a few notable examples. One site generated an extensive list of subcategories for each condition based on a keyword search using a metathesaurus. Two sites prompted the entry of condition-specific information related to associated symptoms, etiology, diagnosis, and treatment. Sites that did not make use of lists relied on free-text entry.

The range of descriptive information requested for each medical condition was limited. Eight sites asked patients to enter the date of onset of each medical condition, four asked about the physician or provider responsible for treating each condition, and three asked about the actual treatment prescribed for each condition.

## Medications

Three sites directed patients to select medications from lists, with two generating listings based on keyword searches. Sites that did not make use of lists relied on free-text entry. A wide range of descriptive information was requested for each medication. Ten sites asked patients to enter the prescribed dose for each medication, seven asked about the frequency of administration, and five asked about starting dates for each medication. Four sites asked about the pharmacy that issued each medication, four asked about the provider responsible for prescribing each medication, and three asked whether each medication was a past or current prescription.

## Laboratory Tests

Nine sites allowed patients to enter information about laboratory tests. Two sites were set up to import results from outside sources, although only one was fully functional at the time of review. Six sites directed patients to select laboratory tests from lists. Sites that did not make use of lists relied on free-text entry. A limited range of descriptive information was requested for each laboratory test. Six sites asked patients to enter a date and result for each test. Results were entered as free text without quantification of units or reference ranges. Only one site asked

patients to identify the provider responsible for ordering each test.

## Diagnostic Studies

Four sites allowed patients to enter information about diagnostic studies. One site directed patients to select diagnostic studies from a list, whereas the others relied on free-text entry. All four sites asked patients to enter a date and result for each study. Results were entered as free text. Only one site asked patients to identify the provider responsible for ordering each study.

## Immunizations

Each site allowed patients to enter information related to immunizations. Seven sites directed patients to select different types of immunizations from lists, whereas the others relied on free-text entry. Nine sites asked patients to enter a date for each immunization. Three sites allowed patients to indicate whether a specific dose was part of a series. Three sites asked patients to identify the provider responsible for administering each immunization. None of the sites requested any information about specific antibody titers.

## Utility

At a basic level of representation, 5 of the 11 PHRs selected for review incorporated all the data elements needed to manage a simple problem based on the results of objective laboratory tests. Two of these sites were plagued by technical problems that hampered the display of medication information. One was unable to express doses of prescribed medications in micrograms or fractions of milligrams, whereas the other failed to display any values at all. One PHR that relied on the importation of laboratory test results from an outside source was unable to display the full range of results entered in its profile. Four of the remaining PHRs presented accurate medication information without any associated test results. One PHR failed to incorporate any of the essential data elements.

At a more comprehensive level of representation, only 1 of the 11 PHRs selected for review incorporated all the elements needed to provide a complete clinical history. Each of the others was missing at least one critical element. The most uniformly represented elements were listings of immunizations that appeared in designated profiles. Nine PHRs included listings that reported hepatitis A and hepatitis B immunizations, although only four allowed for specification of doses in a series. Five PHRs incorporated complete sets of laboratory test and diagnostic study results, including scanned or entered summaries of biopsy and radiographic study reports. Six PHRs documented a history of treatment with interferon-alpha. Only one PHR included temporal information that linked treatment with interferon-alpha to the development of autoimmune thyroiditis.

## Discussion

Overall, the patient-entered PHRs we selected for evaluation demonstrated limited functionality. At a basic level, each site did manage to provide Web-based access to personal medical information. A minority of these sites extended this capacity to provide access to information in emergency situations. This finding was surprising in light of the emphasis placed on this mode of access in the promotion of these applications.

Many of the functions we evaluated were compromised by limitations related to the process of data entry and validation. Each site required patients to select entries from lists or to type information into text fields without much in the way of guidance or explanation. There were no mechanisms to direct patients through the process of selecting appropriate diagnoses. None of the sites provided any directions to help guide patients through the process of abstracting relevant information from prescription labels or test reports. Even simple functions that might ensure greater accuracy, such as spell-checking typed entries or identifying normal dose and reference ranges, were notably lacking. With few exceptions, there were no systems to verify information abstracted from test and study reports. Limited ranges of descriptive information further compromised entries that might be called into question.

Evaluation from a clinical perspective using the example of a test case demonstrated that the PHRs we selected for review provided varying representations of information at increasing levels of complexity. Given the range of information that could be entered, it was surprising that most of these records failed to include the basic data elements needed to manage one of the simpler problems encountered in outpatient medicine. Evaluation at a comprehensive level demonstrated that any inherent deficiencies of representation became magnified in proportion to the number of data elements included in a clinical history. Those PHRs that included listings of infor-

mation kept different elements segregated in discrete sections without problem-based integration. Actual use of information in clinical practice would require abstraction and rearrangement of elements to provide context for analysis.

The criteria for evaluation outlined in this review set high standards for accuracy and validation. Questions might arise as to whether patient-oriented applications need to be this exacting. Although PHRs may primarily be viewed as an extension of the technologic capacity of the Internet, in truth they appear to embody a new representation of medical information. Despite claims that point to their potential for use in tracking and guiding personal health care, their status as an informational resource is yet to be defined.

When held to the rigorous standards of provider-entered records, PHRs reveal deficiencies and limitations that cast doubt on whether they will ever be able serve as effective primary resources. Of principal concern is the fact that the entire process of data entry assumes that individuals can accurately categorize and prioritize their own medical information. No documented studies have examined the question of whether this strategy is feasible or efficacious.

Additional concerns may be raised by the potential for misrepresentation of patient-entered information. Most currently available PHRs are organized along the lines of standard provider-entered charts. Lists presented for selection use standard medical terminology to describe diagnoses, medications, and laboratory tests. Printed summaries convey an air of medical sophistication. In many respects they appear to be indistinguishable from standardized records used by service agencies and chronic care facilities. There are no signifiers that indicate that the information presented is entirely patient-entered. This lack of distinction raises the serious issue of whether printed summaries of PHRs may be mistaken for provider-entered records.

Strategies to improve performance may vary, depending on the intended uses of future applications. If PHRs are scaled back to provide limited medical history and prescription information, efforts might focus on methods of registering information. At one extreme, providers might be asked to work with patients to supervise the creation of individual profiles. Other approaches might focus on abstraction of information from billing records or pharmacy databases. If PHRs continue to be promoted as entities that mirror the full content of standard institutional records, challenges for refinement will be much greater. At a basic level, patients will need to be guided through the process of sorting through information to determine which elements warrant inclusion. Methods will need to be developed to verify the accuracy of entered information. Logical approaches might focus on optimizing user interfaces to increase accuracy.

The approach we adopted in completing this assessment had certain limitations. Our evaluation of clinical utility was based on a single test case that focused on specialized domains of endocrinology and hepatology. In an effort to overcome the limitations of this approach, output was stratified and analyzed at different levels of representation to reflect the concerns of primary care providers and medical subspecialists.

Questions might arise as to whether information entry performed by a clinically experienced operator provided a realistic simulation of the prospective use of these applications by real patients. Our goal in adopting this approach was directed toward optimizing the accuracy and efficiency of information entry to provide a reliable standard for comparison of representations of data elements. This may have led to overestimation of the functionality of these applications, since the accuracy of information entered by real patients would probably vary to a greater extent with differing levels of knowledge and experience.

Further research should focus on the evaluation of test cases explicitly limited to the entry of data elements that patients are likely to be able to self-report with acceptable degrees of accuracy. It remains to be seen whether PHRs generated by real patients can provide enough reliable information to serve as basic representations of medical information.

## Conclusion

The data entry, validation, and information display methods employed by currently available PHRs may limit their ability to serve as adequate representations of medical information for use in clinical practice. Future development of PHRs should be guided by patient-oriented research targeted to evaluate the performance and usability of evolving applications.


*References* ■

1. Spragins E. Get it in writing. Newsweek. Aug 24, 1998:62.
2. Personal and Family Health History. AMA Health Insight Web site. 1997. Available at: http://www.ama-assn.org/insight/yourhlth/per_ hlth/per_hlth.htm. Accessed Jul 2000.
3. Maintaining a treasure chest: your health record. University of Nebraska Cooperative Extension Web site. 1999. Available at: http://www.ianr.unl.edu/pubs/consumered/hef481.htm. Accessed Jul 2000.
4. Savard M. The Savard Health Record: A Six-Step System for Managing Your Healthcare. Alexandria, Va.: Time-Life, 2000.
5. Ryan MA. Maintain your medical records. Today's Chemist at Work. 1999;8(8):49–50, 52–53.
6. MyBodyBook.com Web site. Available at: http://www.mybodybook.com. Accessed Sep 2000.
7. CancerOption.com Web site. Available at: http://www.canceroption.com/capmed/index.asp. Accessed September 2000.
8. Putting patients at the center. Internet Health Care Web site. 2000. Available at: http://www.internethealthcaremag.com/html/current/050100_1.htm. Accessed Jul 2000.
9. Winters R. Your vital signs online. Time. Feb 28, 2000:G4.
10. Rashbass J. The patient-owned, population-based electronic medical record: a revolutionary resource for clinical medicine. JAMA. 200;285(13):1765.
11. Personal communication with Nelson Hazeltine, iVista Group. Oct 24, 2000.
12. Waegermann CP. Consumer-driven health care records [lecture]. Presented at: TEPR 2001; Boston, Mass.; May 11, 2001.
13. Permanent record: allowing patients to post their own medical records on the Internet is becoming big business. American Medical News Web Site. 1999. Available at: http://www.ama-assn.org/sci-pubs/amnews/pick_99/biza1108.htm. Accessed Feb 2001.
14. Online Consumer Health Records: Revolution or Confusion? Journal of AHIMA Web site. 2000. Available at: http://www.ahima.org/journal/features/feature.0003.2.html. Accessed Sep 2000.
15. California emergency physicians medical group and PersonalMD introduce online medical records to state's emergency departments. PersonalMD, Inc. Web site. 2001. Available at: http://www.personalmd.com/pressCEP_article.shtml. Accessed Mar 2001.
16. Can the Web save disease management? Healthcare Informatics Online Web site. 2000. Available at: http://www.healthcareinformatics.com/issues/2000/03_00/cover.htm. Accessed Sep 2000.
17. Tsai CC, Starren J. Patient participation in electronic medical records. JAMA. 2001;285(13):1765.
18. Cohn W. PM Health Heritage: development and evaluation of a family health history collection and assessment tool [lecture]. Presented at: TEPR 2001; Boston, Mass.; May 11, 2001.
19. Hertz CG, Bernheim JW, Perloff TN. Patient participation in the problem-oriented system: a health care plan. Med Care. 1976;14(1):77–9.
20. Hetzel MR, Williams IP, Shakespeare RM. Can patients keep their own peak-flow records reliably? Lancet. 1979;1(8116):597–9.
21. Miller SA. A trial of parent held child health records in the armed forces. BMJ. 1990;300(6731):1046.
22. Dickey LL, Petitti D. A patient-held minirecord to promote adult preventive care. J Fam Pract. 199;34(4):457–63.
23 Cimino JJ, Li J, Mendonca EA, Sengupta S, Patel VL, Kushniruk AW. An evaluation of patient access to their electronic medical records via the World Wide Web. Proc AMIA Symp. 2000:151–5.
24. Jones R, Pearson J, McGregor S, et al. Randomised trial of personalised computer based information for cancer patients. BMJ. 1999;319(7219):1241–7.
25. Masys DR, Baker DB. Patient-Centered Access to Secure

Systems Online (PCASSO): a secure approach to clinical data access via the World Wide Web. Proc AMIA Annu Fall Symp. 1997:340-3.

26. Schneider JH. Online personal medical records: Are they reliable for acute/critical care? Crit Care Med. 2001;29(8 suppl):196-201.

27. Koh LK, Greenspan FS, Yeo PP. Interferon-alpha induced thyroid dysfunction: three clinical presentations and a review of the literature. Thyroid. 1997;7(6):891-6.

28. Fernandez-Soto L, Gonzalez A, et al. Increased risk of autoimmune thyroid disease in hepatitis C vs. hepatitis B before, during, and after discontinuing interferon therapy. Arch Intern Med. 1998;158(13):1445-8.

29. Pianko S, McHutchison JG. Treatment of hepatitis C with interferon and ribavirin. J Gastroenterol Hepatol. 2000;15(6): 581-6.

# Building a Controlled Health Vocabulary in Japanese

Y. Liu, Y. Satomura
Division of Medical Informatics, Chiba University Hospital, Japan

## Summary

*Objectives:* This study is aimed at developing a controlled clinical vocabulary for use in electronic patient record (EPR) systems.

*Methods:* In this paper, we propose a model for building the vocabulary. The model is composed of a Canonical Term Dictionary, an Atom Dictionary, a Composite Atom Dictionary, and an Index. Parsing and composing functions are included in this model. Canonical terms were extracted from reference terminologies. Atoms were extracted from the Canonical Term Dictionary and reduced to a set from which the Composite Atom Dictionary can be built. The index was built to link these two dictionaries. For testing the model, we compiled a sample vocabulary and applied the model to a SNOMED translation system (English to Japanese) and a term similarity estimation system.

*Results:* The sample vocabulary consisted of 15,600 atomic terms and 4,450 composite terms. 33,441 SNOMED terms were translated by the SNOMED translation system. The system gave adequate Japanese candidates in 56.3% of cases. The similarity estimation system found an average of 5.4 candidates when the equality ratio was over 50%.

*Conclusions:* The trial applications produced good results. The model seems promising for building a standard clinical vocabulary system. This system can be applied in certain other Asian countries, such as China and Korea.

## Keywords

Controlled Vocabulary, Medical Dictionary, Terminology, Translations, Standards

Method Inform Med 2001; 40: 307–14

## 1. Introduction

Standard health terminology is an essential platform for advanced health information systems, particularly for the application of electronic health records (EHR) [1]. Several dominating methods to establish general health terminology and nomenclature exist in the USA and UK, such as SNOMED, UMLS and Read [2-4]. Although the Japanese medical society has taken measures to standardize health terminology in the last fifty years, the focus has been on nomenclature alone, without semantic structure, for coordination with English representation.

The Ministry of Health and Welfare (MHW) launched a project in 1994, to promote the use of electronic health record systems and has supported the development of a standardized terminology. This has led to the compilation of terminology sets, such as a disease terminology, procedure and clinical examination classifications, and drug and medical materials coding systems. These sets, however, are not consistent in their representation or semantic relationships [5-6]. To use electronic health record systems, users will need access to a consistent generalized vocabulary systems for their ease-of-use and efficient EHR data exchange.

In this paper, the authors propose a structured vocabulary system based on this Japanese health terminology environment.

## 2. Terminology Model

The model is composed of a Canonical Term Dictionary, an Atom Dictionary, a Composite Atom Dictionary and an Index. The functions of parsing and composing are included in this model. The general structure of this model is shown in Fig. 1.

## 2.1 Dictionaries and Index

1) Canonical Term Dictionary: We collected canonical terms from a number of reference terminology sources and linked them to original references. The terms, stemming from reference terminologies (diagnosis, procedure, examination, drug & pharmacology and healthcare materials), were compiled into a standardized representation under rules normalizing the character code and the use of punctuation and parentheses.

2) Atomic Term Dictionary (Atom Dictionary): An atomic term (atom) is a language element that identifies a single idea. Such an entity can not be broken down further without losing meaning [5]. The atoms were selected from the Canonical Term Dictionary.

3) Composite Atom Dictionary: Multiple atoms are compounded to represent a concept in a particular domain. We selected composite atoms that are frequently used in medical texts to build this dictionary.

4) Index: Canonical terms can be broken into atoms and composite atoms. The Index is a set of permutations of these elements (atoms and composite atoms), as shown in Fig. 2. The Index inherits classification information from original reference terminology (e.g. ICD-10). In this model, we call this information the Class Code.

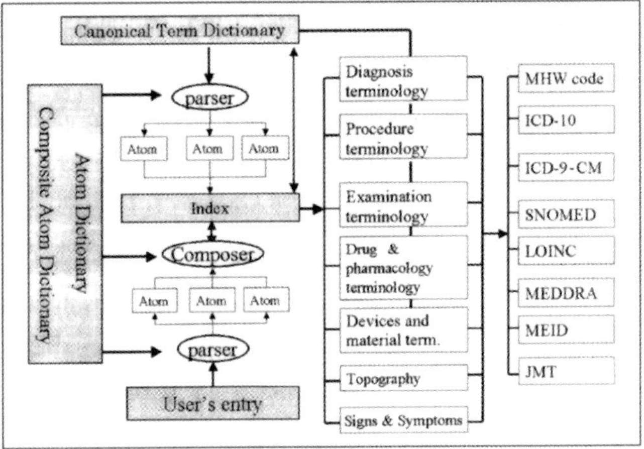

**Fig. 1** The structure of the system (Model)
The Model is composed of an Atom Dictionary, a Composite Atom Dictionary, a Canonical Term Dictionary and an Index. The canonical terms are extracted from reference terminologies. Atoms are extracted from the Canonical Term Dictionary. The combinations of Atoms, which are frequently used in medical texts, are collected to build a Composite Atom Dictionary. Canonical term can be separated into Atoms and composite atoms. The Index is a set of permutations of these elements. There are two functions in this model: parsing and composing. They work to relate these dictionaries.

## 2.2 Functions

1) Parsing: Parsing divides the object term into atoms and composite atoms.
2) Composing: When users enter a certain medical concept, they will use a familiar term without thinking whether it is a canonical term. In order to exchange data and to access reference terminology, the entry should be altered to a canonical term. In this system, the entry is divided to atoms, which are then combined and matched in the Index.

## 3. Resources

1) SNOMED (Ver. 3.4): SNOMED (Systematized Nomenclature of Human and Veterinary Medicine) is a nomenclature that allows comprehensive patient description [7]. It can be considered relatively domain-complete. SNOMED terms are assigned to one of eleven independent systematized modules. Within each module, terms are placed in their natural hierarchies and are assigned a five-or six-digit alphanumeric code.

The SNOMED separates terms into "atomic" units. The units are organized into chapters or "axes", which can be combined to form complex concept [4].
2) MEID: The Medical Intelligent Dictionary (MEID) is a bilingual dictionary (Japanese-English) of medical terms, containing medical and linguistic information and about 230,000 terms. The MEID was compiled with the cooperation of a diverse range of experts (physicians, computer scientists, library and publishing professionals, etc.) in 1989 [8].
3) Japan Medical Terminology (JMT): This terminology set was completed by the Japanese Association of Medical Sciences in 1994. The terminology set took about 10 years to develop and includes about 64,000 terms relevant to the medical and other scientific fields, such as pharmacology, physics, agriculture, engineering. It provides the formal representation of Japanese medical terms [9].
4) Japanese Diagnosis Terminology is in accordance with ICD-10 (ICD-10J): This terminology set was put together by the Medical Information System Development Center (MEDIS) for representing clinical disease names. It includes 28,000 diagnostic identifiers in ICD10 class code. It was published in 1997 [10].

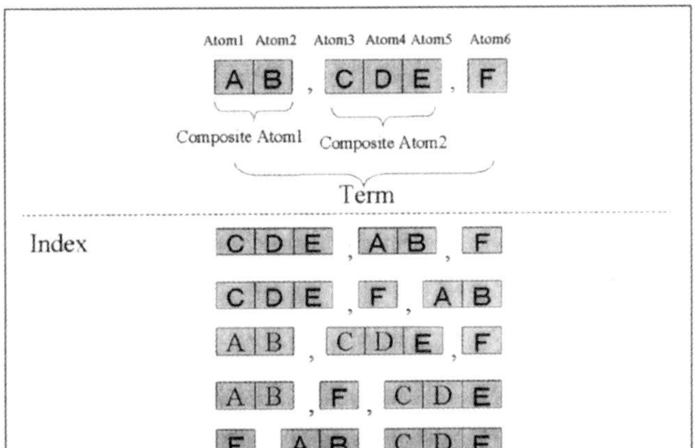

## 4. Japanese Health Terms

1) The Japanese written language uses three sets of characters. Also, texts frequently contain words written in both the Latin and Japanese alphabet. The three Japanese character sets are kanji, hiragana, and katakana. Kanji characters are the ideograms that originally came from China. They are quite similar to contemporary Chinese hanzi. There are about two thousand kanji used in daily Japanese, plus about three thousand used in technical-scientific Japanese. Kanji are mostly roots of verbs, nouns, adjectives, and adverbs. There are about fifty hiragana. These are mainly conjunctions and prepositions

**Fig. 2**
A term is parsed into possible permutations of elements (Atoms and composite atoms) to create the Index.

(which are known as "jyoshi" and are placed after nouns) and in verb conjugations. There are also about fifty katakana, which are used mainly for the Japanese representation of foreign words [27].

2) Spaces are not used to separate words.

3) A Japanese term composed entirely of kanji (80% medical terms are of this type) can be divided into atoms by character. Every kanji character has its own meaning. A Kanji character is the same as a word in English. Several characters or compound characters are used to represent one concept. Sometimes the meaning of individual characters may change when part of such a composition. The same concept can also be represented by several different compositions of characters.

4) Japanese medical concepts primarily come from western medicine, although some come from eastern medicine (Chinese medicine).

# 5. Atom Dictionary

## 5.1 The Function of Atoms

When analyzing a Latin alphabetic sentence, the parser can easily identify words, because they are separated by spaces. In Japanese, however, the parser must analyze character by character, concatenating with the next character, and then look at dictionaries to see if it is a meaningful basic unit, or atom. A term is composed of several atoms, which are composed to represent one concept. For example:

Term1 = A + B + C (A, B, C are atoms)

Term2 = B + C + A' (A ≑ A') (A and A' are synonymous)

Term3 = C + B' + A (B ≑ B')

All three terms represent the same single concept, even though the positions of the atoms differ between terms. The meanings of the atoms are composed to create a single concept [11].

## 5.2 Properties of Atom Dictionary

a. Atoms represent the basic concept of a unit.

b. Atoms retain the information inherited from the original reference terminology.

c. Atoms include speech information.

d. Atoms have domain information (Domain Code).

e. Atoms include information about inflection or conjugation for the English language, however, this is not necessary for the Japanese language.

f. Atoms hold both English and Japanese representations.

g. Atoms have synonyms in the dictionary, including abbreviations, colloquialisms, and acronyms. Priority terms should be defined.

# 6. Composite Atom Dictionary

Composition is an important and necessary part for a controlled vocabulary system. Atoms are usually composed to represent a concept in a particular domain [13]. These composite atoms can be expressed through these atoms. For example, the concept "言語中枢" (language center) is divided into two atoms; "言語" (language) and "中枢" (center). The term "language center" may be used often, whereas the individual atoms may occur only rarely, if at all. To build this dictionary, we selected composite atoms that are used frequently in medical texts.

# 7. Specific Terms: Group and Table

a. Linking terms: There are many linking terms such as "by," "and," and "for," (in Japanese; 〜による，〜と，〜ために that link one word to another. We collected these linking terms into a special group. Some of these terms are semantically redundant when a term is parsed or atoms are composed into a new term [14].

b. Character Exchange Table: In Japanese, one meaning may be represented by different compositions of characters, each with different kanji (i.e. Shift-Jiscode or Unicode). Thus, a priority character should be defined to represent a given concept. (It is necessary to check if a particular kanji is used correctly to represent an intended concept.) As similar meanings with different character compositions are frequently used in texts, when parsing a term, this table should be checked and any non-standard characters should be exchanged with the priority characters [11-12].

# 8. Trial Applications

When users input an entry freely into an EPR system, the vocabulary system should translate the entry into canonical terms. If the action fails, a list of possible alternatives should be generated. Therefore, we developed two applications for testing the reliability of the model; the SNOMED translation system and the similarity estimation system.

## 8.1 Sample Vocabulary

Before the test systems were developed, we constructed a sample vocabulary. The sample vocabulary consisted of an Atom Dictionary (15,600 atomic terms), a Composite Atom Dictionary (4,450 terms), 220,800 MEID terms (English and Japanese), and 84 linking terms.

### 8.1.1 Building the Atom Dictionary

a. Atoms from SNOMED
We selected SNOMED as the main resource to build the Atom Dictionary.

1) Why SNOMED?: a) It allows comprehensive patient description. b) It has an alphabetic index with terms separated into atomic units. c) It has domain information. d) SNOMED, version 2, has been partly translated into Japanese in the MEID. There are about 50,000 terms included in the MEID [8].

**Table 1** The result of SNOMED translation (English to Japanese). 33,441 SNOMED records were entered. 9,438 terms were found in the MEID dictionary, the system found single or plural candidates in 56.3%.

| Type of hit | Number of hits | Rate(%) |
|---|---|---|
| Identical | 9,438 | 28.2 |
| Presented candidates | 18,836 | 56.3 |
| Failed | 5,167 | 15.5 |
| Total | 33,441 | 100 |

2) Methods: First, we divided the SNOMED records (D-Axis) into words and then sorted them in order of their frequency of use in SNOMED. There were 9500 words that were used more than 4 times in SNOMED (D-Axis). These were selected as a tentative atom set. English words were assumed to be atoms, which is not entirely correct because some English words do not retain their medical connotation when taken out of context. On the contrary, some English words can be separated into two or more atoms when translated into Japanese. Therefore, the English words selected are tentative. These words were then translated into Japanese. They may be translated into several different Japanese representations according to the context in which they are used. Therefore, medical experts should review the translations. Each translation was given the following contextual information: a) Domain Code, (identical to the SNOMED module), such as D – Disease, F – Function, b) speech representation, and c) priority sequence, which was used to list the Japanese translation according to priority.

b. Atoms from other sources
As some special Japanese terms (such as some Chinese medicine concepts) do not exist in SNOMED, they should be obtained from other resources. We assembled some atoms from ICD-10J, JMT. We took 1,890 terms from ICD-10J and 3,410 terms from JMT.

### 8.1.2 Building the Composite Atom Dictionary and Index

Composite Atoms were selected automatically from the MEID and JMT, consisting of two to four atoms and used in over five different medical concepts. Additionally, 220,800 MEID Japanese terms were parsed and permuted into combinations of atoms and composite atoms. They were then linked to the original terms and their classification information. The product of this process was the Index.

## 8.2 SNOMED Translation (into Japanese) System

### 8.2.1 Translation Process (as shown in Fig. 3)

a. The terms are divided into atoms and composite atoms.
b. The system translates these terms using the Atom Dictionary and the Composite Atom Dictionary. As each atom may have several different Japanese translations, the best translation is selected by referring to priority, speech, and classification information.
c. As the word order in English and Japanese differs, the words and phrases are transposed into Japanese word order.
d. When the computer outputs more than one option, a human expert selects the best translation and adjusts the word order if necessary.

### 8.2.2 Translation Results

This system was used to translate 33,441 SNOMED terms (D-Axis). 28.2% of the translations were found in the MEID. The system gave adequate Japanese candidates in 56.3% of cases, however, 15.5% terms failed to produce a result (Table 1). The

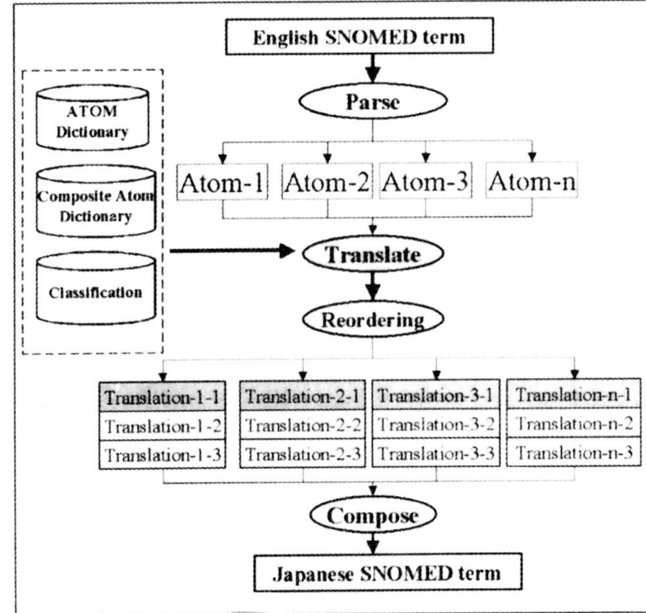


**Fig. 3** SNOMED translation system (process)
(1) The terms are divided into elements (atoms and composite atoms). (2) The system translates these terms using the Atom Dictionary and Composite Atom Dictionary. As each atom may has several different Japanese translations, the best one is selected by referring to the priority, speech and classification information. (3) As the word orders in English and Japanese, the words and phrases are transposed into Japanese word order. (4) Should the computer output more than one candidate, a human expert selects the best translation and the word order is adjusted if necessary.

translation rate was increased by about 56% over simply finding a term in the MEID.

We applied the system to a random sample of 100 cases in order to evaluate how correctly the system works when checked by medical experts. The results were as follows: 62 cases were translated correctly without human intervention, 17 cases needed adjustment by manual selection of appropriate Japanese terms from a list of candidates. New Japanese words were required in 21 cases, because the system did not provide appropriate Japanese terms in correspondence to the English elements (atom and composite atoms).

A sample of the output is shown in Fig. 4.

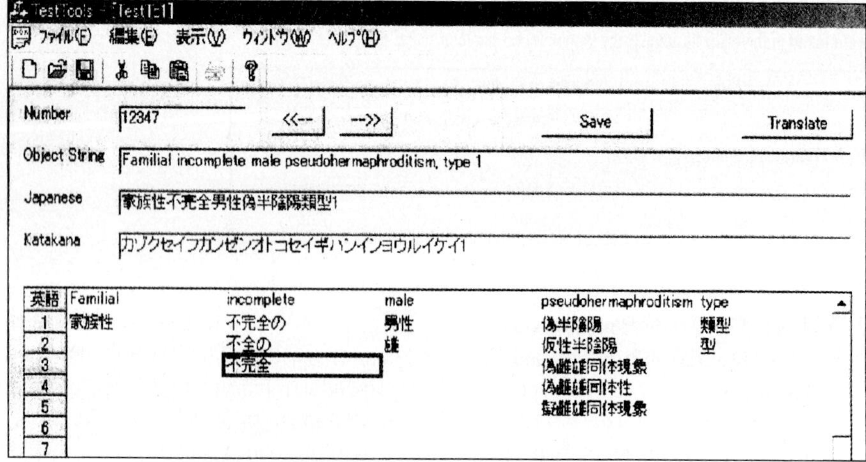

**Fig. 4**   A sample output of SNOMED translation
The string-"Familial incomplete male pseudohermaphroditism, type1" was translated to what is displayed in the third line (Japanese), the fourth line (Katakana) shows the phonetic representation, and several different translations are given in each English words (Atoms).

## 8.3 Similarity Estimation System

Similarity estimation is an essential tool for editing a dictionary by which the editor can find hidden similar terms from a tremendous number of terms. When a useful canonical term or atom is selected for presenting a particular concept from references, it is necessary to find all similar terms and estimate their similarity in order to help experts easily find the best translation. Furthermore, when a user entry is parsed, similar terms should be found and exchanged with the free entry to provide a canonical term. We developed a similarity estimation system and applied it to disease names in order to test the model.

### 8.3.1 Algorithm for Similarity Estimation

Before estimating the similarity of an object term, a number of preparatory steps are necessary:

1) Processes such as checking the Character Exchange Table should be completed. 2) The object term should be divided into atoms by referring to the Atom Dictionary. 3) All terms that have at least one atom in common with the object term are selected from the Index. These terms comprise the basic group, or preliminary candidates. 4) The similarity of each term in the basic group to the object term is estimated by the following algorithm [15]:

Step 1. By Morphology: The characters of the two terms are compared. A higher ratio of matching characters in both terms corresponds to a higher similarity.

Step 2. By Atom: The atoms of the two terms are compared. A higher ratio of matching atoms in both terms corresponds to a higher similarity.

Step 3. By Classification: The Class Code of the two terms is compared. If a high similarity between the terms was confirmed in step 1 or 2, and they have a Class Code (SNOMED code or ICD10 code), the parent and brother code in SNOMED or ICD10 are selected.

### 8.3.2 Results of Similarity Estimation

Ten thousand disease names of the Chiba University Hospital System were taken to estimate similarity using the above algorithm.

a. Estimating similarity by morphology (Table 2)

When the equality ratio between two terms was over 40% and less than 50%, the average number of candidates generated was 59.1 terms. For equality ratios over 50%, the average number of candidates dropped to 6.3. For ratios over 60%, an average of 4.7 was found, while, for ratios over 70%, the average number decreased to 1. The minimum adequate equality ratio appears to be > 60% for efficiently estimating similarity by morphology.

b. Estimating similarity by atom (Table 3)

On average, 6.6 candidates were generated when not less than two atoms common to both terms were available. An average of 5.4 candidates was found when the equality ratio was over 50%. When the equality ratio exceeded 50% and there were two or more common atoms, 3.2 candidates were generated on average. In this trial, terms with more than 5 atoms were excepted.

c. Estimating similarity by classification

Terms with equality ratios of over 70% by morphology and more than two common atoms were chosen. The class

**Table 2**

Morphological analysis applied to 10,000 Chiba-University disease terminology terms. Average number of candidates is reduced by higher threshold ratio.

| The equality ratio(%) | Average number of candidates |
|---|---|
| >40 | 59.1 |
| >50 | 6.3 |
| >60 | 4.7 |
| >70 | 1.0 |

| The equality ratio(%) | Average number of candidates |
|---|---|
| >=2* | 6.6 |
| >50% | 5.4 |
| >50% & >=2 | 3.2 |

*Not less than two atoms existing in both terms.

**Table 3**
Composed Atom analysis applied to 10,000 Chiba-University disease terminology terms. These three ratios give a practical number of candidate terms.

| Condition | | Miss ratio(%) |
|---|---|---|
| Morphology (%) | Atom | |
| >60 | >=2* | 28.78 |
| >50 | >=2 | 25.92 |
| >40 | >=2 | 7.07 |

*Not less than two atoms existing in both terms.

**Table 4**
The result of the ratio of missing candidate. The miss ratio was listed according to the condition (the equality ration in morphology and the equal numbers in atom).

code was obtained for these terms (if they had classification information) and the parents and brothers were generated as candidates. Averages of 21.4 candidates were generated per object term.

d. Miss Ratio (Table 4)
We estimated the ratio of instances for which the system found no candidate under several conditions. Conditions we applied were: not less than two common atoms and several morphological equality ratios. The miss rate was 28.8% for morphological equality ratios over 60% and 25.9% for those over 50%. When we applied ratios over 40%, the miss rate was reduced to 7.1%.

e. As shown in Fig. 5, we applied these estimation processes in this trial, given a certain condition. The result is the average number of extracted candidate for one term was 5.3, and one or more candidates were presented in 70%.

# 9. Discussion

## 9.1 Comparison to other Models

a. Conceptual graph: Concept-oriented models represent complex relationships between concepts and map conceptual graphs [16-20]. However, the selection of an adequate and useful concept is an exhaustive issue. Building a full relationship between concepts, as well as bridging the gap between the "language of the texts" and "the language of concepts", might require tremendous expert effort.

b. Semantic network: Cimino et al. have developed a knowledge-based representation for a controlled terminology of clinical information called the Medical Entities Dictionary (MED). The MED utilizes a semantic network model that

includes a classification hierarchy. Each concept is a node and relates to other nodes in the network [21-24]. The MED is a complex data structure that might require extensive effort to create and maintenance.

## 9.2 Features of this Model

a. Facilitating creation and vocabulary maintenance
The Atom Dictionary is relatively compact and easier to build than a conceptual graph or semantic network. The vocabulary system of this model does not require definitions of semantic relationships between atoms, and combinations of atoms can be made to correspond to the original terms. It contains no intentionally generated semantic information, passively inheriting from the source reference terminology. Canonical terms in the controlled vocabulary are extracted from many reference terminology sources. When new reference terminology is added to the vocabulary, the records of the new reference terms are matched in the existing vocabulary and new canonical terms are added if they are not found. These new canonical terms are also parsed and divided to atoms. If a new atom is found, it will be added to the Atom Dictionary. The index is then rebuilt and linked with the new reference terminology. This process could be completed almost automatically.

b. Practicality for Japanese language
Speech information is very important in an English vocabulary, whereas it is not in Japanese. Almost all medical concepts can be represented by nouns, without declension. After a Japanese term is parsed, the fundamental meaning can easily be obtained by referring to the Atom Dictionary. In Japanese, each kanji character in a term has an autonomous meaning. It is difficult to assess the similarity of these characters by checking character-by-character as many similar terms will be generated. However, if terms are analyzed by referring to the Atom Dictionary, the fundamental meaning can easily be obtained and an

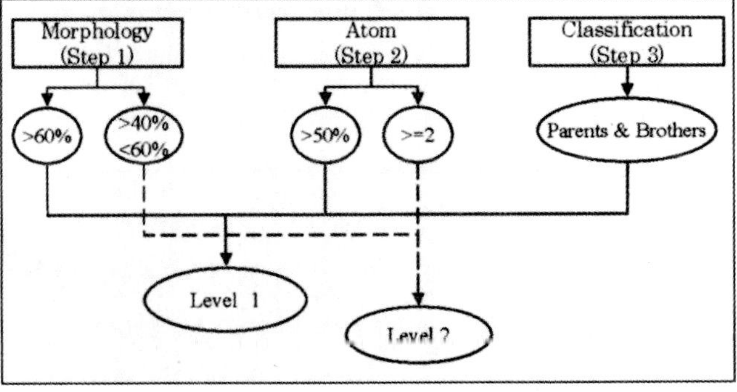


**Fig. 5**
Algorithm for estimating the similarity
The conditions given to each of the three steps for extracting similar terms from sample vocabulary are presented. The test was executed on 10,000 disease names used in the Chiba University Hospital.

effective set of similar terms will be presented.

## 9.3 Existing Problems

1) Atom Selection

There are several problems in selecting atoms. Every Japanese kanji character has an autonomous meaning, however a concept is commonly represented by a composition of several characters. Different kanji characters can also represent the same concept. The same composition of characters can also have a different meaning in a different domain.

There are two methods for solving these problems:

a. If a term has a different meaning in another domain, it is difficult to make the differentiation while parsing the term. Therefore, this kind of term should not be selected as an atom. Such a character is accepted in connection with neighbor characters to make a concrete and unique concept.

b. Priority order: It is necessary to select the most appropriate option, since several different atoms can represent a single medical concept in a particular domain. Therefore, an order of priority should be given to these atoms. This process requires the intervention of medical experts.

2) Limitation

Atoms do not contain cross-reference information or conceptual relationships. The Index contains only links to original reference terminology [25]. The SNOMED and ICD-10 class code is simply linked to the Index. The limitations of the original class code also limit the classification information used in this model. The developer of SNOMED (CAP) has entered into a collaboration with NHS to combine SNOMED and Clinical Terms Version 3 (Read Codes V3). The new project, SNOMED CT [28], may provide a tremendous amount of semantic information, as this model will be able to fully reflect source knowledge.

## 9.4 Expected Applications

a. Use in EPR: Clinical data stored in an EPR system should be described using standardized terminology. Free user entry can be translated into canonical terms when sufficient sets of synonyms have been prepared in the Atom Dictionary.

b. A literature retrieval system: This model can be applied to key word selection for scientific literature retrieval. It can also parse the entered term and generate several appropriate or similar key words in the retrieval system.

c. Translation of a terminology in accordance with one classification scheme to a new terminology under another scheme. For example, from ICD9 to ICD10 [14].

## 10. Conclusion

The system defined by this model will contain less semantic information than other systems. The depth of semantic information will be enriched, however, when new reference terminology or classification schemes are entered. The vocabulary of this model can easily be created and maintained using established reference terminologies. There are many terminologies and classifications for specific areas, which are needed to produce a comprehensive document like an EPR. A standard vocabulary system, as proposed by this model, is a promising way to solve these problems [26].

This system can be applied in certain other Asian countries, such as China and Korea, where kanji-based medical terms are used.

## References


1. Hammond WE. Call for a Standard Clinical Vocabulary. JAMIA 1997; 4: 254-5.
2. O'Neil MJ, Payne C, Read JD. Read Codes Version 3: A User Led Terminology. Meth Inform Med 1995; 34: 187-92.
3. National library of medicine. Unified Medical Language System 11th edition. NLM; 2000.
4. Cote RA, Rothwell DJ, Palotay JL, Beckett RS, Brochu L, eds. The Systematized Nomenclature of Human and Veterinary Medicine: SNOMED International. College of American Pathologists 1993.
5. Satomura Y, Liu YB, et al. A structured Japanese medical Terminology aiming at CPR system. AMIA WG6 conference Washington D.C. 1999.
6. American Society for Testing and Materials. Standard Guide for Construction of a Clinical Nomenclature for Support of Electronic Health Records. ASTM E-1284-97.
7. Campbell JR, Carpenter P, et al. Phase II Evaluation of Clinical Coding Schemes: Completeness, Taxonomy, Mapping, Definitions, and Clarity. JAMIA 1997; 4: 238-51.
8. Oshima M. Medical Dictionary. Tokyo: Nichigai Associates Inc 1989.
9. Japanese Association of Medical Sciences Committee of Medical Terminology. Japan Medical Terminology. Tokyo: Nanzando Company Limited 1994.
10. Department of MHW Statistical Information. According to the ICD-10 Classification of Mental and Behavioural Disorders. MHW Statistical Association 1995.
11. Liu YB, Satomura Y, et al. Development of Structured Medical Terminology. The 19th Joint Conference on Medial Informatics. Yokohama 1999; 760-1.
12. Satomura Y, Sasaki T. Standard Disease Name Terminology according to ICD-10. Japan Medical Journal 1998; 3876: 23-7.
13. Elkin PL, Tuttle M, Keck K, Campbell K, Atkin G, Chute CG. The Role of Compositionality in Standardized Problem List Generation. MEDINFO 98; 660-4.
14. Satomura Y, Yamazaki S, Sasaki T. According to ICD10 Disease Name Terminology and Auto-coding System. The 15th Joint Conference on Medial Informatics. 1995; 957-60.
15. Liu YB, Satomura Y. Development of the Editing Tools of Medical Terminology. The 18th Joint Conference on Medial Informatics. Kobe, 1998; 372-3.
16. Evans DA, Cimino JJ, Hersh WR, Huff SM, Bell D. Toward a Medical-concept Representation Language. JAMIA 1994; 1: 207-7.
17. Rassinoux AM, Miller RA, Baud RH, Scherrer JR. Modeling Concepts in Medicine for Medical Language Understanding. Meth Inform Med 1998; 37: 361-72.
18. Johnson SB. Conceptual Graph Grammar- A Simple Formalism for Sublanguage. Meth Inform Med 1998; 37: 345-52.
19. Sowa JP. Conceptual Graphs: information processing in mind and machine. Reading MA: Addison Wesley 1984.
20. Rassinoux AM, Miller RA, Baud RH, Scherrer JR. Modeling Concepts in Medicine for Medical Language Understanding. Meth Inform Med 1998; 37: 361-72.
21. MacGregor R. The evolving technology of classification-based knowledge representation systems. Principles of Semantic Networks: Explorations in the Representation of Knowledge. San Mateo, CA: Morgan Kaufmann, 1991; 385-400.

22. Cimino JJ, Clayton PD, Hripcsak G, Johnson SB. Knowledge-based approaches to the maintenance of a Large Controlled Medical Terminology. JAMIA 1994; 1: 35-50.
23. Campbell KE, Das AK, Musen MA. A Logical Foundation for Clinical Data. JAMIA 1994: 1: 218-32.
24. Scherrer JR. Concepts, Knowledge and Language in Healthercare Information Systems: Follow-up 30 Months Later. Meth Inform Med 1998; 37: 312-4.
25. Wiederhold G. Objects and Domains for Managing Medical Data and Knowledge. Method Inform Med 1995; 34: 40-6.
26. Cimino JJ. Desiderata for Controlled Medical Vocabularies in the Twenty-First Century. Method Inform Med 1998; 37: 394-403.
27. Amaral MB, Satomura Y. Processing Natural Language at Chiba University Hospital. M Computing Silver Springs, 1993; 1(4): 6-15.
28. SNOMED CT. http://www.snomed.org/snomedct_txt.html.

Correspondence to:
Ya-bin Liu, M.D.
Division of Medical Informatics
Chiba University Hospital
Inohana 1-8-1, Cyuou-ku, Chiba city
Chiba Province
Japan 260-8677
E-mail: lybmn@ho.chiba-u.ac.jp

# Section 3:



*Reprinted by kind permission of:*
*American Medical Informatics Association (406, 420),*
*Elsevier Science (391, 431)*

**L. de Assis Moura, Jr.**

Business Development - Health Care
Atech Foundation
São Paulo, Brazil

# Synopsis

# *Health Information Systems*

In recent years the concept of Health Information Systems has evolved from organization-centered to patient-centered systems. There are several reasons for this, but two deserve special attention: a) the need for integration and inter-operability and b) the advent and development of the Internet.

The need for integration at all levels is very clear today, but a long and strenuous pathway had to be opened and paved before it became evident that software applications in healthcare share a common kernel that is essentially centered on the patient and patient data.

Till recently, several good Hospital Information Systems were mostly directed towards administrative and billing purposes. There has been a very distinct but misleading division into clinical and administrative systems. Although for those unfamiliar with health care information that division may make things clear, it applies only to the use people will make of data, but unfortunately usually defines how to collect data, in detriment of other possible and desirable uses.

Collecting and storing data should be done just once, whatever the final purpose may be. Proper data collection is essential for an integral and integrated Health Information System. Applica-

tions within a health care organization must access data from a unified data-repository and use it to generate new data. However, each individual datum should not be entered or stored twice.

Data collection and storage must be assessed carefully and somehow unified if the information system is to fulfill the needs of all stakeholders in the health care organization. This task is not simple. In particular, it requires strategic planning.

The Internet has brought above all a new state-of-mind. Although Health Information Systems have not been able to make full use of all potential aroused by the Internet and its technologies it is self-evident, today, that the patient must be somehow considered when designing Health Information Systems.

Classically, from the 70's to the mid 90's, Information Systems tended to be used internally for organizations to deal with their demands for production automation and enterprise management. The typical systems of that era were designed to be used only by the staff. Clients, partners and suppliers were kept away from the corporate Information System. The Information System was centered on the organization and the organization tended to be self-centered.

A revolution started with the Internet. At first, customers were able to purchase goods from websites that "recognized" the client from previous purchases. Then banks started stimulating "people like us" to use the same Information Systems they used to deny clients only few years ago. Nowadays it is possible to use our own bank's Information System, via the Internet, to assess the profitability of investment funds and then decide what to do.

Healthcare organizations in general recognize the need to treat patients and partners as an active part of the organization and providing proper room for them within their Information Systems.

One interesting point to consider is that there is a difference in view between the healthcare organization and the patient. From the Hospital point of view, a patient-centered heath care Information System is one which is designed around the patient, the data they provide, their needs and their well-being. Most data are available to the patient on line and at their request. However, from the patient viewpoint, a patient-centered system is one which will give them a view of all health Information related to them, wherever such information may be available from.

The Internet provides the means for

making such an Information System available, and that IS a revolution. We are years away from having nationwide fully integrated multi-institution Health Information Systems. However the *seed* has been sown. The combination of Internet concepts, standards and technologies with the awareness that the Health Information System must remain adherent to the organization's needs means a deep change in the way we think, design and deploy Information Systems.

Not surprisingly, the four papers in this section deal directly or indirectly with the concepts outlined above.

The paper by Beuscart-Zephir, Anceaux, Crinquette and Renard, entitled *Integrating Users' Activity Modeling in the Design and Assessment of Hospital Electronic Patient Records: The Example of Anesthesia*, explores the need for revitalizing methods (and concerns) for extracting information from the user that will lead to an Electronic Patient Record that meets the requirements for practical use.

*Generation and Evaluation of Intraoperative Inferences for Automated Health Care Briefings on Patient Status After Bypass Surgery,* by Jordan, McKeown, Concepcion, Feiner and Hatzivassiloglou is a fine example of a system that takes knowledge from the literature and data from the Information System to bring in the information where it is required for decision making.

The paper *Giving Patients Access to Their Medical Records via the Internet: The PCASSO Experience,* by Masys, Baker, Butros and Cowles, deals with the problem of giving patients access to their data. Not only do the technical aspects deserve a great deal of thought but also legal, ethical and moral aspects are very complex indeed. The paper unveils pathways and outlines guidelines for patients to be in control of the data available on themselves. Just for the record, as the paper discusses matters related to denial of access to patient's own data, the reader may like to know that the Brazilian legislation clearly states that all patient data *belongs to the patient* and the health care provider guards the data on the patient's behalf.

Finally, the paper *Strategic Information Management Plans: the Basis for Systematic Information Management in Hospitals,* by A. F. Winter and co-workers, tackles the need for planning strategic, tactical and operational actions in order to cope with a Hospital's complexity and diversity.

The papers in this section are decisive examples that Health Information Systems are increasingly more adherent to results and progressively distant from technical and technological aspects. There is a long way to go till Hospital Information Systems reach the maturity and the integration that has been achieved by IS in other areas, but, then, other areas are not as complex as health care!

Address of the author:
Lincoln de A. Moura Jr.; MSc, PhD
Business Development - Health Care
Atech Foundation
President of SBIS - Brazilian Health Informatics Foundation
President of IMIA-LAC - Regional Federation of Health Informatics for Latin America and the Caribbean
Av Macuco 550, Apartment 72
São Paulo SP 04523-001
Brazil
E-mail:    lamoura@uol.com.br

# Integrating users' activity modeling in the design and assessment of hospital electronic patient records: the example of anesthesia

M.C. Beuscart-Zéphir [a,*], F. Anceaux [b], V. Crinquette [c], J.M. Renard [a]

[a] *Cerim, Faculté de Médecine, Université de Lille 2, Place de Verdun, 59041 Lille, Cedex, France*
[b] *CNRS-UVHC, LAMIH-Equipe Percotec, BP311, F-59304 Valenciennes, Cedex, France*
[c] *Centre Hospitalier Régional et Universitaire de Lille, 59041 Lille, Cedex, France*

**Abstract**

As computers become more and more an aid in the management of medical information, some specialists, such as anesthesiologists, demand tuned applications to support their own activity. The development of these specific applications is based upon the user's requirements analysis, and functional and technical specifications. But some failures show that a better understanding of human factors of acceptance could improve the usability and utility of these tools. In this study, we demonstrated that when the management of medical information is closely intertwined with the physician's activity, it is necessary to perform a precise analysis of this activity in order to identify the cognitive and organizational constraints that affect the usability and acceptance of the tool. We focused our study on the pre-operative anesthetic consultation. After recording and analyzing 50 consultations, we were able to identify the key points to fulfill in order to meet users' acceptance. From this study, we propose some strong recommendations to handle the constraints imposed by the anesthesiologists' activity in their daily working environment. We applied this method to evaluate an electronic patient record (EPR) for the pre-anesthetic consultation. The results of this evaluation validate our hypotheses and the importance of the activity constraints. In conclusion, human factors, and particularly those linked with the activity of healthcare professionals, have to be carefully studied before any development and installation of an EPR into a specialty domain. © 2001 Elsevier Science Ireland Ltd. All rights reserved.

*Keywords:* Usability; Electronic patient record; Anesthesia; Activity modeling; Cognitive ergonomics

## 1. Introduction

In many hospitals, departments, such as emergency, intensive care and anesthesiology, tend to remain cut from the general development of hospital information systems (HIS): they are still badly or not well computerized, at least from the medical information management point of view. However, on the other hand, most of the intensive care or anesthesiology machines (respirators, moni-

---

* Corresponding author.
*E-mail address:* mcbeuscart@univ-lille2.fr (M.C. Beuscart-Zéphir).

tors) have been working with computers for several years. Then, most of the companies providing these machines: Datex-Ohmeda*, Agilent Technology* (Care-Vue), Drager*, Picis* (Care-Suite), Thermaco* (Idacare), progressively developed software applications designed to automatically record the physiological parameters gathered by the machines during intensive care episodes. In the past 10 years, those software were progressively adapted for the anesthetic process during surgery, thus providing the anesthesiologists with an elementary anesthetic patient record, reduced to an archive containing the main physiological parameters automatically recorded during the anesthesia.

Following users' requirements, most of these tools now try to incorporate in their software, some parts devoted to handling medical information during the other phases of the anesthetic process, especially the anesthetic consultation, which takes place 1 week before the surgery. But, according to the vendors of those tools themselves, these parts of the software are difficult to use and meet acceptance problems. Thus, the users who cannot integrate them properly in their daily working environment often reject them.

On the other hand, some prototypes have been developed on a smaller scale, specifically to handle medical information during the anesthetic consultation. These tools are usually developed by a user cooperating with a small company, following a specific demand of a single department of anesthesia. These anesthetic computerized records are usually successfully utilized by the anesthesiologists who created them, but they often fail to spread to other departments of anesthesiology and remain confined to a small amount of users [1,2].

Some evaluation studies have been per-formed in order to assess the efficiency and usability of software applications in intensive care units (ICU) or during the pre-operative anesthetic process [3–5]. Most of these studies focus primarily on establishing time saving due to automated data recording; their methodology relies mainly on task decomposition, allowing them to compare the time spent in performing each elementary task with and without the computer. The results usually confirm time savings [4,5] for the tasks devoted to physiological parameters recording, but they also emphasize usability problems for the sub-tasks dealing with medical information management, such as drug prescriptions and shift changeovers [4]. Then, these authors call for a deeper behavioral and cognitive analysis of users' activity, in order to properly design or redesign the applications.

Probably because they are more recent and not yet disseminated in many anesthesiology departments, software applications specifically designed for the preoperative phase of anesthesia (pre-evaluation or consultation) have hardly been assessed and when they are [1,2,6], the evaluation reveals deep usability or transferability problems.

For example, in a previous study [6], we performed the usability assessment of a prototype named Anesthesia Mobile System (AMS) specifically designed to support direct data entry during the anesthetic consultation. The AMS was developed within the context of a European project (Isar-T), following a standard conception cycle, including an extensive users requirements phase performed by both engineers and consultants of the project. Moreover, two expert anesthesiologists participated in the phase of elicitation of expertise, which was performed by an expert physician specialized in hospital information systems databases. Unfortunately, this software application proved to be totally unusable. Part of the failure was due to the poor ergonomic quality of the graphic user interface (GUI) and to the slow rate of the application, which were assessed through a standard heuristic evaluation [7]. But, some more fundamental problems could be identified as well. As with most similar products, the AMS was unable to deal with human factors and especially with the cognitive aspects of the users' activity [6].

The applications that are intended to handle medical data are closely intertwined with the physician's medical activity. This close physician–machine cooperation involves complex cognitive processes: the medical and anesthetic expertise of physicians is deeply involved in dialog with the interface. Under those circumstances, standard usability methods, such as heuristic evaluation or cognitive walkthrough [7], which are mostly task-oriented, do not allow the identification of the major cognitive problems the physicians will encounter when dealing with the interface. Then, those complex cognitive processes underlying the actual activity must be carefully analyzed to ensure proper usability and acceptance of the software. This dynamic and cognitive approach constitutes a new trend in the design and assessment of new software [8], especially in the domain of anesthesia and emergency [9,10]. This paper comes within the scope of this cognitive approach and presents an analysis and modeling of the physician's activity during the anesthetic consultation. From this model, we identify some constraints the software must respect and we draw up some recommendation for the human–machine interface. We then illustrate these specific points with the assessment of an anesthetic computerized record developed in one of the departments of anesthesiology in the University Hospital of Lille.

## 2. Analysis and modeling of the anesthesiologists' activity during their consultation

### 2.1. Background

According to Gaba [11], Nyssen and Javaux [12] and Xiao et al. [13] the anesthetic process mainly involves a dynamic situation management (DSM) activity [14,15]. The characteristics of this situation are complexity, time pressure and risks (the patient's life may be at stake). The main goal of the anesthesiologists is to ensure that the patient survives the surgery. It is important for the anesthesiologist to be able to anticipate and to plan the anesthetic process for each patient. This planning activity relies on the elaboration and adjustment of a schematic representation of the patient's medical case, which acts as a 'conductor' of the activity [15,16]. Gaba [11] shows that for each particular anesthesia, the physician elaborates a plan from a preoperative evaluation. This plan includes a representation of the patient's physiological and medical state, the goal of the surgery and an evaluation of the available mental, physical and material resources. All through the anesthetic process, this plan guides the anesthesiologist's activity and supports his decisions. The representation supporting the plan (and thus the plan itself) may be continuously adjusted according to the patient's evolving physiological state.

The whole anesthetic process can be divided into four phases: (i) pre-operative preparation; (ii) induction; (iii) maintenance; and (iv) survey of the recovery phase [9,10].

The pre-operative phase is devoted to the planning of the three remaining phases. The anesthesiologists try to anticipate the potential problems and to assess the risks of the anesthesia for the patient. In this respect, the anesthesiologist has to exhaustively scan the patient's medical background.

In many countries, the pre-operative phase is set on legal grounds. The patient has a medical consultation with an anesthesiologist $\approx 1$ week ($\not< 2$ days) before the actual surgical operation. The anesthesiologist who performs this consultation may not be the same person in charge of the remaining phases. Therefore, the anesthetic file completed by the physician during the consultation is of major importance because:

- it is a legal medical record
- it has the important function of transmitting the relevant medical information to the anesthesiologist on duty during surgery.

Thus, it conveys all necessary medical information to manage the induction and maintenance tasks and it allows the anesthesiologist in charge to assess those plans and eventually to modify them according to the evolution of the patient's medical status during the surgery.

The following section is dedicated to the analysis and modeling of the anesthesiologist's activity during this pre-operative phase.

## 2.2. Material and methods

We performed the observation, description and analysis of the anesthesiologists' activity during the consultation with a special focus on the interview of the patient and on data acquisition. The methods were interviews, video and audio recording and auto-facing interviews.

Thirteen anesthesiologists participated in this specific phase of the study; 11 were experienced anesthesiologists and two were novices. They were observed and audio- or video-taped while performing a consultation with real patients volunteering to participate in the study or with trained actors playing the patient's part. Each anesthesiologist had to face at least one simple and one complex case. Up to 50 consultations could be recorded.

The main objective of this analysis was to identify the procedures for searching, selecting and writing down the relevant information. From the analysis of the patient/anesthesiologist dialogs and of the corresponding paper files, we reported for each consultation, the order of the questions asked by the physician, the answers of the patient and the resulting written data.

## 2.3. Results

The medical data collected by the anesthesiologists during the interview with the patient are written down on a specific one-page sheet of paper. Those paper files ordinarily contain nine fields (administrative data, medical and surgical antecedents, etc.); each field is divided into several zones, each zone devoted to one main physiological system. Throughout the interview of the patient, the anesthesiologist fills in the given fields and zones.

### 2.3.1. Information recording (hand writing)

Relevant data are handwritten on the anesthetic consultation one-page paper-file. A lot of abbreviations are used to quicken handwriting; important information and recommendation are underlined. The data are written down as the corresponding information occur in the dialog, leading the anesthesiologist to frequently jump from one field to another of the paper sheet. Those handwritten files are sometimes very difficult to read. In a statistical study, covering 261 completed consultation files coming from five different anesthetic departments of the University Hospital of Lille, we found 21 files (8%) containing at least one undecipherable data; for one of the departments, the percentage came up to 24% (12 out of 50); those illegible data may belong to any field, including crucial ones. Moreover, a lot of files are incomplete, although the missing data may vary significantly from one department to another: for example, the ASA score is systematically missing (100%) in one department and systematically completed (100%) in another, the percentage of missing scores being 11, 16 and 68%, respectively in the three other departments. However, all the anesthesiologists claim this data to be positively required in the consultation files. Those results are coherent with Falcon's extended study of the quality of anesthetic records [17].

The observation of the anesthesiologist's activity during the consultation demonstrated that most of them tend to emphasize important data and eventually to set alerts in some cases. Out of the 261 completed files which were analyzed, 32 (12.26%) contained explicit 'alarm' signs, 52 (20%) had highlighted data, some of them acting like an alert (for example, circled in red) and 126 (48%) contained emphasized data (underlined) (Fig. 1).

These observations show that it is not only raw data that are transmitted to the anesthesiologist on duty for the surgery: the consultation file also conveys interpreted data which are parts of the representation of the patient's medical case and elements of the planning for the anesthetic process.

### 2.3.2. Strategies for information gathering

All patients are asked the same general set of questions, but the interview does not usually go through the successive fields in a systematic way. We observed that the order of the questions differs from one case to another. This order depends on two independent factors: the degree of complexity of the case and the procedure for exploring the patient's medical background. We could identify three different procedures for the exploration of the patient's medical case.

Each procedure accounts for an observed order of the questions. All three procedures can be used alternately during the same examination.

- *Procedure 1*: the anesthesiologist follows a standard and systematic order when questioning the patient, field by field and system by system.
- *Procedure 2*: from an answer given by the patient, the anesthesiologist infers some further relevant information and sets specific questions to confirm this hypothesis. This procedure leads to significant short cuts in the exploration of the patient's medical framework.
- *Procedure 3*: at times, the anesthesiologist may allow the patient to 'tell his story' as far as it is relevant to the purpose of the consultation.

Procedures 2 and 3, for which the order of the questions is no longer the standard and systematic order, are not used by novice anesthesiologists.

### 2.3.3. Expert/novice comparison

There are important differences between expert and novice anesthesiologists in the way they gather and record relevant information.

*The novice anesthesiologists:*

- Follow the systematic order of the paper file, whatever the complexity of the medical case.
- Ask all the questions
- Write down all the answers
- Do not interpret the data and make no differences according to their importance for the anesthetic process
- Never underline, nor circle or emphasize any information
- Do not provide any element for the planning of the anesthesia itself
- Try to reassure the patient at the end of the interview

- Are unable to question the patient in the form of a natural dialog.

*The expert anesthesiologists:*

- Do not follow the standard order of the paper file, except sometimes for simple cases
- Jump from one field to another following significant expert inferences
- Write down only relevant data
- Interpret the data collected and categorize them according to their importance for the anesthetic process.
- Underline or emphasize crucial information
- Give significant clues for the planning of the anesthesia itself, sometimes set alarms

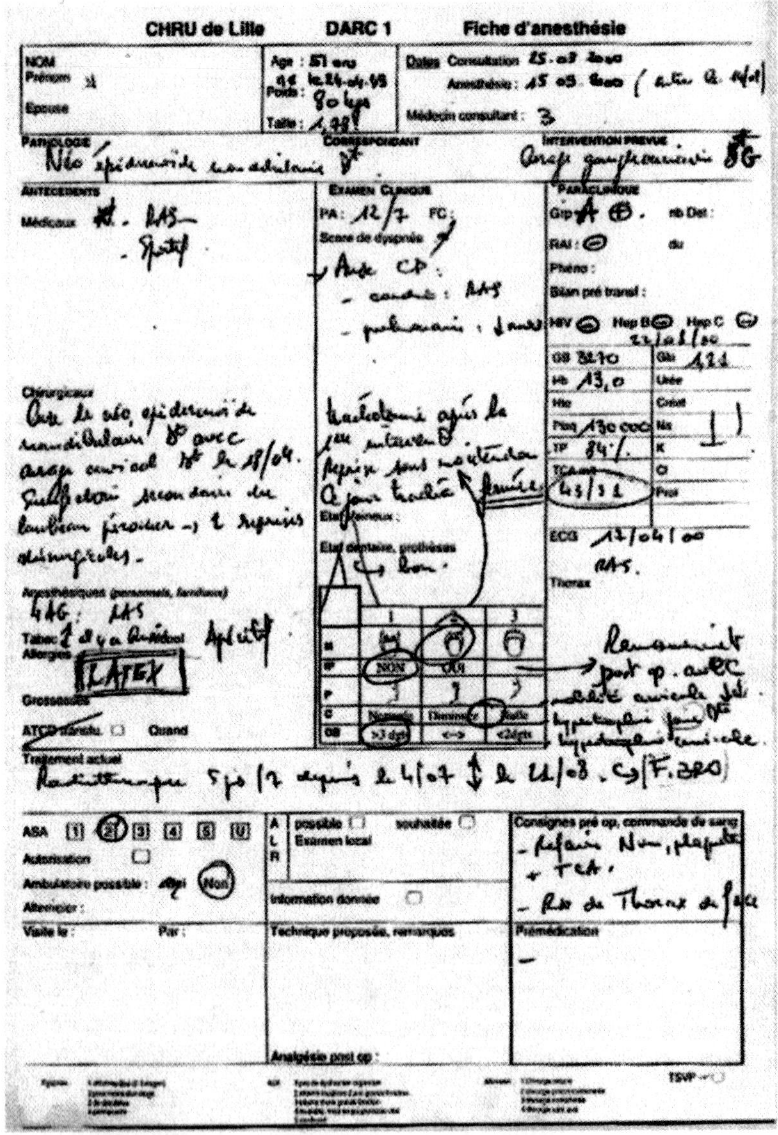

Fig. 1. An example of a typical anesthetic consultation paper file completed by an expert anesthesiologist. It contains explicit alarm signs, emphasized data and it is somehow uneasy to read.

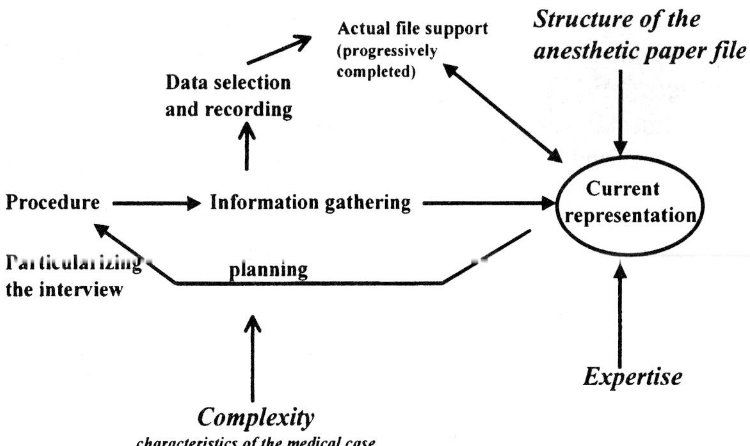


Fig. 2. Model of the anesthesiologist's activity for information gathering and recording during the consultation.

- Pay attention to the patient's anxiety and reassure him all along the consultation
- Are able to give the clinical interview the form of a natural dialog.

When presented with this analysis of their activity, all the anesthesiologists, experts as well as novices, acknowledged its authenticity. But unfortunately, only two novices participated in that part of the study. Then, one must be careful when trying to generalize from the results obtained here: the succeeding model will need further experiments for broader verification.

### 2.4. Interpretation and elaboration of the model

The three different procedures identified in the expert medical interviews (described in Section 2.3.2) reveal specific strategies and thus planning activities for information gathering. The expert alternate use of these three procedures constitute a mixed bottom-up/top-down planning [16], usually called opportunistic planning [18], which is partly supported by the actual acquisition of data. We can draw up a model representing this particular activity; this model relies on the Rasmussen's general architecture, modified by Hoc and Amalberti [19] to adapt to planning activities in dynamic environments. This approach emphasizes the role of the current representation and can be represented as shown in Fig. 2.

The anesthesiologist always begins the interview in a standard way, with the administrative data and the type of surgery expected. Then, he usually goes through the patient's medical history. He then begins to gather relevant information and this information feeds the emerging representation of the patient's medical case, which allows the anesthesiologist to identify significant patterns in the information given by the patient. Relying on the representation of the patient's medical framework, the anesthesiologist begins to plan the search for further information and ends up particularizing the procedure for the interview and adapting it to the characteristics of the patient's medical case. Amongst the information given by the patient, the anesthesiologist selects and writes down the relevant data on the paper file. This file becomes a kind of external support for the representation, which is an important point given the limited capacity of the human memory. In this model, the current representation of the patient's medical case is a key concept, acting as a kind of conductor of the activity, as in an orchestra.

The construction of this representation is influenced by three main factors. (1) The anesthesiologist's expertise, which allows him to interpret and assemble the data in significant patterns and to select, record and emphasize relevant or important information. (2) The structure of the anesthetic paper file, which leads to a specific categorization of the data. (3) The complexity of the medical case, which orients the planning of information gathering and influences the adjustment of the interview.

## 3. Constraints for the software and recommendations for the man–machine interface

From the analysis of the activity and its modeling, we can identify some constraints the software should respect in order to ensure proper usability and acceptance of the tool. Taking into account these cognitive constraints implies some specific developments for the human machine interface. In Table 1, we present the more important of these recommendations.

Obviously, Table 1 can be used as a basis for the assessment of any software application designed to handle medical data synchronously during the anesthetic consultation. This evaluation of the interface must take place between the technical verification and the functional assessment phase [20–23]. It must be performed with end users and in real work environment or in closely simulating situations. As far as possible, the key variables, identified by the model as influencing the performance, must be controlled. In Section 4, we present an example of such

an assessment of a software application for the anesthetic consultation.

## 4. Evaluation of a software application for anesthetic consultation

Tabellar* is a computerized medical record specific for the anesthetic consultation. It was developed on behalf of an anesthesiologist in charge of a department of anesthesiology in the University Hospital of Lille. It has been used routinely for 3 years in this specific anesthetic department, but at the time of the evaluation study (1997/1998), the main user (if not the only one) remained the author of the tool.

Tabellar* fulfills the strong users' requirements for the exhaustiveness of the database: the anesthesiologists want to be able to enter any relevant information. Thus, the software contains a lot of catalogs comprising lists of numerous items. The structure of the database is close to the structure of the anesthetic paper file; it is then divided into six domains, each containing several fields.

The interface can be characterized as follow:
- it is closely linked to the database; the natural (by default) order of appearance of the screens follows the structure of the database;
- the resulting interface is made up of more than ten screen pages. There is a synthesis screen dynamically updated as the data are entered, but this screen is unavailable while the user goes through the successive catalogs devoted to medical and surgical antecedents, which concerns the major part of the medical interview. The user has to quit (shutdown) these screen-pages to retrieve the synthesis screen;
- the anesthesiologist may choose not to follow the order set by the interface to

Table 1
Constraints for the software and recommendations for the GUI

| Constraints | Consequences | Recommendations |
| --- | --- | --- |
| The anesthesiologist relies on the progressing representation of the patient's medical framework to drive the clinical interview. The paper file acts as an external support for this representation. | All along the clinical interview, the anesthesiologist must have before his eyes all the data already gathered. At least, he must be able to access this information very rapidly. | The software must provide the physician with a summary screen page, continuously updated with each new data and always available while he questions the patient and enters new data. |
| The anesthesiologist relies partly on the structure of the paper file to plan the clinical interview and to categorize the items. | The anesthesiologist must have this structure before his eyes all along the interview. | The summary screen page must include this structure. Each new data must be entered in the proper field or zone of the structure. The order of data gathering set by default should follow this structure. |
| Expert anesthesiologists particularize the interview according to the characteristics of the patient's medical framework. | The anesthesiologist must be able to jump from one field to another in order to enter a new data easily and rapidly enough to deal with the speed of a natural dialog. | The software must allow the physician to enter the data randomly and very rapidly. If the software contains several screens and catalogs, the shift from one screen to the other must be easy and fast. |
| Expert anesthesiologists may transmit to the anesthesiologist on duty for the surgery interpreted data, part of their representation of the medical case and elements of planning. | Expert anesthesiologists underline, circle or emphasize important data, sometimes they add alarms. | The software must allow the anesthesiologist to emphasize crucial data and to set specific alarms. |

enter the data and is thus allowed to jump from one field to another. But, then he has to shutdown the actual catalog and/or screen page to open the targeted one and this procedure is quite slow;

- there is no specific procedure to allow the anesthesiologist to emphasize crucial data or to add personal remarks, recommendations or warnings.

### 4.1. A priori assessment of the Tabellar* application

The comparison of these characteristics with the recommendations listed above provides the a priori evaluation in Table 2.

This a priori evaluation allows some forecasts for the usability and acceptance of this software application:

- Due to the synthesis screen and the visibility of the structure, the anesthesiologists should be able to gather and record the relevant data while performing their consultation; the resulting anesthetic record should be of satisfactory quality.
- Due to the poor capacity of the tool to adapt to different orders for data gathering, the expert anesthesiologists should feel uncomfortable with the interface because

Table 2
A priori assessment of the Tabellar application

| Recommendation | Tabellar interface |
| --- | --- |
| Dynamically updated synthesis screen page | Medium |
| Possibility of particularizing the order of data gathering | Low |
| Visibility of the structure for data gathering | Good |
| Possibility to emphasize crucial data | Low |

they will be unable to rely on their expertise to drive the interview of the patient. Conversely, novice anesthesiologists should not be disturbed by the order set by the interface for data gathering; they should rely on the interface for driving the medical interview.

- The expert anesthesiologists should be less disturbed with the interface for simple cases than for complex cases.

### 4.2. Experimental assessment of the Tabellar* application

In order to validate the above hypotheses, we performed an experimental evaluation of the Tabellar* application, which involved three independent variables corresponding to the three main influencing factors of the model of activity: expertise, complexity of the medical case and the structure of the file.

- Subjects (Expertise):
  - One expert anesthesiologist, unfamiliar with the Tabellar* application
  - Two novice anesthesiologists, unfamiliar with the application.
  - One expert anesthesiologists, familiar with the application (author of Tabellar*), who represents the optimal performance that can be obtained with the application after a 2-year period of daily utilization. Each subject (unfamiliar) had three 1-h training sessions.

- Experimental design (complexity, structure): Each anesthesiologist performed four consultations corresponding to the combination of a two degrees of complexity variable (Simple × Complex cases) and a two conditions variable (Paper file × Tabellar*).
- Quantitative results (Fig. 3;; Table 3)):The consultation with the paper file and for simple cases is always faster than the con-

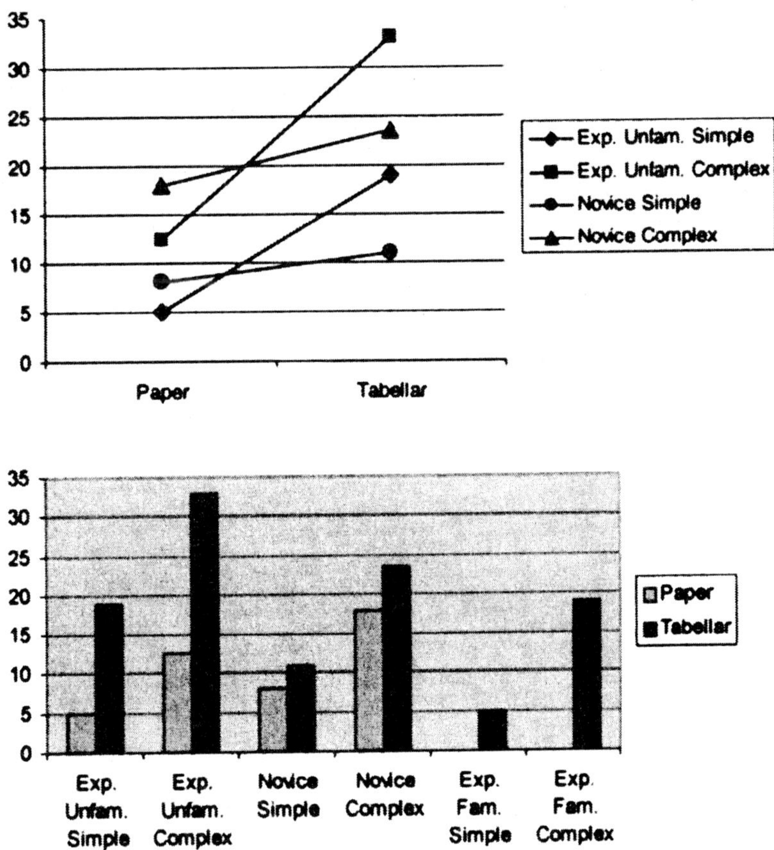



Fig. 3. Duration of the consultation (minutes) according to the type of support for the record (Tabellar × Paper), the complexity of the medical case (Simple × Complex) and the expertise of the anesthesiologists (Expert × Novice).

sultation with the computer and for complex cases. The expert anesthesiologists are faster than the novices, but as we expected, they are much more disturbed by the computer condition, where they become even slower than the novices. But this main effect is not influenced by the complexity of the case. For simple cases, the anesthesiologist familiar with the tool is as fast as the other experts with the paper file, but for complex cases, she remains slower than any of the other experts working with the paper file.

- Qualitative results:The expert anesthesiologists enter the same data (same number,

same quality) on the paper file and on the computer. But the novices tend to enter less data on the computer and these data are less precise. Expert anesthesiologists feel uneasy whenever the summary screen is not available and they have some difficulties with the categorization of the items and data or with the catalogs each time this categorization is slightly different from the one they are used to (paper file and personal expertise). As expected, expert anesthesiologists feel 'less in control' in the computer condition and they get the impression they cannot drive the interview of the patient exactly the way they want, that they are compelled to follow the order set by the computer. They usually end the session claiming that 'their personal habits do not fit the computer way' and they are reluctant toward the utilization of this tool in their daily working environment. In summary, the experimental results validate the a priori evaluation of the Tabellar* application, which demonstrates medium usability and poor acceptance, at least from the experts point of view.

When faced with the completed Tabellar* consultation files (edited on paper), anesthetic nurses in charge of the induction phase with the anesthesiologists find it easier and faster to read than the previous paper file because it is typewritten. But they complain about the lack of explicit categorization of the data and their non-differentiation; they ask for important data to be highlighted.

## 5. Discussion

### 5.1. The 'usability' problem

The quantitative and qualitative results of the experimental evaluation of Tabellar* are coherent with the hypothesis derived from the model of activity and the a priori assessment. The problems of usability are actually due to the incompatibility between the software application and the main characteristics of the anesthesiologist's activity, especially if we consider the complex cognitive aspects of this activity:

- Strategies for information gathering in order to elaborate a proper representation of the patient's medical case and to set preliminary elements for the planning of the anesthetic process.

- Strategies for transmitting the relevant information to the anesthesiologist and anesthetic nurse in charge of the per-operative phase of the anesthesia. In this highly complex communication process, the particularization of data notation acts as a specialized operative language.

Understanding these essential features of the anesthesiologists activity helps to interpret correctly the usability problems. It is then possible to give reliable recommendations for the design of new tools or for the redesign and improvement of existing tools.

Such recommendations were provided for the Tabellar* software, which has hence been significantly enhanced:

Table 3
Duration of the consultation (in minutes) according to the expertise, the complexity and the file support

| Conditions/ subjects | Expert anesthesiologist familiar with the application | Expert anesthesiologists unfamiliar with the application | Novice anesthesiologists unfamiliar with the application |
|---|---|---|---|
| Simple case Paper file | | 5 min = max = 5 | 8 min: 7; max: 9 |
| Simple case Tabellar | 5 | 19 min: 14; max: 28 | 11 min: 9; max: 13 |
| Complex case Paper file | | 12.5 min: 4.5; max: 18.5 | 17.5 min: 17; max: 18 |
| Complex case Tabellar | 19 | 33 min: 20; max: 46 | 23.5 min: 22; max: 25 |

Table 4
Differential efficiency of the computer and paper files according to the functionalities considered

| Functionalities/support | Paper | Computer |
|---|---|---|
| *To support the activity:* | | |
| Elaboration of the representation | + + | − − |
| Information gathering | + + | − − |
| Transmission of interpreted information (representation) | + | − |
| Transmission of raw information | + − | + + |
| *Data management:* | | |
| Archiving | − − | + + |
| Statistics | − − | + + |
| Data retrieving and data availability | + − | + + |
| Editions, complementary services | − − | + + |

- Improvement of the synthesis screen: more fields are visible altogether; the synthesis screen now includes complementary data such as laboratory results.
- When a user searches a catalog, the corresponding field and the items already entered in this field remain in view.
- The GUI is faster.

All those amendments support the elaboration of the current representation and allow the user to browse more easily among the fields of the consultation file. Therefore, the usability of the application seems positively improved. It is currently utilized routinely by all the expert anesthesiologists of the department (three) and by the novices as well.

### 5.2. Usability versus efficacy

When they claim that the paper file is 'easier to use', the anesthesiologists express the fact that this paper file suitably supports their activity in the preoperative phase of the anesthetic process (Table 4). But the software application somehow helps solve some usability and quality problems induced by the use of handwritten paper files, such as the legibility and the missing information problems. Moreover, if we consider the quality of the anesthetic patient record and the quality of information management, the software application becomes unavoidable (Table 4).

For example, Tabellar* includes a sophisticated and accurate intubation's score [24] which is automatically computed; in case of a difficult intubation, the appropriate anesthetic technique is suggested. Similar to most of the current EPR, the Tabellar* application entails an automatic check for the completeness of the critical fields, automatic loading of the previous anesthetic file in case of repeated anesthesia, a specific link with the nurses' file and so on. Most of these functionalities could be considered as 'another way' of supporting the anesthesiologists' activity.

### 6. Conclusion

The continuous extension of HIS, as well as the increase in quality requirements for anesthesiology, allows the consideration of the anesthetic computerized record as very probable in most hospitals within the next 10 years. Then, these software applications must be readily acceptable in the anesthesiologist's daily working environment. The acceptance of these tools will rely on their ability to support both essential functions:

- To provide a reliable archive;
- To support the users' activity by providing them with an adequate external support of the current representation that allows a proper management of dynamic situations.

Most of the existing tools actually reach the first target. But, they still have to improve their capacity to deal with the second target.

This statement could be extended to most of the major applications proposed to the physicians. This paper demonstrated the usefulness of the activity modeling approach in this domain.

## References


[1] M.C. Beuscart-Zéphir, F. Anceaux, J.M. Renard, Integrating user's activity analysis in the design and assessment of medical software applications: the example of anesthesia, in: A. Hasman, B. Blobel, J. Dudeck, R. Engelbrecht, G. Gell, H.U. Prokosch (Eds.), Medical Infobahn for Europe, vol. 77, Proceedings of MIE 2000 and GMDS 2000, IOS Press, Health, Technology and Informatics, Amsterdam, 2000, pp. 234–238.

[2] M.C. Beuscart-Zéphir, J.M. Renard, F. Anceaux, Activity analysis for designing an anesthesia record system, in: J.M. Fouke, R.M. Nerem, S.M. Blanchard, A.P. Yoganathan (Eds.), Proceedings of the First Joint Meeting of BMES and EMBS, Twenty-first Annual International Conference of the IEEE Engineering in Medicine and Biology Society, IEEE, Piscataway, NJ, 1999, p. 1221.

[3] X. Wang, R.M. Gardner, P.R. Seager, Integrating computerized anesthesia charting into a hospital information system, International Journal of Clinical Monitoring and Computing 19 (1995) 61–70.

[4] J. Ramsay, J. Popp, B. Thull, G. Rau, The evaluation of an information system for intensive care, Behavior and Information Technology 16 (1) (1997) 17–24.

[5] D. Piazza, S. Largillière, Système d'information de bloc opératoire: le projet du CHU d'Amiens, RBM 20 (2) (1998) 25–30.

[6] F. Anceaux, M.C. Beuscart-Zéphir, P. Sockeel, Human–machine cooperation in the anesthetic consultation: importance of planning activities for information gathering, in: J.M. Hoc, P. Millot, E. Hollnagel, P.C. Cacciabue (Eds.), Proceedings of CSAPC '99 Valenciennes, Presses Universitaires de Valenciennes, 1999, pp. 15–20.

[7] J. Nielsen, R.L. Mack, Usability Inspection Methods, Wiley, New York, 1994.

[8] R. Amalberti, F. Deblon, Cognitive modeling of fighter aircraft process control: a step towards an intelligent on-board assistance system, The International Journal of Man–Machine Studies 36 (1992) 639–671.

[9] Y. Xiao, P. Milgram, D.J. Doyle, Capturing and modelling planning expertise in anaesthesiology: results of a field study, in: C.E. Zsambok, G.A. Klein (Eds.), Naturalistic Decision Making, LEA, Mahwah, NJ, 1997, pp. 197–205.

[10] Y. Xiao, P. Milgram, D.J. Doyle, Planning behaviour and its functional role in interactions with complex systems, IEEE Transactions on Systems, Man and Cybernetics—Part A: Systems and Humans 27 (3) (1997) 313–324.

[11] D.M. Gaba, S. Howard, K. Fish, Crisis Management in Anesthesiology, Churchill Livingstone, New York, 1994.

[12] A.S. Nyssen, D. Javaux, Analysis of synchronization constraints and associated errors, Ergonomics 39 (10) (1996) 1249–1264.

[13] Y. Xiao, C.F. Mackenzie, The Lotas Group, Decision making in dynamic environments: fixation errors and their causes, in: Proceedings of Human Factors and Ergonomic Society, Thirty-Ninth Annual Meeting, Human Factors and Ergonomic Society, Santa Monica, CA, 1995.

[14] J.M. Hoc, R. Amalberti, Modeling NDM cognitive activities in dynamic situations: the role of a coding scheme, Proceedings of the NDM5 Meeting, Tammsvik, Sweden, May 2000.

[15] J.M. Hoc, Supervision et Contrôle de Processus—la Cognition en Situation Dynamique, Presses Universitaires de Grenoble, Grenoble, 1996.

[16] J.M. Hoc, Cognitive Psychology of Planning, Academic Press, London, 1988.

[17] D. Falcon, P. François, C. Jacquot, J.F. Payen, Evaluation de la tenue du dossier d'anesthésie, Ann. Fr. Anesth. Réanim. 18 (1999) 360–367.

[18] B. Hayes-Roth, F. Hayes-Roth, A cognitive model of planning, Cognitive Science 3 (1979) 275–310.

[19] J.M. Hoc, R. Amalberti, Diagnosis: some theoretical questions raised by applied research, Current Psychology of Cognition 14 (1995) 73–100.

[20] J. Brender, P. McNair, User requirements in a system development and evaluation context, in: A. Hasman, B. Blobel, J. Dudeck, R. Engelbrecht, G.

Gell, H.U. Prokosch (Eds.), Medical Infobahn for Europe, vol. 77, Proceedings of MIE 2000 and GMDS 2000, IOS Press, Health, Technology and Informatics, Amsterdam, pp. 203–207.

[21] J. Brender, Methodology for constructive assessment of IT-based systems in an organisational context, Internation Journal of Medical Informatics 56 (1999) 67–86.

[22] M.C. Beuscart-Zéphir, J. Brender, R. Beuscart, I. Ménager-Depriester, Cognitive evaluation: how to assess the usability of information technology in healthcare, Computer Methods and Programs in Biomedicine 54 (1–2) (1997) 19–28.

[23] M.C. Beuscart-Zéphir, P. Sockeel, B. Bossard, R. Beuscart, Activity modeling for assessing the usability of telematics applications in healthcare, in: B. Cesnik et al. (Eds.), Medinfo '98, IOS Press, IMIA, Amsterdam, 1998, pp. 832–836.

[24] V. Crinquette, G. Dumenil, E. Kipnis, Intubation difficile et informatisation, actes de la SFIM@R Société Francophone d'Informatique et de Monitorage en Anesthésie-Réanimation, 6–7 Octobre, 2000, http://www.univ-lille2.fr/sfimar2000/actes/

# Generation and Evaluation of Intraoperative Inferences for Automated Health Care Briefings on Patient Status After Bypass Surgery

DESMOND A. JORDAN, MD, KATHLEEN R. MCKEOWN, PHD,
KRISTIAN J. CONCEPCION, MS, STEVEN K. FEINER, PHD,
VASILEIOS HATZIVASSILOGLOU, PHD

**Abstract** Objective: The authors present a system that scans electronic records from cardiac surgery and uses inference rules to identify and classify abnormal events (e.g., hypertension) that may occur during critical surgical points (e.g., start of bypass). This vital information is used as the content of automatically generated briefings designed by MAGIC, a multimedia system that they are developing to brief intensive care unit clinicians on patient status after cardiac surgery. By recognizing patterns in the patient record, inferences concisely summarize detailed patient data.

**Design:** The authors present the development of inference rules that identify important information about patient status and describe their implementation and an experiment they carried out to validate their correctness. The data for a set of 24 patients were analyzed independently by the system and by 46 physicians.

**Measurements:** The authors measured accuracy, specificity, and sensitivity by comparing system inferences against physician judgments, in cases where all three physicians agreed and against the majority opinion in all cases.

**Results:** For laboratory inferences, evaluation shows that the system has an average accuracy of 98 percent (full agreement) and 96 percent (majority model). An analysis of interrater agreement, however, showed that physicians do not agree on abnormal hemodynamic events and could not serve as a gold standard for evaluating hemodynamic events. Analysis of discrepancies reveals possibilities for system improvement and causes of physician disagreement.

**Conclusions:** This evaluation shows that the laboratory inferences of the system have high accuracy. The lack of agreement among physicians highlights the need for an objective quality-assurance tool for hemodynamic inferences. The system provides such a tool by implementing inferencing procedures established in the literature.

Affiliation of the authors: Columbia University, New York, New York.

This research was supported in part by contract R01 LM06593-01 from the National Library of Medicine and by the Columbia University Center for Advanced Technology in High Performance Computing and Communications in Healthcare (funded by the New York State Science and Technology Foundation).

Correspondence: Desmond A. Jordan, MD, Department of Anesthesiology, 622 West 168th Street, PH-5, New York Presbyterian Hospital, New York, NY 10032; e-mail: <daj@columbia.edu>. Reprints: Kathleen R. McKeown, 450 Computer Science Building, Department of Computer Science, 1214 Amsterdam Avenue, Columbia University, New York, NY 10027; e-mail: <kathy@cs.columbia.edu>.

When a caregiver needs to act quickly because of a patient's clinical status, a succinct overview highlighting important events (e.g., that the patient was hypertensive) can communicate information more efficiently than an exhaustive log of every vital sign, procedure, and laboratory result over a length of time. For example, a single sentence that mentions an inferred episode of hypertension occurring during a bypass operation could effectively summarize what would otherwise be an overwhelming number of low-level raw blood pressure readings gathered during the operation (1,080 readings for the average five-hour bypass operation).[1,2] Both brevity and

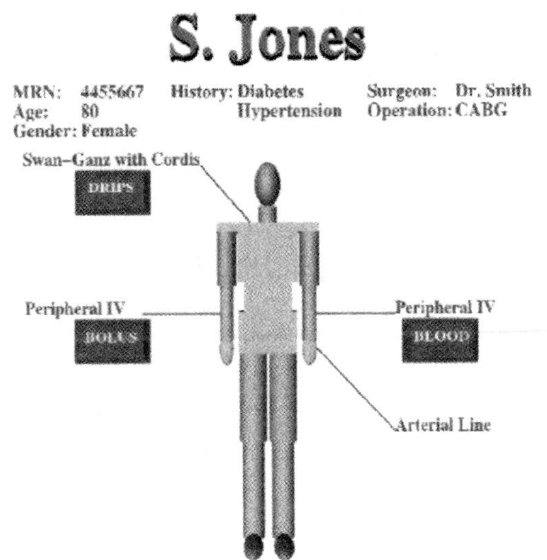



Voice: ... Ms. Jones is an 80-year-old, diabetic, hypertensive, female patient of Dr. Smith's who is undergoing CABG.... Before start of bypass, she had two episodes of bradycardia. After coming off bypass, she had two episodes of hypocalcemia, relative anemia, and hypokalemia.

**Figure 1** MAGIC-generated response including graphics and speech.

identification of important events can be achieved by recognizing relevant patterns in the patient's record that represent illness severity. However, if these inferences are wrong, the summary can be useless or even harmful. The research we describe here addresses the development and evaluation of inference rules that identify important information about the patient's status to include in a summary.

We are carrying out our work on inferences in the context of MAGIC (multimedia abstract generation of intensive care data), an experimental system that generates multimedia presentations automatically to explain a cardiac patient's postoperative status to caregivers.[1,2] These presentations are based on detailed medical data obtained during the patient's cardiac surgery and are intended to inform personnel in the cardiac intensive care unit (ICU) of the patient's status prior to their arrival from the operating room (OR). The transfer of an anesthetized and ventilated patient is a critical event that entails a high degree of risk. Notifying ICU personnel in advance of the patient status and impending transfer minimizes delays in therapy.[3]

Patient status at critical points[4] represents information that is necessary for continued care of the patient in the ICU and for improvement in individual patients' outcomes, as shown by mortality studies[5] and the resultant severity of illness measurements developed by the New York State Heart Association.[6] Without such information, care may be inappropriate or

delayed.[3] Because patients are aggressively treated in the OR, those with derangements in physiologic values should be considered nonresponders to therapy, or "treatment failures," heightening the need to convey problems to subsequent care providers.[7]

A key component of MAGIC is its set of medical inference rules. These rules identify patterns in the patient's record, from which they infer information that can be used to describe the patient's status more concisely, as shown in Figure 1.[1,2] In this paper, we present the inference rules that we designed and describe an experiment to validate their correctness. Our inference rules operate in real time, identifying abnormal events from numeric data in current cases, but they can also be used on historical cases. Our experiment compares system performance on a set of historical cases with performance of a group of residents and attending physicians on the same cases. The physicians were provided with the same patient data given to the system and asked to identify whether the abnormal conditions that the system tracks occurred.

## Background

While many researchers study the integration of individual abnormalities to judge the overall severity of patients' conditions,[8] our focus is on communication of abnormalities and severity to clinicians. When a cardiac patient arrives in the ICU after surgery, a variety of information about the patient's condition and status must be summarized for the ICU medical team. This summary is usually given orally by a physician from the OR, the anesthesia resident, to another physician and nurse in the ICU. Some critical information about the patient is provided by telephone during the operation, but this information is cursory and OR physicians are rushed. In current practice, the information that has been conveyed is not easily accessible to a clinician who is responsible for the patient's care but was not present at the briefing. Therefore, as nursing shifts change and new medical staff are added, these clinicians must review the anesthesia chart along with other material in the patient record.

Our goal in developing MAGIC is to replace the telephone call from the OR with an automatically generated briefing that provides the full information given in the ICU briefing. This will supplement, rather than replace, the ICU briefing, providing information earlier so that ICU clinicians have time to prepare.[3] MAGIC can also be used to replay the briefing for clinicians who missed it. MAGIC offers the potential to provide a consistent, standard set of information for each patient, offsetting the possibility that a resident may forget to report to the ICU staff critical incidents that require postoperative follow-up.

MAGIC is unique in its ability to determine automatically the content and form of a briefing on patient status, including the sentence structure and wording of the language,[9] the graphic representations,[10] the intonation of the speech,[11] and the coordination of the different media in a single briefing.[1,12] Figure 1 shows a portion of MAGIC's multimedia output. In this context, inferencing plays a critical role in determining what is important to communicate. Given that the resulting briefing must be concise, MAGIC must select from a large quantity of information on the patient only information that is critical to the patient's ongoing care. This places demands on the inferencing process above and beyond those placed on traditional expert systems, requiring reasoning over time, limiting information, and linking it to events that can be communicated (i.e., critical time points). In the past, medical inferencing has been used primarily to suggest diagnoses, recommend practice, and provide decision support rather than to select information to communicate.[13,14]

Although communicating the existence and degree of abnormalities in physiologic parameters is important at any time during cardiac surgical procedures, there are several critical points at which transmitting the status of this information to subsequent caregivers is vital.[5,15] The four critical points investigated here are induction, skin incision, start of bypass, and end of bypass. *Induction* (or intubation) is when the patient is anesthetized and mechanically ventilated. *Skin incision* initiates the onset of surgical stimulation and stress. During cardiopulmonary bypass, the heart is stopped and blood pressure is controlled by a mechanical pump. *Start of bypass* refers to the point when this begins, and *end of bypass* is the time when the patient is taken off the pump. These milestones constitute reference points[4] at which surgical processes commonly induce lability in heart rate, blood pressure, and laboratory test results.

Other researchers have developed systems to scan electronic surgical records and report incidents.[15] However, their focus was on outcome instead of communication. They did not link incidents to critical points, and they used higher thresholds for abnormality than we do. In our experience, this approach misses events that, although more difficult to detect, should be communicated when they occur at a critical point. For example, hypocalcemia following bypass is far more important than hypocalcemia at any other

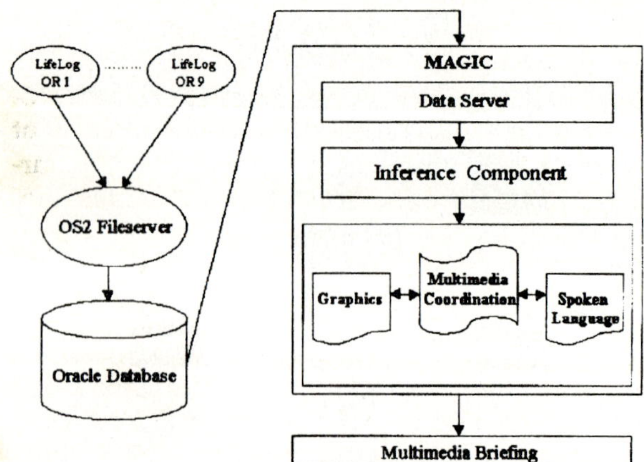


**Figure 2** MAGIC system architecture.

point in the case.[16] An ionized calcium concentration below 0.7 mcg/dL is considered hypocalcemic.

To determine when an event is abnormal, we use severity-of-patient-illness scores developed previously, such as the Acute Physiologic and Chronic Health Status Evaluation (APACHE III),[5,8] Multi-organ System Illness Score (MSIS),[7] and the therapeutic Intervention Severity Score (TISS).[17] These scores have been used individually or in combination for many years for the prognostic scoring of surgical and critically ill patients as well as for stratification of patient illness severity.[18] In this paper, the existence and extent of physiologic derangement during bypass surgery was assessed using APACHE III, MSIS, and intraoperative thresholds[19] representing abnormality for blood pressure, heart rate, arterial blood oxygen (both $PO_2$ and saturation), pH, potassium, glucose, hematocrit, and ionized calcium (see Table 1). Our use of these multiple scores is similar to the use of composite outcome scales, such as the American Society of Anesthesiology (ASA) Physical Status[16] and the MSIS,[7] which allow quantification of complex clinical phenomena that cannot be adequately described by a single clinical or biochemical measure.

### System Description

The system architecture for MAGIC, shown in Figure 2, shows that during the course of a cardiac operation, information is automatically collected using the LifeLog data acquisition system (Modular Instruments Inc.), which is part of the existing information infrastructure in the cardiac OR at New York Presbyterian Hospital. It polls medical devices (Hewlett Packard Merlin monitors, Ohmeda anesthesia machines, and saturation monitors) every 50 seconds, recording indicators of patient status, including vital signs, inhaled anesthetics, and ventilation parameters. Bolus drugs, postoperative drugs, laboratory results, intravenous lines, information about devices such as a pacemaker, and data from echocardiograms are manually entered by the anesthesiologist using the LifeLog interface. Surgical events such as time of intubation, skin incision, and start and stop of bypass are also entered manually.

At the end of the operation, the collected data are downloaded into an Oracle database, for easy access using a standard query language. MAGIC's inference engine, which we developed for the purpose of generating multimedia briefings, scans heart rate and blood pressure readings, for which values are available at 50-second intervals, and laboratory results, for which values for one to ten tests are available before the start of bypass and after the end of bypass. The inference engine applies a set of inference rules to determine whether any abnormal events occurred within a 20-minute window before or after any of the four critical time points, determining the time interval of the event (i.e., start and stop times) and identifying drugs that were given. Any database entry labeled as DRUG is extracted; typical drugs include pressors (e.g., phenylephrine, ephedrine) and depressors (e.g., esmolol, nitroglycerine). This yields eight possible time periods (one before and one after each critical point) during which abnormalities are detected and reported, if they occur.

For the rare cases in which the patient goes on and off bypass multiple times, we currently use the first on-bypass and the last off-bypass times, although it would be relatively easy to include all on and off bypass times if we found that this were preferable. This inferred information is then stored in MAGIC's database, along with other extracted data such as demographics, medical history, and drugs given, to be used as the content for a multimedia briefing. At the time of the inferencing experiments reported here, there were no facilities for automatically transferring data from the OR to the Oracle database at the end of each operation. Instead, information for a set of patients could be transferred periodically.

For the experiment, information on a test group of a month's worth of concurrent patients was stored in the database once, and we evaluated MAGIC on this test set. MAGIC has since been integrated into the online information infrastructure in the cardiac OR at New York Presbyterian Hospital, although it is not yet deployed. It runs in a networked environment with full access to the OR database. Information on a patient is automatically stored in the database as soon as the operation is complete.

The inference engine can find two classes of abnormal events: those relating to hemodynamics and those indicated by laboratory results, both described below. Hemodynamic inferences identify episodes of hypotension, hypertension, bradycardia, and tachycardia. Laboratory inferences identify acidosis, alkalosis, hypercardia, hypoxia, low saturation, hyponatremia, hypernatremia, hypokalemia, hyperkalemia, hypocalcemia, hypercalcemia, anemia, hypoglycemia, and hyperglycemia. The algorithms used for each class are rule-based and use thresholds based on severity of illness scores developed and extensively tested in previous work,[5,7,8,19] as described below. However, the algorithms differ because of differences in the amount of information available. For hemodynamics (i.e., arterial blood pressure and heart rate), there is a tremendous amount of data, since heart rate and systolic, diastolic, and mean blood pressures are recorded every 50 seconds. In contrast, laboratory results are reported sporadically, usually before and after bypass. As a result, hemodynamic inference rules operate over temporal intervals, using temporal abstraction to determine abnormality from a set of frequent readings, whereas laboratory inference rules test a specific point in time.

### Hemodynamic Inferences

These inferences look for intervals of time when blood pressure or heart rate rises above or falls below a predetermined threshold for a length of time. We developed rules that directly encode standard thresholds for bradycardia, tachycardia, hypotension, and hyper-

*Table 1* ∎

Threshold Values of the Inference Engine

|  | Hypo/Low | Hyper/High |
| --- | --- | --- |
| Blood pressure | 100 | 150 |
| Heart rate | 50(pre)/60(post) | 120 |
| Calcium | 0.8 | 1.5 |
| K+ | 3.5 | 5 |
| Carbon dioxide | N/A | 45 |
| Oxygen | 60 | N/A |
| pH | 7.35 | 7.45 |
| Sodium | 135 | 145 |
| Saturated oxygen | 90 | N/A |
| Glucose | 90 | 200 |
| Hematocrit | 32(pre)/30(post) | N/A |

tension,[20,21] shown in Table 1. Berger et al.[20] and Block[21] based these thresholds on experiments using extensive data and statistical models. For example, our rules detect hypotension when blood pressure falls below 100 for 250 seconds (five 50-second intervals).

To smooth over temporal variations in data, we use a sliding scale average,[15] looking at a window of five consecutive values of blood pressure and heart rate. If the average does not meet the threshold, MAGIC drops the oldest value and slides forward in time to add a new value. If the average meets the threshold, the start of an abnormal episode is recorded and we continue calculating sliding averages across the window until the average returns to a normal value, marking the end of the episode. Once the time period for each episode has been calculated, MAGIC then records the drugs and amounts that were given so that the briefing can describe treatment. After all abnormal episodes have been found, MAGIC links each episode with one of the four critical time points (induction/intubation, skin incision, start of bypass, end of bypass), noting whether it occurred within a window of 20 minutes before or after that point. Since the anesthesiologist manually enters the critical time points during the operation, this window also helps compensate for errors in charting.

In almost all cases, we found artifacts in the data. For example, a spike may occur in the heart rate or blood pressure because of electric cautery, blood draws, catheter flushing, or other reasons. To avoid making false inferences, MAGIC automatically filters the data before beginning inferencing, to retain only data in cases both where values remain within valid ranges and where changes in one value (e.g., heart rate) are accompanied by an appropriate change in the other (e.g., blood pressure). More specifically, our algorithm for filtering artifacts is as follows:

1. Filter any values that fall within the following invalid ranges:

    A. All three blood pressures (mean, systolic, and diastolic) are equal. This usually occurs when the LifeLog controls are incorrectly set.

    B. Any systolic blood pressure greater than 250.

    C. Both blood pressure and heart rate are zero. This happens when the machine was not turned on immediately. Zeros are replaced by average heart rate and blood pressure, provided that the patient was not currently on bypass.

2. Remove cases in which one parameter's change is not accompanied by a change in another parameter.

If the patient had a change in heart rate greater than 50 within a 50-second interval, MAGIC retains the spike if there is a corresponding change of 10 in blood pressure. If blood pressure did not change, then the spike is replaced with the last good heart rate value. The reverse is also true; spikes in blood pressure are retained when accompanied by changes in heart rate.

### Laboratory Inferences

Thresholds for laboratory values were taken directly from APACHE scores.[8] To accurately report abnormal values, our system separately inspects data obtained before and after bypass. If laboratory tests were performed during bypass, we ignore the results because of the difference between "normal" values and "on-bypass" values. Results of laboratory tests taken during bypass are not known to be indicative of patient postoperative status and are used only to control bypass settings.[16] For each set of laboratory results, we apply the corresponding APACHE threshold (listed in Table 1) to calculate whether or not the results were abnormal.

## Methods

The performance of an automated system for medical inferencing should, in principle, be evaluated against a set of correct decisions on the same input data. If such a gold standard were available, then measures such as specificity, sensitivity, and accuracy could be used to measure quantitatively system performance. It could be argued that the carefully calculated decision thresholds and associated rules that are part of methodologies such as APACHE[5,8] would provide such a standard for hemodynamic and laboratory inferences. This is problematic, though, since MAGIC itself incorporates these rules, so using the APACHE rules as a standard would give very high scores to our automated system and would not determine whether system output was useful in practice.

Instead of using APACHE, we relate the evaluation to actual physicians' decisions in the ICU. Consequently, we collected data from physicians on a set of historical patients and compared their decisions to those automatically produced by our system. One of the goals of our study was to establish whether the physicians' answers are consistent enough across different physicians to be used to evaluate the automated system, or whether the automated system should be used as a quality assurance tool in the face of significant physician uncertainty about the correct answer.

## Selection of Human Judges

We obtained LifeLog data for input to MAGIC and the corresponding human-readable charts for a set of 24 concurrent adult patients, aged 36 to 78 years, at New York Presbyterian Hospital, who had undergone cardiac surgery, performed by a variety of surgical teams, during February and March 1998.

A standard questionnaire was prepared and handed out to physicians participating in the study, along with each patient record; this questionnaire is given in Appendix A. For each of the four critical time points discussed previously, the questionnaire asked the physician to determine, using a checklist, the presence or absence, within 20 minutes before or after that point, of each of the conditions that MAGIC can identify. For pre-bypass and post-bypass, a list of laboratory results was provided, each of which was to be marked by the subject if it was abnormal. Again, the physicians made a binary ("yes"/"no") decision on each potential abnormality. No definition of abnormal was provided; subjects used their own judgment. This deliberate design decision was made to avoid forcing physicians to use a definition that was not their own and to learn how abnormalities can be identified in practice. A final question asked the subject to identify any other abnormality not covered and to indicate its temporal relationship to the nearest critical time point.

Each individual patient's chart (see Figure 3) was given to three different physicians, yielding three responses per patient. Most physicians saw more than one chart. No physician reviewed their own patient's chart. A total of 46 physicians affiliated with New York Presbyterian Hospital participated in the experiment, of whom 18 were residents in anesthesiology and 28 were attending physicians in anesthesiology, ranging in age from 28 to 63 years. The residents were in their third or fourth year of training. Using attending physicians in addition to residents means that the accumulated responses may be of higher accuracy than responses in practice, where the residents may be the only ones who report on the patient's intraoperative course. Monitoring of a patient in the OR and the ICU is performed by anesthesiologists, and thus they may be more qualified than the other physicians involved in the case (e.g., the thoracic surgeon or cardiologist) to make decisions about laboratory and hemodynamic abnormalities. Anesthesiologists manually record these data in the OR and may have the highest skill level required to read the surgical record.

The experiment was conducted over a $2\frac{1}{2}$-day period, and assignment of cases to physician subjects was done on a first-come first-served basis. Each physician was allowed to spend as much time as desired on the questionnaire for a given patient (average, 20 minutes), and the patient's record was available during the entire time.

Both the physicians and the system produced judgments on 60 variables for each patient whose chart they examined. Each of these binary variables represents the presence or absence of a particular abnormal condition at a particular time (e.g., hypotension before the start of bypass). Hemodynamic inferences include four conditions and four critical time points, with time periods both before and after, giving a total of 32 variables. Laboratory inferences include 14 conditions and two time periods (before and after bypass), giving a total of 28 variables.

We collected judgments for 24 patients; however, it was impractical to have a physician produce judgements on all 1,440 combinations of patients and potential inferences (24 patients times 60 variables), because of the time required (about 20 minutes per review of each case). Instead, each of the 46 physicians processed the entire set of data for a limited number of patients (three or fewer per physician), and we ensured that each patient received three sets of judgments from three different physicians. In this way, we were able to create three composite judges, whose assessments of the patients' conditions we analyzed and compared with the system's output.

## Measuring Agreement among Human Judges

In the analysis that follows, we first look at the average agreement between the three composite judges, as a means of determining the types of decisions for which the physicians can be considered correct and thus for which their responses can form a gold standard for evaluation. We measure the average rate of agreement between the three human judges in each case, which provides a measure of the validity of their responses as a gold standard.[22,23] The average rate of agreement between three binary decision sets is defined as the average of the three percentages of pairwise agreement, calculated on each of the three possible pairs of decision sets.

We also calculate the average agreement rate between the system and the judges when any one of the latter is replaced by the system. Three replacement operations are performed (in each case, one human judge is left out), the average agreement between the remaining two physicians and the system is calculated as described earlier, and the three resulting numbers are averaged. Rates of agreement in these pools of three sets of decisions (two by humans and one by the system) that are similar to the inter-agreement rate in the original pool of three human judges validate that the system's performance is comparable with that of the physicians.

### Comparing System Output with a Reference Standard

Whenever the agreement analysis provides evidence that the three physicians' judgments can form the basis for an objective gold standard, we need to create a single "best" set of responses, which becomes the reference standard and can be compared with the system's output. We considered two methods for constructing the standard:

- *Full agreement standard.* We consider only the cases in which all three physicians agree. These cases are most likely to be truly correct, but may also be the easiest ones to judge. Of the 1,440 patient–inference pairs, 1,156 fall into this category.

- *Majority evaluation standard.* We take the majority opinion as the ground truth in each case. This may increase the number of errors in the evaluation standard; two rather than three physicians must misinterpret the same data to cause an error. Since the cases in which disagreement arises are likely to be more difficult to judge, we expect a lower accuracy for the system if it is evaluated against that standard and increased uncertainty in the quality of the evaluation than what we get by use of the first method. On the other hand, this approach covers all 1,440 samples.

For each of these evaluation standards, we measured sensitivity, the percentage of abnormal situations correctly identified by the system among all abnormal situations in the reference model; specificity, the percentage of correctly avoided false positives among all non-abnormal situations in the model; and accuracy, the percentage of identical decisions between the system and the gold standard across all cases.

## Results

### Agreement between Human Judges

We measured the average agreement between the three composite judges for each type of inference, and for classes of inferences (hemodynamic vs. laboratory); the results are shown in Table 2. We note that

*Table 2* ■

Average Agreement (%) Between Human Subjects and Between System and Human Subjects

| Inference | Human Subjects | System and Human Subjects |
|---|---|---|
| Hemodynamic: | | |
| Hypotension | 75.35 | 71.41 |
| Hypertension | 86.11 | 85.42 |
| Bradycardia | 83.33 | 79.40 |
| Tachycardia | 86.46 | 85.07 |
| AVERAGE ACROSS ALL HEMODYNAMIC INFERENCES | 82.81 | 80.32 |
| Laboratory: | | |
| Acidosis | 91.67 | 93.52 |
| Alkalosis | 83.33 | 83.80 |
| Hypercardia | 91.67 | 93.98 |
| Hypoxia | 98.61 | 99.07 |
| Lowsaturation | 91.67 | 94.44 |
| Hypernatremia | 100.00 | 100.00 |
| Hyponatremia | 98.61 | 98.61 |
| Hyperkalemia | 95.83 | 96.30 |
| Hypokalemia | 93.06 | 93.06 |
| Anemia | 80.56 | 81.02 |
| Hyperglycemia | 68.06 | 73.61 |
| Hypoglycemia | 100.00 | 100.00 |
| Hypercalcemia | 93.06 | 95.37 |
| Hypocalcemia | 94.44 | 95.83 |
| AVERAGE ACROSS ALL LABORATORY INFERENCES | 91.47 | 92.76 |

NOTE: Sample sizes were 192 for each hemodynamic inference, 48 for each laboratory inference.

the percentage of agreement is much higher in the case of laboratory inferences (91.47 percent) than in hemodynamic ones (82.81 percent). This can be attributed to two possible causes—laboratory inferences involve the assessment of a single number (rather than a curve on the chart) and thresholds for abnormal conditions are routinely reinforced in practice by the laboratory results. When the system takes the place of one of the physicians, the inter-agreement rate consistently decreases for hemodynamic inferences but increases for laboratory inferences. If the physicians were making their decisions at random according to the observed rate of "yes" answers

*Table 3* ■

Results for Laboratory Inferences

| Inference | Full Agreement Reference Standard | | | Majority Reference Standard | | |
|---|---|---|---|---|---|---|
| | Sensitivity (%) | Specificity (%) | Accuracy (%) | Sensitivity (%) | Specificity (%) | Accuracy (%) |
| Acidosis | 100.00 (6) | 100.00 (36) | 100.00 | 100.00 (8) | 95.00 (40) | 95.83 |
| Alkalosis | 100.00 (3) | 90.91 (33) | 91.67 | 100.00 (6) | 88.10 (42) | 89.58 |
| Hypercardia | 100.00 (4) | 100.00 (38) | 100.00 | 100.00 (5) | 97.67 (43) | 97.92 |
| Hypoxia | N/A (0) | 100.00 (47) | 100.00 | 100.00 (1) | 100.00 (47) | 100.00 |
| Lowsat | N/A (0) | 100.00 (42) | 100.00 | 100.00 (1) | 100.00 (47) | 100.00 |
| Hypernatremia | N/A (0) | 100.00 (48) | 100.00 | N/A (0) | 100.00 (48) | 100.00 |
| Hyponatremia | N/A (0) | 100.00 (47) | 100.00 | N/A (0) | 97.92 (48) | 97.92 |
| Hyperkalemia | N/A (0) | 100.00 (45) | 100.00 | 100.00 (1) | 95.74 (47) | 95.83 |
| Hypokalemia | N/A (0) | 97.67 (43) | 97.67 | 0.00 (2) | 97.83 (46) | 93.75 |
| Anemia | 86.67 (15) | 94.74 (19) | 91.18 | 77.27 (22) | 92.31 (26) | 85.42 |
| Hyperglycemia | 66.67 (6) | 100.00 (19) | 92.00 | 56.25 (16) | 100.00 (32) | 85.42 |
| Hypoglycemia | N/A (0) | 100.00 (48) | 100.00 | N/A (0) | 100.00 (48) | 100.00 |
| Hypercalcemia | N/A (0) | 100.00 (43) | 100.00 | N/A (0) | 100.00 (48) | 100.00 |
| Hypocalcemia | N/A (0) | 100.00 (44) | 100.00 | 50.00 (2) | 100.00 (46) | 97.92 |
| Average (micro-averaged) | 8.24 (34) | 99.09 (552) | 98.46 | 76.56 (64) | 97.70 (608) | 95.68 |
| Average (macro-averaged) | 90.67 | 98.81 | 98.04 | 78.36 | 97.47 | 95.69 |

NOTE: The sample size is 48 for all individual inferences under the majority standard and varies between 25 and 48 for inferences under the full agreement standard. The number of abnormal and normal events is listed in parentheses in the sensitivity and specificity columns respectively (their sum equals the sample size).

(13 percent for hemodynamic inferences and 11 percent for laboratory inferences), their expected rate of agreement would be much closer to their actual rate of agreement for hemodynamic inferences (77.2 vs. 82.8 percent) than for laboratory inferences (80.7 vs. 91.5 percent).

Given the lower overall values of agreement in the class of hemodynamic inferences, we conclude that the physicians are not reliable enough to be used as a gold standard for such inferences. This is further supported by the fact that our system (which applies a decision process established in the literature) agrees more with the average human judge than the other judges do in the case of laboratory inferences, but less so in the case of hemodynamic inferences.

## Comparison Between Human Judges and Our System on Laboratory Inferences

Given the above analysis, it is possible, for laboratory inferences only, to compare the decisions of the three composite judges, taken collectively, with those of the system. We constructed the majority and full

agreement models, as described earlier, and calculated measures of sensitivity, specificity, and accuracy for our system. Table 3 shows the results of this evaluation. Averages for each inference class are calculated by either micro-averaging, which gives each sample equal weight, or macro-averaging, which calculates the result for each inference and averages those, giving the same weight to each inference. Different inferences have different sample sizes in the case of the full agreement reference standard, because there are different numbers of patients for which all physicians agree. We report only micro-averaged results for each separate inference, in the interest of brevity.

The evaluation indicates that our system performs with high sensitivity and specificity compared with the physicians on laboratory inferences, for an average of 88 and 91 percent (micro- and macro-averaging, respectively) sensitivity and 99 percent specificity (both micro- and macro-averaging) against the full agreement model, and 77 and 78 percent sensitivity (micro- and macro-averaging, respectively) and 97 and 98 percent specificity (micro- and macro-averaging, respectively) against the majority model. In almost all cases of individual inferences, the performance scores are in the high 90s; the few cases in which our system displayed poor sensitivity are associated with extremely low counts of abnormal findings (e.g., the system found none of the two cases of hypokalemia according to the majority model). The results in Table 3 confirm our expectation of slightly worse scores against the majority model, compared with the full agreement model (especially on sensitivity), since the former is likely to contain more marginal or harder cases.

## Discussion

These results show that physicians are consistent in identifying abnormal events indicated by laboratory test results, and thus, both the full agreement and majority models can be used as a gold standard against which to evaluate the performance of MAGIC on laboratory inferences.

MAGIC performs quite well in comparison with physicians, achieving perfect accuracy on 10 of 14 inferences in the full agreement model and 7 of 14 in the majority model. Average accuracy is 98 percent for the full agreement model and 96 percent for the majority model.

For the purposes of our study, physicians cannot be used as a gold standard for the more difficult hemodynamic events. In fact, physicians agree only 83 percent of the time, while a chance assignment of results with the same proportion of abnormal results would yield a 77 percent rate of agreement. As we discuss below, our examination of discrepancies between system and physician performance revealed cases in which the physicians were clearly in error. Physicians did not identify abnormal events even when therapy was given to correct for the event. These are clear indications that the event was considered abnormal by the attending physician.

The lack of a viable gold standard in practice indicates the need for a quality assurance tool that can consistently identify and report hemodynamic problems. Given that MAGIC is based on the APACHE thresholds, it could provide a predictable means for reporting events over time. Currently, no existing tool can perform this same service. Once we have modified MAGIC's rules as suggested by our experiments and verified that they produce quality results, our plan is to install MAGIC as a quality assurance tool and do further testing.

Given that the consistency of physician decisions on hemodynamic inferences appears low, and only marginally better than chance, we carried out further analysis of the discrepancies to identify causes of the differences. We re-examined the charts of the patients for whom the physicians reported a hemodynamic anomaly that the system did not report (false negative results, if we consider the physicians a gold standard) and cases in which the system reported a hemodynamic anomaly but the physicians did not (false positive results). This was performed by the first author, as knowledge of MAGIC's inferencing procedure in addition to medical expertise was essential for this comparative analysis.

### False Negative Findings

There are 46 cases in which the physicians report an abnormality that the system missed under the majority model (out of decisions for hemodynamic inferences), of which 8 also appear in the full agreement model. By examining the charts, we found five major causes for the discrepancies:

- *Artifact errors.* An artifact in the chart caused the physician to label an event abnormal when, in fact, it was not. The system correctly screened out these artifacts. (4 cases total, 0 in the full agreement model.)

- *Charting errors.* The relevant critical time point (e.g., intubation or skin incision) was not charted by the anesthesiologist in the OR. It was missing from the LifeLog data and was not shown on the chart. The system misses all inferences around such time points. Physicians, however, could sometimes infer the approximate time of such events by observing changes in the blood pressure and heart rate lines. (18 cases, 0 in the full agreement model.)

- *Window errors.* An abnormal event occurred and was reported by the physicians, but outside the 20-minute window around the critical time point. Despite directions that clearly instruct physicians to identify abnormal events within the 20 minutes before and after a time point (Appendix A), physicians did not always follow these instructions consistently. (7 cases, 0 in the full agreement model.)

- *Threshold errors.* The physicians used lower thresholds than those established in the literature and used by the system, usually by a small margin. (7 cases, 1 in the full agreement model.)

- *Corresponding changes.* The physicians used a lower threshold, as above, but were also influenced by another curve in the chart that also increased or decreased simultaneously (e.g., an increase in the heart rate along with a below-threshold increase in blood pressure may lead to their reporting of hypertension). This merits further analysis, and may lead to the consideration of dependencies between curves in the chart for events that just missed the threshold, something MAGIC currently does not do. (10 cases, 7 also in the full agreement model.)

This analysis shows that 29 of the 46 discrepancies (63 percent) that fall into the categories of artifacts, charting errors, and window mismatches are ones in which the system should not be penalized. None of these errors occurred in the full agreement model. In the case of charting errors, if data are missing from the database, there is no way that the system can compensate. For future experiments, we may want to remove both artifact and charting discrepancies from the set of test cases for evaluation. In the case of window discrepancies, we may be able to provide better instructions to physicians. Instead of providing directions only once at the beginning of the set of instructions, we may want to highlight the appropriate time period around each critical time point.

The remaining 17 cases may indicate system omissions of abnormal conditions. For threshold errors, given the small differences between physician and system thresholds, it is possible that the system should use a small window around the APACHE thresholds, but it is equally possible that the physicians were incorrect. More experimentation is required.

Finally, correlated changes account for the largest discrepancy in missed abnormalities in the full agreement model, and these are second only to charting errors in the majority model. We will experiment with relaxing the thresholds when parallel changes in corresponding measurements occur, investigating the effect on both false negatives and false positives.

**False Positive Findings**

Analysis of the discrepancies that occurred when the system identified an abnormal event that the physician missed revealed seven categories of differences. Four of these—at threshold, above threshold, charting errors, and artifacts—are similar to problems identified for false negative results and are described again below. The new categories are related to the duration of an event and where exactly in relation to a critical time point it occurred. Of the total 102 false positive findings, 60 occurred in the full agreement model. In a few cases, there were two reasons for the discrepancy (e.g., artifact and short duration), and in these cases each reason was assigned 0.5 in determining counts.

- *Charting errors.* The critical time point was entered manually after it actually occurred. For example, if start of bypass is entered too late, the system detects hypotension in the interval before the start of bypass instead of after. (13 cases total, 11 in the full agreement model.)

- *Artifacts.* An artifact occurred, which the system did not screen out, whereas the physicians did. (1.5 cases total, also in the full agreement model.)

- *At threshold.* An event occurred right at the threshold specified by APACHE. The system caught these cases, whereas the physicians did not count them. (30.5 cases total, 18.5 of which occurred in the full agreement model.)

- *Above threshold.* These events were well above the APACHE threshold but, depending on duration, were missed by physicians. For example, when a parameter (e.g., blood pressure) remained low or high for a long duration, physicians often did not call it abnormal, perhaps reasoning that it must not be serious if the physicians on the case opted not to treat it. In contrast, if the parameter stayed at the same low or high rate but then had a quick rise or dip, physicians would label it abnormal. (24.5 cases total, of which 10 occurred in the full agreement model.)

- *Short duration at specific time points.* When systolic blood pressure or heart rate crossed a threshold for a short period of time at start or end of bypass, physicians ignored the abnormality. We suspect that physicians expect abnormalities briefly around bypass and do not report them. (28.5 cases total, 15 in the full agreement model.)

- *Fixed time points.* While the system always uses an interval of 20 minutes before and after a critical time point, it appears that physicians use different time intervals, depending on the critical time point. For example, they use a narrower time interval than the system for skin incision and a wider time interval for induction. (3 cases total, all in the full agreement model.)

- *Chart difficult to read.* The chart is difficult to read in cases where the hemodynamics change quickly, such as after going off bypass (e.g., distinguishing heart rate graph line from the blood pressure line can be difficult). Readability for physicians is made even more difficult by the presence of artifacts in the chart, but for the system these are screened out. A portion of a chart, illustrating these difficulties, is shown in Figure 3. (1 case total, also in the full agreement model.)

The system should not be penalized for charting errors. Both categories of threshold discrepancies show that MAGIC is in line with APACHE scores but in disagreement with the physicians. Furthermore, addressing "at threshold" discrepancies would conflict with addressing the "threshold" discrepancies identified for the false negative findings. We suggested that for false negative discrepancies, adding a window around the threshold would allow the system to identify missed cases, but this would cause an increase in the number of "at threshold" false positives. Conversely, adjusting the threshold for the false positive discrepancies would increase the number of false negatives. More experimentation with thresholds needs to be done.

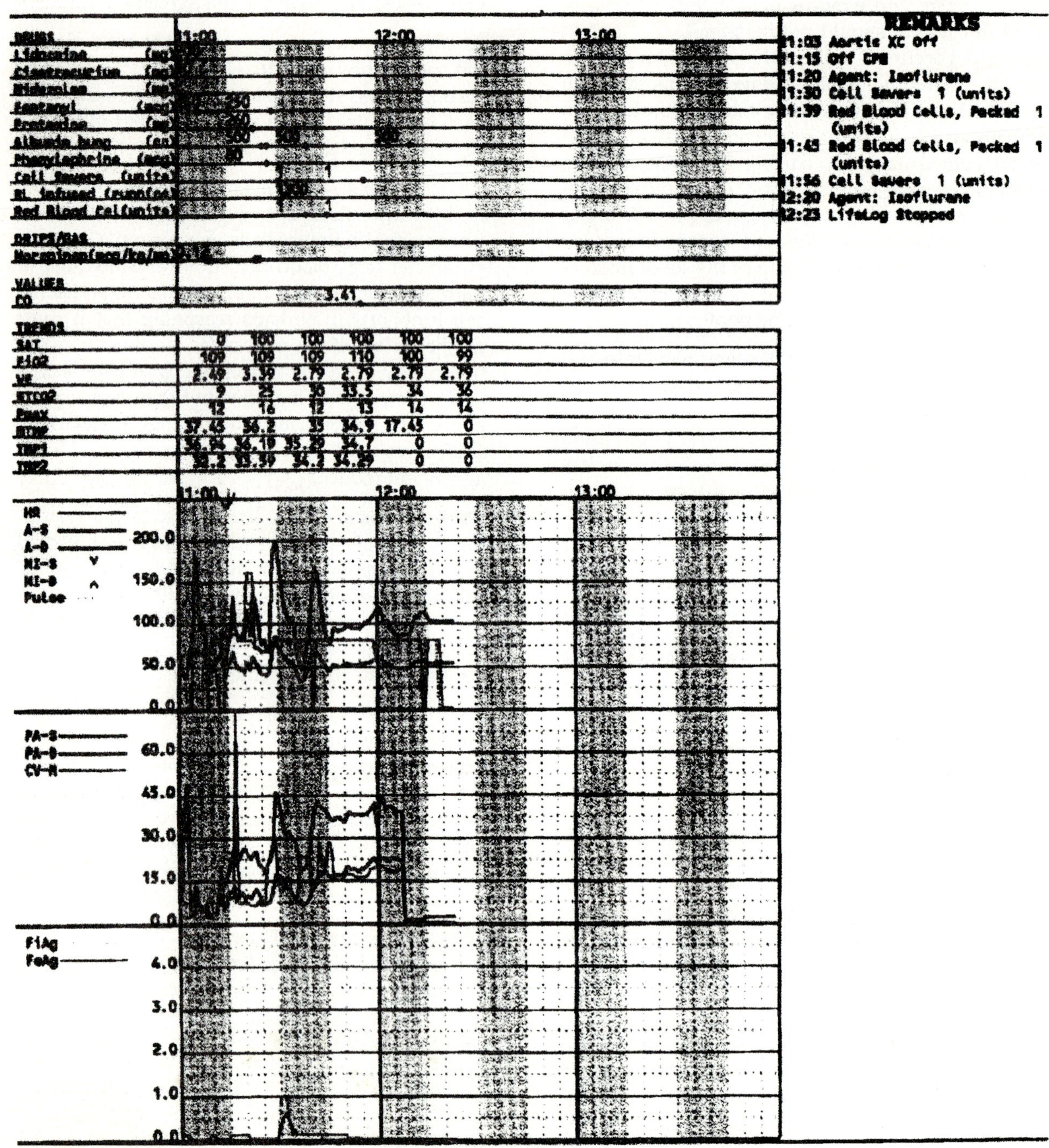

**Figure 3** A portion of the chart showing end of bypass at 11:15.

In multiple cases in the set of discrepancies, the physicians were clearly in error. For example, in several cases, the patient experienced bradycardia or tachycardia before end of bypass. Therapy was given, and this was indicated on the chart. For bradycardic incidents, a pacemaker was placed, while for tachycardic incidents, cardioversion was given. In cases in which therapy has been given on the basis of abnormal physiologic parameters, this should be communicated to subsequent caregivers (e.g., the patient is on a pacemaker because he had bradycardia before the end of bypass).

On the other hand, the categories "short duration" and "fixed time point" suggest some changes that could be made to the system design. We may want to modify MAGIC so that it ignores abnormal events that occur for a short period of time immediately before or after bypass. Similarly, we may need to modify the length of the window in which we check for abnormal events around critical points such as skin incision and induction.

**Study Limitations**

The primary limitation of the study is the lack of data. A set of 24 patients is a small sample size. Furthermore, the interdependence of the inference decisions, which all involve the same set of patients, does not allow the computation of statistical significance levels for comparing the observed agreement with the agreement expected by chance. Nonetheless, this initial study allowed us to determine the viability of using physicians as a gold standard before going on to large-scale studies. It also allowed us to identify places where we can experiment with changes to MAGIC. In addition, it allowed us to critique and improve possible plans for conducting a real-time, prospective study.

It is extremely difficult to obtain adequate data without seriously interfering with normal physician practice in the stressful environment of the ICU. When we are ready to do a large-scale, prospective study with patients, it is important that our experimental methodology place minimal demands on their time and measure accuracy efficiently.

**Future Work**

Our analysis of discrepancies yielded some good insights into changes that we can institute in MAGIC and test in future studies. We found three rules used by the physicians that seem to us to be justified and that could be easily implemented. These include

checking for correlated changes (when a parameter is close to a threshold and a corresponding parameter also changes, count this as an abnormal event), short duration (when a parameter crosses a threshold for a short duration immediately after going on or coming off bypass, ignore the abnormality, as it likely related to bypass), and flexible time periods (use different windows for different critical time points). Our study also shows the need for a follow-up study on the use of thresholds. It is unclear whether the physician or the system is correct when discrepancies in the use of thresholds occur, and we need more experimentation to determine when and how to change thresholds.

One major issue for future work, in particular when investigating disagreement about thresholds, is finding a good gold standard. Some alternatives that have been suggested include using experienced physicians only (but this seriously limits the supply of judges and does not reflect actual practice), using only physicians present during the operation (but this limits us to two or less per case), and using a panel of physicians who discuss the results and come to agreement among themselves as to what constitutes an abnormal hemodynamic event. Given that clear standards for abnormal hemodynamic events are not routinely taught or discussed, having a panel of physicians who spend time resolving disagreements seems the most promising alternative. Given time constraints, this would be most feasible if limited to the questionable cases identified by our current study.

Finally, we plan to test MAGIC as a quality assurance tool. Once it is used on a daily basis, we will conduct a study based on a task analysis and subjective questioning to determine whether use of MAGIC demonstrates the usefulness of the inferences. For example, we will study whether identification of abnormalities leads to differences in patient care and, through questioning, whether physicians find the identification of abnormalities useful in practice.

## Conclusions

We have presented an implemented system that can detect abnormal events during cardiac surgery and, thus, can identify information that is critical to the provision of responsible care for patients arriving in the ICU. Furthermore, inferencing allows the system to summarize large amounts of collected but otherwise unexamined data in a meaningful way. Evaluation shows the system to be quite accurate for laboratory inferences, with an average accuracy of 98 percent (full agreement) and 96 percent (majority model). An analysis of inter-rater agreement, however, showed that physicians do not agree on hemodynamic abnormal events; thus, we were left with no viable gold standard for evaluating hemodynamic events.

Examination of discrepancies between the system and physicians yielded several suggestions for future changes to MAGIC but also revealed cases in which physicians were clearly in error. For example, physician judges reported no abnormality when attending physicians on a case treated an abnormality. More important, the lack of a viable gold standard suggests that MAGIC should be tested as a quality assurance tool, providing a service that is currently lacking in practice. Such a tool could help physicians better learn how to identify abnormal events.

MAGIC is an ongoing group project that has benefited from the design and development work of Elizabeth Chen, Shimei Pan, James Shaw, and Michelle Zhou.

*References* ∎


1. Dalal M, Feiner S, McKeown K, Jordan D, Allen B, alSafadi Y. MAGIC: an experimental system for generating multimedia briefings about post-bypass patient status. Proc AMIA Annu Fall Symp. 1996:684–8.
2. Dalal M, Feiner S, McKeown K, et al. Negotiation for automated generation of temporal multimedia presentations. Proceedings of the 4th ACM International Conference on Multimedia; Nov 18–22, 1996; Boston, Massachusetts, pp 55–64.
3. Insel J, Weissman C, Kember M, Askanazi J, Hyman AI. Cardiovascular changes during transport of critically ill and postoperative patients. Crit Care Med. 1986;14(6):539–42.
4. DiNardo JA, Schwartz M. Anesthesia for cardiac surgery. Norwalk, Conn: Appleton & Lang, 1990.
5. Becker RB, Zimmerman JE, Knaus WA, et al. The use of APACHE III to evaluate ICU length of stay, resource use, and mortality after coronary artery by-pass surgery. J Card Surg. 1995;36(1):1–11.
6. Dept. of Health (NY State), Cardiac Advisory Committee. Cardiac Surgery Report. Feb 1999. Report DOH-2243A.
7. Jordan D, Miller C, Kubos K, Rogers M. Evaluation of sepsis in a critically ill surgical population. Crit Care Med. 1987;15:897–904.
8. Knaus WA, Wagner DP, Draper EA. The APACHE III prognostic system: risk prediction of hospital mortality for critically ill hospitalized adults. Chest. 1991;100:1619–36.
9. McKeown K, Pan S, Shaw J, Jordan D, Allen B. Language generation for multimedia healthcare briefings. Proc Applied NLP. 1997:277–82.
10. Zhou M, Feiner S. Automated production of visualizations: from heterogeneous information to coherent visual discourse. J Intell Info Sys Dec. 1998;11(3):205–34.
11. McKeown K, Pan S. Prosody modeling in concept-to-speech generation: methodological issues. Phil Trans R Soc Lond. 2000; 358(1769):1419–31.
12. McKeown K, Feiner S, Dalal M, Chang S-F. Generating multimedia briefings: coordinating language and illustration. Artif Intell J. 1998;103:95–116.
13. Hripcsak G, Clayton PD, Jenders RA, Cimino JJ, Johnson SB. Design of a clinical event monitor. Comput Biomed Res. 1996;29:194–221.
14. Clancey WJ, Shortliffe EH (ed). Readings in Medical Artificial Intelligence: The First Decade. Reading, Mass: Addison-Wesley, 1984.
15. Sanborn KV, Castro J, Kuroda M, Thys DM. Detection of intraoperative incidents by electronic scanning of computerized anesthesia records. Anesthesiology. 1996;85(5): 977–87.
16. Miller P. Anesthesia. New York: Churchill Livingstone, 1981.
17. Cullen DJ, Keene R, Waternaux C, et al. Objective, quantitative measurement of severity of illness in critically ill patients. Crit Care Med. 1984; 5:137.
18. Zimmerman JE, Knaus WA, Sun X, Wagner DP. Severity stratification and outcome prediction for multisystem organ failure and dysfunction. World J Surg. 1996;20(4):401–5.
19. van Oostrom J, Gravenstein C, Gravenstein J. Acceptable ranges for vital signs during general anesthesia. J Clin Monit. 1993;9:321–5.
20. Berger J, Donchin M, Morgan L, van der Aa J, Gravenstein J. Perioperative changes in blood pressure and heart rate. Anesth Analg. 1984;63:647–52.
21. Block F. Normal fluctuation of physiologic cardiovascular variables during anesthesia and the phenomenon of "smoothing". J Clin Monit. 1991;7:141–5.
22. Hripcsak G, Kuperman GJ, Friedman C, Heitjan DF. A reliability study for evaluating information extraction from radiology. J Am Med Inform Assoc. 1999;6:143–50.
23. Friedman C, Hripcsak G. Evaluating natural language processors in the clinical domain. Methods Inf Med. 1998;37:334–44.


*The Appendix appears on the following page.*

*Appendix*

QUESTIONNAIRE GIVEN TO PHYSICIANS FOR THE EXPERIMENT

Your Name: _______________________________

MRN of Patient:  00000000

1)  Please look over the following patient record and become familiar with the case.

2) Given the following list of critical points, please check all abnormalities (blood pressure and heart rate) that occurred during the procedure before or after each critical point. Please check the "Nothing" slot if none of the listed abnormalities took place. Please check the "Not Documented" slot and continue if the critical point was not documented in the patient report. (NOTE: "Before" and "after" should be interpreted as "up to 20 minutes before" and "up to 20 minutes after," respectively. Please do not indicate abnormalities that occurred outside this range.)

**Induction**—There was:  __Nothing  __Not Documented

| Hypotension | Hypertension | Bradycardia | Tachycardia |
|---|---|---|---|
| __before __after | __before __after | __before __after | __before __after |

**Skin Incision**—There was:  __Nothing  __Not Documented

| Hypotension | Hypertension | Bradycardia | Tachycardia |
|---|---|---|---|
| __before __after | __before __after | __before __after | __before __after |

**Start of Bypass**—There was:  __Nothing  __Not Documented

| Hypotension | Hypertension | Bradycardia | Tachycardia |
|---|---|---|---|
| __before __after | __before __after | __before __after | __before __after |

**End of Bypass**—There was:  __Nothing  __Not Documented

| Hypotension | Hypertension | Bradycardia | Tachycardia |
|---|---|---|---|
| __before __after | __before __after | __before __after | __before __after |

3)  Please indicate whether or not the following abnormal labs occurred during the time period listed, where pre-bypass means the entire time recorded before the start of bypass and post-bypass means the entire time after the end of bypass. Labs taken during bypass can be ignored.

**Pre-bypass**—There was:  __Nothing  __No labs documented

| __Acidosis | __Alkalosis | __Hypercarbia | __Hypoxia |
|---|---|---|---|
| __Low saturation | __Hypernatremia | __Hyponatremia | __Hyperkalemia |
| __Hypokalemia | __Anemia | __Hyperglycemia | __Hypoglycemia |
| __Hypercalcemia | __Hypocalcemia | | |

**Post-bypass**—There was:  __Nothing  __No labs documented

| __Acidosis | __Alkalosis | __Hypercarbia | __Hypoxia |
|---|---|---|---|
| __Low saturation | __Hypernatremia | __Hyponatremia | __Hyperkalemia |
| __Hypokalemia | __Anemia | __Hyperglycemia | __Hypoglycemia |
| __Hypercalcemia | __Hypocalcemia | | |

4) If there are any abnormalities, not covered above, that you feel are important, please list them here along with where they fall with respect to the critical points.

# Giving Patients Access to Their Medical Records via the Internet:

## The PCASSO Experience

DANIEL MASYS, MD, DIXIE BAKER, PHD, AMY BUTROS, MLS, KEVIN E. COWLES

**Abstract** Objective: The Patient-Centered Access to Secure Systems Online (PCASSO) project is designed to apply state-of-the-art-security to the communication of clinical information over the Internet.

**Design:** The authors report the legal and regulatory issues associated with deploying the system, and results of its use by providers and patients. Human subject protection concerns raised by the Institutional Review Board focused on three areas—unauthorized access to information by persons other than the patient; the effect of startling or poorly understood information; and the effect of patient access to records on the record-keeping behavior of providers.

**Measurements:** Objective and subjective measures of security and usability were obtained.

**Results:** During its initial deployment phase, the project enrolled 216 physicians and 41 patients; of these, 68 physicians and 26 patients used the system one or more times. The system performed as designed, with no unauthorized information access or intrusions detected. Providers rated the usability of the system low because of the complexity of the secure login and other security features and restrictions limiting their access to those patients with whom they had a professional relationship. In contrast, patients rated the usability and functionality of the system favorably.

**Conclusion:** High-assurance systems that serve both patients and providers will need to address differing expectations regarding security and ease of use.

The Patient-Centered Access to Secure Systems Online (PCASSO) project is designed to apply state-of-the-art security to the communication of clinical information over the Internet. When the project began in 1996, several prototype Web-based clinical information systems existed,[1-3] but these were explicitly designed to serve only health professionals, and most used security "firewalls" to filter queries originating from outside an organization's private network.

PCASSO was conceived with the premise that the full potential of a ubiquitous national information infrastructure (NII) lies in its catalysis of new and expanded opportunities for communication, not simply in the acceleration of existing lines of communication. A key theme of the NII is individual empowerment, a focus on the "customer" as a participant and partner in the flow of information. In a medical environment, this customer is the patient, who is empowered by PCASSO technology to access his or her own health information.

The PCASSO security model explicitly recognizes the rights and responsibilities of providers and their patients, and implements those rights and responsi-

Affiliation of the authors: University of California, San Diego, La Jolla, California.

Correspondence and reprints: Daniel Masys, MD, Director, Biomedical Informatics, UCSD School of Medicine, 9500 Gilman Drive, Mailcode 0602, La Jolla, CA 92093-0602; e-mail: <dmasys@ucsd.edu>.

bilities through a role-based access-control scheme that enforces confidentiality, integrity, and accountability rules compatible with public data networks such as the Internet. The technical details of the system design, including the overall architecture,[6] the security model and concept of operations,[7] the approach to overcoming client-side vulnerabilities,[8–10] and methods for attaining high assurance of correct operations[11] have been described elsewhere. Here we report the legal and regulatory issues associated with deploying the system, and the results of its use by providers and patients associated with the University of California, San Diego (UCSD) Healthcare, during calendar year 1999.

## Legal and Regulatory Context

The legal and regulatory context for the PCASSO project included existing and emerging federal and state laws and regulations regarding health information security and patient privacy, as well as Institutional Review Board (IRB) regulations regarding the use of human subjects in research activities.

The PCASSO vision, as described in the initial project plan, was to capitalize on state-of-the-art security technologies and the ubiquity of the Internet to enable patients and their providers to view patients' medical records from virtually anywhere. The legislative authority and mandate for doing this in the State of California is contained in the California Health and Safety Code, which states that:

> The Legislature finds and declares that every person having ultimate responsibility for decisions respecting his or her own health care also possesses a concomitant right of access to complete information respecting his or her condition and care provided.[11]

The Code defines both a general right of access and several special circumstances for denying or restricting patients' access to their health records, including health records of minors, alcohol and drug abuse treatment records, mental health records, and records describing communicable disease carriers. The California statutes entitling patients to full access to their records are similar to statutes found in approximately 20 other states, but the variability among states' laws also extends to the opposite extreme, where seven states specifically deny patients the right to see medical records, and three additional states allow patients to see only mental health records.[12]

Since the start of the PCASSO project, health care has experienced significant change in the areas of infor-

mation security and patient privacy, primarily prompted by the Health Insurance Portability and Accountability Act (HIPAA) of 1996,[13] which called for the development and implementation of a number of standards, including security and privacy. The Privacy Standard,[14] which went into effect in April 2001, set forth the rights of individual patients with respect to the access to and use of their protected health information, thus establishing a uniform, minimum set of patient rights nationwide. However, because states still may enact laws that extend the rights to patients beyond what is specified in the Privacy Standards, variability remains.

The draft Security Standard issued pursuant to HIPAA[15] specified requirements covering administrative practices, physical safeguards, and technical services and mechanisms. The draft standard was issued in August 1998; the Department of Health and Human Services has announced final issuance by the end of 2001.

In November 1998, the U.S. Centers for Medicare and Medicaid Services (CMS, formerly Health Care Financing Administration) released technical guidelines for the acceptable use of the Internet to communicate person-identifiable health information.[16] The guidelines specify that all CMS information protected by the Privacy Act and other sensitive CMS information may be transmitted over the Internet so long as an acceptable method of encryption is used to protect confidentiality and integrity, and authentication or identification procedures are employed to ensure that both the sender and the recipient of the data are known to each other and are authorized to receive and decrypt such information.

## Methods

### The PCASSO Model and User Experience

The PCASSO model was built using high-assurance methods that have been described previously.[10] The architecture includes an application server to which the UCSD clinical information systems pass data in HL7 messages. These messages are parsed and stored in PCASSO's clinical data repository (CDR), labeled at one of five sensitivity levels—low, standard, public-deniable, guardian-deniable, and patient-deniable. "Low" data are not patient-identifiable, such as data that have been de-identified in accordance with the HIPAA Privacy Standard. "Standard" data are routine health information; that is, identifiable health information that does not fall into any of the "deniable" categories. "Public-deniable" includes information about conditions specifically addressed by state law, such as mental health, HIV/AIDS, abortion, adoption, sexually transmitted diseases, and substance abuse. "Guardian-deniable" is health information that by law can be withheld from a guardian, such as (in some states) information about a teenager's abortion. "Patient-deniable" is information that the patient's primary care physician considers capable of causing harm to the patient were it disclosed to that patient. The HIPAA Privacy Standard recognizes three types of "patient-deniable" information—psychotherapy notes; information compiled for use in a civil, criminal, or administrative action or proceeding; and certain information that is subject to or exempted from the Clinical Laboratory Improvements Amendments (CLIA) of 1988. No data were specifically excluded from the PCASSO system.

The client application is contained in a Java applet that communicates with the PCASSO server over a TCP/IP link. The PCASSO server performs security mediation in accordance with the role-based security policy. A firewall stands behind the PCASSO server to protect the university's information systems, while the PCASSO host sits directly on the Internet. Host hardening and internal firewall functions protect the PCASSO server from external threats to its data and services. The architecture combines a protected Java client, a secure communication protocol, a trusted application server, and secure administration services to enable authorized persons to view specific information in the clinical data repository, or to perform privileged actions such as relabeling data or assigning and revoking access rights. All actions on the PCASSO host are audited.

Because this paper reports the results of our evaluation of the model with our test users, we describe here the experience of using the PCASSO system. The user logs in using multi-factor authentication involving a password, a challenge-response token, and a public–private key pair. The graphical image of a keyboard is used to enter all security-critical information, such as the user's password and patients' names. The user starts a Web browser (Netscape Navigator or Microsoft Internet Explorer) and enters the PCASSO URL, which retrieves a file containing the Java code for the PCASSO graphical user interface and displays the login screen shown in Figure 1.

The user enters her user ID and password through the graphical keyboard, after which the client asks the user to insert a personal read-only, encrypted diskette containing her private key. The client and server use their respective public–private key pairs to

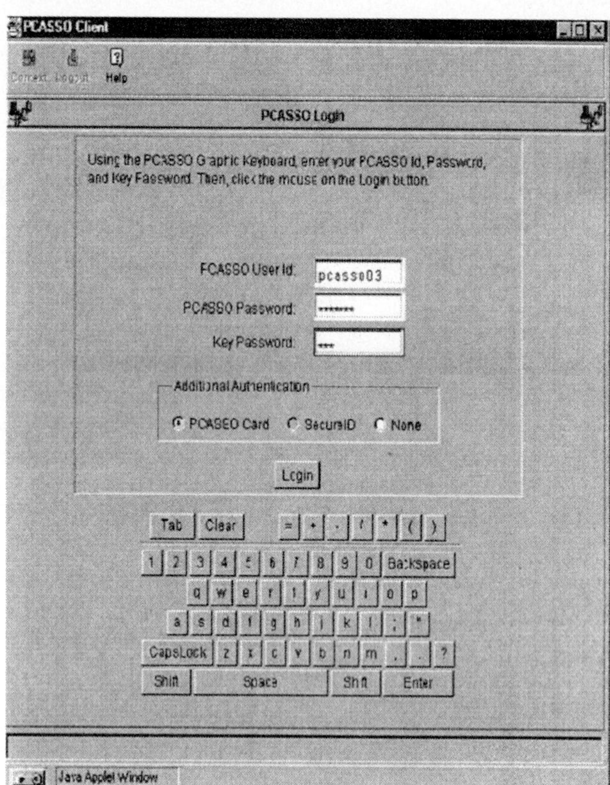

**Figure 1** PCASSO login screen.

mutually authenticate each other ("handshake"), and the application notifies the user that a secure connection has been established. The user then is asked to input the next character string that appears on her "PCASSO card," a laminated card containing random numbers that are synchronized with a corresponding list stored on the server. The PCASSO model system provides all the security services required by the HIPAA security standard and the HCFA Internet security **policy.**[*]

Following authentication, a screen customized for the user's context (patient or provider) is displayed. If the user is both a patient and a provider, she is asked to select which context she wants to use for the current session. The server receives the user's requests, determines what data she can see and what actions she may perform, and returns the results. If the user is a provider, the server prompts her to select a patient. She may type either a name or a non-zero character string to return a list of patients whose names begin with that string and for whom she has

---

*For a detailed description of the PCASSO architecture and operations concept, see Baker.[17]

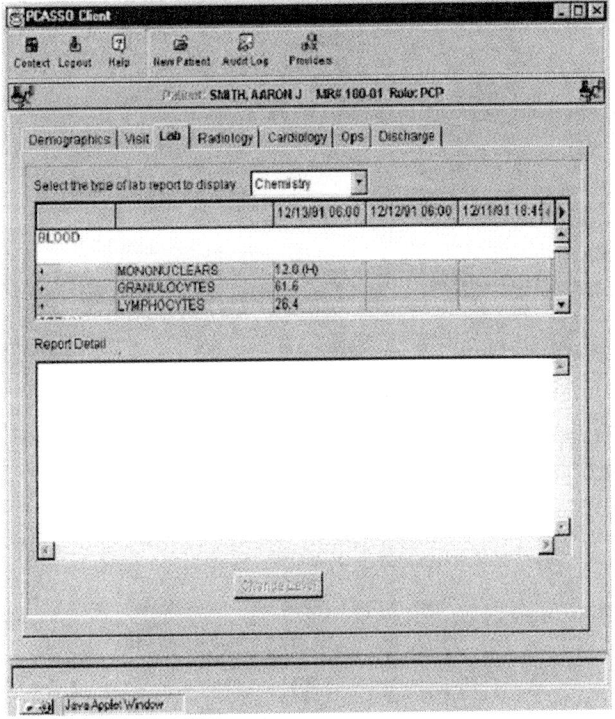

**Figure 2**  Sample results screen.

been authorized a provider role. A results screen for laboratory data is shown in **Figure 2**.

At the completion of each usage session, users are prompted but not required to fill out a user response form regarding the just-completed session, which is shown in **Figure 3**. Feedback from the response forms was used to assess user perceptions and behaviors.

## Evaluation Criteria

The PCASSO system was evaluated using the same criteria used by the Food and Drug Administration to evaluate medial devices—Is it safe and is it effective? Safety was judged using both qualitative and quantitative measures. Qualitative measures were evaluated using feedback from users regarding their perceptions of the security provided by the PCASSO system. Data sources for quantitative evaluation included access logs and system penetration activities. The system is instrumented to detect a wide variety of attempts to intrude or misuse the system, including unauthorized login attempts; attempts to modify data; and misuse of the "emergency" role. System penetrations were measured both through formal penetration testing exercises ("white hat" hacking) and ad hoc penetration attempts from the Internet at large. Effectiveness was judged using feedback from samples of both providers and patients.

## Pilot Deployment

The model system was first released as a pilot to credentialed UCSD faculty physicians to judge its safety and efficacy, as well as its suitability for use by patients. A total of 210 faculty physicians were enrolled as users during the pilot. At the time of the pilot deployment, the system contained demographic, clinical laboratory, radiology, and dictated transcribed reports for 178,000 patients for whom care was provided in the UCSD Healthcare network, dating from mid 1998. The clinical data repository was continuously updated with copies of new data sent by the operational UCSD clinical information system. Although the PCASSO system provided neither the "open" access nor the features of the internal clinical information systems interface at UCSD, the benefit to physicians was the ability to securely access their patients' data from any Internet-connected PC, essentially from anywhere in the world. The data acquired from the pilot deployment to physicians showed the system to be operating according to its security design principles, without any penetrations, intrusions, or other breeches of information security and confidentiality being detected.

## Full Deployment

Using the results of the system usage by providers as an indicator of system safety and efficacy, application was made to the UCSD IRB in May 1999 to open the system for use by patients. Patients were eligible to participate if the following conditions were met:

- They were active UCSD Healthcare patients (i.e., had at least one clinic visit or hospitalization within the previous year)

- They had pre-existing Internet access, and a compatible computer (the project did not support the costs of computers or online access for participants)

- Their primary care physician agreed to their participation and co-signed the informed consent document acknowledging the patient's participation in the project and its implications.

Patients who met these criteria completed a computer use and demographics survey, and a user account was created for them by the PCASSO user support staff. The support staff included members of the UCSD biomedical library staff who have extensive experience in helping persons use PC technology and find answers to health-related questions from a variety of sources. PCASSO's multiple complementary

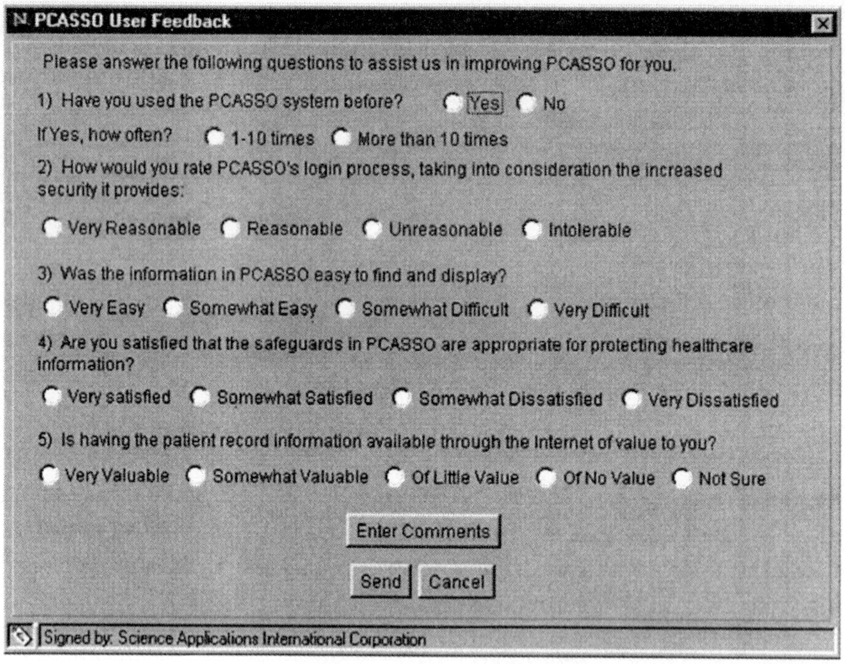

**Figure 3** Feedback form.

security mechanisms ensured that patients could view only their own medical data, excluding any data that the patient's primary care provider had specifically labeled **"patient-deniable."**[†]

Each new user received a security diskette containing that user's private key, a user guide with a tutorial on how to use the system, and a PCASSO card, as described above. New users were also given a toll-free number to call in case they had either technical or medical questions that arose as a result of using the system. This number connected them to the PCASSO support staff at the UCSD biomedical library. The library support staff were expected to answer technical questions related to use of the system, and a triage protocol was used to handle inquiries related to medical information received by patients.

### Human Subjects Research Issues

As noted above, the PCASSO project required review by the UCSD IRB before patients could be involved in the research. The IRB required clarification of several issues before approving participation by patients, and may have been sensitized to issues of health information privacy by our providing a background description of Internet-associated security threats. These issues and our approaches to dealing with them are presented here because we believe they are a harbinger of concerns that will arise in health care organizations generally as a result of HIPAA-mandated access to medical records by patients and the increasing use of electronic medical records.

Human subject protection concerns focused on three areas—unauthorized access to information by persons other than the patient; the effect of patients' seeing startling or poorly understood information; and the effect of patient access to records on the record-keeping behavior of providers. These issues and our approach to dealing with them are described below.

The IRB was concerned about the scenario of theft of information access, such as by a family member of a patient participating in the clinical trial of the system. The response to this concern noted that electronic information security requires that access be granted only after user authentication (i.e., proving that one is who he claims to be) that is based on some combination of "something the user knows" (e.g., password), "something the user has" (e.g., token), and "something the user is" (e.g., fingerprint).

PCASSO uses something the user knows (user ID and password pair) and something the user has (an encrypted, read-only security diskette and a PCASSO key). Also, PCASSO account creation involves physical validation of the user's identity by a trusted party (i.e., physician). Thus, although it is possible to give away one's identity, this would require that the authorized PCASSO user actually train a family member in how to assume his identity, as well as give the family member

---

[†]The HIPAA Privacy Standards do not allow for denial of patient access to any of their medical information.

the necessary security diskette and PCASSO card. PCASSO does not allow information to be saved to disk on the user's PC and does not allow information to be copied to other applications. Thus, the risk of theft is substantially lower than the risk that would be associated, for example, with paper health records maintained by the patient or with a password-protected Web site for which the patient had saved the password locally via their Web browser.

Several IRB questions related to the potential psychological harm of startling or poorly understood information. Because the PCASSO system makes information available to providers and patients simultaneously, the scenario of a patient's gaining access to a particular laboratory result or dictated note before his providers see it is a genuine concern. However, the content the patient would view is identical to the information that he would receive if he requested a photocopy of his clinical records. The issue is further clouded by the fact that what patients may find startling is "in the eye of the beholder" and cannot be predicted a priori, just as medical emergencies are generally defined by patients and not by providers.

The IRB asked what would happen if the record contained a new diagnosis of a disease such as cancer and, because of timing or scheduling difficulties, the physician had not had an opportunity to get back to the patient personally before the patient read it on the computer. The PCASSO team called this the "out-of-the-blue diagnosis" scenario, in which a completely unexpected result appears and the physician and patient have had no prior discussion of possible outcomes.

An analysis of this scenario reveals that definitive diagnoses virtually always follow a specific test or procedure ordered by a provider, rather than a screening test. For example, a routine chest x-ray report might note a previously unreported mass, and a routine complete blood count may reveal a high white cell count, but the initial reports of these abnormalities do not state conclusive diagnoses, and uniformly comment on the need for further evaluation. Cancer requires a tissue diagnosis and a procedure to obtain that tissue.

The PCASSO project relies on the premise that consent for diagnostic procedures has included a discussion of the reasons for those procedures. Stated otherwise, if a patient could truly say, "I never knew they wanted to do a biopsy because one of the possibilities was that I might have cancer," then both PCASSO and the patient would fall victim to a prior failure to obtain fully informed consent for clinical care.

To address the concerns of the IRB, the PCASSO project incorporated the following four elements into the system design:

- The PCASSO system filters those results transactions labeled "pending" or "interim" and displays only final results. Subsequent amendments and revised results replace any clinical data found to be in error.

- The project's informed consent language was amended to read:

  The information you will be able to access via the PCASSO system is technical and contained in systems that were originally designed for trained health professionals' use only. As a result, there is a possibility that you will be exposed to information that you do not understand or find startling. PCASSO is not intended to place on you the burden of interpreting your medical record, nor to cause you to act on the information received without first discussing it with your physician. One of the risks associated with this study is that "a little knowledge is a dangerous thing." By agreeing to participate, you agree to contact your physician to help resolve any questions or problems that may arise as a result of viewing your medical data online. If you have difficulty contacting your physician, you may contact the PCASSO project staff, who will assist you in contacting your physician.

- A toll-free phone "hotline" was established and a formal triage mechanism created for inquiries from distraught patients. The primary user support for the project was provided by the UCSD biomedical library and staffed by a librarian with extensive experience in assisting patients with cancer and other serious diseases. The triage protocol included contacting a patient's primary care physician to make the physician aware of patient concerns, and immediate referral to the psychiatry service crisis intervention team if circumstances warranted.

- By study design, all such instances would be considered "information toxicity" and reported to the IRB as adverse events. The project staff looked to the IRB as a pro-active data and safety monitoring group that could help represent the balance of interests of participants and UCSD Healthcare providers.

The IRB also questioned whether physicians' knowing that their patients would have computer access to their health records would discourage the physicians from recording candid and detailed observations and impressions. The project response to this issue was that physicians create their records with the knowledge that those records may be subject to review in the future for a variety of purposes, including quality assurance, risk management, and legal inquiry. In addition, patients can and do request copies of their paper-based records, including provider notes. Indeed, the PCASSO security technology enables providers to raise the sensitivity level of specific information in the record to the "patient-deniable" sensitivity level, which enables other authorized providers to view the information but removes it from view by the patient. Individual results and reports can also be given this label via a set of rules used by the system's import function. For example, one loading rule stated that all notes originating from the psychiatry department would default to the patient-deniable category.

The IRB required that the project plan be reviewed by the risk management office of the UCSD Medical Center and by the Office of General Counsel of the University of California. Among these advisors, the general consensus was that the benefits of providing patients with online access to medical records far outweighed the risks. Given the technical capabilities provided by a high-assurance system like PCASSO and the growing ubiquity of the Internet, it could be argued that a liability might more likely derive from delaying patient access to information to which they are entitled than from providing it to them under the terms of consent used in the project. The advisors also noted that PCASSO could reduce the institution's liability by virtually ensuring that results would receive expeditious review by someone. Legal counsel also emphasized the imperative to direct patients to contact their physicians to discuss the specific implications of test results and other information viewed using the system.

## Results

The prototype PCASSO system was installed at UCSD for 12 months. During that time, our audit detected a number of attempted intrusions, but to our knowledge the system was never penetrated. In March 1999, the operational system was subjected to an intense and comprehensive simulated attack by a computer security "penetration team" from a division of SAIC (Science Applications International Corporation, San Diego, California) that was not involved in the PCASSO development. This team used more than 300 "hacker" tools and penetration techniques acquired from commercial sources, obtained from the hacker "underground," or developed by the company. The system passed this test flawlessly; results of this testing have been published.[11]

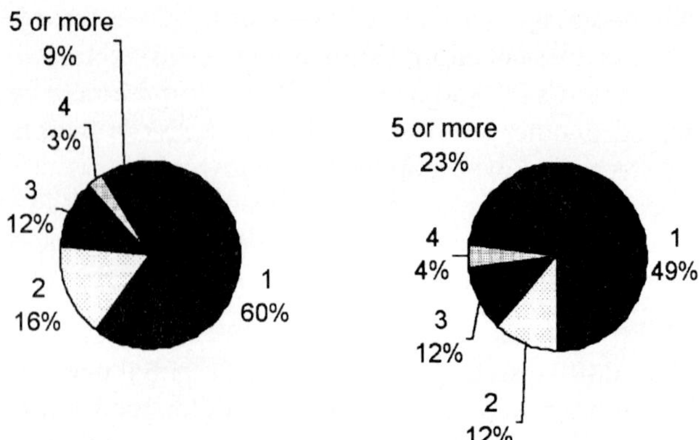



**Figure 4** Comparison of numbers of sessions. *Left,* number of provider sessions; *right,* number of patient sessions.

A total of 216 physicians and 41 patients were enrolled as users of the system, of whom 68 physicians and 26 patients logged in one or more times. At the time of the full trial, the PCASSO clinical data repository contained clinical data for more than 178,000 patients. The typical physician enrollee was male (78 percent) and had good computer skills (53 percent) and good knowledge of the Internet (48 percent). The typical patient enrollee was female (73 percent), was well educated (71 percent with college degree), and had excellent computer skills (49 percent) and excellent Internet knowledge (54 percent). The vast majority of enrollees had well-equipped PCs, with 47 percent having Pentium II or Pentium Pro processors with clock speeds of 90 MHz or higher (77 percent) and at least 64 MB of RAM (57 percent).

A considerably larger percentage of patient enrollees actually used the system than did physicians—26 of the patient enrollees (61 percent) compared with 68 physicians (31 percent). Of those who used the system, more patients logged in at least five times (23 percent) than did physicians (9 percent), despite the fact that most of the physicians had access to the system for at least 10 months, whereas PCASSO was accessible to patients for only 6 months. An informal sampling of patients who enrolled but did not use the system revealed that the most common reason for not accessing the system was that they had not had a recent clinic visit. The distribution of the numbers of sessions for physicians and patients is shown in **Figure 4**.

The user feedback form asked for feedback in several areas—reasonableness of the PCASSO security features, effectiveness of the system, ease of use, and usefulness of the data. As described earlier, logging

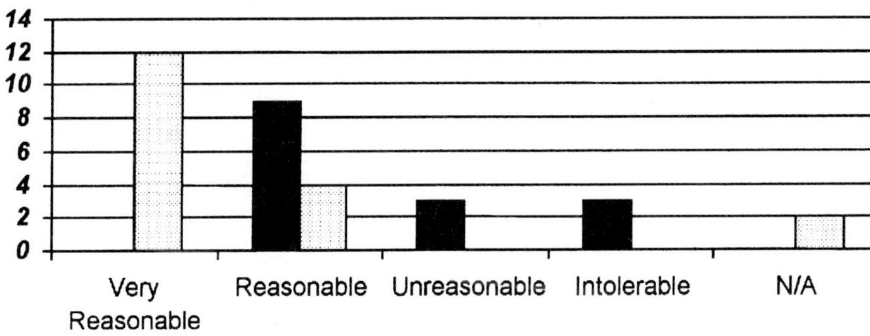

**Figure 5** Perceptions of PCASSO login process. *Dark columns,* physicians' ratings; *light columns,* patients' ratings.

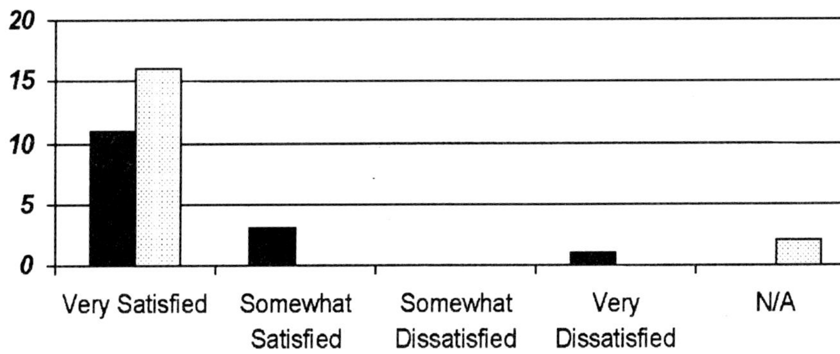

**Figure 6** Perceptions of PCASSO safeguards. *Dark columns,* providers ratings; *light columns,* patients' ratings.

into the PCASSO system is a multi-step process requiring the use of a user ID, a password, a diskette, and a PCASSO card. This multi-step process is designed to provide a high level of assurance that users are indeed who they claim to be and that they are authorized to use the system.

Patients and physicians judged this process quite differently, as shown in **Figure 5.** Sixty-eight percent of the patients who provided feedback (18 users) considered this process "very reasonable," whereas none of the physicians who provided feedback (15 users) considered it so. Indeed, fully 88 percent of the patients who provided feedback rated the login process either "very reasonable" or "reasonable," 11 percent rated it "not applicable," and none considered it either "unreasonable" or "intolerable."

Although 60 percent of the physicians who provided feedback rated it "reasonable," the remainder of the physicians who provided feedback rated it either "unreasonable" (20 percent) or "intolerable" (20 percent). The differences between patient and physician ratings of the acceptance of the login process were statistically significant, with a two-tailed *P* value of less than 0.0001 as measured by the Mann-Whitney test.

Despite the negative perceptions of the physicians, when asked to rate their degree of satisfaction with the PCASSO safeguards, both physicians and patients said they were "very satisfied." **Figure 6** shows a comparison of the physicians' and patients' ratings of the PCASSO safeguards.

With respect to effectiveness, we also asked the users to rate the overall value of having records available to them over the Internet. As shown in **Figure 7**, a majority of both physicians and patients rated the value as "very high." No one said they found no value in having medical records available, and only one physician rated Internet accessibility of "little value."

Users were also given the opportunity to provide free-text feedback. A number of physicians and patients commented that some specific information they were looking for was not available. This resulted from several circumstances. First, the PCASSO clinical data repository was populated with real-time data sent from active clinical systems; it was not preloaded with data recorded before PCASSO was installed. Second, some data types (e.g., urinalysis serology) were simply not implemented in the model system. Finally, some data may not yet have been sent to PCASSO at the time a user logged in.

The primary comment from the physicians was that the role-based access controls did not allow them to view all the data in the system, as they currently can using the operational clinical system. Also, some security features, such as the multi-step challenge-

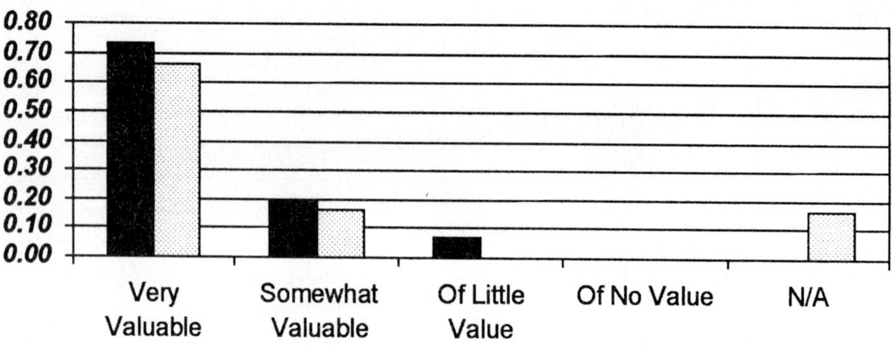



**Figure 7** Perceptions of value of having records accessible on the Internet. *Dark columns, physicians' ratings; light columns, patients' ratings.*

response user authentication and use of a graphical keyboard in place of the physical keyboard, generated a substantial number of negative reactions.

Some comments from patients suggested that the IRB's initial concern that patients might overreact or panic if they saw results without having their physicians there to explain them was not an issue in this group of users, although one patient asked for a "key to understand the notation in my lab report." Other comments simply expressed appreciation for having the information available:

> I was at the lab this morning and some results are posted already…very impressed!!

> It was great to be able to read my lab results, as my physician has not reported them to me.

We also saw indications that PCASSO influenced patients' behaviors and assisted clinicians in providing care. One user said that he or she "caught the lab doing the wrong test and had it corrected." Another noted that his or her lab results were not yet in the system, so he or she would "wait a few days before I call the office."

We received positive comments from both physicians and patients. Here is a sampling:

> As a demonstration of "SSO" part of the acronym, it seems very secure—certainly much more so than most e-commerce transactions (including stock trades) I've done. It's incredibly handy to have this stuff available on the Internet. Nice work. (From a physician)

> Thank you for this "peek" into our own medical records. So often patients seem to feel at the mercy of the HMOs, and at least this may alleviate some of that distrust.

> Love this program and it really is super easy to use! Did notice that I have 3 PCPs, when actually two of them are specialists. …Nice to get to read reports of special tests. Thanks!

> As one who has always been involved in my health care decisions, I value that I have access to this infor-

mation. Great system. I find it very user friendly and feel very confident that my privacy is maintained at all times. Thank you for allowing me the opportunity to use it.

## Discussion and Conclusions

The qualitative data we collected from our users and the quantitative audit and penetration data revealed that the PCASSO system is both perceived to be safe and is safe. Both physicians and patients gave PCASSO very high ratings on its safety, and the system has continually resisted attack. One unsolicited comment came to us from a person who approached one of the investigators following a talk about the project, handed the investigator a business card, and identified himself as a "professional hacker." He said that he had been targeting the PCASSO server for some months and to that point had been unsuccessful in penetrating it. We were gratified by his observation that "you guys really know what you're doing."

However, this safety has come with a price in usability. The PCASSO system clearly is more difficult to use than the systems to which most people are accustomed. Our data suggest that, for patients, some "challenge" is acceptable and may even have value, in that it contributes to the perception of safety. However, some features, while contributing to PCASSO's safety, may be overly burdensome, particularly for providers, to the point of affecting PCASSO's effectiveness. Our data suggest that our patients may value security over convenience, whereas our providers' values may be quite the reverse.

A clear majority of our users found value in having patient information accessible over the Internet. But that effectiveness is moderated by a user experience that may discourage its use. Our findings suggest that security features need to be flexible and configurable, based on the needs and expectations of users and the risks an enterprise is willing to assume.

*Table 1* ■

PCASSO meets HIPAA's Requirements for
Technical Security Services to Guard Data,
Integrity, Confidentiality, and Availability

| Requirement | PCASSO Model |
| --- | --- |
| Emergency access | Yes |
| Context-based, role-based, or user-based access control | Role-based |
| Encryption over public networks | Yes |
| Audit controls | Yes |
| Role-based or user-based authorization control | Role-based |
| Data authentication | Encryption ensures integrity of data passed over the Internet; importer rejects malformed messages |
| Automatic logoff | Yes |
| Unique user identification | Yes |
| Biometric, password, PIN, telephone callback, or token | Password and token |

*Table 2* ■

PCASSO meets HIPAA's Requirements for
Technical Security Mechanisms to Guard
Against Unauthorized Access to Data That is
Transmitted over a Communication Network

| Requirement | PCASSO Model |
| --- | --- |
| Integrity controls | Encryption protects integrity of data; label-based access control protects integrity of executable code |
| Message authentication | Encryption authenticates message integrity; no MAC or digital signature |
| Access controls or encryption | Access controls and encryption |
| Alarm | Server senses loss of client |
| Audit trail | Yes |
| Entity authentication | Both server and client are authenticated |
| Event reporting | Detection/reporting of intrusion attempts and misuse of "emergency" role |

We are often asked whether the PCASSO model is "HIPAA compliant." Our first response is to observe that the final HIPAA Security Standard has not yet been released. However, evaluating PCASSO against the final Privacy Standard, we observe that PCASSO empowers patients consistent with the letter and spirit of the standard, including support for its "minimum necessary" mandate. Evaluating PCASSO against the August 1998 Security Standards Proposed Rule, we find that PCASSO contains all the features specified for technical services and mechanisms, as shown in **Tables 1 and 2**.

Through our experience in building and evaluating the PCASSO model, we have shown that a system can be built that is strong enough to provide safe access to highly sensitive personal health information over the Internet. However, building systems that meet both patients' expectations for privacy and safety and their providers' expectations for convenience and usability remains a substantial challenge. Work to achieve these goals is currently under way.

*References* ■


1. Cimino JJ, Socratous S, Clayton PD. Internet as clinical information system: application development using the World Wide Web. J Am Med Inform Assoc. 1995;2(5):273–83.
2. Chute CC, Crowson DL, Buntrock JD. Medical information retrieval and WWW browsers at Mayo. Proc Annu Symp Comput Appl Med Care. 1995:903–7.
3. Jagannathan V, Reddy YV, Srinivas K, et al. An overview of the CERC ARTEMIS project. Proc Annu Symp Comput Appl Med Care. 1995:12–6.
4. Kahn CE, Bell DS. WebSTAR: platform-independent structured reporting using World Wide Web technology. In Hripcsak G. ed. Proc AMIA Spring Congress. 1995:86.
5. Masys DR, Baker DB. Patient-centered access to secure systems online (PCASSO): a secure approach to clinical data access via the World Wide Web. Proc AMIA Annu Fall Symp. 1997:340–3.
6. Baker D, Barnhart R, Buss T. PCASSO: applying and extending state-of-the-art security in the healthcare domain. Presented at: 13th Annual Computer Security Applications Conference; San Diego, California; Dec 12, 1997. Available at http://medicine.ucsd.edu/pcasso/.
7. Masys DR, Baker DB, Barnhart R, Buss T. PCASSO: A secure architecture for access to clinical data via the Internet. Medinfo. 1998;9 pt 2:1130–4.
8. Masys DR, Baker DB. Protecting clinical data on Web client computers: the PCASSO approach. Proc AMIA Symp. 1998:366–70.
9. Baker DB, Masys DR. PCASSO: a design for secure communication of personal health information via the internet. Int J Med Inf. 1999;54(2):97–104.
10. Baker DB, Masys DR. Assurance: the power behind PCASSO security. Proc AMIA Symp. 1999:666–70.
11. Health Care Financing Administration Internet Security Policy. Nov 24, 1998. HCFA Web site. Available at: http://www.hcfa.gov/security/isecplcy.htm
12. Pritts JJ, Goldman J, Hudson Z, Berenson A, Hadley E. The

State of Health Privacy: An Uneven Terrain. Washington, DC: Health Privacy Project, Georgetown University, 1999:22.

13. National Committee on Vital and Health Statistics. Uniform Data Standards for Patient Medical Record Information. Report to Secretary of U.S. Department of Health and Human Services. Health Insurance Portability and Accountability Act (HIPAA) of 1996. Washington, DC: DHHS, 2000.

14. Department of Health and Human Services. Standards for Privacy of Individually Identifiable Health Information.

Billing Code 4150-04M. Federal Register, Dec 28, 2000, pp 82461–82829 (45 CFR parts 160-164).

15. Department of Health and Human Services. Security and Electronic Signature Standards: Proposed Rule. Federal Register, Aug 12, 1998, pp 43241–43280 (45 CFR part 142).

16. California Health and Safety Code, Section 123100. Available at: http://www.leginfo.ca.gov/calaw.html

17. Baker DB. PCASSO: a model for safe use of the Internet in health care. J AHIMA. 2000;71(3):33–6.

# Strategic information management plans: the basis for systematic information management in hospitals

A.F. Winter [a,*], E. Ammenwerth [m], O.J. Bott [c], B. Brigl [a], A. Buchauer [b],
S. Gräber [d], A. Grant [e], A. Häber [a], W. Hasselbring [f], R. Haux [m],
A. Heinrich [g], H. Janssen [h], I. Kock [i], O.-S. Penger [j], H.-U. Prokosch [k],
A. Terstappen [c], A. Winter [l]

[a] *Institute for Medical Informatics, University of Leipzig, Statistics, and Epidemiology, Liebigstraße 27, D-04103 Leipzig, Germany*
[b] *Institute for Medical Biometry and Informatics, University of Heidelberg, Heidelberg, Germany*
[c] *Institute for Medical Informatics, Technical University of Braunschweig, Braunschweig, Germany*
[d] *Institute for Medical Biometry, Epidemiology and Medical Informatics, Saarland University Hospital, Homburg, Germany*
[e] *Department of Clinical Biochemistry, University of Sherbrook, Quebec, Canada*
[f] *Department of Software Engineering, Faculty of Computer Science, C.v.O. University of Oldenburg, Oldenburg Germany*
[g] *Network Department GmbH, Berlin, Germany*
[h] *Central Hospital Reinkenheide, Bremerhaven, Germany*
[i] *Kock, Arnold & Partner Business Consulting, Hamburg, Germany*
[j] *SMS Dataplan, Hamburg, Germany*
[k] *Institute for Medical Informatics and Biomathematics, University of Münster, Münster, Germany*
[l] *Institute for Software Technology, University of Koblenz–Landau, Landau, Germany*
[m] *University for Health Informatics and Technology, Tyrol, Innsbruck, Austria*

## Abstract

Information management in hospitals is a complex task. In order to reduce complexity, we distinguish strategic, tactical, and operational information management. This is essential, because each of these information management levels views hospital information systems from different perspectives, and therefore uses other methods and tools. Since all these management activities deal only in part with computers, but mainly with human beings and their social behavior, we define a hospital information system as a sociotechnical subsystem of a hospital. Without proper strategic planning it would be a matter of chance, if a hospital information system would fulfil the information strategies goals. In order to support strategic planning and to reduce efforts for creating strategic plans, we propose a practicable structure. © 2001 Published by Elsevier Science Ireland Ltd.

*Keywords:* Hospital information system; Hospital information system management; Information management; Organizational issues; Strategic plan

* Corresponding author.
*E-mail address:* winter@imise.uni-leipzig.de (A.F. Winter).

## 1. Introduction

High quality healthcare depends on extensive and carefully planned information processing. The expenses associated with information processing have been subjected to cost analysis and already in 1993 it was estimated that within the European Union about 3.5 billion Euro were spent on the computer supported parts of hospital information systems, with a projected 15 billion Euro in 2000 ([1], p. 2). A more recent investigation states, that 'the current European market size for hospital information systems is 2.4 billion $US compared to 2.7 billion $US in US' [2]. To this amount, the costs of conventional/manual information processing must be added. This indicates the paramount importance of information processing (regardless if computer-based or conventional/manual) and information management for hospitals. At the same time it indicates that information management is developing from a secondary to a primary subject of institutional management [3,4].

Success of information systems implementations does not only depend on the quality of hard- and software used. Berg cites in [5] that some 75–98% of computer supported management information systems 'should be considered as failures' and argues similarly as [6] that organizational issues are and have been the key factors for success, precisely unsuccessfulness. As a consequence, Aarts et al. propose in [7] a model for describing the stages involved in information and systems changes. Knaup et al. report on a method for planning and executing projects for introducing information systems' components properly and systematically [8]. Hence these papers concentrate on tactical tasks of information management.

The costs and 'success'-rates mentioned make obvious, that organizational issues in health informatics and especially the quality of information management are important factors for hospitals to gain a competitive edge. In the USA for example, the Joint Commission on Accreditation of Healthcare Organizations (JCAHO)[1] includes 10 information management standards in its accreditation process to assess the quality of an organization as a whole. For a review of the information management standards the healthcare organizations have to present a strategic information management plan [9]. So JCAHO stresses the strategic aspects of information management. Similarly, professional consultants on healthcare emphasize the important role of a systematic information management and the necessity of strategic plans [10]. This corresponds to the personal experiences of the authors who are working as information managers in large hospitals, as consultants, and in software industries.

These considerations in mind the aim of this paper is

- to clarify the difference between strategic, tactical, and operational information management in hospitals,
- to explain the significance of strategic information management plans for *all* information management activities and
- to give support for the construction of strategic plans by proposing a practicable structure.

We will define the terms *information management in hospitals* and *hospital information system* and differentiate *strategic, tactical,* and *operational information management*. We will show, that tactical and operational management depend on strategic information management and especially on strategic information management plans. The proposed structure of strategic plans should serve as a basic guideline for drawing up such plans.

---

[1] http://www.jcaho.org

## 2. Information management in hospitals

### 2.1. Definition of information management in hospitals

Interpreting the term management in a functional manner, management contains all leadership activities that determine the enterprise's goals, structures, and behavior. According to [11] (p. 21), we define:

Information management in hospitals is the sum of all management activities in a hospital that transpose the potential contribution of information processing to fulfill the strategic hospital goals into hospital's success.

Therefore, it manages the maintenance and operation of an appropriate information system for the hospital. When a new hospital is planned and constructed the hospital information system's initial construction has also to be managed.

### 2.2. Definition of hospital information systems

Hospital information systems can be characterized by their functions, their types of processed information and their types of services offered. In order to support patient care and the associated administration, the tasks of hospital information systems are to provide:

- information, primarily about patients, in a way that it is correct, pertinent and up to date, accessible to the right persons at the right location in a usable format. It must be correctly collected, stored, processed, and documented;
- knowledge, primarily about diseases—but also for example about drug actions and adverse effects-to support diagnosis and therapy;

- information about the quality of patient care and about hospital performance and costs.

This highlights, that hospital information systems have to provide high quality communication between the various hospital sectors in terms of both information and knowledge related functions [12].

In addition to patient care, university hospitals undertake research and teaching to gain medical knowledge and deepen understanding. New knowledge is gained from specific experiences in patient care through careful data collection.

A hospital is itself a system, precisely a sociotechnical system, in which human beings and machines carry out specific actions following established rules. In this context, it is not surprising, that introducing components of a hospital information system needs a sociotechnical approach [5]. Therefore, we should consider a hospital information system as a sociotechnical subsystem of a hospital [13] and we define similar to [14]:

A *hospital information system* is that sociotechnical subsystem of a hospital, which comprises all information processing actions as well as the associated human or technical actors in their respective information processing role.

That part of the hospital information system in which computer systems are used as tools for information processing is referred to as the computer-supported part of the hospital information system; the remaining part is referred to as the non-computer-supported part.

### 2.3. Classification of information management tasks in hospitals

Because each hospital has a hospital information system from its very beginning we must not question whether a hospital should be equipped with a hospital information system or not. The question of information management rather focuses on the issue, whether the performance should be enhanced, for example by using computer-supported information processing tools. Accordingly, information management engages in the following objects ([15], p. 1):

- information,
- application systems,
- computer-supported and non-computer-supported information and communication techniques.

The general tasks of management are planning, directing, and monitoring [11]. For information management in hospitals this means

- *planning* the hospital information system, respectively its architecture,
- *directing* its establishment and its operation, and
- *monitoring* its development and operation with respect to the planned objectives.

With respect to its scope information management can be differentiated into strategic, tactical, and operational management [11]. The corresponding activities will be specified in the next sections.

In summary, activities of information management can be classified by a three dimensional classification as depicted in Fig. 1.

### 2.4. Strategic information management in hospitals

Strategic information management deals with the hospital's information processing as a whole. It depends strictly on the hospital's business strategy and strategic goals and has to translate these into a well fitting information strategy.

The result of strategic information management *planning* activities is a strategic in-

formation management plan [16]. The plan includes the direction and strategy of information management and gives directives for the construction and development of the hospital information system by describing its intended architecture. A proposal for the structure and content of strategic information management plans will be presented in Section 3.

The strategic plan is the basis for strategic project portfolios. They contain concrete projects, which implement the objectives of the strategy, and shall be revised regularly.

*Directing* a hospital information system as part of strategic information management means to transform the strategic plan into action, i.e. to systematically manipulate the hospital information system in order to make it conform to the strategic plan. The system's manipulation is done by the initiation of the projects of the strategic project portfolio. The projects deal with the construction or further development and the maintenance of components of the hospital information system.

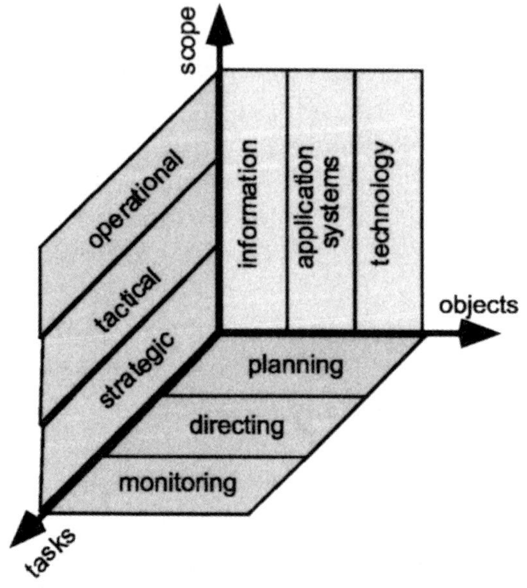


Fig. 1. Three-dimensional classification of information management activities.

Planning, directing and monitoring these projects are the tasks of tactical information management. Operational management will be responsible for the proper operation of the components.

*Monitoring* a hospital information system as part of the strategic information management means continuously auditing its quality as defined by means of its strategic plan's directives and goals. It should be audited, whether the hospital information system is able to fulfill its tasks. In order to be able to audit the information system's quality the management task is to install 'sensors'. They have to receive information from the projects running, from operational management, from users and from the various stakeholders. Additional information can be gained by evaluation projects (e.g. [17]).

Strategic information management and in result the strategic plan are the vital requirement for tactical and operational information management in a hospital.

## 2.5. Tactical information management in hospitals

Tactical management deals with certain enterprise functions [18], i.e. with hospital functions as for example the planning and documentation of operations. It aims to construct or to maintain components of the hospital information system. According to the example above, this could be an application system for planning and documentation of operations. Related activities are usually executed as projects; they have to be initiated as part of an information strategy, which is formulated in the project portfolio of a strategic plan as drawn up by the information management.

*Planning* in tactical information management means planning of projects and all resources needed. Even though projects of tactical information management are based on the strategic plan they need a specific i.e. tactical project plan. This plan has to describe the project's subject and motivation, the problems to be solved, the aims to be achieved, the tasks to be performed, and the activities to be undertaken to reach the aims [8]. Based on that *directing* in tactical management means the execution of such projects of tactical information management in hospitals. Therefore, it includes typical tasks of project management like resource allocation and coordination, motivation and training of the personnel etc. *Monitoring* means continuously checking, whether the initiated projects are running as planned and whether they will still produce the expected results.

## 2.6. Operational information management in hospitals

Operational information management is responsible for maintaining the installed hospital information system and its components. It has to care for its operation in accordance with the strategic plan.

*Planning* in operational information management means planning of all resources like organizational structures, finance, personnel, rooms, buildings that are necessary to ensure the faultless operation of all components of the hospital information system. These resources need to be available for a longer period of time. Therefore, they should be allocated as part of a strategic plan. Moreover, planning in this context concerns the allocation of personnel resources on a day-to-day basis (e.g. planning of shifts).

*Directing* means the sum of all management activities, which are necessary to ensure proper reactions to operating faults of components of the hospital information system i.e. to provide back-up facilities, to operate a helpdesk, to maintain servers, to keep ready task forces for repairing of network components, servers, personal computers, printers etc. Directing in this context deals with engaging the resources planned by the strategic plan in such a way that faultless operation of the hospital information system is ensured.

*Monitoring* deals with verifying the proper working and effectiveness of all components of the hospital information system. For example, a messaging infrastructure must be installed, which enables a quick transmission of users' error notes to the responsible services.

### 3. Strategic information management plans in hospitals

A strategic information management plan documents, how the goals of a particular hospital shall be supported by information technology. Therefore, it describes how information management will be organized, what the different working groups have to do and how the various stakeholders are concerned (Fig. 2). The strategic plan defines direction and schedule for all tactical and operational information management activities in the hospital.

As a result of our experiences in drawing up strategic information management plans for a municipal hospital in Bremerhaven and for university hospitals in Utrecht (Netherlands) [19], Heidelberg,[2] Homburg,[3] and Leipzig[4] we want to make some recommendations concerning structure and content of such plans [20].

---

<sup></sup>[2] http://www.med.uni-heidelberg.de/mi/department/service/rahmenko.zip

[3] http://www.med-rz.uni-sb.de/zik/rahmenkonzept2000.pdf

[4] http://www.imise.uni-leipzig.de/ ~ gabi/KAS/Ueber sichten/rahmenkonzept.html

### 3.1. Stakeholders and their concerns

There are various stakeholders[5] involved in the creation, updating, approval, and use of strategic plans:
- top management,
- funding institutions,
- employees, e.g. physicians, nurses, administrative staff,
- clinical, administrative, and service departments,
- information management department (IM department),
- consultants,
- hardware and software vendors.

It has also been suggested to involve patients or patient organizations as stakeholders [19]. These stakeholders may have different expectations from a strategic plan and are involved in different life-cycle phases of strategic plans:

*Creation*, i.e. writing a first plan,

*Approval*, i.e. making some kind of contract among the stakeholders,

*Deployment*, i.e. asserting that the plan is put into practice,

*Use*, i.e. the involved stakeholders refer to the plan whenever needed,

*Updating* when a new version is required (because of new requirements, new available technologies, failure to achieve individual tasks, or adjusting the time frame of the plan). After the first version, the creation and update phases merge into a cyclic, evolutionary development of the plan.

Top management is interested in seamless and cost-effective operation of the hospital. They approve the plans, probably together with the funding institutions, which are pri-

---

[5] The term stakeholder is used to refer to everyone who may have some direct or indirect influence on the system requirements [21] (p. 80).

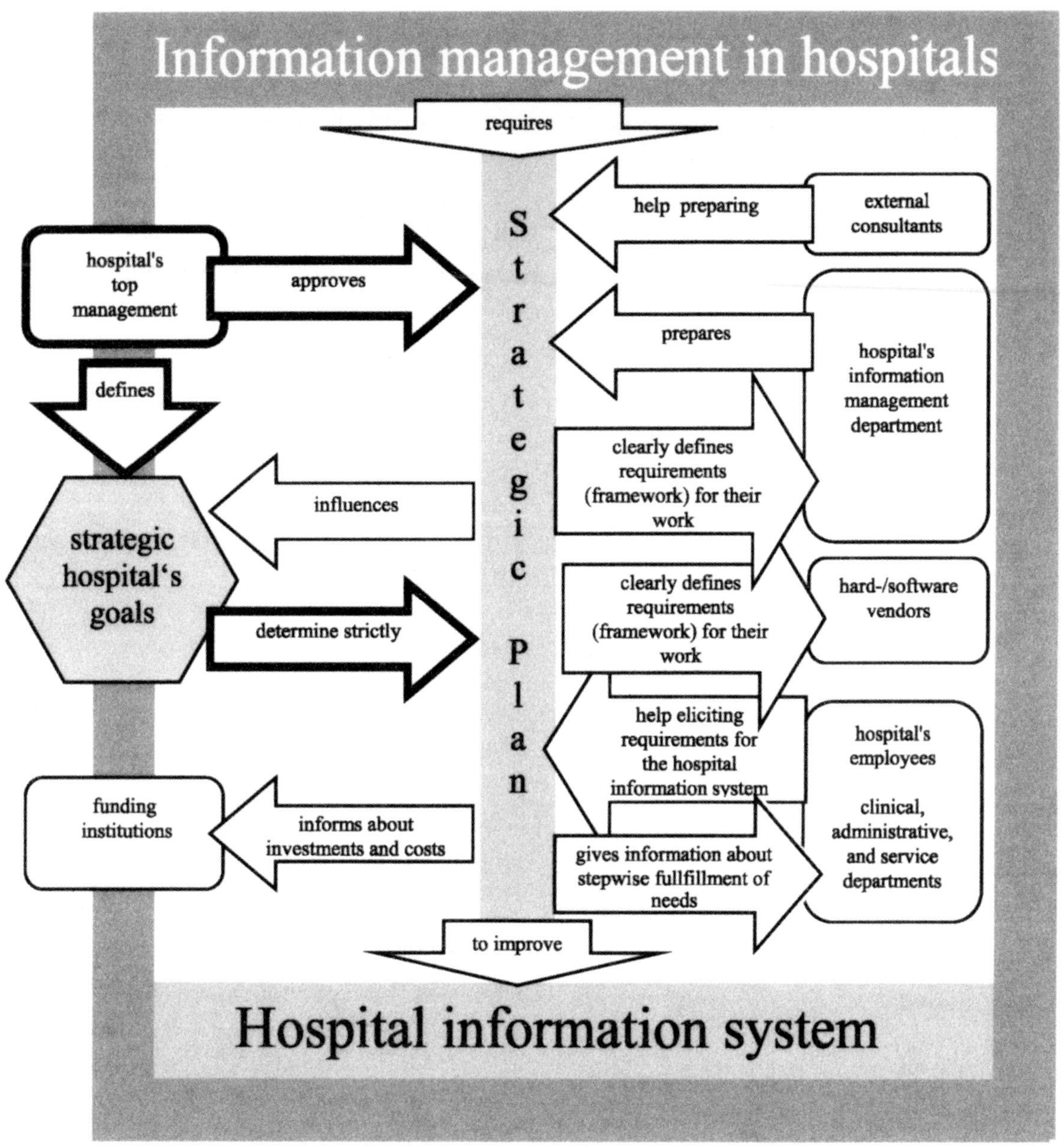


Fig. 2. Strategic plans for information management in hospitals.

marily interested in the financial consequences. Employees as well as the different hospital departments should be involved in eliciting the requirements, since they will use the resulting information systems. IM departments will usually create and maintain proposals for the plans. They are interested in clearly defined requirements for their work,

reflecting tactical management issues. Additionally the IM department usually has to deploy the plan, which cannot be done without effective backing from the top management. Due to technological and market changes and the development of the hospital over time, the validity of a strategic plan is temporal limited. Therefore, after a period of

3–5 years the IM department will initiate the update of the plan. External consultants may help creating or updating plans, but can also be effective in negotiations for the approval. The actual strategic plans will be used by the IM departments as well as by software or hardware vendors when constructing or maintaining components of hospital information systems.

### 3.2. Structure and content of strategic information management plans

The most essential purpose of a strategic plan is to improve a hospital's information system in a way it better contributes to the hospital's goals. This purpose determines its structure, i.e. it should show a path from the current situation to an improved situation, in which the hospital's goals are achieved as far as possible and reasonable.

A strategic plan should encompass the hospital business strategy or strategic goals, the resulting information management strategies, the current state of the hospital information system, and an assessment on how far the current information system fits to the strategies. The planned architecture should be derived as a conclusion of this assessment.

The strategic plan also has to deal with the resources needed to realize the planned architecture, and has to include a strategy for the operation of the resulting hospital information system and a description of appropriate long term organizational structures. Examples for resources are money, personnel, soft- and hardware, energy, rooms for servers and (paper-based) archives, and for training. The resources should fit to the architecture and vice versa.

The general structure of strategic plans for information management in hospitals can be summarized as follows:

- Strategic goals of the hospital and of the information management
- Description of the current state of the hospital information system
- Assessment of the current state of the hospital information system
- Description of the planned state of the hospital information system
- Path from the current to the planned state

This is only a basic structure that may be adapted to the specific requirements of individual hospitals. Particularly, a short management summary and appendices describing the organizational structure, personnel resources, the building structure, the network architecture, etc. are likely to complement a strategic plan.

### 3.2.1. Strategic goals of the hospital and of the information management

Hospitals aim at providing health care. However, these goals may be further refined. For instance, specific goals could be to increase the number of outpatients, to decrease the average duration of inpatient stays, to perform best quality patient treatment, to improve collaboration with healthcare institutions in the nearer region, to be more competitive by an image of being a modern hospital with all the latest technical means, to offer wholesome patient care by less technical but more personal engagement, to increase profit, and so on. Obviously, such very different and partly conflicting goals can result in different and conflicting information management strategies and different architectures of hospital information systems.

### 3.2.2. Description of the current state of the hospital information system

Before any planning is commenced, the hospital information system's current state should be described. This may require some discipline, because some stakeholders may be more interested in the planned (new) state than in the current (obsolete) state.

The description of the current state will be the basis for identifying those functions [18] of the hospital that are supported well—e.g. by information technology—and those functions that are not (yet) well supported. Thus, application systems as well as existing information and communication technology have to be described including their contribution to the overall performance of the hospital's functions. The functions having to be considered here can be derived from the goals of the hospital.

Problems in information processing do not always have technical reasons only, but may also be caused by shortcomings in organizing information management [6]. Thus, the description of the current state should be completed by the description of the current organizational structure of information management.

### 3.2.3. Assessment of the current state of the hospital information system

When the current state is described, it should be assessed with respect to the achievement of the hospital's strategic goals and the related information management strategies. Note that missing computer support for a certain function may not be assessed in all cases as being a bad support for that function. For example, missing computers in patient rooms and in consequence a paper-based documentation of clinical findings may be more conforming to the goal of being a patient-oriented hospital than the use of computers and handheld digital devices in this area.

### 3.2.4. Description of the planned state of the hospital information system

Based on the assessment of the current state, a new state should be described that achieves the goals better, provided that the current state does not already achieve the hospital's goals. Note that beside of technical aspects also organizational aspects have to be discussed. In many cases this is an opportunity for introducing a chief information officer (CIO) or to clarify its role respectively.

### 3.2.5. Path from the current to the planned state

This section should describe a project portfolio as a step-by-step path from the current to the planned state. It should include assigned resources, i.e. personnel, estimated investment costs as well as future operation cost, etc. and concrete deadlines for partial results of the portfolio's projects. This path could also assign priorities to individual projects as well as dependencies between projects.

## 4. Conclusion

Information management in hospitals is a complex task. In order to reduce complexity, we distinguish strategic, tactical, and operational information management. This is essential, because each of these information management levels views hospital information systems from different perspectives, and therefore uses other methods and tools. While strategic information management focuses on strategic plans, tactical management needs methods for project management, user requirements analysis, software development or customizing, etc. Operational management requires methods and tools for topics, which range from intra-enterprise marketing of services to helpdesk management and network management.

All these management activities deal only in part with machines and computers, but mainly with human beings and their social behavior. As a consequence we proposed to define a hospital information system as a sociotechnical subsystem of a hospital.

We showed, that without a strategic information management plan, neither tactical nor operational management would work appropriately. A strategic information management plan is the 'plot' for planning, directing, and monitoring the hospital information system. It should be written and approved by the hospital management. Without proper strategic planning it would be a matter of chance, if a hospital information system would fulfil the information strategies goals.

But obviously, considerable efforts have to be made for creating strategic plans. Therefore, we propose a practicable structure, which might help information managers organizing their work.

Though we stated, that hospitals, which have a properly organized information management and especially an adequate strategic information management plan, gain better hospital information systems, we could not empirically prove this assertion so far. There are some arguments, which support this hypothesis:

- As cited in [22] (p. xxi), a study amongst practitioners, educators, and consultants determined 'improving information systems strategic planing' as one of the three most important issues of information management (out of 25).
- U.S. funding institutions seem to rely more on those hospitals, which are certified by the JCAHO and therefore have an adequate strategic information management plan.
- It is argued in [5,6] that bad information management leads to bad information systems.

The latter studies may be possible since it will not be so difficult to define what a really

'bad' information system is. But what are criteria for 'good' hospital information systems? So future work has to define such criteria, which enable us to compare 'chaotically' developed hospital information systems with systematically developed hospital information systems based on strategic plans.

## References


[1] J.H. van Bemmel, An international perspective on information management and technology in health care, in: Proceedings of Conference on Clinical Information, London, 1993.

[2] I. Iakovidis, Towards a Health Telematics Infrastructure in the EU, Information Technology Strategies from US and the European Union: Transferring Research to Practice for Health Care Improvement, IOS press, Amsterdam, 2000, pp. 23–33.

[3] C.J. Austin, J.M. Trimm, P.M. Sobczak, Information systems and strategic management, Health. Care. Manage. Rev. 20 (3) (1995) 26–33.

[4] A.L. Lederer, V. Sethi, Guidelines for strategic information planning, J. Bus. Strategy 12 (6) (1991) 38–43.

[5] M. Berg, Patient care information systems and health care work: A sociotechnical approach, Int. J. Med. Inf. 55 (1999) 87–101.

[6] N.M. Lorenzi, R.T. Riley, Organizational Aspects of Health Informatics: Managing Technological Change, Springer, New York, 1995.

[7] J. Aarts, V. Peel, G. Wright, Organizational issues in health informatics: a model approach, Int. J. Med. Inf. 52 (1998) 235–242.

[8] P. Knaup, R. Haux, A. Häber, A. Lagemann, F. Leiner, Teaching the fundamentals of information systems management in health care-Lecture and practical training for students of Medical Informatics (Heidelberg/Heilbronn), Int. J. Med. Inf. 50 (1998) 195–206.

[9] M. Thomas, G. Vaughan, Preparing for the joint commission survey: the information systems perspective, HIMSS. Proceedings 3 (1998) 369–382.

[10] Gartner Group, Three Documents for Healthcare IT Planning, Gartner Group's Healthcare Executive and Management Strategies Research Note, KA-03-5074, 1998.

[11] L.J. Heinrich, Informationsmanagement: Planung, Überwachung und Steuerung der Informations-Infrastruktur (Information Management: planning, monitoring, and directing of information infrastructure), Oldenbourg, München, 1999. (in German).

[12] H.U. Prokosch, Hospital information systems: a pragmatic definition, in: H.U. Prokosch, J. Dudeck (Eds.), Hospital Information Systems: Design and Development Characteristics; Impact and Future Architecture, Amsterdam, Elsevier, 1995, pp. XI–XIII.

[13] E. Lang, O.J. Bott, D.P. Pretschner, Specification of an Information System for Ophthalmology using Modelling and Simulation Techniques, in: R.A. Greens, H. Peterson, D. Protti (Eds.) MEDINFO'95—Proceedings of the 8th World Congress on Medical Informatics, 1995, 1092.

[14] A. Winter, R. Haux, A Three-Level Graph-Based Model for the Management of Hospital Information Systems, Methods Inf. Med. 34 (4) (1995) 378–396.

[15] H. Krcmar, Informationsmanagement (Information management), Springer, Berlin, 1997 (in German).

[16] J. Ward, P. Griffiths, Strategic Planning for Information Systems, John Wiley & Sons, Chichester, 1996.

[17] E.M.S.J. van Gennip, F. Grémy, Challenges and Opportunities for technology Assessment in Medical Informatics. Report of MEDINFO'92 workshop, Med. Inform. 18 (3) (1993) 179–184.

[18] J. Martin, Information Engineering, Book II: Planning & Analysis, Prentice Hall, Englewood Cliffs, 1990.

[19] W. Hasselbring, R. Peterson, M. Smits, R. Spanjers, Strategic information management for a Dutch University Hospital, in: A. Hasman, B. Blobel, J. Dudeck, R. Engelbrecht, G. Gell, H.-U. Prokosch (Eds.), Medical Infobahn for Europe, IOS Press, Amsterdam, 2000, pp. 885–889.

[20] A. Winter, B. Brigl, A. Buchauer, C. Dujat, S. Gräber, W. Hasselbring, R. Haux, A. Heinrich, H. Janssen, I. Kock, A. Winter, Purpose and structure of strategic plans for information management in hospitals, in: A. Hasman, B. Blobel, J. Dudeck, R. Engelbrecht, G. Gell, H.-U. Prokosch (Eds.), Medical Infobahn for Europe, IOS Press, Amsterdam, 2000, pp. 880–884.

[21] I. Sommerville, Software Engineering, Addison-Wesley, Reading, MA, 1996.

[22] S.H. Spewak, S.C. Hill, Enterprise Architecture Planning, John Wiley & Sons, New York, 1992.

# *Section 4:*

**B. Tilg**

University for Health Informatics and
Technology Tyrol (UMIT)
Innsbruck, Austria

# Synopsis

## *Biomedical Signal Processing*

## Introduction

In biomedical signal processing, major progress has been made due to a better understanding of the underlying physiological processes, due to the further development of high-quality measurement techniques, and due to novel mathematical algorithms, which have recently evolved. Significant improvements were achieved with regard to the measurement of biomedical signals. For example, high-quality biopotential amplifier and recording systems have been developed for a signal-to-noise ratio up to 40 Decibel. Also, today, we have a better understanding of the "source-field-relationship", in particular for the human brain and heart. Such an understanding is very important in order to apply the proper mathematical tools and to understand the limitations of the applied approaches. Beside statistical approaches, model-based signal processing techniques have been developed. In general, these approaches are based on a biophysical model of the underlying physiological process. Formulating a linear or a nonlinear input-output relationship is the basis for these model-based approaches, which are powerful techniques also in the case of very complex and noisy signals, like the magneto- (MEG) and electroencephalogram (EEG).

Today, biomedical signal processing is further developed at an organ level and, in particular, on a cellular and subcellular level. Traditional signal processing techniques, like time-frequency domain or wavelet analysis, are these days also applied to biomolecular data. For instance in microarray analysis or in the analysis of mass spectrometric data, statistical and model-based approaches are just on the way to be introduced for a better and more specific analysis. Here, classification and pattern recognition algorithms play a fundamental role.

## Selected papers of excellence

Five outstanding papers were selected for this section [1-5]. The papers are dedicated to the analysis of transcranial Doppler ultrasound data for embolus identification, to the segmentation of the EEG signal waves, to the analysis of spinal somatosensory evoked potentials, to the determination of the complexity of EEG signals for measuring the depth of anesthesia, and to the reconstruction of neural activity from MEG data. All five papers deal with biomedical signal processing at an organ level.

In the following, these five papers of excellence are summarized and shortly discussed:

Blood flow in the middle cerebral artery can be monitored by transcranial Doppler ultrasound. It may be used to detect cerebral emboli in patients with an increased stroke risk and during invasive cardiovascular examinations and operations. The paper by Fan et al. [1] describes an interesting approach for a quantitative interpretation and analysis of transcranial Doppler ultrasound data for automated embolus identification. An automatic system was developed that replaces the so-called "Human Expert" (HE). Doppler signal patterns were analyzed in both the time domain and frequency domain. The system was trained and tested on Doppler signals recorded during the dissection and recovery phases of carotid endarterectomy. The results were compared with the results obtained by HEs. The automatic system displayed a high sensitivity and specificity.

From a technical point of view, the applied frequency and time domain evaluation has several advantages. It makes pattern recognition much more stable than a pure time domain approach. Also, this approach can handle noisy ultrasound data, which often is the case in a clinical environment. From a clinical perspective, transcranial Doppler ultrasound has several significant benefits. The technique is noninasive, painless and safe. The procedure is quick and with training, 30-40 minutes is sufficient for acquisition and analysis. The instrumentation is inexpensive and portable. The most crucial aspect in applying transcranial Doppler ultrasound is achieving good operator technique. With training and experience, however, reproducibility between operators is good.

The work by Gharieb et al. [2] involves segmentation of EEG data for tracking the delta, theta, alpha, sigma, beta and the gamma wave. An adaptive recursive bandpass filter is employed for estimating and tracking the center frequency associated with each of these waves. The main advantage is that the employed adaptive filter has only one unknown coefficient to be updated. This coefficient represents an efficient distinct feature for each EEG specific wave. The proposed approach is simple and accurate in comparison with existing multivariate adaptive approaches. It can be applied to on-line EEG data and was used for the detection of sleep spindles.

Evoked potentials have been used to detect the integrity of spinal cord function during spinal surgery to minimize the possibility of spinal cord injury. Traditional methods for evoked potential monitoring use only amplitude and latency measurements to indicate potential injury to the spinal cord. However, spectral changes in evoked potentials also occur during neurological injury. Hu et al. [3] conducted an investigation of various time-frequency analysis techniques to detect both temporal and spectral changes in spinal somatosensory evoked potentials waveforms. The time-frequency distributions (TFDs) computed using these methods were assessed and compared. As shown, short-term Fourier transform with a 20-point length Hanning window provides the best result for spinal somatosensory evoked signals. The authors demonstrated the applicability and validity of time frequency analysis of evoked potentials to detect spinal cord function.

The monitoring of depth of anesthesia is an important aspect for patients during interventions and operations. Several methods for automatic segmentation, classification and compact presentation of suppression patterns in the EEG have been developed. A new approach for quantifying the relationship between brain activity patterns and depth of anesthesia is presented by Zhang et al. [4]. The authors analyzed the spatio-temporal patterns in the EEG using Lempel-Ziv complexity analysis. Twenty-seven patients undergoing vascular surgery were studied under general anesthesia. The EEG was recorded and patients' anesthesia states were assessed according to the responsiveness component of the observer's assessment of alertness/sedation score. Complexity of the EEG was quantitatively estimated by the Lempel-Ziv complexity measure $C(n)$. The study shows that $C(n)$ is a very useful and promising EEG-derived parameter for characterizing the depth of anesthesia under clinical situations.

The analysis of the MEG for purpose of reconstructing neural electrical activity and for pattern recognition in the temporal or frequency domain has been a subject of research in the last years. The work by Sekihara et al. [5] involves the analysis of MEG data and is an important contribution to enhance contrast in the reconstructed images. The basic idea of applying the beamformer technique to this approach is very promising and might give a significant improvement for source localization. A method for reconstructing spatio-temporal activities of neural sources by using MEG data is presented. The method extends the adaptive beamformer technique to incorporate the vector beamformer formulation in which a set of three weight vectors is used to detect the source activity in three orthogonal directions. Both spatial resolution and output signal-to-noise ratio of the proposed beamformer are significantly higher than those of the minimum-variance-based vector beamformer. The authors also applied the proposed beamformer to two sets of auditory-evoked MEG data. The results clearly demonstrated the method's capability of reconstructing spatio-temporal activities of neural sources. In reconstructing neural electrical activity, one of the key problems is that we still not have a proper and physically based source model available. The beamformer technique may overcome this limitation, in particular for the imaging of independent electrical sources.

On an organ level there are various research areas in which novel methodology is developed [1-7]. Examples are the imaging of electrical function within the human brain and heart from observations on the body surface (from electric potential (e.g., EEG) or magnetic field mapping (e.g., MEG) data), the non-invasive and real-time beat-to-beat monitoring of stroke volume, blood pressure, total peripheral resistance and for assessment of autonomic function by measuring ECG, blood pressure and thorax impedance, and the classification of biosignals like EEG or MEG.

## Future perspectives

Today, signal processing methods developed at an organ level are further developed also for the application to biomolecular data [7-10]. Recently, in the signal processing community, terms like genomic signal processing came up [8-10]. Under genomic signal processing we understand solving problems in making use of the well established theory, tools, and methodologies from the field of biomedical signal processing. Fields of research are clustering, detection, prediction, and classification of gene expression data, signal transforms and statistical models for the interpretation of biological sequences and statistical and dynamical modeling of gene networks. Sequence analysis techniques including Hidden Markov models, wavelet analysis, and artificial neural networks are on the way being introduced.

From a biomedical signal processing point of view it is very challenging to see that mathematical approaches developed for "traditional" signals like the EEG are now further developed for the application to data on a molecular level [7-10]. In a couple of years it will be fascinating to see the wide spectrum of biomedical signal processing from an organ to a sub-cellular level and the similarities of the signal processing approaches used for these different scaling dimensions.

## References


1. Fan L, Evans DH, Naylor AR: Automated embolus identification using a rule-based expert system. Ultrasound Med Biol 2001;27(8):1065-77.
2. Gharieb RR, Cichocki A. Segmentation and tracking of the electro-encephalogram signal using an adaptive bandpass filter. Med Biol Eng Comput 2001;39:237-48.
3. Hu Y, Luk KDK, LU WW, Holmes A, Leong JCY. Comparison of time-frequency distribution techniques for analysis of spinal somatosensory evoked potential. Med Biol Eng Comput 2001;39:375-80.
4. Zhang X, Roy RJ, Jensen EW. EEG complexity as a measure of depth of anesthesia for patients. IEEE Trans Biomed Eng 2001;48(12):1424-33.
5. Sekihara K, Nagarajan SS, Poeppel D, Marantz A, Miyashita Y. Reconstruction spatio-temporal activities of neural sources using an MEG vector beamformer technique. IEEE Trans Biomed Eng 2001;48(7):760-71.
6. Akay M. Nonlinear biomedical signal processing: Fuzzy logic, neural networks, and new algorithms. Vol. 1. New York: IEEE Press; 2000.
7. Akay M. Nonlinear biomedical signal processing: Dynamic analysis and modeling. Vol. 1. New York: IEEE Press; 2000.
8. Zhang W, Shmulevich I. Computational and statistical approaches to gnomics. Amsterdam: Kluwer Academic Publishers; 2002.
9. http://sigwww.cs.tut.fi/TICSP/GenomicSP; Signal processing, Special issue on genomic signal processing, December 2002.
10. http://www.gensips.gatech.edu/; Workshop on genomic signal processing and statistics, IEEE Signal Processing Society Raleigh, North Carolina, USA, October 12-13, 2002.



Address of the author:
Bernhard Tilg, PhD, Professor
University for Health Informatics and Technology Tyrol (UMIT)
Institute for Medical Signal Processing and Imaging
Innrain 98, 6020 Innsbruck
Austria
Tel:      +43 512 586 734 0
Fax:      +43 512 586 734 850
E-mail:   bernhard.tilg@umit.at
http://www.UMIT.at

# AUTOMATED EMBOLUS IDENTIFICATION USING A RULE-BASED EXPERT SYSTEM

LINGKE FAN,* DAVID H. EVANS* and A. ROSS NAYLOR[†]

Departments of *Medical Physics and [†]Surgery, Leicester Warwick Medical School, University of Leicester, Leicester, UK

(*Received* 19 *February* 2001; *in final form* 17 *May* 2001)

**Abstract**—Transcranial Doppler ultrasound (US) can be used to detect microemboli in the cerebral circulation, but is still limited because it usually relies on "human experts" (HEs) to identify signals corresponding to embolic events. The purpose of this study was to develop an automatic system that could replace the HE and, thus, make the technique more widely applicable and, potentially, more reliable. An expert system, based around a digital signal-processing board, analysed Doppler signal patterns in both the time domain and frequency domain. The system was trained and tested on Doppler signals recorded during the dissection and recovery phases of carotid endarterectomy. It was tested with 74 separate 2.5-min recordings that contained at least 575 artefacts in addition to 253 s of diathermy interference. The results were compared with the results obtained by three HEs. Using a "gold-standard" that classified any event detected by the majority of HEs as an embolus, the automatic system displayed a sensitivity of 94.7% and a specificity of 95.1% for 1151 candidate events 7 dB or more above the clutter (signal-to-clutter ratio, SCR, $\geq$ 7 dB), and 89.6% and 95.3%, respectively, for 2098 candidate events with SCR $\geq$ 5 dB. The system had a very similar performance to individual HEs for SCR $\geq$ 7dB, and was only marginally worse for SCR $\geq$ 5 dB. (E-mail: dhe@le.ac.uk) © 2001 World Federation for Ultrasound in Medicine & Biology.

*Key Words:* Carotid artery disease, Cerebral embolism, Doppler ultrasound, Emboli detection, Expert systems, Signal processing, Transcranial Doppler sonography.

## INTRODUCTION

Transcranial Doppler ultrasound (US) or TCD is now widely used to detect microemboli entering the cerebral circulation. Several clinical applications for this technique have been reported, including the detection of emboli from mechanical heart valves (Georgiadis et al. 1994, 1998; Rams et al. 1993), of embolization occurring during (Ackerstaff et al. 1995b, 1996; Smith et al. 1995) and after (Lennard et al. 1997; Levi et al. 1997; Van Zuilen et al. 1995) carotid artery surgery, and during cardiac surgery (Braekken et al. 1998; Pugsley et al. 1994; Sylivris et al. 1998). The methodology consists of fixing a Doppler probe, with a frequency of approximately 2 MHz, over the temporal bone and adjusting its position, orientation, and the Doppler sample volume depth (to approximately 50 to 55 mm) to obtain a good signal from blood flow within the ipsilateral middle cerebral artery (Aaslid et al. 1982; Santalucia and Feldmann 1999). Because a microembolus has different acoustic properties than that of the blood in which it is travelling, there is a transient increase in the backscattered ultrasonic power as it passes through the Doppler sample volume and, therefore, careful monitoring of the Doppler signal provides a means of detection (Evans 1999). Subjectively, Doppler signals from emboli are described as sounding like a "snap," a "chirp," or a "moan" (Ackerstaff et al. 1995a) and appearing on the Doppler sonogram as a short-duration unidirectional high-intensity signal within the Doppler flow spectrum, occurring at random in the cardiac cycle (Spencer 1992; Georgiadis et al. 1994). More objectively, they may be described as short-duration (usually between 8 and 80 ms) amplitude-modulated sine waves that exceed the level of the background blood flow signal by anywhere between 3 dB and 60 dB (Evans et al. 1997). For reasons that are not fully understood, they may also exhibit significant frequency modulation (Smith et al. 1997a). An example of an embolus signal that is approximately 14-dB higher than the background signal is shown in Fig. 1.

Address correspondence to: Prof. D. H. Evans, Department of Medical Physics, Leicester Royal Infirmary, Leicester LE1 5WW UK. E-mail: dhe@le.ac.uk

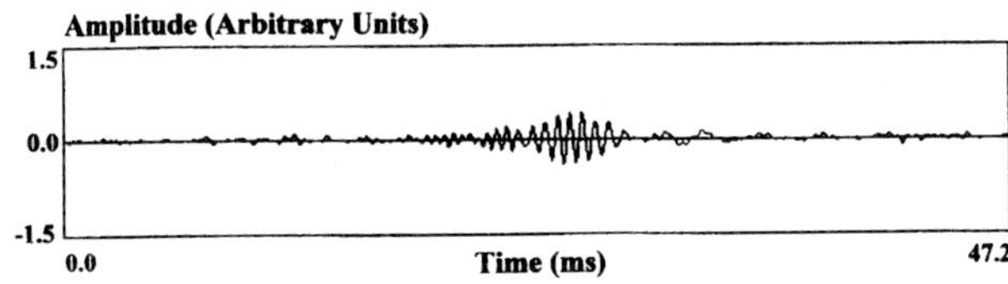

Fig. 1. Example of an embolus signal that can easily be heard and also seen on a Doppler sonogram.

Although there was originally some debate about the significance of microemboli detected by TCD, recent studies have shown that they provide valuable clinical information in several areas. They are an independent predictor of future stroke risk in patients with both symptomatic and asymptomatic carotid stenosis (Molloy and Markus 1999), high numbers of particulate emboli detected during carotid artery surgery predict deterioration in postoperative cognitive function (Gaunt et al. 1994a) and are correlated with perioperative cerebral complications and with new ischaemic lesions on magnetic resonance (MR) images of the brain (Ackerstaff et al. 1996). Furthermore, TCD monitoring helps significantly reduce the amount of microembolisation during carotid surgery (Smith et al. 1998) and improves the safety of the procedure (Van Zuilen et al. 1998). In the postoperative phase, TCD can be used to detect emboli that precede incipient carotid occlusion (Gaunt et al. 1994b), and to help to tailor preventative therapy (Lennard et al. 1997).

To date, most studies of embolic signals have relied on trained human observers (human experts = HEs) to identify candidate events, and to distinguish between true embolic signals and those due to other mechanisms, but there are a number of drawbacks associated with this (in terms of both cost and reliability) and, if the technique is to become widely accepted in clinical practice, then some form of automatic recognition will become mandatory. The current method is very costly because it requires a trained observer to both listen to the TCD audio output and to observe the analysis screen for as long as each study continues, which may be many h. Also, the reliability of the HE under clinical conditions must be questioned. It is known that there is quite poor interobserver agreement, particularly for low-intensity signals, even under idealised laboratory conditions (Markus et al. 1997) but, in clinical situations, there is often considerable background noise, and the observer may well become fatigued over the long observation periods necessary. In some situations, there may also be a very low prevalence of embolic signals (perhaps as few as one or two per h) (Droste et al. 1996; Molloy et al. 1998), which will lead to operator inattention and the missing of important signals. Clearly, what is needed is a system capable of automatically detecting and classi-

fying embolic signals, and a number of attempts have been made to implement such systems in commercial devices. Three such systems have been described by Van Zuilen et al. (1996), who concluded that these systems could not reach the level of agreement shown by HEs and that further research and development in this area was necessary. Two years later, Ringelstein et al. (1998) concluded, in an international consensus statement, that the systems then available were not yet able to automatically discriminate artefacts from signals due to microemboli. Very recently, Cullinane et al. (2000) have reported an evaluation of a detection algorithm that appears to give much better results than previous methods. We report here the details of a new Fast fourier transform (FFT)-based expert system that uses both the time domain and frequency domain signatures of the Doppler signal to discriminate embolic signals from artefact signals, and present a preliminary evaluation of performance that suggests that it displays both a very high sensitivity and specificity.

*System design*

At first sight, the automatic detection of embolic signals may appear to be a fairly straightforward problem; however, this is not the case because there are many events that give rise to transient increases in Doppler power that may easily be mistaken for embolic events. Such events include patient movement, including swallowing or talking in the conscious patient or movements caused by the anaesthetist or surgeon in the unconscious patient, slight movements of the probe or cable, and electrical pickup from other equipment including diathermy. In addition, the Doppler power from an artery fluctuates significantly in the short term due to the random nature of the signal scattered from blood (Angelsen 1980; Mo and Cobbold 1986). The problem, thus, is not so much that of detecting transient increases in power conforming to the characteristics described above but, rather, that of rejecting all the increases in power due to other events. It must also be noted that, because recording time can be very long and the prevalence of emboli very low, the system must exhibit a remarkable specificity. If a recording lasts for 1 h and can, just for illustrative purposes, be regarded as being made up of a series of segments of Doppler signals lasting 80 ms, each of which has to be analysed, then a system with a "raw" specificity of 99% would detect approximately 450 false-positive results. For this reason, we later define specificity in terms of the number of (approximately) 80-ms data segments that contain signals of greater than a given energy threshold.

The system described was designed to detect particulate emboli occurring during the dissection phase of carotid endarterectomy and during the postoperative pe-

Table 1. "Public knowledge" concerning signals from emboli and artifacts

1. Embolic signals are narrow band within a limited time window
2. The energy levels of embolic signals are generally higher than those of the neighbourhood background
3. The maximum spectral peak of an embolic signal carries most of the signal energy and, therefore, should have a high magnitude
4. Signals from large artifacts usually have low central frequencies, high amplitudes, and relatively large band-widths
5. Signals from large artefacts tend to have time-domain envelopes that change more dramatically than embolic signals over short time intervals
6. Low-frequency embolic signals tend to have a longer duration than high-frequency embolic signals and, therefore, a higher signal energy within a given observation window
7. Signals from emboli may have a time-varying central frequency, but the rate of frequency change is significantly slower than for some artifacts

riod of the same operation, because our clinical interests lie in this area, but it should be noted that these embolic signals are considered to be the most difficult to detect because they have a relatively low intensity compared with signals that are due to gaseous emboli (Evans 1999). The system is the culmination of several years of development in this area, during which we employed a number of strategies for detection, and eventually concluded that the simpler the "front-end" of the system, the more reliable the result was likely to be in clinical practice. Thus, we opted for a single-gate system and only processed one channel (representing flow toward the transducer) of the bidirectional Doppler signal.

Due to the highly complicated nature of embolic signals, the different types of artefact and the background (clutter) Doppler signal, the detection system was designed as a knowledge-based (expert) system rather than a conventional algorithm-based system. It was designed in accordance with the development procedures for a diagnosis-type expert system (Hayes-Roth et al. 1983), in which a number of high-level qualitative assumptions (see Table 1) are regarded as the "public knowledge" of the specialized problem-solving expertise, and the corresponding quantitative training information derived from practical experiments is used as the "private knowledge." The basic design procedure is illustrated in Fig. 2. The process is initiated within the "problem identification" block by combining basic information about embolic signals (the "public knowledge") with the detection results of an HE, to derive quantitative information about the characteristics of embolic signals. This information is sent to the "conceptualization" and "formalization" blocks, where corresponding reasoning rules are generated (or modified during subsequent iterations). The reasoning rules are implemented and tested, and a prototype detector constructed (or revised). The experimental data are then updated (by the addition of previously unseen signals) and the new data set analysed by both the prototype detector and the HE. The results of these analyses are sent back to the "problem identification" block and the entire process repeated in an iterative

fashion. A high-level block diagram of the system resulting from this process after a number of iterations is shown in Fig. 3. Further details of each of these blocks are given below. The rules are described in very general terms but, because of their complexity, cannot be given in detail, although a specific example of a rule is given in Appendices 1 and 2.

*Signal preconditioning*

The analogue signal outputs from the DAT recorder are digitised at a sampling frequency of 12.5 kHz, using a real-time system based on an AT&T DSP32C digital signal-processing board (Blue Wave Systems, Loughborough, UK). The digital data are then saved into data files, each containing about 2.5 min of data for further off-line processing.

*Spectral analysis*

Spectral analysis is carried out using a digital implementation of the classical spectrogram-based time-

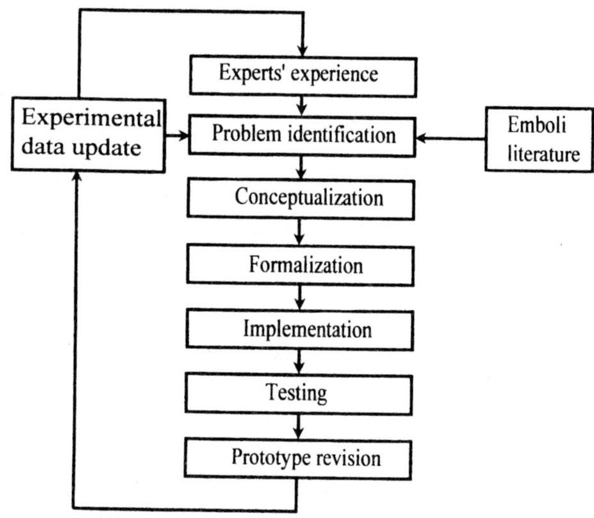


Fig. 2. Flow diagram illustrating the basic design procedure for the expert system.

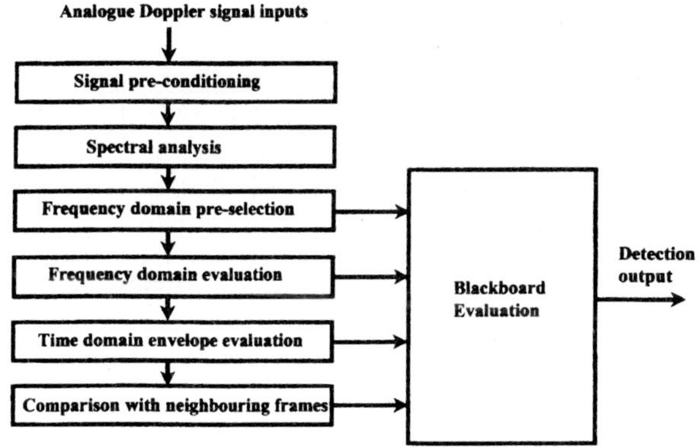



Fig. 3. Block diagram of the expert system.

frequency analyser (Cohen 1989). The estimate of the power in each 10.24-ms data window centred around the sample index $n_0$ and at frequency index $k$ is given by:

$$\hat{P}(n_0, k)$$

$$= \left| C_0 \sum_{n=n_0-63}^{n_0+64} \exp(-j2\pi nk/128) \times s(n)h(n-n_0) \right|^2 , \quad (1)$$

where $s(n)$ is the sampled signal, $h(n - n_0)$ is a sampled 10.24-ms Hanning window, and $C_0$ is a scaling constant. The data window is shifted forward by 2.56 ms (*i.e.*, 32 samples) after each spectral calculation is completed to provide a 75% overlap between adjacent frames.

### Frequency domain preselection

The calculated signal spectra are processed to pre-select candidate narrow-band signals, which have a dominant frequency peak with a 3-dB bandwidth no greater than $W_{\text{dom (3 dB)}}$. [$W_{\text{dom (3 dB)}}$ is initially set to 300 Hz, but is dynamically altered following a preliminary relative energy evaluation, similar to that described under in the Frequency domain evaluation section 4.] These candidate signals are further evaluated in the frequency and time domains.

### Frequency domain evaluation

The frequency domain evaluation can be divided into the following expert system symbolic structure groups:
1. Single-peak magnitude evaluation. The magnitude of the dominant peak is compared with other parts of the signal spectrum, to ensure that it is significantly higher than the magnitude of the next highest peak.
2. Summed peak magnitude evaluation. The magnitude of the dominant peak is compared with the sum of the magnitudes of the next three highest peaks, to further ensure its significance.
3. Dominant peak frequency evaluation. The frequency of the dominant peak $F_{\text{dom}}$ is compared with a "threshold frequency" $F_{\text{thresh}}$ to identify low-frequency artefacts ($F_{\text{thresh}}$ is dynamically altered according to signal duration).
4. Relative energy evaluation. The energy contained within the dominant peak must exceed a certain percentage compared with the energy contained in the rest of the spectrum. The percentage threshold is determined according to the value of $F_{\text{dom}}$.
5. High-frequency component evaluation. The magnitudes of the frequency components higher than 2 $F_{\text{dom}}$ must be very small. The threshold is determined according to the value of $F_{\text{dom}}$.
6. Peak number evaluation. The spectrum must contain a limited number of spectral peaks (currently not more than five) that have magnitudes higher than a certain level (currently 5% of the maximum magnitude), and have significant attack and decay rates around the peaks.
7. Frequency grouping evaluation. All significant frequency components (currently 12% of the maximum magnitude or greater) must be grouped around $F_{\text{dom}}$ within a certain range (currently $F_{\text{dom}} \pm 600$ Hz).

### Time domain envelope evaluation

Time domain evaluation is carried out to obtain information about the envelope shape of the signal. It is carried out on the same segment of signals as the frequency domain evaluation, but the window function in this case is merely rectangular.

The evaluation can be divided into the following expert system symbolic structure groups:
1. Envelope attack and decay evaluation. The attack and decay of the time domain envelope is evaluated to eliminate artefacts, which often contain dramatic changes.
2. Envelope shape evaluation. The signal envelope body is evaluated and heavily modulated signals are eliminated.
3. Signal frequency-duration evaluation. This group evaluation combines frequency domain and time domain information, and sets a duration threshold derived from $F_{\text{dom}}$. For example, when $F_{\text{dom}} < 500$ Hz, the signal duration of an embolus is usually longer than 8 ms. Because most signals occupy more than one frame, this evaluation is also combined with the comparison with neighbouring frames (see next section).
4. Overloaded signal evaluation. The signal envelope and bandwidth become abnormal when the signal is overloaded in the time domain; therefore, overloaded

signals have to be given special attention. When an overload is detected, a number of thresholds are automatically altered (such as that in the frequency domain evaluation of high-frequency components).

*Comparison with neighbouring frames*

*Relative total energy evaluation.* The relative total energy $E_{\text{ratio}}$ is evaluated from time domain signals using the following energy relationship:

$$E_{\text{ratio}} = \frac{E_{\text{current}}}{E_{\text{neighbor}}}, \qquad (2)$$

where $E_{\text{current}}$ is the total signal energy and $E_{\text{neighbour}}$ is a neighbourhood energy. The value of $E_{\text{current}}$ is calculated using the time domain signal samples $s(n)\{n = 0, 1, 2, ..., 127\}$ within the current 128-point (10.24-ms) data window:

$$E_{\text{current}} = \sum_{n=0}^{127} s^2(n). \qquad (3)$$

The calculation of $E_{\text{neighbour}}$ is normally based on a formula similar to eqn (3), but it uses two 51.2-ms moving-average type finite impulse response (FIR) filters centred at a data point 76.8 ms before and 76.8 ms after the centre of the detection data window, to provide a stable estimate of the neighbourhood energy. However, the calculation of $E_{\text{neighbour}}$ is automatically switched to an alternative source (an infinite impulse response (IIR) filter applied to a different region) if the system detects that there are strong artefacts or emboli in the FIR windows. This prevents high FIR outputs from "blinding" the detection temporarily.

The energy evaluation is satisfied if:

$$E_{\text{ratio}} \geq E_{\text{thresh}} \qquad (4)$$

where $E_{\text{thresh}}$ is an energy threshold. Its value can be set according to different signal-to-clutter ratio (SCR) detection requirements.

*Relative peak energy evaluation.* The relative peak energy $M_{\text{ratio}}$ is evaluated from frequency domain signals using the following energy relationship:

$$M_{\text{ratio}} = \frac{M_{\text{current}}}{M_{\text{neighbor}}} \qquad (5)$$

where $M_{\text{current}}$ is the magnitude of the dominant spectral peak within the current data window, and $M_{\text{neighbour}}$ is a neighbourhood maximum peak energy. Its value is again

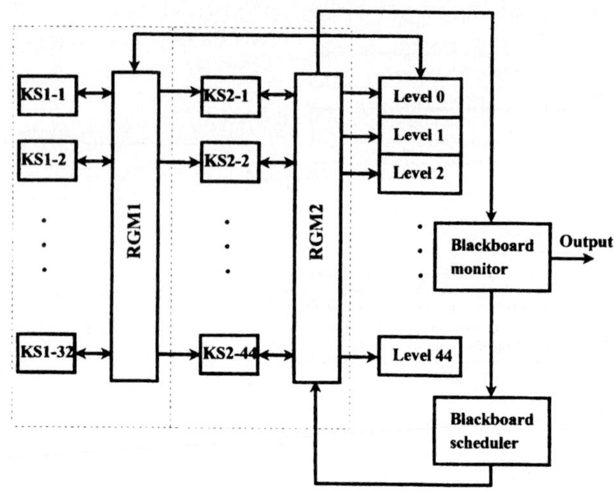


Fig. 4. Block diagram of the blackboard structure used in the expert system. KS1-N, ($n$ = 1,2, ..., 32) represent 32 knowledge sources in stage 1; KS2-N, ($n$ = 1,2, ..., 44) represent 44 knowledge sources in stage 2; RGM1 and RGM2 represent the two activated source regroup managers used.

calculated either from the two 51.2-ms FIR filter regions or from the IIR filter region, depending on whether there are strong artefacts or emboli in the FIR regions.

The maximum spectral peak evaluation is satisfied if:

$$M_{\text{ratio}} \geq M_{\text{thresh}} \qquad (6)$$

where $M_{\text{thresh}}$ is a magnitude threshold.

Combined with $E_{\text{thresh}}$, the value of $M_{\text{thresh}}$ can be set according to different SCR detection requirements.

*Signal duration evaluation.* The signal is evaluated within a neighbourhood of 25 ms to obtain duration information (beyond 25 ms, any further information is regarded as redundant becsause it does not aid the classification process).

*Blackboard evaluation*

Altogether 76 knowledge sources are derived from the above 14 knowledge source groups in two stages. All these knowledge sources are then linked to a blackboard-type intermediate hypotheses and decision base (Jackson 1999), before a signal can be detected or rejected at the output of the system. There are 164 reasoning rules and 45 blackboard levels involved in the processing, which evaluates signals as belonging to one of three classes: possible emboli, artefacts and background signals. A simplified block diagram of the blackboard architecture used in the detection system is as shown in Fig. 4.

Although it is difficult to write down or formalize the empirical knowledge used in expert systems (Jackson

1999), examples are given in Appendices 1 and 2 to demonstrate how the rule-based processing is carried out.

*Clinical data acquisition and interpretation*

Training and test data were derived from the same data library of routine clinical recordings (together with a few recordings from healthy subjects). These library recordings were made using a Scimed PC Dop 842 pulsed Doppler unit equipped with a 2-MHz transducer. The receive gate width was set to 1.16 cm, and the sample depth adjusted to give the optimal signal from the ipsilateral middle cerebral artery (between 4 cm and 5.8 cm). The high pass filter was normally set in the "off" position but, for four recordings in the test set, had been set to either 300 Hz or 600 Hz to remove wall thump signals.

Following initial work that made use of an arbitrary selection of 28 transcranial Doppler recordings, the system was trained with 81 separate 2.5-min Doppler recordings of middle cerebral artery blood flow from 41 carotid endarterectomy patients. These comprised 9 recordings made from 9 patients during the predissection phase of endarterectomy, 55 recordings made from 38 patients during the dissection phase, and 17 recordings made from 4 patients in the recovery room (some patients contributed records from more than one phase of the operation).

The system was tested with 74 separate Doppler recordings of middle cerebral artery blood flow from 29 carotid endarterectomy patients and 4 healthy volunteers, each lasting approximately 2.5 min (total recording time 185 min). These comprised 1 recording made from 1 patient during the predissection phase, 40 recordings made from 23 patients during the dissection phase (one of whom also contributed the predissection recording), 29 recordings made from 6 patients in the recovery room, and 4 recordings made from 4 healthy volunteers. The patient test recordings were chosen at random from a subset of recordings that had previously been analysed subjectively for clinical purposes. The subset consisted of records that had been noted to contain at least one embolic signal, and excluded recordings that had been used as training data for the expert system or had been previously noted as being "too poor to analyse" (a classification given to between 10% and 15% of our TCD recordings due to problems of penetrating the temporal bone with US). Different patients contributed a different number of recordings, with one contributing 11, one 8, one 6, one 4, two 3 each, twelve 2 each, and 11 one each (and the four healthy volunteers one each). Of the 74 recordings, 20 contained one or more periods of diathermy and the total duration of diathermy during these records was 253 s. With regard to other artefacts catalogued at the time of clinical analysis, 12 records con-

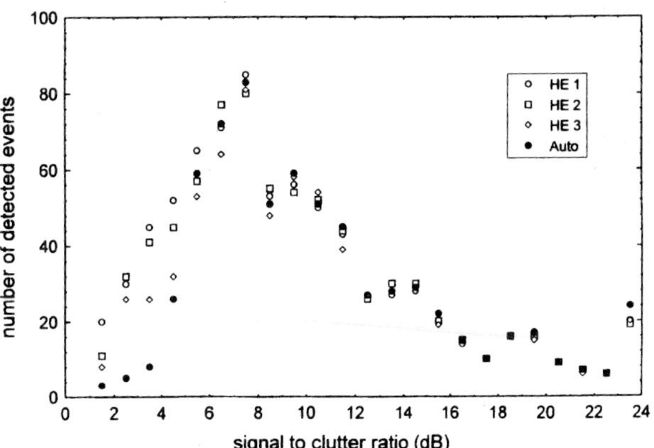

Fig. 5. The distribution of all detected events classified as embolic by each of the HEs and the automatic system, plotted as a function of SCR. The final set of points plotted as 23 dB < SCR < 24 dB represent all events with SCR > 23 dB.

tained a total of 163 artefacts identified at the time of recording (44 due to the patient moaning, 37 due to snoring, 31 due to head movement, 26 due to speech, 20 due to probe tapping, 4 due to probe adjustment, and 1 due to jaw movement), and 47 records (including all 12 records mentioned above) contained artefacts (a total of 414) of unknown origin. A total of 27 records, including all those from the healthy volunteers, appeared to be artefact-free. All recordings were digitised as described in the System design section of this paper.

Each of the test recordings was analysed by the automatic embolus identification system, and by each of three "expert" technicians with considerable experience of embolus detection and analysis. The HEs were blinded to the results of the automatic system, to the previous subjective analysis for clinical purposes, and to each other's results. They were asked to note the exact position of each signal they believed to correspond to an embolic event. The automatic system was programmed to store the position of signals classified as embolic, and also the position of any event with a significantly increased SCR (> 5 dB) not classified as embolic. The formal definition of SCR used in these studies is given in Appendix 3.

## RESULTS

In total, the three HEs classified 813, 787 and 714 events as being due to an embolus, and the automatic system classified 499 events as embolic using a threshold of 7 dB, 630 as embolic using a threshold of 5 dB, and 672 as embolic when no threshold was used. The distribution of all the detected events as a function of their measured SCR is shown in Fig. 5. It can be seen that the numbers of events detected by the automatic system

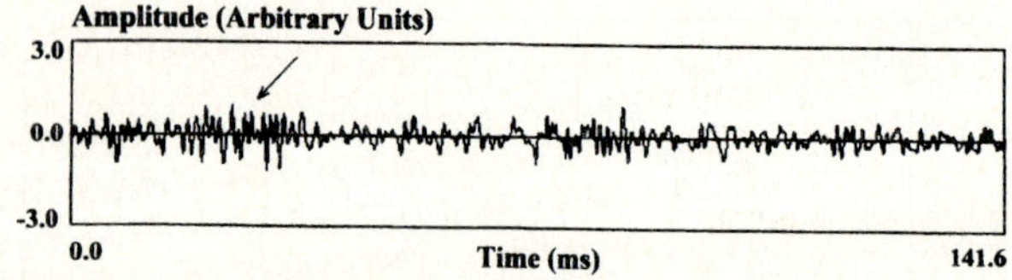



Fig. 6. Example of a signal classified as embolic by one of the HEs, but not detected by the automatic system. The central frequency of the signal is 1.27 kHz, and the SCR 4.9 dB. This event was classified as positive using the CSD proxy standard.

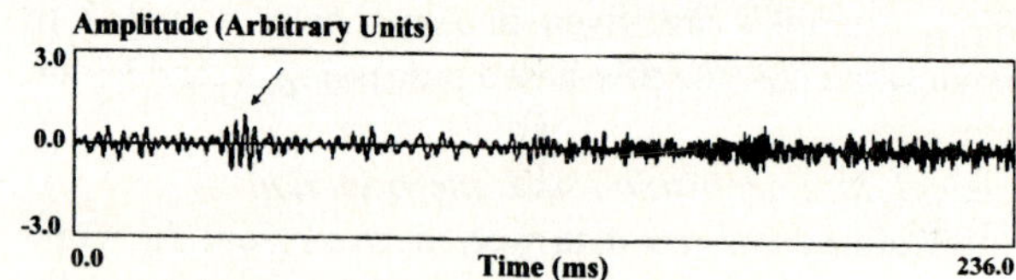



Fig. 7. Example of a signal detected by the automatic system, but not heard by any of the HEs. The central frequency of the signal is 390 Hz, and the SCR 7.9 dB. This event was classified as positive using the CSD proxy standard.

were very similar to the numbers of events detected by the individual HEs (although frequently very slightly higher) at high SCRs, and became progressively less in comparison below 5 dB.

To make a meaningful comparison between the automatic system and the HEs, it is necessary to quantify the agreement with regard to specific events. Unfortunately there is no "gold standard" for the detection of embolic events because there is no way of knowing if individual Doppler events really correspond to the passage of a microembolus through the sample volume. Furthermore, even experienced HEs will disagree about the interpretation of many events, especially if they are of low amplitude. To try and overcome this problem, we have adopted three different "gold standards" to compare the performance of the automatic system with HEs: the "human expert absolute detection" (HEAD) method, the

"human expert majority detection" (HEMD) method and the "case study detection" (CSD) method.

The HEAD method classifies any event detected by any HE as a true positive, and all other events are classified as negative. The HEMD method classifies any event detected by the majority of HEs (at least two in the current evaluation) as a true positive and all others as negative (*i.e.*, if an event is detected by only one HE in this study it is regarded as a false-positive). The CSD method is based on a careful re-examination of each candidate event by a fourth HE, who is able to replay the events *ad lib* and also to examine the time domain signal and high-resolution spectral display before arbitrating on the classification of the signal. The essential criteria used during this process are reproduced in Appendix 4. Examples of two signals classified as emboli by the CSD method (one detected by one HE only, and one detected

Table 2. Detection results using the "Human Expert Absolute Decision" standard

| Classifier | All SCRs* | | SCR ≥ 5 dB[†] | | SCR ≥ 7 dB[‡] | |
|---|---|---|---|---|---|---|
| | Sensitivity (%) | Specificity (%) | Sensitivity (%) | Specificity (%) | Sensitivity (%) | Specificity (%) |
| Expert 1 | 86.1 | 100 | 92.3 | 100 | 94.9 | 100 |
| Expert 2 | 83.4 | 100 | 92.4 | 100 | 95.5 | 100 |
| Expert 3 | 75.6 | 100 | 88.4 | 100 | 93.6 | 100 |
| Automatic | 63.1 | 99.95 | 86.7 | 96.8 | 93.0 | 96.4 |

* 944 embolic events 144234 candidate events.
[†] 674 embolic events, 2098 candidate events.
[‡] 512 embolic events, 1151 candidate events.

Table 3. Detection results using the "Human Expert Majority Decision" standard

| Classifier | All SCRs* | | SCR ≥ 5 dB[†] | | SCR ≥ 7 dB[‡] | |
|---|---|---|---|---|---|---|
| | Sensitivity (%) | Specificity (%) | Sensitivity (%) | Specificity (%) | Sensitivity (%) | Specificity (%) |
| Expert 1 | 95.4 | 99.94 | 96.3 | 98.7 | 97.4 | 99.1 |
| Expert 2 | 94.6 | 99.95 | 96.5 | 98.7 | 97.8 | 98.9 |
| Expert 3 | 89.9 | 99.98 | 93.6 | 99.3 | 95.9 | 99.1 |
| Automatic | 74.5 | 99.93 | 89.6 | 95.3 | 94.7 | 95.1 |

* 760 embolic events 144234 candidate events;
[†] 626 embolic events, 2098 candidate events;
[‡] 493 embolic events, 1151 candidate events.

Table 4. Detection results using the "Case Study Decision" standard

| Classifier | All SCRs* | | SCR ≥ 5 dB† | | SCR ≥ 7 dB‡ | |
| | Sensitivity (%) | Specificity (%) | Sensitivity (%) | Specificity (%) | Sensitivity (%) | Specificity (%) |
| --- | --- | --- | --- | --- | --- | --- |
| Expert 1 | 84.0 | 99.97 | 90.2 | 99.4 | 95.3 | 99.2 |
| Expert 2 | 82.1 | 99.98 | 89.3 | 98.9 | 94.3 | 98.0 |
| Expert 3 | 75.5 | 99.99 | 86.2 | 99.4 | 93.3 | 98.8 |
| Automatic | 69.9 | 99.98 | 89.9 | 98.7 | 95.8 | 97.7 |

* 921 embolic events, 144234 candidate events;
† 681 embolic events, 2098 candidate events;
‡ 505 embolic events, 1151 candidate events.

by the automatic system only) are shown in Figs. 6 and 7, respectively. To implement this method, the fourth HE needed access to the previous results and, therefore, was not blinded. Although this technique is potentially subject to operator bias, we would regard it as possibly the most reliable of the three proxy "gold standards" because of the detailed examination of each candidate event that took place.

The sensitivity and specificity of each of four methods of detection, when compared with each of the three proxy "gold standards" are presented in Tables 2–4. Additionally, the sensitivity of each of the HEs and the automatic system, using the CSD method, are plotted as a function of SCR (Fig. 8). Sensitivity was defined as the number of true positive detections above a given SCR threshold, divided by the number of events above the threshold classified as embolic by the "gold standard." Specificity was defined as one minus the number of false-positive detections above the specified SCR threshold, divided by the number of events above the threshold classified as nonembolic by the proxy "gold standard." In

the case of the 5-dB and 7-dB thresholds, there were 2098 and 1151 events, respectively, that exceeded the threshold and these numbers were taken as the total number of events (*i.e.*, true-positives + false-positives + true-negatives + false-negatives). In the case where no SCR threshold was used, the total recording was regarded as being comprised of 144,234 76.8-ms segments of Doppler signal, each of which might contain an independent embolic event. The value of 76.8 ms was chosen because this period proved (subject to sampling rate constraints) to be the best compromise for the "shut-down" period following each detected embolic event, when no detected event could be regarded as a separate embolic event.

The use of HE detection results to define proxy "gold standard" results inevitably biases the comparison of the automatic system with individual human performance and, therefore, an alternative way to analyse the data was also adopted. The proportion of specific agreement between each of the several methods of detecting embolic events, ($p_{\text{row, column}}^{\text{SCR range}}$, defined as the probability for a specified range of SCRs, that the method defined by the column heading would classify a signal as embolic, if the method defined by the row had classified the event as embolic (Cullinane et al. 2000)), was calculated and the results are shown in Tables 5 to 7.

## DISCUSSION

A significant difficulty in interpreting the results of an automatic embolus detection system is the lack of a true "gold standard." To partially overcome this difficulty, we have compared the performance of our system both with the results from individual HEs, and with three proxy "gold standards."

The results for the HEAD "gold standard" are shown in Table 2, where it can be seen that the three HEs always have a specificity of 100%, because any event detected by even one of them is regarded as a true-positive. Although the automatic system cannot compete with such a high specificity, its results are actually quite promising, reaching 96.8% and 96.4% for potential em-

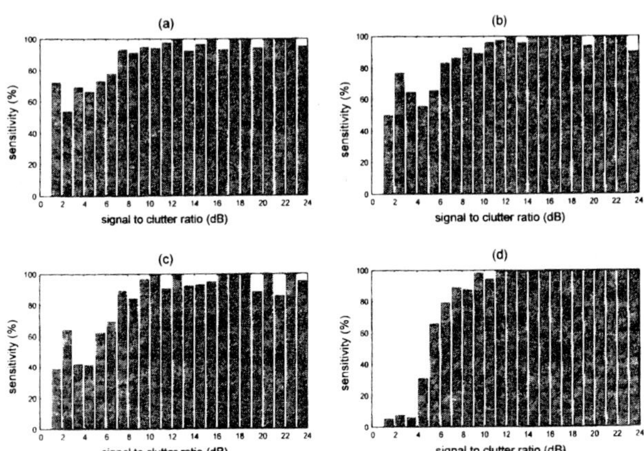

Fig. 8. Histograms of the sensitivity achieved by each of the HEs and the automatic system when using the CSD proxy, plotted as a function of SCR. (a)–(c), HEs 1 to 3; (d) automatic system.

Table 5. Proportion of specific agreement for SCR $\geq$ 7 dB

| $p^{SCR \geq 7\,dB}_{row,column}$ | Expert 1 | Expert 2 | Expert 3 | Automatic |
|---|---|---|---|---|
| Expert 1 | 1 | 0.96 | 0.94 | 0.95 |
| Expert 2 | 0.96 | 1 | 0.94 | 0.94 |
| Expert 3 | 0.95 | 0.96 | 1 | 0.95 |
| Automatic | 0.93 | 0.92 | 0.91 | 1 |

bolic events with SCRs of greater than 5 dB and 7 dB, respectively. Note that the specificity actually increases as the value of SCR reduces due to the progressively greater number of candidate events. With regard to sensitivity, the automatic system does not perform as well as any of the HEs but, in the case of the 5-dB threshold, is only marginally worse than HE 3 and, in the case of the 7-dB threshold, is only marginally worse than any of the HEs. It should be noted that, because of the definition of the HEAD standard, the automatic system has to detect each event declared as embolic by any one of three HEs to achieve 100% sensitivity, but each of the three HEs has only to detect each event declared as embolic by one of the remaining two HEs to achieve 100% sensitivity, so that the results are biased in favour of the HEs.

The results for the HEMD proxy standard are shown in Table 3. The automatic system shows better sensitivity than for the HEAD proxy standard because events are only regarded as embolic if at least two HEs classify them as such, which means there are fewer potentially equivocal events that are classified as embolic in origin. The specificity is, however, marginally lower because some weaker events detected by only a single HE, and therefore classified as artefacts, are also detected by the automatic system and classified as embolic in nature. Further examination of the data showed that of the 69 "false-positives" detected by the automatic system using a threshold of 5 dB, 23 were also classified as

embolic by a single HE. Note that the HEs also display better sensitivity and poorer specificity when compared with this proxy standard.

Careful examination of the embolic data, including replaying short segments of data several times and examining the time-domain and frequency-domain displays, convinced us that both the HEAD and the HEMD method produced some classifications for individual events that were incorrect and, therefore, a fourth observer replayed and examined every event classified by any of the HEs or the automatic system as embolic in nature. As already mentioned, this method is open to observer bias but, nevertheless, was considered a useful adjunct because it compared the performance with our best estimate of the origin of each event (and the results that would be used for further training of the system if a further update were considered necessary). Using the CSD proxy standard, the sensitivity of the automatic system was as good as any of the HEs for thresholds of both 5 dB and 7 dB, but was significantly worse for lower SCRs. The specificity was in all cases similar to that of the HEs.

Tables 5 to 7 show individual comparisons between the detections achieved by the three HEs and the automatic system. Above 7 dB, any event called positive by one HE was just as likely to be called positive by the automatic system as by any of the remaining HEs. On the other hand, there seems to be a slightly smaller proba-

Table 6. Proportion of specific agreement for SCR $\geq$ 5 dB

| $p^{SCR \geq 7\,dB}_{row,column}$ | Expert 1 | Expert 2 | Expert 3 | Automatic |
|---|---|---|---|---|
| Expert 1 | 1 | 0.93 | 0.90 | 0.89 |
| Expert 2 | 0.93 | 1 | 0.90 | 0.89 |
| Expert 3 | 0.94 | 0.94 | 1 | 0.89 |
| Automatic | 0.88 | 0.88 | 0.85 | 1 |

Table 7. Proportion of specific agreement for all SCRs

| $p^{all\,SCR}_{row,column}$ | Expert 1 | Expert 2 | Expert 3 | Automatic |
|---|---|---|---|---|
| Expert 1 | 1 | 0.84 | 0.79 | 0.69 |
| Expert 2 | 0.87 | 1 | 0.81 | 0.71 |
| Expert 3 | 0.90 | 0.89 | 1 | 0.75 |
| Automatic | 0.84 | 0.83 | 0.80 | 1 |

bility that an event called positive by the automatic system will also be called positive by any of the HEs, which means that either the automatic system is more sensitive or less specific than the HEs with respect to some events. Reference to Fig. 8 suggests that, if the CSD proxy standard is reliable, then the automatic system is, in fact, more sensitive than the HEs at high SCRs where it appears that individual HEs may miss events that even the rest of their peers detect, presumably due to a lapse in concentration (see, for example, the sensitivities achieved by HE 1 between 16 dB and 17 dB or those achieved by HE 3 between 11 dB and 12 dB).

There is a similar pattern above 5 dB (Table 6), although in this instance both the automatic system and HE 3 seem less likely to confirm an event previously called as positive. Once again, the HEs are less likely to detect an event classified as embolic by the automatic system, presumably because of falling specificity. If the results for all SCRs are considered, then there is clear reduction in the number of events called positive by the HEs that the automatic system is able to confirm, an effect that is also clearly visible in Fig. 8d.

Overall, the results of the automatic system appear to be extremely good for SCRs of above 5 dB. Below this value, performance deteriorates very rapidly so that few events with a SCR of below 4 dB are detected (see Fig. 5). However, we and others (Markus et al. 1997) have found that the agreement between HEs also deteriorates rapidly at these levels and so, even if it were possible to detect embolic events with much lower SCRs, the difficulty of finding a suitable "gold standard" would become even more challenging. It should also be remembered that the HE results have been obtained under ideal conditions; they were only required to analyse 2.5-min of recording at a time in quiet laboratory conditions. Under more normal clinical conditions, it is likely that their performance would decline significantly but, of course, the automatic system is unaffected by such considerations. Also, embolic signals recorded during the dissection and recovery phases of carotid artery surgery are relatively more difficult to detect than signals from gaseous emboli, which suggests that the present system should be able to cope with a wide variety of emboli.

The philosophy behind the design of the automatic system has been to keep the requirements for the Doppler front-end as simple as possible. The use of two or more Doppler sample volumes at different depths along the middle cerebral artery has proved a useful method of classifying signals as embolic or artefact by human observers (Georgiadis et al. 1996; Smith et al. 1996), but further experience has shown that, for the method to work reliably, the SCR needs to be relatively large and the Doppler gates placed very carefully to derive the most benefit from the technique. In practice, the auto-

matic system already works well at high SCRs and, if it is to be reliable in routine clinical use, it must be relatively insensitive to gate placement and applicable to as many patients as possible (some of whom will have relatively short segments of artery suitable for insonation). Reference to Fig. 6 illustrates the difficulty in defining the start of an event with a low SCR and, thus, the difficulty of using time delay as a method of distinguishing embolic from artefact signals. One further difficulty with the dual-gate technique is that a significant proportion of embolic signals only appear in a single channel (Lindner et al. 1997; Smith et al. 1997b).

We have also avoided the use of the reverse channel because, although large artefacts often appear in the reverse channel, these are, in general, easy to reject but, at lower levels, the situation is much less clear-cut. It is possible that simultaneous processing of the reverse channel could improve our results, but it is questionable if the added complexity of the system would justify any small gains.

The approach used in our system is very computationally intensive and currently has not been implemented in real-time. This is clearly a limitation, but we have calculated that, using new high-speed hardware, it should be possible to develop an online version of the system, and we are currently working on this.

## CONCLUSION

We have designed and implemented an expert system capable of automatically detecting Doppler signals believed to arise from cerebral emboli, at the same time successfully rejecting artefact signals from a wide variety of sources. Because it is difficult to define a "gold standard" for embolic events, it is also difficult to determine exact values for the sensitivity and specificity of the system, but it appears to deal well with signals down to a level of 5 dB above the background clutter, a level below which human performance begins to deteriorate rapidly. In practice, if an automatic system can perform almost as well as a HE in an ideal laboratory setting, it is likely to perform relatively better in a clinical situation where it has the advantages that it is not affected by the environment and does not fatigue, and can be used to provide an objective and reproducible estimate of embolic load.

*Acknowledgements*—The authors gratefully acknowledge the financial support of the UK Stroke Association, the NHS Executive Trent Research and Development Group and the University Hospitals of Leicester NHS Trust. They also thank Emma Angell, Harry Hall, Simon Hartley, Fatima Patel, Kate Randle and Sarah Steel, who acted as "human experts" at various stages during the development of the automatic expert system.

# REFERENCES

Aaslid R, Markwalder T, Nornes H. Noninvasive transcranial Doppler ultrasound recording of flow-velocity in basal cerebral arteries. J Neurosurg 1982;57:769–774.

Ackerstaff RGA, Babikian VL, Georgiadis D, Russell D, Siebler M, Spencer MP, Stump D. Basic identification criteria of Doppler microemboli signals: Consensus committee of the 9th International Cerebral Hemodynamics Symposium. Stroke 1995a;26:1123.

Ackerstaff RGA, Jansen C, Moll FL, Vermeulen FEE, Hamerlijnck RPHM, Mausr HW. The significance of microemboli detection by means of transcranial Doppler ultrasonography monitoring in carotid endarterectomy. J Vasc Surg 1995b;21:963–969.

Ackerstaff RGA, Jansen C, Moll FL. Carotid endarterectomy and intraoperative emboli detection: Correlation of clinical, transcranial Doppler, and magnetic resonance findings. Echocardiography 1996;13:543–550.

Angelsen BAJ. A theoretical study of the scattering of ultrasound from blood. IEEE Trans Biomed Eng 1980;BME-27:61–67.

Braekken SK, Reinvang I, Russell D, Brucher R, Svennevig JL. Association between intraoperative cerebral microembolic signals and postoperative neuropsychological deficit: Comparison between patients with cardiac valve replacement and patients with coronary artery bypass grafting. J Neurol Neurosurg Psychiat 1998;65:573–576.

Cohen L. Time-frequency distributions—a review. Proc IEEE 1989; 77:941–981.

Cullinane M, Reid G, Dittrich R, Kaposzta Z, Ackerstaff R, Babikian V, Droste DW, Grossett D, Siebler M, Valton L, Markus HS. Evaluation of new online automated embolic signal detection algorithm, including comparison with panel of international experts. Stroke 2000;31:1335–1341.

Droste DW, Decker W, Siemens H-J, Kaps M, Schulte-Altedorneburg G. Variability in occurrence of embolic signals in long term transcranial Doppler recordings. Neurol Res 1996;18:25–30.

Evans DH. Detection of microemboli. In: Babikian VL, Wechsler LR, eds. Transcranial Doppler ultrasonography. 2nd ed. Boston: Butterworth Heinemann, 1999:141–155.

Evans DH, Smith JL, Naylor AR. Characteristics of Doppler ultrasound signals recorded from cerebral emboli. Ultrasound Med Biol 1997; 23(Suppl. 1):S140.

Gaunt ME, Martin PJ, Smith JL, Rimmer T, Cherryman G, Ratliff DA, Bell PRF, Naylor AR. Clinical relevance of intraoperative embolization detected by transcranial Doppler ultrasonography during carotid endarterectomy: A prospective study of 100 patients. Br J Surg 1994a;81:1435–1439.

Gaunt ME, Ratliff DA, Martin PJ, Smith JL, Bell PRF, Naylor AR. On-table diagnosis of incipient carotid artery thrombosis during carotid endarterectomy by transcranial Doppler scanning. J Vasc Surg 1994b;20:104–107.

Georgiadis D, Grosset DG, Kelman A, Faichney A, Lees KR. Prevalence and characteristics of intracranial microemboli signals in patients with different types of prosthetic cardiac valves. Stroke 1994;25:587–592.

Georgiadis D, Goeke J, Hill M, König M, Nabavi DG, Stögbauer F, Zunker P, Ringelstein EB. A novel technique for identification of Doppler microembolic signals based on the coincidence method. In vitro and in vivo evaluation. Stroke 1996;27:683–686.

Georgiadis D, Lindner A, Zierz S. Intracranial microembolic signals in patients with artificial heart valves: Drowning in numbers. Eur J Med Res 1998;3:99–102.

Hayes-Roth F, Waterman DA, Lenat DB. An overview of expert systems. In: Hayes-Roth F, Waterman DA, Lenat DB, eds. Building expert systems. London: Addison-Wesley, 1983:3–29.

Jackson P. Introduction to expert systems. 3rd ed. Harlow, UK: Addison-Wesley, 1999.

Lennard N, Smith JL, Dumville J, Abbott R, Evans DH, London NJM, Bell PRF, Naylor AR. Prevention of post-operative thrombotic stroke after carotid endarterectomy: The role of transcranial Doppler ultrasound. J Vasc Surg 1997;26:579–584.

Levi CR, O'Malley HM, Fell G, Roberts AK, Hoare MC, Royle JP, Chan A, Beiles BC, Chambers BR, Bladin CF, Donnan GA. Trans-

cranial Doppler detected cerebral microembolism following carotid endarterectomy: High microembolic signal loads predict postoperative cerebral ischaemia. Brain 1997;120:621–629.

Lindner A, Georgiadis D, Fischer G, Zerkowski HR, Zierz S. Identification of Doppler microembolic signals with a bigate probe in patients with prosthetic heart valves. Eur J Med Res 1997;2:299–301.

Markus HS, Ackerstaff R, Babikian V, Bladin C, Droste D, Grosset D, Levi C, Russell D, Siebler M, Tegeler C. Intercenter agreement in reading Doppler embolic signals: A multicenter international study. Stroke 1997;28:1307–1310.

Mo LYL, Cobbold RSC. A stochastic model of the backscattered Doppler ultrasound from blood. IEEE Trans Biomed Eng 1986; BME-33:20–27.

Molloy J, Markus HS. Asymptomatic embolization predicts stroke and TIA risk in patients with carotid artery disease. Stroke 1999;30: 1440–1443.

Molloy J, Khan N, Markus HS. Temporal variability of asymptomatic embolization in carotid artery stenosis and optimal recording protocols. Stroke 1998;29:1129–1132.

Pugsley W, Klinger L, Paschalis C, Treasure T, Harrison M, Newman S. The impact of microemboli during cardiopulmonary bypass on neuropsychological functioning. Stroke 1994;25:1393–1399.

Rams JJ, Davis DA, Lolley DM, Berger MP, Spencer M. Detection of microemboli in patients with artificial heart valves using transcranial Doppler: Preliminary observations. J Heart Valve Dis 1993;2: 37–41.

Ringelstein EB, Droste DW, Babikian VL, Evans DH, Grosset DG, Kaps M, Markus HS, Russell D, Siebler M. Consensus on microembolus detection by TCD. International Consensus Group on Microembolus Detection. Stroke 1998;29:725–729.

Santalucia P, Feldmann E. The basic transcranial Doppler examination: Technique and anatomy. In: Babikian VL, Wechsler LR, eds. Transcranial Doppler ultrasonography. 2nd ed. Boston: Butterworth Heinemann, 1999:13–31.

Smith JL, Evans DH, Fan L, Bell PRF, Naylor AR. Differentiation between emboli and artefacts using dual-gated transcranial Doppler ultrasound. Ultrasound Med Biol 1996;22:1031–1036.

Smith JL, Evans DH, Fan L, Gaunt ME, London WJM, Bell PRF, Naylor R. Interpretation of embolic phenomena during carotid endarterectomy. Stroke 1995;26:2281–2284.

Smith JL, Evans DH, Gaunt ME, London NJM, Bell PRF, Naylor AR. Experience with transcranial Doppler monitoring reduces the incidence of particulate embolization during carotid endarterectomy. Br J Surg 1998;85:56–59.

Smith JL, Evans DH, Naylor AR. Analysis of the frequency modulation present in Doppler ultrasound signals may allow differentiation between particulate and gaseous cerebral emboli. Ultrasound Med Biol 1997a;23:727–734.

Smith JL, Evans DH, Naylor AR. Signals from dual gated TCD systems: Curious observations and possible explanations. Ultrasound Med Biol 1997b;23:15–24.

Spencer MP. Detection of cerebral arterial emboli. In: Newell DW, Aaslid R, eds. Transcranial Doppler. New York: Raven Press, 1992:215–230.

Sylivris S, Levi C, Matalanis G, Rosalion A, Buxton BF, Mitchell A, Fitt G, Harberts DB, Saling MM, Tonkin AM. Pattern and significance of cerebral microemboli during coronary artery bypass grafting. Ann Thorac Surg 1998;66:1674–1678.

Van Zuilen EV, Mess WH, Jansen C, Van Der Tweel I, Van Gijn J, Ackerstaff RGA. Automatic embolus detection compared with human experts. A Doppler ultrasound study. Stroke 1996;27:1840–1843.

Van Zuilen EV, Moll FL, Vermeulen FEE, Mauser HW, van Gijn J, Ackerstaff RGA. Detection of cerebral microemboli by means of transcranial Doppler monitoring before and after carotid endarterectomy. Stroke 1995;26:210–213.

Van Zuilen EV, Van Gijn J, Ackerstaff RGA. The clinical relevance of cerebral microemboli detection by transcranial Doppler ultrasound. J Neuroimag 1998;8:32–37.

## APPENDIX 1

The Activating Condition of Rule No. 61 is:

**IF**
[I_MAXFRQ61] **AND**
[I_SNR61] **AND**
[I_ENG61] **AND**
{([G_ENGW] **AND** [G_ENGPK] **AND** [G_SPSHP] **AND** [G_PKIDX]
**AND**
[G_NTFRM] **AND** [G_FQPKEV]) **OR**
([G_ENGW] **AND** [G_ENGPK] **AND** [G_SPSHP] **AND**
[G_PKIDX] **AND**
[G_NTFRM] **AND** [G_FQPKEV]) **OR**
([G_ENGW] **AND** [G_ENGPK] **AND** [G_SPSHP] **AND**
[G_PKIDX] **AND**
[G_NTFRM] **AND** [G_FQPKEV]) **OR**
([G_ENGW] **AND** [G_ENGPK] **AND** [G_SPSHP] **AND**
[G_PKIDX] **AND**
[G_NTFRM] **AND** [G_FQPKEV]) **OR**
([G_ENGW] **AND** [G_ENGPK] **AND** [G_SPSHP] **AND**
[G_PKIDX] **AND**
[G_NTFRM] **AND** [G_FQPKEV]) **OR**
([G_ENGW] **AND** [G_ENGPK] **AND** [G_SPSHP] **AND**
[G_PKIDX] **AND**
[G_NTFRM] **AND** [G_FQPKEV]) **OR**
([G_ENGW] **AND** [G_ENGPK] **AND** [G_SPSHP] **AND**
[G_PKIDX] **AND**
[G_NTFRM] **AND** [G_FQPKEV]) **OR**
([G_ENGW] **AND** [G_ENGPK] **AND** [G_SPSHP] **AND**
[G_PKIDX] **AND**
[G_NTFRM] **AND** [G_FQPKEV]) **OR**
([G_ENGW] **AND** [G_ENGPK] **AND** [G_SPSHP] **AND**
[G_PKIDX] **AND**
[G_NTFRM] **AND** [G_FQPKEV])
}
Then

See following "output consequence."
Else

Blackboard level 12 is deactivated and all parameters on the level
are set to zero.

The output consequence for rule No. 62:
1. Blackboard level 12 is activated.
2. The mixed incremental counter mix_ct12 is updated.
3. The maximum value of SNR is searched and stored as max_snr12
   while blackboard level 12 is activated.
4. An averaged SNR is calculated and stored as ave_snr12 while the
   blackboard level 12 is activated.
5. The maximum value of the relative peak energy (RPE) is searched
   and stored as max_tot12 while the blackboard level 12 is activated.
   The relative peak energy is defined as the value of the maximum
   spectral peak energy relative to the total frame energy.
6. The maximum frequency index value of the maximum spectral peak
   is searched and stored as max_fb12 while the blackboard level 12 is
   activated.
7. The maximum number of sastisfied general conditions is recorded
   and stored as max_mark12 while the blackboard level 12 is activated.
8. The number of those frames in which the relative peak energy is
   higher than 80% is recorded and stored as tot_h_12 while the
   blackboard level 12 is activated.
9. **IF**

   9-1. The parameter mix_ct12 $\geq$ 4 (frames), and
   9-2. The parameter max_snrl12 $\geq$ 7.0 (dB), and
   9-3. The parameter ave_snrl12 $\geq$ 5.0 (dB), and
   9-4. The parameter max_tot12 $\geq$ 95%, and
   9-5. The parameter max_fb12 $\geq$ 1.07 (kHz), and
   9-6. The parameter max_mark12 $\geq$ 6 (non-dimensional), and
   9-7. The parameter tot_h_12 $\geq$ 2 (frames)

   **Then**

   The signal contained in these several frames is detected as an
embolus.

*Parameter denotations*

[condition]: condition satisfied.
[condition]: condition not satisfied.
I_MAXFRQ61: Individual maximum frequency peak condition
for Rule No. 61.
I_SNR61: Individual signal to noise ratio condition for Rule No.
61.
I_ENG61: Individual energy condition for Rule No. 61.
G_ENGW: General energy condition for the whole frame eval-
uation.
G_ENGPK: General energy condition for the maximum peak of
the spectrum evaluation.
G_SPSHP: General condition for the basic spectral shape of
current frame evaluation.
G_PKIDX: General condition for the index of the maximum
spectral peak evaluation
G_NTFRM: General condition for the next frame evaluation.
G_FQPKEV: General shape condition for the current maximum
frequency peak evaluation.

To avoid tedious and tangled explanations, the details of above
conditions are not listed one-by-one. As an example, however, the
details of the general condition G_FQPKEV are given in Appendix 2,
to show how information is obtained and further processed.

## APPENDIX 2

*Details of an example general condition*

The general shape condition for the current maximum frequency
peak evaluation G_FQPKEV would be satisfied if:
1. The normalized spectrum should have at least one peak that has a
   height rising rate higher than 0.05/point.
2. The peak number should not be more than 5.
3. No peak except the maximum peak should have a magnitude higher
   than 0.2.
4. No peak should have a magnitude higher than 0.12 and also a
   distance more than 391 Hz from the maximum spectral peak.
5. The 3-dB bandwidth of the maximum spectral peak should not be
   wider than 300 Hz.
6. The maximum spectral peak should contain at least 55% of the
   energy of the whole frame.
7. The bandwidth of the maximum spectral peak that is defined using
   two $-5.2$ dB points should not be wider than 490 Hz.

Magnitudes are normalized to the maximum peak unless otherwise
stated.

## APPENDIX 3

*Definition of signal-to-clutter ratio (SCR)*

To estimate the signal-to-clutter ratio (SCR) for a frame centred
at time index $p$, the signal energy contained in a 10.24-ms processing
frame is calculated as:

$$E(p) = \sum_{n=p-63}^{p+64} s^2(n) \qquad (1A)$$

where $s(n)$ is the signal magnitude at time index $n$.

Two different definitions of clutter energy are used, depending
on whether or not emboli ar artefacts have been found in the neighbourhood of the processing frame, which leads to two separate definitions of SCR, *i.e.*:

*Case 1.* No emboli or artefacts detected in the $[p + 640$ to $p +
1248]$ and $[p - 640$ to $p - 1248]$ regions.:

$$SCR_{p(case1)} = 10\log[[E(p)/E_{FIR}(p)]] \qquad (2A)$$

where

$$E_{FIR}(p) = \frac{1}{40}\left[\sum_{m=0}^{19} E(p + 640 + 32m)\right.$$

$$\left. + \sum_{m=0}^{19} E(p - 640 - 32m)\right] \quad (3A)$$

*Case 2.* Emboli or artefacts detected in the $[p + 640$ to $p + 1248]$ or $[p - 640$ to $p - 1248]$ regions:

$$SCR_{p(case2)} = 10\log[E(p)/E_{IIR}(p)] \quad (4A)$$

where

$$E_{IIR}(p) = 0.8E_{IIR}(p - 1) + 0.2E(p - 32) \quad (5A)$$

Review of the detection results showed that, in fact, the second criterion was only used for 8 of the 672 embolic events detected.

## APPENDIX 4

*General criteria used to classify events using the CSD method*
    A signal is classified as an embolus, if:
1. It was detected by most HEs and the checker, and its central frequency is higher than 300 Hz, OR
2. it ws detected by one HE and is also vaguely heard by the checker, AND its central frequency appears higher than 300 Hz, although its time domain waveform and its energy level are very similar to those of its neighbourhood, OR
3. it was detected by one HE only, AND its central frequency seems higher than 300 Hz, AND its time domain waveform OR its evergy level is different from those of its neighbourhood, OR
4. it was detected by the automated system, AND can be vaguely heard by the checker, AND its time domain waveform appears like a narrow-band sigmal with a central freauency not lower than 300 Hz, AND its energy level is clearly higher than those of its neighbourhood, OR
5. it was detected by the automated system, but cannot be heard; hoever, the time domain waveform is that of a short narrow-band signal with a central frequency higher than 300 Hz, and an energy level much higher than that of its neighbourhood.

The method is biased toward classifying an event as embolic if any of the human observers believe this to be the case.

## Table of symbols and abbreviations

| | |
|---|---|
| CSD = | case study detection |
| $C_0$ = | scaling constant |
| $E_{current}$ = | total signal energy for the current data window |
| $E_{neighbour}$ = | neighbourhood energy |
| $E_{ratio}$ = | energy ratio (current frame to neighbourhood) |
| $E_{thresh}$ = | energy ratio threshold |
| FIR = | finite impulse response (filter) |
| FFT = | fast Fourier transform |
| $F_{dom}$ = | frequency of dominant spectral peak |
| $F_{thresh}$ = | frequency threshold |
| HE = | human expert |
| HEAD = | human expert absolute detection |
| HEMD = | human expert majority detection |
| $h(n)$ = | discrete Hanning window signal at time index $n$ |
| IIR = | infinite impulse response (filter) |
| $k$ = | discrete frequency index |
| $M_{current}$ = | magnitude of dominant spectral peak in current data window |
| $M_{neighbour}$ = | neighbourhood dominant peak magnitude |
| $M_{ratio}$ = | dominant peak magnitude ratio (current frame to neighbourhood) |
| $M_{thresh}$ = | magnitude threshold |
| $n$ = | discrete time index |
| $n_0$ = | discrete time index |
| $\hat{P}(n_0,k)$ = | estimate of power around sample index $n_0$ and at frequency index $k$ |
| $P^{SCR\ range}_{row,column}$ = | proportion of specific agreement |
| SCR = | signal-to-clutter ratio |
| $s(n)$ = | discrete input signal at time index $n$ |
| TCD = | transcranial Doppler |
| $W_{dom(3\ dB)}$ = | 3 dB bandwidth threshold for dominant spectral peak |

# Segmentation and tracking of the electro-encephalogram signal using an adaptive recursive bandpass filter

**R. R. Gharieb[1,2]**     **A. Cichocki[1,3]**

[1]Laboratory for Advanced Brain Signal Processing, Brain Science Institute, RIKEN, Wako-Shi, Saitama, Japan
[2]Assiut University, Assiut, Egypt
[3]Warsaw University of Technology, Warsaw, Poland

**Abstract**—*An adaptive filtering approach for the segmentation and tracking of electro-encephalogram (EEG) signal waves is described. In this approach, an adaptive recursive bandpass filter is employed for estimating and tracking the centre frequency associated with each EEG wave. The main advantage inherent in the approach is that the employed adaptive filter has only one unknown coefficient to be updated. This coefficient, having an absolute value less than 1, represents an efficient distinct feature for each EEG specific wave, and its time function reflects the non-stationarity behaviour of the EEG signal. Therefore the proposed approach is simple and accurate in comparison with existing multivariate adaptive approaches. The approach is examined using extensive computer simulations. It is applied to computer-generated EEG signals composed of different waves. The adaptive filter coefficient (i.e. the segmentation parameter) is −0.492 for the delta wave, −0.360 for the theta wave, −0.191 for the alpha wave, −0.027 for the sigma wave, 0.138 for the beta wave and 0.605 for the gamma wave. This implies that the segmentation parameter increases with the increase in the centre frequency of the EEG waves, which provides fast on-line information about the behaviour of the EEG signal. The approach is also applied to real-world EEG data for the detection of sleep spindles.*

**Keywords**—*Electro-encephalogram analysis, Non-stationarity, Adaptive tracking of centre frequency of biomedical signals*

## 1 Introduction

COMPUTER-AIDED ANALYSIS of the electro-encephalogram (EEG) signal, especially during sleep, is essential to facilitate the analysis of a great number of recorded data (AMIR and GATH, 1989; ANDERSON *et al.*, 1998; NIEDERMEYER and LOPES DA SILVA, 1999; KIM *et al.*, 2000; GATH *et al.*, 1992; WRIGHT *et al.*, 1990; BLINOWSKA and MALINOWSKI, 1989; ARNOLD *et al.*, 1998; DING *et al.*, 2000; ROSIPAL *et al.*, 1998; GOTO *et al.*, 1995; NING and BRONZINO, 1989). Various computer procedures employ a preliminary stage of feature extraction, followed by decision-making for classification and segmentation tasks. A classical procedure is to apply the Fourier transform to successive windows of the EEG signal to investigate variation of the frequency spectrum over time.

The main assumption associated with these procedures is that the EEG signal recorded during sleep or the waking stage (e.g. performing different mental tasks) is piecewise and stationary. However, owing to the strong non-stationarity of the EEG signals, the use of either stationarity-based methods or block-wise adaptive methods is often not satisfactory for the analysis of the EEG signal.

Various time-varying autoregressive (TVAR) modelling-based approaches have been used for the analysis and segmentation of the EEG signal (AMIR and GATH, 1989; ANDERSON *et al.*, 1998; WRIGHT *et al.*, 1990; ARNOLD *et al.*, 1998; DING *et al.*, 2000; GOTO *et al.*, 1995). In these approaches, the EEG signal is assumed to be the output of a linear filter fed by a white-noise process. Thus the EEG signal is modelled as an AR process of unknown coefficients. These coefficients could be computed by applying the linear prediction framework (KAY and MARPLE, 1981; HAYKIN, 1996) to the EEG signal, in addition to an adaptive algorithm, to achieve on-line computation of the AR coefficients. However, such TVAR modelling-based approaches suffer from tedious, heavy computation as they try to update all the coefficients of the AR model and to use these coefficients for the on-line computation of the EEG signal spectrum (ANDERSON *et al.*, 1998; ARNOLD *et al.*, 1998; DING *et al.*, 2000; GOTO *et al.*, 1995).

In this paper, an alternative, efficient approach is described for the segmentation and tracking of the EEG signal waves. In this approach, an adaptive recursive bandpass filter is used to track the centre frequency of the EEG signal. The adaptive bandpass

Correspondence should be addressed to Dr R. R. Gharieb;
e-mail: rada@hsp.brain.riken.go.jp

First received 22 September 2000 and in final form 2 January 2001

MBEC online number: 20013559

filter employed has only one unknown coefficient to be updated. This coefficient is updated to adjust the centre frequency of the adaptive bandpass filter to be matched with that of the input signal. Thus the proposed wave segmentation is based on on-line estimation of the centre frequency of the EEG signal, and the segmentation parameter is described by the unique adaptive filter coefficient. Therefore the advantage of the presented approach is to make the segmentation and tracking process a function of only one parameter, providing a simpler and more accurate approach in comparison with multivariate adaptive approaches.

## 2 EEG segmentation based on adaptive AR modelling

To apply the AR framework (KAY and MARPLE, 1981; HAYKIN, 1996) to the EEG signal, it is assumed that the EEG signal is modelled as the output of a linear filter fed by a white-noise process. To compute the AR coefficients given the noisy observed EEG signal, the linear prediction (LP) theory is applied (HAYKIN, 1996). In the LP theory, an estimate $\hat{x}(n)$ of the current sample $x(n)$ is obtained as a weighted linear combination of the past samples, i.e.

$$\hat{x}(n) = \sum_{i=1}^{P} a_i x(n-i) \tag{1}$$

The prediction error of the estimated sample is given by

$$e(n) = x(n) - \hat{x}(n) \tag{2}$$

Minimising the sum of squared errors results in the well-known Yule–Walker (YW) equations, which should be solved for the parameters $\{a_i\}$ (KAY and MARPLE, 1981; HAYKIN, 1996). The recursive least squares algorithm (RLS) is the tool commonly used for finding the on-line solution of the YW equations. Thus the RLS algorithm enables us to compute the AR coefficients on-line (adaptively). In this case, the adaptive AR coefficients $\{a_i(n)\}$ can follow the time varying of the EEG signal model. Unfortunately, the only distinct feature that can be formulated using the AR coefficients is the power spectrum of the EEG signal. This on-line power spectrum against the frequency $f$ at time $n$ can be expressed as

$$S(f|n) = \frac{1}{\left| 1 - \sum_{i=1}^{P} a_i(n) \exp(-j2\pi f i) \right|^2} \tag{3}$$

There are some difficulties associated with the AR modelling-based segmentation approach. The first is the unavailability of order $P$ of the AR model. The second is that the RLS algorithm consists of matrix computations, which increases the computational cost. The third is the huge computations required for eqn 3 at every instant of time $n$, in addition to a three-dimensional plotter that is also required to show the power spectrum values on the frequency–time grid.

## 3 Bandpass adaptive filter

### 3.1 *Filter structure*

The bandpass filter applied to track the centre frequency of a bandpass signal can be the fourth-order Butterworth filter, whose transfer function is expressed as (RAJA KUMAR and PAL, 1985; 1986; 1990)

$$H(z)$$
$$= \frac{a_0 + a_2 z^{-2} + a_4 z^{-4}}{1 + b_1 w(n) z^{-1} + (b_2 w^2(n) + b_2') z^{-2} + b_3 w(n) z^{-3} + b_4 z^{-4}} \tag{4}$$

where

$$a_0 = a_4 = 1/(k^2 + \sqrt{2}k + 1)$$
$$a_2 = -2a_0$$
$$a_1 = a_3 = -4a_0$$
$$b_1 = -2k(2k + \sqrt{2})a_0$$
$$b_2 = 4k^2 a_0$$
$$b_2' = 2(k^2 - 1)a_0$$
$$b_3 = 2k(-2k + \sqrt{2})a_0$$
$$b_4 = (k^2 - \sqrt{2}k + 1)a_0$$
$$k = \cotan(\pi B)$$

$$w(n) = \frac{\cos(\pi(f_1(n) + f_2(n))}{\cos(\pi B)} \tag{5}$$

$f_1(n) =$ normalised lower cutoff frequency as a function of discrete time $n$; $f_2(n) =$ normalised higher cutoff frequency as a function of discrete time $n$; and $B =$ normalised bandwidth of the filter.

From the expressions given by eqn 5, it is obvious that, with the assumption that the bandwidth $B$ is a constant, $w(n)$ is an only-centre frequency-dependent parameter. That is, the bandpass adaptive filter $H(z)$ has only a centre frequency-dependent coefficient to be updated. It is worthwhile mentioning that the stability constraints on $H(z)$ are provided if

$$k > 0 \quad \text{and} \quad |w(n)| < 1 \tag{6}$$

Fig. 1 shows the amplitude spectrum $|H(e^{j2\pi f})|$ against the frequency $f$ for different values of $w(n)$. It is apparent that the spectrum moves on the frequency axis to the higher frequency with the decrease of $w(n)$. This implies that $w(n)$ is inversely proportional to the centre frequency of the input signal.

Figs 2a–c show the filter coefficient $w(n)$ against the frequency $(f_1(n) + f_2(n))$ for the filter bandwidth $B$ equal to 0.15, 0.10 and 0.05, respectively. It is obvious that, for low- and high-frequency ranges, the filter can be unstable. Relationship $|w(n)| \geqslant 1$ extends with the increase of the bandwidth $B$. Also, it is evident that this instability occurs for normalised frequency ranges from 0.0 to 0.1 and from 0.9 to 1.0 for $B = 0.1$, as an example. Although the frequency range for which the instability problem occurs decreases with the decrease in the bandwidth $B$, a very small bandwidth is not recommended. To avoid this problem, we propose to shift the frequency of the observed signal to the

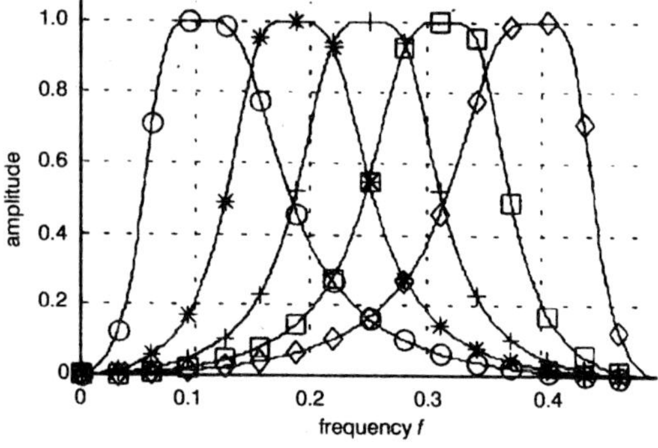

**Fig. 1** *Amplitude spectrum of adaptive recursive bandpass filter at different values of w(n) (i.e. different values of centre frequencies): (○) w(n) = 0.8; (∗) w(n) = 0.4; (+) w(n) = 0.0; (□) w(n) = −0.4; (◇) w(n) = −0.8*

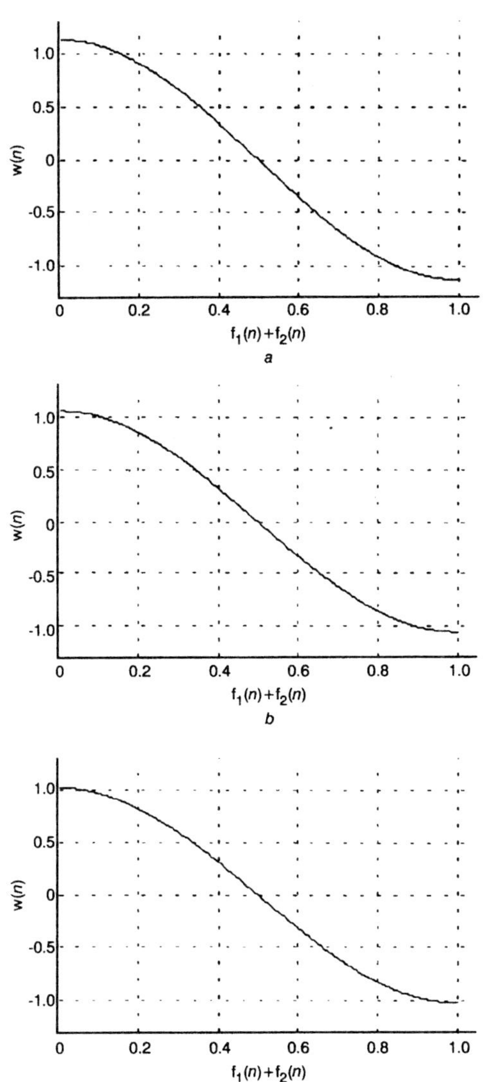

Fig. 2 *Segmentation parameter w(n) against twice centre frequency for different filter bandwidths B: (a) B = 0.15; (b) B = 0.1; (c) B = 0.05*

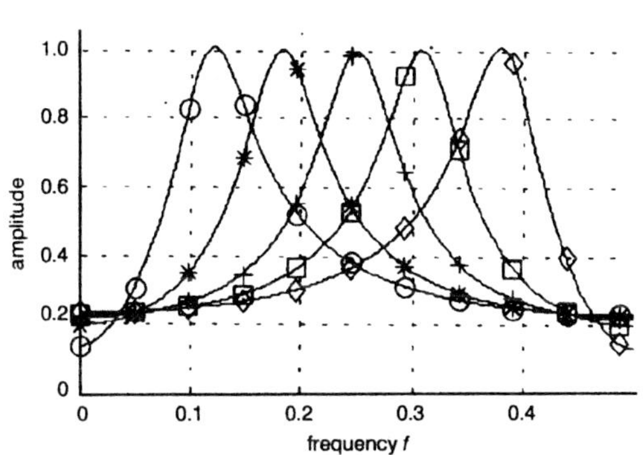

**Fig. 3** *Amplitude spectrum of second-order adaptive line enhancer at different centre frequencies*

stable frequency range before it is applied to the adaptive filter.

To show the advantage of the fourth-order Butterworth filter in comparison with other filters, Fig. 3 shows the amplitude spectrum of the exemplary second-order adaptive filter with transfer function given by (RAJA KUMAR and PAL, 1990).

$$H_{ALE}(z) = (1 - r^2)\frac{w(n)z^{-1}/(r + r^2) - 1}{1 - w(n)z^{-1} + r^2 z^{-2}} \qquad (7)$$

where $w(n) = 2r\cos(2\pi f_o n)$ is the only centre frequency term in eqn 7. The parameter $r$ is a fixed design one related to the frequency bandwidth $B$, as follows:

$$B = (1 - r)/2 \qquad (8)$$

Investigating the amplitude spectrum for a bandwidth $B = 0.1$ and for different centre frequencies $f_o$ shows that the filter is not a normal bandpass filter. It provides unity amplitude at the centre frequency alone. Therefore, by choosing a very narrow bandwidth, this filter can be applied for tracking and enhancement of a single sinusoid in white noise. This approach has been referred to as the adaptive line enhancer (ALE), owing to the fact that the spectrum of the filter input signal shows only one line at the sinusoidal frequency, as does the ALE spectrum.

### 3.2 Adaptive algorithm

Maximising the output power of the filter $H(z)$ makes its centre frequency self-adjusted to that of the input bandpass signal (RAJA KUMAR and PAL, 1986; 1990). That is, the adaptive filter coefficient $w(n)$ is updated for the maximisation of the expected output power $E\{y^2(n)\}$. A standard gradient-ascending approach could be used for achieving such maximisation. The resulting algorithm, called the recursive maximum mean-square (RMXMS) algorithm for updating $w(n)$ can be described as follows: From eqn 4, the filter output $y(n)$ is given by the following difference equation:

$$y(n) = a_0 x(n) + a_2 x(n - 2) + a_4 x(n - 4)$$
$$- b_1 w(n)y(n - 1) - (b_2 w^2(n) + b_2')y(n - 2)$$
$$- b_3 w(n)y(n - 3) - b_4 y(n - 4) \qquad (9)$$

The update equation in order for $w(n)$ to maximise $E\{y^2(n)\}$ is given by (LJUNG, 1977; RAJA KUMAR and PAL, 1985; 1986).

$$w(n + 1) = w(n) + 0.5\mu_n \nabla(E\{y^2(n)\}) \qquad (10)$$

where $\mu_n > 0$ is a normalised step-size and $\nabla(E\{y^2(n)\})$ is the gradient with respect to the adaptive coefficient $w(n)$. It is worthwhile mentioning that the well-known recursive

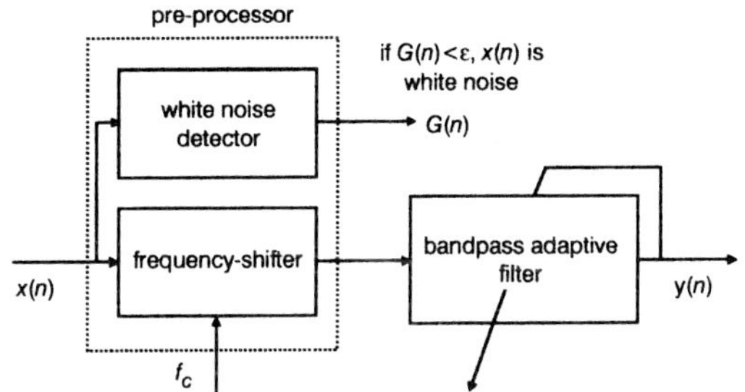


**Fig. 4** *Conceptual scheme of adaptive approach for segmentation and tracking of EEG signal*

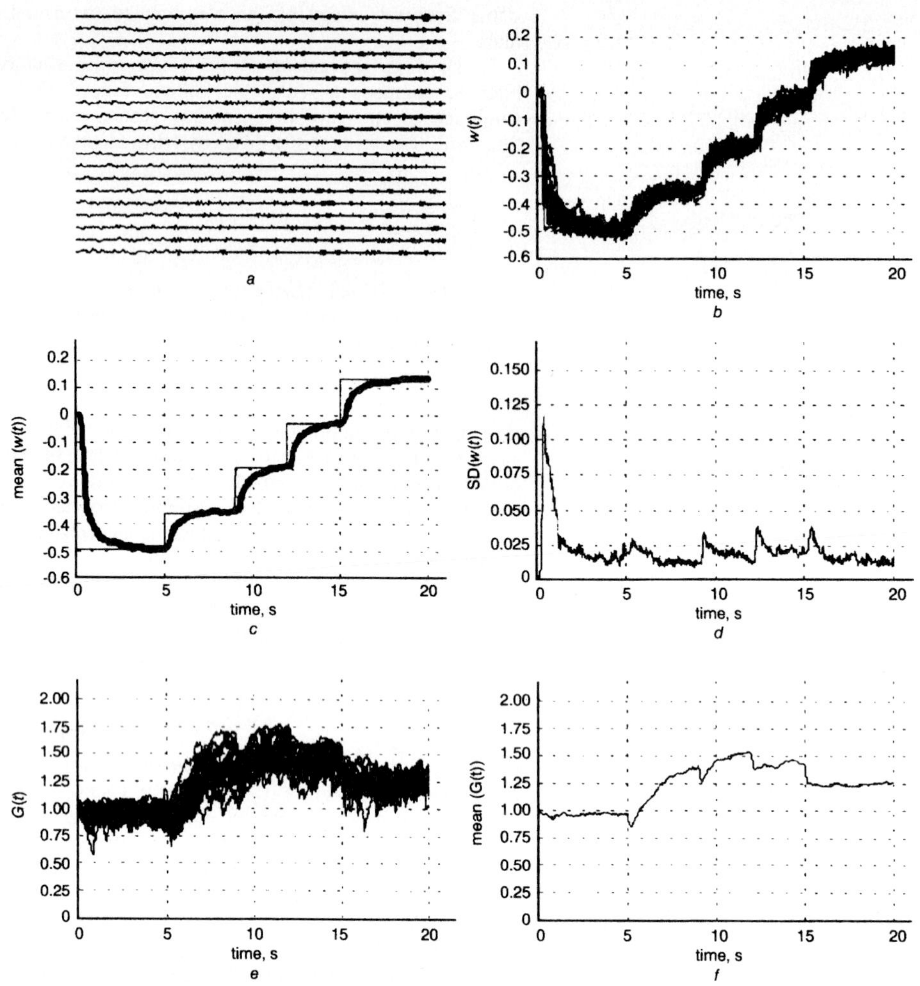

**Fig. 5** *Results of proposed approach for tracking waves given in Table 1 in 10.0 dB SNR case: (a) 20 realisations of EEG signal; (b) time function w(t) of segmentation parameter; (c) (——) mean and (——) true values of w(t); (d) standard deviation of w(t); (e) time function of G(t); (f) mean of G(t)*

minimum mean-square (RMMS) algorithm is also given by eqn 10 but by changing the sign of the gradient. As the mean-square output $E\{y^2(n)\}$ is unknown, the instantaneous gradient $\nabla\{y^2(n)\}$ can be used as a stochastic approximate for the true gradient. Thus eqn 10 can be written as

$$w(n+1) = w(n) + \mu_n y(n)\alpha(n) \tag{11}$$

where $\alpha(n) = \nabla(y(n))$. To guarantee the stability of the filter, we impose an on-line constraint $w(n+1) = w(n)$ if $|w(n+1)| \geq 1$. From eqn 9, the gradient $\alpha(n)$ can be computed as

$$\alpha(n) = \frac{\partial y(n)}{\partial w(n)} = -b_1 y(n-1) - 2b_2 w(n)y(n-2)$$
$$- b_3 y(n-3) - b_1 w(n)\alpha(n-1)$$
$$- (b_2' + b_2 w^2(n))\alpha(n-2) - b_3 w(n)\alpha(n-3)$$
$$- b_4 \alpha(n-4) \tag{12}$$

The normalised step-size $\mu_n$ is given by

$$\mu_n = \mu/r(n) \tag{13}$$

where $\mu$ is a fixed positive step-size and $r(n)$ is a recursive estimate of the power of the gradient given by

$$r(n) = \lambda r(n-1) + \alpha^2(n) \tag{14}$$

with $0 \ll \lambda < 1$ as the so-called forgetting factor.

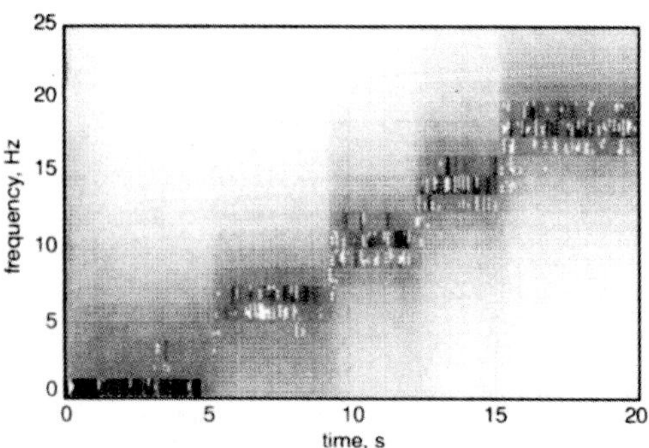

**Fig. 6** *Results of adaptive AR modelling-based approach for tracking waves given in Table 1 in 10.0 dB SNR case*

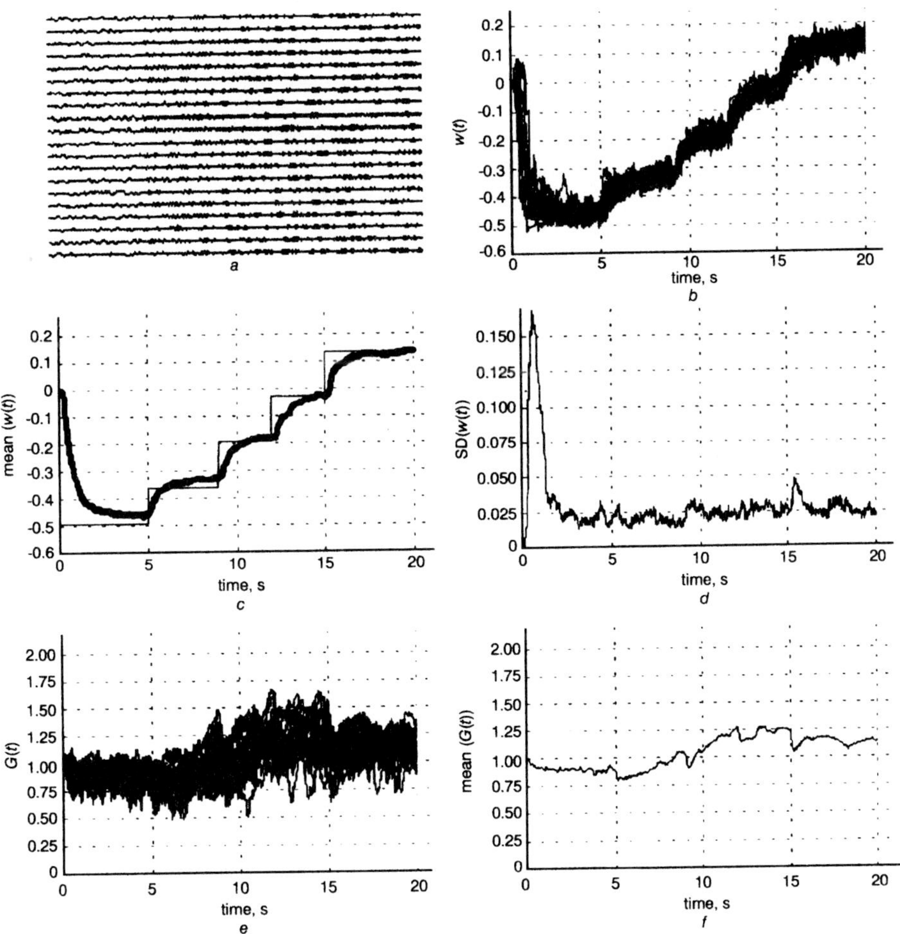

**Fig. 7** *Results of proposed approach for tracking waves given in Table 1 in 5.0 dB SNR case: (a) 20 realisations of EEG signal;(b) time function w(t) of segmentation parameter; (c) (———) mean and (——) true values of w(t); (d) standard deviation of w(t); (e) time function of G(t); (f) mean of G(t)*

## 4 Proposed approach and its practical implementation

To track the centre frequency of the EEG waves, the EEG signal can be processed by the adaptive bandpass filter described in the preceding Section and given by eqn 4. The adaptive filter coefficient $w(n)$ is then a function of the centre frequency $(f_1(n) + f_2(n))/2$ of each EEG wave, as the bandwidth of the filter is chosen to be constant. This implies that the time function of $w(n)$ reflects the spontaneity of the EEG signal and can be used as a segmentation parameter.

As is evident from Fig. 2 for a filter bandwidth of 0.1, $w(n)$ decreases with the increase of the frequency $(f_1(n) + f_2(n))$, and it is highly non-linear in the frequency ranges from 0.0 to 0.3 and from 0.7 to 1.0. Moreover, it should be noted that, for the low-frequency range from 0.0 to 0.1, $w(n) \geqslant 1$ and, for the high-frequency range from 0.9 to 1.0, $w(n) \leqslant -1$, causing the adaptive filter to be unstable for these ranges. It is also evident from Fig. 2 that the frequency providing the high-stability condition and, approximately, a linear function for $w(n)$ is in the range from 0.3 to 0.7. Unfortunately, the frequencies associated with the EEG signal are low frequencies ranging from 0.5 Hz to 40 Hz. Therefore, with a sampling frequency equal to or greater than the Nyquest rate, i.e. $F_s > 80\,Hz$, the corresponding normalised frequencies of the EEG signal exist in the instability and non-linear low-frequency range.

To clarify that, let the sampling frequency be 102.4, for example, and the filter bandwidth $B$ be 0.1; then $w(n)$ is 1.044 for the delta wave (from 0.5 to 3.5 Hz) and 0.992 for the theta wave (from 4 to 7 Hz), thus causing an instability problem for the delta wave, and there is no clear distinction between both waves owing to the small variation in the segmentation parameter $w(n)$. Therefore, to overcome the instability and non-linear problems, we can shift the EEG signal frequencies to the range from 0.3 to 0.7. Another objective of this frequency shifting is to ensure that $w(n)$ increases almost

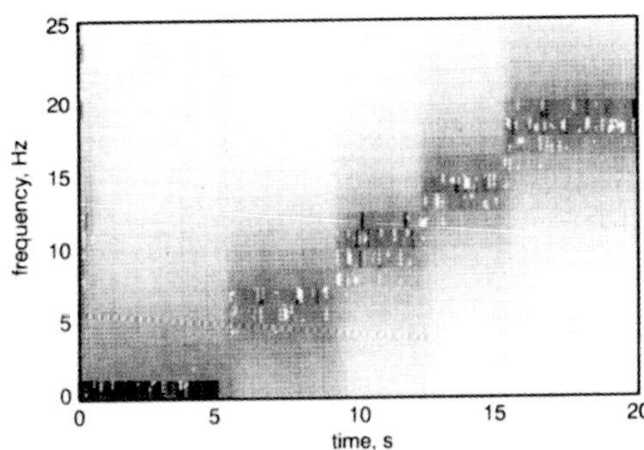

**Fig. 8** *Results of adaptive AR modelling-based approach for tracking waves given in Table 1 in 5.0 dB SNR case*

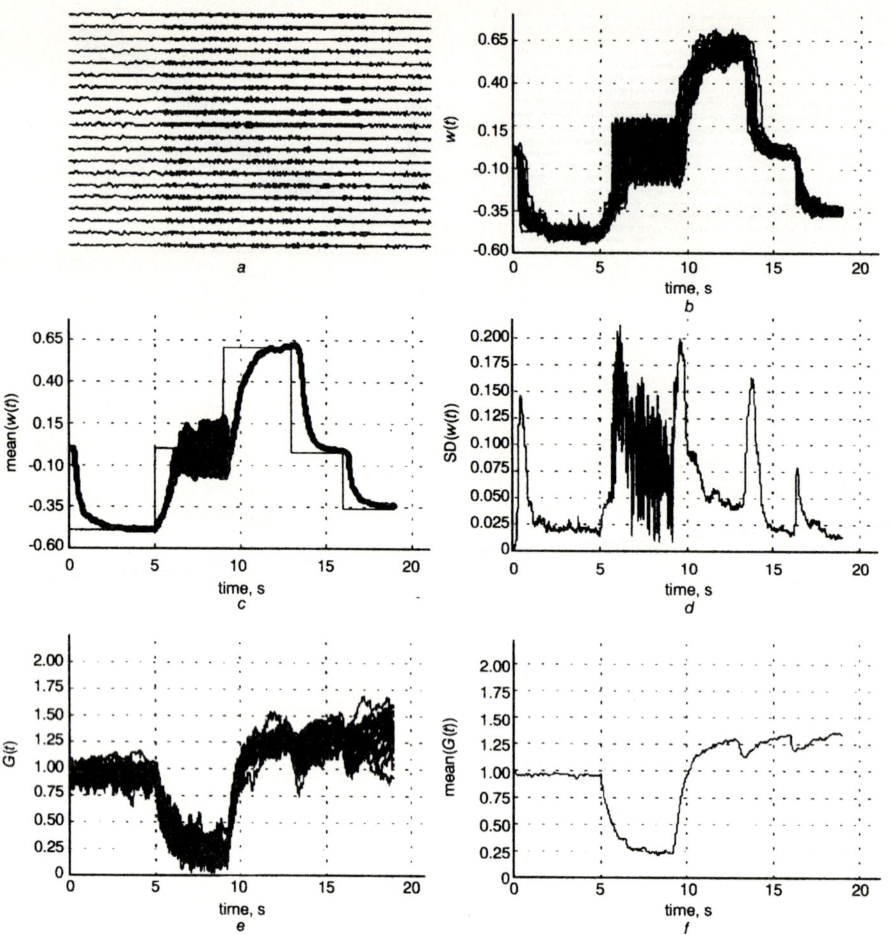

**Fig. 9**  *Results of proposed approach for tracking waves given in Table 2 in 10.0 dB SNR case: (a) 20 realisations of EEG signal; (b) time function w(t) of segmentation parameter; (c) (———) mean and (———) true values of w(t); (d) standard deviation of w(t); (e) time function of G(t); (f) mean of G(t)*

linearly with the increase in the normalised frequency $(f_1(n) + f_2(n))$ of the EEG signal. A simple high-frequency shifter is implemented by modulating the amplitude of a single tone (a carrier signal) using the EEG signal and only passing the lower sideband modulated signal. This can be accomplished by multiplying the observed EEG signal by $\cos(2\pi f_c n)$ and passing the resulting signal through a bandpass filter whose normalised frequency bandwidth is from $(f_c - 40/F_s)$ to $(f_c - 0.5/F_s)$.

It should be noted that 0.5 Hz and 40 Hz, respectively, represent the lowest and highest possible frequencies that can exist in the observed EEG signal. Therefore such a bandpass filter is suitable for all the EEG waves when there is no *a priori* knowledge about the observed EEG signal. Intuitively, if we expect the lowest and highest frequency associated with the observed EEG signal, we can determine the appropriate bandwidth, which indeed efficiently improves the signal-to-noise ratio. If the carrier frequency is $f_c$, and $(f_1(n) + f_2(n))$ is (twice) the centre frequency associated with the observed (modulating) EEG signal, then $(2f_c - f_1(n) - f_2(n))$ will describe (twice) the new centre frequency associated with the modulated signal used as the input of the adaptive bandpass filter. Therefore, with the increase of $(f_1(n) + f_2(n))$, the new centre frequency associated with the input signal of the adaptive filter will decrease, thus causing $w(n)$ to be increased and *vice versa*. Also, the highest new centre frequency exists if the raw EEG signal contains the lowest centre frequency wave (delta wave), and the lowest new

centre frequency exists in the gamma wave case. It is very important to transfer both the lowest and highest frequencies into the stable frequency range. It should be mentioned that choosing the appropriate sampling and the carrier frequencies enables us to achieve this task and thus to localise $w(n)$ within the stable and linear range.

We assume that additive noise is white noise. Therefore, in a certain wave and after convergence, if the forthcoming wave has no specific EEG wave, we need another classifier to detect this signal-free noise case. This detector can be achieved as follows.

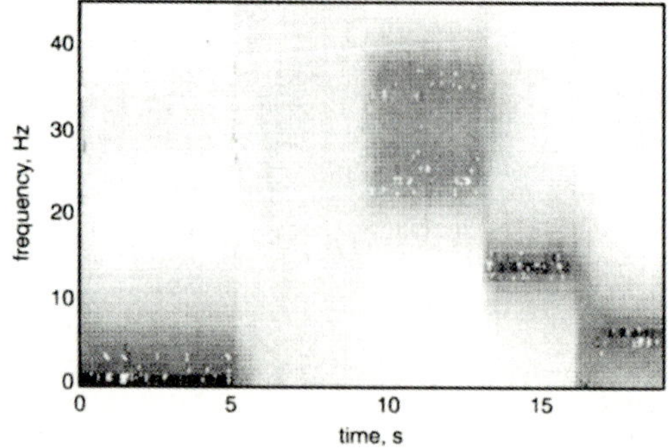

**Fig. 10**  *Results of adaptive AR modelling-based approach for tracking waves given in Table 2 in 10.0 dB SNR case*

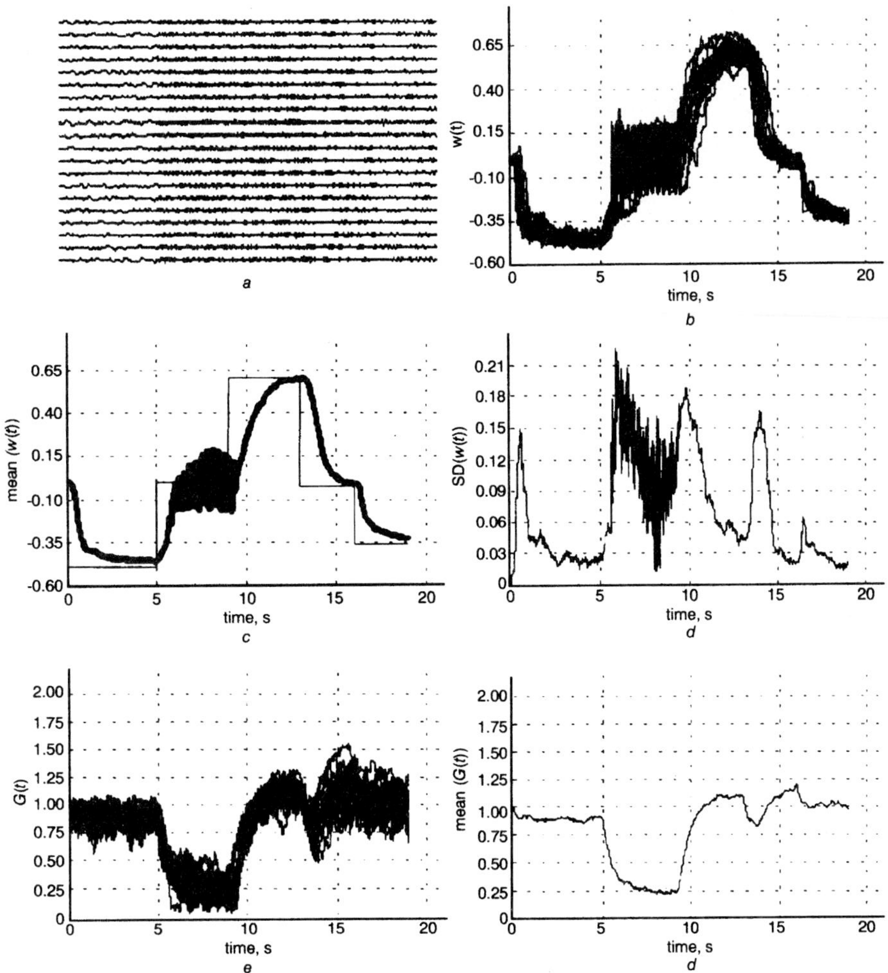

**Fig. 11** *Results of proposed approach for tracking waves given in Table 2 in 5.0 dB SNR case: (a) 20 realisations of EEG signal; (b) time function w(t) of segmentation parameter; (c) (——) mean and (——) true values of w(t); (d) standard deviation of w(t); (e) time function of G(t); (f) mean of G(t)*

We pass the raw EEG signal through an adaptive $M$th-order linear predictor. The output error of the $M$th-order linear prediction error (LPE) filter is given by

$$e(n) = x(n) + \sum_{i=1}^{M} g_i(n)x(n-i) \qquad (15)$$

The coefficients $\{g_i(n)\}$ are updated using the standard normalised least-mean square (NLMS) algorithm given by (HAYKIN, 1996)

$$g_i(n+1) = g_i(n) - \gamma e(n)x(n-i) \Big/ \left(\sum_{i=1}^{M} x^2(n-i)\right) \qquad (16)$$

where $\gamma > 0$ is a step-size. It should be mentioned that, for convergence improvement, it is also possible to use other more sophisticated linear predictors, such as the lattice structure.

If the measured EEG signal represents only random white noise, then the LPE filter coefficients $\{g_i(n)\}$ are close to zero, and a coefficient $G(n)$, expressed as

$$G(n) = \sum_{i=1}^{M} |g_i(n)| < \varepsilon \qquad (17)$$

is taken as a whiteness detector. Then, if $G(n)$ is less than a small positive threshold value $\varepsilon$, $x(n)$ can be considered to be white noise. In this case, we propose to impose the segmentation parameter to be $w(n) = A\cos(2\pi f_c n)$. Therefore oscillation of the segmentation parameter indicates that the observed signal is only a signal-free noise. This oscillation may provide

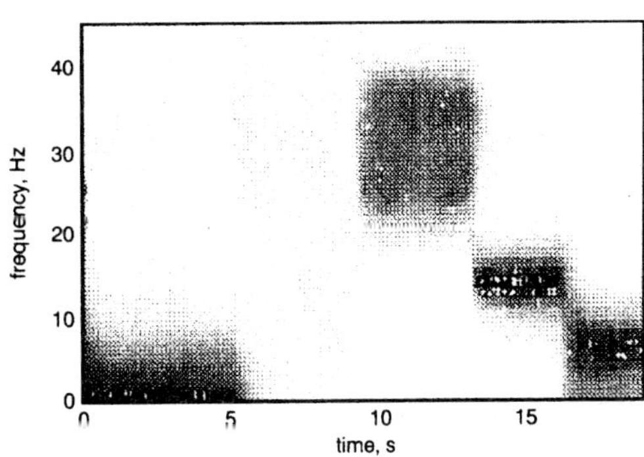

**Fig. 12** *Results of adaptive AR modelling-based approach for tracking waves given in Table 2 in 5.0 dB SNR case*

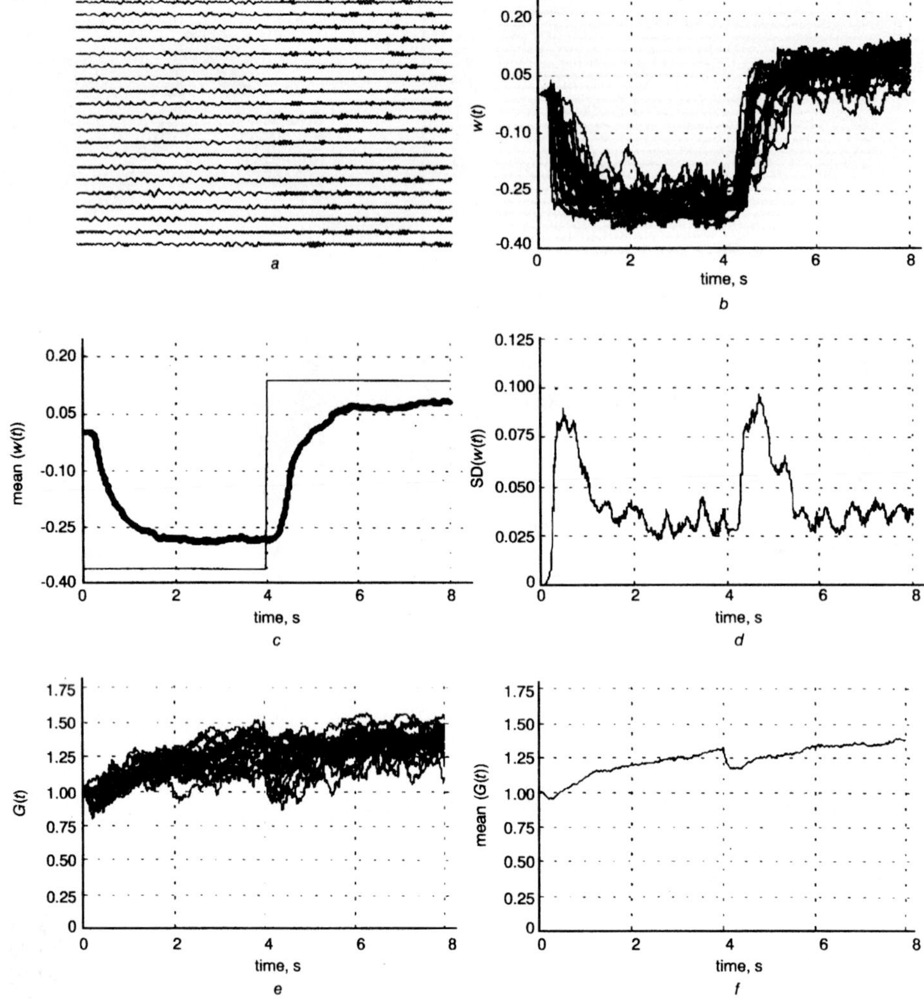

**Fig. 13**   *Results of proposed approach for tracking dominant waves given in 10.0 dB SNR case: (a) 20 realisations of EEG signal; (b) time function w(t) of segmentation parameter; (c) (——) mean and (——) true values of w(t); (d) standard deviation of w(t); (e) time function of G(t); (f) mean of G(t)*

indication of the absence of any of the EEG waves in the observed signal.

Fig. 4 shows a conceptual scheme of the proposed adaptive filtering approach for segmentation and tracking of the EEG signal waves.

## 5  Simulation results

### 5.1  *Computer-generated data*

To obtain a qualitative evaluation of the presented adaptive segmentation approach, we track 20 simulated realisations of different EEG signals. Each EEG signal is composed of different waves, such as alpha, beta (see Tables 1 and 2), etc. Each wave is generated by passing a zero-mean white Gaussian noise through a Hamming-weighted FIR filter of length 64, whose bandwidth is equal to the corresponding wave bandwidth. The power of each wave is adjusted to unity. We add a zero-mean white Gaussian noise to achieve 10.0 and 5.0 dB signal-to-noise ratios (SNRs). The parameters associated with the proposed adaptive approach are adjusted as follows. The sampling frequency $F_s$ and the normalised carrier frequency $f_c$ are 160.0 and 0.34 Hz, respectively. These sampling and carrier frequencies make the

lowest and highest frequencies of $(2f_c - f_1(n) - f_2(n))$ be 0.305 and 0.655, respectively, i.e. the values of the adaptive filter

*Table 1   Tracking different EEG waves: computer-generated EEG signal waves and corresponding true values of adaptive coefficient w(t)*

| Wave | Bandwidth, Hz | Time range, s | True value $w(t)$ |
| --- | --- | --- | --- |
| Delta | 0.5–3.5 | 0–5 | −0.492 |
| Theta | 4.0–7.0 | 5–9 | −0.360 |
| Alpha | 7.5–12.0 | 9–12 | −0.191 |
| Sigma | 12.5–15.0 | 12–15 | −0.027 |
| Beta | 15.5–20.0 | 15–20 | 0.138 |

*Table 2   Tracking different EEG waves: computer-generated EEG signal waves and corresponding true values of adaptive coefficient w(t)*

| Wave | Bandwidth, Hz | Time range, s | True value $w(t)$ |
| --- | --- | --- | --- |
| Delta | 0.5–3.5 | 0–5 | −0.492 |
| WGN | – | 5–9 | – |
| Gamma | 20–40 | 9–13 | 0.60 |
| Sigma | 12.5–15.0 | 13–16 | −0.027 |
| Theta | 4.0–7.0 | 16–19 | −0.360 |

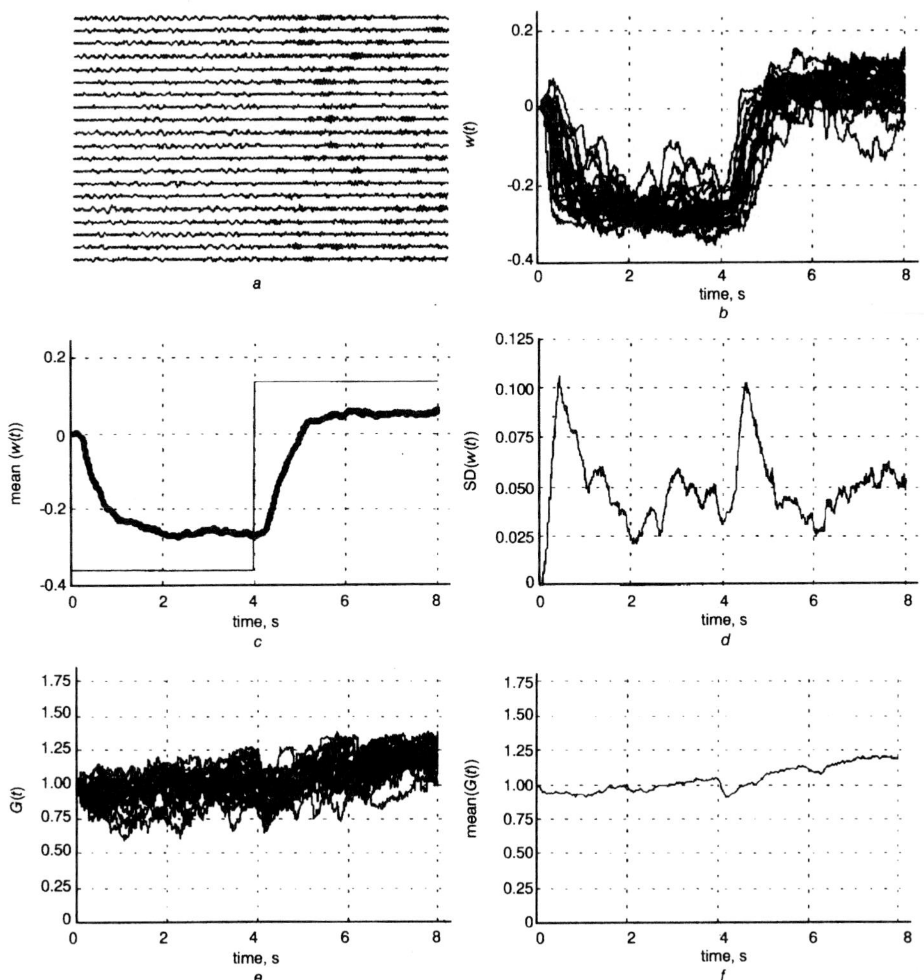

**Fig. 14** *Results of proposed approach for tracking dominant wave in 5.0 dB SNR case: (a) 20 realisations of EEG signal; (b) time function w(t) of segmentation parameter; (c) (——) mean and (- - -) true values of w(t); (d) standard deviation of w(t); (e) time function of G(t); (f) mean of G(t)*

coefficient $w(n)$ will be within the stable and nearly linear range. The normalised bandwidth of the frequency shifter filter is then from 0.09 to 0.3369. The normalised bandwidth $B$ of the adaptive bandpass filter is 0.1. The initial values of the coefficients of the adaptive approach are adjusted to zero, except the first coefficient of the whiteness detector, which is adjusted to 1.0. The forgetting factor and the step size associated with the adaptive algorithm are 0.95 and 0.95, respectively. The step size has been selected experimentally to achieve fast convergence and low fluctuations. The initial value for $r(0)$ is 100.0. Regarding the white-noise detector, we take the step-size $\gamma$, the order $M$ and the threshold value $\epsilon$ to be 0.03, 4 and 0.3, respectively. The amplitude $A$ of the oscillation associated with the whiteness detector is 0.2. Some results of the TVAR modelling-based segmentation approach are used for comparisons. The AR model (with zero initial coefficients) order $P$ and the forgetting factor of the adaptive RLS algorithm have been experimentally selected to be 8 and 0.98, respectively.

5.1.1 *Tracking different EEG waves:* To examine the proposed approach for tracking different EEG waves, the approach is applied to the EEG signals composed of the waves given in Tables 1 and 2. It should be noted that the EEG signal given by Table 2 contains a signal-

free white noise in the time range from 5 to 9 s. Figs 5, 7, 9 and 11 show the EEG data and the results of the presented approach. The panels *a–f* of each figure show the 20 realisations of the EEG signals, the time function $w(t)$, the mean value $\bar{w}(t)$ and the standard deviation (SD) of $w(t)$, the time function of the whiteness detector $G(t)$ and the mean value $\bar{G}(t)$, respectively. Investigating $w(t)$ and its mean values confirms that we can efficiently recognise the different waves of the EEG signal. Also, the time function $w(t)$ and its mean values give us information about the sequence of the EEG waves. Comparing the true values of $w(t)$ given in Tables 1 and 2 and the values of $\bar{w}(t)$ shows that the adaptive approach provides good convergence properties. In the 5.0 dB SNR case, the mean value $\bar{w}(t)$ shows a small bias for delta and theta waves. This is because the filter of the frequency shifter has been adjusted to the widest bandwidth, whereas both waves have narrower bandwidths, which does not improve the SNR so much. It is also obvious that, after convergence, the SD of the segmentation parameter $w(t)$ is less than 0.05 and decreases with the increase of the SNR. From Figs 9 and 11 it is apparent that the whiteness detector provides efficient performance. It is also obvious that the segmen-

 

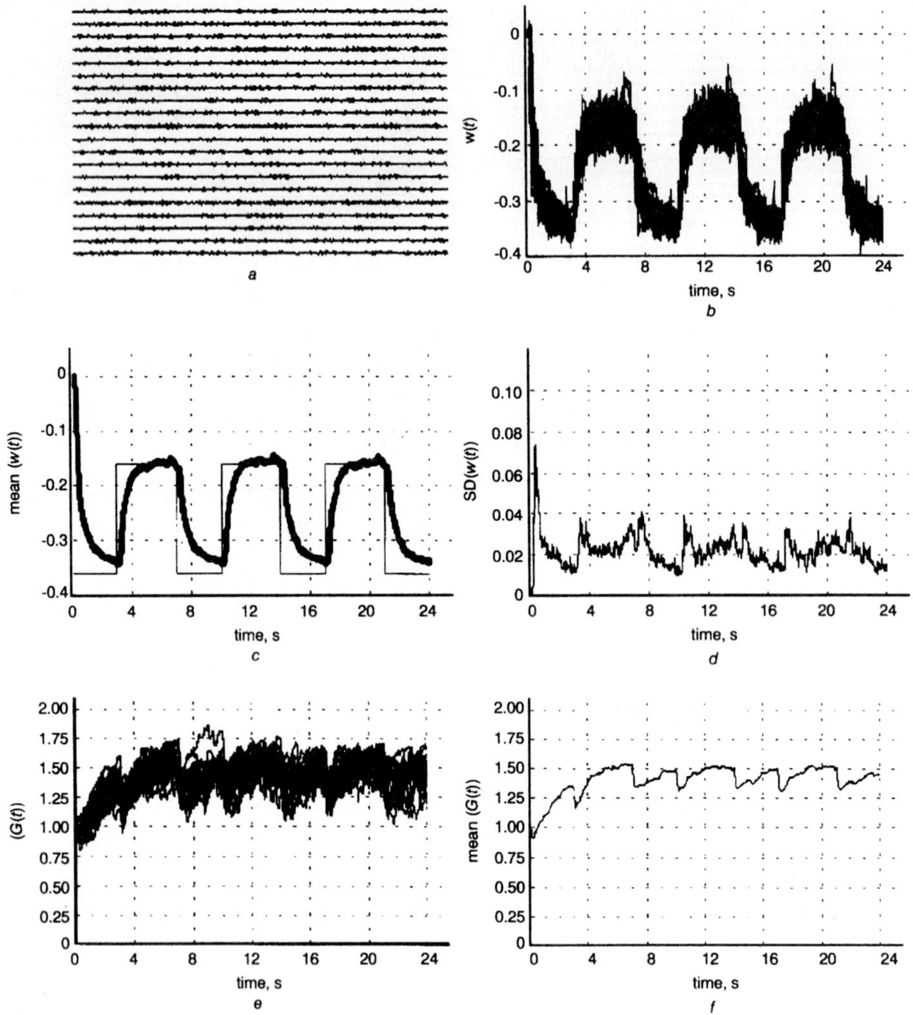

**Fig. 15** *Results of proposed approach for detection of computer-generated sleep spindles in 10.0 dB SNR case: (a) 20 realisations of EEG signal; (b) time function w(t) of segmentation parameter; (c) (———) mean and (- - -) true values of w(t); (d) standard deviation of w(t); (e) time function of G(t); (f) mean of G(t)*

tation parameter $w(t)$ and its mean value oscillate somewhat in the time where the free-signal white noise exists. Figs 6, 8, 10 and 12 show the 256 grey levels of the average power spectrum, in decibels, for the EEG signals obtained using the adaptive AR approach. Although it is obvious that we can recognise the sequence of the EEG waves, the bandwidth and the centre frequency associated with each wave are biased owing to the additive noise, especially in the low SNR such as 5.0 dB SNR.

5.1.2 *Tracking dominant wave:* To show the capability of our approach in tracking the dominant wave existing in the EEG signal, we carry out the following simulation. The observed signal is composed of theta and beta waves for a period of 10 s. In the first 5 s, the power ratio of the theta wave to the beta wave is 1.00 : 0.16. In the last 5 s, the power ratio of the theta wave to the beta wave is 0.16 : 1.00. Fig. 13 shows the EEG data and the results for the 10.0 dB SNR case, whereas Fig. 14 stands for the 5.0 dB SNR case. Investigating the segmentation parameter $w(t)$ and its mean value shows that the EEG signal is

segmented as a theta wave in the first 5 s and as a beta wave in the last 5 s. It is also obvious that the whiteness detector shows that no signal-free noise is observed.

5.1.3 *Sleep-spindle detection:* To examine the capability of the proposed adaptive approach to detect sleep spindles, we carry out the following simulation example. In this example, each realisation of the computer-generated EEG signals is organised as given in Table 3. The wave whose bandwidth is 6–15 Hz corresponds to the sleep spindle. Fig. 15 illustrates the EEG data and the results for the 10.0 dB SNR case, whereas Fig. 16 shows the 5.0 dB SNR case. Panels *b*, *c* and *d* of each Figure show the time function $w(t)$, its mean and its standard deviation, respectively. It is obvious that we can

*Table 3 Sleep spindle detection: computer-generated EEG signal waves and corresponding true values of adaptive coefficient w(t)*

| Wave | Bandwidth, Hz | Time range, s | True value $w(t)$ |
|---|---|---|---|
| Theta | 4–7 | 0–3,7–10,14–17,21–24 | −0.360 |
| Sleep spindle | 6–15 | 3–7,10–14,17–21 | −0.160 |

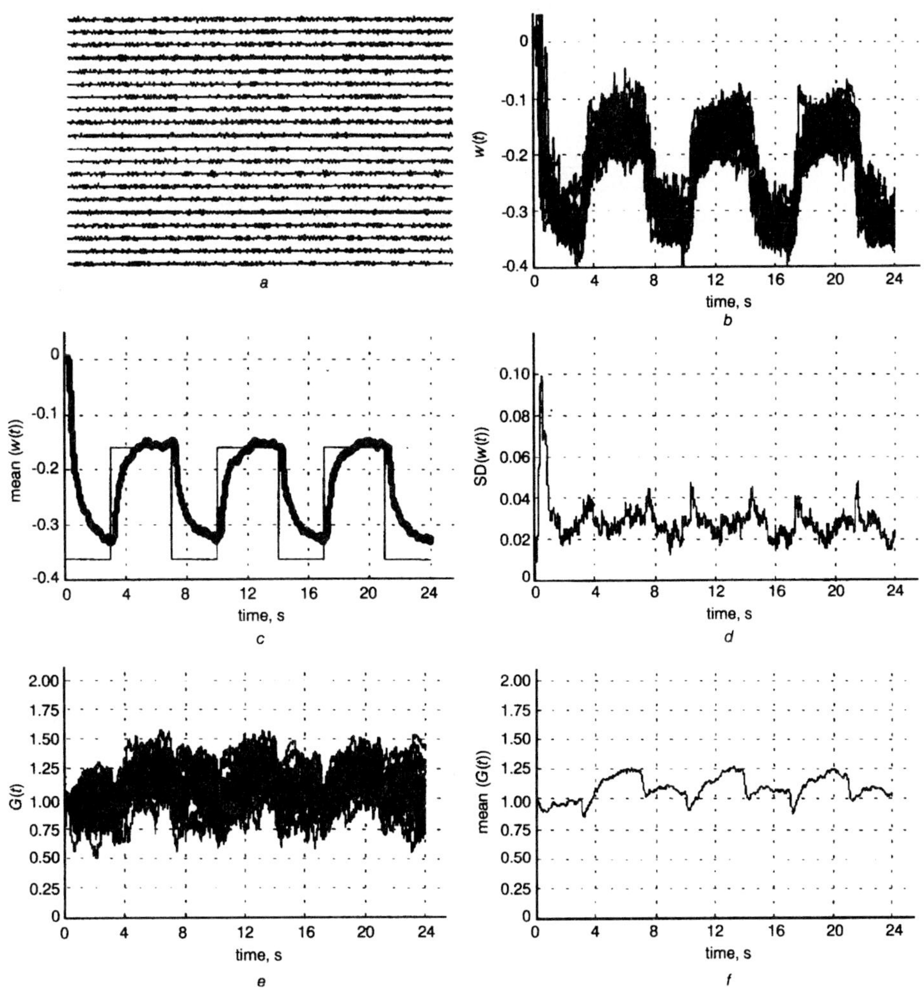

**Fig. 16** *Results of proposed approach for detection of computer-generated sleep spindles in 5.0 dB SNR case: (a) 20 realisations of EEG signal; (b) time function w(t) of segmentation parameter; (c) (——) mean and (- - -) true values of w(t); (d) standard deviation of w(t); (e) time function of G(t); (f) mean of G(t)*

efficiently recognise sleep spindles and another wave of the EEG signal by investigating either the segmentation parameter $w(t)$ or its mean. It is apparent that, after convergence, the standard deviation is less than 0.03, even in the 5.0 dB SNR case. The function of the mean value $\bar{w}(t)$ shows that the adaptive algorithm needs less than 1 s to reach the steady state. Panels $e$ and $f$ of each figure show the whiteness detection function $G(t)$ and its mean value, respectively. It is clear that both $G(t)$ and its mean show that there is no level equal to or less than 0.3, which confirms that there is no signal-free noise existing in the observed signal.

### 5.2 Real world data

*Sleep spindle detection:* About 12 s recording of 18 channels of EEG (Fp1, F8, F4, Fz, F3, F7, T4, C4, Cz, C3, T3, T6, P4, Pz, P3, T5, 02, 01) was used for demonstrating the performance of the approach presented for the detection of sleep spindles. Electrodes were placed according to the international 10–20 system. The data were sampled with a sampling frequency of 102.4 Hz. The measured signals were filtered by a Butterworth bandpass filter between 10 and 20 Hz. The signals were passed forward and backward through the filter to avoid phase distortion (ROSAPIL *et al.* 1998).

The parameters of the adaptive filtering approach are taken as follows. The normalised carrier frequency is 0.29, the forgetting factor is 0.9, the step-size is 0.95, and the initial values for $r(0)$ and $w(0)$ are 100.0 and 0, respectively. The normalised frequency bandwidth of the adaptive bandpass filter is taken to be 0.15. Fig. 17$a$ shows the first ten channels of the measured EEG signals after filtering by the 10–20 Hz bandpass filter. Fig. 17$b$ shows the corresponding time function of the adaptive coefficient $w(t)$ of these channels. It is evident that we can detect the sleep spindles by investigating the time function of $w(t)$.

## 6 Conclusion

In this paper, a novel adaptive approach for the segmentation and tracking of EEG signal waves has been presented. In this approach, an adaptive recursive bandpass filter implemented as a fourth-order Butterworth filter is employed for tracking the centre frequency of each EEG wave. This filter has only one unknown coefficient to be updated. This coefficient, having an absolute value less than 1, represents an efficient distinct feature for each EEG specific wave, and its time function reflects the nonstationarity behaviour of the EEG signal. Therefore the main advantage of this approach is that

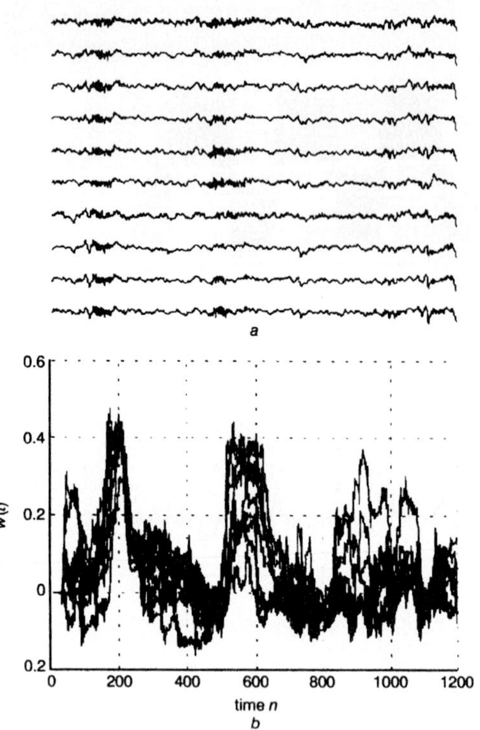

**Fig. 17** *Results of proposed approach for detection of sleep spindles from real-world data: (a) observed EEG signals; (b) time function w(t) of segmentation parameter*

the segmentation and tracking processes are achieved using only one parameter, which facilitates the analysis of the EEG signal. Another advantage of the approach is that the segmentation parameter increases with the increase in the centre frequency of the input signal. This enables us to track the sequence of the EEG signal waves just by investigating the behaviour of the segmentation parameter.

A white–noise detector has also been introduced to investigate the only noise hypothesis. The proposed approach has been applied to computer-generated data for tracking different waves and for sleep-spindle detection. It has also been applied to real-world EEG data for the detection of sleep spindles and has been shown to be capable of achieving this task.

*Acknowledgment*—The revised version of this paper was produced in National Saitama Hospital (NSH), where R. R. Gharieb stayed for about one and half months. The authors would like to thank the staff of the fourth floor of the NSH, especially Dr E. Sekizuka, Dr Y. Hosoda, Dr T. Tamai and Dr Takagi, for their kind help and the friendly environment offered to the R. R. Gharieb during his stay.



## References

AMIR, N., and GATH, I. (1989): 'Segmentation of EEG during sleep using time-varying autoregressive modeling', *Biol. Cybern.*, **61**, pp. 447–455

ANDERSON, C. W., STOLZ, E. A., and SANYOGITA, S. (1998): 'Multivariate autoregressive models for classification of spontaneous electroencephalographic signals during mental tasks', *IEEE Trans.*, **BME-45**, pp. 277–286

ARNOLD, M., MILTNER, W. H. R., WITTE, H., BAUER, R., and BRAUN, C. (1998): 'Adaptive AR Modeling of nonstationary time series by means of Kalman filtering', *IEEE Trans.*, **BME-45**, pp. 553–562

BLINOWSKA, K. J., and MALINOWSKI, M. (1989): 'Non-linear and linear forecasting of the EEG time series', *Biol. Cybern.*, **66**, pp. 159–165

DING, M., BRESSLER, S. L., YANG, W., and LIANG, H. (2000): 'Short-window spectral analysis of cortical event-related potentials by adaptive multivariate autoregressive modeling: data processing, model validation and variability assessment', *Biol. Cybern.*, **83**, pp. 35–45

GATH, I., FEUERSTEIN, C., PHAM, D. T., and RONDOUIN, G. (1992): 'On the tracking of rapid dynamic changes in seizure EEG', *IEEE Trans.*, **BME-39**, pp. 952–958

GOTO, S., NAKAMURA, M., and UOSAKI, K. (1995): 'On-line spectral estimation of nonstationary time series based on AR model parameter estimation and order selection with a forgetting factor', *IEEE Trans. Signal Process.*, **43**, pp. 1519–1522

HAYKIN, S. (1996): 'Adaptive Filter Theory' (Prentice Hall, Inc., Englewood Cliffs, N.J.)

KAY, M., and MARPLE, S. L. (1981): 'Spectrum analysis – A modern perspective', *Proc. IEEE*, **69**, pp. 1380–1418

KIM, H., KIM, T., CHOI, Y., and PARK, S. (2000): 'The prediction of EEG signals using a feedback-structured adaptive rational function', *Biol. Cybern.*, **83**, pp. 131–138

KONG, X., BRAMBRINK, A., HANLEY, D. F., and THAKOR, N. V. (1999): 'Quantification of injury-related EEG signal changes using distances measures', *IEEE Trans.*, **BME-46**, pp. 899–901

LJUNG, L. (1977): 'Analysis of recursive stochastic algorithms', *IEEE Trans. Automat. Contr.*, **AC-22**, pp. 551–575

NIEDERMEYER, E., and LOPES DA SILVA, F. (1999): Electroencephalography: basic principles, clinical applications and related fields, 4th edn. (Williams & Wilkins)

NING, T., and BRONZINO, J. D. (1989): 'Bispectral analysis of the rate EEG during various vigilance states', *IEEE Trans.*, **BME-36**, pp. 497–499

RAJA KUMAR, R. V., and PAL, R. N. (1985): 'A gradient algorithm for center-frequency adaptive recursive bandpass filters', *Proc. IEEE*, **73**, pp. 371–372

RAJA KUMAR, R. V., and PAL, R. N. (1986): 'The recursive center-frequency adaptive filters for the enhancement of bandpass signals', *IEEE Trans. Acoust. Speech Signal Process.*, **34**, pp. 633–637

RAJA KUMAR, R. V., and PAL, R. N. (1990): 'Tracking of bandpass signals using center-frequency adaptive filters', *IEEE Trans. Acoust. Speech signal Process.*, **38**, pp. 1710–1721

ROSIPAL, R., DORFFINER, G., and TRENKER, E. (1998): 'Can ICA improve sleep spindles detection?', *Neural Netw. World*, **5**, pp. 539–547

WRIGHT, J., KYDD, R. R., and SERGEJEW, A. A. (1990): 'Autoregressive models of EEG', *Biol. Cybern.*, **62**, pp. 201–210





## Authors' biographies

REDA R. GHARIEB received his BSc, MSc and PhD in Electrical Engineering in 1985, 1993 and 1997, respectively, from Assiut University, Assiut, Egypt. From 1988 to 1997, he was at the Faculty of Engineering, Assiut University, working as an Assistant Lecturer. Since 1997 he has been a lecturer. From July 1999 to January 2000, he was a Post-Doctoral Fellow with the Faculty of Engineering, Toyama University, Japan. Since January 2000, he has been a Scientist at the Laboratory for Advanced Brain Signal Processing, RIKEN Brain Science Institute, RIKEN, Japan. His research interests include adaptive filters, statistical signal processing, and higher-order statistics.

ANDRZEJ CICHOCKI received his MSc (Hons), PhD, and Habilitate Doctorate (DrSc) in Electrical Engineering from Warsaw University of Technology, Poland, in 1972, 1975, and 1982, respectively. Since 1972, he has been with the Institute of Theory of Electrical Engineering and Electrical Measurements at the Warsaw University of Technology, where he became a full professor in 1991. He is the co-author of two books and more than 150 scientific papers. He has spent several years as an Alexander Humboldt Research Fellow and Guest Professor at the University of Erlangen, Germany. He is currently working at the Brain Science Institute RIKEN, Japan, as a Head of the Laboratory for Advanced Brain Signal Processing. More details about his research can be found at: http://www.bsp.brain.riken.go.jp

# Comparison of time-frequency distribution techniques for analysis of spinal somatosensory evoked potential

**Y. Hu    K. D. K. Luk    W. W. Lu    A. Holmes    J. C. Y. Leong**

Department of Orthopaedic Surgery, The University of Hong Kong, Hong Kong

**Abstract**—*Spinal somatosensory evoked potential (SSEP) has been employed to monitor the integrity of the spinal cord during surgery. To detect both temporal and spectral changes in SSEP waveforms, an investigation of the application of time–frequency analysis (TFA) techniques was conducted. SSEP signals from 30 scoliosis patients were analysed using different techniques; short time Fourier transform (STFT), Wigner–Ville distribution (WVD), Choi–Williams distribution (CWD), cone-shaped distribution (CSD) and adaptive spectrogram (ADS). The time–frequency distributions (TFD) computed using these methods were assessed and compared with each other. WVD, ADS, CSD and CWD showed better resolution than STFT. Comparing normalised peak widths, CSD showed the sharpest peak width ($0.13 \pm 0.1$) in the frequency dimension, and a mean peak width of $0.70 \pm 0.12$ in the time dimension. Both WVD and CWD produced cross-term interference, distorting the TFA distribution, but this was not seen with CSD and ADS. CSD appeared to give a lower mean peak power bias ($10.3\% \pm 6.2\%$) than ADS ($41.8\% \pm 19.6\%$). Application of the CSD algorithm showed both good resolution and accurate spectrograms, and is therefore recommended as the most appropriate TFA technique for the analysis of SSEP signals.*

**Keywords**—*Spinal somatosensory evoked potential (SSEP), Time–frequency analysis (TFA), Intraoperative spinal cord monitoring, Short time Fourier transform (STFT), Wigner–Ville distribution (WVD), Choi–Williams distribution (CWD), Cone shaped distribution (CSD), Adaptive spectrogram (ADS)*

## 1 Introduction

SPINAL SURGERY is a common and effective method of correcting deformities of the spine, but also carries the risk of spinal cord injury. To avoid this, various evoked potential techniques have been used for intraoperative spinal cord monitoring. Spinal somatosensory evoked potential (SSEP) is a useful technique for intraoperative spinal cord monitoring, and is relatively resistant to the influence of the popular anaesthetic agents (NASH *et al.*, 1989).

Current intraoperative monitoring techniques measure only the latency and amplitude of the SSEP. This technique cannot represent the precise characteristics of SSEP, as the signals usually possess polyphasic waveforms reflecting different activation thresholds and conduction velocities within the spinal cord (JONES *et al.*, 1982; RYAN and BRITT, 1986; MACCABEE *et al.*, 1986; FUJIOKA *et al.*, 1994).

Theoretically, the power spectrum can show the entire characteristics of a signal in the frequency field (THAKOR *et al.*, 1993; BASAR-EROGLU *et al.*, 1993; LOENING-BAUCKE

*Correspondence should be addressed to: Dr Y. Hu,
email: yhud@hkusua.hku.hk*

*First received 15 May 2000 and in final form 20 February 2001*

*MBEC online number: 20013573*

and YAMADA, 1993), and therefore localised changes (at various time instances or delays) in the SSEP waveform due to spinal cord injuries will cause changes in the spectrum. Previous studies have proved that SSEP appears over a finite duration after stimulation, and the waveform varies in time as well as frequency (JONES *et al.*, 1982; MACCABEE *et al.*, 1986; FUJIOKA *et al.*, 1994). Therefore information from both the time and the frequency domain should be considered in analysis of SSEP signals. To obtain information on the frequency domain as well as time domain, time–frequency analysis (TFA) methods must be used. TFA of EP waveforms has demonstrated that the peak energy in the TFD may be of particular diagnostic value in assessing neurological injury (HU *et al.*, 2000). The energy of the EP waveforms is normally found to be concentrated in a certain time–frequency space, and this can be used to interpret the character of the EP signal in greater detail and more reliably than in the time domain alone (BRAUN *et al.*, 1997; HU *et al.*, 2000). Injury is known to cause localised changes in the morphology of the SSEP waveform, and therefore in the time–frequency spectrum of the EP waveforms (BRAUN *et al.*, 1997; HU *et al.*, 2000).

Different methods can be used to transform signals into time–frequency distributions (TFD) with different fitting conditions, however, the most appropriate method should match the definitive characteristics of the SSEP signal. The purpose of this paper is to assess the applicability of different TFA methods to SSEP signals and their potential for clinical use.

## 2 Materials and methods

### 2.1 Data acquisition

Thirty patients undergoing scoliosis surgery were selected for this study. SSEP signals were recorded intraoperatively with an intraoperative evoked potential measurement system.*

A pair of stimulating electrodes were applied over the posterior tibial nerve behind the medial malleoli to obtain the SSEP signal. The stimulation current was set at the minimum current required to produce a small movement of the toes, typically 10 to 30 mA. Single pulse stimulation at a rate between 5.1 and 5.7 Hz and a duration of 300 μs was applied. When the spine was exposed during surgery, a bipolar epidural electrode† was inserted into the epidural space one or two levels above the surgical region, and the SSEP signal was collected from this electrode. The responses were continuously recorded with a 20–3000 Hz band-pass filter, and were averaged 100 times at a sampling rate of 5 kHz.

### 2.2 Data processing

SSEP signals were analysed using a processing programme with Labview 5.0.‡ Several different time–frequency distributions were used.

#### 2.2.1 Short time Fourier transform (STFT):
The short time Fourier transform (STFT) spectrogram is a commonly used method of time–frequency analysis. For a recorded SSEP signal $s(t)$, the STFT spectrogram is defined by the following equation:

$$\text{STFT}(t, \omega)|_{t=n\Delta t, \omega=\frac{2k\pi}{N\Delta t}} = \text{STFT}(n, k)$$
$$= \sum_{i=0}^{N-1} s(i)w(i-n)e^{-\frac{j2ki\pi}{N}} \qquad (1)$$

where $\Delta t$ denotes the time sampling interval, and $N$ is the block length of the window function. In the present study, rectangular Hanning, Hamming and Blackman windows were used to process the SSEP signals.

#### 2.2.2 Wigner–Ville distribution (WVD):
The Wigner–Ville distribution (WVD) is a quadratic time–frequency distribution. SSEP waveforms were analysed using a discrete WVD, defined below:

$$\text{WVD}(n, k) = \sum_{i=0}^{N-1} R(n, i)e^{-\frac{j2ki\pi}{N}} \qquad (2)$$

where $R(n, i)$ is a time-dependent auto-correlated function given by

$$R(n, i) = Z(n+i)Z(n-i) \qquad (3)$$

and $Z(n)$ denotes the analytical sequence corresponding to $s(n)$. The analytical sequence is obtained by the equation

$$Z(n) = s(n) + jH\{s(n)\} \qquad (4)$$

where $H\{\}$ denotes the Hilbert transform.

#### 2.2.3 Choi–Williams distribution (CWD):
CHOI and WILLIAMS (1989) introduced a distribution using an exponential kernel function. The CWD can be defined in discrete formulation as

$$\text{CWD}(n, k) = \sum_{i=0}^{N-1} \frac{1}{4\pi\alpha i^2} \sum_{l} R(n-l, i)e^{-\frac{l^2}{4\alpha i^2}} \qquad (5)$$

where $\alpha$ is a parameter that controls the decay speed of the kernel function.

#### 2.2.4 Cone-shaped distribution (CSD):
The cone-shaped distribution (CSD) was developed to reduce the interference distribution (ZHAO *et al.*, 1990). The CSD also uses an exponential weighting term with parameter $\alpha$ to introduce smoothing in an attempt to control spurious terms. Its discrete formulation is represented by

$$\text{Cone}(n, k) = \sum_{i=0}^{N-1} e^{-\alpha i^2} \sum_{l} R(n-l, i)e^{-\frac{j2ki\pi}{N}} \qquad (6)$$

#### 2.2.5 Adaptive spectrogram (ADS):
Adaptive spectrogram (ADS) is a new technique which adaptively selects the parameters of the kernel function at each point in time to match the signal. In this study, an adaptive Gabor spectrogram algorithm was applied to the EP signals, as described by the following equation.

$$\text{AS}(n, k) = \sum_{p=0}^{P-1} B_p^2 e^{-(\frac{n-n_p}{\sigma_p})^2 - (\frac{2\pi\sigma_p}{N})^2(k-k_p)^2} \qquad (7)$$

The coefficients were determined by optimal Gaussian basis functions using an algorithm developed by QIAN and CHEN (1994).

### 2.3 Assessment and comparison

The SSEP signal was interpreted in practice by displaying a two-dimensional TFA distribution, and three parameters previously found to be indicative of spinal cord injury were recorded: peak time, peak frequency and peak power (BRAUN *et al.*, 1997; HU *et al.*, 2000). The accuracy of spinal cord monitoring therefore depends on the clear interpretation of the time–frequency distribution and accurate energy representation. As such, the resolutions of the peaks in the time–frequency distribution were used as the criteria for comparison between methods. Pilot studies have shown that the lower frequency peak in the time–frequency plot of SSEP is a more reliable indicator of injury-related TFA change than the higher frequency peaks (HU *et al.*, 2000) and therefore this peak was used as the basis for comparison between the methods. To choose a practical TFA method for intraoperative SSEP monitoring, all the signals were analysed with the various algorithms, including different window functions and lengths. The results were compared by assessment of the three following parameters:

(a) Time and frequency resolutions (peak widths in time and frequency). The time–frequency properties of SSEP signals are distinct for each individual, and therefore only relative comparisons can be made between TFA resolutions. To evaluate the resolution of the spectrogram, the peak width (which denotes 80% energy density of the main power peak in the TFA distribution) was measured in both time and frequency dimensions. A narrow peak indicates a relatively high resolution, whereas a wide peak means low resolution. The peak width values were normalised by 10 points rectangular-windowed STFT to minimise individual difference across subjects. The results for the various distributions were analysed by one-way parametric analysis of variance (ANOVA).

---

* Nicolet Viking IV, Nicolet Biomedical Inc. Madison, WI, USA.
† IMC-KG-102, Inter Medical Co. Ltd., Nagoya, Japan.
‡ National Instruments Co., Texas, USA.

*Table 1   Comparison of peak width in STFT spectrograms of SSEP with different windows and different window lengths*

| | | Window length (sampling points) | | | |
| | Window form | 10 | 20 | 40 | 64 |
| --- | --- | --- | --- | --- | --- |
| Peak width in time (ms) | Rectangular | | $1.58 \pm 0.01$ | $1.97 \pm 0.23$ | $3.12 \pm 0.24$ |
| | Hanning | $0.78 \pm 0.1$ | $1.1 \pm 0.13$ | $1.96 \pm 0.15$ | $2.75 \pm 0.21$ |
| | Hamming | $0.89 \pm 0.13$ | $1.15 \pm 0.11$ | $1.89 \pm 0.19$ | $2.26 \pm 0.23$ |
| | Blackman | $0.87 \pm 0.13$ | $1.04 \pm 0.17$ | $1.6 \pm 0.15$ | $2.45 \pm 0.16$ |
| Peak width in frequency (Hz) | Rectangular | | $0.58 \pm 0.2$ | $0.44 \pm 0.23$ | $0.26 \pm 0.12$ |
| | Hanning | $0.84 \pm 0.18$ | $0.51 \pm 0.15$ | $0.34 \pm 0.13$ | $0.24 \pm 0.1$ |
| | Hamming | $0.80 \pm 0.13$ | $0.53 \pm 0.12$ | $0.38 \pm 0.1$ | $0.24 \pm 0.12$ |
| | Blackman | $0.97 \pm 0.14$ | $0.56 \pm 0.1$ | $0.40 \pm 0.1$ | $0.31 \pm 0.1$ |

(b) Accuracy of time–frequency distribution. If false peaks appear in the TFA distribution they may interfere with the measurement of the energy peak. The time–frequency distribution was evaluated qualitatively, and the peak power calculated by various algorithms was compared with that of STFT to determine whether the peak power reflects the magnitude of the signal or not.

(c) Speed of computation. The calculation times of various TFA algorithms were observed, and related to that of the STFT.

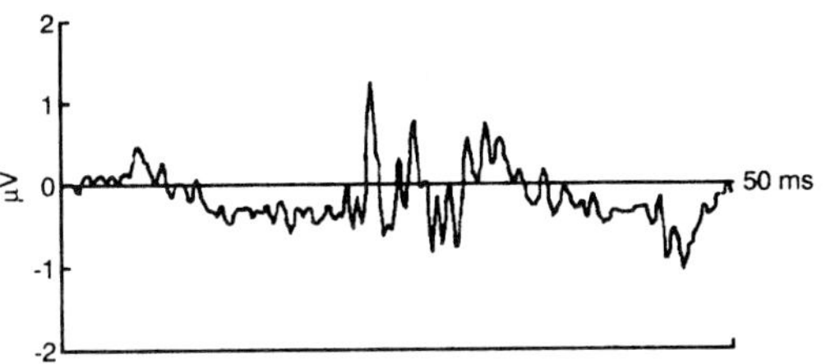

**Fig. 1**   *Example of SSEP signal for time–frequency analysis*

## 3 Results

The normalised peak widths in the time and frequency domains of the different STFT windows on the SSEPs of all 30 patients are shown in Table 1. Generally, increasing window length will result in a decrease in time resolution but an increase in frequency resolution. Considering both time and frequency resolution, the corresponding peak in the SSEP signal (Fig. 1) can be obtained with good resolution in both time and frequency dimensions when the window length is set to 20 sampling points.

The STFT distributions of the sample SSEP signal with rectangular, Hanning, Hamming and Blackman windows, each 20 sampling points long, are shown in Fig. 2. Using the same window length, a rectangular-windowed STFT shows wider peaks in both time and frequency dimensions than the STFTs by other windows, meaning that the rectangular-windowed STFTs resulted in lower resolution distributions than those produced by other windows. For a 20 sampling point window length, the time-dimension peak widths of Hanning, Hamming and Blackman windowed STFT spectrograms did not show any significant differences ($p > 0.05$, Table 1). However, the Hanning-windowed STFT showed a significantly sharper peak width in the frequency dimension than the other windows ($p < 0.001$, Table 1).

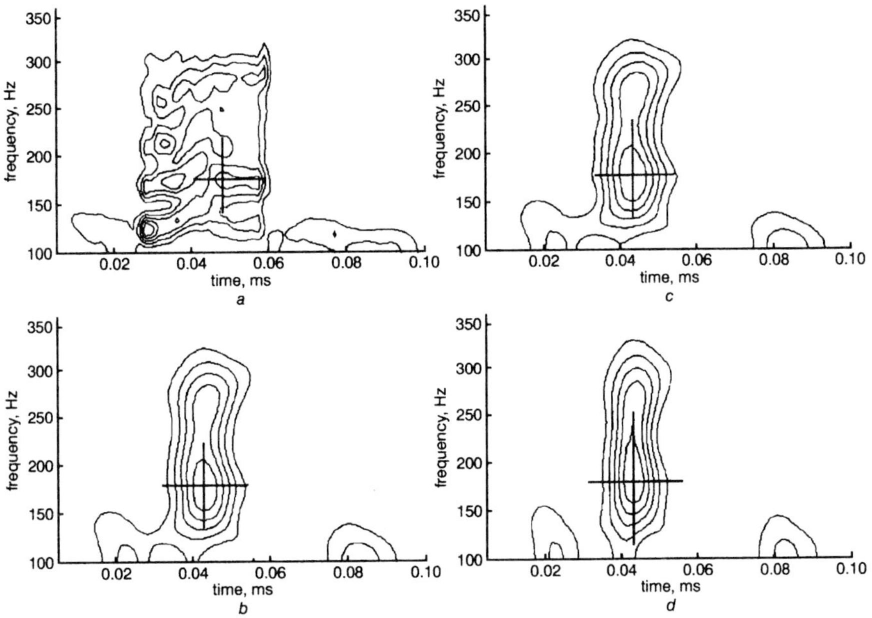

**Fig. 2**   *Illustration of SSEP time–frequency distribution by STFT with 20 sampling points length window in different function. The contours are marked in 20% intervals from minimum to maximum power (peak), and the cross indicate the measurement point of peak time, peak frequency and peak power. (a) Rectangular window; (b) Hanning window; (c) Hamming window; (d) Blackman window*

*Table 2   Comparison of peak width in SSEP TFA distribution with WVD, ADS, CSD and CWD*

|  | WVD | ADS | CSD | CWD |
|---|---|---|---|---|
| Width in time (ms) | 0.6±0.14 | 2.58±0.4 | 0.70±0.12 | 0.49±0.14 |
| Width in frequency (Hz) | 0.47±0.15 | 0.30±0.17 | 0.13±0.1 | 0.42±0.21 |

*Table 3   Bias (%) of peak power in SSEP TFA distribution by WVD, ADS, CSD and CWD compared with STFT*

|  | WVD | ADS | CSD | CWD |
|---|---|---|---|---|
| Percentage difference from STFT power | 9.2±3.4 | 41.8±19.6 | 10.3±6.2 | 14.9±7.4 |

The comparison of peak widths of SSEP by CSD, CWD, WVD and ADS are given in Table 2. The TFA of SSEP appears to offer very good time resolution for these four distributions (Fig. 3), and consequently, the standard deviation of the frequency peak width is comparatively high, particularly for CWD and WVD. The value for the peak frequency using ADS is significantly different from that of the other algorithms, believed to be due to the finding of a false peak.

The main peak of the SSEP signal was not easily identified in CWD and WVD due to cross-term interference (Fig. 3*b* and *c*). The large standard deviation of the time-dimension peak width in ADS suggests that its use in conjunction with SSEP signals is highly variable and unreliable.

Table 3 shows the mean bias of peak power by various TFA methods in comparison with STFT, and Fig. 4 shows three-dimensional plots of various TFA methods. Negative peaks were seen in WVD, CWD and CSD, and this negative energy may cause false peaks in the time–frequency distribution (AKAY, 1998).

In addition to the above observations, the speeds of different TFA algorithms were compared during data processing. STFT is the fastest algorithm, irrespective of the window function or size used, while ADS is the slowest algorithm, and WVD, CSD and CWD are ranked between these two. However, the calculation time for each SSEP signal was in the range of a few minutes, making them all acceptable for intraoperative spinal cord monitoring in practice.

## 4 Discussion

Previous studies have applied TFA to visual evoked potentials (VEPs) or event-related potentials (ERPs) to aid in the identification of specific components of the signal (MORGAN and GEVINS, 1986; NORCIA *et al.*, 1986). Another earlier study specifically examined the optimum trade-off between time and frequency resolution by using STFT on somatosensory, visual, and brainstem auditory evoked potentials (DE WEERD and KAP, 1981). The application of TFA to SSEP signals can provide a reliable indication of spinal cord function (HU *et al.*, 2000). However, different TFA algorithms have their own fitting conditions, and algorithms should be adapted to match the definitive characteristics of the signal.

From the results of this study, WVD, CWD and CSD showed the highest resolution in time–frequency analysis of SSEP, following by ADS and STFT. WVD showed the most severe cross-term interference, while CSD depressed the interference in the TFA distribution. ADS and STFT did not present any evident cross-term interference. The peak power calculated by STFT is linearly correlated to the actual energy distribution in the signal. In comparison with the peak power calculated by STFT, a larger bias was shown with ADS than with the other methods. The calculation speed of all the algorithms tested is sufficient for practical intraoperative spinal cord monitoring.

STFT is a conventional fast Fourier transform with a short block length, sliding along with full or partial overlap. In STFT, it is important to calculate each spectral component using a time window of minimal length around the analysed data point.

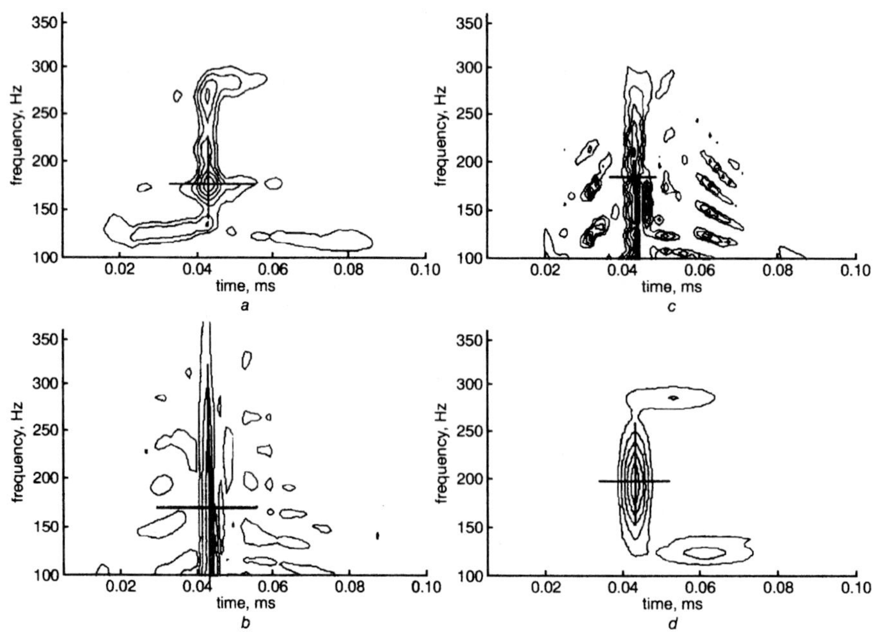

**Fig. 3**   *Time–frequency analysis of SSEP by different algorithms. The contours are marked in 20% intervals from minimum to maximum power (peak), and the cross indicate the measurement point of peak time, peak frequency and peak power. (a) Cone-shaped distribution; (b) Choi–Williams distribution; (c) Wigner–Ville distribution; (d) adaptive spectrogram*

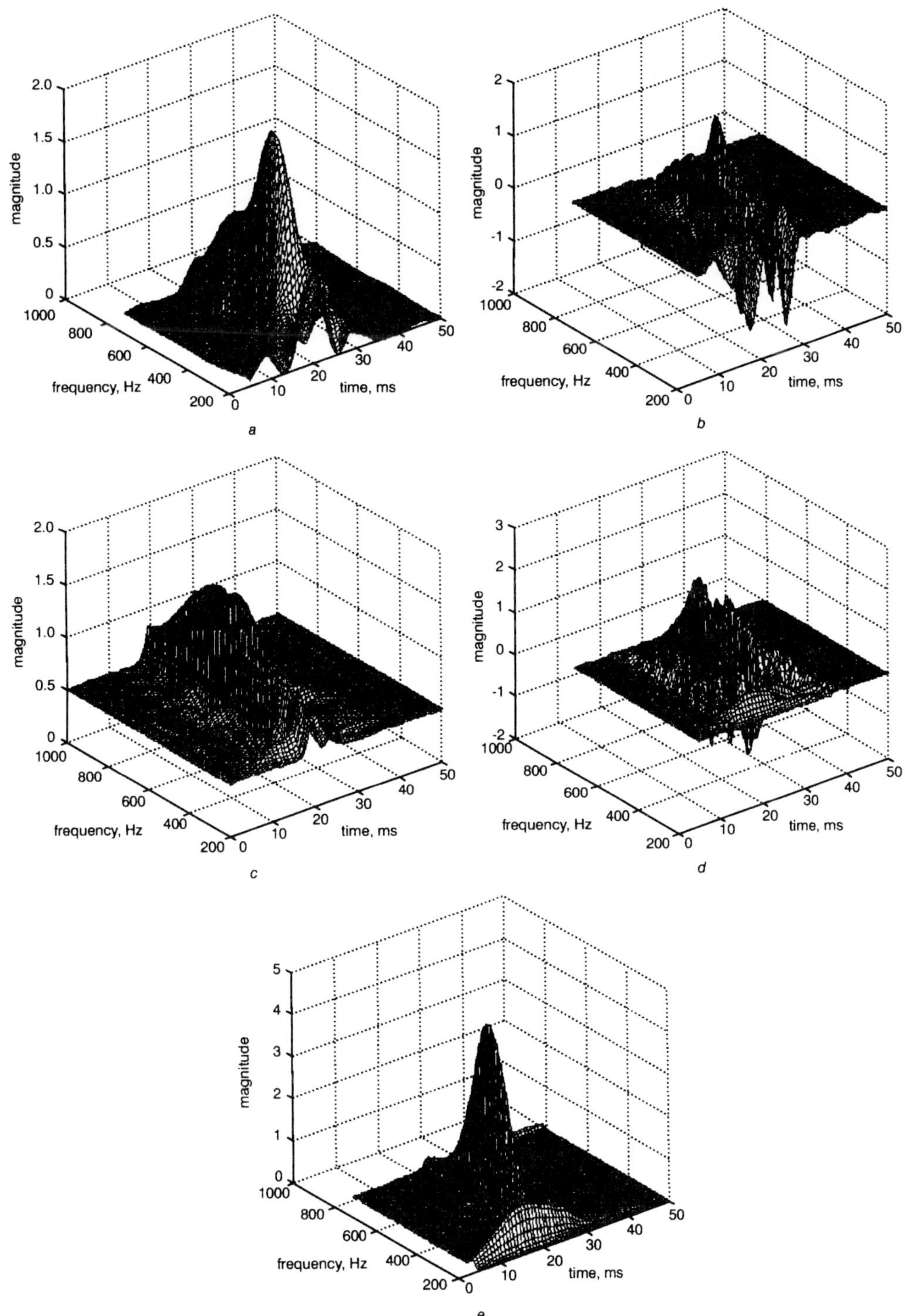

**Fig. 4** *Comparison of time–frequency distribution of SSEP by different algorithms. The three-dimensional surface plots show (a) STFT distribution; (b) Choi–Williams distribution; (c) cone-shaped distribution; (d) Wigner–Ville distribution, and (e) adaptive spectrogram*

However, all the windows have an inherent trade-off between the extent of time resolution and the extent of frequency resolution (DE WEERD and KAP, 1981). According to the present study, a Hanning window function 20 points long appears to be the best choice. Nevertheless, the performance of the STFT in terms of simultaneous time–frequency resolution is still modest compared with the other algorithms.

WVD, CWD and CSD are three of the best-known transforms of the large, more general class of bilinear transform. WVD provides high-resolution representations in time and frequency for non-stationary signals, and importantly satisfies the time and frequency borders in terms of the instantaneous power in time and energy spectrum in frequency. However, its energy distribution is partially negative and it often possesses severe cross-terms, or interference terms potentially leading to confusion and misinterpretation. BRAUN *et al.* (1997) noted the poor time–frequency resolution of STFT analysis of cortical somatosensory evoked potential, and also found cross-term effects when using WVD. Although they considered this interference to be negligible, they suggested that the interference could be considered significant in different experimental situations. The results of this present study show that the interference incurred using WVD can cause confusion and misinterpretation, and is by no means negligible in the analysis of SSEP signals.

CHOI and WILLIAMS (1989) introduced the CWD, which has an exponential-type kernel, and as such is more computationally intensive than the WVD as it adds an extra parameter which controls the degree of smoothing in the spectrogram. This new distribution overcomes several drawbacks of WVD; providing high resolution with suppressed interference. However, the results of the present study indicated that use of the CWD in the analysis of SSEP signals resulted in high levels of cross-term interference.

Another TFD method that has received a lot of attention in recent years is the cone-shaped kernel distribution (CSD) introduced by ZHAO, ATLAS and MARKS (1990). The CSD is spectrogram-like in some aspects, but it overcomes several drawbacks of the spectrogram and offers high resolution with sharp time delineation and good frequency resolution of segmented sine waves. The CSD also uses an exponential weighting term with a parameter to introduce smoothing in an attempt to control spurious terms. The work presented here proved that the CSD can provide good resolution in time and frequency with little cross-term interference in time–frequency distributions of SSEP signals.

The adaptive algorithm places the kernel function adaptively, adjusting their variance and position in the time–frequency plane to best model the signal (AKAY, 1998). The adaptive spectrogram offers the best time–frequency resolution of all the above algorithms and does not cause cross-term interference. However, its application to TFA of SSEP signals is limited for two reasons. First, ADS will adjust the kernel function for every signal so that the transform may change the time–frequency characteristics of the SSEP signals at different surgical stages, in turn affecting the reliability of the monitoring. Secondly, ADS will change the peak power seen in the time–frequency distributions of SSEP signals.

## 5 Conclusion

The results of this study indicated that TFA preserves the time and frequency information of SSEP signals. Both WVD and CWD produce cross-product terms that are not present in the original SSEP signal. These cross-terms distorted the measurements of the energy peak for intraoperative SSEP monitoring, and WVD and CWD are therefore not recommended for TFA of SSEP signals. STFT, ADS and CSD can be applied to SSEP signal processing for intraoperative spinal cord monitoring as cross-term interference was not incurred. However, ADS did not show any discernible improvement over CSD for time–frequency analysis of EP signals. STFT is fast and easy to obtain, but its poor resolution limits its application to the clinical analysis of SSEP signals. The CSD algorithm shows good resolution and a smooth spectrogram, and despite having a little slower processing speed than the STFT algorithm, CSD is recommended as a practical algorithm for the time–frequency analysis of SSEP signals.

*Acknowledgement*—This project was supported by a grant from the Hong Kong Research Grant Council (RGC No. 227/95M and 553/96M).

## References

AKAY, M. (1998): 'Time frequency and wavelets in biomedical signal processing' (IEEE Inc., New York)

BASAR-EROGLU, C., WARECKA, K., SCHURMANN, M., and BASAR, E. (1993): 'Visual evoked potentials in multiple sclerosis: frequency response shows reduced alpha amplitude', *Int. J. Neurosci.*, **73**, pp. 235–258

BRAUN, J. C., HANLEY, D. F., and THAKOR, N. V. (1997): 'Detection of neurological injury using time-frequency analysis of the somatosensory evoked potential', *Electroenceph. Clin. Neurophysiol.*, **100**, p. 310

CHOI, H. I., and WILLIAMS, W. J. (1989): 'Improved time-frequency representation of multicomponent signals using exponential kernels', *IEEE Trans. Acoust., Speech, Signal proc.*, **ASSP-37**, pp. 862–871

DE WEERD, J. P. C., and KAP, J. I. (1981): 'Spectro-temporal representations and time-varying spectra of evoked potentials: a methodological investigation', *Biol. Cybern.*, **41**, pp. 101–117

FUJIOKA, H., SHIMOJI, K., TOMITA, M., DENDA, S., TAKADA, T., HOMMA, T., UCHIYAMA, S., TAKAHASHI, H., TOBITA, T., and BABA, H. (1994): 'Spinal cord potential recordings from the extradural space during scoliosis surgery', *Br. J. Anaesth.*, **73**, pp. 350–356

HU, Y., LUK, K. D. K., LU, W. W., HOLMES, A., and LEONG, J. C. Y. (2000): 'Prevention of spinal cord injury with Time-Frequency analysis of evoked potentials: an experimental study', Proceedings of Asia-Pacific Congress on BME, pp. 634–635

JONES, S. J., EDGAR, M. A., and RANSFORD, A. O. (1982): 'Sensory nerve conduction in the human spinal cord: epidural recordings made during scoliosis surgery', *J. Neurol. Neurosurg. Psychiatry*, **45**, pp. 446–451

LOENING-BAUCKE, V., and YAMADA, T. (1993): 'Cerebral potentials evoked by rectal distention in humans', *Electroenceph. Clin. Neurophysiol.*, **88**, pp. 447–452

MACCABEE, P. J., HASSAN, N. F., CRACCO, R. Q., and SCHIFF, J. A. (1986): 'Short latency somatosensory and spinal evoked potentials: power spectra and comparison between high pass analog and digital filter', *Electroenceph. Clin. Neurophysiol.*, **65**, pp. 177–187

MORGAN, N. H., and GEVINS, A. S. (1986): 'Wigner distributions of human event-related potentials', *IEEE Trans. Biomed. Eng.*, **33**, pp. 66–70

NASH-CL Jr. (1989): 'Spinal cord monitoring', *J. Bone Joint Surg. Am.*, **71**, pp. 627–630

NORCIA, A. M., SATO, T., SHINN, P., and MERTUS, I. (1986): 'Methods for the identification of evoked response components in the frequency and combined time-frequency domains', *Electroenceph. Clin. Neurophysiol.*, **65**, pp. 212–226

QIAN, S., and CHEN, D. (1994): 'Signal representation via adaptive normalized Gaussian function', *Signal Processing*, **36**, pp. 1–12

RYAN, T. P., and BRITT, R. H. (1986): 'Spinal and cortical somatosensory evoked potential monitoring during corrective spinal surgery with 108 patients', *Spine*, **11**, pp. 352–361

THAKOR, N. V., GUO, X. R., SUN, Y. C., and HANLEY, D. F. (1993): 'Multiresolution wavelet analysis of evoked potentials', *IEEE Trans. Biomed. Eng.*, **40**, pp. 1085–1094

ZHAO, Y., ATLAS, L. E., and MARKS, R. (1990): 'The use of cone shaped kernels for generalized time-frequency representations of nonstationary signals', *IEEE Trans. Acoust., Speech, Signal Process.*, **ASSP-38**, pp. 1084–1091

## Authors' biographies

YONG HU received his BSc and MSc in Biomedical Engineering from Tianjin University, Tianjin, China in 1985 and 1988, respectively, and his PhD from The University of Hong Kong in 1999. He is currently a postdoctoral research fellow in the Department of Orthopaedic Surgery, The University of Hong Kong. His research interests include neural engineering, clinical electrophysiology, biomedical signal measurement and processing.

KEITH DK LUK is Professor at the Department of Orthopaedic Surgery, The University of Hong Kong, and the President of the Hong Kong College of Orthopaedic Surgeons. At present, his research interests include intraoperative spinal cord monitoring, biomechanics of the lumbosacral spine, real-time analysis of human lumbar motion, developing fast evoked potential measurement methods and correction of spinal deformities.

# Reconstructing Spatio-Temporal Activities of Neural Sources Using an MEG Vector Beamformer Technique

Kensuke Sekihara*, *Member, IEEE*, Srikantan S. Nagarajan, David Poeppel, Alec Marantz, and Yasushi Miyashita

*Abstract*—We have developed a method suitable for reconstructing spatio-temporal activities of neural sources by using magnetoencephalogram (MEG) data. The method extends the adaptive beamformer technique originally proposed by Borgiotti and Kaplan to incorporate the vector beamformer formulation in which a set of three weight vectors are used to detect the source activity in three orthogonal directions. The weight vectors of the vector-extended version of the Borgiotti–Kaplan beamformer are then projected onto the signal subspace of the measurement covariance matrix to obtain the final form of the proposed beamformer's weight vectors. Our numerical experiments show that both spatial resolution and output signal-to-noise ratio of the proposed beamformer are significantly higher than those of the minimum-variance-based vector beamformer used in previous investigations. We also applied the proposed beamformer to two sets of auditory-evoked MEG data, and the results clearly demonstrated the method's capability of reconstructing spatio-temporal activities of neural sources.

*Index Terms*—Beamformer, biomagnetism, functional neuroimaging, magnetoencephalography, MEG inverse problems, neuromagnetic signal processing.

## I. INTRODUCTION

**A**MONG the various kinds of functional neuroimaging methodologies, the major advantage of magnetoencephalography (MEG) is its ability to provide fine time resolution of the millisecond order [1]. Neuromagnetic imaging can thus be used to visualize neural activities with such a fine time resolution, and to provide functional information about brain dynamics [2]. Toward this goal, a number of algorithms for reconstructing spatio-temporal source activities have been developed. Well-known approaches for this reconstruction employ the model of the equivalent current dipole (ECD) [3], which assumes a highly localized source. Although this ECD

Manuscript received March 17, 2000; revised April 6, 2001. The work of S. S. Nagarajan was supported by a grant from the Whitaker Foundation. This work was carried out as part of the MIT-JST International Cooperative Research Project "Mind Articulation." *Asterisk indicates corresponding author.*

*K. Sekihara is with the Department of Electronic Systems and Engineering, Tokyo Metropolitan Institute of Technology, Asahigaoka 6-6, Hino, Tokyo 191-0065, Japan (e-mail: ksekiha@cc.tmit.ac.jp).

S. S. Nagarajan is with the Department of Bioengineering, University of Utah, Salt Lake City, UT 84112-9202 USA.

D. Poeppel is with the Department of Linguistics and Biology, University of Maryland, College Park, MD 20742 USA.

A. Marantz is with the Department of Linguistics and Philosophy, Massachusetts Institute of Technology, Cambridge, MA 02139 USA.

Y. Miyashita is with the Department of Physiology, The University of Tokyo, School of Medicine, Hongo, Tokyo 113-0033, Japan.

Publisher Item Identifier S 0018-9294(01)05134-5.

model has successfully been applied to neuromagnetic data, we cannot rely on ECD modeling when the source is distributed or when no information on the spatial extent of the source is available.

Another approach for spatio-temporal reconstruction is based on the linear estimation method [4]; it assumes voxels in the reconstruction region and attempts to estimate the moment of a source assigned to each voxel by using least-squares fitting. Although this approach does not impose any models on the neuromagnetic source, a naive form of such an approach has a serious problem in that the estimation becomes severely ill posed. This is because the number of voxels generally reaches, at least, a few thousand, so several thousand parameters need to be estimated from the measured data obtained at only one to two hundred points on the scalp surface. To reduce the influence from this ill-posed condition, an efficient method of constraining the least-squares solution should be developed. This has been an area of active research, and many kinds of investigations in this direction have been reported [5]–[7].

In this paper, we explore the possibility of applying a class of techniques called the adaptive beamformer to this reconstruction problem. The adaptive beamformer provides a versatile form of spatial filtering suitable for processing data from an array of sensors. Adaptive-beamformer-type techniques were originally developed in the fields of array signal processing, including radar, sonar, and seismic exploration [8], and they have been already applied to the MEG/EEG source-reconstruction problem [9]–[12]. In these investigations, the minimum-variance beamformer, which is one of most popular adaptive beamformer techniques, was modified to incorporate the detection of three-dimensional (3-D) vector sources. Particularly, in [9], [10], [12], a vector beamformer technique has been developed on the basis of the minimum-variance beamformer; the vector beamformer uses a set of three weight vectors for detecting the source activity in three orthogonal directions such as $x$, $y$, and $z$, thereby reconstructing not only the source magnitude but also the source orientation.

This paper develops a vector beamformer technique on the basis of the Borgiotti–Kaplan beamformer [13]. The developed beamformer performs significantly better than the minimum-variance beamformer used in the previous investigations, with respect to the spatial resolution and the output signal-to-noise ratio (SNR). In Section II, after a brief introduction to the minimum-variance-based beamformer technique, we formulate our proposed vector beamformer. In Section III, a series of numerical experiments verify the effectiveness of the proposed beamformer. In Section IV, we apply the proposed beamformer to two sets of auditory MEG data. The results of these applications demonstrate its capability of reconstructing spatio-temporal activities of neural sources. Throughout this paper, plain italics indicate scalars, lower-case boldface italics indicate vectors, and upper-case boldface italics indicate matrices.

## II. METHOD

### A. Definitions and Problem Formulation

Let us define the magnetic field measured by the $m$th detector coil at time $t$ as $b_m(t)$, and a column vector $\boldsymbol{b}(t) = [b_1(t), b_2(t), \ldots, b_M(t)]^T$ as a set of measured data where $M$ is the total number of detector coils and the superscript $T$ indicates the matrix transpose. A spatial location $(x, y, z)$ is represented by a 3-D vector $\boldsymbol{r}$: $\boldsymbol{r} = (x, y, z)$. A total of $Q$ current sources are assumed to generate the neuromagnetic field, and the locations of these sources are denoted as $\boldsymbol{r}_1, \boldsymbol{r}_2, \ldots, \boldsymbol{r}_Q$. The moment magnitude of the $q$th source at time $t$ is defined as $s_q(t)$, and the source magnitude vector is defined as $\boldsymbol{s}(t) = [s_1(t), s_2(t), \ldots, s_Q(t)]^T$.

To express the orientation of the $q$th source, we define the angles between its moment vector and the $x$, $y$, and $z$ axes as $\beta_q^x(t)$, $\beta_q^y(t)$, and $\beta_q^z(t)$, respectively. The orientation of the $q$th source is defined as a vector $\boldsymbol{\eta}_q(t) = [\eta_q^x(t), \eta_q^y(t), \eta_q^z(t)]^T$, where $\eta_q^\mu(t) = \cos[\beta_q^\mu(t)]$ and $\mu$ is equal to $x$, $y$, or $z$ throughout this paper. We define a $3Q \times Q$ matrix that expresses the orientations of all $Q$ sources as $\boldsymbol{\Psi}$ such that

$$\boldsymbol{\Psi} = \begin{bmatrix} \boldsymbol{\eta}_1 & 0 & \cdots & 0 \\ 0 & \boldsymbol{\eta}_2 & & \vdots \\ \vdots & & \ddots & 0 \\ 0 & \cdots & 0 & \boldsymbol{\eta}_Q \end{bmatrix}.$$

We assume in this paper that the orientation of each source is time independent.

The lead field vector for the $\mu$ component of a source at $\boldsymbol{r}$ is defined as $\boldsymbol{l}_\mu(\boldsymbol{r}) = [l_1^\mu(\boldsymbol{r}), l_2^\mu(\boldsymbol{r}), \ldots, l_M^\mu(\boldsymbol{r})]^T$. Here, $l_m^\mu(\boldsymbol{r})$ expresses the $m$th sensor output induced by the unit-magnitude source that is located at $\boldsymbol{r}$ and directed in the $\mu$ direction. We define the lead field matrix as $\boldsymbol{L}(\boldsymbol{r}) = [\boldsymbol{l}_x(\boldsymbol{r}), \boldsymbol{l}_y(\boldsymbol{r}), \boldsymbol{l}_z(\boldsymbol{r})]$, which represents the sensitivity of the sensor array at $\boldsymbol{r}$. The lead field vector representing the sensitivity of a sensor array in the $\boldsymbol{\eta}$ direction at $\boldsymbol{r}$ is denoted as $\boldsymbol{l}(\boldsymbol{r}, \boldsymbol{\eta})$, which is calculated from $\boldsymbol{l}(\boldsymbol{r}, \boldsymbol{\eta}) = \boldsymbol{L}(\boldsymbol{r})\boldsymbol{\eta}^T$. The composite lead field matrix for the entire set of $Q$ sources is defined as

$$\boldsymbol{L}_c = [\boldsymbol{L}(\boldsymbol{r}_1), \boldsymbol{L}(\boldsymbol{r}_2), \ldots, \boldsymbol{L}(\boldsymbol{r}_Q)]. \tag{1}$$

The relationship between $\boldsymbol{b}(t)$ and $\boldsymbol{s}(t)$ is then expressed as

$$\boldsymbol{b}(t) = (\boldsymbol{L}_c \boldsymbol{\Psi})\boldsymbol{s}(t) + \boldsymbol{n}(t) \tag{2}$$

where $\boldsymbol{n}(t)$ is the additive noise. We define, for later use, the covariance matrix of the measured magnetic field as $\boldsymbol{R}_b$ such that $\boldsymbol{R}_b = \langle (\boldsymbol{b}(t) - \langle \boldsymbol{b}(t) \rangle)(\boldsymbol{b}(t) - \langle \boldsymbol{b}(t) \rangle)^T \rangle$ where $\langle \cdot \rangle$ indicates the ensemble average.

To estimate the source moment from the measured magnetic field, we focus on the class of techniques referred to as a beamformer [8]. The beamformer technique estimates the moment

magnitude of a source located at $\boldsymbol{r}$ and directed in the $\boldsymbol{\eta}$ direction using the following linear spatial filter operation:

$$\hat{s}(\boldsymbol{r}, \boldsymbol{\eta}, t) = \boldsymbol{w}^T(\boldsymbol{r}, \boldsymbol{\eta})\boldsymbol{b}(t) \tag{3}$$

where $\hat{s}(\boldsymbol{r}, \boldsymbol{\eta}, t)$ is the estimated moment magnitude. In (3), the column vector $\boldsymbol{w}(\boldsymbol{r}, \boldsymbol{\eta})$ represents a set of weights that characterizes the property of the beamformer. It should be pointed out that according to (3), the power of the output noise due to the additive white noise $\boldsymbol{n}(t)$ is proportional to $\langle |\boldsymbol{w}^T \boldsymbol{n}(t)|^2 \rangle = \sigma^2 \boldsymbol{w}^T \boldsymbol{w}$ where $\boldsymbol{n}(t)$ is assumed to be the white Gaussian noise and $\sigma^2$ is its variance. That is, the power of the output noise is proportional to $\boldsymbol{w}^T \boldsymbol{w}$, which is called the white noise gain for this reason.

### B. Existing Beamformer Techniques for Reconstructing Neural Source Activities

*1) Minimum-Variance Distortionless Beamformer:* One well-known beamformer technique is the minimum-variance distortionless beamformer [14], in which the weight vector $\boldsymbol{w}$ is obtained by minimizing $\boldsymbol{w}^T \boldsymbol{R}_b \boldsymbol{w}$ with the constraint of $\boldsymbol{w}^T \boldsymbol{l}(\boldsymbol{r}, \boldsymbol{\eta}) = 1$. (Although the weight vector depends on the pointing location $\boldsymbol{r}$, we omit the explicit notation of $\boldsymbol{r}$ unless this omission causes ambiguity.) This weight vector is

$$\boldsymbol{w}(\boldsymbol{r}, \boldsymbol{\eta}) = \frac{\boldsymbol{R}_b^{-1}\boldsymbol{l}(\boldsymbol{r}, \boldsymbol{\eta})}{\boldsymbol{l}^T(\boldsymbol{r}, \boldsymbol{\eta})\boldsymbol{R}_b^{-1}\boldsymbol{l}(\boldsymbol{r}, \boldsymbol{\eta})}. \tag{4}$$

This minimum-variance beamformer is widely used in various signal-processing fields. One problem arises when we apply it to reconstructing neural sources. That is, to calculate the beamformer weight by using (4), we must first determine the source orientation $\boldsymbol{\eta}$ at each $\boldsymbol{r}$. This determination is not straightforward, although a method have been proposed for this purpose [15].

*2) Vector-Extension of Minimum-Variance Beamformer:* Instead of estimating the source orientation and magnitude separately, the minimum-variance beamformer can be modified to estimate not only the source magnitude but also the source orientation. Such a beamformer simultaneously estimates the source moment in three orthogonal directions such as $x$, $y$, and $z$. Let us denote the unit vectors in the $x$, $y$, and $z$ directions, as $\boldsymbol{f}_x$, $\boldsymbol{f}_y$, and $\boldsymbol{f}_z$, respectively, i.e., $\boldsymbol{f}_x = [1, 0, 0]^T$, $\boldsymbol{f}_y = [0, 1, 0]^T$, and $\boldsymbol{f}_z = [0, 0, 1]^T$. Let us also denote the weight vectors that estimate $\hat{s}_x(t)$, $\hat{s}_y(t)$, and $\hat{s}_z(t)$ as $\boldsymbol{w}_x$, $\boldsymbol{w}_y$, and $\boldsymbol{w}_z$. Then, these weight vectors can be derived by the following minimizations with multiple constraints:

$$\min_{\boldsymbol{w}_x} \boldsymbol{w}_x^T \boldsymbol{R}_b \boldsymbol{w}_x$$

subject to

$$\boldsymbol{w}_x^T \boldsymbol{l}_x(\boldsymbol{r}) = 1, \quad \boldsymbol{w}_x^T \boldsymbol{l}_y(\boldsymbol{r}) = 0, \quad \text{and} \quad \boldsymbol{w}_x^T \boldsymbol{l}_z(\boldsymbol{r}) = 0,$$

$$\min_{\boldsymbol{w}_y} \boldsymbol{w}_y^T \boldsymbol{R}_b \boldsymbol{w}_y$$

subject to

$$\boldsymbol{w}_y^T \boldsymbol{l}_x(\boldsymbol{r}) = 0, \quad \boldsymbol{w}_y^T \boldsymbol{l}_y(\boldsymbol{r}) = 1, \quad \text{and} \quad \boldsymbol{w}_y^T \boldsymbol{l}_z(\boldsymbol{r}) = 0,$$

$$\min_{\boldsymbol{w}_z} \boldsymbol{w}_z^T \boldsymbol{R}_b \boldsymbol{w}_z$$

subject to

$$w_z^T l_x(r) = 0, \quad w_z^T l_y(r) = 0, \quad \text{and} \quad w_z^T l_z(r) = 1. \quad (5)$$

The minimum-variance beamformer with multiple linear constraints, referred to as the linearly constrained minimum-variance beamformer, is known to have the following solution [9], [10]:

$$[w_x, \, w_y, \, w_z] = R_b^{-1} L(r) \left[ L^T(r) R_b^{-1} L(r) \right]^{-1} \Phi \quad (6)$$

where $\Phi$ is defined as $\Phi = [f_x, \, f_y, \, f_z]$.

Equation (5) indicates that, when estimating one of the three orthogonal components of the source moment, we need to suppress the other two components. This is because when estimating one of the three components, the other two components behave like perfectly correlated virtual sources. Therefore, without this suppression, considerable amount of signal cancellation should arise. By applying these null constraints, however, we can avoid this signal cancellation, and the beamformer can detect the source moment projected in three orthogonal directions. Such a beamformer is referred to as a vector beamformer.

There are two problems when applying (6) to actual MEG/EEG source reconstruction problems. First, the beamformer output has erroneously large values near the center of the sphere used for the forward calculation. This is because $\|L(r)\|$ becomes very small when $r$ approaches the center of the sphere. To avoid these $\|L(r)\|$-dependent artifacts, the use of the normalized lead field matrix $L(r)/\|L(r)\|$ has been suggested [10], [12].

Second, the performance of the beamformer in (6) is very sensitive to errors in calculating the lead field matrix, when applied to the spatio-temporal reconstruction of the source activities [15]. This problem is known to be partly solved by replacing $R_b^{-1}$ in (6) with its regularized inverse $(R_b + \gamma I)^{-1}$ [11], [12], [16], [17] where the parameter $\gamma$ is the regularization parameter. Such replacement, however, is known to degrade the spatial resolution, providing a tradeoff between the SNR and the spatial resolution [11]. In the following section, we propose a beamformer that is free from this tradeoff and can attain an inherently higher spatial resolution.

*C. Formulation of the Proposed Method*

The proposed beamformer is formulated on the basis of the beamformer developed by Borgiotti and Kaplan [13]; its weight vector is derived by minimizing $w^T R_b w$ with the constraint of $w^T w = 1$. Because the Borgiotti–Kaplan beamformer has the unit white noise gain, the output power of the Borgiotti–Kaplan beamformer is equal to the power of the signal normalized by the power of the noise [13]. The weight vectors of the proposed beamformer are derived by a two-step procedure. The first step extends the Borgiotti–Kaplan beamformer to the vector-type beamformer. The second step further extends this vector-extended version of the Borgiotti–Kaplan beamformer to an eigenspace-projected beamformer.

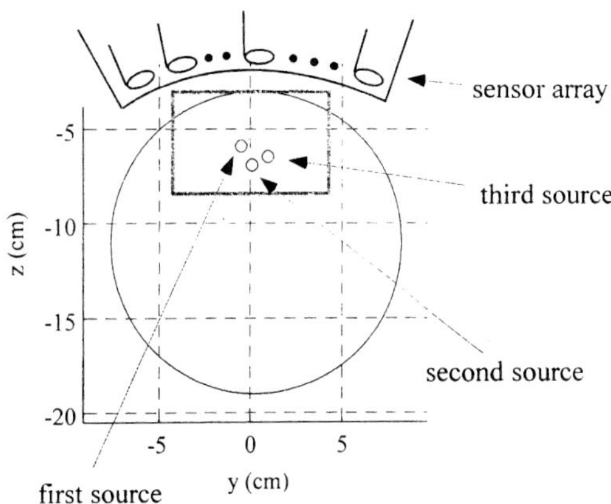



Fig. 1. The coordinate system and the source-detector configuration used in the numerical experiments. The coordinate origin was set at the center of the detector coil located at the center of the coil array. The cross section at $x = 1.0$ is shown. The circle shows the cross section of the sphere used for the forward calculation. The square shows the reconstruction region for the experiments whose results are shown in Figs. 3–6.

TABLE I

SOURCE PARAMETER VALUES USED FOR THE NUMERICAL EXPERIMENTS IN SECTION III

| source number | location (cm) | orientation |
|:---:|:---:|:---:|
| 1 | (1.0, −0.5, −5.9) | (1.0, 0., 0.) |
| 2 | (1.0, 0.1, −6.9) | (0.7, 0.7, 0.) |
| 3 | (1.0, 0.8, −6.7) | (1.0, 0., 0.) |

*1) Vector-Type Borgiotti–Kaplan Beamformer:* The vector-extended Borgiotti–Kaplan beamformer is obtained by using the following constrained minimizations:

$$\min_{w_x} w_x^T R_b w_x$$

subject to

$$w_x^T w_x = 1, \quad w_x^T l_y(r) = 0, \quad \text{and} \quad w_x^T l_z(r) = 0,$$

$$\min_{w_y} w_y^T R_b w_y$$

subject to

$$w_y^T l_x(r) = 0, \quad w_y^T w_y = 1, \quad \text{and} \quad w_y^T l_z(r) = 0,$$

$$\min_{w_z} w_z^T R_b w_z$$

subject to

$$w_z^T l_x(r) = 0, \quad w_z^T l_y(r) = 0, \quad \text{and} \quad w_z^T w_z = 1. \quad (7)$$

We first derive the expression for $w_x$. Let us introduce a scalar constant $\xi$ such that $w_x^T l_x(r) = \xi$ where $\xi$ can be determined from the relationship $w_x^T w_x = 1$. Then, the constrained optimization problem in (7) is changed to

$$\min_{w_x} w_x^T R_b w_x \quad \text{subject to} \quad L^T(r) w_x = \xi \begin{bmatrix} 1 \\ 0 \\ 0 \end{bmatrix} = \xi f_x. \quad (8)$$

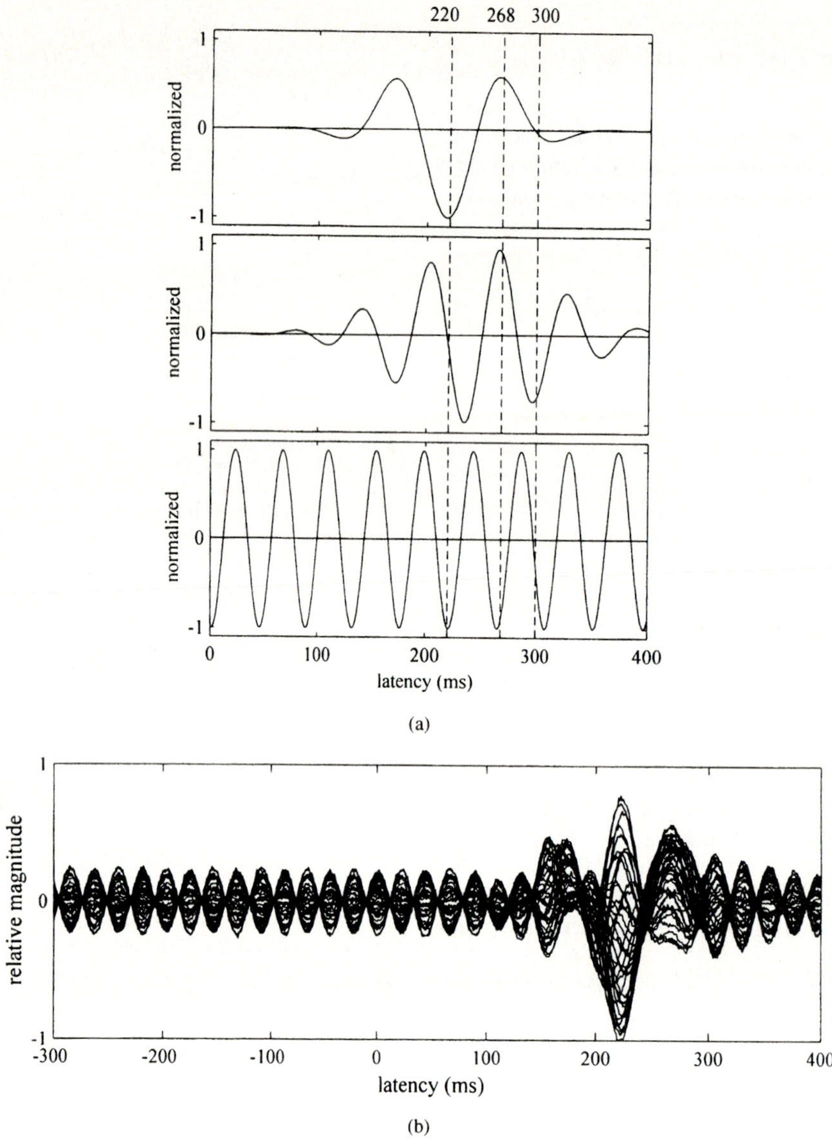

Fig. 2. (a) Time courses of the three sources assumed in the numerical experiments. Time courses from the first to the third sources are shown from the top to the bottom, respectively. The time courses are shown for the time window between 0 and 400 ms. Each time course is normalized by its maximum value. Three vertical broken lines indicate the time instants 220, 268, and 300 ms at which the source-moment magnitude is displayed in Figs. 3(a)–6(a). (b) The generated magnetic field used for the numerical experiments.

The solution of this optimization problem is known to have the form

$$\boldsymbol{w}_x = \xi R_b^{-1} L(\boldsymbol{r}) \left[ L^T(\boldsymbol{r}) R_b^{-1} L(\boldsymbol{r}) \right]^{-1} \boldsymbol{f}_x. \tag{9}$$

Then, we have

$$\boldsymbol{w}_x^T \boldsymbol{w}_x = \xi^2 \boldsymbol{f}_x^T \Omega \boldsymbol{f}_x \tag{10}$$

where

$$\Omega = \left[ L^T(\boldsymbol{r}) R_b^{-1} L(\boldsymbol{r}) \right]^{-1} L^T(\boldsymbol{r}) R_b^{-2} L(\boldsymbol{r}) \\ \cdot \left[ L^T(\boldsymbol{r}) R_b^{-1} L(\boldsymbol{r}) \right]^{-1}.$$

Thus, we get $\xi = 1/\sqrt{\boldsymbol{f}_x^T \Omega \boldsymbol{f}_x}$ from the relationship $\boldsymbol{w}_x^T \boldsymbol{w}_x = 1$. Using exactly the same derivation, the weights $\boldsymbol{w}_y$ and $\boldsymbol{w}_z$ can be derived, and a set of the weights is expressed as

$$\boldsymbol{w}_\mu = \frac{R_b^{-1} L(\boldsymbol{r}) \left[ L^T(\boldsymbol{r}) R_b^{-1} L(\boldsymbol{r}) \right]^{-1} \boldsymbol{f}_\mu}{\sqrt{\boldsymbol{f}_\mu^T \Omega \boldsymbol{f}_\mu}}. \tag{11}$$

It can be shown that the above beamformer retains the property of the Borgiotti–Kaplan beamformer, and its output power is equal to the power of the source activity normalized by the power of the output noise due to the additive sensor noise.

*2) Extension to an Eigenspace-Projection Beamformer:* The extension to an eigenspace-projection beamformer is attained by projecting the weight vectors in (11) onto the signal subspace of the measurement covariance matrix. The eigenspace projection improves the output SNR without sacrificing the spatial resolution. The general analysis regarding how this eigenspace projection improves the output SNR has been reported [18].

Unless the source activities are perfectly correlated with each other, $R_b$ has $Q$ eigenvalues greater than $\sigma^2$ and $M - Q$ eigenvalues equal to $\sigma^2$ where $\sigma^2$ is the variance of the additive noise. Assuming that the eigenvalues are numbered in decreasing order, let us define the matrix $E_S$ as $E_S = [e_1, \ldots, e_Q]$, where $\{e_j\}$ with $j = 1, 2, \ldots, M$ are the eigenvectors of $R_b$. The column span of $E_S$ is the maximum-likelihood estimate of the signal subspace of $R_b$ [19]. The weight vectors of the eigenspace-projected beamformer is obtained by using [20]

$$\overline{w}_\mu = E_S E_S^T w_\mu. \tag{12}$$

The projection onto the signal subspace using the above equation, however, invalidates the null constraints imposed on the orthogonal components. This can be understood by considering, for example, the case of $\overline{w}_x$. The null constraints in this case should be $\overline{w}_x^T l_y(r) = 0$ and $\overline{w}_x^T l_z(r) = 0$. However, let us consider

$$\overline{w}_x^T l_y(r) = \left(E_S E_S^T w_x\right)^T l_y(r) = w_x^T E_S E_S^T l_y(r)$$

$$\overline{w}_x^T l_z(r) = \left(E_S E_S^T w_x\right)^T l_z(r) = w_x^T E_S E_S^T l_z(r). \tag{13}$$

Because $l_y(r)$ and $l_z(r)$ are not necessarily in the signal subspace, we generally have $E_S E_S^T l_y(r) \neq l_y(r)$ and $E_S E_S^T l_z(r) \neq l_z(r)$ and, therefore, $w_x^T E_S E_S^T l_y(r) \neq 0$ and $w_x^T E_S E_S^T l_z(r) \neq 0$, leading to the relationships $\overline{w}_x^T l_y(r) \neq 0$ and $\overline{w}_x^T l_z(r) \neq 0$. Consequently, we conclude that the signal subspace projector $E_S E_S^T$ does not preserve the null constraints.

It can, however, be shown that the eigenspace-projection beamformer in (12) can detect the three orthogonal components of the source moment even though the null constraints are not preserved. Omitting the time notation, let us decompose the measured magnetic field $b$ into two parts, $b = b^{\text{tar}} + b^{\text{oth}}$ where $b^{\text{tar}}$ is the magnetic field generated from the target source at $r$, and $b^{\text{oth}}$ is the contribution from other sources. The magnetic field $b^{\text{tar}}$ can be expressed as $b^{\text{tar}} = (\eta_x l_x(r) + \eta_x l_y(r) + \eta_z l_z(r))s(t)$, where $[\eta_x, \eta_y, \eta_z]$ expresses the orientation of the target source, and $s(t)$ is its moment magnitude. Then, the estimated $x$ component of the source moment, $\hat{s}_x(t)$, is expressed as $\hat{s}_x(t) = \overline{w}_x^T(r)b(t) = \overline{w}_x^T(r)b^{\text{tar}} + \overline{w}_x^T(r)b^{\text{oth}}$. Since the weight $\overline{w}_x^T(r)$ does not pass the signal other than that from $r$, we have $\overline{w}_x^T(r)b^{\text{oth}} = 0$ and, consequently

$$\hat{s}_x(t) = \overline{w}_x^T(r)b^{\text{tar}}$$
$$= w_x^T E_S E_S^T (\eta_x l_x(r) + \eta_x l_y(r) + \eta_z l_z(r))s(t). \tag{14}$$

Because the vector $(\eta_x l_x(r) + \eta_r l_y(r) + \eta_z l_z(r))$ is in the signal subspace, we get

$$E_S E_S^T (\eta_x l_x(r) + \eta_x l_y(r) + \eta_z l_z(r))$$
$$= (\eta_x l_x(r) + \eta_x l_y(r) + \eta_z l_z(r)). \tag{15}$$

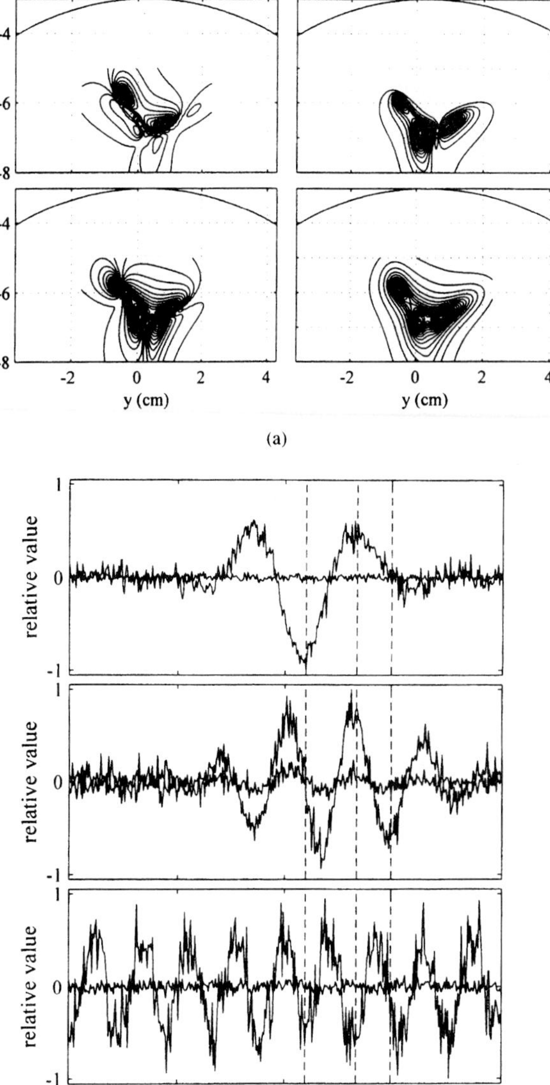



Fig. 3. (a) Results of the spatio-temporal reconstruction obtained using the minimum-variance-based vector beamformer in (6). The upper-left, upper-right, and lower-left maps respectively show the snapshots of the source-moment magnitude at 220, 268, and 300 ms. The lower-right map shows the time-averaged reconstruction. (b) Estimated time courses from the first to the third sources are shown from the top to the bottom, respectively. The three vertical broken lines indicate the time instants of 220, 268, and 300 ms.

Therefore, we finally get

$$\hat{s}_x(t) = \overline{w}_x^T(r)b^{\text{tar}}$$
$$= w_x^T (\eta_x l_x(r) + \eta_x l_y(r) + \eta_z l_z(r))s(t)$$
$$= \eta_x s(t) \left(w_x^T l_x(r)\right) \propto \eta_x s(t). \tag{16}$$

Similarly, we can also obtain $\hat{s}_y(t) = \overline{w}_y^T b(t) \propto \eta_y s(t)$ and $\hat{s}_z(t) = \overline{w}_z^T b(t) \propto \eta_z s(t)$. Thus, the eigenspace-projection beamformer in (12) can detect the three orthogonal components of the source moment, even though the null constraints are not preserved.

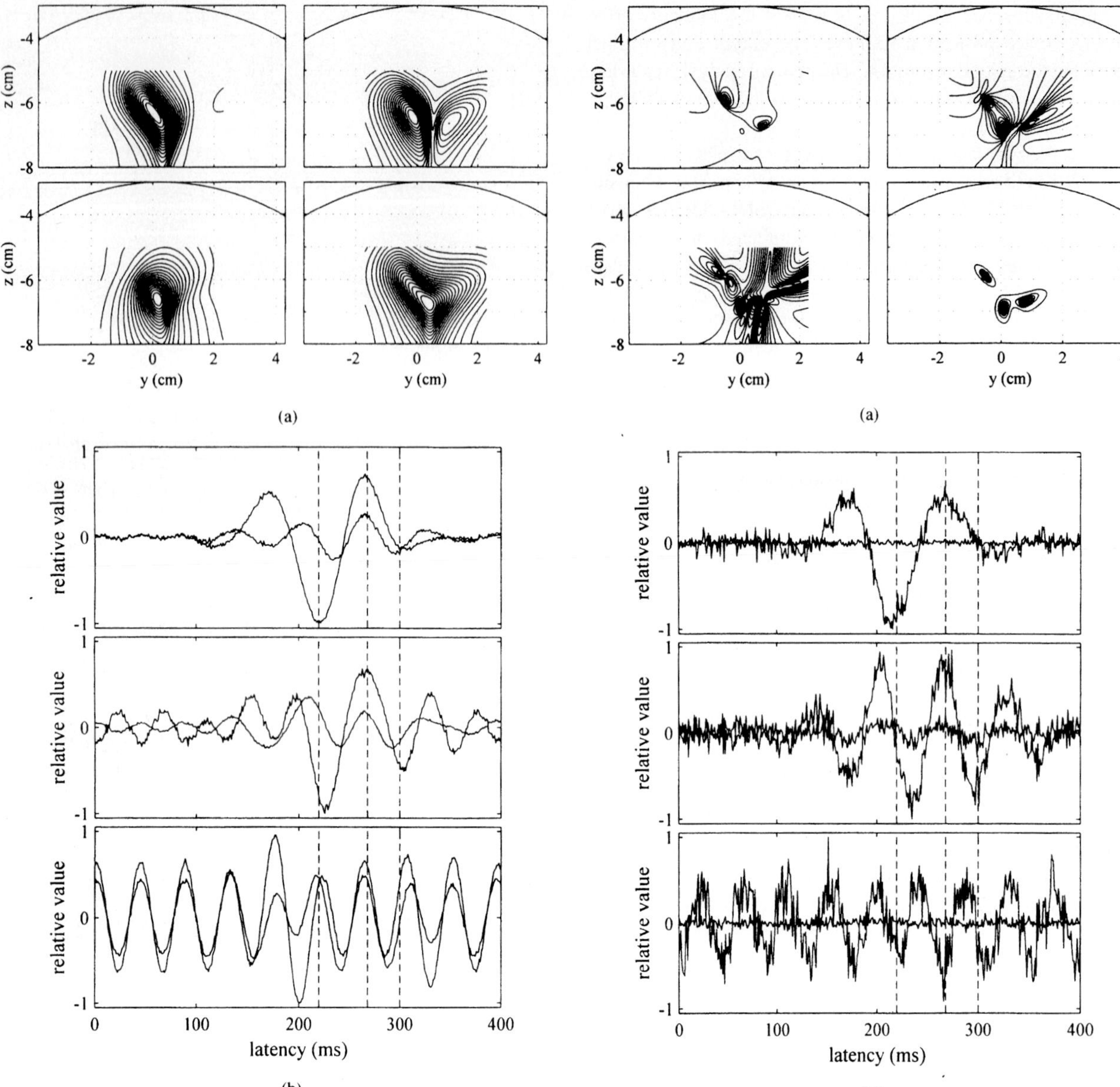

Fig. 4. (a) Results of the spatio-temporal reconstruction obtained using the minimum-variance-based vector beamformer in (6) together with the use of the regularized inverse $(\boldsymbol{R}_b + \gamma\boldsymbol{I})^{-1}$. The parameter $\gamma$ was set at $0.003\lambda_1$, where $\lambda_1$ is the largest eigenvalue of $\boldsymbol{R}_b$. The upper-left, upper-right, and lower-left maps respectively show the snapshots of the source-moment magnitude at 220, 268, and 300 ms. The lower-right map shows the time-averaged reconstruction. (b) Estimated time courses from the first to the third sources are shown from the top to the bottom, respectively. The three vertical broken lines indicate the time instants of 220, 268, and 300 ms.

Fig. 5. (a) Results of the spatio-temporal reconstruction with the weight vectors obtained using (11) alone. The upper-left, upper-right, and lower-left maps respectively show the snapshots of the source-moment magnitude at 220 ms, 268 ms, and 300 ms. The lower-right map shows the time-averaged reconstruction. (b) Estimated time courses from the first to the third sources are shown from the top to the bottom, respectively. The three vertical broken lines indicate the time instants of 220, 268, and 300 ms.

## III. NUMERICAL EXPERIMENTS

### A. *Data Generation*

We conducted a series of numerical experiments to test the effectiveness of the proposed method. A coil alignment of the 37-channel Magnes biomagnetic measurement system (Biomagnetic Technologies Inc., San Diego, CA) was used in these experiments. The coordinate system used in our numerical experiments is illustrated in Fig. 1. The values of the spatial coordinates $(x, y, z)$ were expressed in centimeters. Three signal sources were assumed to exist on a plane defined as $x =$ 1.0. The locations as well as the orientations of the sources are listed in Table I. Because a spherical homogeneous conductor [3] with the origin set at $(1, 0, -11)$ was used, we express the source-moment vector using the two tangential components $(\theta, \phi)$.

The magnetic field was generated at a 1-ms interval from $-300$ to 400 ms. The moment time courses of the three sources are shown in Fig. 2(a) for the time window between 0 and 400 ms. The white Gaussian noise was added to the generated magnetic field, and the SNR, defined as the ratio of the Frobenius norm of the signal-magnetic-field data matrix to that of

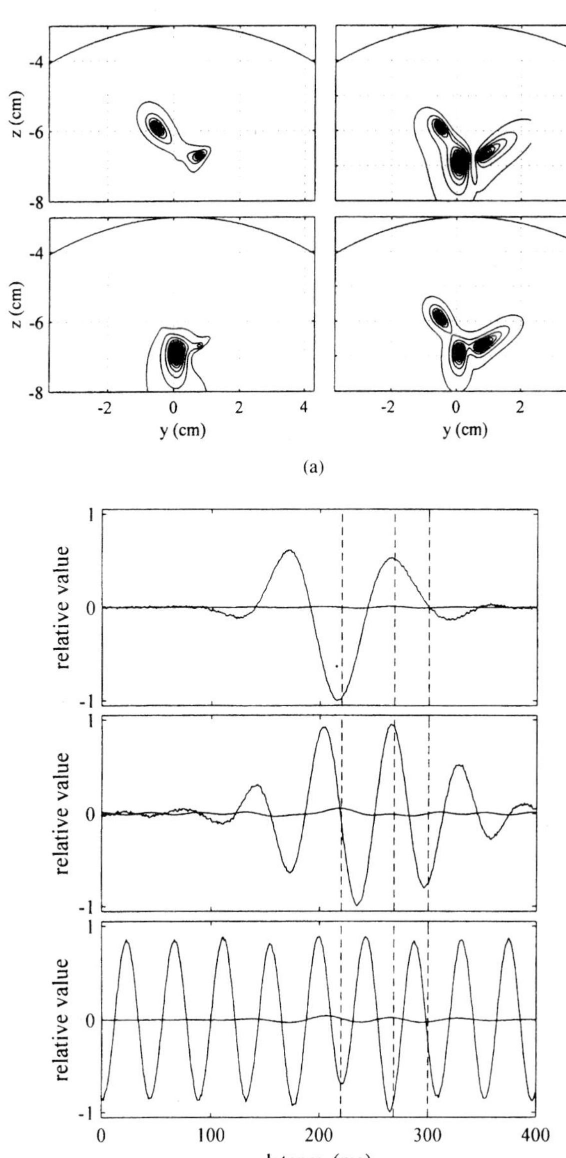

(a)

(b)

Fig. 6. (a) Results of the spatio-temporal reconstruction obtained using the proposed vector beamformer technique [(11) and (12)]. The upper-left, upper-right, and lower-left maps respectively show the snapshots of the source-moment magnitude at 220, 268, and 300 ms. The lower-right map shows the time-averaged reconstruction. (b) Estimated time courses from the first to the third sources are shown from the top to the bottom, respectively. The three vertical broken lines indicate the time instants of 220, 268, and 300 ms.

the noise matrix, was set to 18. The generated magnetic field is shown in Fig. 2(b). This SNR is higher than that in typical cases of actual MEG measurements. We used such a high SNR value because the differences in the source estimation results obtained using tested beamformer techniques can be more easily observed under such high SNR conditions; such differences might otherwise be obscured by noise effects.

### B. Spatio-Temporal Reconstruction Experiments

The spatio-temporal reconstruction was performed by using

$$\hat{s}_\phi(\boldsymbol{r},\,t) = \boldsymbol{w}_\phi^T(\boldsymbol{r})\boldsymbol{b}(t) \quad \text{and} \quad \hat{s}_\theta(\boldsymbol{r},\,t) = \boldsymbol{w}_\theta^T(\boldsymbol{r})\boldsymbol{b}(t). \quad (17)$$

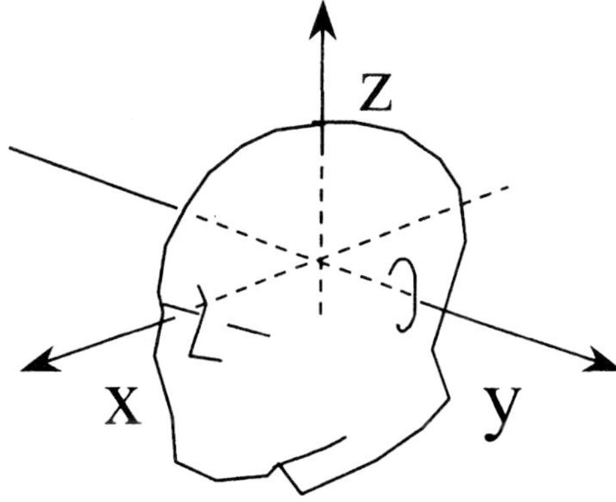



Fig. 7. The $x$, $y$, and $z$ coordinates used to express the reconstruction results in Section IV. The midpoint between the left and right preauricular points was defined as the coordinate origin. The axis directed away from the origin toward the left preauricular point was defined as the $+y$ axis, and that from the origin to the nasion was the $+x$ axis. The $+z$ axis was defined as the axis perpendicular to both these axes and was directed from the origin to the vertex.

Note that since these weight vectors are calculated for any spatial location $\boldsymbol{r}$, the source-moment distribution at any location can be reconstructed in a perfectly post-processing manner. The reconstruction region was set as an area defined by $-4 \leq y \leq 4$ and $-8 \leq z \leq -3$ on the plane $x = 1$ (as indicated by the square in Fig. 1), and the reconstruction interval was 1 mm in the $y$ and $z$ directions.

Once $\hat{s}_\phi(\boldsymbol{r},\,t)$ and $\hat{s}_\theta(\boldsymbol{r},\,t)$ were obtained, an angle representing the mean source direction in the $\phi - \theta$ plane, $\rho$, was calculated using

$$\rho = \arctan\left(\sqrt{\frac{\langle \hat{s}_\theta(t)^2 \rangle}{\langle \hat{s}_\phi(t)^2 \rangle}}\right), \quad \text{if} \quad \frac{\langle \hat{s}_\theta(t) \rangle}{\langle \hat{s}_\phi(t) \rangle} \geq 0$$

$$\rho = -\arctan\left(\sqrt{\frac{\langle \hat{s}_\theta(t)^2 \rangle}{\langle \hat{s}_\phi(t)^2 \rangle}}\right), \quad \text{if} \quad \frac{\langle \hat{s}_\theta(t) \rangle}{\langle \hat{s}_\phi(t) \rangle} < 0 \quad (18)$$

where $\langle \cdot \rangle$ indicates the average over the time window with which $R_b$ was calculated. Then, the time course expressed in the mean source direction, $\hat{s}_\parallel(\boldsymbol{r},\,t)$, and that in its orthogonal direction, $\hat{s}_\perp(\boldsymbol{r},\,t)$ were given by

$$\hat{s}_\parallel(\boldsymbol{r},\,t) = \hat{s}_\phi(\boldsymbol{r},\,t)\cos(\rho) + \hat{s}_\theta(\boldsymbol{r},\,t)\sin(\rho)$$

$$\hat{s}_\perp(\boldsymbol{r},\,t) = \hat{s}_\theta(\boldsymbol{r},\,t)\cos(\rho) - \hat{s}_\phi(\boldsymbol{r},\,t)\sin(\rho). \quad (19)$$

In the following experiments, we used $\hat{s}_\parallel(\boldsymbol{r},\,t)$ and $\hat{s}_\perp(\boldsymbol{r},\,t)$ when displaying the time course of a source activity.

To display the results of the spatio-temporal reconstruction, three time points at 220, 268, and 300 ms [marked in Fig. 2(a)] were selected. The amplitude of the second source happened to be zero at 220 ms, all the sources had nonzero amplitudes at 268 ms, and only the second source had a nonzero amplitude at 300 ms. The snapshots of the source magnitude distribution $|\hat{s}(\boldsymbol{r},\,t)| = \sqrt{\hat{s}_\phi^2(\boldsymbol{r},\,t) + \hat{s}_\theta^2(\boldsymbol{r},\,t)}$ at these three time points, and the time averaged reconstruction $\sqrt{\langle \hat{s}(\boldsymbol{r},\,t)^2 \rangle}$ were displayed in the following experiments.

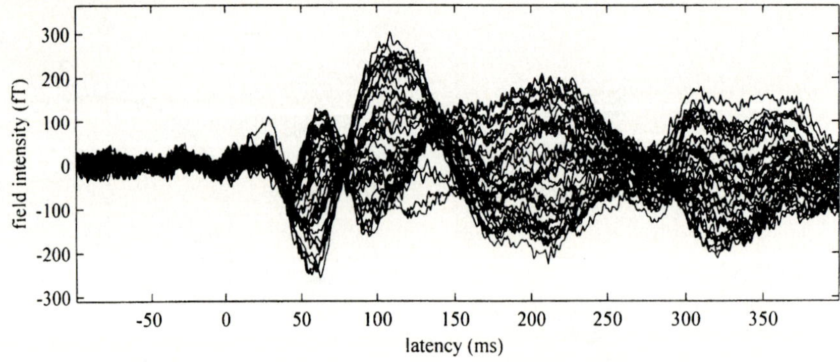

Fig. 8. The auditory-somatosensory combined response measured by simultaneously applying an auditory stimulus and a somatosensory stimulus. The auditory stimulus was a 1-kHz pure tone delivered to the subject's right ear and the somatosensory stimulus was a 30-ms-duration tactile pulse delivered to the distal segment of the right index finger. A total of 256 epochs were averaged.

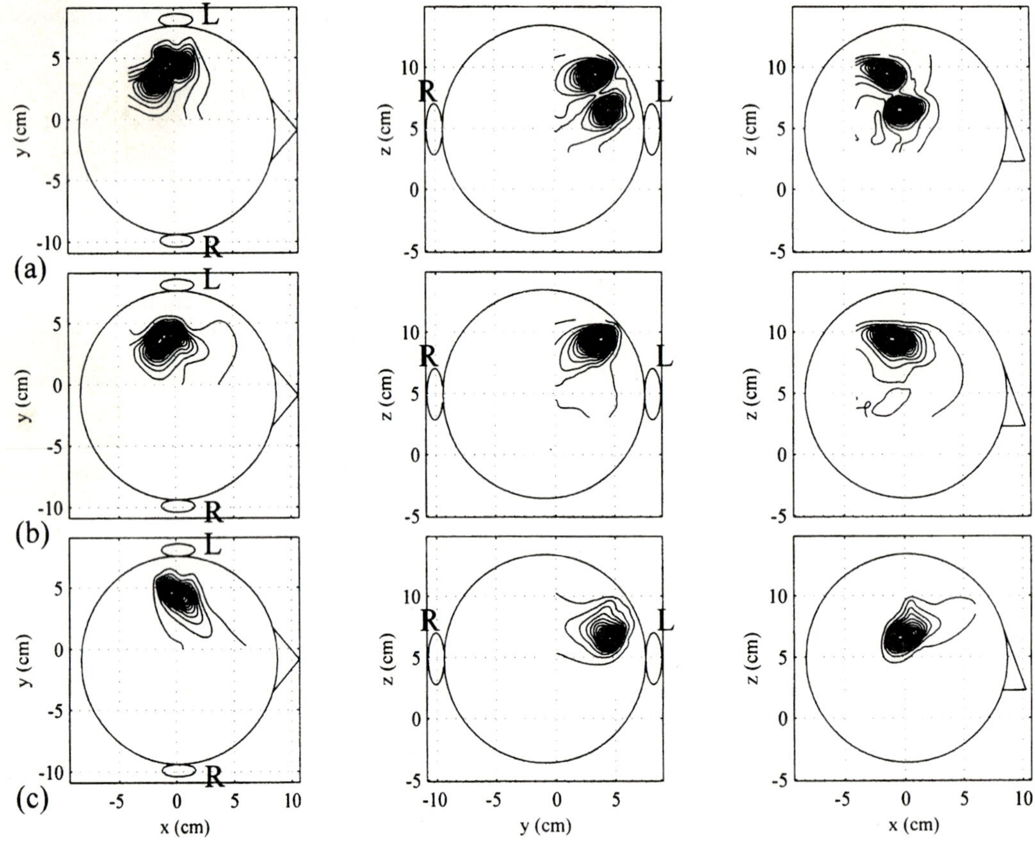

Fig. 9. Results of the spatio-temporal reconstruction from the auditory-somatosensory combined response in Fig. 8. The reconstruction was obtained using the proposed beamformer. The maximum intensity projection of the source-moment magnitude onto the axial (left), coronal (middle), and sagittal (right) slices are displayed. The source-magnitude distributions are shown at latencies of (a) 65 ms, (b) 138 ms, and (c) 194 ms. These time instants are shown by the vertical broken lines in Fig. 10.

### C. Results from Minimum-Variance Vector Beamformer

The results of the spatio-temporal reconstruction obtained using the minimum-variance vector beamformer in (6) with the normalized lead field matrix are shown in Fig. 3(a). The estimated time courses at the pixels nearest to the three source locations are shown in Fig. 3(b). These results show that the reconstruction at each instant in time was fairly noisy: the snapshot at 220 ms showed some influence from the second source, and the snapshot at 300 ms contained the activities of the first and third sources. The time-averaged reconstruction, however, clearly resolved three active sources. Note that this time-averaged reconstruction is equal to the map of the neural activity index proposed in [10],

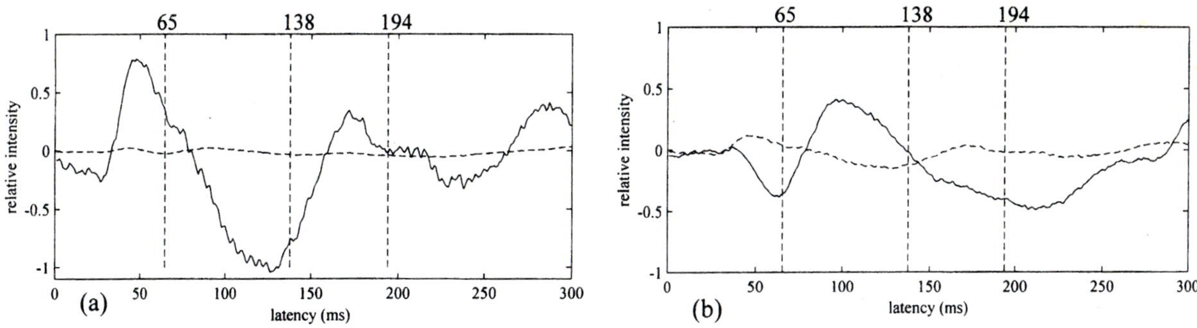

Fig. 10.   Time courses of the points nearest to (a) the primary somatosensory cortex and (b) the primary auditory cortex. The solid and broken plotted lines correspond, respectively, to $\hat{s}_\parallel(\boldsymbol{r}, t)$ and $\hat{s}_\perp(\boldsymbol{r}, t)$. Three vertical broken lines indicate the time instants of 65, 138, and 194 ms.

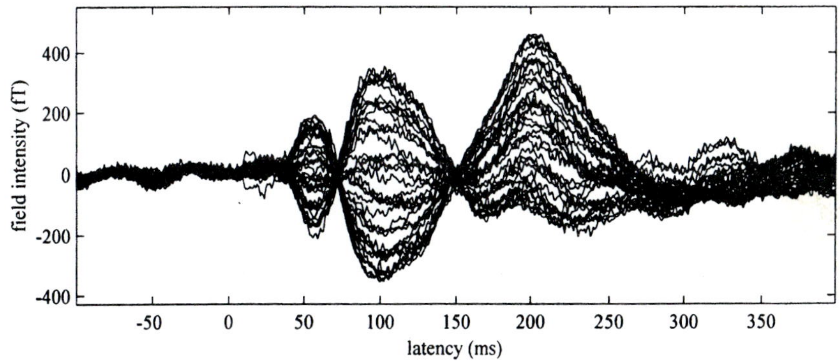

Fig. 11.   The auditory-button-press response. The data was measured with a subject who pressed a response button with his left index finger when he heard the 1-kHz pure tone delivered to his right ear. A total of 256 epochs are averaged.

because the noise was white Gaussian and the noise co-variance matrix was expressed as the unit matrix in these numerical experiments.

It is known that this poor output SNR is due to the use of the direct matrix inversion $\boldsymbol{R}_b^{-1}$ [11], [12], [16]. Thus, we next tested the minimum-variance beamformer together with the use of the regularized inverse $(\boldsymbol{R}_b + \gamma\boldsymbol{I})^{-1}$ instead of $\boldsymbol{R}_b^{-1}$. The regularization parameter was set at $0.003\lambda_1$, where $\lambda_1$ is the largest eigenvalue of $\boldsymbol{R}_b$. The results in Fig. 4(a) show that a considerable amount of blur was introduced. The estimated time courses are shown in Fig. 4(b). Fig. 4 shows that the SNR of the beamformer output was considerably increased in this case, although each time course shows some influence from neighboring sources. The results here demonstrated that the regularization leads to a tradeoff between the spatial resolution and the SNR of the beamformer output.

### D. Results from Proposed Vector Beamformer

We first show the reconstruction results from weight vectors obtained using (11) alone. This is equivalent to the vector-extended Borgiotti–Kaplan beamformer without the eigenspace projection. The results are shown in Fig. 5. Comparison between the time-averaged reconstruction in Fig. 3(a) and that in Fig. 5(a) confirms that the Borgiotti–Kaplan-type beamformer has a spatial resolution much higher than the minimum-variance beamformer. The spatio-temporal reconstruction, however, is very noisy for both cases.

We then applied the proposed vector beamformer obtained using (11) and (12) to the same computer-generated data set. The reconstructed source distributions are shown in Fig. 6(a), and the estimated time courses are shown in Fig. 6(b). Comparison between Figs. 5 and 6 confirms that the eigenspace projection can improve the SNR with almost no sacrifice of the spatial resolution. Comparing the results in Fig. 6 with the minimum-variance results in Fig. 3, we can clearly see that the proposed beamformer technique significantly improved both spatial resolution and output SNR.

### IV.  Application to Auditory-Evoked MEG Data

We applied the proposed beamformer technique to two sets of auditory-evoked MEG data to demonstrate its spatio-temporal reconstruction capability. The auditory-evoked fields were measured using the 37-channel Magnes biomagnetometer installed at the Biomagnetic Imaging Laboratory, University of California, San Francisco. The auditory stimulus was presented to the subject's right ear. The sensor array was placed above the subject's left hemisphere with the position adjusted to optimally record the N1m auditory-evoked field. The average inter-stimulus interval was 2 s, with the interval randomly varied between 1.75 s and 2.25 s. The sampling frequency was set at 1 kHz. An on-line filter with a bandwidth from 1 to 400 Hz was used, and no post-processing digital filter was applied. To express the results of reconstructing source activities in this section, we used the head coordinate system illustrated in Fig. 7.

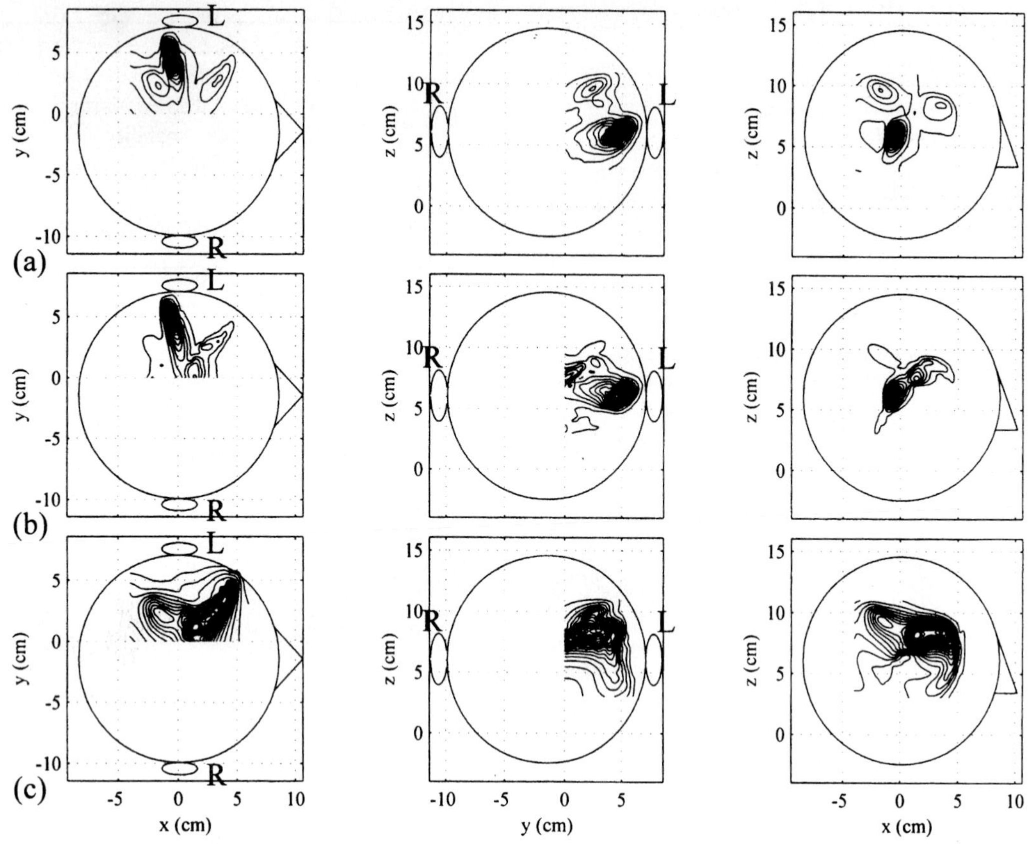

Fig. 12.    Results of the spatio-temporal reconstruction from the auditory-button-press response in Fig. 11. The maximum intensity projection of the source-moment magnitude onto the axial (left), coronal (middle), and sagittal (right) slices are displayed. The source-magnitude distributions are shown at latencies of (a) 100 ms, (b) 170 ms, and (c) 200 ms. These time instants are shown by the vertical broken lines in Fig. 13.

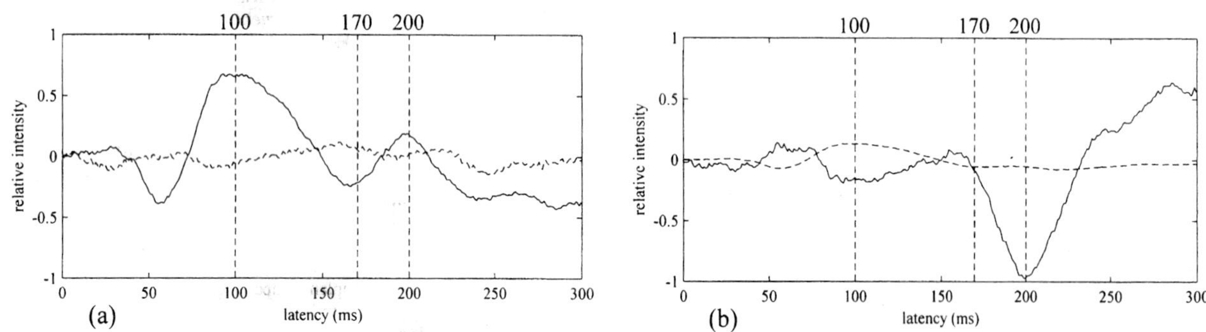

Fig. 13.    Time courses of the points nearest to (a) the primary auditory cortex and (b) the center of the motor activities. The solid and broken plotted lines correspond, respectively, to $\hat{s}_{\parallel}(\boldsymbol{r}, t)$ and $\hat{s}_{\perp}(\boldsymbol{r}, t)$. Three vertical broken lines indicate the time instants of 100, 170, and 200 ms.

The first data we tested was the auditory-somatosensory combined response measured by simultaneously applying an auditory stimulus and a somatosensory stimulus to a male subject. The auditory stimulus was a 1-kHz pure tone with a 200-ms duration, and the somatosensory stimulus was a 30-ms-duration tactile pulse (17 psi) delivered to the distal segment of the right index finger. These two stimuli started at the same time. A total of 256 epochs were measured, and the response averaged over all the epochs is shown in Fig. 8. We applied the proposed beamformer to this aver-

aged data. The data in the time window ranging from 0 to 300 ms was used for calculating the covariance matrix $\boldsymbol{R}_b$. The signal subspace dimension $Q$ was set at two because the eigenvalue spectrum of $\boldsymbol{R}_b$ showed two distinctly large eigenvalues.

The reconstructed source-magnitude maps at three latencies, 65, 138, and 194 ms, are shown in Fig. 9. The source magnitude map at 138 ms [Fig. 9(b)] contains a source activity presumably at the primary somatosensory cortex. The source magnitude map at 194 ms [Fig. 9(c)] shows a source activity at the primary auditory cortex. The map at 65 ms [Fig. 9(a)] contains both of these activities.

The time courses of the points at the primary somatosensory and auditory cortices are shown in Fig. 10(a) and (b), respectively. The coordinates of these cortices were determined from the maximum points in Fig. 9(b) and (c). Both $\hat{s}_\|(t)$ and $\hat{s}_\perp(t)$ were plotted in Fig. 10 so that we could check whether the orientation of the source was fixed or changed during the time window with which $R_b$ was calculated. In Fig. 10(a) the P50 peak, which is known to represent activity of the primary somatosensory cortex, is observed near the latency of 50 ms. In Fig. 10(b), the auditory N1m peak is observed near the latency of 100 ms. These time course plots also show that both sources were active at 65 ms, that only the primary somatosensory area was active at 138 ms, and that only the primary auditory area was active at 194 ms. These observations are consistent with the source-activity behavior shown in Fig. 9(a)–(c).

We next applied the proposed beamformer to auditory-button-press data. When we measured this data set, the subject pressed a response button with his left index finger when he heard the 1-kHz pure tone. Thus, the data should contain motor activities fairly closely time-locked to the auditory stimulus. The results obtained by averaging a total of 256 epochs are shown in Fig. 11. The proposed beamformer was applied to this averaged auditory-button-press data. The data from a time window ranging from 0 to 300 ms was used for calculating $R_b$ and the signal subspace dimension was set at two. The results of the reconstruction are shown in Fig. 12. Here, the reconstructed source-magnitude distribution at 100 ms is shown in Fig. 12(a), that at 170 ms is shown in Fig. 12(b), and that at 200 ms is shown in Fig. 12(c). The reconstructed results at 100 ms contained clear activity near the primary auditory cortex in the left temporal area. The results at 170 ms showed that the activity at the primary auditory area was still dominant. The results at 200 ms showed wide-spread activities, presumably around motor and premotor areas.

We determined the location of the primary auditory area by choosing the maximum point in Fig. 12(a), and the location of the center of the motor activities by choosing the maximum point in Fig. 12(c). The time course of the activity in the primary auditory area is shown in Fig. 13(a). The time course forms a peak near the latency around 100 ms, clearly showing the auditory N1m component. The auditory activity was relatively weak, but still dominant at the latency of 170 ms. The time course of the motor activities is shown in Fig. 13(b), which indicates that the motor activity formed a peak near 200 ms. These plots are also consistent with the results in Fig. 12.

## V. Conclusion

We have developed a novel MEG vector beamformer technique suitable for reconstructing spatio-temporal activities of neural sources. The developed beamformer is formulated in a two-step procedure: the first step extends the Borgiotti–Kaplan heamformer to the vector-type beamformer and the second step projects its weight vectors onto the signal subspace of the measurement covariance matrix. The proposed beamformer has the spatial resolution and the output SNR, both significantly higher

than those of the minimum-variance vector beamformer used in the previous investigations. Our numerical experiments verified the superiority of the proposed method, and its application to two sets of auditory MEG data demonstrated the method's spatio-temporal reconstruction capability.

### Acknowledgment

The authors would like to thank Dr. T. Roberts and S. Honma for their help in performing the auditory MEG measurements.

### References

[1] M. Hämäläinen, R. Hari, R. J. Ilmoniemi, J. Knuutila, and O. V. Lounasmaa, "Magnetoencephalography-theory, instrumentation, and applications to noninvasive studies of the working human brain," *Rev. Mod. Phys.*, vol. 65, pp. 413–497, 1993.

[2] T. P. L. Roberts, D. Poeppel, and H. A. Rowley, "Magnetoencephalography and magnetic source imaging," *Neuropsychiatry, Neuropsych... Behavioral Neurol.*, vol. 11, pp. 49–64, 1998.

[3] J. Sarvas, "Basic mathematical and electromagnetic concepts of the biomagnetic inverse problem," *Phys. Med. Biol.*, vol. 32, pp. 11–22, 1987.

[4] M. S. Hämäläinen and R. J. Ilmoniemi, "Interpreting measured magnetic fields of the brain: Estimates of current distributions," Helsinki Univ. Technol., Helsinki, Finland, Tech. Rep. TKK-F-A559, 1984.

[5] R. D. Pascual-Marqui and C. M. Michel, "Low resolution electromagnetic tomography: A new method for localizing electrical activity in the brain," *Int. J. Psychophysiol.*, vol. 18, pp. 49–65, 1994.

[6] K. Uutela, M. Hämäläinen, and E. Somersalo, "Visualization of magnetoencephalographic data using minimum current estimate," *NeuroImage*, vol. 10, pp. 173–180, 1999.

[7] I. F. Gorodnitsky and B. D. Rao, "Sparse signal reconstruction from limited data using FOCUSS: A re-weighted minimum norm algorithm," *IEEE Trans. Signal Processing*, vol. 45, pp. 600–616, Mar. 1997.

[8] B. D. Van Veen and K. M. Buckley, "Beamforming: A versatile approach to spatial filtering," *IEEE Acoust. Speech, Signal Processing Mag.*, vol. 5, pp. 4–24, Apr. 1988.

[9] M. E. Spencer, R. M. Leahy, J. C. Mosher, and P. S. Lewis, "Adaptive filters for monitoring localized brain activity from surface potential time series," in *Proc. 26th Annu. Asilomer Conf. Signals, Systems, and Computers*, Nov. 1992, pp. 156–161.

[10] B. D. Van Veen, W. van Drongelen, M. Yuchtman, and A. Suzuki, "Localization of brain electrical activity via linearly constrained minimum variance spatial filtering," *IEEE Trans. Biomed. Eng.*, vol. 44, pp. 867–880, Sept. 1997.

[11] S. E. Robinson and J. Vrba, "Functional neuroimaging by synthetic aperture magnetometry (SAM)," in *Recent Advances in Biomagnetism*, T. Yoshimoto, et al., Eds. Sendai, Japan: Tohoku Univ. Press, 1999, pp. 302–305.

[12] J. Gross and A. A. Ioannides, "Linear transformations of data space in MEG," *Phys. Med. Biol.*, vol. 44, pp. 2081–2097, 1999.

[13] G. Borgiotti and L. J. Kaplan, "Superresolution of uncorrelated interference sources by using adaptive array technique," *IEEE Trans. Antennas Propagat.*, vol. AP-27, pp. 842–845, 1979.

[14] J. Capon, "High-resolution frequency wavenumber spectrum analysis," *Proc. IEEE*, vol. 57, pp. 1408–1419, 1969.

[15] K. Sekihara, D. Poeppel, and Y. Miyashita, "Application of eigenspace beamformer to virtual depth-electrode measurement using MEG," in *Proc. 2nd Int. Symp. Noninvasive Functional Source Imaging Within the Human Brain and Heart (Biomedizinische Technik)*, S. Supek, Ed., Zagreb, Croatia, Sept. 1999, pp. 127–130.

[16] H. Cox, R. M. Zeskind, and M. M. Owen, "Robust adaptive beamforming," *IEEE Trans. Signal Process.*, vol. SP–35, pp. 1365–1376, 1987.

[17] B. D. Carlson, "Covariance matrix estimation errors and diagonal loading in adaptive arrays," *IEEE Trans. Aerosp. Electron. Syst.*, vol. 24, pp. 397–401, July 1988.

[18] L. Chang and C. C. Yeh, "Performance of DMI and eigenspace-based beamformers," *IEEE Trans. Antennas Propagat.*, vol. 40, pp. 1336–1347, Nov. 1992.

[19] L. L. Scharf, *Statistical Signal Processing: Detection, Estimation, and Time Series Analysis.* New York: Addison-Wesley, 1991.

[20] D. D. Feldman and L. J. Griffiths, "A constrained projection approach for robust adaptive beamforming," in *Proc. Int. Conf. Acoust., Speech, and Signal Processing*, Toronto, Canada, May 1991, pp. 1357–1360.

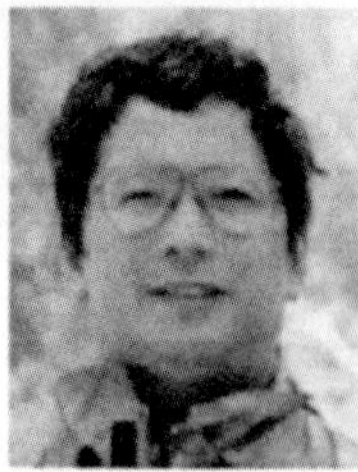

**Kensuke Sekihara** (M'88) received the M.S. degree in 1976 and the Ph.D. degree in 1987 both from Tokyo Institute of Technology, Tokyo, Japan.

From 1976 to 2000, he worked with Central Research Laboratory, Hitachi, Ltd., Tokyo, Japan. He was a visiting Research Scientist at Stanford University, Stanford, CA, from 1985 to 1986, and at Basic Development, Siemens Medical Engineering, Erlangen, Germany, from 1991 to 1992. From 1996 to 2000, He worked with "Mind Articulation" research project sponsored by Japan Science and Technology Corporation. He is currently Professor at Tokyo Metropolitan Institute of Technology, Tokyo, Japan. His research interests include the biomagnetic inverse problems, and statistical estimation theory, especially its application to noninvasive functional neuroimaging.

Dr. Sekihara is a member of the IEEE Medicine and Biology Society, and the IEEE Signal Processing Society.

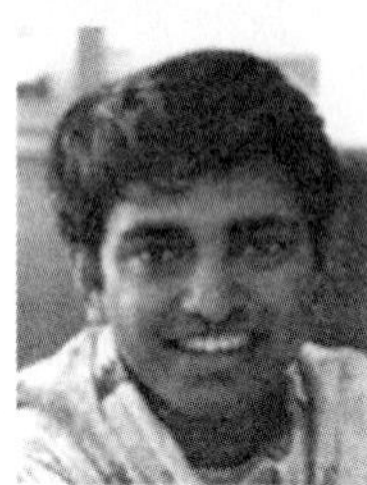

**Srikantan S. Nagarajan** received the B.S. degree in electrical engineering from the University of Madras, Madras, India, and the M.S. and Ph.D degrees from the Department of Biomedical Engineering at Case Western Reserve University, Cleveland, OH, in 1993 and 1995, respectively.

From 1995-1998, he was a Post-doctoral Fellow in the Keck Center for Integrative Neuroscience at the University of California, San Francisco (UCSF). In 1999, he was a full-time Research Scientist at Scientific Learning Corporation, Berkeley, CA, and an Adjunct Assistant Professor in the Department of Otolaryngology at UCSF. He is currently an Assistant Professor in the Department of Bioengineering at the University of Utah, Salt Lake City. His research interests in neural engineering include bioelectromagnetism, systems and computational neuroscience, and statistical signal processing.

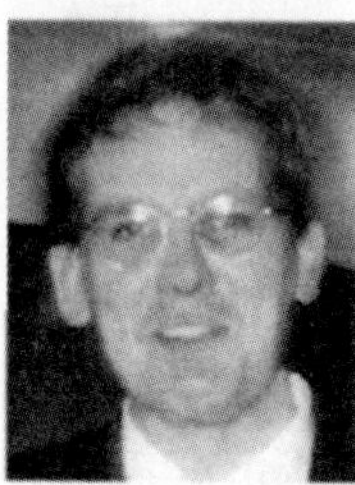

**David Poeppel** received the B.S. and Ph.D degrees in cognitive neuroscience from Massachusetts Institute of Technology, Cambridge, in 1990 and 1995, respectively.

He is currently an Assistant Professor in the Departments of Linguistics and Biology at the University of Maryland at College Park. His research uses the functional neuroimaging methods magnetoencephalography (MEG), electroencephalography (EEG, positron emission tomography (PET), and functional magnetic resonance imaging (fMRI) to investigate the neural basis of speech and language processing.

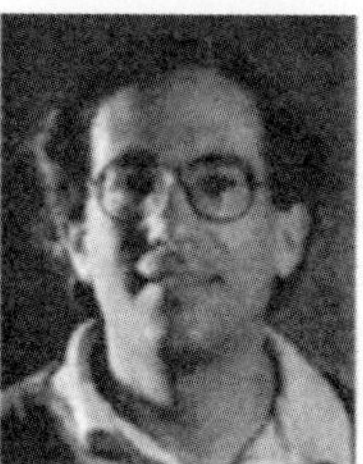

**Alec Marantz** received the B.A. degree in psycholinguistics from Oberlin College, Oberlin, OH, in 1978 and the Ph.D. degree in linguistics from the Massachusetts Institute of Technology (M.I.T.), Cambridge, MA, in 1981.

He joined the faculty at M.I.T. in 1990, where he is currently Professor of Linguistics and Head of the Department of Linguistics and Philosophy. His research interests include the syntax and morphology of natural languages, linguistic universals, and the neurobiology of language. He is currently involved in revising morphological theory within linguistics and in exploring MEG techniques to uncover how the brain process language.

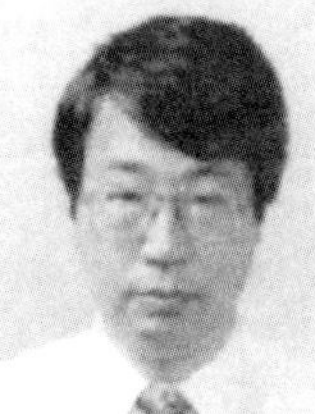

**Yasushi Miyashita** received the Ph. D. degree in physiology from the University of Tokyo, Tokyo, Japan, in 1979.

He is currently Professor and Chairman of the Physiology Department, the University of Tokyo School of Medicine, Tokyo, Japan. His reserach interests include neural basis of cognition in primates, functional imaging, and image processing with MRI, MEG, and optical devices.

# EEG Complexity as a Measure of Depth of Anesthesia for Patients

Xu-Sheng Zhang, *Senior Member, IEEE*, Rob J. Roy*, *Life Senior Member, IEEE*, and Erik Weber Jensen

*Abstract*—A new approach for quantifying the relationship between brain activity patterns and depth of anesthesia (DOA) is presented by analyzing the spatio-temporal patterns in the electroencephalogram (EEG) using Lempel–Ziv complexity analysis. Twenty-seven patients undergoing vascular surgery were studied under general anesthesia with sevoflurane, isoflurane, propofol, or desflurane. The EEG was recorded continuously during the procedure and patients' anesthesia states were assessed according to the responsiveness component of the observer's assessment of alertness/sedation (OAA/S) score. An OAA/S score of zero or one was considered asleep and two or greater was considered awake. Complexity of the EEG was quantitatively estimated by the measure $C(n)$, whose performance in discriminating awake and asleep states was analyzed by statistics for different anesthetic techniques and different patient populations. Compared with other measures, such as approximate entropy, spectral entropy, and median frequency, $C(n)$ not only demonstrates better performance (93% accuracy) across all of the patients, but also is an easier algorithm to implement for real-time use. The study shows that $C(n)$ is a very useful and promising EEG-derived parameter for characterizing the (DOA) under clinical situations.

*Index Terms*—Complexity analysis, depth of anesthesia, electroencephalogram (EEG), nonlinear dynamics, spatio-temporal pattern.

## I. Introduction

DURING surgery, reliable and noninvasive monitoring of depth of anesthesia (DOA) is highly desirable for administering the minimal amount of drugs needed to maintain adequate anesthesia and avoid intraoperative awareness [1]. Since a principal action of general anesthetic agents takes place in the brain [2], it would be reasonable to monitor the brain activity by examining the electroencephalogram (EEG) to assess the DOA [3]. However, the raw EEG is difficult to interpret. Therefore, an adequate quantitative interpretation of the EEG recordings is of great importance for the recognition of different anesthesia states. To this end, numerous efforts have been made to develop and test various EEG-derived parameters in the time-domain [4], [5], frequency-domain [6], [7], time-frequency domain [8], and bispectral domain [9]–[11]. Except for bispectral analysis, these methods use only linear computational algorithms. Nevertheless, none of these techniques have been shown to be sufficiently reliable for assessing anesthetic efficacy during routine procedures. More sophisticated signal processing technique is still required to extract information from the raw EEG for continuously evaluating the DOA.

Electrical activity of the brain (EEG) exhibits significant complex behavior with strong nonlinear and dynamical properties [12], [13]. This behavior takes the form of EEG activity patterns with different complexities. Considering this, nonlinear dynamics theory may be a better approach than traditional linear methods in characterizing the intrinsic nature of the EEG. The first important nature of the EEG lies in its dynamic "complexity," which can be characterized quantitatively by complexity analysis. Recently, there is an increasing study in this field. Correlation dimension ($D_2$) [14], a measure of system dimensional complexity, has been extensively investigated in EEG studies, such as characterization of brain function [15], evolution of human brain maturation [16], emotional processing [17], divergent and convergent thinking [18], EEG analysis for stroke patients [19] and for epileptic patients [20], brain dynamics [21], [22], and EEG complexity analysis [23]–[25]. Other complexity measures were also proposed for EEG study, such as approximate entropy ($ApEn$)[26], [27], neural complexity [28], [29], and $KL$-complexity [30]. However, off-line EEG analysis of these studies show that these measures are useful for a specific use and may not be useful for real-time clinical use, such as DOA estimation, since they usually lack effective computational methods for implementation.

Watt and Hameroff [31] found that the EEG correlation dimension ($D_2$) was different for awake and anesthetized states during anesthesia. This was further proved by Kumpf *et al.* [32]. On-line use of $D_2$ in a clinical situation is still impractical, since reliable estimation of $D_2$ requires a large quantity of data and a long calculation time. Fortunately, the Lempel–Ziv complexity measure $C(n)$ [33] can act as an alternative tool for EEG analysis, since it is well suited for characterizing the development of spatio-temporal activity patterns in high-dimensionality nonlinear systems [34], like brain and heart. Moreover, the concept of $C(n)$ is simpler to understand and its computation is easier to implement. It has been applied to study the brain function [35], brain information transmission [36], ECG dynamics study [37], epileptic seizure study [38], and movement prediction during anesthesia in animals [39].

In this study, clinical tests with humans show that, compared with other EEG-derived parameters, $C(n)$ is suitable for characterizing the EEG under anesthesia and that it can help estimate

Manuscript received July 3, 2000. This work was supported by the National Science Foundation (NSF) under Grant BES-9522639 and by the Whitaker Foundation. *Asterisk indicates corresponding author.*

X.-S. Zhang is with Siemens Medical Solutions USA, Inc., Danvers, MA 01923 USA.

*R. J. Roy is with the Department of Biomedical Engineering, Rensselaer Polytechnic Institute, Troy, NY 12180 USA, and also with the Department of Anesthesiology, Albany Medical College A-131, Albany, NY 12208 USA (e-mail: robjroy@worldnet.att.net).

E. W. Jensen is with the Center of Research in Biomedical Engineering, Polytechnic University of Barcelona, Barcelona 08028, Spain.

Publisher Item Identifier S 0018-9294(01)10236-3.

TABLE I
RESPONSIVENESS SCORES OF THE MODIFIED OBSERVER'S ASSESSMENT OF ALERTNESS/SEDATION SCALE (OAA/S) [40]

| Responsiveness | Score |
|---|---|
| Responds readily to name spoken in normal tone | 5 (alert) |
| Lethargic response to name spoken in normal tone | 4 |
| Responds only after name is called loudly and/or repeatedly | 3 |
| Responds only after mild prodding or shaking | 2 |
| Responds only after painful trapezius squeeze | 1 |
| Does not respond to painful trapezius squeeze | 0 |

the DOA in real-time on a continuous scale between the awake and asleep states. The effectiveness and feasibility of $C(n)$ for clinical use are validated by 27 human cases under four anesthesia regimens.

## II. MATERIALS AND METHODS

### A. Protocol Design and Data Collection

The patients were drawn from two different populations. Fifteen patients came from Albany Medical Center (AMC) and another 12 patients' EEG data were supplied by Dr. Erik W. Jensen of the Polytechnic University of Barcelona. The AMC patients (11 men and four women) scheduled for vascular surgery under general anesthesia were studied according to a protocol approved by the institutional review board. The Spanish patients (nine men and three women) were also scheduled for vascular surgery. Patients ranged in age from 28 to 87 years ($59 \pm 14$ year; mean $\pm$ SD) and in weight from 40 to 109 kg ($74 \pm 17$ kg). Written informed consent was obtained from all the study patients.

The concept of this study was to determine if the Lempel–Ziv complexity analysis technique, which had performed well during animal studies, was robust for different anesthetic techniques with human studies. The anesthetic technique was chosen by the anesthesiologist as fitting for that patient. Consequently, a number of different anesthetic techniques were employed. For the AMC patients there were nine etomidate, four pentothal, and two propofol inductions. Maintenance was with either isoflurane (12 cases) or desflurane (three cases). For the Spanish patients there were six sevoflurane and six propofol inductions, with maintenance by the induction agents.

For the AMC patients, they received 1–2 mg of midazolam prior to being brought into the operating room. Once in the operating room they received 50–250 $\mu$g of fentanyl, followed by 0.1–0.2 mg/kg of etomidate, or 3–4 mg/kg of pentothal, or 2 mg/kg of propofol. Five patients, received succinylcholine 0.15 mg/kg, eight received vecuronium 0.1 mg/kg, one received atracurium 0.5 mg/kg, followed by orotracheal intubation. One patient had a laryngeal mask placed.

For the Spanish patients, all patients were premedicated with 0.02 mg/kg of midazolam. Six patients had induction with 8% sevoflurane, followed by maintenance with 1%–1.6% sevoflurane. The six propofol patients were induced using a Diprifusor on a syringe pump with a target concentration of 5 $\mu$g/ml to be achieved within 5 min.

The DOA was assessed using the responsiveness component of the observer's assessment of alertness/sedation (OAA/S) rating scale (Table I) [40]. This assessment procedure involves introduction of progressively more intense stimulation, ranging from a moderate speaking voice to physical shaking or moderate noxious stimuli (trapezius squeeze), until a response is observed. If the score is greater than one (i.e., larger or equal to two), the state is awake-state, otherwise, asleep-state (i.e., the score is one or zero). All assessments of sedation level were performed by one investigator at each institution to minimize inter-observer variability.

For the AMC patients, EEG electrodes (silver/silver chloride disposable electrodes, Nicolet Biomedical, Inc., Madison, WI) were positioned at $F_{p1}$ and $F_{p2}$, with the reference electrode at Fpz (positive at left forehead, negative at right forehead, reference at middle forehead). The impedance of each electrode was less than 4 k$\Omega$. The EEG was recorded continuously using an Axon Systems Sentinel-4 EEG/EP monitor. From the postamplifier port of the Axon monitor, after anti-aliasing filter the analog EEG signals were continuously digitized (sampling rate 200 Hz) into a computer by an analog-to-digital card (Data Translation TM DT2801) with 12-bit resolution. At the same time, time-synchronized markers describing all clinical assessment events were also collected.

The Spanish EEG data were recorded by a Danmeter monitor (Odense, Denmark) at a sampling rate of 880 Hz, with a 1–200 Hz bandpass filter. The EEG electrodes were placed at $F_z - T_5$ with reference electrode at $F_{p1}$ (positive at middle forehead, negative at left mastoid, reference at left forehead). In order to have the same sampling frequency with AMC data, the raw Spanish data was down-sampled to 200 Hz after the anti-aliasing filtering.

In this study, only one channel was used for analysis, since previous studies [5], [8], [39] have shown that using only one channel is sufficient for estimating DOA.

The values of $C(n)$ at each OAA/S score were calculated by averaging all the values during the 30-s interval immediately before assessment.

After signal processing a total of 487 data sets were obtained including 231 awake and 256 asleep, each set having the EEG-derived parameter values and the corresponding state (asleep or awake). The data obtained from different anesthetic techniques were processed separately. The AMC data and the Spanish data were also processed separately and then both data sets were combined and processed together.

### B. Lempel–Ziv Complexity Analysis

Lempel–Ziv complexity analysis is based on a coarse-graining of the measurements, i.e., the signal to be analyzed is transformed into a sequence whose elements are only a few symbols. The complexity counter $c(n)$ measures the number of distinct patterns contained in the given sequence. Briefly described, a sequence $P = s_1, s_2, s_3, \ldots, s_n$ (where, $s_1$, $s_2$, etc. denote characters, for example, zero or one) is scanned from left to right and the complexity counter $c(n)$ is increased by one unit every time a new subsequence of consecutive characters is encountered in the scanning process. After normalization, the complexity measure reflects the rate of new pattern occurrences with time.

*Algorithm:* The basic idea of Lempel–Ziv complexity analysis is as follows. Let $S$ and $Q$ denote, respectively, subsequence of the sequence $P = s_1, s_2, s_3, \ldots, s_n$ and $SQ$ be the concatenation of $S$ and $Q$, while sequence $SQ\pi$ is derived from $SQ$ after its last character is deleted ($\pi$ means the operation to delete the last character in the sequence). Let $\nu(SQ\pi)$ denote the vocabulary of all different subsequences of $SQ\pi$. At the beginning, $C(n) = 1$, $S = s_1$, $Q = s_2$, therefore, $SQ\pi = s_1$. For generalization, now suppose $S = s_1, s_2, \ldots, s_r$, $Q = s_{r+1}$, then $SQ\pi = s_1, s_2, \ldots, s_r$; if $Q \in \nu(SQ\pi)$, then $Q$ is a subsequence of $SQ\pi$, not a new sequence. $S$ needn't change and now renew $Q$ to be $s_{r+1}, s_{r+2}$, then judge if $Q$ belongs to $\nu(SQ\pi)$ or not; and continue until $Q \notin \nu(SQ\pi)$, now $Q = s_{r+1}, s_{r+2}, \ldots, s_{r+i}$ is not a subsequence of $SQ\pi = s_1, s_2, \ldots, s_r, s_{r+1}, \ldots, s_{r+i-1}$, so increase $c(n)$ by one. Thereafter, combine $S$ with $Q$ and $S$ is renewed to be $S = s_1, s_2, \ldots, s_r, s_{r+1}, \ldots, s_{r+i}$, at the same time take $Q$ as $Q = s_{r+i+1}$. Repeat these procedures until $Q$ is the last character. At this time, the number of different subsequences is $c(n)$, i.e., the measure of complexity. This algorithm uses only two simple operations, comparison and accumulation, which makes the computation of $c(n)$ easy to implement.

In order to obtain a complexity measure which is independent of the sequence length, we use a normalized complexity measure $C(n)$.

Suppose the number of different symbols in a symbol set $A$ is $\alpha$ and the length of sequence $P \in A^*$ is $l(P) = n$, where $A^*$ denotes the set of all finite length sequences over the finite symbol set $A$. In [33], it has been proved that the upper bound of $c(n)$ is given by

$$c(n) < \frac{n}{(1 - \varepsilon_n) \log(n)}, \qquad (1)$$

where, $\varepsilon_n$ is a small quantity and $\varepsilon_n \to 0 \quad (n \to \infty)$. Therefore, in general $n/\log(n)$ is the upper bound of $c(n)$, where $n = l(P)$ and the base of the logarithm log is $\alpha$. i.e.,

$$\lim_{n \to \infty} c(n) = b(n) \equiv \frac{n}{\log_\alpha(n)}$$

For a 0–1 sequence, $\alpha = 2$, therefore

$$b(n) \equiv \frac{n}{\log_2(n)} \qquad (2)$$

and $c(n)$ can be normalized via this limit

$$C(n) = \frac{c(n)}{b(n)}. \qquad (3)$$

Due to the pattern formation in the given sequence, $C(n)$ is usually less than one. It reflects the arising rate of new pattern

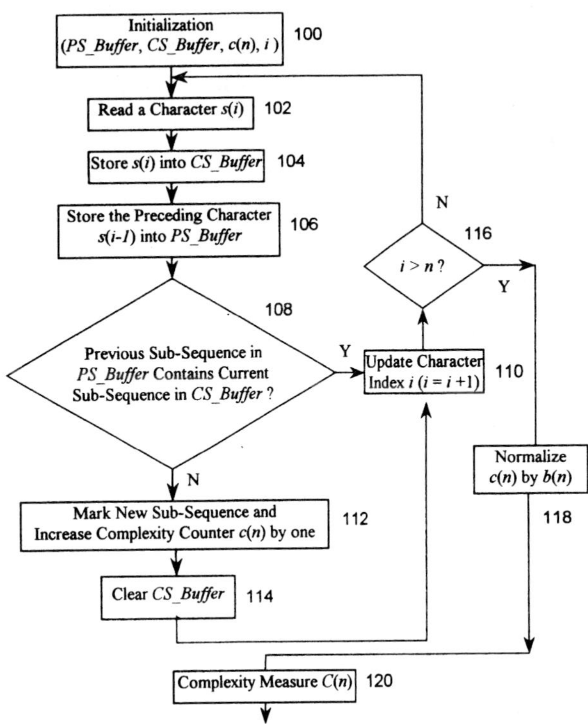


Fig. 1. A general flow diagram for the algorithm to calculate the complexity measure $C(n)$ of a sequence $P = s_1, s_2, \ldots, s_n$.

along with the sequence. For the details on the mathematical proofs of this measure see [33] and [34].

A general flow diagram for the algorithm to calculate the $C(n)$ of a sequence $P = s_1, s_2, \ldots, s_n$ is depicted in Fig. 1, where two character buffers, previous subsequence buffer ($PS_Buffer$) and current subsequence buffer ($CS_Buffer$), are used to hold two subsequences of $P$. At the initialization step 100, $PS_Buffer$ and $CS_Buffer$ are cleared to null, complexity counter $c(n)$ is cleared to zero, and character index ($i$) is set to one. In step 102, a character $s(i)$ is read from the sequence $P$, starting from the first character $s(1)$. In step 104, the character $s(i)$ is stored into $CS_Buffer$ and concatenated with the subsequence already in the buffer. In step 106, the character $s(i - 1)$, preceding $s(i)$, is stored into $PS_Buffer$ and concatenated with the subsequence already in the buffer. If $i = 1$ (i.e., for the first character $s(1)$), $s(i - 1)$ (i.e., $s(0)$) is null. In step 108, the current subsequence located in the $CS_Buffer$ is compared to the previous subsequence located in the $PS_Buffer$. If the previous subsequence does contain the current subsequence (i.e., the current subsequence can be copied from the previous one), then the current subsequence is not a new sequence and step 110 just updates the character index $i(i = i + 1)$ for reading the next character. If the previous subsequence does not contain the current subsequence, then the current subsequence is a new one and in step 112 the new subsequence is marked and the complexity counter $c(n)$ is increased by one and $CS_Buffer$ is cleared to null in step 114 and then the process continues with step 110 to update the character index $i$. In step 116, the current index $i$ is compared to $n$ (the length of the sequence $P$). If $i$ is not larger than $n$,

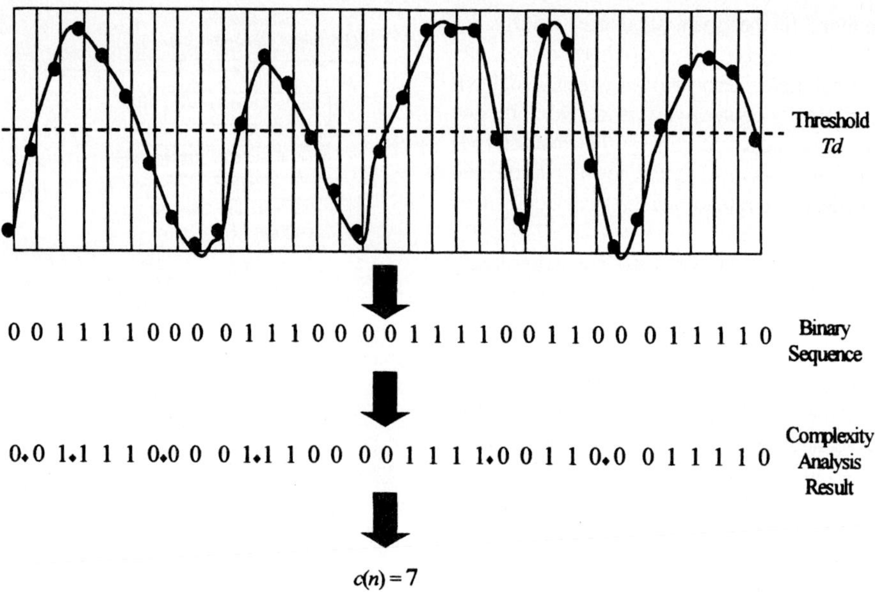



Fig. 2. An illustration showing how to transform a segment of EEG signal series into a binary sequence by threshold method and the result of complexity analysis on the binary sequence.

then a new character $s(i)$ is read in step 102. If $i$ is larger than $n$ (i.e., out of the length of the sequence $P$), then the scanning process is terminated. In step 118, the complexity counter $c(n)$ is normalized by the upper boundary value $b(n)$ to the complexity measure $C(n)$ in step 120. As can be seen, the $c(n)$ calculation which is the key part of the algorithm uses just two simple operations: character comparison and number accumulation. Therefore, the algorithm is very easy to implement by software or hardware (either in digital electronics, or with low computational overhead on a microprocessor).

*Example:* In order to easily understand the calculation of complexity measure, one example is given as follows in details. Fig. 2 shows one segment of an analog EEG signal waveform represented by a solid curve. After filtering, the signal is digitized at every sampling interval of the grid. The solid dots "•" on the waveform denote the digital data samples. The horizontal dashed line, across the figure, denotes a threshold $Td$. Using $Td$, the data series is transformed into the sequence $P$ which contains EEG activity patterns. In this sequence, $P$, if the corresponding dot "•;" is above the $Td$, then the character $s(i)$ corresponding to the "•" is "1", otherwise, it is "0". The resulting sequence is $P = 001\,111\,000\,011\,100\,001\,111\,001\,100\,011\,110$ (length $n = 33$). From this sequence $P$, the number of different subsequences (as determined by the complex counter $c(n)$) contained in $P$ are calculated by complexity analysis as follows. Symbol "♦" denotes the end of each different subsequence.

1) First character (i.e., in this case zero) is always a new one. Therefore, the first subsequence is $\rightarrow 0$♦.

2) The second character of $P$ is zero and this is identical to the first subsequence. In this case, old subsequence $S = 0$, the current subsequence $Q = 0$, concatenated subsequence $SQ = 00$ and previous subsequence $SQ\pi = 0$. Therefore, $SQ\pi$ contains $Q$, so $Q$ is not a new subsequence $\rightarrow 0$♦$0$.

3) The third character of $P$ is one. The old subsequence (before "♦") is zero and, therefore, $S = 0$, the current subsequence $Q = 01$, concatenated subsequence $SQ = 001$ and previous subsequence $SQ\pi = 00$. Therefore, $SQ\pi$ does not contain $Q$, so $Q$ is a new subsequence $\rightarrow 0$♦$01$♦.

4) The fourth character of $P$ is one. The old subsequence (before the second "♦") $S = 001$, the current subsequence $Q = 1$, concatenated subsequence $SQ = 0011$ and previous subsequence $SQ\pi = 001$. Therefore, $SQ\pi$ contains $Q$, so $Q$ is not a new subsequence $\rightarrow 0$♦$01$♦$1$.

5) The fifth character is a one. The old subsequence (before the second "♦") $S = 001$. The current subsequence $Q = 11$. $SQ = 00111$ and previous subsequence $SQ\pi = 0011$. Therefore, $SQ\pi$ contains $Q$, so $Q$ is not a new subsequence $\rightarrow 0$♦$01$♦$11$.

6) The sixth character is a one. The old subsequence (before the second "♦") $S = 001$. The current subsequence $Q = 111$. $SQ = 001\,111$ and previous $SQ\pi = 00\,111$. $SQ\pi$ contains $Q$, so $Q$ is not a new subsequence $\rightarrow 0$♦$01$♦$111$.

7) The seventh character is a zero. The old subsequence (before the second "♦") $S = 001$. The current subsequence $Q = 1110$. $SQ = 0011\,110$, $SQ\pi = 001\,111$. $SQ\pi$ does not contain $Q$, so $Q$ is a new subsequence $\rightarrow 0$♦$01$♦$1110$♦.

8) The eighth character is a zero. The old subsequence (before the third "♦") $S = 0011\,110$. The current subsequence $Q = 0$. $SQ = 00\,111\,100$, $SQ\pi = 0011\,110$. $SQ\pi$ contains $Q$, so $Q$ is not a new subsequence $\rightarrow 0$♦$01$♦$1110$♦$0$.

9) The ninth character is a zero. The old subsequence (before the third "♦") $S = 0011\,110$. The current subsequence $Q = 00$. $SQ = 001\,111\,000$, $SQ\pi =$

00 111 100. $SQ\pi$ contains $Q$, so $Q$ is not a new subsequence $\rightarrow$ 0◆01◆1110◆00.

10) The tenth character is a zero. The old subsequence (before the third "◆") $S = 0\,011\,110$. The current subsequence $Q = 000$. $SQ = 0\,011\,110\,000$, $SQ\pi = 001\,111\,000$. $SQ\pi$ contains $Q$, so $Q$ is not a new subsequence $\rightarrow$ 0◆01◆1110◆000.

11) The eleventh character is a one. The old subsequence (before the third "◆") $S = 0\,011\,110$. The current subsequence $Q = 0001$. $SQ = 00\,111\,100\,001$, $SQ\pi = 0\,011\,110\,000$. $SQ\pi$ does not contain $Q$, so $Q$ is a new subsequence $\rightarrow$ 0◆01◆1110◆0001.

12) The 12th character is a one. The old subsequence (before the fourth "◆") $S = 00\,111\,100\,001$. The current subsequence $Q = 1$. $SQ = 001\,111\,000\,011$, $SQ\pi = 00\,111\,100\,001$. $SQ\pi$ contains $Q$, so $Q$ is not a new subsequence $\rightarrow$ 0◆01◆1110◆0001◆1.

By this process the, sequence $P$ is scanned and segmented as follows:

$$P = 0◆01◆1110◆0001◆1\,100\,001\,111◆00\,110◆0\,011\,110$$

The number of subsequence (i.e., distinct patterns) divided by "◆" in $P$ is seven and this is the complexity counter $c(n)$. The corresponding complexity measure $C(n)$ can be further obtained by normalization.

*Comments on $C(n)$ Calculation:* In this study, the simplest way is selected to convert EEG samples $\{x_i | i = 1, 2, \ldots, n\}$ into a sequence of characters (zero and one), $n$ is the length of data segment to be analyzed (i.e., the window length): within the window, the mean $x_m = (1/n)\sum_{i=1}^{n} x_i$ is estimated as a threshold $Td$. By comparison with the threshold, EEG data samples are converted into a 0–1 sequence $P = s_1, s_2, \ldots, s_n$: if $x_i < x_m$, $s_i = 0$, otherwise $s_i = 1$. From the sequence $P$, $C(n)$ can be estimated using the previous algorithm. Fig. 3(A) shows one curve of $C(n)$ against the length of $n$ obtained by making complexity analysis on one EEG recording under awake state for one patient via this 0–1 sequence conversion. It can be seen that $C(n)$ declines quickly at the beginning, oscillates and tends to a final stable value (about 0.78) at one certain $n$, which is different for different EEG recordings. For all the available EEG recordings, the average of this $n$, where $C(n)$ attains stability, is 6000. Therefore, $n = 6000$ is used as the window length for all the calculation of $C(n)$ throughout this study.

For comparison, another sequence conversion method is also tested. Within the window, from the EEG samples, the mean $x_m$, maximum $x_{max}$ and minimum $x_{min}$ are calculated. Two thresholds are obtained: $Td1 = x_m - |x_{min}|/16$ and $Td2 = x_m + |x_{max}|/16$. Then the EEG data are converted into a 0–1–2 sequence $P = s_1, s_2, \ldots, s_n$: if $x_i \leq Td1$, $s_i = 0$; if $Td1 < x_i < Td2$, $s_i = 1$; if $x_i >= Td2$, $s_i = 2$. Fig. 3(B) shows the curve of $C(n)$ against the length of $n$ obtained from the same EEG recording as used in Fig. 3(A) via this 0–1–2 sequence conversion. It can be seen that when $n$ is 10 000 the $C(n)$ is still not stable and oscillates around 0.78. Running the algorithm through the available EEG recordings, statistics show that for this case the $n$ needs to be larger than 12 000 to obtain a stable $C(n)$ value. However, the calculation time of $C(n)$ exponen-

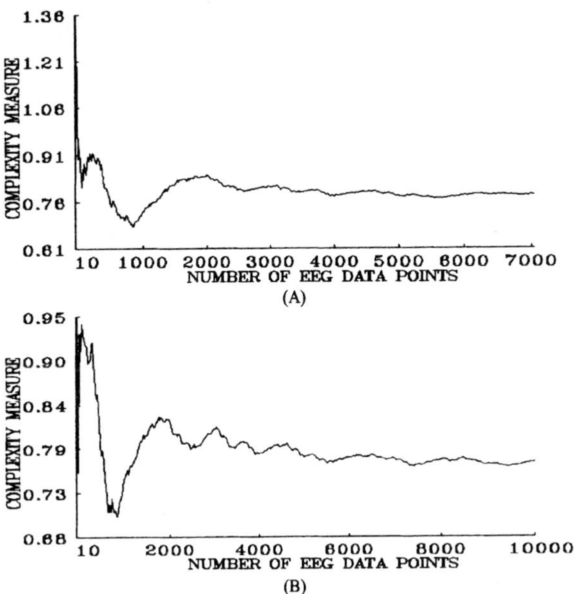

Fig. 3. The curve of $C(n)$ against the length of $n$ obtained by making complexity analysis on the same EEG recording under awake state for one patient via different sequence conversion methods: (A) 0–1 sequence conversion and (B) 0–1–2 sequence conversion.

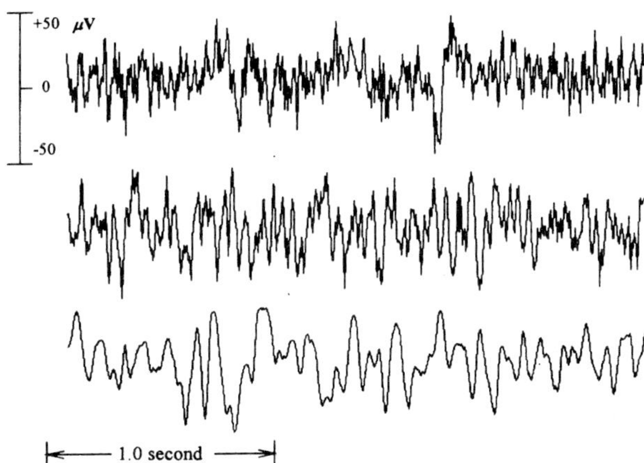


Fig. 4. Raw EEG waveform recorded from one patient under sevoflurane at around 10, 80, and 150 s, respectively, corresponding to awake state, intermediate state and asleep state [the corresponding figure of $C'(n)$ against time see Fig. 5(A)].

tially increases with $n$. Although 0–1–2 conversion can keep more information of the EEG than a 0–1 conversion during the coarse-graining process, the 0–1 conversion method is selected in this study, considering that it is simpler, easier to implement and needs less data and time for calculation. Moreover, previous studies [35]–[39] show that 0–1 conversion is enough to study the dynamic complexity of a system.

## III. RESULTS

### A. On-Line Operation of the Complexity Analysis

On-line operation is used to investigate, by EEG complexity analysis, brain dynamic behavior under anesthesia. In addition to displaying the raw EEG data, by consecutively shifting the

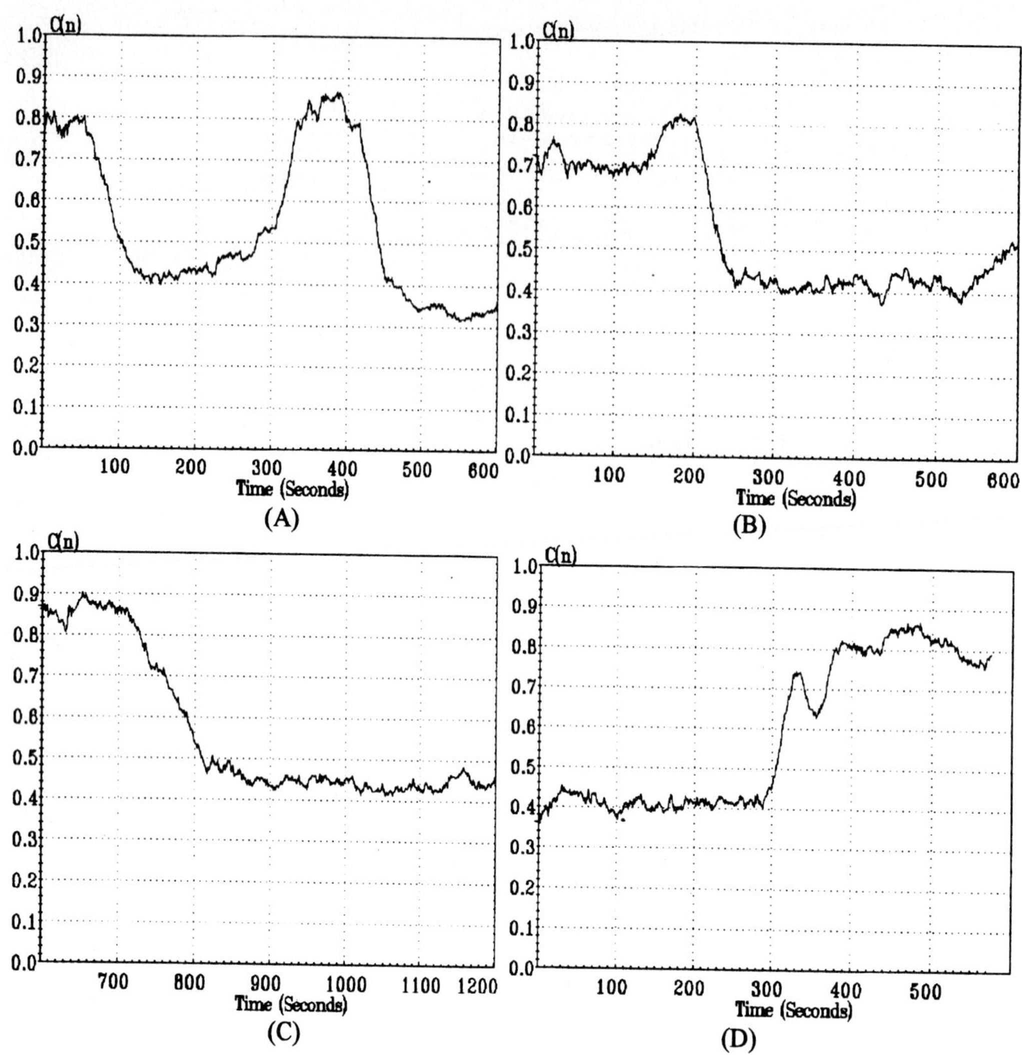

Fig. 5. Complexity measure $C(n)$ against time (part of the whole case) during different cases with different anesthetic regimens. (A) under sevoflurane anesthesia, patient entered asleep- state from awake-state at 1.5 min (i.e., 90 s), returned into awake-state at 5.3 min (i.e., 318 s), and re-entered asleep-state at 7.6 min (i.e., 456 s); (B) under isoflurane anesthesia, patient entered asleep-state from awake-state at 4 min (i.e., 240 s); (C) under propofol anesthesia, patient entered asleep-state from awake-state at 13.3 min (i.e., 798 s); and (D) under desflurane anesthesia, patient woke from asleep-state at 5.4 min (i.e., 324 s).

analysis window 200 points (i.e., ones) forward for the next analysis of the patient's brain activity patterns, the EEG signal is converted into a DOA number between 0.0 (indicating asleep) and 1.0 (fully awake), represented by $C(n)$. The average time needed for estimating $C(n)$ is about 120 ms on our DELL PC (with Intel 266-MHz Pentium II processor). Therefore, it is computationally fast and can be easily implemented for real-time use. The EEG raw signal is not easy to interpret quantitatively. Fig. 4 illustrates three raw EEG waveforms recorded from one patient under sevoflurane at around 10, 80, and 150 s, respectively, corresponding to awake state, intermediate state and asleep state. [corresponding figure of $C(n)$ against time see Fig. 5(A)]. Fig. 5 demonstrates $C(n)$ against time (part of the whole case) for four different patients under different anesthetic techniques.

It can be seen that $C(n)$ works very well in tracking a patient's depth and trend of anesthesia, especially at the state-turning points (from awake to asleep or from asleep to awake). During the procedure, the state of the anesthesia changed with the adjustment of the amount of anesthetic. The complexity measure $C(n)$ continuously demonstrates different values. The deeper the DOA, the smaller the value of $C(n)$. $C(n)$ increases while decreasing the DOA (from asleep to awake) and decreases while increasing the DOA (from awake to asleep). As can be seen, $C(n)$ can not only capture subtle changes in the different EEG spatio-temporal patterns during the same state, but also capture changes between different states (asleep and awake). Transitions between stages may be very gradual, making it difficult to pinpoint their occurrence, however, $C(n)$ clearly and quickly tracks this transition in a timely manner. Moreover, $C(n)$ is sensitive enough to the pattern changes in the EEG caused by the anesthetic agent, which indicates the usefulness of $C(n)$ as a feature for characterizing the DOA.

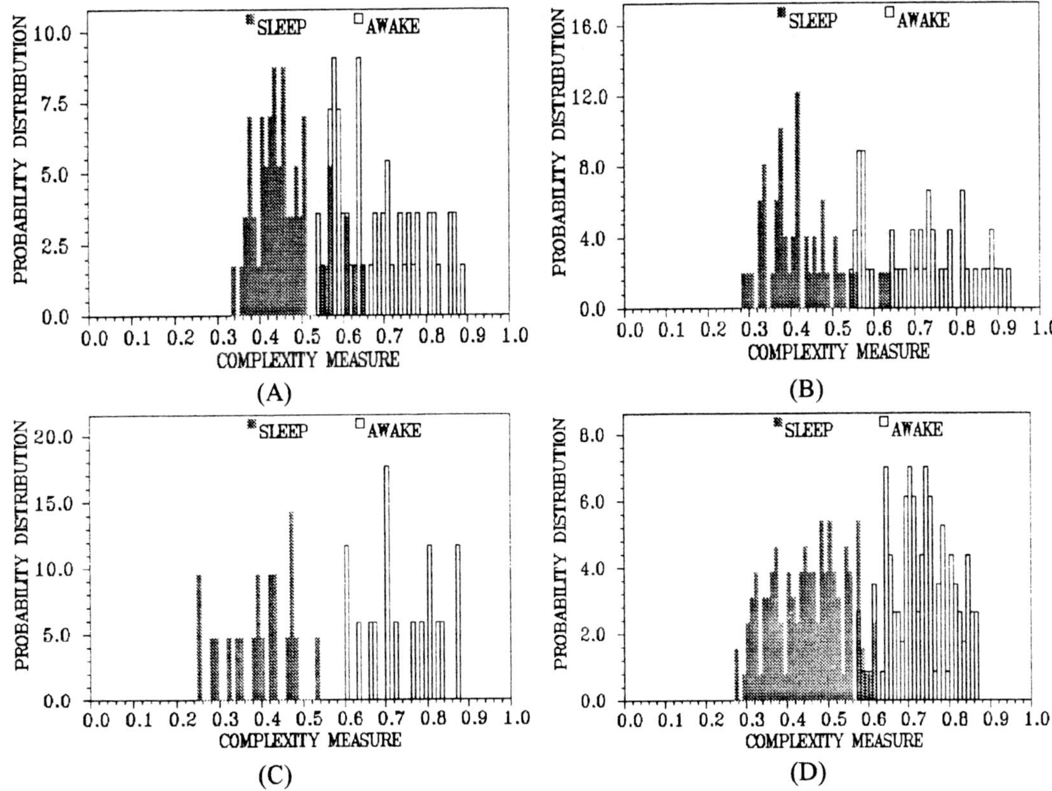

Fig. 6. $C(n)$ PDFs for different anesthetic techniques. (A) Propofol: 57 asleep-state and 55 awake-state data sets from six Spanish patients. (B) Sevoflurane: 49 asleep-state and 45 awake-state data sets from six Spanish patients. (C) Desflurane: 21 asleep-state and 17 awake state data sets from three AMC patients. (D)Isoflurane: 129 asleep-state and 114 awake-state data sets from 12 AMC patients.

TABLE II

TEST RESULTS ON DIFFERENT ANESTHETIC TECHNIQUES BY "THRESHOLD METHOD" TO DISCRIMINATE THE AWAKE AND ASLEEP STATES USING $C(n)$

| Anesthetic Technique | Threshold | State | Sensitivity (%) | Specificity (%) | Accuracy (%) |
|---|---|---|---|---|---|
| Sevoflurane | 0.562 | Awake | 93 | 94 | 94 |
| | | Asleep | 94 | 93 | 94 |
| Isoflurane | 0.590 | Awake | 96 | 96 | 96 |
| | | Asleep | 96 | 96 | 96 |
| Propofol | 0.569 | Awake | 91 | 91 | 91 |
| | | Asleep | 91 | 91 | 91 |
| Desflurane | 0.565 | Awake | 100 | 100 | 100 |
| | | Asleep | 100 | 100 | 100 |

Sensitivity = TP/(TP/FN); Specificity =TN/(TN + FP); Accuracy = (TP + TN)/(TP + FN + TP +FN), where TP: true positive; FN = false negative, TN + true negative, and FP =false positive.

### B. For Different Anesthetic Techniques

The overall results of testing $C(n)$ on the patients under sevoflurane, isoflurane, propofol, and desflurane anesthesia using a threshold method to distinguish between awake and asleep states are listed in Table II. The criterion for selecting the threshold is that it can simultaneously optimize the sensitivity and specificity in identifying these two states. probability distributions (PDFs) of $C(n)$ for different anesthetic techniques under asleep and awake states are shown in Fig. 6.

### C. For Different Patient Populations

The overall results of testing $C(n)$ on AMC patients, Spanish patients and AMC plus Spanish patients using a threshold method to distinguish between awake and asleep states are listed in Table III. A confidence estimation method suggested by Highleyman [41] was used to determine the 95% confidence intervals. For the sample size of 487, the 95% confidence interval of the identification rate of 93% is 90%~95%.

PDFs of $C(n)$ for different patient populations under asleep and awake states are shown in Fig. 7.

From the distribution for all of patients, we obtain the following statistics:

For Awake: Max = 0.929, Min = 0.534, Mean = 0.722, SD(standard deviation) = 0.094

For Asleep: Max = 0.644, Min = 0.249, Mean = 0.443, SD(standard deviation) = 0.084

TABLE III
TEST RESULTS ON DIFFERENT PATIENT POPULATIONS BY "THRESHOLD METHOD" TO DISCRIMINATE THE AWAKE AND ASLEEP STATES USING $C(n)$

| Patient Source | Threshold | State | Sensitivity (%) | Specificity (%) | Accuracy (%) |
|---|---|---|---|---|---|
| AMC | 0.600 | Awake | 96 | 97 | 97 |
| | | Asleep | 97 | 96 | 97 |
| Spain | 0.565 | Awake | 90 | 92 | 91 |
| | | Asleep | 92 | 90 | 91 |
| AMC + Spain | 0.574 | Awake | 93 | 93 | 93 |
| | | Asleep | 93 | 93 | 93 |

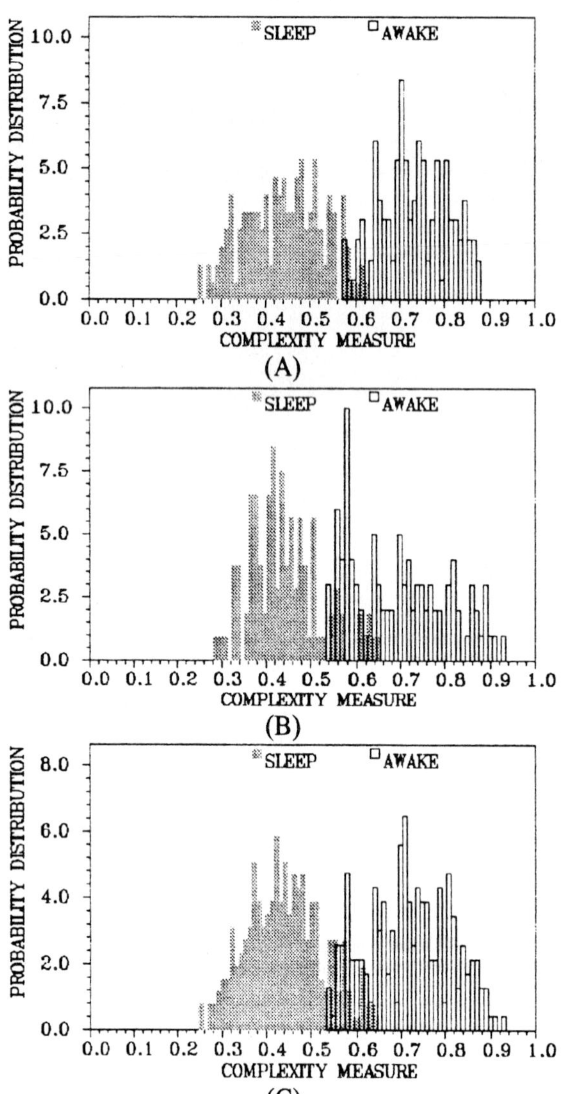


Fig. 7. $C(n)$ PDFs for different patient populations. (A) AMC patients: 150 asleep-state and 131 awake-state data sets from 15 patients. (B) Spanish patients: 106 asleep-state and 100 awake-state data sets from 12 patients. (C) AMC and Spanish patients: 256 asleep-state and 231 awake-state data sets from 27 patients.

### D. Comparison With Other Analyses

It would be insightful to briefly compare the $C(n)$ complexity analysis with other methods over the same human EEG database. Therefore, another emerging complexity measure, *ApEn* proposed by Pincus [26], [27], which has been studied for DOA

estimation [42], [43], was selected to compare with $C(n)$ analysis. Moreover, the commonly used spectral analysis methods, spectral entropy (*SE*) [45] and median frequency (*MF*) [6], [7] are also used for comparison.

*ApEn* measures the logarithmic likelihood that runs of patterns in the EEG, that are close, remain close on the next incremental comparisons. It is a nonnegative number with larger numbers indicating more complexity, unpredictability and randomness (for a detailed algorithm, see [26], [27]n and [44]).

*SE* quantifies the spectral complexity of the EEG signal and can be estimated from the normalized power spectral density by fast Fourier transform (FFT) [45].

Median frequency (*MF*) is the frequency below which 50% of the energy of the signal contained. *MF* can be estimated by FFT [6], [7].

Test results on the database from AMC plus Spanish patients by these analyses are listed in Table IV, respectively.

Only the performance (89%) of *ApEn* is comparable with the one (93.0%) of $C(n)$. However, the time needed for computation of *ApEn* is about 50 times more than that needed for $C(n)$. Moreover, the algorithm of *ApEn* is much more complex than the one of $C(n)$.

### IV. DISCUSSION

As can be seen, the $C(n)$ complexity analysis method is intuitively pleasing. In the awake-state, the brain is active, so the complexity of EEG dynamics is high. In the asleep-state, the brain activity is depressed by the anesthetic and results in a loss of complexity, so the complexity is low. States between awake and asleep have an intermediate complexity value with gradual scaling (see Fig. 5). The EEG test database used in this study were obtained from 27 patients from two different populations under four different anesthetic techniques. Nevertheless, the $C(n)$ threshold values for discriminating awake and asleep states were quite similar for different populations or for different anesthetic techniques. The accuracy obtained with the AMC patients was 97% whereas the accuracy obtained with the Spanish patients was 91% and the overall accuracy of 93% for all patients is still quite good (see Table III). For the four different anesthetic techniques, the accuracy is 94%, 96%, 91%, and 100% for sevoflurane, isoflurane, propofol and desflurane, respectively (see Table II). The measure $C(n)$ is better than *ApEn* and traditional spectral measures (e.g., *SE* and *MF*) in discriminating anesthesia states (see Table IV). This demonstrates that the $C(n)$ is a useful parameter in characterizing EEG dynamics during anesthesia. This measure can be an important supplement to other domain EEG information for estimating DOA.

TABLE IV

TEST RESULTS ON THE DATABASE FROM AMC PLUS SPANISH PATIENTS, BY "THRESHOLD METHOD" TO DISCRIMINATE THE AWAKE
AND ASLEEP STATES USING THE DERIVED MEASURES (*ApEn*, *SE* AND *MF*)

| Measure | Threshold | State | Sensitivity(%) | Specificity(%) | Accuracy(%) |
|---|---|---|---|---|---|
| **ApEn** | 0.967 | Awake | 89 | 89 | 89 |
| | | Asleep | 89 | 89 | 89 |
| **SE** | 3.810 | Awake | 76 | 75 | 76 |
| | | Asleep | 75 | 76 | 76 |
| **MF** | 7.420 | Awake | 64 | 63 | 64 |
| | | Asleep | 63 | 64 | 64 |

The mathematical operations needed for estimating $C(n)$ are just sequence comparison and number accumulation, which are more easier to implement in hardware or software than the operations needed by *ApEn* and FFT-based *SE* and *MF*. Therefore, such a measure is very suitable for a simple detection scheme for implementation in a practical medical device.

The results clearly show the ability of $C(n)$ in measuring the DOA and its on-line implementation feasibility. These are crucial for a measure to be accepted in clinical situations. In the future, $C(n)$ can also be used in an anesthetic delivery system to help more rapid and accurate control of the administered amounts of anesthetics.

From Fig. 5 and statistical results, it also can be seen that, by use of a "higher threshold" (e.g., 0.65), $C(n)$ has the ability to predict the awake-state during anesthesia. This is of important clinical significance since avoiding movement during surgery is a major concern. Furthermore, monitoring the trend of $C(n)$ also allows the clinician to anticipate when the patient will recover. In the similar way, by the use of a "lower threshold" (e.g., 0.30) we can avoid having the patient too deeply anesthetized. The target $C(n)$ number for an anesthetized patient is approximately 0.35–0.50.

One important feature of $C(n)$ is model-independence. Only those differences between activity patterns that make a difference to the underlying system itself is considered, no matter whether the system is dominated by deterministic chaos or a stochastic process. A stochastic process is a random experiment for which the result is a function of time instead of simply a number or a set of numbers. Model-independence is very useful in analyzing a biological system, such as the electrical activity of the brain. The EEG may not be simply generated by a purely deterministic or stochastic process, but rather by some combination of both [46]. While applying $C(n)$ to the EEG, we are not testing for a particular model form, such as deterministic chaos, but attempting to distinguish among the EEG data sets on the basis of complexity. Such complexity can be seen in both deterministic and/or stochastic processes, similar to brain activity. The use of the quantitative complexity measure can help us gain a better insight into the system dynamics.

The study also demonstrates that the concept of complexity is valuable for EEG studies, especially for DOA estimation. This finding is consistent with previous findings that complexity analysis, derived from nonlinear dynamics theory, having certain advantages over linear analyses in EEG studies [17], [18], [47] and agrees with the prediction of B.L. Grundy that "analysis of deterministic chaos of the EEG may well replace spectral analysis early in the 21st century" [48].

In summary, this study shows that EEG complexity measure $C(n)$ is a good candidate for characterizing patients' brain activity under different depths of anesthesia. This measure will help better our understanding of the complex levels of consciousness during anesthesia and enhance our ability to assess the DOA. More patient cases are needed to further confirm the statistical results obtained in this study.

## ACKNOWLEDGMENT

The authors would like to thank the reviewers for their many useful comments and suggestions.

## REFERENCES


[1] S. O. V. Ranta, R. Laurila, J. Saario, T. Ali-Melkkila, and M. Hynynen, "Awareness with recall during general anesthesia: Incidence and risk factors," *Anesth. Analg.*, vol. 86, pp. 1084–1089, 1998.

[2] D. R. Stanski, "Monitoring depth of anesthesia," in *Anesthesia*, R. D. Miller, Ed. New York: Churchill Livingstone, 1994, pp. 1127–1159.

[3] I. J. Rampil, "A primer for EEG signal processing in anesthesia," *Anesthesiology*, vol. 89, pp. 980–1002, 1998.

[4] C. E. Thomsen, K. N. Christensen, and A. Rosenflack, "Computerized monitoring of depth of anesthesia with isoflurane," *Br. J. Anaesthesia*, vol. 63, pp. 36–43, 1989.

[5] A. Sharma and R. J. Roy, "Design of a recognition system to predict movement during anesthesia," *IEEE Trans. Biomed. Eng.*, vol. 44, pp. 505–511, June 1997.

[6] J. C. Drummond, C. A. Brann, D. E. Perkins, and D. E. Perkins, "A comparison of median frequency, spectral edge frequency, a frequency band power ratio, total power and dominance shift in the determination of depth of anesthesia," *Acta Anaesthesiologica Scandinavica*, vol. 35, pp. 693–699, 1991.

[7] H. S. Traast and C. J. Kalkman, "Electroencephalographic characteristics of emergence from Propofol/Sufentanil total intravenous anesthesia," *Anesth. Analg.*, vol. 81, pp. 366–371, 1995.

[8] A. Nayak, R. J. Roy, and A. Sharma, "Time-frequency spectral representation of the EEG as an aid in the detection of depth of anesthesia," *Ann. Biomed. Eng.*, vol. 22, pp. 501–513, 1994.

[9] T. P. Barnett, L. C. Johnson, P. Naitoh, N. Hicks, and C. Nute, "Bispectrum analysis of electroencephalogram signals during waking and sleeping," *Science*, vol. 172, pp. 401–402, 1971.

[10] P. S. Sebel, S. M. Bowles, V. Saini, and N. Chamoun, "EEG bispectrum predicts movement during thiopental/isoflurane anesthesia," *J. Clin. Monit.*, vol. 11, pp. 83–91, 1995.

[11] J. Muthuswamy and R. J. Roy, "The use of fuzzy integrals and bispectral analysis of the electroencephalogram to predict movement under anesthesia," *IEEE Trans. Biomed. Eng.*, vol. 46, pp. 291–302, Mar. 1999.

[12] N. Hazarika, A. C. Tsoi, and A. A. Sergejew, "Nonlinear considerations in EEG signal classification," *IEEE Trans. Signal Processing*, vol. 45, pp. 829–836, Apr. 1997.

[13] I. Yaylali, H. Kocak, and P. Jayakar, "Detection of seizures from small samples using nonlinear dynamic system theory," *IEEE Trans. Biomed. Eng*, vol. 43, pp. 743–751, July 1996.

[14] P. Grassberger and I. Procaccia, "Characterization of strange attractors," *Phys. Rev. Lett.*, vol. 50, pp. 346–349, 1983.

[15] P. Grassberger, T. Schreiber, and C. Schaffrath, "Nonlinear time sequence analysis," *Int. J. Bifurcation Chaos*, vol. 1, pp. 521–548, 1991.

[16] A. Meyer-Lindenberg, "The evolution of complexity in human brain development: An EEG study," *Electroenceph. Clin. Neurophysiol.*, vol. 99, pp. 405–411, 1996.

[17] L. I. Aftanas, N. V. Lotova, V. I. Koshkarov, V. P. Makhnev, Y. N. Mordvintsev, and S. A. Popov, "Non-linear dynamic complexity of the human EEG during evoked emotions," *Int. J. Psychophysiol.*, vol. 28, pp. 63–76, 1998.

[18] M. Molle, L. Marshall, B. Wolf, H. L. Fehm, and J. Born, "EEG complexity and performance measures of creative thinking," *Psychophysiology*, vol. 36, pp. 95–104, 1999.

[19] M. Molnar and Y. Z. Nag, "Dimensional complexity of the EEG and ERPS in stroke patients," *Int. J. Psychophysiol.*, vol. 33, p. 161, 1999.

[20] R. Hornero, P. Espino, A. Alonso, and M. Lopez, "Estimating complexity from EEG background activity of epileptic patients," *IEEE Eng. Med. Biol. Mag.*, pp. 73–79, Nov./Dec. 1999.

[21] W. S. Tirsch, M. Keidel, S. Perz, H. Scherb, and G. Sommer, "Inverse covariation of spectral density and correlation dimension in cyclic EEG dynamics of the human brain," *Biol. Cybern.*, vol. 82, pp. 1–14, 2000.

[22] A. P. Anokhin, W. Lutzenberger, A. Nikolaev, and N. Birbaumer, "Complexity of electrocortical dynamics in children: Developmental aspects," *Develop. Psychobiol.*, vol. 36, pp. 9–22, 2000.

[23] N. Pradhan and P. K. Sadasivan, "Validity of dimensional complexity measures of EEG signals," *Int. J. Bifurcation Chaos*, vol. 7, pp. 173–186, 1997.

[24] H. Preissl, W. Lutzenberger, F. Pulvermuller, and N. Birbaumer, "Fractal dimensions of short EEG time series in humans," *Neurosci. Lett.*, vol. 225, pp. 77–80, 1997.

[25] A. Accardo, M. Affinito, M. Carrozzi, and F. Bouquet, "Use of the fractal dimension for the analysis of electroencephalographic time series," *Biol. Cybern.*, vol. 77, pp. 339–350, 1997.

[26] S. M. Pincus, "Approximate entropy as a measure of system complexity," in *Proc. Nat. Acad. Sci. USA*, vol. 88, 1991, pp. 2297–2301.

[27] ——, "Approximate entropy (ApEn) as a complexity measure," in *Chaos*, vol. 5, 1995, pp. 110–117.

[28] G. Tononi, O. Sporns, and G. M. Edelman, "A complexity measure for selective matching of signals by the brain," in *Proc. Nat. Acad. Sci. USA*, vol. 93, 1996, pp. 3422–3427.

[29] G. Tononi and G. M. Edelman, "Consciousness and complexity," *Science*, vol. 282, pp. 1846–1851, 1998.

[30] W. Klonowski, W. Jernajczyk, K. Niedzielska, A. Rydz, and R. Stepien, "Quantitative measure of complexity of EEG signal dynamics," *Acta Neurobiologiae Experimentalis*, vol. 59, pp. 315–321, 1999.

[31] R. C. Watt and S. R. Hameroff, "Phase space electroencephalography (EEG): A new mode of intraoperative EEG analysis," *Int. J. Clin. Monit. Comput.*, vol. 5, pp. 3–13, 1988.

[32] K. Kumpf, W. Nahm, E. Kochs, and W. Miltner, "Dynamic complexity of the EEG predicts movement during anesthesia," *J. Psychophysiol.*, vol. 12, p. 210, 1998.

[33] A. Lempel and J. Ziv, "On the complexity of finite sequences," *IEEE Trans. Inform. Theory*, vol. IT-22, pp. 75–81, 1976.

[34] F. Kaspar and H. G. Schuster, "Easily calculable measure for the complexity of spatiotemporal patterns," *Phys. Rev. A.*, vol. 36, pp. 842–848, 1987.

[35] X. Wu and J. Xu, "Complexity and brain function," *Acta Biophysica Sinica*, vol. 7, pp. 103–106, 1991.

[36] J. Xu, Z. R. Liu, R. Liu, and Q. F. Yang, "Information transformation in human cerebral cortex," *Physica D*, vol. 106, pp. 363–374, 1997.

[37] X.-S. Zhang, Y.-S. Zhu, and X.-J. Zhang, "New approach to studies on ECG dynamics: Extraction and analyses of QRS complex irregularity time series," *Med. Biol. Eng. Comput.*, vol. 35, pp. 467–474, 1997.

[38] N. Radhakrishnan and B. N. Gangadhar, "Estimating regularity in epileptic seizure time-series data," *IEEE Eng. Med. Biol. Mag.*, pp. 89–94, May/June 1998.

[39] X.-S. Zhang and R. J. Roy, "Predicting movement during anesthesia by complexity analysis of the EEG," *Med. Biol. Eng. Comput.*, vol. 37, pp. 327–334, 1999.

[40] D. A. Chernik, D. Gillings, H. Laine, J. Hendler, J. M. Silver, A. B. Davidson, E. M. Schwam, and J. L. Siegel, "Validity and reliability of the observer's assessment of alertness/sedation scale: Study with intravenous midazolam," *J. Clin. Psychopharmacol.*, vol. 10, pp. 244–251, 1990.

[41] W. H. Highleyman, "The design and analysis of pattern recognition experiments," *Bell Syst. Tech. J.*, vol. 41, pp. 723–744, 1962.

[42] J. Bruhn, H. Roepcke, B. Rehberg, T. W. Bouillon, and A. Hoeft, "EEG approximate entropy, but not median EEG frequency or SEF 95, correctly classifies burst suppression pattern as deep anesthesia," *Anesthesiology*, vol. 91, no. 3A, p. A604, 1999.

[43] J. W. Sleigh and J. Donovan, "Comparison of bispectral index, 95% spectral edge frequency and approximate entropy of the EEG, with changes in heart rate variability during induction of general anaesthesia," *Br. J. Anaesth.*, vol. 82, pp. 666–671, 1999.

[44] J. Bruhn, H. Ropcke, and A. Hoeft, "Approximate entropy as an electroencephalographic measure of anesthetic drug effect during desflurane anesthesia," *Anesthesiology*, vol. 92, pp. 715–726, 2000.

[45] I. A. Rezek and S. J. Roberts, "Stochastic complexity measures for physiological signal analysis," *IEEE Trans. Biomed. Eng.*, vol. 45, pp. 1186–1191, Sept. 1998.

[46] N. Pradhan and P. K. Sadasivan, "Validity of dimensional complexity measures of EEG signals," *Int. J. Bifurcation Chaos*, vol. 7, pp. 173–186, 1997.

[47] G. Widman, T. Schreiber, B. Rehberg, A. Hoeft, and C. E. Elger, "Quantification of depth of anesthesia by nonlinear time series analysis of brain electrical activity," *Physical Review E.*, vol. 62, pp. 4898–4903, 2000.

[48] B. L. Grundy, "The electroencephalogram and evoked potential monitoring," in *Monitoring in Anesthesia and Critical Care Medicine*, 3rd ed, C. D. Blitt and R. L. Hines, Eds. New York: Churchill Livingstone, 1995, ch. 16 , p. 435.

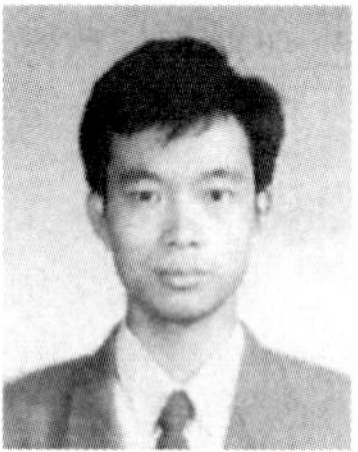

**Xu-Sheng Zhang** (M'98–SM'01) received the B.S. degree from Chongqing University, Chongqing, China, in 1992, the M.S. degree from Harbin Institute of Technology, Harbin, China, in 1995, both in electrical engineering, the Ph.D. degree from Shanghai Jiao Tong University, Shanghai, China, in 1997, in biomedical engineering, and the M.E. degree from Rensselaer Polytechnic Institute (RPI), Troy, NY, in 1999, in electrical, computer and systems engineering.

From October 1997 to February 2000, he worked at RPI as a Post-doctoral Research Associate in biomedical engineering and then he worked at Cardiac Science, Inc, Irvine, CA, as an Algorithm Software Engineer until February 2001. Since then he has been working at Siemens Medical Solutions USA, Inc., Danvers, MA, as a Project Engineer. His research interests include digital signal processing, nonlinear time series modeling, cardiac tachyarrhythmia detection, depth of anesthesia estimation, and control and mechanical fault diagonosis.

Dr. Zhang is a recipient of All-China Excellent Doctoral Thesis for the year 2000.

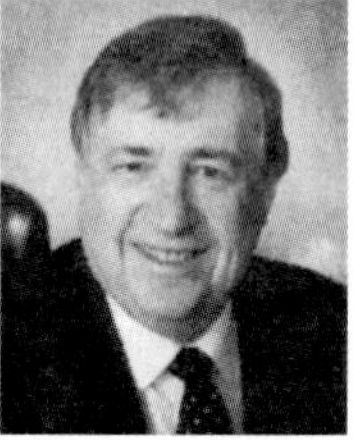

**Rob J. Roy** (S'56–M'57–SM'73–LS'97) received the B.S.E.E. degree from Cooper Union, New York, the M.S.E.E. degree from Columbia University, New York, the D.Eng.Sc. degree from Rensselaer Polytechnic Institute (RPI), Troy, NY, and the M.D. degree from Albany Medical College, Albany.

He has been Professor of Electrical Engineering and Chairman of Biomedical Engineering at RPI and is now Active Profesor Emeritus. He is currently Professor of Anesthesia and Attending Anesthesiologist at Albany Medical Center, where he is Director of Vascular Anesthesia. His research interests are in biological signal processing and adaptive control systems. He has published extensively in the areas of pattern recognition, control systems, radar signal processing, process identification, cardiac output measurement, closed circuit anesthesia delivery systems, multiple drug delivery systems, and depth of anesthesia monitoring.

Dr. Roy was recently chosen as one of the Best Doctors in America.

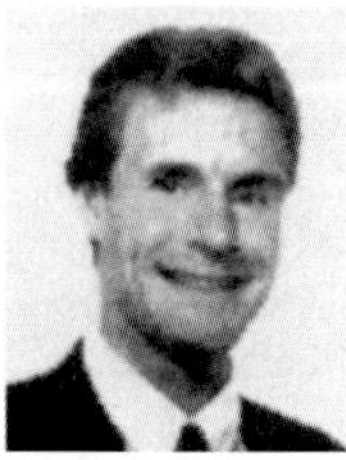

**Erik Weber Jensen** received the M.Sc. degree in electronics engineering from Technical University of Denmark, Lyngby, Demnark, in 1992 and the Ph.D. degree in medicine from University of Southern Denmark, Odense, Denmark, in 2000

He worked as a Biomedical Engineer at Odense University hospital, Department of Anaesthetics and Intensive Care, Odense, from 1992 to 1997. His research interests are time series analysis and fuzzy inductive reasoning. Currently, he is a Research Fellow at the Center of Research in Biomedical Engineering, Polytechnic University of Catalonia, Catalonia, Spain, where he works with analysis of auditory evoked potentials for monitoring depth of anaesthesia. He is also a Sientific Advisor for the bioinstrumentation company, Danmeter A/S, Odense.

# Section 5:

## *Image Processing*

*Reprinted by kind permission of:*
*Elsevier Science (518, 530),*
*Lippincott Williams & Wilkins (506),*
*Wiley & Sons (509)*

**H. Handels**

Institute for Medical Informatics
University of Lübeck
Germany

# Synopsis

# *Medical Image Processing: New Perspectives in Computer Supported Diagnostics, Computer Aided Surgery and Medical Education and Training*

Medical image processing has become one of the most important fields in medical informatics. In the past, with the introduction of tomographic imaging techniques like computer tomography, magnetic resonance imaging, positron emission tomography etc. the amount of digital medical images has increased rapidly. Moreover, the availability of the DICOM standard for medical images has facilitated image handling and image exchange, especially between radiological departments and scientific image processing groups. Nowadays, basic image processing and visualisation techniques are used in daily routine. However, high-level image processing methods are needed to analyse and visualise anatomical and pathological image structures in a user-oriented mode, especially if a large number of images for one patient containing spatial, anatomical and functional information are available. Moreover, 4D image processing algorithms are required to analyse the temporal signal changes in a whole body volume, if temporal 3D image sequences have been generated.

In the last years, 3D image processing has become a key technology for operation planning and computer aided surgery. The rapid development of computer hardware in combination with the enormous decrease in hardware prices significantly facilitated the development and introduction of 3D image processing techniques in clinical environments. Image processing tools will be an essential part of the operation room of the future: Operations will be planned in the virtual patient body and interventions will be done using image based navigation systems as well as surgical robots. In [1] the fascinating possibilities of the use of an image based tele-robot system in surgery are demonstrated in the field of urology.

High-level image processing techniques are needed to improve medical diagnostics, operation planning and image guided surgery. The impact of new developments in image processing on these fields can be illustrated by the development of registration algorithms. Registration algorithms have offered new possibilities for the analysis and visualisation of multimodal image data sets. Using these algorithms, image data from different imaging modalities like radiography, ultrasound, computer tomography, magnetic resonance imaging, functional magnetic resonance imaging, positron emission tomography etc. can be matched and represented in a common coordinate system of a reference body. Hence spatial, anatomical, and functional image information usually distributed over a huge number of images can be visualised in one common 3D scene showing key anatomical structures, pathological tissue changes, functional brain regions, and their spatial correlation to each other. These new image processing methods enable completely new insights into the patients image data improving medical diagnostics and patient treatment. Impressive results of the clinical use of registration algorithms in neurosurgery are given in [2].

Furthermore, image based 3D models of human organs and tissues can be used to develop and to verify biophysical models describing the state and behaviour of tissues and organs in terms of quantitative parameters like strain, elasticity, and so on. These models can provide the physician with a new quality of information. An interesting example illustrating the value of simulation models is given in [3], where the regional cardiac deformation from 3D ultrasound image sequences is described using a bio-mechanical model. Alternatively, 3D models of the human body in combination with anatomical knowledge can be used to generate a digital anatomical atlas of the human body. In [4] an impressive description of an atlas based 3D learning environment is given, which offers new possibilities to study the human anatomy in virtual bodies with fascinating photo-realistic 3D images.

The development of image analysis systems for diagnostic support, operation planning and computer aided surgery is a very complex interdisciplinary process. On the one hand, new image processing methods have to be developed to support the physician during the diagnostic and therapeutic process. On the other hand, methods of different scientific fields have to be adapted and used in combination: Image analysis algorithms need to be applied in combination with methods of pattern recognition, mathematics, computer graphics, simulation, and robotics. The four selected papers give an impression of the breadth and heterogeneity of new developments in the field of medical image processing.

The paper by Abbou et al. [1] describes the use of the robotic system DA VINCI during a laparoscopic radical prostatectomy in urology. The DA VINCI system consists of two main parts: a slave unit placed by the patient in the operation room and a master unit located in an area adjacent to the operating room. Both are connected by a computer based system. The slave unit consists of a surgical cart with a camera arm, instrument arms

and a vision cart. The surgeon directs the robot at the master unit consisting of the surgeon console and an integrated 3-dimensional display stereo viewer. A stereo camera generates stereo images of the inner organs for image based navigation of the surgeon. The instrument tips viewed in the display are aligned with the master to ensure natural and predictable instrument movements. The authors show that the system has proven to be ideal not only for remote surgical demonstration and practical teaching, but also for tele-robotic surgery. A special advantage of the system was that hand tremor was eliminated during the operation. In summary, it was demonstrated by the authors that robotically assisted laparoscopic radical prostatectomy is feasible and that the robot provided an ergonomic surgical environment and remarkable dexterity enhancement.

In the paper by Gering et al. [2] an image processing system for surgical planning and guidance using an open interventional MR system is described. This paper is a fascinating report on the integration and the use of high level image processing tools in neuro-surgery. It describes the possibilities and advantages for patient treatment, if 3D image processing algorithms including segmentation, registration and 3D visualisation algorithms become available in clinical routine. Registration algorithms are applied to align multimodal image sequences in one common coordinate system. In the considered application, pre-operative data (T1- and T2-weighted MR images, MR angiography images, functional MR images) are fused. Each of these image sequences contains different information about the patient: While T1- and T2-weighted images show the same brain tissues with different contrast, in MR angiographies the vessel system of the brain is strongly enhanced. Furthermore, in fMR images the

individual localisation of the patient's brain functions can be displayed.

Key anatomical structures like tumour, vessels, ventricles, skin, brain, and functional regions have to be segmented. This is done in different data sets, e.g. the vessels are extracted in the MR angiography while the functional regions are separated in the functional MR data set. A 3D surface model can be generated automatically for each segmented structure. After the registration step, it is possible to visualise the segmented vessels, functional regions, brain, tumour etc. in one 3D scene. Furthermore, pre-operative images are aligned to images generated by an open MRI during the intervention. In the application, only rigid registration methods compensating rotations and translations between the data sets are applied, and local deformations like brain shift effects are not taken into account. However, Gering et al. report that rigid registration was sufficient in the considered cases. The system has been applied in 45 neurosurgical cases and found to have beneficial utility for planning and guidance.

The paper by Papademetris et al. [3] deals with a new approach for the model based estimation of quantitative parameters to describe the regional cardiac deformation from 3D ultrasound image sequences. In a first step, the images are segmented interactively and a dense displacement field is estimated using a Bayesian estimation framework. The dense motion field is in turn used to calculate the deformation of the heart wall in terms of strains in cardiac specific directions using a biomechanical model. The computed strain data are compared with data measured in open-chest dogs with implanted sonomicrometers, which were considered to be the gold standard. The strains computed in the 3D ultrasound image sequence exhibit a high correlation to the measured sonomicrometer derived strains. With this innovative approach the authors open up new perspectives to model the biomechanical behaviour of the left ventricle.

The system presented by Pommert et al. [4] has been developed to support medical education and training. A high-resolution, digital 3D atlas of the human body was described based on the visible human image data set of the National Library of Medicine. Three-dimensional models of anatomical structures have been generated and visualised in high quality to give a fascinating insight into the spatial inner structure of the human body. In the paper, an excellent survey on the methods applied in the 3D atlas system is given. A symbolic description is used to give the user information about the relationships of anatomical structures to each other. Hence, image processing methods and knowledge representation methods are applied in combination. The authors describe the techniques to make anatomical knowledge available during the photo-realistic 3D visualisation of anatomical structures. Through the combination of anatomical and radiological image information with anatomical knowledge, the atlas opens up a new intuitive way to a deeper understanding of the structure of the human body as well as to the interpretation of radiological image data.

## References


1. Abbou CC, Hoznek A, Salomon L, Olsson LE, Lobontiu A, Saint F, et al. Laparoscopic radical prostatectomy with a remote controlled robot. J Urol 2001;165(6 Pt 1):1964-6.

2. Gering DT, Nabavi A, Kikinis R, Hata N, O'Donnell LJ, Grimson WE, et al. An integrated visualization system for surgical planning and guidance using image fusion and an open MR. J Magn Reson Imaging 2001;13(6):967-75.

3. Papademetris X, Sinusas AJ, Dione DP, Duncan JS. Estimation of 3D left ventricular deformation from echocardiography. Med Image Anal 2001;5(1):17-28.

4. Pommert A, Höhne KH, Pflesser B, Richter E, Riemer M, Schiemann T, et al. Creating a high-resolution spatial/symbolic model of the inner organs based on the Visible Human. Med Image Anal 2001 Sep;5(3):221-8.



Address of the author:
PD Dr. rer. nat. habil. Heinz Handels
Institute for Medical Informatics
University of Lübeck
Ratzeburger Allee 160
23538 Lübeck
Germany
E-mail: handels@medinf.mu-luebeck.de

# LAPAROSCOPIC RADICAL PROSTATECTOMY WITH A REMOTE CONTROLLED ROBOT

CLÉMENT-CLAUDE ABBOU, ANDRÁS HOZNEK, LAURENT SALOMON, LEIF ERIC OLSSON, ADRIAN LOBONTIU, FABIEN SAINT, ANTONY CICCO, PATRICK ANTIPHON AND DOMINIQUE CHOPIN

*From the Service d'Urologie, Hôpital Henri Mondor, Créteil, France*

## ABSTRACT

Purpose: Robotics in surgery is a recent innovation. This technology offers a number of attractive features in laparoscopy. It overcomes the difficulties with fixed port sites by restoring all 6 degrees of freedom at the instrument tips, provides new possibilities for miniaturization of surgical tasks and allows remote controlled surgery. We investigated the applicability of remote controlled robotic surgery to laparoscopic radical prostatectomy.

Materials and Methods: Our previous experience with laparoscopic prostatectomy served as a basis for adapting robotic surgery to this procedure. A surgeon at a different location who activated the tele-manipulators of the da Vinci* robotic system performed all steps of the intervention. A scrub nurse and second surgeon who stood at patient side had limited roles to port and instrument placement, exposure of the operative field, assistance in hemostasis and removal of the operative specimen. Our patient was a 63-year-old man presenting with a T1c tumor discovered on 1 positive sextant biopsy with a 3+3 Gleason score and 7 ng./ml. preoperative serum prostate specific antigen.

Results: The robot provided an ergonomic surgical environment and remarkable dexterity enhancement. Operating time was 420 minutes, and the hospital stay lasted 4 days. The bladder catheter was removed 3 days postoperatively, and 1 week later the patient was fully continent. Pathological examination showed a pT3a tumor with negative margins.

Conclusions: Robotically assisted laparoscopic radical prostatectomy is feasible. This new technology enhances surgical dexterity. Further developments in this field may have new applications in laparoscopic tele-surgery.

KEY WORDS: robotics, feasibility studies, laparoscopy, prostatectomy, prostatic neoplasms

Robotics have been commonly used in numerous industrial fields for several decades. However, application of this technology to surgery is only a recent innovation. It provides new possibilities for performing certain special surgical tasks, especially in the field of laparoscopy. In 1994 Kavoussi et al demonstrated the feasibility of tele-mentoring laparoscopic surgery and remote robotic control of the camera.[1] Partin et al reported 17 miscellaneous solo surgical urological interventions in which surgical assistance was exclusively provided by robotic technology.[2]

One main factor limiting performance of laparoscopy is the loss of 2 of the 6 degrees of freedom. To overcome these spatial restrictions, more elaborate robots, including remote activated dexterous manipulators, were developed. Such tele-robotic units were successfully used by Sung et al during pyeloplasty in swine.[3] To date, only a few cases have been reported in the fields of heart surgery and gynecology.[4-6] We report our first case of laparoscopic radical prostatectomy with a remote controlled robot.

### MATERIALS AND METHODS

Our patient was a 63-year-old man presenting with a T1c tumor discovered on 1 positive sextant biopsy, with a 3+3 Gleason score and 7 ng./ml. (normal less than 4 ng./ml) pre-

Accepted for publication December 15, 2000.
*Intuitive Surgical, Inc., Mountain View, California.

***Editor's Note: Editor's Note:*** **This article is the fifth of 5 published in this issue for which category 1 CME credits can be earned. Instructions for obtaining credits are given with the questions on pages 2034 and 2035.**

operative serum prostate specific antigen.† After staging, which included pelvic magnetic resonance imaging and bone scan, the decision to perform laparoscopic, computer enhanced, robotically assisted radical prostatectomy was made. Informed consent was obtained from the patient.

Our technique of laparoscopic radical prostatectomy has already been described elsewhere.[7] The particular features of this case included 5 trocars placed through the abdominal wall, 1, 12 mm. trocar inserted through the lower margin of the umbilicus for the laparoscope and 2, 8 mm. trocars located at the lateral border of the rectus sheath. The instruments passed through these trocars were connected to the robot. These instruments included Cadiere and DeBakey forceps, 2 large needle drivers, long and round tip forceps, scalpel, electrocautery, and a prototype of bipolar forceps. There were 2 additional 5 mm. trocars inserted in the iliac position for the assistant who had sufficient practice in laparoscopy to create the access sites. During the rest of the procedure the assistant was limited to exposing the operative field, assisting with hemostasis, including suction and irrigation, and application of clips and electrocautery. At the end of the procedure, the prostate was removed through the umbilical port site and the port sites were closed. At no time during the procedure was it required for the surgeon to scrub.

The da Vinci system is a master slave type of surgical robot. It consists of a slave or work unit and a master or control unit, which are connected by a computer based system (see figure). The slave unit is placed near the patient and includes a surgical cart with a camera arm, 2 instrument arms and a vision cart. The master unit is located in an area

†Hybritech, Inc., San Diego, California.

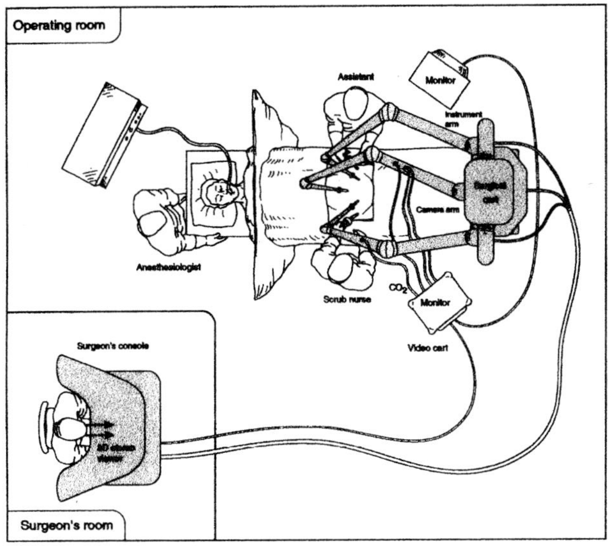

da Vinci system in operating room

adjacent to the operating room. It consists of a surgeon console with an integrated 3-dimensional (3-D) display stereo viewer. The surgeon sitting at the console holds master grips for remote control of the instruments and laparoscope, which are attached to the arms of the surgical cart near the patient. The head of the surgeon rests between sensors on either side of the view port so that he can see the 3D display in the stereo viewer. The instrument tips viewed in the display are aligned with the master to ensure natural and predictable instrument motion. Motion scaling reduces hand movements to correspondingly smaller instrument tip movements in the surgical field.

The manipulators have a total of 6 degrees of freedom plus the grip, and at the tip, 2 more degrees than traditional endoscopic instruments. Tip articulations mimic the wrist up and down and side-to-side flexibility. With these features, the surgeon is able to perform the entire procedure, including dissection, intracorporeal suturing and knot tying.

### RESULTS

We performed bilateral nerve sparing without pelvic lymphadenectomy. Vesicourethral anastomosis was performed with a single circumferential 3-zero polyglactin running suture. All steps in the operation were completed with the da Vinci robotic system, which placed instrument movements under direct real-time control, and provided great dexterity and precision. Hand tremor was eliminated, and the master range of motion allowed full, natural movements that were transmitted accurately to the surgical arms.

Operating time was 420 minutes. Assembly of the robot required 30 minutes and disengaging it required 15 minutes. Vesicourethral anastomosis time was 30 minutes. Total anesthesia time was 8 ½ hours, and blood loss was 300 ml. Postoperative hospitalization lasted 4 days, and the bladder catheter was removed after 3 days. One week later the patient was fully continent. The pathological examination showed an extracapsular stage pT3a, grade G2 tumor, with a 3+3 Gleason score and negative surgical margins.

### DISCUSSION

Currently, in the present era of telecommunication technology laparoscopy, a technique based primarily on images, has proved ideal not only for remote surgical demonstration and practical teaching, but also for tele-robotic surgery. The possibility of transmitting real-time video images with videoconferencing or the Internet allows remote teaching and tele-assistance. In 1994 Kavoussi et al demonstrated the feasibility of laparoscopic nephrectomy by an inexperienced surgeon tele-mentored by a surgeon at a remote site.[1] The same experience was successfully conducted between Baltimore and Innsbruck.[8]

Currently, videoconferencing is routinely used at several training centers for urological laparoscopy, and has the advantage of reducing costs and saving time by eliminating unnecessary travel. Tele-surgical mentoring can improve the safety of surgery during the learning curve and can potentially provide patients with global access to surgical specialists.[9] In addition to the transmission of video, remote control of spatial motion itself has today become a reality. Voice commanded robotic camera control has been clinically investigated and is routinely used by several laparoscopic teams.[1, 8, 10, 11] Robotic camera holding has the advantage of providing a steadier image and enables the reduction of the number of assistants necessary for the procedure. Similarly, the feasibility of several ablative or reconstructive solo surgical laparoscopies has also been documented. Thus, Partin et al reported 17 complete robot assisted laparoscopic procedures, including nephrectomy, retroperitoneal or pelvic lymph node sampling, varix ligation, pyeloplasty, Burch procedure, orchidopexy, ureterolysis and nephropexy.[2]

A further development in robotic surgery was the elaboration and clinical application of dexterous robotic manipulators in a "master-slave" configuration. In fact, conventional laparoscopy with rigid instruments provides only 4 of the 6 degrees of freedom required for free handling of objects in space. This result is the main inherent limitation of laparoscopic surgery, which contributes to the steep learning curve.

The most elaborated currently available tele-robotic unit permits restoration of all 6 degrees of freedom by adding flexibility to the instrument tips. These devices also allow activation of the manipulators by a surgeon geographically remote from the patient, provide new possibilities for the miniaturization of surgical tasks, and filter hand tremor, thus permitting additional precision and dexterity. Two computer enhanced systems with these characteristics have been clinically investigated. With the Zeus‡ robotic system, Sung et al performed laparoscopic pyeloplasty in a porcine model, with results closely resembling those of open surgery.[3] The da Vinci system was successfully used in obstetrical and cardiovascular surgery.[4-6]

In 1998 we started performing laparoscopic radical prostatectomy for localized prostate cancer.[7] The difficulties inherent with laparoscopy, which we encountered during this advanced reconstructive surgery, prompted us to explore the applicability of robotics to this procedure. In our present feasibility study the remote controlled dexterous manipulators, combined with the 3-D video imaging, offered a user-friendly ergonomic surgical platform that proved to be beneficial for all phases of the operation, including vesicourethral anastomosis and preservation of the neurovascular bundles. Only a few in vitro and animal training sessions were required for the robot to be safely used in our patient.

Besides all of these advantages, the method has drawbacks, including lack of tactile feedback, which is even greater than with conventional laparoscopy. However, this difficulty may be overcome with some practice before robotics are applied to humans. Another limitation is the high cost of the necessary equipment. The cost of the da Vinci system is approximately 1 million dollars. The cost of disposables for our laparoscopic prostatectomy was $1,800 but this might be decreased once the procedure becomes standardized. Currently, robotic surgery can only be viewed in the framework of research protocols at large centers in which several spe-

‡Computer Motion, Goleta, California.

cialties, such as cardiovascular, gynecological, urological and general surgery, share the robot. Further progress in miniaturization and the growth of data flow through public lines will presumably help to propagate this technology and eventually lead to implementation of true tele-surgery.

The operating time for our first tele-robotic procedure was significantly longer than usual because of the special circumstances. Specifically, this procedure represents our initial human case with the da Vinci system, and there undoubtedly exists a learning curve. During this procedure, we tested miscellaneous instruments with the robotic arm before selecting the optimal instrument sets for the different steps. This testing necessitated frequent changes of instruments, which can be avoided once the procedure is standardized. In addition, this first procedure was not performed at our operative suite nor with our regular team of nurses. An equally long operating time was observed during our first traditional laparoscopic prostatectomy, which required 9 hours but has currently decreased to 3 ½ hours.[7] Surgical results were similar to those obtained to date with our standard laparoscopic radical prostatectomy.

### CONCLUSIONS

Our first laparoscopic radical prostatectomy with a remote controlled robot demonstrates the feasibility of dissociating surgeon and patient even for one of the most challenging current urological procedures. The robot permits operation with a 3D display and improves surgical dexterity and precision. The results of the present robotically assisted surgery in regard to local cancer control, hospitalization and postoperative course were similar to those of standard laparoscopic radical prostatectomy. Future developments in the application of tele-robotic surgery to urological laparoscopy should allow urologists to perform surgical procedures at a remote site and surpass the current limitations of human performance.

### REFERENCES

1. Kavoussi, L. R., Moore, R. G., Partin, A. W. et al: Telerobotic assisted laparoscopic surgery: initial laboratory and clinical experience. Urology, **44**: 15, 1994
2. Partin, A. W., Adams, J. B., Moore, R. G. et al: Complete robot-assisted laparoscopic urologic surgery: a preliminary report. J Am Coll Surg, **181**: 552, 1995
3. Sung, G. T., Gill, I. S. and Hsu, T. H.: Robotic-assisted laparoscopic pyeloplasty: a pilot study. Urology, **53**: 1099, 1999
4. Falk, V., Diegeler, A., Walther, T. et al: Total endoscopic computer enhanced coronary artery bypass grafting. Eur J Cardiothorac Surg, **17**: 38, 2000
5. Loulmet, D., Carpentier, A., d'Attellis, N. et al: Endoscopic coronary artery bypass grafting with the aid of robotic assisted instruments. J Thorac Cardiovasc Surg, **118**: 4, 1999
6. Cadiere, G. B., Himpens, J., Vertruyen, M. et al: The world's first obesity surgery performed by a surgeon at a distance. Obes Surg, **9**: 206, 1999
7. Abbou, C. C., Salomon, L., Hoznek, A. et al: Laparoscopic radical prostatectomy: preliminary results. Urology, **55**: 630, 2000
8. Janetschek, G., Bartsch, G. and Kavoussi, L. R.: Transcontinental interactive laparoscopic telesurgery between the United States and Europe. J Urol, **160**: 1413, 1998
9. Schulam, P. G., Docimo, S. G., Saleh, W. et al: Telesurgical mentoring. Initial clinical experience. Surg Endosc, **11**: 1001, 1997
10. Kavoussi, L. R., Moore, R. G., Adams, J. B. et al: Comparison of robotic versus human laparoscopic camera control. J Urol, **154**: 2134, 1995
11. Guillonneau, B. and Vallancien, G.: Laparoscopic radical prostatectomy: the Montsouris technique. J Urol, **163**: 1643, 2000

### EDITORIAL COMMENT

This article demonstrates that advanced urological procedures can be accomplished with the aid of robotic devices. These machines can facilitate the performance of complex surgical maneuvers, particularly suturing, which is an integral part of urological reconstructive surgery. The potential for complete remote surgical intervention is intriguing. It is noteworthy that this robot is designed to be operated from a workstation. Therefore, the surgeon, by necessity, is already removed from the operative field, and all visual information is obtained from the surgical console. However, the critical steps to allow complete remote surgery will involve complex modification of the current robotic control systems to allow signals to be transmitted through telephone lines. This procedure is feasible but will not be a simple engineering feat due to the complex analog signals currently used to control this robot. Moreover, an active surgical assistant needs to be at the operating table to help replace instrumentation and help with retraction, instrument exchange, suction, extraction and passage of suture material into the abdomen. Complete robotic surgery will require this individual be replaced with an even more complex robot than the da Vinci system.

Robotic surgery will be an integral part of complex, minimally invasive surgical procedures. The precision and versatility of these machines will allow novel surgical approaches to urological pathology. As technical refinements evolve and prices of such devices decrease, robots will become an important part of the urological armamentarium.

*Louis R. Kavoussi*
*Department of Urology*
*James Buchanan Brady Urological Institute*
*The Johns Hopkins University of Medicine*
*Baltimore, Maryland*

# An Integrated Visualization System for Surgical Planning and Guidance Using Image Fusion and an Open MR

David T. Gering, MS,[1][*] Arya Nabavi, MD,[3] Ron Kikinis, MD,[2] Noby Hata, PhD,[2]
Lauren J. O'Donnell, BS,[1] W. Eric L. Grimson, PhD,[1] Ferenc A. Jolesz, MD,[2]
Peter M. Black, MD,[3] and William M. Wells III, PhD[1,2]

A surgical guidance and visualization system is presented, which uniquely integrates capabilities for data analysis and on-line interventional guidance into the setting of interventional MRI. Various pre-operative scans (T1- and T2-weighted MRI, MR angiography, and functional MRI (fMRI)) are fused and automatically aligned with the operating field of the interventional MR system. Both pre-surgical and intra-operative data may be segmented to generate three-dimensional surface models of key anatomical and functional structures. Models are combined in a three-dimensional scene along with reformatted slices that are driven by a tracked surgical device. Thus, pre-operative data augments interventional imaging to expedite tissue characterization and precise localization and targeting. As the surgery progresses, and anatomical changes subsequently reduce the relevance of pre-operative data, interventional data is refreshed for software navigation in true real time. The system has been applied in 45 neurosurgical cases and found to have beneficial utility for planning and guidance. J. Magn. Reson. Imaging 2001; 13:967–975. © 2001 Wiley-Liss, Inc.

**Index terms:** neurosurgical planning; image guided surgery; image fusion; 3D visualization; interventional MRI

IMAGE-GUIDED SURGERY SYSTEMS strive to enhance the surgeon's capability to utilize medical imagery to decrease the invasiveness of surgical procedures and increase their accuracy and safety. These systems can be categorized into performing one or more of the following functions: data analysis (2,3,4), surgical planning (2,3,4),

surgical guidance (5,6,7,8,9,10), and surgical guidance with intra-operative updates (11,12,13,14). The systems focused on surgical guidance tend to present the surgeon with data that was gathered prior to surgery, track surgical instruments within the operating field, and render the tracked devices along with the data. For more difficult surgeries, it is beneficial to present the surgeon with not just one diagnostic scan, but with an array of information derived from fusing data sets with information on morphology, cortical function, and metabolic activity. These varied data sets are acquired in different coordinate systems and need to be aligned, or registered, to a common framework for surgical planning before that framework is in turn registered to the patient for surgical guidance. The latter registration allows the surgeon to establish a correspondence between the patient lying on the operating table and the images rendered on a nearby computer screen.

The major shortcoming of image guided surgery systems is that the use of pre-surgically acquired data does not account for intra-operative changes in brain morphology. The systems with intra-operative updates have been introduced to fill that void, but they have fallen short of achieving perfect interactivity and full information disclosure to the surgeon. In particular, the benefits of interventional MRI could be amplified by focusing on five issues: image quality, imaging time, multi-modal fusion, faster localization, and three-dimensional visualization. The need for better image quality arises because some anatomical structures are difficult to distinguish on interventional MR images, but are clearer on conventional, diagnostic MRI that benefits from a higher magnetic field and longer imaging times. Our goal is to provide both in surgery. Imaging time is a critical constraint because in order for surgical guidance to be interactive, images must be acquired quickly enough to be utilized without disrupting or slowing down the procedure. Multi-modal fusion is desirable considering that functional and metabolic data that is acquired pre-operatively could deliver increased benefit if integrated with intra-operative, anatomical information. Faster localization is needed because interventional MR provides the capability of planning approach trajectories by maneuvering a

[1]Artificial Intelligence Laboratory, Massachusetts Institute of Technology, 200 Technology Square, Cambridge, MA 02139.
[2]Department of Radiology, Brigham and Women's Hospital and Harvard Medical School, 75 Francis Street, Boston, MA 02115.
[3]Department of Surgery, Brigham and Women's Hospital and Harvard Medical School.

Contract grant sponsor: GE Medical Systems; Contract grant sponsor: W.A. Rosenblith; Contract grant sponsor: Whitaker Foundation; Contract grant sponsor: NIH; Contract grant number: P41 RR13218-01; Contract grant sponsor: NIH; Contract grant number: P01 CA67165-03; Contract grant sponsor: NIH; Contract grant number: R01 RR11747-01A; Contract grant sponsor: NSF; Contract grant number: IIS-9610249.

This paper was presented at ISMRM 2000 in Denver as An Integrated Visualization System for Surgical Planning and Guidance.

*Address reprint requests to: D.G., NE43-739, 545 Technology Square, Cambridge, MA 02139. E-mail: gering@ai.mit.edu

Received June 7, 2000; Accepted November 27, 2000.

Table 1
Population for Craniotomies by Histopathology

| Pathology | Age range | No. females | No. males |
|---|---|---|---|
| Astrocytoma I–II | 4–63 | 8 | 6 |
| Astrocytoma III anaplastic | 35–67 | 0 | 2 |
| AVM | 37 | 0 | 1 |
| Ganglioglioma | 26 | 1 | 0 |
| Glioblastoma | 29–67 | 4 | 6 |
| Metastasis | 13–31 | 2 | 0 |
| Oligodendroglioma | 27–49 | 4 | 1 |
| Other | 6–67 | 6 | 3 |

tracked surgical instrument and collecting images at the rate of 6–20 seconds per image, but an ideally interactive system needs an update rate of 0.1 seconds per image. Lastly, three-dimensional visualization would free the surgeon from needing to mentally map the two-dimensional interventional images seen on a computer screen to the three-dimensional operating field.

Any attempt to improve interventional MRI by using the combination of several currently available data analysis and surgical planning systems can be cumbersome and time-consuming, making it impractical for clinical applications. Therefore, the aim of this study was to integrate all facets of image guided medicine (data analysis, surgical planning, surgical guidance, and intra-operative updates) into a single environment. Our system is the first to augment the functionality of an open MR scanner (15,16) with various pre-operative data sets featuring information on morphology (MR, CT, MR angiography), cortical function (fMRI), and metabolic activity (PET, SPECT), as well as to offer the same level of analysis previously reserved for pre-operative data to interventional data. The 3D Slicer is the software package we developed to address the five aforementioned issues. Image quality, visualization time, and localization are improved by performing real-time re-slicing of both pre-operative and intra-operative data sets, and displaying them for simultaneous review. Multi-modal information is aligned using automatic registration for visualizing in the same scene. Three-dimensional visualization is accomplished with a computer graphics display that offers the flexibility to see the situation from viewpoints not physically possible, in order to facilitate the understanding of complex situations and to aid in avoiding damage to healthy tissue.

## MATERIALS AND METHODS

### *Patient Population*

Over a one-year period, the system was applied to 45 patients (25 female, 20 male), ages 4 to 67. All patients received craniotomies with the exception of one biopsy. Table 1 aggregates the population for craniotomies by histopathology.

### *Pre-procedural Imaging*

MRI examination was performed in a 1.5-Tesla clinical scanner (Signa Horizon; GE Medical Systems, Milwaukee, WI). The standard protocol in our hospital includes ac-

quiring a T1-weighted, spoiled gradient echo (SPGR) volume (124 1.5mm sagittal slices, TR=35msec, TE=5msec, Flip angle=45, FOV=24cm, matrix=256×192, NEX=1), a T2-weighted fast spin echo (FSE) volume (124 axial slices, TR=600msec, TE=19msec, FOV=22cm, matrix=256×192, NEX=1), and a phase-contrast MR angiogram (60 axial slices, TR=32msec, Flip angle=20, FOV=24cm, matrix=256×128, NEX=1). Patients whose pathology was located within the vicinity of eloquent cortex additionally received an fMRI exam (HORIZON EPI-BOLD sequence, 21 contiguous 7mm coronal slices, TE=50msec, TR=3sec, FOV=24cm, matrix=64×64, 6 alternating 30-second epochs of stimulus and control tasks).

### *Augmented Interventional MR System*

All procedures were performed in an open-configuration MRI system (Signa SP; GE Medical Systems, Milwaukee, WI). The location of the imaging plane was specified with an optical tracking system (Flashpoint; Image Guided Technologies, Boulder, CO), referred to hereafter as the *locator*. The spatial relationship of the locator relative to the scanner was reported as both a position and an orientation with an update rate of 10 Hz.

We added a visualization workstation (Ultra 30; Sun Microsystems, Mountain View, CA) with a TCP/IP network connection to the SP imaging workstation. Whenever the locator's position or orientation changed, or a new image was acquired, a server process we created on the SP imaging workstation sent the new data to our 3D Slicer software resident on the visualization workstation. The visualization workstation contained two Sun Creator three-dimensional graphics accelerator cards. One drove the 20-inch display placed in the control area of the surgical suite, and the other output the three-dimensional view to color LCD panels inside the scanner gantry.

### *Key Features of the 3D Slicer That Enable This Application*

#### *Open Source Design*

The 3D Slicer is an application package we developed which comprises the Visualization Toolkit (VTK) (17) for processing, OpenGL (18) for graphics acceleration, and Tcl/Tk (19) for the user interface. The architecture of the 3D Slicer is crafted around a modular paradigm that optimizes extendability. Adding a new module (for interfacing with a robot, for example) consists of adding only one new Tcl file containing the user-interface code and optionally adding new VTK objects for processing. The mechanisms for controlling that module's behavior with respect to the data already exist within the framework. The 3D Slicer is a freely available, open source tool for clinicians and scientists (20).

#### *Multi-Volume Reformatting*

Volume data is commonly visualized through multiplane reformatting (MPR). We made novel extensions to MPR to allow the three slices to:

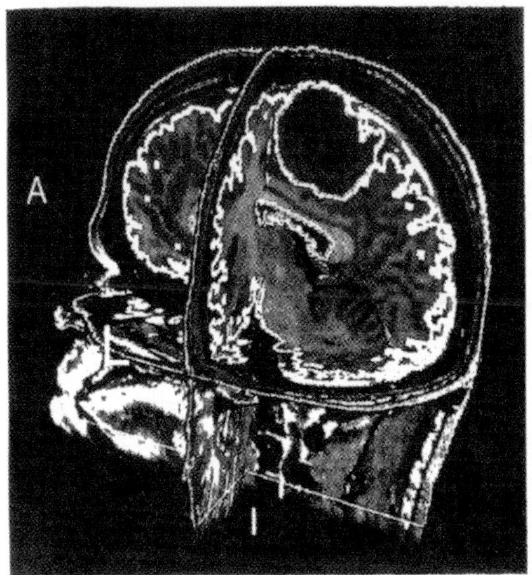

**Figure 1.** Multiple layers are displayed on each slice, allowing the fusion of data from different times or modalities. MR phase contrast angiography information (red and yellow) is overlaid on grayscale SPGR data. Also, the boundaries created through segmentation are displayed: the tumor is outlined in green, the skin in pink, the brain in white, and the ventricles in blue. [Color figure can be viewed in the online issue, which is available at www.interscience.wiley.com.]

- be orthogonal or independently oblique,
- orient orthogonal slices relative to either the scanner (mm space) or the data (voxel space),
- follow either the user's pointing device in the operating room,
- slice through multiple volumes simultaneously: each slice is the composite of a background layer, a foreground layer, and a label layer.

Typically, functional information is presented in color on the foreground layer, which is overlaid with an adjustable opacity on a gray background layer. Additionally, the output of the segmentation process is funneled into the label layer to draw a boundary around key structures, such as the tumor and vessels, as illustrated in Figure 1.

### Segmentation

Volumetric data can be semi-automatically segmented using the 3D Slicer's suite of editing tools. Effects such as thresholding, morphological operations (erosion, dilation), island removal (erasing small groupings of similar pixels), measuring the size of islands, cropping, and free-hand drawing of polygons, lines, or points can be applied to the data. Each effect can be administered on either a three-dimensional or slice-by-slice basis. One strength of our system is that effects can be visualized by overlaying the edited volume translucently on the original volume and exploring both in the three-dimensional view, as shown in Figure 2.

### Three-Dimensional Surface Models

Surface models of key anatomical structures (usually tumor, vessels, ventricles, skin, brain, and functional regions when applicable) are generated from the segmentations using Marching Cubes (21) and decimation (22). Surface models are visualized in the three-dimensional view along with the reformatted slices. Our surgeons prefer to view a portion of the skin as a landmark, so we allow for the slice planes to selectively clip away the skin model to reveal other unclipped models beneath, such as a tumor or critical structures like blood vessels, as well as the respective image planes. Each model is colored differently (and consistently between cases), and rendered with adjustable opacity as presented in Figure 3. As an alternative to generating mod-

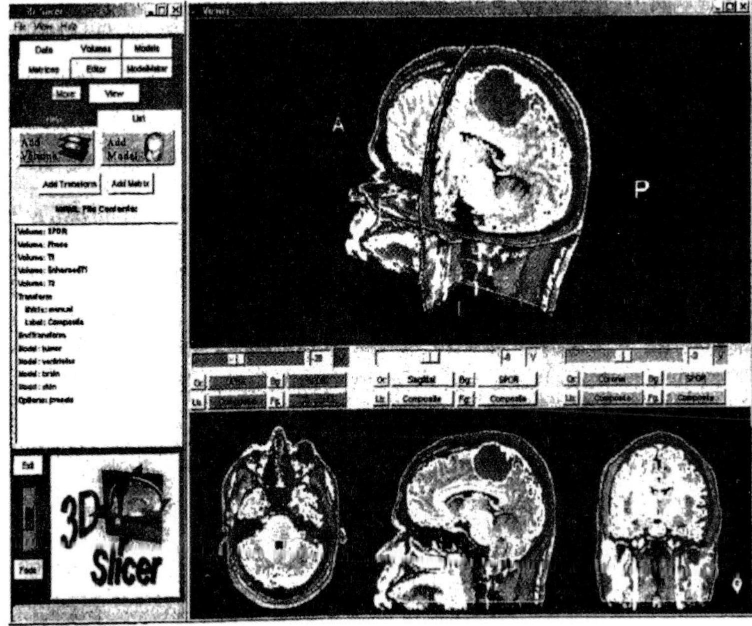

**Figure 2.** The output of a segmentation is displayed with variable opacity over the original grayscale SPGR images. The three slices on the bottom of the screen correspond to those shown above in the three-dimensional view. [Color figure can be viewed in the online issue, which is available at www.interscience.wiley.com.]

and transformations obtained through three-dimensional registrations of both the volumes and models. We have found that the proper coordination of these items is easiest to obtain by the use of a hierarchical paradigm as exemplified by the modeling systems and languages of graphics and CAD/CAM. Toward this end, we created the MRML as a format for describing scenes that consist of various types of data sets collected in various geometric locations and fused using multiple registrations.

### Trajectory Assistance

A key component of neurosurgical planning is plotting an approach trajectory that avoids critical structures such as blood vessels or the motor cortex. The 3D Slicer facilitates trajectory planning by automatically orienting slice planes relative to a trajectory specified by entry and target points. The plane perpendicular to the candidate trajectory may be slid along its path to visualize the structures that will be encountered en route. Additionally, the other two orthogonal planes allow views through the tissue that lines the approach. This feature can help prevent unfortunate surprises during surgery, as we detail below with an actual biopsy.

### Pre-Operative Procedure in the Open MR

A volume scan (same parameters as below) is collected while the patient is being prepped in the operating room. In cases where pre-procedural anatomical or functional imaging is relevant and not obtainable intra-operatively, the new volume scan serves as an intermediate registration reference that relates the pre-operative data sets to the coordinate frame of the interventional MR scanner. The relation is expressed as a transformation matrix that is inserted into the MRML file for the case. The MR scanner is treated as the reference frame to preserve the highest accuracy for the measurements of intra-operative movements relative to earlier intra-operative data. To assure the surgeon that the volume, as rendered in the 3D Slicer, is aligned with the patient's actual position, external anatomical landmarks are touched with the locator while observing whether the real-time graphics rendering agrees.

In cases where pre-procedural imaging is not required for guidance, the new volume scan is utilized for reformatting during trajectory planning, or as a pre-operative reference for comparative evaluation of contrast diffusion or brain shift as the surgery progresses.

### Intra-Operative Imaging Protocol

The radiologist involved in intra-operative imaging in our institution routinely specifies two-dimensional acquisitions to answer questions asked by the surgeon. Additionally for this study, data volumes were collected for reformatting, and updated 3–5 times throughout the duration of every craniotomy at the request of the surgeon. These volumes are 3D SPGR (12–60 2.5mm thick axial slices, TR=28.6, TE=12.8, FOV=24, matrix=256×128, NEX=1), with imaging times ranging from 0:55 to 3:55 minutes.

A summary of the complete pre- and intra-operative procedure is listed below:

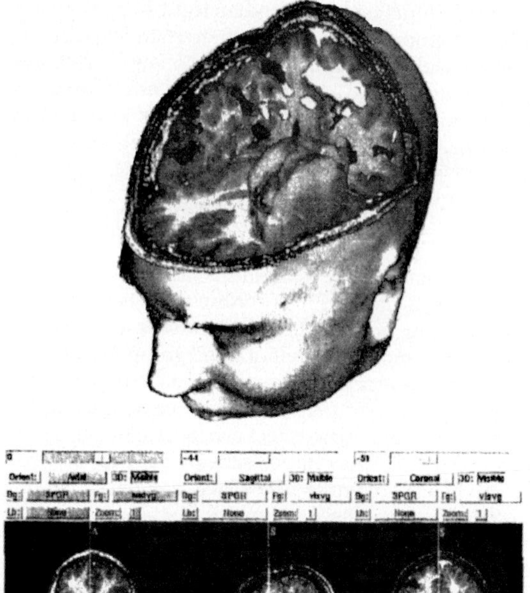

**Figure 3.** Surface models of key anatomical structures can be visualized in the three-dimensional view along with the reformatted slices. Shown here are models of skin, tumor (green), motor cortex (yellow), auditory verb generation (red), and visual verb generation (blue). [Color figure can be viewed in the online issue, which is available at www.interscience.wiley.com.]

els with the 3D Slicer, the system also possesses the capability to import models created externally by experimental programs.

### Multi-Modal Registration

The various volumes being segmented and reformatted in the 3D Slicer are acquired in different coordinate systems and need to be registered to a common framework in order to correctly view all components in a single, unified scene. The 3D Slicer supports manual rigid registration as well as automatic registration by maximization of mutual information (MI) (23,24). This method is of general utility, and other implementations of it have performed well in an NIH-sponsored test (25). MI is more robust than conventional correlation techniques that use a mean squared error. For example, when registering T1-weighted MRI to T2-weighted MRI, tissue that appears hypointense in one image can be hyperintense in the other, and therefore correlation is an incorrect metric for multi-contrast alignment.

### Medical Reality Modeling Language (MRML)

Visualizing medical data involves combining various data sets into a single scene, and exploring the scene interactively. The usage of the 3D Slicer typically involves the creation of a scene from a variety of volume data sets, surface models derived from those volumes,

1. Collect diagnostic anatomical scans (MR, CT, angiography).
2. For cases near eloquent cortex, conduct functional exams (fMRI).
3. Use the 3D Slicer to segment the scans and generate three-dimensional surface models of key structures, both anatomical and functional.
4. Automatically register all pre-operative data together using the 3D Slicer.
5. Position patient in the interventional MR, collect a volume scan, and set up the 3D Slicer.
6. Automatically register pre-operative data to intra-operative data using the 3D Slicer.
7. Use the fusion of all data to plan the optimal trajectory. Guide the initial resection by aiming the locator while viewing the 3D Slicer's display on the in-bore monitor.
8. As surgery progresses, periodically acquire intra-operative volumes for visualization within the 3D Slicer. Drive the location of reformatted slices with the tracked locator device.
9. Re-register if necessary due to patient movement.

## RESULTS

The open MR scanner, complemented by the 3D Slicer, has been applied as a navigational tool in 45 neurosurgical procedures over the course of a year.

### Registration With Pre-Procedural Data

In two of the cases, pre-surgical studies were relevant regarding functional or structural data that could not be obtained intra-operatively. Registration performed between pre- and intra-operative data during craniotomy was completed within five minutes to be ready for use when needed by the surgeon. Although intra-operative brain deformation is non-rigid, rigid registration was sufficient in these cases, since the primary use of the pre-surgical data was to guide the initial approach.

### Trajectory Planning

In many cases, the optimal trajectory from the skin surface to the tumor was obvious from the two-dimensional images. However, the 3D Slicer became helpful in cases where the tumor was deeply situated or dangerously near critical functional tissue or vasculature. Prior to the opening of the skull, the surgeon maneuvered the locator to point at his intended craniotomy at various angles. The pointer and its trajectory were rendered in true real time with the anatomy, a feat presently achievable only with computer reformatting. As the tracked pointer moved within the surgical field, the reformatted slice planes followed its position, sweeping through the volumes. The surgeon verified, and in one case altered, the planned approach by visualizing it on the display relative to all the surface models of critical structures.

The biopsy case depicted in Figure 4 is the prime example of the surgeon altering the approach following examination with the 3D Slicer. According to a conventional examination of MRI on a light box outside the operating room, an access hole was created near the top

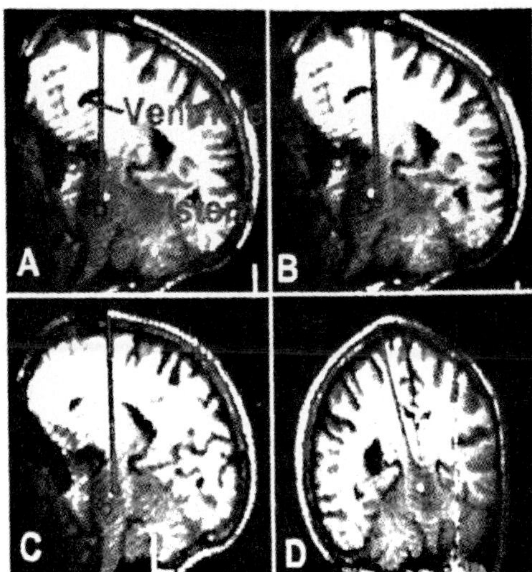

**Figure 4.** Altering the surgical tactic during biopsy planning. (A) Trajectory planning using the original access hole, but hitting the cistern. (B) Avoiding the cistern and ventricle, but missing the two targets (marked with red and yellow spheres). (C) Trajectory planning using a new hole that allows reaching the targets while missing both the cistern and ventricle. (D) Actual biopsy with coronal and sagittal reformatted slices. [Color figure can be viewed in the online issue, which is available at www.interscience.wiley.com.]

of the head to reach a deep tumor in the brain stem. Then the locator was held at the site of the craniotomy by a Buckwalter clamp and oriented to try various trajectories. The locator, normally a handpiece with a needle of known length protruding from its center, was used *without* the needle in order to visualize penetration in the 3D Slicer. The 3D Slicer was used to reformat images in the plane of the locator, and the biopsy targets were clearly marked using red and yellow spheres. The surgeon needed to reach the tumor while avoiding the ventricle and the peripeduncular cistern with the basilar artery. The 3D Slicer revealed that the surgeon would pierce either the ventricle or cistern (Fig. 4A). Avoiding both hazards would require missing the tumor as well (Fig. 4B).

Therefore, a new access hole was drilled in the skull. Figure 4C shows the same planning exercise being executed with the new hole. With the 3D Slicer's guidance, the tumor was reached while avoiding damage to both the ventricle and cistern. Figure 4D shows the actual biopsy with a real needle in place. Here, two slices are being reformatted in perpendicular planes so that both hazards may be seen simultaneously, since a single two-dimensional view cannot reveal all hazards.

### Augmenting Intra-Operative Images With Pre-Operative Images

Of the 45 patients in this study, nine had tumors in the immediate vicinity of the motor, speech, or visual cortices. Therefore, navigation with respect to pre-surgically acquired fMRI was a helpful tool in defining the surgical goal and preventing morbidity. In the case depicted in Figure 5, the locator was maneuvered to the

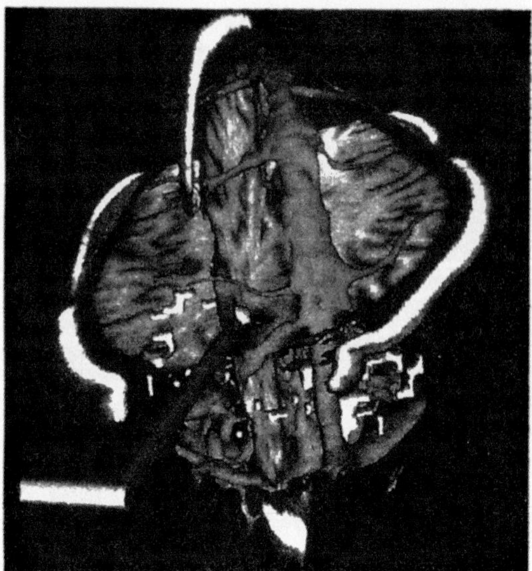

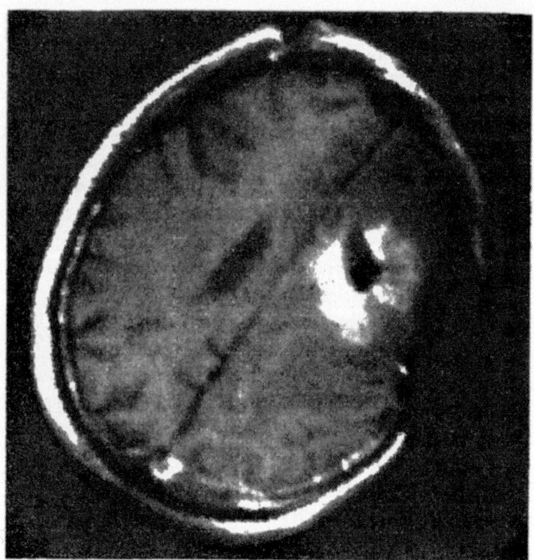

**Figure 5.** Pre-surgical information emphasizes three-dimensional spatial relationships between critical structures, with vessels in pink and results of functional MRI in yellow. Slices are reformatted according to the position of the tracked locator, which is shown following a safe path to the cavernoma. [Color figure can be viewed in the online issue, which is available at www.interscience.wiley.com.]

cavernoma while avoiding hazards consisting of vessels and visual cortex.

### Progressive Intra-Operative Imaging Updates

Once trajectory planning was complete, the 3D Slicer assisted in monitoring the progress of the resection. Since the positions of anatomical structures changed throughout the time course of the procedures, 3–5 new slabs of data were acquired for reformatting during each craniotomy.

We experimented with exploiting overlays to relate the intra-operative changes to the higher-resolution definition of tumor location. A lower-resolution T1-weighted slab acquired quickly during resection was overlaid semi-transparently on an SPGR that was scanned after craniotomy but prior to resection. Figure 6 depicts one of these cases with a fronto-temporal glioma where the SPGR was contrast-enhanced. Figure

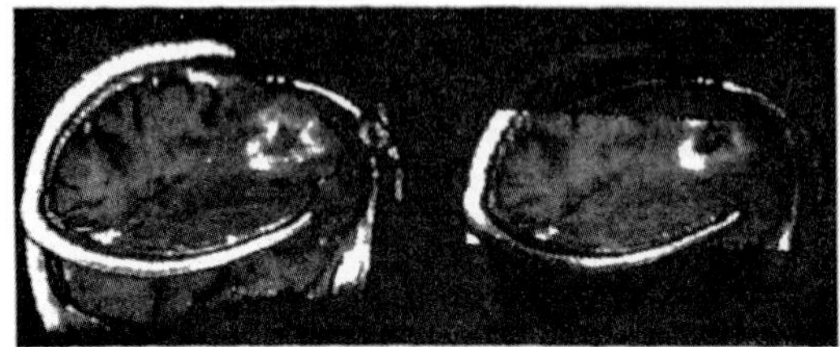

**Figure 6.** The image on the left is from an SPGR scan of a fronto-temporal glioma taken prior to resection. The image on the right shows data from a lower-resolution T1 scan acquired during resection, overlaid on the earlier SPGR scan for comparison.

**Figure 7.** Surgeons are able to characterize the intra-operative shift by transparently overlaying recent images on previously acquired images.

7 displays a reformatted axial slice overlaid on a reformatted slice from the same location prior to resection. The collapse of brain tissue during the resection is indicated by the pronounced shadow.

### Post-Resection Validation

The 3D Slicer offered assistance with anatomy that appeared normal to the eye but displayed abnormal signal intensities in the applied sequences (T1 or T2). In these circumstances, the 3D Slicer was used to create real-time, reformatted images through an intra-operatively acquired slab of images. Near the end of the procedures, the surgeon steered the locator around the perimeter of the cavity that was vacated through resection, and noted the boundary between the non-enhanced normal tissue and the enhanced diseased tissue after resection of the lesion. By viewing the location of the locator's tip on the display, the surgeon had a direct correlation between his visual impression of the tissue and the MR definition of the tissue, as illustrated in Figure 8. The attending neuroradiologist also examined the reformatted images for evidence of residual, diseased tissue to be removed.

In two cases we experimented with affixing the locator's handle to the ultrasonic aspirator so that the surgeon could directly correlate the aspirator's position to the information present in the dynamically reformatted images.

### DISCUSSION

In this paper, we have presented an integrated software tool, called the 3D Slicer, that, when used in conjunction with an open configuration MR scanner, has the capability to beneficially address the issues of interventional image quality, imaging time, multi-modal fusion, faster localization, and three-dimensional visualiza-

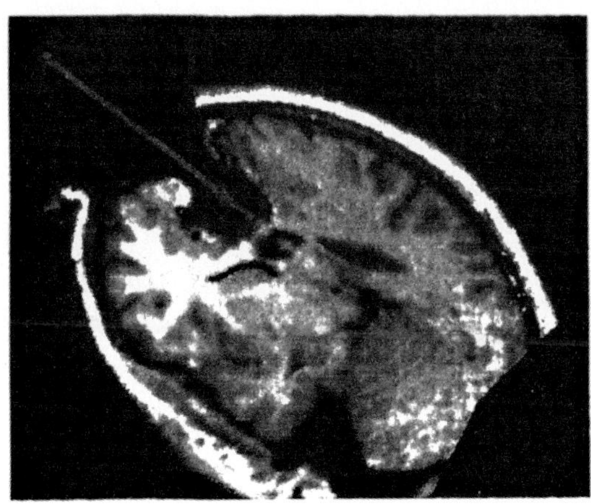

**Figure 8.** Virtual real-time imaging: the surgical instrument (red) is tracked, and two orthogonal planes are shown reformatted relative to the instrument tip's position and updated at 10 frames per second. [Color figure can be viewed in the online issue, which is available at www.interscience.wiley.com.]

tion. This initial feasibility phase has been an experiment to determine the utility of various features, and the results have been strictly qualitative so far. The 3D Slicer has proved to be a stable and reliable application, as highlighted by the variety of histopathology in the 45 cases. As we apply the 3D Slicer on a routine basis, a clinical evaluation of its influence on surgical decision-making and resection control is being conducted. Our neurosurgical colleagues have found the 3D Slicer helpful for blending data sets together that differ in information-type and time. First, it can merge functional information, anatomical information, and information from contrast agents into a single view. Second, it can fuse images serially distributed throughout the course of surgery. This carries two important benefits. First, surgeons are given the ability to distinguish between the diffusion of an intra-operatively administered contrast agent over a prolonged period into regions exterior to the pathology, and the shifting of the pathology itself. Second, since the warping of pre-surgical data to account for intra-operative shift has yet to reach a clinically acceptable level of accuracy, data that is not easily acquired interventionally (fMRI, MRA) needs to be mentally warped by the surgeon to account for morphological changes. The 3D Slicer's overlay capability conveniently facilitates this process.

The 3D Slicer has been shown by case study to be critically beneficial in biopsies. Biopsy localization is much better facilitated when imaging and tracking are in real time. If the needle's trajectory is only slightly incorrect, the needle's tip veers off target. To provide interactive trajectory planning, a small volume is acquired for software reformatting. Positioning is critical because negative histopathological results can indicate either that the tumor is benign, or that the needle missed the mark. The surgeon watches the 3D Slicer's display to help prevent the latter while simultaneously avoiding repeated needle repositioning. In this way, the importance of the 3D Slicer increases for the deeper tumors, since the risks associated with tissue damage rise with repeated penetrations and maneuvering. Al-

though surgeons are accustomed to viewing two-dimensional images, a single two-dimensional view cannot reveal all hazards.

Another very important application of the 3D Slicer is in cavernoma cases, because the lesion is benign, small, and difficult to find. Before the existence of interventional imaging, such lesions could be found only through following the blood after an episode of bleeding. Even with imaging, experienced surgeons have trouble pinpointing the lesion. Invasion of the brain always carries the risk of side effects such as paresis or bleeding, complications which may be unavoidable in cases of malignant tumors that must be removed completely for survival. Cavernomas seldom occur, but they are benign, which reduces the tolerance of error. The 3D Slicer could potentially reduce the risk of damage by guiding the surgeon more directly toward small lesions.

In cases with low-grade gliomas, for which total resection is correlated with a prolonged survival time and even total cure, precise margin definition was of utmost importance. Visual differentiation of tissue in these tumors was difficult, whereas T2-weighted images gave a good estimate of the tumor extent. The display of these pre-surgical images allowed more careful control of total tumor resection.

Other JMRI articles (26) have cited "software limitations" as barriers to trajectory optimization, and have expressed the need for fusing and transferring three-dimensional models derived from different MR sequences to the operating field of the interventional MR system. The 3D Slicer satisfies that need and is freely available for researchers to use in their own interventional environments. Furthermore, due to its modular design and open source nature, the 3D Slicer is a useful platform for bootstrapping development of image-analysis algorithms. In addition, our novel file format, MRML, can be adopted for describing three-dimensional medical scenes for any application.

Besides these positive implications for impacting planning and guidance, there are limitations pertaining to the surgeon's learning curve, the applicability of pre-surgical models throughout the procedure, the efficacy of the overhead display, and registration problems due to magnetic field inhomogeneity. Although the 3D Slicer has the capability to present the surgeon with a vast array of information, we found that all available information was extremely beneficial for planning in practice, but overwhelming for on-line guidance. As a result, we presented the surgeon with one or two reformatted planes and one key surface model at a time. Surgeons are gradually becoming more accustomed to three-dimensional guidance, but require more time to fully embrace the technology. The use of three-dimensional models during surgery is limited, because intra-operative shift inaccurately renders surfaces created from pre-operative data. Creating new models on-line from intra-operative data was attempted during this study, but was found to be too time-intensive to be useful. Future progress in automatic segmentation may enable this approach. Caveats of registering intra-operative MR data stem from magnetic field inhomogeneity and patient movement. Patients are typically positioned in the magnet to optimize the surgeon's access to the area of interest, which sometimes leaves features near the extremities, such as the tip of the skull, near the boundary for homogeneity. This can present a problem for fully automatic registration algorithms that rely on the strong signal present in the skin. In particular, we found that patients who are positioned according to a worst-case scenario experience a flattening of the head in the interventional images. This usually does not present a problem for accurate tracking of the locator, since the tumor tends to be positioned near the center of the magnetic field. Proper patient positioning is presently used to avoid this situation. Patient movement has not posed a problem in our cases; complete reregistration was required in only one case, in which the patient moved during seizure. As one final present limitation, the display screen in the gantry, though useful, is not ergonomically sound, as it forced the surgeon to frequently look up from the patient in order to view the images.

Our future plans are to work toward automatic segmentation and deformable registration. As automatic and faster semi-automatic segmentation algorithms are invented, more rapid model generation will become possible. Potential applications are in surgery where models could be created from intra-operative data, and also in surgical planning, where model generation would become less labor-intensive. Since model deformation has yet to achieve a sufficiently dependable accuracy for surgeons, we often stop using pre-operative models once resection is well underway. Deformable registration being developed (27,28) holds promise in being able to warp pre-operative data to match the intra-operative changes. Existing algorithms are not yet accurate enough to be relied upon by surgeons, but when ready, such tools can be incorporated in the 3D Slicer.

In conclusion, we have presented here an integrated visualization tool that allows the incorporation of multiple data sets into a single display environment. Tools are available in this environment for data fusion, segmentation, three-dimensional model generation, and tracking of instrumented sensors. We have utilized this tool in 45 neurosurgical procedures, and have found its integrated functionality to be critical in providing the surgeon with full access to all available imaging data. The 3D Slicer achieves the objectives established in the introduction as an end-to-end solution that bundles different aspects of analysis into a single visualization framework. The system has been used in the most difficult cases where precise margin definition is of utmost importance, and where updated navigation is a valuable tool to define the surgical goal and prevent morbidity. Feedback from clinical users suggests that they most appreciate its ability to help them navigate a complicated assembly of information. The system's flexible design will allow it to expand as a highly integrated suite for analysis and visualization.

## ACKNOWLEDGMENTS

David Gering is grateful for the generous support of GE Medical Systems. Lauren O'Donnell was supported by a W.A. Rosenblith Fellowship. William Wells III was supported by a Whitaker Foundation Biomedical Engineering Research Grant. Ron Kikinis and Ferenc Jolesz received partial support from NIH grants P41 RR13218-01, P01 CA67165-03, and R01 RR11747-01A. Eric Grimson received partial support from NSF grant IIS-9610249.

## APPENDIX

### *Medical Reality Modeling Language*

MRML files essentially describe three aspects of data:

Disk Location: MRML files are not a copy of the data in another format. Instead, a MRML file describes where the data is stored so the data can remain in its original format and location.

Geometric Position: A MRML file describes how to position the data sets relative to each other in three-dimensional space.

Appearance: A MRML file describes how to display the data by specifying parameters for rendering and coloring.

### *XML Syntax*

MRML is implemented as a type of XML document where new tags have been defined to handle medical data types such as volumes, models, and the coordinate transforms between them. XML (29) is the next generation of HTML for use as the document language of the World Wide Web. HTML tags data with instructions of how a browser should interpret the data. Example tags are images, links, and tables. XML extends this functionality by allowing users to define their own tags.

There are several advantages to building on the XML standard, as opposed to an original format. The World Wide Web has popularized markup languages so that the XML structure is immediately familiar to computer scientists everywhere. There are off-the-shelf XML parsers available in several programming languages. Double-clicking on any XML file in Windows opens the file in Microsoft Internet Explorer, where it can be viewed.

### *Design*

A three-dimensional scene is represented in MRML as a tree-like graph where volumes, models, and other items are the nodes in the graph. Each node has attributes for specifying its data. We introduce the most important MRML nodes here, and more details can be found at the 3D Slicer Web site (20).

### *Volume*

Volume nodes describe data sets that can be thought of as stacks of two-dimensional images that form a three-dimensional volume. Volume nodes describe where the images are stored on disk, how to render the data (window and level), and how to read the files. This information is extracted from the image headers (if they exist) at the time the MRML file is generated. Consequently, MRML files isolate MRML browsers from needing to understand how to read the myriad of file formats for medical data.

### Model

Model nodes describe polygonal data. They indicate where the model is stored on disk, and how to render it (e.g., color, opacity). Models are assumed to have been constructed with the orientation and voxel dimensions of the original segmented volume.

### Matrix

The output of a rigid-body registration is a rotation and translation expressed mathematically as a transformation matrix. These transforms can be inserted into MRML files as matrix nodes. Each matrix affects volumes and models that appear inside its transform node in the MRML file. Multiple matrices can be concatenated.

### Transform

A transform is not a node with attributes, but a construct for building MRML files. A transform encapsulates the matrix nodes inside it such that they are invisible to nodes outside the transform.

### Color

Color nodes define colors by describing not only the actual color value, but also their names and a list of label values. One attribute of a model node is the name of its color. When the 3D Slicer displays label maps, it colors each voxel by looking up the color associated with that label value. Thus, when label maps are displayed on reformatted slices, their colors match the corresponding surface models in the three-dimensional view.

### Option

Option nodes allow browser-specific information to be stored in a MRML file. For example, the 3D Slicer uses option nodes to store the user's three-dimensional viewpoint information.

### REFERENCES


1. Jolesz FA. Image-guided procedures and the operating room of the future. Radiology 1997;204:601–612.
2. ANALYZE Software. http://www.mayo.edu/bir/analyze/ANALYZE_Main.html
3. MEDx Software. http://www.sensor.com/medx_info/medx_docs.html
4. MNI Software. http://www.bic.mni.mcgill.ca/software/
5. Grimson WEL, Leventon M, Ettinger G, et al. Clinical experience with a high precision image-guided neurosurgery system. In: Wells III WM, Colchester A, Delp S, editors. First international conference on medical image computing and computer-assisted intervention. Boston: Springer-Verlag; 1998. p 63–73.
6. Colchester ACF, Zhao J, Holton-Tainter KS, et al. Development and preliminary evaluation of Vislan, a surgical planning and guidance system using intra-operative video imaging. Med Image Anal 1996; 191:73–90.
7. Galloway RL. Stereotactic frame systems and intraoperative localization devices. In: Maciunas RJ, editor. Interactive image-guided neurosurgery. American Association Neurological Surgeons; 1993. p 9–16.
8. Maciunas RJ, Fitzpatrick J, Galloway RL, Allen G. Beyond Stereotaxy: Extreme levels of application accuracy are provided by implantable fiducial markers for interactive image-guided neurosurgery. In: Maciunas RJ, editor. Interactive image-guided neurosurgery. American Association Neurological Surgeons; 1993. p 261–270.
9. Peters T, Davey B, Munger P, Comeau R, Evans A, Olivier A. Three-dimensional multimodal image-guidance for neurosurgery. IEEE Trans Med Imaging 1996;15:121–128.
10. Ryan MJ, Erickson RK, Levin DN, Pelizzari CA, Macdonald RL, Dohrmann GJ. Frameless stereotaxy with real-time tracking of patient head movement and retrospective patient-image registration. J Neurosurgery 1996;85:287–292.
11. Schenk JF, Jolesz FA, Roemer PB, et al. Superconducting open-configuration MR imaging system for image-guided therapy. Radiology 1995;195:805–814.
12. Black PM, Moriarty T, Alexander III E, et al. The development and implementation of intraoperative MRI and its neurosurgical applications. Neurosurgery 1997;41:831–842.
13. Lunsford LD, Parrish R, Albright L. Intraoperative imaging with a therapeutic computed tomographic scanner. Neurosurgery 1984; 15:559–561.
14. Bucholtz RD, Yah DD, Trobaugh J, et al. The correction of stereotactic inaccuracy caused by brain shift using an interaoperative ultrasound device. In: First Joint CVRMED/MRCAS. Genoble: Springer-Verlag; 1997. p 459–466.
15. Hata N, Dohi T, Kikinis R, Jolesz FA, Wells III WM. Computer assisted intra-operative MR-guided therapy: pre and intra-operative image registration, enhanced three-dimensional display, deformable registration. In: 7th Annual Meeting of Japan Society of Computer Aided Surgery. Sapporo, Japan, 1997. p 119–120.
16. Gering D, Nabavi A, Kikinis R, et al. An integrated visualization system for surgical planning and guidance using image fusion and interventional imaging. In: Taylor C, Colchester A, editors. Second International Conference on Medical Image Computing and Computer-Assisted Intervention. Cambridge: Springer-Verlag; 1999; p 809–819.
17. Schroeder W, Martin K, Lorensen W. The visualization toolkit: an object-oriented approach to 3-D graphics. Upper Saddle River, NJ: Prentice Hall; 1996. p 826.
18. Sun OpenGL for Solaris. http://www.sun.com/software/graphics/OpenGL/
19. Welch BB. Practical programming in Tcl and Tk. Upper Saddle River, NJ: Prentice Hall; 1997. p 630.
20. 3D Slicer. http://www.slicer.org/
21. Lorensen WE, Cline HE. Marching cube: A high resolution 3-D surface construction algorithm. Computer Graphics 1987;21:163–169.
22. Schroeder W, Zarge J, Lorensen W. Decimation of triangle meshes. Computer Graphics 1992;26:65–78.
23. Viola PA, Wells III WM. Alignment by maximization of mutual information. In: International Conference on Computer Vision., 1995. p 16–23.
24. Wells III WM, Viola PA, Atsumi H, Nakajima S, Kikinis R. Multimodalvolume registration by maximization of mutual information. Med Image Anal 1996;1:35–51.
25. West J, Fitzpatrick J. Comparison and evaluation of retrospective intermodality brain image registration techniques. J Comput Assist Tomogr 1997;21:554–566.
26. Kollias SS, Bernays R, Marugg RA, Romanowski B, Yonekawa Y, Valavanis A. Target definition and trajectory optimization for interactive MR-guided biopsies of brain tumors in an open configuration MRI system. J Magn Reson Imaging 1998;8:143–159.
27. Hata N, Dohi T, Warfield S, Wells III W, Kikinis R, Jolesz F. Multimodality deformable registration of pre- and intraoperative images for MRI-guided brain surgery. In: Wells III WM, Colchester A, Delp S, editors. First International Conference on Medical Image Computing and Computer-Assisted Intervention. Cambridge, MA: Springer-Verlag; 1998. p 1067–1074.
28. Warfield S, Robatino A, Dengler J, Jolesz F, Kikinis R. Nonlinear registration and template driven segmentation. In: Toga AW, editor. Brain warping. Academic Press: 1999. p 67–84.
29. Extensible Markup Language. http://www.w3.org/XML/

# Estimation of 3D left ventricular deformation from echocardiography[☆]

Xenophon Papademetris[a,*], Albert J. Sinusas[b,c], Donald P. Dione[c], James S. Duncan[a,b]

[a]*Department of Electrical Engineering, Yale University, PO Box 208042, New Haven, CT 06520-8042, USA*
[b]*Department of Diagnostic Radiology, School of Medicine, Yale University, PO Box 208042, New Haven, CT 06520-8042, USA*
[c]*Department of Medicine, School of Medicine, Yale University, PO Box 208042, New Haven, CT 06520-8042, USA*

Received 14 December 1999; received in revised form 7 April 2000; accepted 12 July 2000

## Abstract

The quantitative estimation of regional cardiac deformation from 3D image sequences has important clinical implications for the assessment of viability in the heart wall. Such estimates have so far been obtained almost exclusively from Magnetic Resonance (MR) images, specifically MR tagging. In this paper we describe a methodology for estimating cardiac deformations from 3D echocardiography (3DE). The images are segmented interactively and then initial correspondence is established using a shape-tracking approach. A dense motion field is then estimated using a transversely isotropic linear elastic model, which accounts for the fiber directions in the left ventricle. The dense motion field is in turn used to calculate the deformation of the heart wall in terms of strain in cardiac specific directions. The strains obtained using this approach in open-chest dogs before and after coronary occlusion, show good agreement with previously published results in the literature. They also exhibit a high correlation with strains produced in the same animals using implanted sonomicrometers. This proposed method provides quantitative regional 3D estimates of heart deformation from ultrasound images. © 2001 Elsevier Science B.V. All rights reserved.

*Keywords:* Left ventricular deformation; Cardiac imaging analysis; Image analysis; Non-rigid motion estimation; Strain estimation

## 1. Introduction

A fundamental goal of many efforts in the cardiac imaging and image analysis communities is to assess the regional function of the left ventricle (LV) of the heart. The general consensus is that the analysis of heart wall deformation provides quantitative estimates of the location and extent of ischemic myocardial injury. Regional left ventricular deformation can be determined using all of the principal imaging modalities, including contrast angiography, echocardiography, radionuclide imaging, cine computed tomography (CT), and magnetic resonance (MR) imaging. There have been considerable efforts within the medical image analysis community aimed at estimating this deformation from each of these imaging modalities. Much of the effort has been confined to analysis of two-dimensional images or projections of the heart. Although, recently significant effort has been directed at a more comprehensive analysis of left ventricular deformation in all three dimensions.

Left ventricular deformation can be assessed in three-dimensional space using ECG-gated single photon emission computed tomography (SPECT) (Shen et al., 1999; Cwajg et al., 1999; Faber et al., 1999; Calnon et al., 1997; Berman and Germano, 1997; Germano et al., 1995; Cooke et al., 1994) or positron emission tomography (PET) (Miller et al., 1994; Yamashita et al., 1989; Buvat et al., 1997). However, both of these radionuclide methods have a restricted ability to assess left ventricular deformation, secondary to the limited spatial and temporal resolution of these approaches. These radionuclide methods have involved both count-based (Shen et al., 1999; Calnon et al., 1997; Cooke et al., 1994) and geometry-based approaches (Cwajg et al., 1999; Faber et al., 1999; Germano et al., 1995).

Cine MR imaging has emerged as a more comprehen-

---

[☆]Electronic Annexes available. See www.elsevier.com/locate/media.
*Corresponding author.
*E-mail address:* papad@noodle.med.yale.edu (X. Papademetris).

sive approach to assess myocardial deformation in three-dimensional space (Moore et al., 2000). MR imaging offers improved spatial resolution. Unique to cine MR imaging is the ability to track deformation of myocardial tissue within the wall as well as on the endocardial and epicardial surfaces. However, the analysis of mid-wall myocardial deformation requires special cine MR imaging sequences, including MR tissue tagging (Amini et al., 1998; Haber et al., 1998; Kerwin and Prince, 1998; Park et al., 1996; Prince and McVeigh, 1992; Young et al., 1995) and others, or MR phase contrast velocity imaging (Pelc, 1991; Duncan et al., 1998; Meyer et al., 1996; Zhu et al., 1997). While these newer MR approaches offer a comprehensive analysis of regional left ventricular deformation, wide application of MR imaging remains limited by cost and the difficulty in routinely applying these MR approaches to critically ill cardiac patients.

Echocardiography offers significant advantages over both radionuclide imaging and MR imaging. Echocardiographic images can be acquired on critically ill patients in an emergency room or at the patient's bedside in the intensive care unit, and this can be accomplished at a reduced cost. Comprehensive analysis of left ventricular deformation is now feasible using echocardiography, with the advent of newer three-dimensional acquisition systems (von Ramm and Smith, 1990). Recently, commercial software has become available to automatically assess global and regional left ventricular function (Lang et al., 1996). However, these newer automated echocardiographic approaches have not been fully validated. Hence, development of automated analysis of echocardiographic images is attracting an increasing amount of attention in the literature (Chuang et al., 1999a,b, 2000; Sheehan et al., 1998; Angelini, 1999; Brandt et al., 1999; Montagnat et al., 1999; Jacob et al., 1999). However, none of these methods is capable of estimating dense maps of three-dimensional deformation from echocardiographic images comparable to those obtained from the analysis of MR tagging images.

In this paper we describe, test and present prelinary validation for an approach to estimate the regional three-dimensional deformation of the left ventricle using echocardiography. We use a biomechanical model to describe the myocardium and shape-based tracking displacement estimates on the endocardial and epicardial walls to generate the initial displacement estimates. These are integrated in a Bayesian estimation framework and the overall problem is solved using the finite element method. This method produces *quantitative regional* 3D cardiac deformation estimates from ultrasound images which up to now was thought to be only possible using magnetic resonance and especially MR tagging. We validate these estimates by comparing them to invasive measurements performed simultaneously using implanted sonomicrometers. The fast improving quality of ultrasound images with the introduction of harmonic imaging (Caidahl et al., 1999) and contrast agents (Porter et al., 1994) should make it

possible to obtain even more accurate estimates of 3D left ventricular deformation in the future.

## 2. Our approach

We estimate a dense displacement field within a Bayesian estimation framework which consists of a data term and a model term. These are described in Sections 2.1 and 2.2, respectively. The data term captures the image-derived information about the problem. We segment the images interactively and then proceed to extract initial displacement estimates using a shape-tracking approach. We then model the noise in these estimates using a Gaussian noise model. The model term captures our prior beliefs about the nature of the displacement field. Since the left ventricle is a single deforming body, we expect the displacements of neighboring points to be related. We capture this relationship using a biomechanical model which is, in turn, used to generate a prior probability density function for the displacement field. Our approach that incorporates a biomechanical model has the advantages of having no arbitrarily set weights and of allowing us to take advantage of forward modeling efforts in the biomechanics literature, see for example the collections in (Hunter et al., 1991; Panfilov and Holden, 1997).

### 2.1. Obtaining initial displacement data

### 2.1.1. Image acquisition

The images were acquired using an HP Sonos 5500 Ultrasound System with a 3D transducer (Transthoracic OmniPlane 21349A (R5012)). The 3D-probe was placed at the apex of the left-ventricle of an open-chest dog using a small ultrasound gelpad (Aquaflex) as a standoff as shown in Fig. 1. Each acquisition consisted of 13–17 frames per cardiac cycle depending on the heart rate. The angular slice spacing was 5 degrees resulting in 36 image slices for each frame. For validation purposes we also implanted arrays of sonomicrometer crystals (Dione et al., 1997; Meoli et al., 1998) at two positions in the left ventricle.

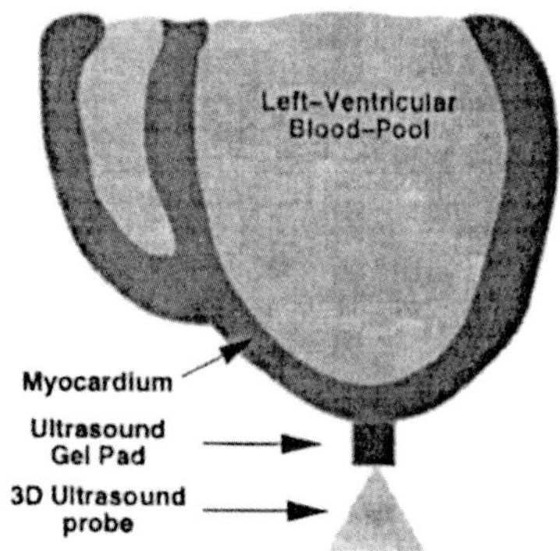


Fig. 1. Image acquisition geometry.

### 2.1.2. Image segmentation

The endocardial and epicardial surfaces were extracted interactively using a software platform (Papademetris et al., 1998) originally developed for MR image data and subsequently modified to allow for the different geometry and image characteristics of ultrasound. For the automated part of the segmentation, for each image slice, we used an integrated deformable boundary method whose external energy function consisted of a standard intensity gradient term and a texture-based term similar to that proposed by Chakraborty (1996). In our approach, however, the contours were parameterized using B-splines (de Boor, 1978) to allow for easy interaction. Clearly detecting the epicardium is the hardest of the two tasks. At this point we are relying on operator intervention and correction of the automatic algorithm to ensure accurate segmentation.

The texture model tries to classify each pixel in one of three classes (blood pool, myocardium, region outside the epicardium) by modeling each class using texture parameters derived from the work of Manjunath (1991). The mean values of these parameters for each class are set interactively by having the user click on one point in each of the three regions. Then the variability of these parameters in each class is modeled as a normal distribution assuming equal variances for all the classes. A first-order Gaussian Markov Random Field (GMRF) model is used to model the class-label for each pixel. The GMRF combines the likelihood of belonging to a class as specified by the texture parameters with a degree of regional smoothness in the classification. A more detailed description can be found in (Papademetris, 2000).

The overall framework produced reasonable results as shown in Figs. 2 and 3. There is clearly room for improvement in this approach, as we are not yet taking advantage of the temporal coherency in the spatial position of surfaces across times. The potential benefits of using such constraints is demonstrated in a number of papers, including (Angelini, 1999; Brandt et al., 1999; Jacob et al., 1999). We are also currently looking into more sophisticated techniques for generating the external energy maps, including those suggested by Mulet-Parada (1998).

### 2.1.3. Shape-tracking displacement estimates

In this work, the original displacements on the surfaces of the myocardium were obtained by using the shape-tracking algorithm whose details were presented in (Shi et al., 2000; Papademetris, 2000). The method tries to track points on successive surfaces using a shape similarity metric which tries to minimize the difference in principal curvatures and was validated using implanted markers (Shi et al., 2000).

For example, consider point $p_1$ on a surface at time $t_1$ which is to be mapped to a point $p_2$ on the deformed surface at time $t_2$, as shown in Fig. 4. First, a search is performed in a physically plausible region $W$ on the deformed surface and the point $\hat{p}_2$ which has the local shape properties closest to those $p_1$ is selected. The shape properties here are captured in terms of the principal curvatures $\kappa_1$ and $\kappa_2$. The distance measure used is the bending energy required to bend a curved plate or surface patch to a newly deformed state. This is labeled as $d_{\mathrm{be}}$ and is defined as

$$d_{\mathrm{be}}(p_1, p_2)$$
$$= \left( \frac{(\kappa_1(p_1) - \kappa_1(p_2))^2 + (\kappa_2(p_1) - \kappa_2(p_2))^2}{2} \right). \tag{1}$$

The displacement estimate vector for each point $p_1$, $u_1^m$ is given by

$$u_1^m = \hat{p}_2 - p_1, \quad \hat{p}_2 = \arg\min_{p_2 \in W} [d_{\mathrm{be}}(p_1, p_2)].$$

#### 2.1.3.1. Confidence measures in the match.
The bending energy measures for all the points inside the search region $W$ are recorded as the basis to measure the *goodness* and *uniqueness* of the matching choice. The value of the minimum bending energy in the search region between the matched points indicates the goodness of the match. Denote this value as $m_{\mathrm{g}}$, we have the following measure for matching goodness:

$$m_{\mathrm{g}}(p_1) = d_{\mathrm{be}}(p_1, \hat{p}_2). \tag{2}$$

On the other hand, it is desirable that the chosen matching

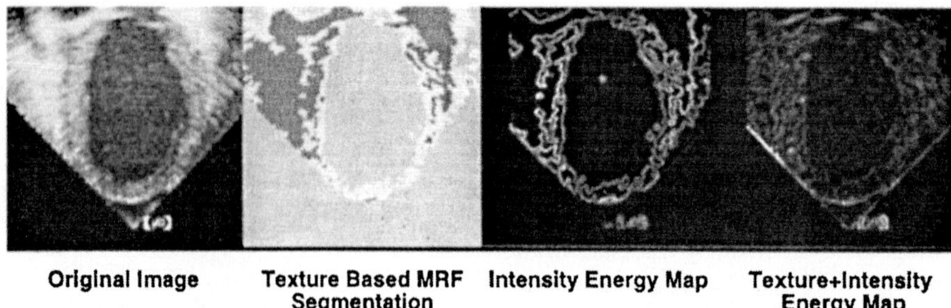



Fig. 2. External energy functions for intensity and intensity+texture snakes. Note that the intensity only energy function is very noisy inside the left-ventricular blood-pool which creates many local minima for the deformable contour. The use of the texture eliminates most of these minima.

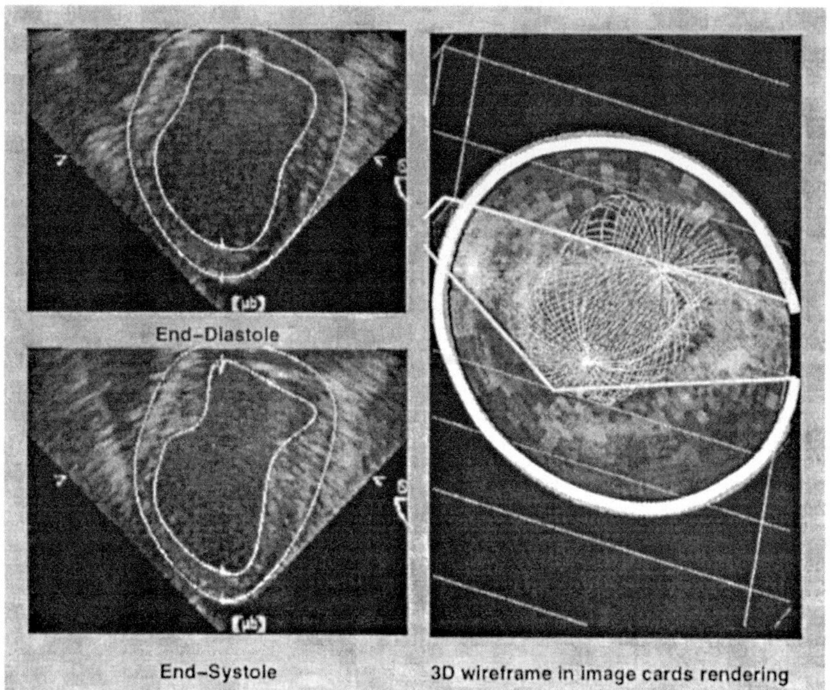



Fig. 3. Left: Images and superimposed extracted contours. Only two of the eight frames are shown. Right: 3D rendering showing all the wire-frame contours superimposed on a long axis (original) and a short-axis (interpolated) image slices.

point is a unique choice among the candidate points within the search window. Ideally, the bending energy value of the chosen point should be an outlier (much smaller value) compared to the values of the rest of the points. If we denote the mean values of the bending energy measures of all the points inside window $W$ except the chosen point as

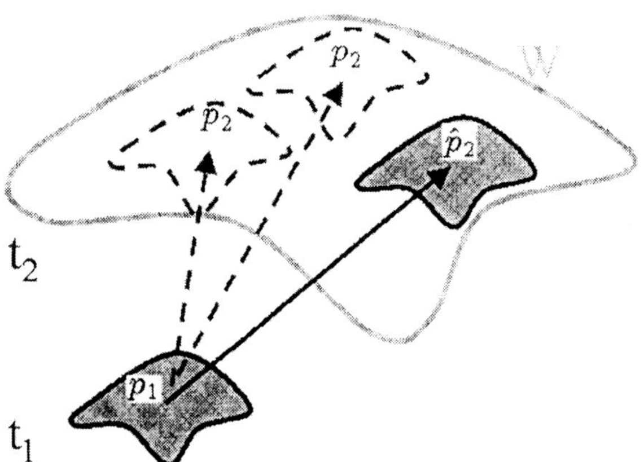



Fig. 4. Example of the shape-tracking approach. The goal here is to map points on the original surface to points on the final surface. For a point $p_1$ on the original surface, we define a search window $W$ on the final surface which contains all plausible corresponding points. Then the point $p_2$ in $W$ which has the most similar shape-properties to $p_1$ is selected as the candidate match point. The distance function for shape-similarity is based on the difference in principal curvatures.

$\bar{d}_{be}$ and the standard deviation as $\sigma_{be}^d$, we define the uniqueness measure as

$$m_u(p_1) = \frac{d_{be}(p_1, \hat{p}_2)}{\bar{d}_{be} - \sigma_{be}^d}. \tag{3}$$

This uniqueness measure has a high value if the bending energy of the chosen point is small compared to some smaller value (mean minus standard deviation) of the remaining bending energy measures. Combining these two measures together, we arrive at one *confidence measure* $c^m(p_1)$ for the matched point $\hat{p}_2$ of point $p_1$,

$$c^m(p_1) = \frac{1}{k_{1,g} + k_{2,g} m_g(p_1)} \times \frac{1}{k_{1,u} + k_{2,u} m_u(p_1)}, \tag{4}$$

where $k_{1,g}$, $k_{2,g}$, $k_{1,u}$ and $k_{2,u}$ are scaling constants for normalization purposes. We normalize the confidences to lie in the range 0–1.

*2.1.3.2. Modeling the initial displacement estimates.* Given a set of displacement vector measurements $u^m$ and confidence measures $c^m$ we model these estimates probabilistically by assuming that the noise in the individual measurements is normally distributed with zero mean and a variance $\sigma^2 = 1/c^m$. In addition, we assume that the measurements are uncorrelated. Given these assumptions we can write the measurement probability for each point as

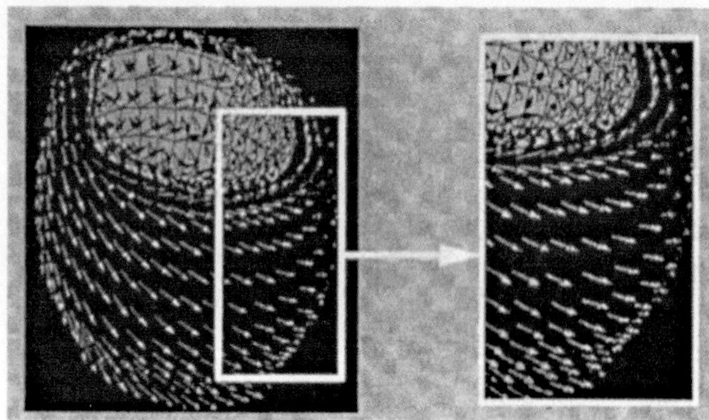

Fig. 5. Fiber direction in the left ventricle as defined in Guccione (1991).

$$p(u^m|u) = \frac{1}{\sqrt{2\pi\sigma^2}}\, e^{-(u-u^m)^2/2\sigma^2}. \tag{5}$$

## 2.2. Modeling the myocardium

The left-ventricular myocardium is modeled using a transversely isotropic linear elastic model which allows us to incorporate information about the preferential stiffness of the tissue along fiber directions from Guccione (1991). These fiber directions are shown in Fig. 5. The model described in terms of an internal or strain energy function of the form

$$W = e^T Ce, \tag{6}$$

where $e$ is the vector form of the strain tensor $\epsilon$ (see next section), $e^T$ is the transpose of $e$ and $C$ is the $6 \times 6$ matrix containing the elastic constants which define the material properties. This is described in more detailed in continuum mechanics textbooks such as Malvern (1969).

### 2.2.1. Deformation and strain

Consider a body $B(0)$ which after time $t$ moves and deforms to body $B(t)$ as shown in Fig. 6. A point $X$ on $B(0)$ goes to a point $x$ on $B(t)$ and the transformation gradient $F$ is defined as $dx = F\, dX$. The deformation is expressed in terms of the strain tensor $\epsilon$. Because the

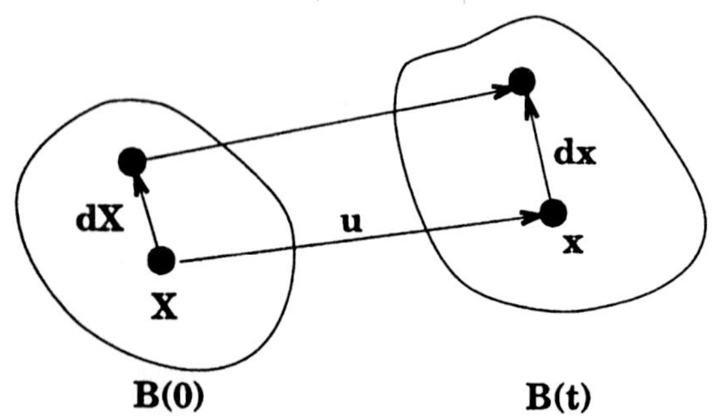


Fig. 6. Geometry of deformation. In this case a body $B(0)$ goes to a body $B(t)$. The deformation operator $F$ is defined as $dx = F\, dX$.

deformations to be estimated in this work are larger than 5%, we use a finite strain formulation implemented using a logarithmic strain $\epsilon^L$, which is defined as: $\epsilon^L = \ln\sqrt{F \cdot F^T}$. Since the strain tensor is a $3 \times 3$ symmetric 2nd-rank tensor (matrix), we can re-write it in vector form as $e = [\epsilon_{11}\ \epsilon_{22}\ \epsilon_{33}\ \epsilon_{12}\ \epsilon_{13}\ \epsilon_{23}]^T$. This enables us to express the tensor equations in a more familiar matrix notation.

### 2.2.2. Strain energy function

The mechanical model can be defined in terms of a strain energy function. The simplest useful continuum model in solid mechanics is the linear elastic one which is of the form $W = e^T Ce$ where $C$ is a $6 \times 6$ matrix and defines the material properties of the deforming body and $e$ is the vector form of the strain tensor. The simplest model is the isotropic linear elastic model used widely in the image analysis literature (Duncan et al., 1998; Haber et al., 1998). In this case the matrix $C$ takes the form

$$C^{-1} = \frac{1}{E}\begin{bmatrix} 1 & -\nu & -\nu & 0 & 0 & 0 \\ -\nu & 1 & -\nu & 0 & 0 & 0 \\ -\nu & -\nu & 1 & 0 & 0 & 0 \\ 0 & 0 & 0 & 2(1+\nu) & 0 & 0 \\ 0 & 0 & 0 & 0 & 2(1+\nu) & 0 \\ 0 & 0 & 0 & 0 & 0 & 2(1+\nu) \end{bmatrix}, \tag{7}$$

where $E$ is the Young's modulus that is a measure of the stiffness of the material and $\nu$ is the Poisson's ratio which is a measure of incompressibility.

In this work, the left ventricle of the heart is specifically modeled as a transversely elastic material to account for the preferential stiffness in the fiber direction. This is an extension of the isotropic linear elastic model which allows for one of the three material axis to have a different stiffness from the other two. In this case the matrix $C$ takes the form

$$C^{-1} = \begin{bmatrix} \dfrac{1}{E_p} & \dfrac{-\nu_p}{E_p} & \dfrac{-\nu_{fp}}{E_f} & 0 & 0 & 0 \\[2ex] \dfrac{-\nu_p}{E_p} & \dfrac{1}{E_p} & \dfrac{-\nu_{fp}}{E_f} & 0 & 0 & 0 \\[2ex] \dfrac{-\nu_{fp}E_f}{E_p} & \dfrac{-\nu_{fp}E_f}{E_p} & \dfrac{1}{E_f} & 0 & 0 & 0 \\[2ex] 0 & 0 & 0 & \dfrac{2(1+\nu_p)}{E_p} & 0 & 0 \\[2ex] 0 & 0 & 0 & 0 & \dfrac{1}{G_f} & 0 \\[2ex] 0 & 0 & 0 & 0 & 0 & \dfrac{1}{G_f} \end{bmatrix}, \tag{8}$$

where $E_f$ is the fiber stiffness, $E_p$ is cross-fiber stiffness and $\nu_{fp}$, $\nu_p$ are the corresponding Poisson's ratios and $G_f$ is the shear modulus across fibers ($G_f \approx E_f/(2(1 + \nu_{fp}))$). If $E_f = E_p$ and $\nu_p = \nu_{fp}$ this model reduces to the more common isotropic linear elastic model. The fiber stiffness was set to be 3.5 times greater than the cross-fiber stiffness (Guccione and McCulloch, 1991). The Poisson's ratios were both set to 0.4 to model approximate incompressibility.[1]

In using a linear elastic model we lose the ability to capture the progressive hardening of the left ventricular myocardium as the strain increases, unlike for example the non-linear models used by Guccione et al. (1991). This is mitigated by the fact that the estimation is done on a frame by frame basis hence the degree of the hardening would be small.

### 2.2.3. A probabilistic description of the model

As previously demonstrated by Geman and Geman (1984) and applied to medical image analysis problems (Christensen et al., 1994; Gee et al., 1997) there is a correspondence between an internal energy function and a Gibbs probability density function. If the mechanical model is described in terms of an internal energy function $W(C, u)$, where $C$ represents the material properties and $u$ the displacement field, then we can write an equivalent prior probability density function $p(u)$ [see Eq. (10)] of the Gibbs form (Geman and Geman, 1984),

$$p(u) = k_1 \exp(-W(C, u)), \qquad (9)$$

where $k_1$ is a normalization constant.

The Markov random field (MRF) then can be thought of as the probabilistic analog of the continuum mechanical model. There are two interesting similarities: (i) both can be defined using energy functions, and (ii) the energy functions at any given point are functions only of the values of that points and its immediate neighbors. In the case of the MRF point (ii) comes from the fact that the Gibbs probability density function is often defined on first and/or second order cliques which are very local neighborhoods of the point. So if the displacement field is modeled as a MRF, the probability of the displacement of a given point effectively only depends on the displacement of its neighbors. In the case of the mechanical model described using a strain energy function, the value of the internal energy function, which via exponentiation in Eq. (9) becomes the probability density function, at a given point depends only on the local strains. These local strains are only dependent on the displacements of the neighbors

of the point and not on the displacements of the whole volume.

The expression of the mechanical model as a MRF allows us to solve the problem within the Bayesian estimation framework. This has the advantage of allowing us to model the noise in the displacement estimates probabilistically and still maintaining the description of the model in the language of continuum mechanics.

### 2.3. Integrating the data and model terms

Having defined both the data term [Eq. (5)] and the model term [Eq. (9)] as probability density functions we naturally proceed to write the overall problem in a Bayesian estimation framework. Given a set of noisy input displacement vectors $u^m$, the associated noise model $p(u^m|u)$ (data term) and a prior probability density function $p(u)$ (model term), find the best output displacements $\hat{u}$ which maximize the posterior probability $p(u|u^m)$. Using Bayes' rule we can write

$$\hat{u} = \arg \max_u \; p(u|u^m) = \arg \max_u \left( \frac{p(u^m|u)p(u)}{p(u^m)} \right). \qquad (10)$$

The prior probability of the measurements $p(u^m)$ is a constant once these measurements have been made and therefore drops out of the minimization process. In this expression we also note that there is an undefined constant. This is the scaling factor that translates the stiffness of the mechanical model to the effective variance of its equivalent probability density function $p(u)$. This constant essentially translates stiffness which is measured in Pascals to confidence in the model which is measured in pixels. The value of this constant sets the relative weight of the data term to the model term. We set this adaptively to be as large as possible (which pushes the optimum towards the data side) subject to solution convergence. In this way we make the following assumption: the best solution is the one which adheres as much as possible to initial estimate of the displacement field but still results in a connected solid. Convergence fails when the Jacobian of the deformation field[2] becomes singular. In this case we lower the value of this weight to produce a smoother displacement field.

### 2.3.1. Model bias and correction

We also note that the mechanical model prior is generated by a passive biomechanical model, that is one which does not capture the active deformation of the left ventricle. This model has a major weakness in that it penalizes all deformations. This model could be thought in some sense as having a mean of zero strain and a variance proportional to the reciprocal of the stiffness. It will tend to underestimate the deformation and hence the strain. As a

---

[1] The value of 0.4 was chosen to model approximate incompressibility. Experience shows that using values greater than 0.4 often causes numerical problems such as mesh locking (Hughes, 1987). Also the myocardium is only approximately incompressible.

[2] The Jacobian of the deformation is the matrix $F$ defined in Fig. 6.

certain amount of deformation *does occur* the use of this model results in an underestimation of the deformation using our approach. A solution to this problem is to incorporate a model of active contraction within the prior, and this is a subject of on-going research within our group (again see (Papademetris, 2000)). At this point the problem is dealt with by forcing the nodes which lie on the endocardial and epicardial surfaces at time $t$ to lie on the segmented surfaces at the time $t + 1$. This corrects for the bias in the estimates of the deformation for those components of the deformation which are perpendicular to the endocardial and epicardial surfaces. The bias in the estimation of deformation parallel to the surfaces remains.

## 2.4. Numerical solution

Taking logarithms in Eq. (10) and differentiating with respect to the displacement field $u$ results in a system of partial differential equations, which we solve using the finite element method (Bathe, 1982). The first step in the finite element method is the division or tessellation of the body of interest into elements; these are commonly tetrahedral or hexahedral in shape. Once this is done, the partial differential equations are written down in integral form for each element, and then the integral of these equations over all the elements is taken to produce the final set of equations. For more information one is referred to standard textbooks such as Bathe (1982). The final set of equations is then solved to produce the output set of displacements. In our case the myocardium is divided into approximately 2500 hexahedral elements, using a custom mesh generation algorithm described in (Papademetris, 2000). A solid mesh of one of the hearts is shown in Fig. 7.

For each frame between end-systole (ES) and end-diastole (ED), a two step problem is posed: (i) solving Eq. (10) normally, and (ii) adjusting the position of all points on the endocardial and epicardial surfaces so they lie on the endocardial and epicardial surfaces at the next frame

using a modified nearest-neighbor technique and solving Eq. (10) once more using this added constraint. This ensures that there is a reduction in the bias in the estimation of the deformation.

## 3. Experimental procedure

### 3.1. Animal experiments

To evaluate the efficacy of using image-derived in vivo deformation estimates to measure regional LV function we conducted experiments on fasting, anesthetized, open chest, adult mongrel dogs with approval of the Yale University Animal Care and Use Committee. In this preliminary work, we report results from four animals. The 3DE images were obtained either before (D1 and D2) or after occlusion of the left anterior descending coronary artery (D3 and D4), using the procedure described in Section 2.1.1. Coronary occlusion created an area of dysfunction which we call the risk area. Also regional blood flow in the myocardium was determined using a radio-labeled microsphere technique. Here, radioactively labeled microspheres were injected into the left atrium and reference blood samples were drawn from the femoral arteries. Regional myocardial blood flow was calculated using a method previously described in (Sinusas et al., 1990). The blood flow measurements are used to identify the risk area and play no further role in this work. Further we implanted sonomicrometers (Sonometrics Corporation, London, Ontario, Canada) at two regions in the myocardium, as shown in the schematic in Fig. 11 (left). We obtain highly accurate invasive measures of the deformation from the analysis of implanted sonomicrometers. Sonomicrometer derived regional strains were considered to be the *gold standard*.

### 3.2. Image analysis

The images were segmented interactively and the surfaces sampled to 0.5 voxel resolution, at which point curvatures were calculated and the shape-tracking algorithm was used to generate initial displacement estimates. The heart wall was divided into 2500 hexahedral elements and the anisotropic linear elastic model was used to regularize the displacements. A commercial finite element solver ABAQUS (Hibbit, Karlsson & Sorencen, 1997) was used to solve the resulting equations. The computational time after the segmentation was of the order of 3–4 h/dog (depending on the heart rate and hence the number of image frames) on a Silicon Graphics Octane with an R10000 195 MHz processor and 128 MB RAM.

### 3.3. Strain analysis

For the purpose of analyzing the results, the left-ventri-

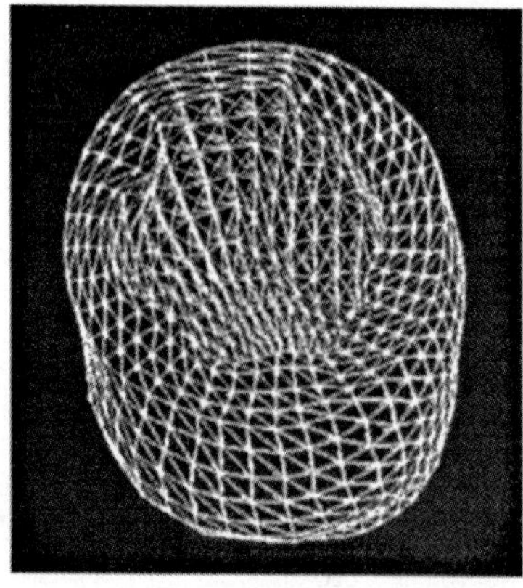

Fig. 7. A 3D mesh generated by interpolating and filling between the endocardial and epicardial boundaries.

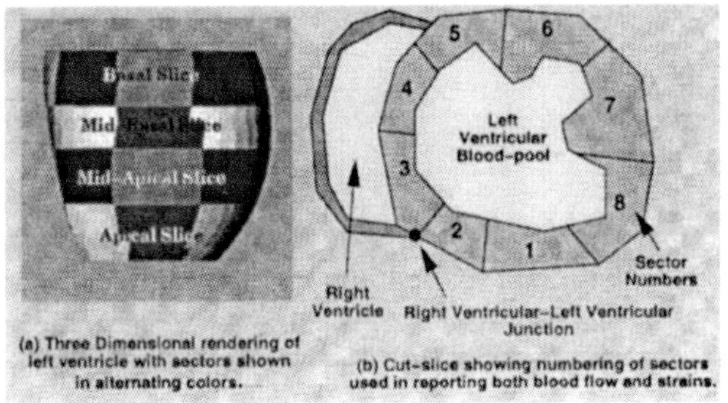



Fig. 8. Division of a slice of the heart for the purpose of reporting results. Each sector consists of approximately 75 elements in the finite element mesh.

cle of the heart was divided into 4 cross-sectional slices, slice 1 being at the apex of the ventricle and number 4 being at the base of the ventricle towards the valve plane. Each slice was further subdivided into 8 sectors, as shown in Fig. 8(b). A sector was labeled as being in the risk area if the endocardial microsphere flow was less than 0.25 ml/min/g. The normal region was defined by 5 transmural sectors located in the posterior lateral wall at the base of the heart (sectors 5, 6, 7 of the basal slice and sectors 6, 7 of the mid-basal slice). We report the average of radial(RR), circumferential(CC) and longitudinal(LL) strains for the risk areas and the normal regions.[3]

## 4. Results

The potential of our methodology is illustrated in Fig. 9, which shows a cut through our tracked 3D mesh overlaid on a slice through the original 3DE image data over time. This could be seen as a form of software-derived, 3DE-based 'tissue tagging' somewhat in the sense of MR tagging. Note the spreading grid lines near the endocardium on the right as the LV thickens from end diastole to end systole.

The quantitative results are summarized in Table 1. Function in the risk area, which was independently defined by microsphere flow, was markedly reduced compared to non-affected regions and the control normal animal. The radial strain is notably smaller in the risk area after coronary occlusion. The circumferential strain becomes less negative also indicating a loss of function. There was a small decrease in the longitudinal strain as well. The

progressive development of regional radial and circumferential strains for 'D3' is shown in Fig. 10.

Croisille (1999) reported similar values (Radial = 23.2±1.9%, Circum = − 10.5±2.0% and Long = − 7.5± 1.0%) for strains in the normal regions of dog hearts using three-dimensional tagged MRI. However, they observed smaller reductions in strains post-occlusion, which can be attributed to coronary reperfusion in their model and significantly delayed imaging after the occlusion (2 days later as opposed to 15–20 minutes in our case). This probably allowed for partial recovery of function in the risk region.

## 5. Validation using implanted sonomicrometers

In an effort to obtain an independent source of in vivo strain values for validation of image-derived strains, we have developed an independent approach for strain measurement using cubic arrays of sonomicrometers implanted in the canine LV myocardium (see details in (Dione et al., 1997)). The efficacy of this technique was illustrated by additional work (Meoli et al., 1998) that showed that the distances obtained with sonomicrometers compared favorably ($r = 0.992$) with those obtained using the more established technique of tracking implanted bead displacements using biplane radiography.

We then compared our image-derived strains to concurrently-estimated sonomicrometer derived strains at several positions in the LV myocardium in the same dogs. The sonomicrometers were located visually from the images and the two nearest sectors of algorithm-derived strains were selected for comparison purposes. The comparison of the principal strain components in two separate regions for a set of 3 studies (the sonomicrometer data was not available for study 'D4') showed a strong correlation ($r^2 = 0.80$). Here we compare the principal strains as it is difficult to estimate the cardiac specific directions in the case of the sonomicrometer data. A scatter plot of algorithm-derived principal strains versus sonomicrometer derived principal strains is shown in Fig. 11.

This validation is still in a preliminary stage and we hope in the future, to also validate strain patterns which are not fully averaged across the wall.

## 6. Conclusions

In this work we have demonstrated that estimates of 3D cardiac deformation can be obtained from ultrasound images. These estimates are generally consistent with values reported in the literature. Further, we validate such estimates of regional deformation directly by comparing them to strains measured concurrently from implanted sonomicrometers. While many problems remain to be

---

[3]Given a strain tensor $\epsilon_1$ in a coordinate frame $c_1$ (e.g. $x$, $y$, $z$) we can map it to a new coordinate frame $c_2$ (e.g. $r$, $c$, $l$) by use of a rotation matrix $R$. If $R$: $c_1 \mapsto c_2$, then the strain transformation is done as: $\epsilon_2 = R\epsilon_1 R^T$. In this way we can rotate the strain tensor to line up with directions of interest. We also note that the principal strains are the eigenvalues of the $3 \times 3$ strain tensor and are invariant to changes in the coordinate frame.

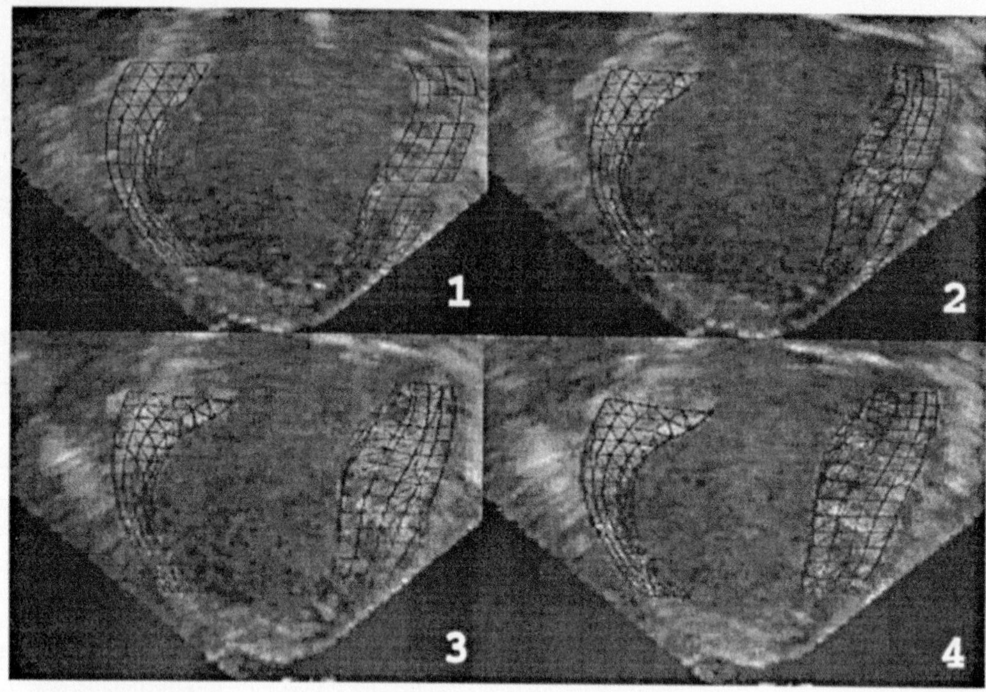

Fig. 9. '3DE-tissue-tagging' – a slice through a 3D visualization with the algorithm-driven deforming mesh overlaid on one slice through a 3DE dataset at four time points between ED and ES. This demonstrates the output of the algorithm which tries to follow (or tag) material points in time, similar to the Magnetic Resonance Tagging approach. Note that thickening (or radial strain) increases from the epicardium to the endocardium as expected. There is also an infarct region in the left half of the image which exhibits bulging instead of contraction. See also the accompanying movie file **papad1.mov** (available as an electronic annex via www.elsevier.com/locate/media).

solved, such as improving and speeding up the segmentation process, we are confident that this approach has the potential to make 3DE a potential source of images for the comprehensive estimation of 3D cardiac deformation.

## 7. Movies

There are three movies included with this paper (available as electronic annexes via www.elsevier.com/locate/media). The first movie, **papad1.mov**, corresponds to Fig.

Table 1
Summary of results for four animal studies. There was no risk area in studies D1 and D2 as the 3DE images, in these cases, were obtained before coronary occlusion

| Study | D1 | D2 | D3 | D4 |
|---|---|---|---|---|
| Normal radial strain | 17.7 | 13.8 | 22.4 | 17.2 |
| Normal circumferential strain | −13.4 | −13.1 | −8.4 | −12.4 |
| Normal longitudinal strain | −4.3 | −3.2 | −3.4 | −3.1 |
| Risk area radial strain | n/a | n/a | −4.3 | −13.7 |
| Risk area circumferential strain | n/a | n/a | 1.9 | −7.3 |
| Risk area longitudinal strain | n/a | n/a | −0.7 | −2.0 |

9. The second and third movies, **papad2.mov** and **papad3.mov**, correspond to the top and bottom parts of Fig. 10, respectively.

## Acknowledgements

The first author would also like to thank professors Turan Onat and Gary Povirk from the Department of Mechanical Engineering at Yale University for many useful discussions. Additional thanks to Farah Janzad, David Meoli, Jason Soares and Jennifer Hu for their help with segmenting the images, processing the sonomicrometer data, tissue processing and surgical preparation respectively. We would like to acknowledge support from the National Institutes of Health under grant NIH-NHLBI RO1-HL44803 and the American Heart Association (Connecticut Affiliate) under grant 9850014T. We would also like to thank Agilent Technologies (formerly part of Hewlett Packard), and especially Dr Karl Thiele, for providing the HP Sonos 5500 Ultrasound System used to acquire the 3DE Images.

An earlier version of this work was presented at MICCAI'99, Cambridge, UK (Conference on Medical Image Computing and Computer Assisted Intervention).

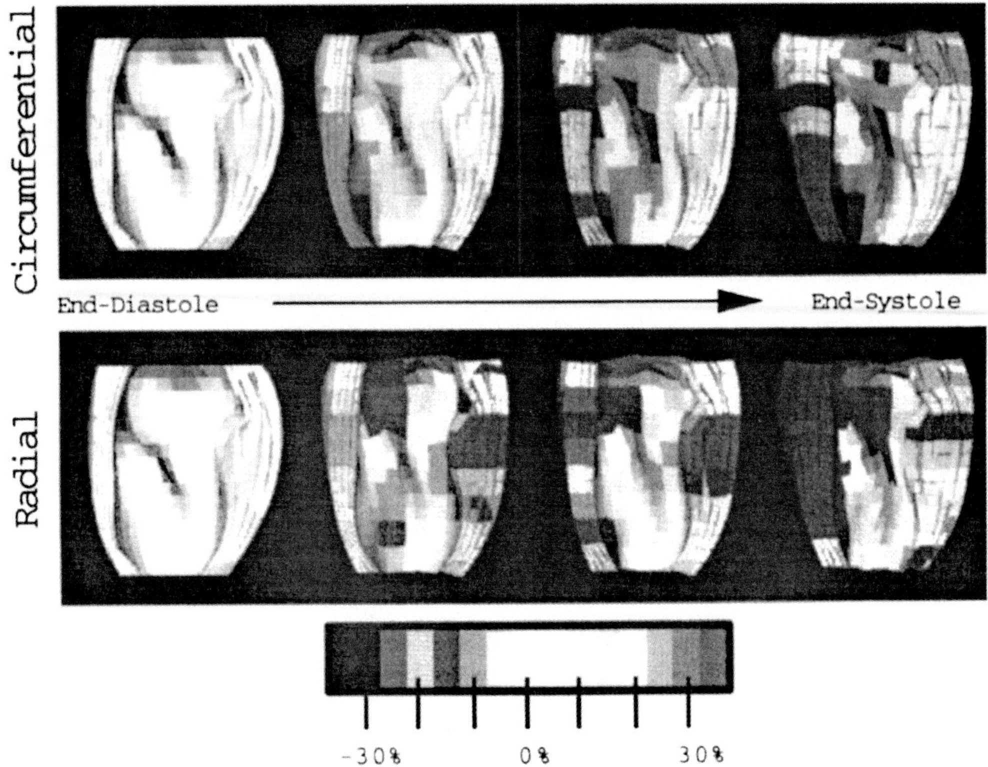



Fig. 10. A long-axis cut-away sectional view of the left ventricle showing circumferential (top) and radial (bottom) strain development in a dog following left anterior descending coronary artery occlusion (on the lower right half of the heart). Note the normal behavior in the left half of the heart. There was positive radial strain (thickening) and negative circumferential strain (shortening) as we move from End Diastole to End Systole. The lower right half of the heart where the affected region was located showed almost the opposite behavior, as expected. See also the accompanying movies **papad2.mov** and **papad3.mov** (available as electronic annexes via www.elsevier.com/locate/media).

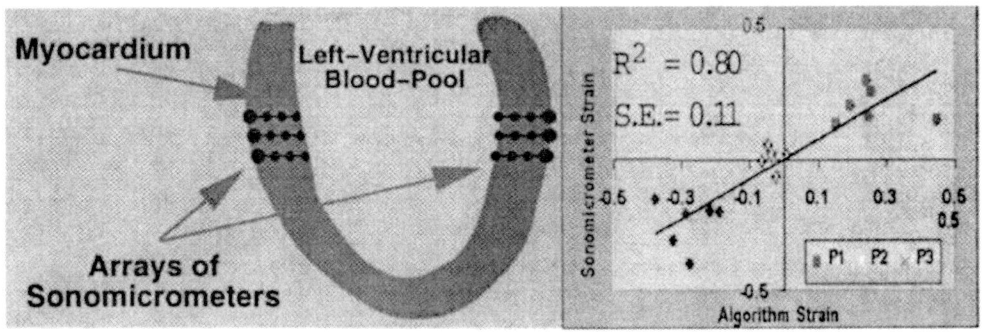



Fig. 11. 3DE Algorithm-Derived Strains versus Sonomicrometer-derived Strains. Scatter plot of principal strains derived from $N=3$ 3DE studies using the algorithm versus same strains derived from sonomicrometer arrays (12 crystals in each cluster) at two positions in the Left Ventricular wall. Note the high correlation between the two sets of strain values ($r^2 = 0.80$).

## References

Amini, A.A., Chen, Y., Curwen, R.W., Manu, V., Sun, J., 1998. Coupled B-snake grides and constrained thin-plate splines for analysis of 2D tissue deformations from tagged MRI. IEEE Trans. Med. Imaging 17 (3), 344–356.

Angelini, E., Laine, A., Takuma, S., Homma, S., 1999. Directional representations of 4D echocardiography for temporal quantification of LV volume, in: Medical Image Computing and Computer Aided Intervention (MICCAI), Cambridge, UK, pp. 430–440.

Bathe, K., 1982. Finite Element Procedures in Engineering Analysis. Prentice-Hall, New Jersey.

Berman, D.S., Germano, G., 1997. Evaluation of ventricular ejection fraction, wall motion, wall thickening, and other parameters with gated myocardial perfusion single-photon emission computed tomography. J. Nucl. Cardiol. 4 (2 Pt 2), S169–271.

Brandt, E., Wigström, L., Wranne, B., 1999. Segmentation of echocardiographic image sequences using spatio-temporal information, in: Medical Image Computing and Computer Aided Intervention (MICCAI), Cambridge, UK, pp. 410–419.

Buvat, I., Bartlett, M.L., Kitsiou, A.N., Dilsizian, V., Bacharach, S.L., 1997. A 'hybrid' method for measuring myocardial wall thickening from gated pet/spect images. J. Nucl. Med. 38 (2), 324–329.

Caidahl, K., Kazzam, E., Lingberg, J., Andersen, G.N., Nordanstig, J., Dahlqvist, S.R., Waldenstro, A., Wikh, R., 1999. New concept in echocardiography: harmonic imaging of tissue without use of contrast agent. The Lancet 352, 1264–1270.

Calnon, D.A., Kastner, R.J., Smith, W.H., Segalla, D., Beller, G.A., Watson, D.D., 1997. Validation of a new counts-based gated single photon emission computed tomography method for quantifying left ventricular systolic function: comparison with equilibrium radionuclide angiography. J. Nucl. Cardiol. 4 (6), 464–471.

Chakraborty, A., Staib, L., Duncan, J., 1996. Deformable boundary finding in medical images by integrating gradient and region information. IEEE Trans. Med. Imaging 15 (6), 859–870.

Christensen, G.E., Rabbitt, R.D., Miller, M.I., 1994. 3D brain mapping using deformable neuroanatomy. Phys. Med. Biol. 39, 609–618.

Chuang, M.L., Parker, R.A., Riley, M.F., Reilly, M.A., Johnson, R.B., Korley, V.J., Lerner, A.B., Douglas, P.S., 1999a. Three-dimensional echocardiography improves accuracy and compensates for sonographer inexperience in assessment of left ventricular ejection fraction. J. Am. Soc. Echocardiography 12, 290–299.

Chuang, M.L., Beaudin, R.A., Riley, M.F., Mooney, M.G., Manning, W.J., Hibberd, M.G., Douglas, P.S., 1999b. Impact of on-line endocardial border detection on determination of left ventricular volume and ejection fraction by transthoracic 3-dimensional echocardiography. J. Am. Soc. Echocardiography 12, 551–558.

Chuang, M.L., Hibberd, M.G., Salton, C.J., Beaudin, R.A., Riley, M.F., Parker, R.A., Douglas, P.S., 2000. Importance of imaging method over imaging modality in non-invasive determination of left ventricular volumes and ejection fraction: Assessment by two- and three-dimensional echocardiography and magnetic resonance imaging. J. Am. Coll. Cardiol. 35, 477–484.

Cooke, C.D., Garcia, E.V., Cullom, S.J., Faber, T.L., Pettigrew, R.I., 1994. Determining the accuracy of calculating systolic wall thickening using a fast Fourier transform approximation: a simulation study based on canine and patient data. J. Nucl. Med. 35 (7), 1185–1192.

Croissile, P., Moore, C.C., Judd, R.M., Lima, J.A.C., Arai, M., McVeigh, E.R., Becker, L.C., Zerhouni, E.A., 1999. Differentiation of viable and nonviable myocardium by the use of three-dimensional tagged MRI in 2-day-old reperfused infarcts. Circulation 99, 284–291.

Cwajg, E., Cwajg, J., He, Z.X., Hwang, W.S., Keng, F., Nagueh, S.F., Verani, M.S., 1999. Gated myocardial perfusion tomography for the assessment of left ventricular function and volumes: comparison with echocardiography. J. Nucl. Med. 40 (11), 1857–1865.

de Boor, C., 1978. A Practical Guide to Splines. Springer, New York, NY.

Dione, D.P., Shi, P., Smith, W., De Man, P., Soares, J., Duncan, J.S., Sinusas, A.J., 1997. Three-dimensional regional left ventricular deformation from digital sonomicrometry, in: 19th Annual International Conference of the IEEE Engineering in Medicine and Biology Society, Chicago, IL, pp. 848–851.

Duncan, J.S., Shi, P., Constable, R.T., Sinusas, A., 1998. Physical and geometrical modeling for image-based recovery of left ventricular deformation. Prog. Biophys. Molec. Biol. 69 (2–3), 333–351.

Faber, T.L., Cooke, C.D., Folks, R.D., Vansant, J.P., Nichols, K.J., DePuey, E.G., Pettigrew, R.I., Garcia, E.V., 1999. Left ventricular function and perfusion from gated spect perfusion images: an integrated method. J. Nucl. Med. 40 (4), 650–659.

Gee, J.C., Haynor, D.R., Le Briquer, L., Bajcsy, R.K., 1997. Advances in elastic matching theory and its implementation, in: CVRMed-MRCAS, Grenoble, France.

Geman, D., Geman, S., 1984. Stochastic relaxation, Gibbs distribution and Bayesian restoration of images. IEEE Trans. Pattern Anal. Machine Intell. 6, 721–741.

Germano, G., Kiat, H., Kavanagh, P.B., Moriel, M., Mazzanti, M., Su, H.T., Van Train, K.F., Berman, D.S., 1995. Automatic quantification of ejection fraction from gated myocardial perfusion spect. J. Nucl. Med. 36 (11), 2138–2147.

Guccione, J.M., McCulloch, A.D., 1991. Finite element modeling of ventricular mechanics. In: Hunter, P.J., McCulloch, A., Nielsen, P. (Eds.), Theory of Heart. Springer, Berlin, pp. 122–144.

Haber, E., Metaxas, D.N., Axel, L., 1998. Motion analysis of the right ventricle from MRI images, in: Medical Image Computing and Computer Aided Intervention (MICCAI), Cambridge, MA, pp. 177–188.

Hibbit, Karlsson & Sorencen, Inc., 1997. Abaqus Version 5. 7, Rhode Island, USA.

Hughes, T.J.R., 1987. The Finite Element Method: Linear Static and Dynamic Finite Element Analysis. Prentice-Hall, Englewood Cliffs, NJ.

Hunter, P.J., McCulloch, A., Nielsen, P., 1991. Theory of Heart. Springer, Berlin.

Jacob, G., Noble, A., Mulet-Parada, M., Blake, A., 1999. Evaluating a robust contour tracker on echocardiographic sequences. Medical Image Analysis 3 (1), 63–75.

Kerwin, W.S., Prince, J.L., 1998. Cardiac material markers from tagged MR images. Medical Image Analysis 2 (4), 339–353.

Lang, R.M., Vignon, P., Weinert, L., Bednarz, J., Korcarz, C., Sandelski, J., Koch, R., Prater, D., Mor-Avi, V., 1996. Echocardiographic quantification of regional left ventricular wall motion with color kinesis. Circulation 15 (93(10)), 1877–1885.

Malvern, L.E., 1969. Introduction to the Mechanics of a Continuous Medium. Prentice-Hall, Englewood Cliffs, New Jersey.

Manjunath, B.S., Chellappa, R., 1991. Unsupervised texture segmentation using markov random field models. IEEE Trans. Pattern Anal. Machine Intell. 13, 478–482.

Meoli, D., Mazhari, R., Dione, D.P., Omens, J., McCulloch, A., Sinusas, A.J., 1998. Three dimensional digital sonomicrometry: comparison with biplane radiography, in: Proceedings of IEEE 24th Annual Northeast Bioengineering Conference, pp. 64–67.

Meyer, F.G., Constable, R.T., Sinusas, A.J., Duncan, J.S., 1996. Tracking myocardial deformation using phase contrast MR velocity fields: a stochastic approach. IEEE Trans. Med. Imaging 15 (4), 453–465.

Miller, T.R., Wallis, J.W., Landy, B.R., Gropler, R.J., Sabharwal, C.L., 1994. Measurement of global and regional left ventricular function by cardiac pet. J. Nucl. Med. 35 (6), 999–1005.

Montagnat, J., Delingette, H., Malandain, G., 1999. Cylindrical echocardiographic images segmentation based on 3D deformable models, in: Medical Image Computing and Computer Aided Intervention (MICCAI), Cambridge, UK, pp. 168–175.

Moore, C.C., Lugo-Olivieri, C.H., McVeigh, E.R., Zerhouni, E.A., 2000. Three-dimensional systolic strain patterns in the normal human left ventricle: Characterization with tagged MR imaging. Radiology 214, 453–466.

Mulet-Pabrada, M., Noble, J.A., 1998. 2D+T acoustic boundary detection in echocardiography, in: Medical Image Computing and Computer Aided Intervention (MICCAI), Boston, MA, pp. 806–813.

Panfilov, A.V., Holden, A.V., 1997. Computational Biology of the Heart. John Wiley & Sons.

Papademetris, X., 2000. Estimation of 3D left ventricular deformation from medical images using biomechanical models, Ph.D. Dissertation, Yale University, New Haven, CT, May 2000 (URL= http://noodle.med.yale.edu/thesis).

Papademetris, X., Rambo, J.V., Dione, D.P., Sinusas, A.J., Duncan, J.S., 1998. Visually Interactive Cine-3D Segmentation of Cardiac MR Images, Suppl. to the J. Am. Coll. of Cardiology 31 (2 Suppl. A).

Park, J., Metaxas, D.N., Axel, L., 1996. Analysis of left ventricular wall motion based on volumetric deformable models and MRI-SPAMM. Medical Image Analysis 1 (1), 53–71.

Pelc, N.J., 1991. Myocardial motion analysis with phase contrast cine MRI, in: Proceedings of the 10th Annual SMRM, San Francisco, p. 17.

Porter, T.R., Xie, F., Kricsfeld, A., Chiou, A., Dabestani, A., 1994. Improved endocardial border resolution using dobutamin stress endocardiography with intravenous sonicated dextrose albumin. J. Am. Coll. Cardiol. 23, 1440–1443.

Prince, J.L., McVeigh, E.R., 1992. Motion estimation from tagged MR image sequences. IEEE Trans. Med. Imaging 11, 238–249.

Sheehan, H., Bolson, E.L., Martin, R.W., Bashein, G., McDonald, J., 1998. Quantitative three dimensional echocardiography: methodology, validation and clinical applications, in: Medical Image Computing and Computer Aided Intervention (MICCAI), Boston, MA, pp. 102–109.

Shen, M.Y., Liu, Y.H., Sinusas, A.J., Fetterman, R., Bruni, W., Drozhinin, O.E., Zaret, B.L., Wackers, F.J., 1999. Quantification of regional myocardial wall thickening on electrocardiogram-gated spect imaging. J. Nucl. Cardiol. 6 (6), 583–595.

Shi, P., Sinusas, A.J., Constable, R.T., Ritman, E., Duncan, J.S., 2000. Point-tracked quantitative analysis of left ventricular motion from 3D image sequences. IEEE Trans. Med. Imaging 19 (1), 36–50.

Sinusas, A.J., Trautman, K.A., Bergin, J.D., Watson, D.D., Ruiz, M., Smith, W.H., Beller, G.A., 1990. Quantification of area of risk during coronary occlusion and degree of myocardial salvage after reperfusion with technetium-99m methoxyisobutyl isonitrile. Circulation 82, 1424–1437.

von Ramm, O.T., Smith, S.W., 1990. Real-time volumetric ultrasound imaging system. J. Digital Imaging 3, 261–266.

Yamashita, K., Tamaki, N., Yonekura, Y., Ohtani, H., Saji, H., Mukai, T., Kambara, H., Kawai, C., Ban, T., Konishi, J., 1989. Quantitative analysis of regional wall motion by gated myocardial positron emission tomography: validation and comparison with left ventriculography. J. Nucl. Med. 30 (11), 1775–1786.

Young, A.A., Kraitchman, D.L., Dougherty, L., Axel, L., 1995. Tracking and finite element analysis of stripe deformation in magnetic resonance tagging. IEEE Trans. Med. Imaging 14 (3), 413–421.

Zhu, Y., Drangova, M., Pelc, N.J., 1997. Estimation of deformation gradient and strain from cine-PC velocity data. IEEE Trans. Med. Imaging 16 (6), 840–851.

# Creating a high-resolution spatial/symbolic model of the inner organs based on the Visible Human[☆]

Andreas Pommert[a,*], Karl Heinz Höhne[a], Bernhard Pflesser[a], Ernst Richter[b],
Martin Riemer[a], Thomas Schiemann[a], Rainer Schubert[a], Udo Schumacher[c], Ulf Tiede[a]

[a]*Institute of Mathematics and Computer Science in Medicine (IMDM), University Hospital Hamburg-Eppendorf, Hamburg, Germany*
[b]*Department of Pediatric Radiology, University Hospital Hamburg-Eppendorf, Hamburg, Germany*
[c]*Institute of Anatomy, University Hospital Hamburg-Eppendorf, Hamburg, Germany*

Received 20 February 2001; received in revised form 19 June 2001; accepted 20 June 2001

## Abstract

Computerized three-dimensional models of the human body, based on the Visible Human Project of the National Library of Medicine, so far do not reflect the rich anatomical detail of the original cross-sectional images. In this paper, a spatial/symbolic model of the inner organs is developed, which is based on more than 1000 cryosections and congruent fresh and frozen CT images of the male Visible Human. The spatial description is created using color-space segmentation, graphic modeling, and a matched volume visualization with subvoxel resolution. It is linked to a symbolic knowledge base, providing an ontology of anatomical terms. With over 650 three-dimensional anatomical constituents, this model offers an unsurpassed photorealistic presentation and level of detail. A three-dimensional atlas of anatomy and radiology based on this model is available as a PC-based program. © 2001 Elsevier Science B.V. All rights reserved.

*Keywords:* Visible Human; Three-dimensional body model; Anatomical atlas; Color-space segmentation; Volume visualization

## 1. Introduction

While in classical medicine, knowledge about the human body is represented in books and atlases, present-day computer science allows for new, more powerful and versatile computer-based representations of knowledge. Their most simple manifestations are multimedia CD-ROMs containing collections of classical pictures and text, which may be browsed arbitrarily or according to various criteria. Although computerized, such media still follow the old paradigm of text printed on pages accompanied by pictures. This genre includes impressive atlases of cross-sectional anatomy, notably from the photographic cross-sections of the Visible Human Project (Ackerman, 1991; Spitzer et al., 1996).

In the past years, however, it has been shown that spatial knowledge, especially about the structure of the human body, may be much more efficiently represented by computerized three-dimensional models (Höhne et al., 1995). These can be constructed from cross-sectional images generated by computer tomography (CT), magnetic resonance imaging (MRI), or histological cryosectioning, as in the case of the Visible Human Project. Such models may be used interactively on a computer screen or in virtual reality environments. If such models are connected to a knowledge base of descriptive information, they can even be interrogated or disassembled by addressing names of organs (Höhne et al., 1995; Brinkley et al., 1999; Golland et al., 1999). They can thus be regarded as a 'self-explaining body'.

Until now, the Visible Human Project has not reported three-dimensional models that reflect the rich anatomical

[☆]Electronic Annexes available. See www.elsevier.com/locate/media.
*Corresponding author. Tel.: +49-40-42803-2300; fax: +49-40-42803-4882.
*E-mail address:* pommert@uke.uni-hamburg.de (A. Pommert).

detail of the original cross-sectional images. This is largely due to the fact that, for the majority of anatomical objects contained in the data, the cross-sectional images could not be converted into a set of coherent realistic surfaces. If we succeed in converting all the detail into a 3D model, we gain an unsurpassed representation of human structure that opens new possibilities for learning anatomy and simulating interventions or radiological examinations.

## 2. Earlier work

Building a comprehensive model of the inner organs of the Visible Human requires both a spatial description consisting of three-dimensional objects, which are displayed using methods of volume visualization, as well as a linked symbolic description of relevant anatomical terms and their relations.

In general, volume visualization may or may not include a segmentation step. In *volume rendering*, transparency values are assigned to the individual voxels according to the intensity values and changes at the object borders (Levoy, 1988). In the case of the Visible Human, this method yields semitransparent views, which are suitable e.g. for visualization of the outer surface and the musculo-skeletal system (Stewart et al., 1996; Tsiaras, 1997). This way, impressive animations could be created (Gagvani and Silver, 2000; Tsiaras, 2000). It fails, however, to display internal structures properly. In addition, organ borders are not explicitly indicated, thus making the removal or exclusive display of an organ impossible.

*Segmentation*, i.e. the exact determination of the surface location of an organ, is therefore crucial for building a realistic model. So far, complete automatic segmentation using methods of computer vision is suitable for very special application areas only, and could not be used to build an extensive model of the human body. The brute force approach to segmentation is manual outlining of objects on the cross-sections (Mullick and Nguyen, 1996; Seymour and Kriebel, 1998). Besides the fact that this procedure is tedious and very time consuming, it is largely observer-dependent and, even more important, does not yield exact and continuous surfaces. Furthermore, despite the high resolution of the dataset, important details such as nerves and small blood vessels cannot be identified clearly, because their size and contrast is too small.

So far, no symbolic description of the inner organs which is suitable for our purposes is available. A general discussion of the problems arising, focusing on the thorax, may be found elsewhere (Rosse et al., 1998).

## 3. Methods and materials

We therefore aimed at a method that yields surfaces for the segmentable organs that are as exact as possible and textured with their original color. In order to arrive at a complete model, we decided to model non-segmentable objects like nerves and small blood vessels artificially on the basis of landmarks present in the image volume. Even though none of the methods presented here is entirely new, building a complex model required a number of substantial improvements.

### 3.1. Data

The original dataset of the male Visible Human consists of 1871 photographic cross-sections with a slice distance of 1 mm and a spatial resolution of 0.33 mm (Fig. 1, left). For reasons of data storage and computing capacity, resolution of the cross-sections was reduced to 1 mm by averaging $3 \times 3$ pixels. From 1049 such slices, an image volume of $573 \times 330 \times 1049$ voxels of 1 mm$^3$ was composed, where each voxel is represented by a set of red, green and blue intensities (*RGB-tuple*). The Visible Human dataset also includes two sets of computer tomographic images of 1 mm slice distance, one taken from the fresh, the other (like the photographic one) from the frozen cadaver. Both were transformed into an image volume congruent with the photographic one, using an interactive, landmark-based registration (Schiemann et al., 1994). Since the frozen body was cut into four large blocks before image acquisition, all these parts had to be aligned individually, leaving some noticeable gaps in the data volume.

### 3.2. Segmentation

The image volume thus created was segmented with an interactive tool, based on classification in color-space (Schiemann et al., 1997). It can be summarized as follows: on one or several cross-sections, an expert marks a typical region of the organ under consideration. All voxels in the volume with similar RGB-tuples are then collected by the program and shown as a painted three-dimensional *mask*. This mask usually needs to be refined by repeating this procedure in order to discriminate the target organ from the surrounding structures more clearly.

A cluster thus defined in color-space usually has an ellipsoidal shape, due to the correlation of the color components. Since a set of tuples is difficult to handle during subsequent visualization, this cluster is approximated by a parameterized *ellipsoid*, which is described by its center and three axis vectors. In general, there are other regions present in the volume which also match this color-space description. If they are not connected to the target organ, it can be isolated easily by a 3D connected component analysis. If not, borders are manually sculptured using a volume editor.

The result of this procedure is a description of an object in terms of an ellipsoid in color-space and a set of voxels, which are marked by object membership labels. Some of

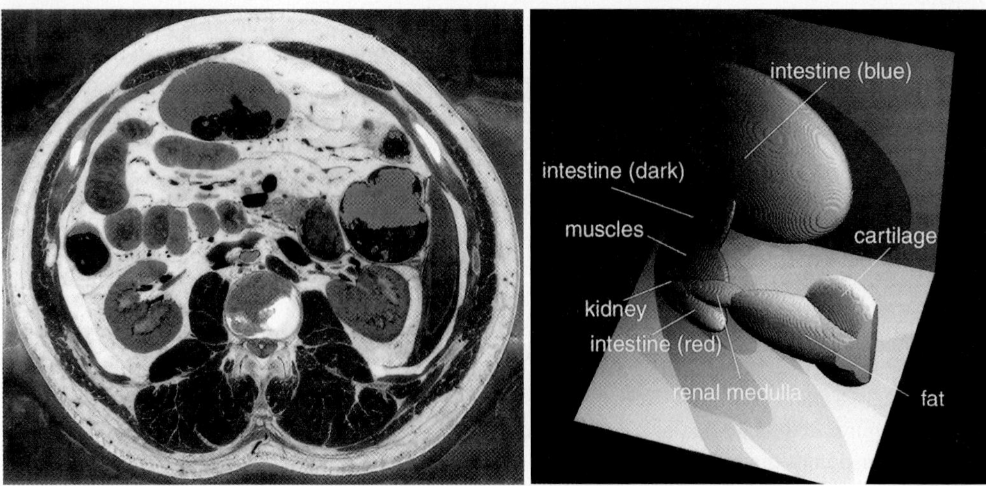



Fig. 1. Left: Photographic cross-section of the abdomen of the male Visible Human. Right: parameterized ellipsoids in color-space, used for classification of various tissue types in the abdomen. Many objects show similar colors, resulting in overlapping ellipsoids.

the ellipsoids defined for segmentation of the abdomen are shown in Fig. 1 (right). As can be seen, there are anatomical constituents like the intestine which could not be described using one ellipsoid only; in this case, actually seven ellipsoids were required. On the other hand, the same ellipsoid may be valid for (parts of) various anatomical constituents, such as small intestine and colon, or even for hundreds of muscles.

As a general strategy, we applied our segmentation procedure going from simple to difficult tasks. This way, borders already defined could be used to facilitate segmentation of other objects. As a first step, several tissue classes such as fat, muscles, cartilage, etc., were defined, for which the ellipsoids could be easily determined within a few minutes. For segmentation of bone, it proved easier to use the frozen CT dataset, applying a threshold value.

Since many objects show similar colors, the resulting ellipsoids are often overlapping (Fig. 1, right). Therefore, some regions such as the anterior parts of the lung or the pericardium could not be segmented this way. In case of

the lung, the missing parts could be determined using the frozen CT dataset and a threshold. For the pericardium and similar cases, the volume editor was used.

### 3.3. Graphic modeling

For several small constituents such as nerves and blood vessels, which were considered essential for a comprehensive anatomical model, our color-space segmentation proved impossible. As regards nerves, this is mostly due to very low contrast between nervous and fat tissues, while many small arteries are collapsed as a post-mortem artifact. Both problems also appear for the full resolution data.

For these cases, we developed a *tube editor* which allows us to include tube-like structures into the model (Fig. 2). Ball-shaped markers of variable diameter are imposed by an expert onto the landmarks still visible on the cross-sections or on the 3D image. These markers are subsequently automatically connected using Overhauser splines (Yamaguchi, 1988). If one of the markers is

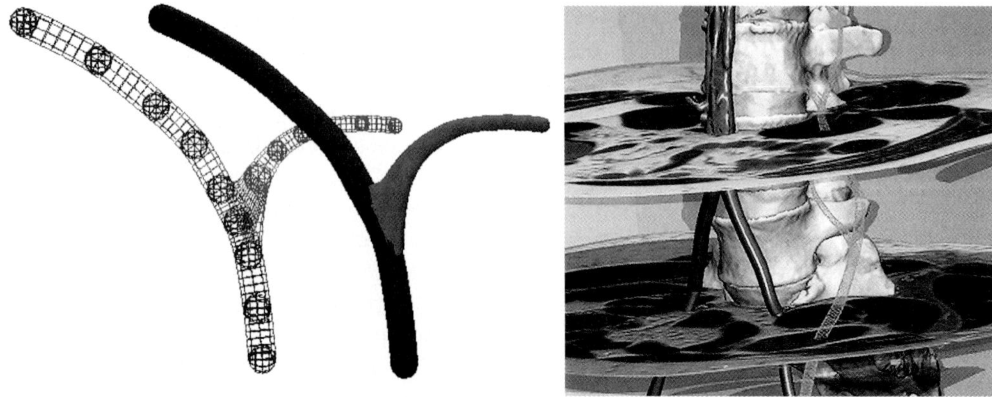

Fig. 2. Small nerves or arteries which could not be segmented were interactively modeled using a tube editor. Tubes are defined by placing spheres of varying diameter into the volume, which are connected by interpolating splines.

moved, these splines will cause only local changes, which makes them easy to handle. Unlike the segmented objects, which are represented as sets of voxels, objects modeled with the tube editor are represented as polygon surfaces.

*3.4. Volume visualization*

The volume visualization algorithm we developed is characterized by the fact that it renders surfaces from volume data, using a ray casting approach (Tiede et al., 1998). Local surface texture (color) and inclination, as needed for surface shading, are calculated from the RGB-tuples at the segmented border line.

A decisive quality improvement is achieved by determining the surface positions with subvoxel resolution. This is done by considering both the ellipsoids (or thresholds, for CT) and the object membership labels. If a surface was created using labels only, it would appear blocky, especially when zooming into the scene. On the other hand, if only the ellipsoids were used, objects usually could not be identified without ambiguity.

In order to avoid these problems, ellipsoids and labels are combined using a color-driven algorithm (Schiemann et al., 1997; Tiede et al., 1998). Depending on the RGB-tuple found at a sampling point on a viewing ray, all ellipsoids enclosing this tuple in color-space are collected, defining a set of 'object candidates'. In a second step, it is tested whether a matching object label is present in the vicinity of the sampling point. In that case, an object has been found. Its subvoxel surface position is determined by interpolating the color at the sampling point (inside the ellipsoid) and the color at the previous sampling point on the viewing ray (outside the ellipsoid), such that the color at the surface is representing the object border (on the surface of the ellipsoid). Since this approach considers colors (or intensities, for CT) before labels, a smooth, continuous surface is obtained, which is not limited by voxel size.

The objects modeled with the tube editor are visualized with standard computer graphics methods within the context of the segmented objects. The visualization program, an extended version of the VOXEL-MAN system (Höhne et al., 1995), runs on Linux workstations. Because of the size and resolution of the model, computation of a single image may take several minutes, even on a high-end workstation.

*3.5. Knowledge modeling*

While segmentation and graphic modeling provide a spatial description of anatomical objects, a comprehensive model also requires a linked symbolic description regarding anatomical terms and their relations. For this purpose, we developed a knowledge base system, using a semantic network approach (Pommert et al., 1994; Höhne et al., 1995). Among others, an object is described by:

- names (preferred terms, synonyms, colloquial terms) in various languages;
- pointers to related medical information (texts, histological images, references, etc.);
- segmentation and visualization parameters (ellipsoid or threshold, object label, shading method, etc.).

For choosing anatomical terms, we built on standardized nomenclature wherever available (Federative Committee on Anatomical Terminology, 1998).

The knowledge base describes not only elementary parts found in the spatial model (e.g. *left rib 3*), but also compositions of these objects (e.g. *true ribs, ribs, thoracic skeleton, thoracic wall, body wall, body*), thus building a part hierarchy. This ontology is composed of several subnets, modeling various 'views' commonly used in anatomy. For example, the kidneys can be seen according to structural or functional criteria:

- *regional anatomy:* in this view, the kidneys are shown as part of the abdominal viscera;
- *systemic anatomy:* in this view, the kidneys are shown as part of the urogenital system;
- *relation to peritoneum*: in this view, the kidneys are shown as part of the primary retroperitoneal organs.

Views are represented as attributes of relations. Besides the 'part of' relation type, our model also contains a 'branching from' type, modeling the arterial blood flow.

As was pointed out earlier, an anatomical constituent may be a combination of several segmented objects, each with an individual name, ellipsoid, and object label. In order to hide these rather technical objects from a user, a relation type 'hidden part of' was introduced, which is extending the part hierarchy. For a user, an anatomical constituent constructed of several hidden parts appears as one single entity.

## 4. Results

Using the methods described above, we built a model of the inner organs of the male Visible Human. It contains more then 650 three-dimensional anatomical constituents and more than 2000 relations between them. The size of segmented anatomical constituents varies between 3.8 million voxels (or $mm^3$, equivalent to 3.8 l) for visceral fat and 124 voxels for the cystic duct. Preparation of the model using the described methods involved up to 10 people and required about 5 man years. Fig. 3 gives an impression of image quality and the level of detail (see also the movie in the electronic annex – available via www.elsevier.com/locate/media).

Since the model is volume-based, cut planes, which can be placed in any number and direction, show the texture of the original photographic images and thus look realistic. This virtual dissection capability not only allows an interactive dissection for learning purposes, but can also be used for the rehearsal of a surgical procedure. In addition,

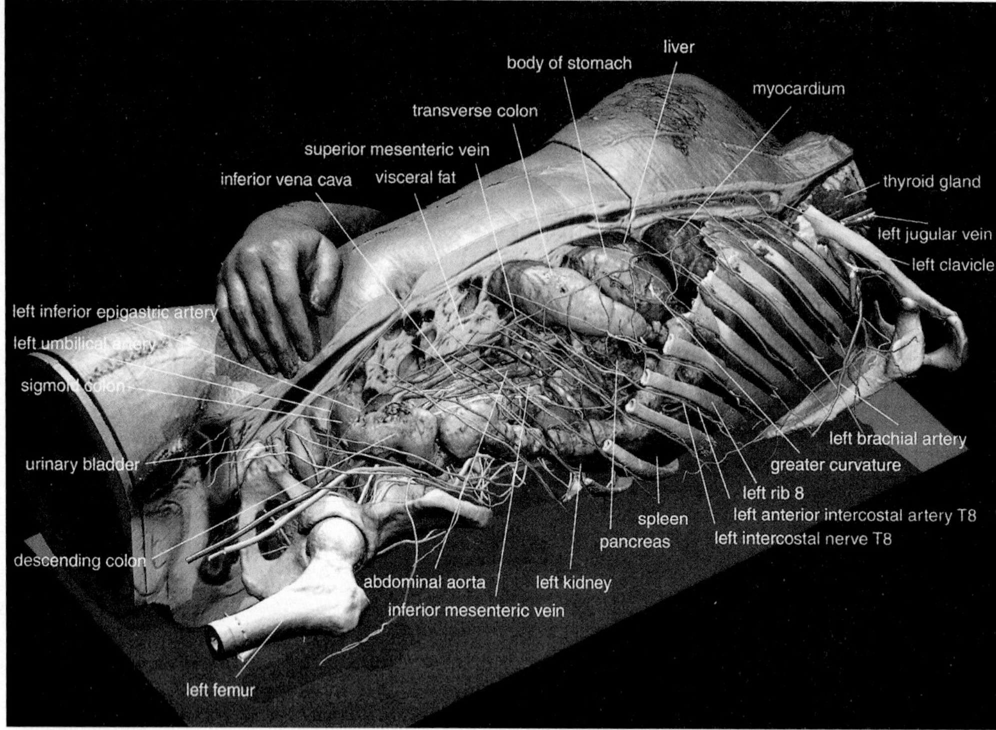



Fig. 3. The model of the inner organs contains more than 650 anatomical constituents, with a spatial resolution of 1 mm$^3$. It can be viewed from any direction, cuts may be placed in any number and direction, and objects may be removed or added. Annotations may be called by mouse click.

the image of a 'self-explaining body' allows us to inquire about complex anatomical facts. The more traditional way of annotating structures of interest is demonstrated within the user-specified scene in Fig. 3. These annotations can be obtained simply by pointing and clicking with the mouse on the structure of interest. Likewise, objects may be painted. Pressing another button of the mouse will call several pop-up menus, which provide structured knowledge about anatomy and function (Fig. 4). Such information is available because every voxel, and therefore any visible point of any user-created 3D scene, is linked to the knowledge base.

Vice versa, the user may navigate through the contents of the knowledge base, going to more general or more specific terms in systemic or regional part hierarchies. Images may be composed by selecting terms from the knowledge base (Fig. 5).

A special feature of the model involves the possibility of simulating radiological examinations. Since the absorption values for every voxel are available in the original tomographic data, artificial X-ray images from any direction can be computed (Fig. 6, left; see also the movie in the electronic annex). Based on the information of the model, both the contributing anatomical structures and the extent of their contribution to the final absorption can be calculated. Similarly, the information present in computer

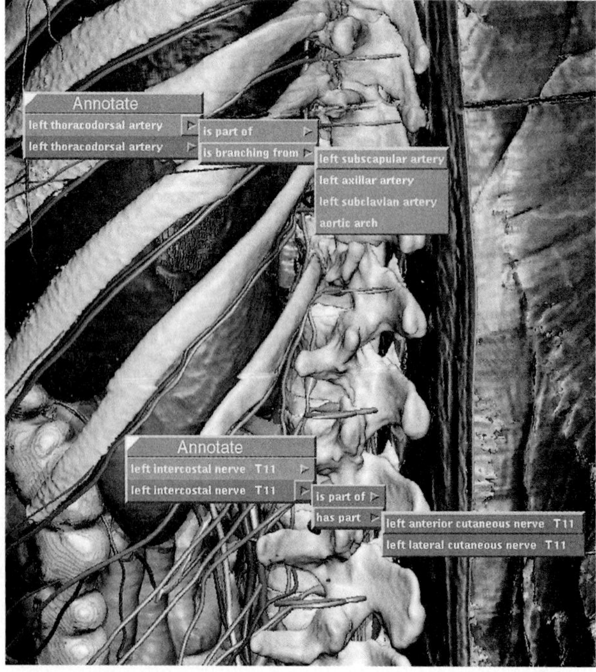



Fig. 4. Exploring the semantic network behind the spatial model. The user has clicked onto a blood vessel and a nerve and received information about systemic (red) and regional (blue) anatomy.

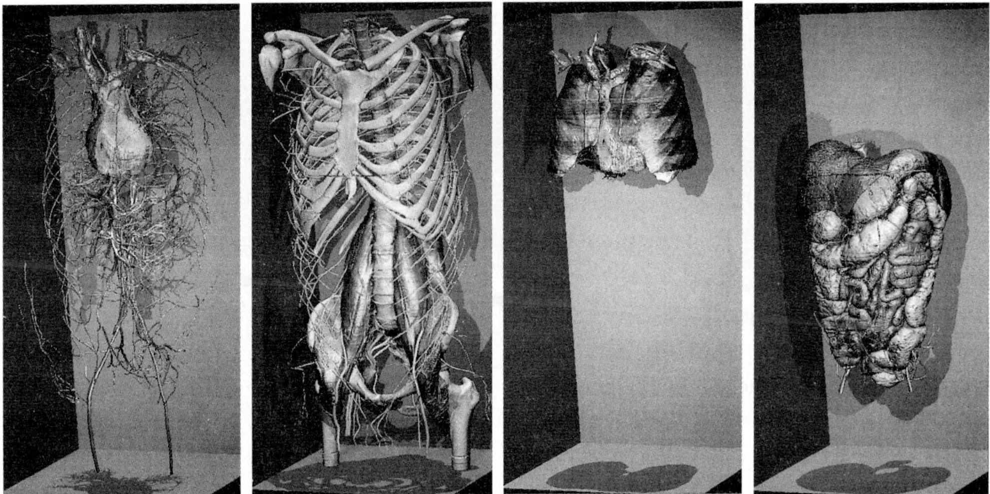

Fig. 5. Visualization of various terms, selected from the knowledge base. Left to right: cardiovascular system; nervous system (with skeleton and iliopsoas muscles); thoracic organs; abdominal viscera.

tomographic images can be clarified by presenting them in the corresponding context of 3D anatomy (Fig. 6, right). For an improved spatial impression, stereoscopic views can also be created.

## 5. Conclusions

In this paper, we presented an approach for creating a high-resolution model of the inner organs, based on the Visible Human data. The following features of this model represent innovations:

- Because of the exact, color-space segmentation and the matched visualization method, the visual impression is one of unsurpassed realism.
- There is, to date, no computer model of the inner organs that contains and describes so many three-dimensional anatomical constituents.

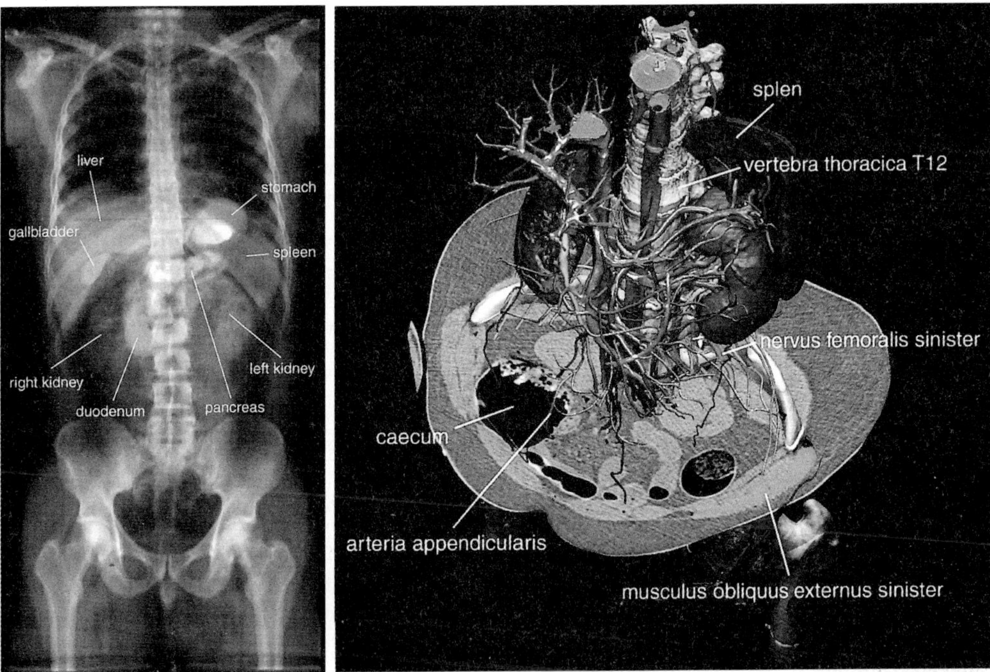


Fig. 6. Different viewing modes such as X-ray imaging (left) or computer tomography (right) may be chosen from any direction and for any part of the model.

- The model is space-filling, i.e. any voxel is labeled as an element of a three-dimensional object.
- The integrated formal organization of spatial and symbolic information allows a virtually unlimited number of ways of using the model.

The model is a general knowledge representation of gross anatomy, from which all classical representations (pictures, movies, solid models) may be derived via mouse click. The versatility of the approach makes it suitable for anatomy and radiology teaching as well as for simulation of interventional procedures. While the general principle was reported earlier (Höhne et al., 1995), the model we describe is the first to offer sufficient detail and comprehensiveness to serve these purposes seriously. A three-dimensional atlas of anatomy and radiology based on this model, called *VOXEL-MAN 3D-Navigator: Inner Organs*, is available as a PC-based program (Höhne et al., 2000).

Yet there are still improvements to be made. First of all, from an anatomist's point of view, an even more detailed segmentation would be desirable for many applications. Currently, improvements are under way. A more serious limitation is the fact that the data is derived from one single individual. The inter-individual variability of organ shape and topology in space and time is thus not yet part of the model. Inclusion of variability into three-dimensional models is a difficult problem not yet generally solved. So far, most progress has been achieved for 3D atlases of the brain (Mazziotta et al., 1995; Styner and Gerig, 2001).

However, the current model should be an excellent basis for further developments. One such development is the inclusion of physiology, e.g. the modeling of blood flow or propagation of electrical fields throughout the body (Spitzer and Whitlock, 1998). Applications such as the computation of body surface potential maps (Sachse et al., 2000) should profit from the increased level of detail. Furthermore, because of the more detailed characterization of tissues, a more realistic surgical simulation involving cutting (Pflesser et al., 2000) and soft tissue deformation (Cotin et al., 1999) can be achieved. This approach is thus an important, albeit early step towards computer models that not only look real, but also act like a real body.


### Acknowledgements

We thank Victor Spitzer and David Whitlock, University of Colorado, and Michael Ackerman, National Library of Medicine (US), for providing the Visible Human dataset. We are also grateful to Jochen Dormeier, Jan Freudenberg, Sebastian Gehrmann, Stefan Noster and Norman von Sternberg-Gospos, who substantially contributed to the segmentation and modeling work. The tube editor was implemented by Klaus Rheinwald. The movie in the electronic annex was produced by Andreas Petersik. The knowledge modeling work was supported by the German Research Council (DFG) under grant number Ho 899/4-1.

An earlier version of this work was presented at *The Third Visible Human Project Conference*, Bethesda, MD, October 2000.


### References

Ackerman, M.J., 1991. Viewpoint: The Visible Human Project. J. Biocommun. 18, 14.

Brinkley, J.F., Wong, B.A., Hinshaw, K.P., Rosse, C., 1999. Design of an anatomy information system. IEEE Comput. Graphics Appl. 19 (3), 38–48.

Cotin, S., Delingette, H., Ayache, N., 1999. Real-time elastic deformations of soft tissues for surgery simulation. IEEE Trans. Visualization Comput. Graphics 5 (1), 62–73.

Federative Committee on Anatomical Terminology (Ed.), 1998. Terminologia Anatomica: International Anatomical Terminology. Thieme, Stuttgart.

Gagvani, N., Silver, D., 2000. Animating the Visible Human Dataset (VHD). In: Banvard, R.A. (Ed.), The Third Visible Human Project Conference Proceedings. National Library of Medicine (US), Office of High Performance Computing and Communications, Bethesda, MD (CD-ROM, ISSN 1524-9008).

Golland, P., Kikinis, R., Halle, M., Umans, C., Grimson, W.E.L., Shenton, M.E., Richolt, J.A., 1999. AnatomyBrowser: A novel approach to visualization and integration of medical information. Comput. Aided Surg. 4 (3), 129–143.

Höhne, K.H., Pflesser, B., Pommert, A., Riemer, M., Schiemann, T., Schubert, R., Tiede, U., 1995. A new representation of knowledge concerning human anatomy and function. Nat. Med. 1 (6), 506–511.

Höhne, K.H., Pflesser, B., Pommert, A., Priesmeyer, K., Riemer, M., Schiemann, T., Schubert, R., Tiede, U., Frederking, H., Gehrmann, S., Noster, S., Schumacher, U., 2000. VOXEL-MAN 3D Navigator: Inner Organs. Regional, Systemic and Radiological Anatomy. Springer Electronic Media, Heidelberg (3 CD-ROMs, ISBN 3-540-14759-4).

Levoy, M., 1988. Display of surfaces from volume data. IEEE Comput. Graphics Appl. 8 (3), 29–37.

Mazziotta, J.C., Toga, A.W., Evans, A.C., Fox, P., Lancaster, J., 1995. A probabilistic atlas of the human brain: theory and rationale for its development. NeuroImage 2 (2), 89–101.

Mullick, R., Nguyen, H.T., 1996. Visualization and labeling of the Visible Human dataset: challenges and resolves. In: Höhne, K.H., Kikinis, R. (Eds.), Visualization in Biomedical Computing, Proc. VBC '96. Lecture Notes in Computer Science, Vol. 1131. Springer, Berlin, pp. 75–80.

Pflesser, B., Tiede, U., Höhne, K.H., Leuwer, R., 2000. Volume based planning and rehearsal of surgical interventions. In: Lemke, H.U., Vannier, M.W., Inamura, K., Farman, A.G., Doi, K. (Eds.), Computer Assisted Radiology and Surgery, Proc. CARS 2000. Excerpta Medica International Congress Series, Vol. 1214. Elsevier, Amsterdam, pp. 607–612.

Pommert, A., Schubert, R., Riemer, M., Schiemann, T., Tiede, U., Höhne, K.H., 1994. Symbolic modeling of human anatomy for visualization and simulation. In: Robb, R.A. (Ed.), Visualization in Biomedical Computing 1994, Proc. SPIE 2359. Rochester, MN, pp. 412–423.

Rosse, C., Mejino, J., Modayur, B., Jakobovits, R., Hinshaw, K., Brinkley, J.F., 1998. Motivation and organizational principles for anatomical knowledge representation: The Digital Anatomist symbolic knowledge base. J. Am. Med. Inform. Assoc. 5 (1), 17–40.

Sachse, F.B., Werner, C.D., Meyer-Waarden, K., Dössel, O., 2000. Development of a human body model for numerical calculation of electrical fields. Comput. Med. Imaging Graph. 24 (3), 165–171.

Schiemann, T., Höhne, K.H., Koch, C., Pommert, A., Riemer, M., Schubert, R., Tiede, U., 1994. Interpretation of tomographic images using automatic atlas lookup. In: Robb, R.A. (Ed.), Visualization in

Biomedical Computing 1994, Proc. SPIE 2359. Rochester, MN, pp. 457-465.

Schiemann, T., Tiede, U., Höhne, K.H., 1997. Segmentation of the Visible Human for high quality volume based visualization. Medical Image Analysis 1 (4), 263–271.

Seymour, J., Kriebel, T.L., 1998. Virtual Human: live volume rendering of the segmented and classified Visible Human Male in a CD-ROM product for PCs. In: Banvard, R.A., Pinciroli, F., Cerveri, P. (Eds.), The Second Visible Human Project Conference Proceedings. National Library of Medicine (US), Office of High Performance Computing and Communications, Bethesda, MD (CD-ROM, ISSN 1524-9808).

Spitzer, V.M., Whitlock, D.G., 1998. The Visible Human data set: the anatomical platform for human simulation. Anat. Rec. 253 (2), 49–57.

Spitzer, V.M., Ackerman, M.J., Scherzinger, A.L., Whitlock, D.G., 1996. The Visible Human Male: a technical report. J. Am. Med. Inform. Assoc. 3 (2), 118–130.

Stewart, J.B., Broaddus, W.C., Johnson, J.H., 1996. Rebuilding the Visible Man. In: Höhne, K.H., Kikinis, R. (Eds.), Visualization in Biomedical Computing, Proc. VBC '96. Lecture Notes in Computer Science, Vol. 1131. Springer, Berlin, pp. 81–85.

Styner, M., Gerig, G., 2001. Medial models incorporating object variability for 3D shape analysis. In: Insana, M.F., Leahy, R.M. (Eds.), Information Processing in Medical Imaging, Proc. IPMI 2001. Lecture Notes in Computer Science, Vol. 2082. Springer, Berlin. pp. 502–516.

Tiede, U., Schiemann, T., Höhne, K.H., 1998. High quality rendering of attributed volume data. In: Ebert, D., Hagen, H., Rushmeier, H. (Eds.), Proc. IEEE Visualization '98. IEEE Computer Society Press, Los Alamitos, CA, pp. 255–262.

Tsiaras, A., 1997. Body Voyage. Time Warner, New York, NY.

Tsiaras, A., 2000. Volumetric imaging for the media. In: Banvard, R.A. (Ed.), The Third Visible Human Project Conference Proceedings. National Library of Medicine (US), Office of High Performance Computing and Communications, Bethesda, MD, (CD-ROM, ISSN 1524-9008).

Yamaguchi, F., 1988. Curves and Surfaces in Computer Aided Geometric Design. Springer, Berlin.

# Section 6:

<table>
<tr><td>

***Knowledge Processing and Decision Support***

<br><br><br><br><br><br>



</td><td>



</td></tr>
</table>

**Y. Shahar**

Medical Informatics Research Center
Department of Information Systems
Engineering
Ben Gurion University
Beer Sheva, Israel

# Synopsis

# *Knowledge-Based Systems: Enhancing the Quality of Care*

Since the early days of medical informatics (when that term, in fact, did not exist as such), there has been a continuing interest in automating medical diagnosis. The clinical-diagnosis task is now considered by the knowledge-modeling community as a very complex, domain-specific version of the generic classification task, not unlike detection of anomalies in digital circuits. The diagnosis task had seemed to often be the first to be tackled enthusiastically by newcomers to the medical-informatics field, especially those from the more mathematical and computational sciences. However, the clinicians themselves did not always equally share that enthusiasm, feeling that *management* of patients, rather then simply *classifying* their initial problem, was the real issue. That feeling was indeed supported by formal and informal surveys regarding the information needs of physicians.

Over the past two decades, it has become increasingly clear that supporting clinical *therapy* and continuous *management*, and in particular, enhancing the *quality* of that therapy by multiple runtime *quality-assurance* and retrospective *quality-assessment* methods, is the major new frontier. The encounter of the overwhelming majority of patients with their clinicians is not the first one. Thus, often the issue at stake is not to classify the patient as a diabetes type II patient, but rather to make the difficult decision, based on past clinical course and present clinical data, how to *manage* that patient. Most of the health-care costs are now spent on management of patients who suffer from chronic conditions such as cardiovascular diseases, diabetes, pulmonary diseases, and chronic infectious diseases (e.g., AIDS).

The four papers in the Knowledge Processing and Decision Support category present four different aspects of tackling the various facets of the clinical-management task:

a. Increasing the use of preventive care in hospitalized patients, by using computerized reminders integrated within an order-entry system [Dexter et al., 2001];
b. Analyzing in depth the relationship between the approach of sharing procedural clinical knowledge regarding continuous, long-term medical care, represented as clinical guidelines in the GLIF3 language, with that of using one-time reminders, represented as individual rules in the Arden syntax [Peleg et al., 2001];
c. Increasing our insight and knowledge regarding the management of patients who have head injuries, by exploiting not only initial, "demographic," data, but also accumulating, time-oriented clinical data; and by discussing the deeper meaning of these data with medical experts, using the structure of decision-trees induced automatically from a database of patients who have had head injuries [McQuatt et al., 2001]; and
d. Continuously assessing the quality of surgical care, using a risk-adjusted cumulative sum method that quickly and graphically zeroes in on changes in surgical outcomes, thus potentially supporting remedial measures [Steiner et al., 2001].

Much of the major progress over the past several years in the task of supporting patient management has occurred in the area of automated support to guideline-based care. Thus, a brief overview of the state of the art in that area would be useful.

**Clinical guidelines** (or **Care Plans**) are a powerful method for standardization and uniform improvement of the quality of medical care. Clinical guidelines are a set of schematic plans, at varying levels of abstraction and detail, for management over extended periods of patients who have a particular clinical condition (e.g., insulin-dependent diabetes). **Clinical protocols** are typically highly detailed guidelines, often used in areas such as oncology and experimental clinical trials. **Reminders** and **alerts** can be viewed as "mini guidelines", useful mostly for representing a single rule that needs to be applied whenever the patient's record is accessed, as opposed to representation of a long-term plan [Peleg et al., 2001]. Their effectiveness (as part of an automated system) in outpatient care has been demonstrated repeatedly, but the paper featured in this section demonstrates forcefully that they are highly effective (especially for promoting preventive care, such as pneumococcal vaccination) also in hospital environments [Dexter et al., 2001]. It is now universally agreed that conforming to state-of-the-art guidelines is the best way to improve the quality of medical care, a fact that had been rigorously demonstrated [Grimshaw and Russel, 1993], while reducing the escalating costs of medical care. Clinical guidelines are most useful at the point of care (typically, when the care provider has access to the patient's record), such as at the time of order entry by the care provider.

The application of clinical guidelines by care providers typically involves collecting and interpreting considerable amounts of data over time, applying standard therapeutic or diagnostic plans in an episodic fashion, and revising those plans when necessary. Clinical guidelines can be viewed as reusable *skeletal plans* that, when applied to a particular patient, need to be refined by a care provider over significant time periods, while often leaving considerable room for flexibility in the achievement of particular goals. Another possible view, however, is that clinical guidelines are a set of

*constraints* regarding the *process* of applying the guideline (i.e., care-provider actions) and its desired *outcomes* (i.e., patient states), that is, process (care-provider *action*) and outcome (patient *state*) **intentions** [Shahar et al., 1998]. These constraints are mostly *temporal*, or at least have a significant temporal dimension, since most clinical guidelines concern the care of chronic patients, or at least specify a care plan to be applied over a significant period.

Most clinical guidelines exist only in free-text format and are inaccessible to the physicians who most need them. Even when guidelines exist in electronic format, and even when that format is accessible online, physicians rarely have the time and means to decide which of the multiple guidelines best pertains to their patient, and, if so, exactly what does applying that guideline to the particular patient entail. Furthermore, recent health-care organizational and professional developments often reduce guideline accessibility, by creating a significant information overload on health care professionals. These professionals need to process more data then ever, in continuously shortening periods of time. Similar considerations apply to the task of assessing the quality of clinical-guideline application.

To support the needs of health-care providers as well as administrators, and ensure continuous quality of care, more sophisticated information processing tools are needed. Due to limitations of state-of-the-art technologies, analyzing unstructured text-based guidelines is not feasible. Thus, there is an urgent need to facilitate guideline dissemination and application using machine-readable representations and automated computational methods.

Several of the major tasks involved in guideline-based care, which would

benefit from automated support, include specification (authoring) and maintenance of clinical guidelines, retrieval of guidelines appropriate to each patient, runtime application of guidelines, and retrospective assessment of the quality of the application of the guidelines.

Supporting guideline-based care implies creation of a *dialog* between a care provider and an automated support system, each of which has its relative strengths. For example, physicians have better access to certain types of patient-specific clinical information (such as their odor, skin appearance, and mental state) and to general medical and commonsense knowledge. Automated systems have better and more accurate access to guideline specifications and detect more easily pre-specified complex temporal patterns in the patient's data. Thus, the key word in supporting guideline-based care is *synergy*.

Several approaches to the support of guideline-based care permit hypertext browsing of guidelines via the World Wide Web [Barnes and Barnett, 1995] but do not directly use the patient's electronic medical record. Several simplified approaches to the task of supporting guideline-based care that *do* use the patient's data encode guidelines as elementary state-transition tables or as situation-action rules dependent on the electronic medical record, as was attempted using the Arden syntax [Sherman et. al., 1995]. An established (ASTM) medical-knowledge representation standard, the Arden Syntax (Hripcsak et al., 1994), represents medical knowledge as independent units called Medical Logical Modules (MLMs), and separates the general medical logic (encoded in the Arden syntax) from the institution-specific component (encoded in the query language and terms of the local database). However, rule-based approaches, such as MLMs, typically do not include an intuitive representation of the guideline's clinical logic, have no semantics for the different types of clinical knowledge represented, lack the ability to easily represent and reuse guidelines and guideline components as well as higher, meta-level problem-solving knowledge, cannot represent intended ambiguity (e.g., when there are several options and several pro and con considerations, but no single action is, or should be, clearly prescribed) [Peleg et al., 2001], and do not support application of guidelines over extended periods of time, [Peleg et al., 2001] as is necessary to support the care of chronic patients. On the other hand, as Peleg et al. also point out, such approaches do have the advantage of simplicity when only a single alert or reminder is called for, and the heavier machinery of higher-level languages is uncalled for and might even be disruptive. Thus, they might be viewed as complementary to complex guideline representations.

During the past 20 years, there have been several efforts to support *complex* guideline-based care over time in automated fashion. Examples of architectures and representation languages include ONCOCIN [Tu et. al., 1989], T-HELPER [Musen et. al., 1992], DILEMMA [Herbert et. al, 1995], EON [Musen et. al., 1996], Asgaard [Shahar et al., 1998], PRO*forma* [Fox et al., 1998], the guideline interchange format (GLIF) [Ohno-Machado et al., 1998; Peleg et al., 2001], the European PRESTIGE project [Gordon and Veloso, 1996], and the British Prodigy project [Johnson et al., 2000].

Most of the approaches can be described as being *prescriptive* in nature, specifying *what* actions need to be performed and *how*. However, several systems, such as Miller's VT-Attending system [Miller, 1986], have used a *critiquing* approach, in which

the physician suggests a specific therapy plan and gets feedback from the program. The Asgaard project [Shahar et al., 1998] uses the *Asbru* language, which supports both an expressive, time-oriented, prescriptive specification of recommended interventions, and a set of meta-level annotations, such as process and outcome intentions of the guidelines, which support also a critiquing approach for retrospective quality assessment. Access to the original process and outcome intentions of the guideline designers supports forming an automated critique of *where*, *when*, and by *how much* the care provider seems to be deviating from the suggested process of applying the guideline, and in *what way* and *to what extent* the care provider's outcome intentions might still similar to those of the author's (e.g., she might be using a different process to achieve the same outcome intention). Thus, effective quality assessment includes searching for a reasonable *explanation* that tries to understand the care provider's rational by comparing it to the *design rational* of the guideline's author. (It is perhaps a specific instance of a rather general observation, that critiquing an agent's actions must always include at least an attempt to understand that agent's reasons for such actions).

Other recent approaches to support guideline use at the point of care enable a Web-based connection from an electronic patient record to an HTML-based set of rules, such as is done in the ActiveGuidelines model [Tang and Young, 2000], which is embedded in a commercial electronic medical record system. However, such approaches have no standardized, sharable, machine-readable representation of guidelines that can support multiple tasks such as automated application and quality assurance, and are not intended for representation of complex care plans over time. A recent

framework, GEM, enables structuring of a text document containing a clinical guideline as an *extensible markup language* (*XML*) document, using a well-defined XML schema [Shiffman et al., 2000]. However, GEM is an application running on a stand-alone computer, and the framework does not support any computational tools that can interpret the resulting semi-structured text, since it does not include a formal language that provides a clear computational model. Thus, it seems that the future lies with architectures that support the full life cycle, from guideline specification by experts, through a computable representation, to a locally customized guideline; GLIF3 is one of the architectures supporting such a life cycle [Peleg et al., 2001].

In summary, there is a clear need for effective guideline-support tools at the point of care and at the point of critiquing, which will relieve the current information overload on both care providers and administrators. To be effective, these tools need to be grounded in the patient's record, must use standard medical vocabularies, should have clear semantics, must facilitate knowledge maintenance and sharing, and need to be sufficiently expressive to explicitly capture the design rational (process and outcome intentions) of the guideline's author, while leaving flexibility at application time to the attending physicians and their local favorite methods.

## References

Barnes M , Barnett GO.  An architecture for a distributed guideline server. In: Gardner RM, editor. Proceedings of the Annual Symposium on Computer Applications in Medical Care (SCAMC-95) (New Orleans, LA). Philadelphia: Hanley & Belfus; 1995. p. 233-7.

Dexter PR, Perkins S, Overhage MJ, Maharry K, Kohler RB, McDonald CJ. A computerized reminder system to increase the use of preventive care for hospitalized patients. N Engl J Med 2001; 345(13): 965-70.

Fox J, Johns N, Rahmanzadeh A. Disseminating medical Knowledge: the PRO*forma* approach. Artif Intell Med 1998; 14:157-81.

Gordon C, Veloso M. The PRESTIGE Project: Implementing Guidelines in Healthcare. Medical Informatics Europe '96: IOS Press. 1996. p. 887-91.

Grimshaw JM, Russel IT. Effect of clinical guidelines on medical practice: A systematic review of rigorous evaluations. Lancet 1993; 342:1317–22.

Herbert SI, Gordon CJ, Jackson-Smale A, Renaud Salis J-L. Protocols for clinical care. Comput Methods Programs Biomed 1995; 48:21-2.

Hripcsak G, Ludemann P, Pryor TA, Wigertz OB, Clayton PD. Rationale for the Arden Syntax. Comput Biomed Res 1994; 27: 291–324.

Johnson PD, Tu SW, Booth N, Sugden B, Purves IN. Using scenarios in chronic disease management guidelines for primary care. In: Overhage MJ, editor. Proceedings of the 2000 AMIA Annual Symposium (Los Angeles, CA, 2000). Philadelphia: Hanley & Belfus; 2000.

Miller PL. Expert Critiquing Systems: Practice-Based Medical Consultation by Computer. New-York, NY: Springer-Verlag; 1986.

McQuatt A, Sleeman D, Andrews PJD, Corruble V, Jones PA. Discussing anomalous situations using decision tres: A head injury case study. Methods Inf Med 2001; 40 (5):373-9.

Musen MA, Carlson RW, Fagan LM, Deresinski SC. T-HELPER: Automated Support for Community-Based Clinical Research. Proceedings of the Sixteenth Annual Symposium on Computer Applications in Medical Care, Washington, D.C.; 1992. p. 719-23.

Musen MA, Tu SW, Das AK, Shahar Y. EON: A component-based approach to automation of protocol-directed therapy. J Am Med Inform Assoc 1996; 3(6): 367–88.

Ohno-Machado L, Gennari JH, Murphy SN, Jain NL, Tu SW, Oliver DE, et al. The guideline interchange format: a model for representing guidelines. J Am Med Inform Assoc 1998; 5:357-72.

Peleg M, Boxwala A, Bernstam E, Tu SW, Greenes R, Shortliffe EH. Sharable representation of clinical guidelines in GLIF: Relationship to the Arden syntax. J Biomed Inform 2001; 34:170-81.

Shahar Y, Miksch S, Johnson P. The Asgaard project: A task-specific framework for the application and critiquing of time-oriented clinical guidelines. Artif Intell Med 1998; (14): 29-51.

Sherman EH, Hripcsak G, Starren J, Jender RA, Clayton P. Using intermediate states to improve the ability of the Arden Syntax to implement care plans and reuse knowledge. In: Gardner RM, editor. Proceedings of the Annual Symposium on Computer Applications in Medical Care (SCAMC-95) (New Orleans, LA, 1995), Philadelphia: Hanley & Belfus; 1995. p. 238-42.

Shiffman RN, Karras BT, Agrawal A, Chen R, Marenco L, Nath S. GEM: a proposal for a more comprehensive guideline document model using XML. J Am Med Inform Assoc 2000; 7(5):488-98.

Steiner SH, Cook RJ, Farewell VT. Risk-adjusted monitoring of binary surgical outcomes. Med Decis Making 2001; 21:163-9.

Tang PC, Young CY. ActiveGuidelines: Integrating Web-Based Guidelines with Computer-Based Patient Records. In: Overhage MJ, editor. Proceedings of the 2000 AMIA Annual Symposium (Los Angeles, CA, 2000), Philadelphia: Hanley & Belfus; 2000.

Tu SW, Kahn MG, Musen MA, Ferguson JC, Shortliffe EH, Fagan LM. Episodic Skeletal-plan refinement on temporal data. Commun ACM 1989; 32:1439–55.

Address of the author:
Yuval Shahar M.D., Ph.D.
Medical Informatics Research Center
Department of Information
Systems Engineering
Ben Gurion University
Beer Sheva, Israel 84105
E-mail:    yshahar@bgumail.bgu.ac.il

# A COMPUTERIZED REMINDER SYSTEM TO INCREASE THE USE OF PREVENTIVE CARE FOR HOSPITALIZED PATIENTS

Paul R. Dexter, M.D., Susan Perkins, Ph.D., J. Marc Overhage, M.D., Ph.D., Kati Maharry, M.A.S., Richard B. Kohler, M.D., and Clement J. McDonald, M.D.

## ABSTRACT

***Background***   Although they are effective in outpatient settings, computerized reminders have not been proved to increase preventive care in inpatient settings.

***Methods***   We conducted a randomized, controlled trial to determine the effects of computerized reminders on the rates at which four preventive therapies were ordered for inpatients. During an 18-month study period, a computerized system processed on-line information for all 6371 patients admitted to a general-medicine service (for a total of 10,065 hospitalizations), generating preventive care reminders as appropriate. Physicians who were in the intervention group viewed these reminders when they were using a computerized order-entry system for inpatients.

***Results***   The reminder system identified 3416 patients (53.6 percent) as eligible for preventive measures that had not been ordered by the admitting physician. For patients with at least one indication, computerized reminders resulted in higher adjusted ordering rates for pneumococcal vaccination (35.8 percent of the patients in the intervention group vs. 0.8 percent of those in the control group, P<0.001), influenza vaccination (51.4 percent vs. 1.0 percent, P< 0.001), prophylactic heparin (32.2 percent vs. 18.9 percent, P<0.001), and prophylactic aspirin at discharge (36.4 percent vs. 27.6 percent, P<0.001).

***Conclusions***   A majority of hospitalized patients in this study were eligible for preventive measures, and computerized reminders significantly increased the rate of delivery of such therapies. (N Engl J Med 2001; 345:965-70.)



ALTHOUGH they are cost effective, preventive care measures are underutilized. Pneumococcal vaccination is associated with decreased rates of hospitalization, decreased rates of bacteremia, and cost savings among patients who are at least 65 years old,[1-3] yet the vaccine is administered to only 45 percent of such patients.[4] Similarly, only 66 percent of patients in this age group are vaccinated against influenza,[4] despite reports that vaccination leads to decreased mortality, hospitalization rates, and medical costs.[5-7] Daily aspirin use reduces the risk of myocardial infarction, stroke, and death in persons who are at high risk for occlusive vascular disease,[8] yet 22 percent of eligible patients may leave the hospital after acute myocardial infarction without an order for aspirin.[9] Similarly, the prophylactic use of subcutaneous heparin reduces the incidence of venous thromboembolism among hospitalized patients with various medical conditions,[10] but only one third of such high-risk patients receive this treatment.[11,12]

Although multiple randomized trials have confirmed that computerized reminders increase the use of preventive care in the outpatient setting,[13-17] a trial among hospitalized patients failed to demonstrate an increase in the use of preventive care measures with this intervention.[14,18] Nevertheless, hospitalization represents an opportunity to target persons who are particularly likely to benefit from preventive care. For example, 1 future hospitalization might be avoided by the simple administration of pneumococcal vaccine to 100 appropriate hospitalized patients.[19] We hypothesized that a computerized reminder system could increase the use of preventive care among hospitalized patients.

## METHODS

### Setting and Eligibility

We obtained approval for this study from the institutional review board of the Indiana University Medical Center. The board did not require informed consent from patients, since computer reminders have been considered routine components of care in the outpatient setting. We included all patients admitted to the general-medicine service of Wishard Memorial Hospital, an urban public teaching hospital in Indianapolis, between May 1, 1997, and October 31, 1998. The organization of the teams of the general-medicine ward has been described previously[18]; at present there are eight independent teams whose staff members (physicians and students) rotate approximately monthly.

### Randomization and Outcomes

Using a blinded system of coin randomization, one of the investigators randomly designated four of the general-medicine teams

From the Department of Medicine, Indiana University School of Medicine (P.R.D., S.P., J.M.O., K.M., R.B.K., C.J.M.); the Regenstrief Institute for Health Care (P.R.D., S.P., J.M.O., C.J.M.); and the Richard L. Roudebush Veterans Affairs Medical Center (P.R.D., R.B.K.) — all in Indianapolis. Address reprint requests to Dr. McDonald at the Regenstrief Institute for Health Care, 1050 Wishard Blvd., Indianapolis, IN 46202, or at clem@regen.rg.iupui.edu.

as intervention teams and four as control teams. All physicians, medical students, and patients associated with a team were assigned that team's intervention status. The same investigator also randomly assigned physicians to teams insofar as practical constraints allowed (e.g., avoiding assignments that might lead to two consecutive nights of overnight on-call duty). When physicians returned for multiple rotations during the study period, we attempted to maintain their original intervention status by assigning them to teams with the same status; most medical students had only one rotation at the hospital during the study period. Patients were admitted to the general-medicine wards with the use of a system that distributed admissions equally among the teams, solely on the basis of the order in which patients required hospitalization. Patients automatically assumed the intervention status of the team to which they were assigned on admission and retained that status for the duration of their hospitalization. Previous studies involving inpatients have shown no material differences in clinical status among patients assigned to different teams.[20]

The primary outcomes of interest were the rates at which the various preventive therapies were ordered. These rates were obtained from routinely stored data.

### Computerized Order Entry and Clinical-Decision Support

Using personal-computer–based order-entry workstations,[18,20-22] resident physicians and medical students on the general-medicine teams wrote all orders (except for do-not-resuscitate orders); these persons were the targets of the intervention. During the order-entry process, the system provided clinical-decision support to physicians and medical students by means of rule-based reminders, which we called Care rules.[18,23] The Care rules generated the reminders in this study as prewritten orders with explanatory text. Physicians could accept or reject the reminders with one or two keystrokes on the computer.

### Generation and Display of Computer Reminders

Using the Care rules, we implemented national guidelines that were current at the time of the study regarding the use of pneumococcal vaccination,[3] influenza vaccination,[24] prophylactic enteric-coated aspirin for cardiovascular disease,[25-27] and prophylactic subcutaneous heparin to reduce the risk of thromboembolic events in patients with certain medical conditions.[28] Computer-generated reminders for all but one of these therapies (subcutaneous heparin) have been a routine part of care in the outpatient setting for more than 15 years. The computer was programmed to suggest influenza vaccination only during the "flu-shot season" from October 1, 1997, through January 31, 1998. Before the study, we tested the appropriateness of the reminders generated by the Care rules (available from NAPS*) by having the practitioners review the rules directly to judge whether they were reasonable and by running the rule-based reminder program on a sample of more than 300 patient records and manually validating the recommendations by reference to the rules and the content of the computerized medical charts.

The Care rules relied on multiple sources of such routinely collected data as demographic characteristics of the patient, lists of medical problems, diagnoses at previous hospital discharge, vital signs, active inpatient orders, previous pharmacy records, and coded radiologic results. In addition, we obtained information from patients on their vaccination status by means of a standard admission questionnaire completed by a research assistant or the admitting nurse. The Care rules generated reminders when the patient's electronic medical record included at least one indication for one of the selected preventive therapies, no evident contraindication to the therapy, no active orders for the therapy, and in the case of the two vaccinations, no record of previous administration within an appropriate time frame.

*See NAPS document no. 05605 for 8 pages of supplementary material. To order, contact NAPS, c/o Microfiche Publications, 248 Hempstead Tpke., West Hempstead, NY 11552.

The Care rules program was used for all study patients (in both the intervention group and the control group) when the physician initiated an order-entry session for daily care, for the transfer of the patient, or for discharge. The program was not run and no reminders were generated when orders were entered at the time of admission; thus, the clinician had one opportunity to order the preventive therapies without receiving a reminder. The computer program logged the following types of data: the names of all the Care rules that were applied, all the resultant messages and orders that were generated, the dates and times of all messages and orders, the physician's identification number and intervention status, and the patient's hospital identification number and intervention status.

In most cases, the physician and the patient had the same intervention status; when physicians were on call or during emergencies, they might write orders for a patient with a different intervention status. When the physician and the patient were both assigned to the intervention group, the computer displayed to the physician all reminders generated by the program. When either the physician or the patient was assigned to the control group, the computer logged the reminders but did not display them. Patients whose data triggered a reminder were considered to be eligible for the specified therapy.

A sample computerized reminder message, as it would appear to a physician assigned to the intervention group, is shown in Figure 1. Physicians indicated their acceptance or rejection of each recommended therapy by choosing "order" or "omit." For the three therapies with few risks (influenza vaccination, pneumococcal vaccination, and subcutaneous heparin), we set the default to "order," so that the physician could accept the item simply by pressing the "enter" key. In the case of daily aspirin prophylaxis against coronary artery disease, we set the default to "omit," thereby requiring a more deliberate effort by the physician to change the status to "order." As a means of capturing the physician's attention briefly, we disabled the "escape" key and presented the reminders in a color scheme different from that used for physician-initiated orders. If a physician ordered the targeted therapy, no more reminders related to that therapy appeared. No reminders were displayed between the fifth hospital day and the time discharge orders were entered, at which time vaccination and prophylactic daily aspirin were suggested again if they were indicated.

### Statistical Analysis

We compared the demographic characteristics of the patients in the intervention and control groups by means of the chi-square test and Student's t-test. The demographic data, including race, used for these comparisons were obtained as part of the routine procedures for hospital registration. The unit of analysis for all models was the individual hospital admission. We used a generalized-estimating-equation method[29] for all estimates of effect. We used a compound-symmetry structure, which assumes that patients are independent of each other and that hospitalizations for a particular patient have a fixed correlation that does not vary over time. Our primary analyses included all hospital admissions, but we also performed analyses that dealt with the effects of crossover by excluding patients and physicians who were part of both the intervention and the control group at different times. We limited these analyses to patients' first hospitalizations during the study period and excluded physicians who were in both the intervention group and the control group during the course of the study.

We modeled the effect of the explanatory variables (intervention status and demographic characteristics) on the binary response variable (therapy ordered or not ordered) with the use of logistic regression, and we considered a P value of 0.05 or less to indicate statistical significance. To account for possible similarities among the ordering rates of physicians working on the same team, we included in the models a variable indicating medical team nested within the intervention status. We created two models for each of the four preventive therapies — one including only the hospitalizations during which a reminder was generated by the computer, and the other including all hospitalizations.

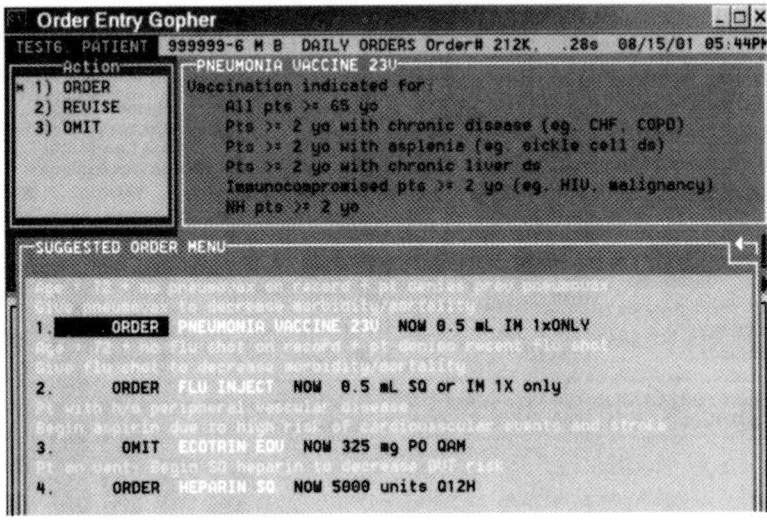

**Figure 1.** Example of a Computerized Reminder as Displayed to Physicians on Intervention Teams.

## RESULTS

### Study Subjects

A total of 6371 patients accounted for 10,065 admissions during the study period; patients were assigned to intervention teams for 4995 hospitalizations and to control teams for 5070 hospitalizations. Twenty-eight percent of the patients were hospitalized more than once. The mean age of the hospitalized patients was 53.2 years, 50 percent were women, and 51 percent were black. There were no significant differences in mean age, race, or sex between the intervention and control groups.

During the 18 months of the study, a total of 202 physicians rotated an average of 2.1 times onto the inpatient service: 96 of these physicians (47.5 percent) were assigned only to intervention teams, 78 (38.6 percent) were assigned only to control teams, and 28 (13.9 percent) were assigned at different times to intervention teams and control teams.

### Computer Reminders and Ordering Rates for Preventive Therapies

Overall, 3416 patients (53.6 percent) were eligible for at least one preventive therapy. The mean number of times that a reminder was displayed to a physician on an intervention team ranged from 3.4 to 5.2 for each hospitalization of an eligible patient in the intervention group.

The display of computer-generated reminders had a significant effect on the use of each of the four preventive therapies (Table 1). The use of the reminders led to a higher ordering rate for pneumococcal vaccination (35.8 percent among eligible patients in the intervention group, as compared with 0.8 percent among eligible patients in the control group) and a higher ordering rate for influenza vaccination (51.4 percent as compared with 1.0 percent) (Table 1). When the total number of hospitalizations was used as the denominator for calculating the ordering rates for each of the preventive therapies, the rates were also significantly higher among patients in the intervention group than among those in the control group (Table 2). There were no important differences in our results when we limited our analyses to the patients' first hospitalizations and excluded the physicians who took part in both intervention and control teams during the study period.

Physicians varied in the frequency with which they accepted these reminders. The distribution of ordering rates among 114 physicians randomly assigned to the intervention group who received computerized reminders for at least 10 patients (range, 10 to 82) is shown in Figure 2.

The rates of physicians' orders for each of the four preventive therapies were positively correlated with the age of the patients (P<0.002 for all comparisons). Physicians also ordered prophylactic aspirin at the time of discharge more frequently for patients who were hospitalized for acute myocardial infarction and unstable angina than for those with other indications (cerebrovascular disease, peripheral vascular disease, and coronary risk factors) (P<0.001 for all comparisons).

## DISCUSSION

The results of this trial provide compelling evidence that computerized reminders can increase the delivery of preventive care to hospitalized patients. For all four preventive therapies, the use of computerized reminders resulted in absolute ordering rates for both eligi-

**TABLE 1.** ADJUSTED ORDERING RATES FOR PREVENTIVE THERAPIES FOR ELIGIBLE PATIENTS.*

| THERAPY | NO. OF ELIGIBLE PATIENTS (% OF ALL PATIENTS) | NO. OF HOSPITALIZATIONS OF ELIGIBLE PATIENTS (% OF ALL HOSPITALIZATIONS) | PERCENTAGE OF HOSPITALIZATIONS DURING WHICH THERAPY WAS ORDERED FOR AN ELIGIBLE PATIENT | | P VALUE |
|---|---|---|---|---|---|
| | | | INTERVENTION GROUP | CONTROL GROUP | |
| Pneumococcal vaccination | 1696 (26.6) | 2314 (23.0) | 35.8 | 0.8 | <0.001 |
| Influenza vaccination | 1033 (16.2) | 1251 (12.4) | 51.4 | 1.0 | <0.001 |
| Subcutaneous heparin | 1083 (17.0) | 1326 (13.2) | 32.2 | 18.9 | <0.001 |
| Aspirin at discharge | 1698 (26.7) | 2240 (22.3) | 36.4 | 27.6 | <0.001 |

*There were a total of 6371 patients and a total of 10,065 hospitalizations; patients were assigned to intervention teams for 4995 hospitalizations and to control teams for 5070 hospitalizations.

**TABLE 2.** ADJUSTED ORDERING RATES FOR PREVENTIVE THERAPIES FOR ALL 6371 HOSPITALIZED PATIENTS DURING 10,065 HOSPITALIZATIONS.

| THERAPY | PERCENTAGE OF HOSPITALIZATIONS WITH AN ORDER FOR THERAPY | | P VALUE |
|---|---|---|---|
| | INTERVENTION GROUP | CONTROL GROUP | |
| Pneumococcal vaccination | 8.5 | 0.9 | <0.001 |
| Influenza vaccination | 5.4 | 0.4 | <0.001 |
| Subcutaneous heparin | 10.5 | 8.2 | <0.001 |
| Aspirin at discharge | 29.7 | 25.4 | 0.005 |

ble patients and all hospitalized patients that were significantly higher than the rates in the control group. In particular, the use of reminders increased the use of pneumococcal and influenza vaccination from practically zero to approximately 35 percent and 50 percent, respectively. (Analyses of data from the 15 months after the completion of the controlled trial revealed that, with continuing reminders, these rates had increased to 50 percent for pneumococcal vaccination and 57 percent for influenza vaccination.) The easy sustainability of computer-based reminder systems contrasts with the weaknesses of such approaches as manual reviewing of charts,[30,31] patient-directed interventions,[32,33] and physician-directed continuing medical education.[30]

Previous studies of computer-generated reminders for preventive care have focused almost exclusively on the outpatient setting.[14] Yet we found that 54 percent of patients hospitalized in general-medicine wards were eligible for preventive care interventions and that physicians' rates of compliance with the reminders were similar to those achieved in outpatient settings.[15] These findings alone would justify focusing greater

attention on preventive care for inpatients, but there are other reasons to do so as well. For one, patients hospitalized because of severe underlying diseases may benefit more from preventive measures (e.g., pneumococcal vaccination[19,34]) than patients who do not require hospitalization. Also, among patients who do not have regular outpatient follow-up, hospitalization may offer the only good case-finding opportunity to provide such care.[35] Other preventive therapies, such as subcutaneous heparin, are specifically indicated in the hospital setting.

The findings of this study contrast with the results of a previous study performed at our institution that did not demonstrate an effect of computerized reminders.[18] We attribute our recent success to relatively small changes in the presentation of these reminders. In our previous study, we relied on physicians to make a deliberate choice to view the reminders and notified them only by means of a banner at the bottom of the screen stating that "there are suggested orders for this patient." By contrast, in the current study, the computer immediately displayed the reminders to the physicians as full, prewritten orders. In this study, we also highlighted the suggested reminders with a distinctive color scheme, disabled the "escape" key, repeated the individual reminders approximately four times per hospitalization, on average, and set the default to "order" for three of the preventive therapies (allowing the physician to accept the item simply by pressing the "enter" key).

We do not have data on the reasons for noncompliance by physicians in the intervention group. In some cases, physicians may have had good reasons for ignoring a reminder; they may have known something that the computer did not — for example, the patient may have told the physician that aspirin had caused bleeding in the past. Furthermore, the compliance rates of physicians in some cases were related to the strength of the indication. For example, physicians complied with reminders for aspirin prophylaxis in 79 percent of the

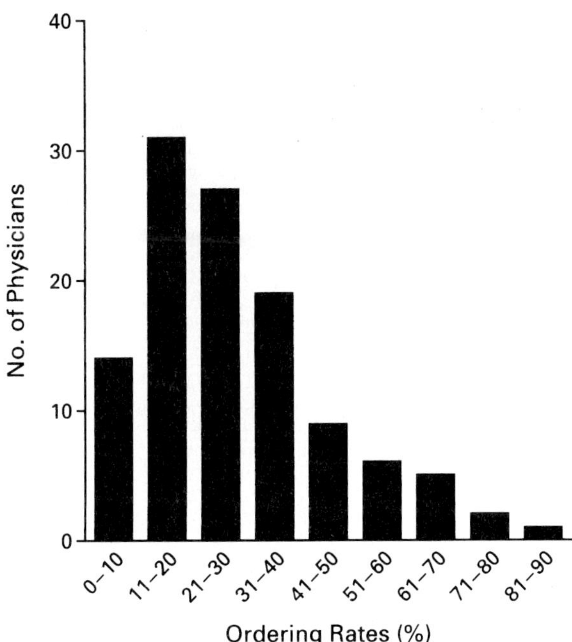



**Figure 2.** Distribution of Ordering Rates for Preventive Therapies among the Physicians in the Intervention Group.
Data are limited to the physicians who had at least 10 patients for whom reminders were displayed.

cases in which a patient was admitted for an acute myocardial infarction but only 22 percent of the cases in which indications were an age of more than 50 years and two or more coronary risk factors.

As in previous studies,[36] there was a great deal of individual variation among physicians in their acceptance of the reminders. This variation suggests that some portion of the overall rate of noncompliance was attributable to very low compliance among some physicians who generally ignored the reminders. The extremely low rate of use of vaccinations in the control group also suggests that some of the noncompliance with vaccination reminders could be attributed to long-established habits of vaccinating patients only in the outpatient setting.

Although the reminders in this study were based on a physician order-entry system and a rich repository of clinical data, neither of these features is necessarily a prerequisite to improving hospital-based preventive care. In the outpatient setting, reminders written on paper encounter forms are effective in increasing the use of preventive care.[16] The daily patient census reports produced for physicians in many hospitals could be as effective a mechanism for delivering reminders in the hospital as an order-entry system. Furthermore, the majority of the reminders generated in our study were triggered by information that is routinely available in hospital information systems. For example, an age of at least 65 years is a valid indication for pneu-

moccal and influenza vaccination. The addition of the diagnosis on admission, past diagnoses, and the service to which the patient was admitted would have been sufficient to identify the majority of patients with indications for vaccinations and many of those with indications for aspirin or subcutaneous heparin. It is likely that with a small amount of computer programming and the creation of nursing or other protocols to check for possible contraindications and previous vaccinations, many hospitals could implement programs that provide simple reminders and thereby improve preventive care for inpatients.

Supported by a grant (HS07719) from the Agency for Healthcare Research and Quality and a grant (N01-LM-6-3546) from the National Library of Medicine.

*We are indebted to the physicians, nurses, and administrators at Wishard Memorial Hospital for their support of the physician order-entry process and this study.*

## REFERENCES

**1.** Sisk JE, Moskowitz AJ, Whang W, et al. Cost-effectiveness of vaccination against pneumococcal bacteremia among elderly people. JAMA 1997; 278:1333-9.
**2.** Fedson DS. The clinical effectiveness of pneumococcal vaccination: a brief review. Vaccine 1999;17:Suppl 1:S85-S90.
**3.** Prevention of pneumococcal disease: recommendations of the Advisory Committee on Immunization Practices (ACIP). MMWR Morb Mortal Wkly Rep 1997;46(RR-8):1-24.
**4.** Influenza and pneumococcal vaccination levels among adults aged ≥65 years — United States, 1997. MMWR Morb Mortal Wkly Rep 1998,47: 797-802.
**5.** Gross PA, Hermogenes AW, Sacks HS, Lau J, Levandowski RA. The efficacy of influenza vaccine in elderly persons: a meta-analysis and review of the literature. Ann Intern Med 1995;123:518-27.
**6.** Nichol KL, Baken L, Nelson A. Relation between influenza vaccination and outpatient visits, hospitalization, and mortality in elderly persons with chronic lung disease. Ann Intern Med 1999;130:397-403.
**7.** McDonald CJ, Hui SL, Tierney WM. Effects of computer reminders for influenza vaccination on morbidity during influenza epidemics. MD Comput 1992;9:304-12.
**8.** Collaborative overview of randomised trials of antiplatelet therapy. I. Prevention of death, myocardial infarction, and stroke by prolonged antiplatelet therapy in various categories of patients: Antiplatelet Trialists' Collaboration. BMJ 1994;308:81-106.
**9.** O'Connor GT, Quinton HB, Traven ND, et al. Geographic variation in the treatment of acute myocardial infarction: the Cooperative Cardiovascular Project. JAMA 1999;281:627-33.
**10.** Geerts WH, Heit JA, Clagett GP, et al. Prevention of venous thromboembolism. Chest 2001;119:Suppl:132S-175S.
**11.** Anderson FA Jr, Wheeler HB, Goldberg RJ, Hosmer DW, Forcier A, Patwardhan NA. Physician practices in the prevention of venous thromboembolism. Ann Intern Med 1991;115:591-5.
**12.** Keane MG, Ingenito EP, Goldhaber SZ. Utilization of venous thromboembolism prophylaxis in the medical intensive care unit. Chest 1994; 106:13-4.
**13.** Fedson DS. Adult immunization: summary of the National Vaccine Advisory Committee Report. JAMA 1994;272:1133-7.
**14.** Hunt DL, Haynes RB, Hanna SE, Smith K. Effects of computer-based clinical decision support systems on physician performance and patient outcomes: a systematic review. JAMA 1998;280:1339-46.
**15.** Shea S, DuMouchel W, Bahamonde L. A meta-analysis of 16 randomized controlled trials to evaluate computer-based clinical reminder systems for preventive care in the ambulatory setting. J Am Med Inform Assoc 1996;3:399-409.
**16.** McDonald CJ, Hui SL, Smith DM, et al. Reminders to physicians from an introspective computer medical record: a two-year randomized trial. Ann Intern Med 1984;100:130-8.
**17.** McDonald CJ. Protocol-based computer reminders, the quality of care and the non-perfectability of man. N Engl J Med 1976;295:1351-5.
**18.** Overhage JM, Tierney WM, McDonald CJ. Computer reminders to

implement preventive care guidelines for hospitalized patients. Arch Intern Med 1996;156:1551-6.

**19.** Fedson DS, Harward MP, Reid RA, Kaiser DL. Hospital-based pneumococcal immunization: epidemiologic rationale from the Shenandoah study. JAMA 1990;264:1117-22.

**20.** Tierney WM, Miller ME, Overhage JM, McDonald CJ. Physician inpatient order writing on microcomputer workstations: effects on resource utilization. JAMA 1993;269:379-83.

**21.** McDonald CJ, Tierney WM. The Medical Gopher — a microcomputer system to help find, organize and decide about patient data. West J Med 1986;145:823-9.

**22.** McDonald CJ, Overhage JM, Tierney WM, et al. The Regenstrief Medical Record System: a quarter century experience. Int J Med Inf 1999; 54:225-53.

**23.** Overhage JM, Mamlin B, Warvel J, Warvel J, Tierney W, McDonald CJ. A tool for provider interaction during patient care: G-CARE. Proc Annu Symp Comput Appl Med Care 1995:178-82.

**24.** Prevention and control of influenza: recommendations of the Advisory Committee on Immunization Practices (ACIP). MMWR Morb Mortal Wkly Rep 1997;46(RR-9):1-25.

**25.** Cairns JA, Lewis HD Jr, Meade TW, Sutton GC, Theroux P. Antithrombotic agents in coronary artery disease. Chest 1995;108:Suppl:380S-400S.

**26.** Sherman DG, Dyken ML Jr, Gent M, Harrison JG, Hart RG, Mohr JP. Antithrombotic therapy for cerebrovascular disorders: an update. Chest 1995;108:Suppl:444S-456S.

**27.** Clagett GP, Krupski WC. Antithrombotic therapy in peripheral arterial occlusive disease. Chest 1995;108:Suppl:431S-443S.

**28.** Clagett GP, Anderson FA Jr, Heit J, Levine MN, Wheeler HB. Prevention of venous thromboembolism. Chest 1995;108:Suppl:312S-334S.

**29.** Zeger SL, Liang KY. Longitudinal data analysis for discrete and continuous outcomes. Biometrics 1986;42:121-30.

**30.** LeBaron CW, Chaney M, Baughman AL, et al. Impact of measurement and feedback on vaccination coverage in public clinics, 1988-1994. JAMA 1997;277:631-5.

**31.** Morrow RW, Gooding AD, Clark C. Improving physicians' preventive health care behavior through peer review and financial incentives. Arch Fam Med 1995;4:165-9.

**32.** Jacobson TA, Thomas DM, Morton FJ, Offutt G, Shevlin J, Ray S. Use of a low-literacy patient education tool to enhance pneumococcal vaccination rates: a randomized controlled trial. JAMA 1999;282:646-50.

**33.** Smith DM, Zhou XH, Weinberger M, Smith F, McDonald RC. Mailed reminders for area-wide influenza immunization: a randomized controlled trial. J Am Geriatr Soc 1999;47:1-5.

**34.** Lipsky BA, Boyko EJ, Inui TS, Koepsell TD. Risk factors for acquiring pneumococcal infections. Arch Intern Med 1986;146:2179-85.

**35.** Spitzer WO, Mann KV. The public's health is too important to be left to public health workers: a commentary on Guide to Clinical Preventive Services. Ann Intern Med 1989;111:939-42.

**36.** Overhage JM, Tierney WM, Zhou XH, McDonald CJ. A randomized trial of "corollary orders" to prevent errors of omission. J Am Med Inform Assoc 1997;4:364-75.

# Discussing Anomalous Situations using Decision Trees:
# A Head Injury Case Study

A. McQuatt [1], D. Sleeman [1], P. J. D. Andrews [2], V. Corruble [1], P. A. Jones [2]
[1] Department of Computing Science, University of Aberdeen, Aberdeen, Scotland
[2] Department of Clinical Neurosciences, Western General Hospital, Edinburgh, Scotland

## Summary

*Objectives:* Predicting the outcome of seriously ill patients is a challenging problem for clinicians.
*Methods:* One alternative to clinical trials is to analyse existing patient data in an attempt to predict the several outcomes, and to suggest therapies. In this paper we use decision tree techniques to predict the outcome of head injury patients. The work is based on patient data from the Edinburgh Royal Infirmary which contains both background (demographic) data and temporal (physiological) data.
*Results:* The focus of this paper is the discussion of the anomalous cases in the decision trees with the domain experts (the clinicians).
*Conclusions:* These analyses led to the detection of several situations where both the data analysis and patient data collection should be enhanced, which in turn should lead to improved patient care.

## Keywords

Anomalies, Decision Tree Analysis, Demographic Data, Traumatic Brain Injuries, Temporal/Physiological Data

Methods Inf Med 2001; 40: 373–9

# 1. Introduction

In most western countries, the treatment of patients with head injuries is very resource intensive and frequently involves the patient staying in a Neurological Intensive Care Unit (NICU) for an extended period. Besides dealing with the initial accident (event), the medical team has to cope with secondary events such as the swelling of the brain. As the brain is encased in the skull, treatment procedures are more limited than for the rest of the body. The primary clinical strategy appears to be alleviating extreme symptoms such as high intra-cranial pressure (ICP) and relying on the self-healing mechanisms of the organ.

Predicting the outcome of seriously ill patients is a challenging problem for clinicians. There are still many situations where it is very hard to predict whether a patient will survive given his or her state on admission to hospital. This makes it difficult to choose the best course of treatment. Head injury has the added complication that it is very difficult to devise effective clinical trials, as the brain is largely inaccessible and experimentation can have serious consequences. One alternative to clinical trials is to analyse existing patient data in an attempt to predict the several outcomes, and to suggest therapies. The focus of this study has been data from head injury patients.

In this paper we will first describe the data that was available to us (section 2). We will then discuss analyses carried out on this data by the Edinburgh NICU group and previous work involving decision tree analysis on head injury data from other researchers (section 3). This is followed by an overview of the decision tree methods used and an evaluation of these methods (section 4). Section 5 describes the analyses and outlines the results. We will then discuss these results in section 6; section 7 discusses the conclusions.

# 2. The Data and Its Use

The full data collected, which describes 121 patients, falls into four distinct categories: demographic data, complication data, temporal data and outcome data. The purpose of these investigations was to determine how well the first three categories, and combinations of them, can be used to predict the fourth, the outcome. Experiments using complication data are not reported here as the outcome of patients with severe complications is fairly straight forward for clinicians to predict. For a variety of logistic and medical reasons complete data-sets were only available for 69 of the patients; some of the analyses were therefore carried out on the full data-set (n = 121) and others on a subset (n = 69).

*Demographic data:* Demographic data describes patients' characteristics and their clinical state on admission to hospital. The following data were used in this analysis: Grade of injury (minor to severe), Glasgow Coma Score, or GCS (a measure of verbal, motor and eye responses), Age, Pupil response, Injury Severity Score (ISS), Sex, Cause of injury, Diagnosis (type of injury to the brain), where the patient was referred from, type of skull fracture (if any).

*Temporal data:* During their stay in the NICU, the bedside monitors for the patients in this study were connected to a data collection system. This recorded the values of various parameters once a minute. These values could then be analyzed to ascertain whether they were indicative of physiological abnormalities, or "insults", depending on their values relative to pre-defined "normal" and "abnormal" values. The degree of abnormality, that is the amount by which the parameter was out of range, was graded on a scale of 0 to being classed as normal and 3 being extremely abnormal.

The number of occurrences and total duration of each of these insult grades could then be calculated, as well as the average length of each insult grade and the percentage of monitored time for each insult, thereby forming a summary of the physiological abnormalities of the patient. It is this summary data which was used in this study. The data are described below:

– *Parameters monitored and recorded:* ICP (Intracranial pressure), BP (Blood pressure), $SaO2_2$ (oxygen content in the arterial blood to the brain), $SvO2_2$ (oxygen content in the venous blood from the brain), $ETCO_2$ (end tidal carbon dioxide), T1 (temperature), HR (heart rate).
– *Insult types derived from recorded data:* Intracranial Pressure (pressure exerted on the brain by the skull), Hypotension (low blood pressure), Hypertension (high blood pressure), Cerebral Perfusion Pressure (cerebral blood flow), Hypoxia (low oxygen content in the arterial blood to the brain), Cerebral Oligaemia (low oxygen content in the venous blood from the brain), Cerebral Hyperaemia (high oxygen content in the venous blood from the brain), Hypocarbia (low end tidal carbon dioxide), Hypercarbia (high end tidal carbon dioxide), Pyrexia (high temperature), Bradycardia (slow heart rate), Tachycardia (fast heart rate), Global cerebral hypoxaemia (low oxygen content in the blood in the brain), Global cerebral hyperaemia (high oxygen content in the blood in the brain).

– *Parameters derived for each insult type:* Duration (total duration in minutes, of a grade 1/2/3 insult, and of all grades taken together), Occurrences (total number of occurrences of a grade 1/2/3 insult, and of all grades taken together), Monitored time (total number of minutes the parameter was recorded), Percentage of monitored time, Percentage of recorded time of a grade 1/2/3 insult, and of all grades taken together, Average insult length (average length, in minutes, of a grade 1/2/3 insult, and of all grades taken together).
– *Outcome data:* Data is generally available concerning the outcome of each patient at 6, 12 and 24 months. Only outcome at 12 months was used in this study. Outcome is graded using the Glasgow Outcome Scale (GOS) (1), which classifies outcome into five categories: 1: Dead; 2: Persistent vegetative state; 3: Severely disabled; 4: Moderately disabled; and 5: Good recovery.

### What Predictions do Clinicians Wish to Make?

Clearly it is desirable to predict the actual GOS (Glasgow Outcome Score) for individual patients. However, given the quantity and the quality of the data available, this has not been possible so far. On the other hand, predicting survival has been achieved reliably. This, however, is not a very useful measure and so most studies have focused their attention, for the moment, on predicting good or poor outcomes on the Glasgow scale. (Good outcome is usually defined as 4 & 5 on this scale and poor as 1, 2 & 3).

# 3. Previous Analyses

## 3.1 Previous Analyses on a Subset of this Data

Details of the statistical analysis (logistic regression) undertaken by the Department of Clinical Neurosciences in Edinburgh are described in (2). This study is basically a statistical analysis of the demographic and time-stamped head-injury data collected by the computerised data collection system in Edinburgh, these analyses were performed on the subset of patients for whom complete data-sets are available (n = 69).

This study found that the important predictors of mortality (death or survival) at 12 months from the date of the injury were the duration of Hypotension (significance, p = 0.0064), the duration of pyrexia (p = 0.0137), and the duration of Hypoxaemia (p = 0.0244). They found these to be "significantly better predictions than the usually described predictive factors of coma score on admission, age, or pupil response." The paper also states: "Previous studies showing important associations between ICP and mortality may be due to the fact that Cerebral Perfusion Pressure (CPP) and Hypotension were not entered into the model."

When predicting morbidity (good or poor outcome), the study found duration of Hypotension (p = 0.0118) and pupil response on admission (p = 0.0226) to be the most significant predictors of outcome.

## 3.2 Previous Decision Tree Analyses Using other Head Injury Data

There have been various studies of data from head injury patients. Two such studies are by Choi et al. in 1991 (3) and by Pilih et al. in 1997 (4). These have been chosen for discussion due to their use of decision tree analysis.

Choi presents a study which predicts the outcome of head-injury patients. Twenty-three prognostic factors were analysed from 555 patients admitted to the Medical College of Virginia hospitals with severe head injuries. The factors used were: age, race, sex, motor response, pupillary response, oculocephalics, eye opening, verbal response, midline shift, intracerebral lesion, extracerebral lesion, intracranial pressure, systolic blood pressure, diastolic blood pressure, pulse, respiration, temperature, hematocrit, $pCO_2$, $pO_2$, pH, blood alcohol. All of these factors were taken at admission, except ICP which was obtained during monitoring in the neurosurgical ICU. The paper compares the result of a decision tree analysis on the data with the results of statistical analysis using logistic regression and discriminant analysis. The decision tree analysis uses the CART methodology (5). All the analyses were to predict outcome on the Glasgow Outcome Score (1) at 12 months after the injury.

The paper claims a predictive accuracy of 77.7% for the decision tree analysis, 74.2% for logistic regression and 74.6% for discriminant analysis (although these figures appear to represent *training* set classification accuracy). The paper argues that, as well as giving a higher predictive accuracy, decision trees are "visually more informative and easier to interpret". The rationale behind this is that when data is represented by a decision tree, patient sub-groups can be identified. This can result in different prognostic indicators being found for different sub-groups of patients and hence higher predictive accuracy.

Of the 23 possible predictive factors, their decision tree includes only four. These are pupillary response, age, motor response and intracerebral lesion. In all, the decision tree contains eight different sub-groups of patients.

A more recent study by Pilih et al. (4), applies decision tree induction to the prediction of outcome of head injured patients six months after admission to hospital. The patient group consisted of 38 patients with severe head injury. Factors used in the study include: Glasgow coma score (GCS) (6), computed axial tomography abnormalities (CT), brain stem syndromes (BSS) (7), age, level of consciousness, motor reactions to sound stimuli, motor reactions to pain stimuli, position and motility of eyes, pupillary size and reactions to light, position of the body and extremities, motility of the body and extremities; the parameters of vegetative functions such as respiration, heart rate, blood pressure and body temperature. The BSS classification separates brain stem dysfunction into seven stages. This classification is estimated from basic clinical attributes. Decision trees were constructed from the data using Magnus Assistant (8) which uses an algorithm based on ID3 (9).

When predicting good or poor outcome, only three factors were used. These were

age, CT score and either GCS or BSS. The first of these analyses, using GCS but not BSS, produced a decision tree with CT score as its root and GCS as one of the sub-nodes. Using each of the 38 patients in turn as a test case and the decision trees generated by the remaining 37 test cases (leave-one-out cross-validation), this produces a prediction accuracy of 82%. Using BSS, but not GCS, produced a tree with BSS as the root note and CT score, BSS and age as sub-nodes. This gives a predictive accuracy of 79%. However, this paper does not present its results as being prognostically reliable, mainly on the grounds of the sample size being so small. It only attempts to show that decision trees can be a useful tool for predicting outcome.

# 4. Decision Tree Methodology

## 4.1 Building Decision Trees

A definition of decision trees and their creation is as follows: "The traditional approach to constructing a decision tree from a training set of cases described in terms of a collection of attributes is based on successive refinement. Tests on the attributes are constructed to partition the training set into smaller and smaller subsets until each subset contains cases belonging to a single class. These tests form the interior nodes of the decision tree and each subset is associated with one of its leaves. An unseen case is classified by tracing a path from the root of the tree to the appropriate leaf and asserting that the case belongs to the same class as the set of training cases associated with that leaf."(10).

The decision trees used in this report were generated using the See5 environment (11). This is a PC application that uses the C5.0 algorithm, an upgraded version of the C4.5 algorithm. As the new facilities of C5.0 have not been utilised in this analysis, the resulting decision trees can be considered as being the same as produced by the C4.5 algorithm. There has been much work done on decision trees since the 70s, both by Quinlan (9, 12) and others in the machine learning and statistics communities (5).

The power of this method lies in its ability to choose the value of the attribute at which the cases can be divided into the lowest entropy categories. Pruning decision trees is useful for simplifying models which have "grown" too much and therefore "overfit" the data. Generally, when generating a decision tree, there will be some misclassifications, i. e., some cases which are assigned to one class by the tree though they belong to another one. These errors are represented in the leaf nodes of the decision trees in the following way:

**(n/m)** where **n** is the total number of cases in the leaf node and **m** is the number of misclassified cases.

## 4.2 Assessing Tree Accuracy

This has been presented using the following measurements:

The *training accuracy* is a measure of how accurately the tree represents all known cases. However, these figures give little indication of how well these decision trees would predict the outcome of a new patient. Predictive accuracy calculated using ten fold cross-validation gives a better measure of predictive accuracy (see below). Also, it could be misleading to consider, for example, an accuracy of 80% as very good, in the situation where one of the classes represents 75% of the population. Therefore, all the results reported in this paper will include the size of the biggest category (as a percentage of population) as a comparison.

*Predictive accuracy* is a measure of how well the tree classifies new cases. The standard method of testing the predictive accuracy of a decision tree is to use a new set of as-yet-unseen cases from the same population. The problem with this is that the predictive accuracy is very much dependent upon which cases are in the test and in the training sets. To avoid this problem, the set of cases is randomly split into a number of equally sized subsets (e. g., 10). Each subset, in turn, becomes the test set, with the remaining 9 subsets forming the training set. This, therefore, requires ten different decision trees to be generated and tested. The overall predic-

**Table 1** Accuracy for the Subset of Patients (CDC) where x/y/z gives Training Accuracy/Test Accuracy/Predictive Accuracy improvement over biggest class (n = 69)

| Outcome | Biggest Category | Demographic | Temporal | Demographic & Temporal |
|---|---|---|---|---|
| Dead/Alive | 78.3 | 85.5 / 73.5 / -4.8 | 94.2 / 87.5 / 9.2 | 94.2 / 87.9 / 9.6 |
| Good/Poor | 62.3 | 95.7 / 60.4 / -1.9 | 87.0 / 67.4 / 5.1 | 89.9 / 64.0 / 1.7 |
| GOS | 39.1 | 78.3 / 39.2 / 0.1 | 88.4 / 41.4 / 2.3 | 85.5 / 37.5 / -1.6 |

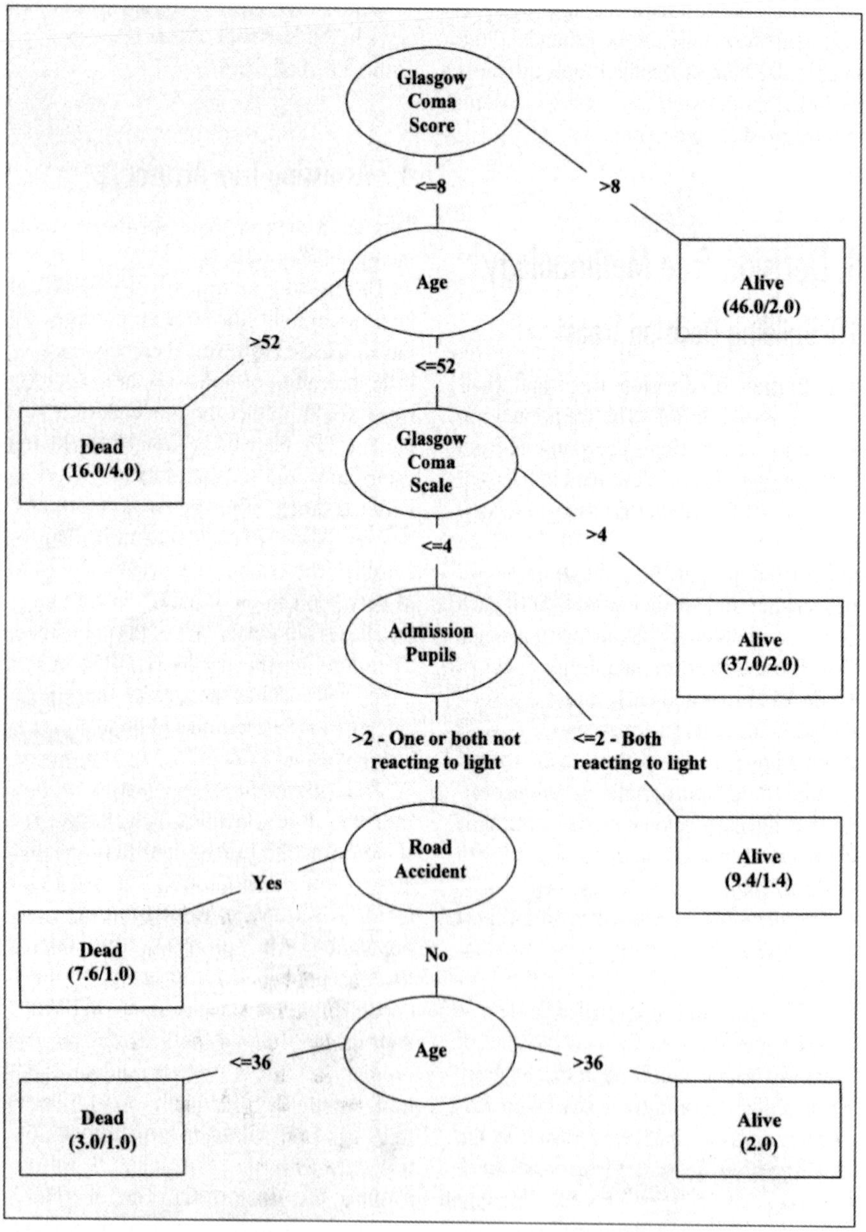

tive accuracy is then the average of all the predictive accuracies. This method is called *cross-validation*, and as it uses 10 subsets, it is referred to as *10-fold cross-validation*. However, when the cross-validation is repeated, it will randomly choose a different 10 subsets and so produce a different overall predictive accuracy. For this reason, the average of ten 10-fold cross validation tests is used for an overall predictive accuracy measurement.

# 5. Analysis and Results

Decision trees were generated for nine different combinations. They were obtained from 3 selections of data-sets (namely demographic, temporal, demographic and temporal) against 3 types of predictions (death/survival, good/poor outcome, the Glasgow Outcome Score [1]). For further details see (13).

As noted in Section 4.1, pruning decision trees can cause some nodes to contain a mixture of classes. If a node contains predominately examples of Class A (e. g., good outcome) and some cases of Class B (e. g., poor outcome) then the later examples are said to be anomalous. In this study, we discussed these anomalous cases with the domain experts in an attempt to find out how such cases differ from the "normal" cases associated with that node. Our hope was that in the course of such discussions, some previously unmentioned descriptors would be identified by the experts. The results of these discussions are reported in Section 6.2.

## 5.1 Accuracy of the Models

The following table gives the results for the nine combinations, in terms of training accuracy (x), test accuracy (y) and predictive accuracy improvement over the biggest class (z), using the format x/y/z.

## 5.2 Decision Trees

As there were a large number of different decision trees generated by this analysis, we



**Fig. 1** Predicting death or survival using only demographic data for the complete set of patients

only show a selection here. The rest are presented in full elsewhere (13). Fig. 1 shows a decision tree for predicting death/survival based only on demographic data for the complete set of patients (n = 121). Fig. 2 predicts good/poor outcome and is based on both demographic and temporal data for a subset of the patients (n = 69).

# 6. Discussion

## 6.1 Predictive Accuracy

**Using only demographic data.** Demographic data, when analysed on its own, consistently produces poor accuracy improvements or a slight reduction in accuracy. Therefore, the decision trees produced are no more accurate than simply predicting the largest outcome category. However, the sub-groups of patients they identify *are* of interest to the medical community. Given a larger sample of data, or perhaps additional demographic data, these accuracies would probably improve.

**Using only temporal data.** This data-set generally produced the best accuracy.

**Using demographic and temporal data together.** This data produced some improvements in accuracy. However, the decision trees produced as a result of this particular analysis are probably of most interest to the medical community, as they show which physiological abnormalities are most useful in summarising cases. For example, the age of a patient appears to affect recovery from a particularly low blood pressure.

## 6.2 Decision Trees and Anomalous Examples

Taking all the decision trees generated (13), there are often *good predictors of outcome* in each of the data categories (demographic, temporal). The best predictors (i.e., those at "high" positions in the decision trees, or those which appear often in decision trees) are as follows:

In the demographic data: Severity of injury, GCS, Grade of injury, Age, Cause of injury,

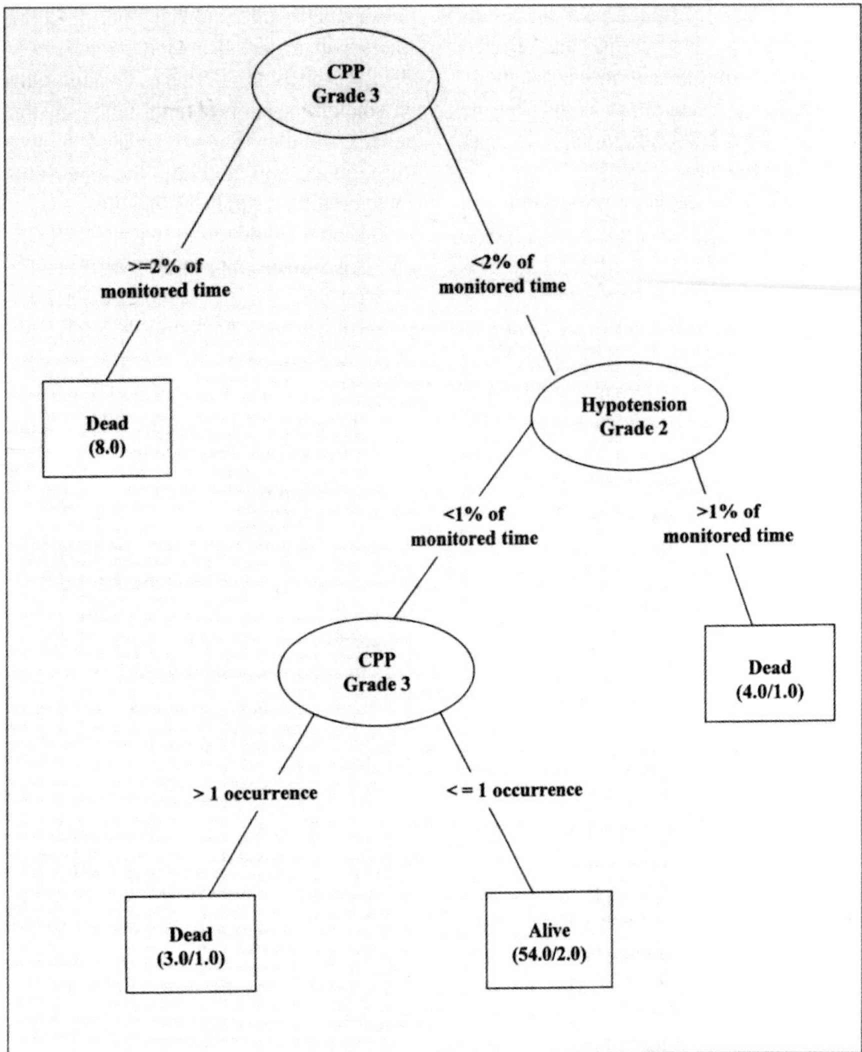



**Fig. 2** Predicting death or survival for a sub-set of patients using both demographic and temporal data

Pupil response on admission, Injury Severity Score (ISS). In the temporal data: Hypotension, Cerebral Perfusion Pressure (CPP), Bradycardia, Intracranial Pressure (ICP).

In general, the decision trees can be viewed as suggesting a series of hypotheses which may explain patient outcomes in a variety of situations. It is the experts' role to confirm, discard and refine these hypotheses. Thus, the form of the decision trees produced, what they predict in a number of concrete situations, and the various anomalous cases inherent in the trees (see Section 5) were discussed with three experts in head injury. The findings are summarised below under three broad headings: those which confirm current medical views, those which challenge them, and those which raise issues to be resolved.

**Views Confirmed.** The decision trees confirm current thinking about *hypotension and pupil response being major predictors of poor outcome* and the management of blood pressure being important in the treatment of head injury patients.

*CPP insults were found to be more significant than ICP insults.* This also mirrors current clinical thinking.

**Views Challenged.** The way that decision trees represent the cases in *sub-groups was of great interest* to the experts. The idea of *hypothesis generation* (suggestion) rather than hypothesis confirmation was also appealing to the experts.

It was suggested that some of the insults (Hypertension, Tachycardia and Bradycardia) are consequences of clinical actions. For example, Tachycardia could be the result of a drug being administered to regulate blood pressure.

*The effect of alcohol and morphine* on the Glasgow Coma Score and pupil response on admission was discussed. If a patient is very drunk when the accident happens, their low coma score or non-reactive pupils may be due to the alcohol rather than being a symptom of brain damage. Similarly, if there have been other bodily injuries to the patient, it is quite common for morphine to be given as a painkiller. This also affects GCS and pupil response. Such medication may make the patient appear to be in a worse state than they actually are and could explain some of the "better than expected" results.

The scale used for measuring *motor response* was also discussed. Point 1 on the scale means no response. This could be due to severe brain damage or possibly to external factors such as alcohol or morphine. However, Point 2 on the scale shows an extension of the limbs response which is always associated with severe brain damage. This means that patients with a motor score of 2 may be more severely brain damaged than those with a score of 1, meaning that the scale is not a continuous one. As this score is a constituent part of the GCS score, it could explain why a patient with a score of 3 (the lowest possible score) may have better outcome that a patient with a score of 4.

**Issues to be resolved.** When considering the different grades of insult in an analysis, it is more realistic to *consider each insult grade to also include insults at a higher grade.* For example, when a patient is suffering grade 2 or grade 3 of an insult, then consider them to be suffering grade 1 of that insult as well (similarly, grade 3 is also grade 2). This would make insult durations and number of occurrences more realistic.

The experts were *interested in "falsely-classified" cases.* Generally, the experts would agree with the sub-groups and expected outcomes given by the decision trees. However, they were interested in those patients who died/had poor outcome when their expected outcome was survival/good outcome. Perhaps if additional parameters (such as alcohol intake of the patient, whether they are sedated or not) were taken into account, the algorithm could better classify these patients.

During the final few hours before death, a patient's heart rate and blood pressure often fluctuates wildly. Usually these parameters will rise to a peak and then fall. This could explain many of the hypotension grade 3 insults and some of the Hypertension, Bradycardia and Tachycardia insults. This "pre-morbid" data is not really useful in predicting outcome of new cases, and so should be removed.

Currently grade 3 of one insult type is not necessarily as bad as grade 3 of a different insult type. For example, grade 3 Hypotension is nearly always fatal, however patients do survive small periods of grade 3 ICP insult. Perhaps the *current thresholds which define the grades of insult need to be adjusted.*

The decision trees for *prediction of Glasgow Outcome Score* were generally thought to be too large to provide useful predictions. Some of the outcome classes contained too few patients to be representative. To improve these decision trees, *more training cases* need to be analysed.

## 7. Conclusions

The use of decision trees to predict outcomes is a useful approach to analysing medical data. The major strength of this approach is the categorisation of patients into sub-groups. Traditional statistical methods tend to treat the patient group as a single population, whereas decision tree analysis considers sub-groups of patients. The identification of subgroups allows predictions to be made for each. The clinicians also found the identification of sub-groups to be interesting and therapeutically relevant.

When comparing the predictive accuracy improvements of decision trees generated using the different types of data (demographic, temporal), experiments show an improvement over using demographic data alone. This investigation clearly shows there are benefits from using minute-by-minute recordings of physiological data when predicting patient outcomes. Moreover, the issues identified in the analyses with the experts should enable the predictive accuracies to be improved further.

## 8. Further Work

This study suggests issues to be considered further both from the perspective of more detailed (data) analyses and from the perspective of collecting additional information from future head injury patients.

**Data analysis perspective:** this study suggests that the evaluation of severity of patient's motor response may not be a continuous scale. In discussing several anomalies, clinicians suggested that a score of 2 might sometimes be more serious than a score of 1. We plan to test this hypothesis on a much larger data-set using standard statistical techniques.

Secondly, there is a pressing need to describe the sequences of events occurring in these patients, and to produce temporal patterns which can be used predictively. An example of such a hypothesis is that a period of raised ICP is always (usually or often) preceded by a period of hypotension. We are building a workbench which will allow clinicians to formulate and test such hypotheses.

**Data collection:** This study suggests that clinicians when they first encounter head injury patients should take care to note their level of blood alcohol, as this can later adversely influence the patient's reaction to standard assessment tests.

We are optimistic that the above activities will, in time, lead to more accurate outcome predictions for this group of patients and, subsequently, to better care. We also believe that this methodology (namely discussion of anomalies detected by decision trees with clinicians) will prove valuable in many other areas of medicine.

# References


1. Jennett B, Bond M. Assessment of outcome after severe brain damage. A practical scale. Lancet 1975; 1: 480-4.
2. Jones PA, Andrews PJD, Midgley S, Anderson SI, Piper IR, Tocher JL, Housley AM, Corrie JA, Slattery J, Dearden NM, Miller JD. Measuring the burden of secondary Insults in Head-Injured Patients during Intensive Care. J Neurosurg Anaesthesiol 1994; 6 (1): 4-14.
3. Choi SC, Muizelaar JP, Barnes TY, Mamarou A, Brooks DM, Young HF. Young. Prediction tree for severely head-injured patients. J Neurosurg 1991; 75: 251-5.
4. Pilih IA, Mladenic D, Lavrac N, Prevec TS. Data analysis of patients with severed head injury. In: Intelligent Data Analysis in Medicine and Pharmacology. Boston: Kluwer Academic Publishers 1997.
5. Breiman L, Friedman JH, Olshen RA et al. Classification and regression trees. Belmont, California: Wadsworth 1984.
6. Teasdale G, Jennett B. Assessment of coma and impaired consciousness. A practical scale. Lancet 1974; 2: 81-4.
7. Gerstenbrand F, Saltuari L, Kofler M, Formisano R. Clinical evaluation of severe head injury. Neurologia 1990; 39 (1): 71-88.
8. Mladenic D. The learning system Magnus Assistant. BSc Thesis. Faculty of Computer and Information Sciences, University of Ljubljana, Slovenia 1990.
9. Quinlan JR. Induction of decision trees. Machine Learning 1986; 1: 81-106.
10. Quinlan JR. Probabilistic Decision Trees. In: Machine Learning: An A. I. Approach. III, Morgan Kaufmann 1990; 140-52.
11. Quinlan JR. Data Mining Tools C5.0 and See5. Rulequest Research, 1997. Web Ref: http://www.rulequest.com/see5-info.html.
12. Quinlan JR. C4.5: Programs for Machine Learning. Morgan Kaufmann 1993.
13. McQuatt A. Using Machine Learning Techniques to Predict Clinical Outcome. MSc Thesis. Computing Science Department, The University of Aberdeen 1999.



**Correspondence to:**
D. Sleeman
Dept. of Computing Science
University of Aberdeen
Aberdeen AB24 3UE
Scotland
E-mail: dsleeman@csd.abdn.ac.uk

# Sharable Representation of Clinical Guidelines in GLIF: Relationship to the Arden Syntax

Mor Peleg,*[,1] Aziz A. Boxwala,† Elmer Bernstam,* Samson Tu,* Robert A. Greenes,†
and Edward H. Shortliffe‡

*Stanford Medical Informatics, Stanford University School of Medicine, Stanford, California 94305-5479;
†Decision Systems Group, Harvard Medical School, Brigham & Women's Hospital, Boston, Massachusetts 02115; and
‡Department of Medical Informatics, Columbia University, New York, New York 10032

*Received June 4, 2001; published online September 20, 2001*

---

Clinical guidelines are intended to improve the quality and cost effectiveness of patient care. Integration of guidelines into electronic medical records and order-entry systems, in a way that enables delivery of patient-specific advice at the point of care, is likely to encourage guideline acceptance and effectiveness. Among the methodologies for modeling guidelines and medical decision rules, the Arden Syntax for Medical Logic Modules and the GuideLine Interchange Format version 3 (GLIF3) emphasize the importance of sharing encoded logic across different medical institutions and implementation platforms. These two methodologies have similarities and differences; in this paper we clarify their roles. Both methods can be used to support sharing of medical knowledge, but they do so in complementary situations. The Arden Syntax is suitable for representing individual decision rules in self-contained units called Medical Logic Modules (MLMs), which are usually implemented as event-driven alerts or reminders. In contrast, GLIF3 is designed for encoding complex multistep guidelines that unfold over time. As a consequence, GLIF3 has several mechanisms for complexity management and additional constructs that may require overhead unnecessary for expressing simple alerts and reminders. Unlike the Arden Syntax, GLIF3 encourages a top–down process of guideline modeling consisting of three levels that are created in order: Level 1 comprises a human-readable flowchart of clinical decisions and actions. Level 2 comprises a computable specification that can be verified for logical consistency and completeness; and Level 3 comprises an implementable specification that includes information required for local adaptation of guideline logic as well as for mapping guideline variables onto institutional medical records. A major emphasis of the current GLIF3 development process has been to create the computable specification that formally represents medical decision and eligibility criteria. We based GLIF3's formal expression language on the Arden Syntax's logic grammar, making the necessary extensions to the Arden Syntax's data structures and operators to support GLIF3's object-oriented data model. We discuss why the process of generating a set of MLMs from a GLIF-encoded guideline cannot be automated, why it can result in information loss, and why simple medical rules are best represented as individual MLMs. We thus show that the Arden Syntax and GLIF3 play complementary roles in representing medical knowledge for clinical decision support. © 2001 Academic Press

*Key Words:* GLIF; Arden Syntax; clinical guidelines; computer-interpretable guidelines; knowledge representation.

---

[1]To whom correspondence should be addressed at Stanford Medical Informatics, MSOB x-208, 251 Campus Drive, Stanford, CA 94305-5479. Fax: (650) 725-7944. E-mail: peleg@SMI.Stanford.edu.

## 1. METHODOLOGIES FOR MODELING SHARED COMPUTER-INTERPRETABLE GUIDELINES AND MEDICAL DECISION RULES

Implementation of computer-interpretable guidelines in decision-support systems that are used at the point of care has been proposed as a way to improve health care safety, quality, and efficiency. Researchers have devised many approaches to this task. Many of the developments have occurred in the context of specific host information-systems platforms. Other workers, who wish to foster sharing and reuse of medical knowledge in guidelines and other decision-support systems, have concentrated on specifying formal methodologies for representing the knowledge.

Hripcsak and colleagues began developing the Arden Syntax for Medical Logic Modules [1, 2] in 1989 to facilitate sharing of single-step alerts (e.g., alert a physician that his patient has hypokalemia) and reminders (e.g., remind a physician to order a test), termed *medical logic modules* or MLMs. The Arden Syntax was initially published as a standard of the American Society for Testing and Materials (ASTM), originally published as such in April 1992 as ASTM E1460-92. Jenders and colleagues developed and published a second version of the Arden Syntax, Arden 2.0 [3], under Health Level Seven, Inc. (HL7), an ANSI-accredited Standards Developing Organization that operates in the health-care arena.

Researchers have built on a variety of approaches to handle representation of multistep clinical guidelines for computer-based decision support. For example, Lobach and colleagues describe a relational database schema for automating the delivery of multistep guidelines [4]. Another model, PRO*forma*, is a logic language with an object-oriented model. In PRO*forma*, guidelines are modeled as constraint-satisfaction graphs, where nodes represent *tasks* (i.e., clinical actions, decisions, enquiries, or complex *plans* that are tasks composed of other tasks). The ordering of tasks reflects logical, temporal, and other constraints [5]. Another guideline-modeling methodology, Asbru [6], emphasizes guideline intentions (e.g., maintain normal blood glucose level), rather than only action prescriptions (e.g., give insulin). Asbru is an expressive language for representing time-oriented actions, conditions, and intentions in a uniform fashion. Asbru models guidelines as plans that can be hierarchically decomposed into (sub)plans or actions. Yet another guideline model, EON, enables the specification of a guideline through a combination of modeling primitives, such as different types of decision-making mechanisms, control-flow constructs, actions, activities, and abstractions [7].

Most of the guideline-modeling methodologies cited have been developed independently from one another. As developers of the GuideLine Interchange Format (GLIF) since the mid-1990s, we have pursued a different goal: to create a shared representation for computer-interpretable guidelines that incorporates features important for a wide variety of applications and can be used as a basis for implementation of

those applications in diverse clinical-systems environments. The GLIF guideline-modeling methodology [8], therefore, was intentionally based on a desire to leverage the work invested in other approaches. Like the Arden Syntax, GLIF is being further examined as a basis for a guideline-representation standard; both the Arden Syntax and GLIF are foci of the Special Interest Groups of the Clinical Decision Support Technical Committee of HL7.

The Arden Syntax has achieved a substantial level of acceptance through standardization. As reported in [3], as of June 2000, four vendors support the Arden Syntax and two others are currently developing applications for it. At least six health care organizations have implemented MLMs. As of March 1997, there were over 150 MLMs in the Columbia-Presbyterian Medical Center. However, the vast majority of them were not used to implement guidelines that unfold over time, but were unconnected MLMs [3]. Because Arden Syntax is relatively well accepted, we decided to explore the feasibility of using it as a basis for the expression language for decision logic in GLIF. In doing so, we identified many required changes and extensions, and identified directions for future evolution of an expression language. This paper describes in detail the relationship between the Arden Syntax and the current version (3.0) of GLIF (GLIF3). The GLIF3 specification is still in development and not yet in operational use.

## 2. BACKGROUND

We developed GLIF3 by augmenting version 2.0 of GLIF (GLIF2) with components that enable computer interpretation of encoded guidelines. A major component of GLIF3 is a formal expression language that enables guideline authors to specify decision criteria formally. This expression language is based on the Arden Syntax's logic grammar. In this section, we provide background material on the Arden Syntax, GLIF2, and GLIF3.

### *The Arden Syntax*

The initial version of the Arden Syntax was based largely on the encoding scheme used for generalized medical decision support in the HELP system [9]. The shared medical knowledge is encoded in the form of individual MLMs, each of which represents a single medical decision. Most MLMs are triggered by clinical events (e.g., admission of a patient, or storage of certain medical data in the electronic medical record (EMR)). Once triggered, MLMs evaluate logical decision criteria (e.g., *potassium < 3.5*), and, if the criteria hold, they perform an action, such as sending an alert to a healthcare provider. An MLM contains slots, grouped into three categories: *maintenance, library,* and *knowledge.* The **maintenance category** is used for knowledge-base maintenance and revision control. The **library category** provides predefined explanatory information and links to the health literature. The **knowledge category** contains the functional components of the MLM. The knowledge category has **evoke, logic,** and **action** slots that specify the events that trigger the MLM, the logical criterion that is evaluated, and the action that is performed if the logical criterion holds, respectively. These knowledge-category components define the logical rule that the MLM specifies.

MLMs separate institution-specific entities, such as the mapping of patient data references to fields in an EMR, from the MLM's decision logic. The mappings between the institution-specific terms and the MLM's variables are specified within another component of the *knowledge category,* called the **data slot.** However, only part of this specification is defined by the syntax. The mapping of the MLM variables to the institutional EMR is defined in a section demarcated by curly braces. Because there is as yet no standard terminology or data model for electronic medical records, there can be no standardized syntax for the content within this section, a difficulty that is called the *curly-braces problem* by the Arden community.

Various authoring tools have been developed for writing MLMs. Jenders and Dasgupta created an MLM authoring tool [10] that guides the author in a stepwise manner. MÉD-AILLE [11] is an application generated by the PROTÉGÉ-II [12] knowledge-acquisition tool that provides support for entering and editing MLMs. MEDAILLE has a syntax checker and an integrated terminology. Translation of MLMs into an executable form can be done by a number of compilers [13, 14].

### GLIF2

We have carried out the development of GLIF [15] through the formation of the InterMed Collaboratory, a consortium of medical-informatics groups at Harvard, Stanford, and Columbia universities. GLIF is designed to allow exchange of computer-interpretable guidelines among institutions and computer-based applications. Unlike the Arden Syntax, which is designed for individual medical alerts and reminders, GLIF is targeted toward complex guidelines that unfold over time. Like the Arden Syntax, GLIF-encoded guidelines

are stored as text files for sharing. GLIF has an object-oriented model that consists of a set of classes for guideline entities, attributes for those classes, and data types for the attribute values. GLIF2, published in 1998 [15], represented guidelines as flowcharts of guideline steps such as clinical actions and decisions. However, the attributes of structured constructs were defined only as free-text strings, and such guidelines could not be used for computer-based execution that requires automatic inference.

### GLIF3

Recent work by the InterMed Collaboratory has concentrated on the development of the subsequent version of GLIF, called GLIF3, hereafter referred to simply as GLIF [8] (http://www.smi.stanford.edu/projects/intermed-web/guidelines/GLIF1.htm). This version of GLIF

1. Supports three different levels of abstraction, to enable specification at conceptual, computable, and implementable levels;

2. Incorporates an expression language based on the Arden Syntax logic grammar for representing logical and temporal decision criteria;

3. Defines an ontology for medical concepts and patient data;

4. Expands GLIF classes to support representation of several new concepts, such as iteration specification, and grade of evidence;

5. Further structures GLIF2 classes by creating hierarchies of action specifications and decision steps to represent more concisely the different forms of clinical actions and decisions found in medical guidelines;

6. Introduces a new guideline step called a patient state step, which can be used as a label or entry point into a guideline.

We have used GLIF to specify guidelines that differ in their clinical domain, stage of the medical problem and its management (e.g., screening, diagnosis, disease management), multiplicity of encounters, setting (e.g., inpatient or outpatient clinic), time frame (emergency, acute, or chronic), and guideline computability (i.e., algorithmic, guiding, or intermediate) [16, 17]. We specified these guidelines at the conceptual and computable levels.

Currently, there are two authoring tools for GLIF: Protégé-2000 [18], which is a general tool for working with knowledge bases, and a GLIF-specific authoring tool developed by the Decision Systems Group at Brigham and Women's Hospital [19]. Both tools help guideline authors to visualize the entire guideline as a flow chart, as well as to manipulate the formal specification of the computable representation level. The execution engine, described by Boxwala and colleagues [20], can execute guidelines that are encoded in an enhanced version of GLIF2, and is used to develop clinical decision-support applications. The enhanced version of GLIF2 includes

1. A patient data model that supports a number of data types, and permits specification of cardinality and temporal and logical constraints on the values of the data;

2. An enhanced action model that allows specifying action-specific parameters for execution of the action;

3. Syntax for logical constraints, influenced by Arden Syntax, enhanced in order to support patient data and action model. However, unlike Arden Syntax it does not support temporal and list operators and data types.

These refinements were not sufficiently rich to enable easy sharing of guidelines across diverse information systems platforms. We are currently in the process of designing a GLIF3 execution engine.

## 3. THE GLIF PROCESS OF GUIDELINE MODELING

GLIF enables a top–down creation of a guideline specification. We envision a multistep process for authoring guidelines. First, a medical expert starts with an informal textual description of the problem, and a set of assembled evidence. She then creates an imprecise, potentially incomplete **conceptual** view of the guideline, in the form of a flowchart that includes guideline steps linked to each other in a temporal order. The guideline steps represent clinical actions (e.g., prescribe aspirin), decisions (should the patient should be placed on a diet?), and patient states (e.g., the patient is receiving a single antihypertensive drug). In addition, branch and synchronization steps can be used to express parallel execution; a branch step can lead to multiple simultaneous execution paths that converge in a synchronization step, thus supporting parallel execution of the steps contained in the different paths or branches (e.g., ordering preoperative laboratory tests and scheduling operating-room time). The information specified in the guideline steps is largely in the form of unstructured text strings. In a second encoding stage, a team consisting of an informatician, aided by a medical expert, refines the flowchart representation to produce a fully detailed, precise, and **computable** specification, in which decision and eligibility criteria, patient data references, action specifications, and control flow are formally specified.

In the third and final stage, an encoding team creates an **implementable** specification, in which data and action specifications are mapped onto specific data and procedures used by the implementing institution. The encoding team performs contextual adaptation of encoded guidelines for local health-care setting and maps encoded guideline variables, concepts, and action specifications to the local clinical information systems. This mapping specification is not yet developed.

GLIF3 is related to the Arden Syntax in three ways. First, GLIF3 logical and temporal decision criteria are specified using an expression language called Guideline Expression Language (**GEL**) that is derived from and enhances the Arden Syntax logic grammar [21]. Second, GLIF's Message__Action action specification is based on the Arden's *write statement*, which enables specification of a text string and its destination. Third, GLIF has a special construct, called an MLM-macro, that guideline authors can use to map guideline declarations onto a procedural specification that defines evoke, logic, and action slots, which correspond to the respective Arden MLM slots.

We use the American College of Cardiology/American Hospital Association/American College of Physicians– American Society of Internal Medicine (ACC/AHA/ACP-ASIM) guidelines for the management of patients with chronic stable angina [22] to demonstrate how we can use GLIF to model a complex guideline, and how GLIF uses constructs derived from the Arden Syntax. Figure 1 shows the top-level flowchart view of the guideline that we created (in this case using Protégé-2000) from the textual description, and the accompanying flowchart supplied by the guideline authors. When a guideline specification is created in GLIF, the flowchart is usually a first approximation of the guideline specification. At this point, the specification is potentially imprecise and incomplete, as the information contained in the guideline steps is only in free-text form.

The top-level flowchart view of the guideline includes steps that represent high-level actions and decisions. GLIF's **nesting** mechanism enables expansion of such steps through the use of subguidelines. For example, the "Empiric Therapy" action step in Fig. 1 can be nested into a subguideline that contains the steps of the treatment algorithm. The *nesting* mechanism is useful in managing the complexity of large, multistep guidelines that contain many pathways.

We refine the conceptual flowchart representation into a *computable* representation by adding a structured specification that corresponds to the text within the guideline steps. Action steps that were described in free text are refined to include well-defined tasks, such as scheduling a procedure, referring a patient, or ordering a test. GLIF has a hierarchy

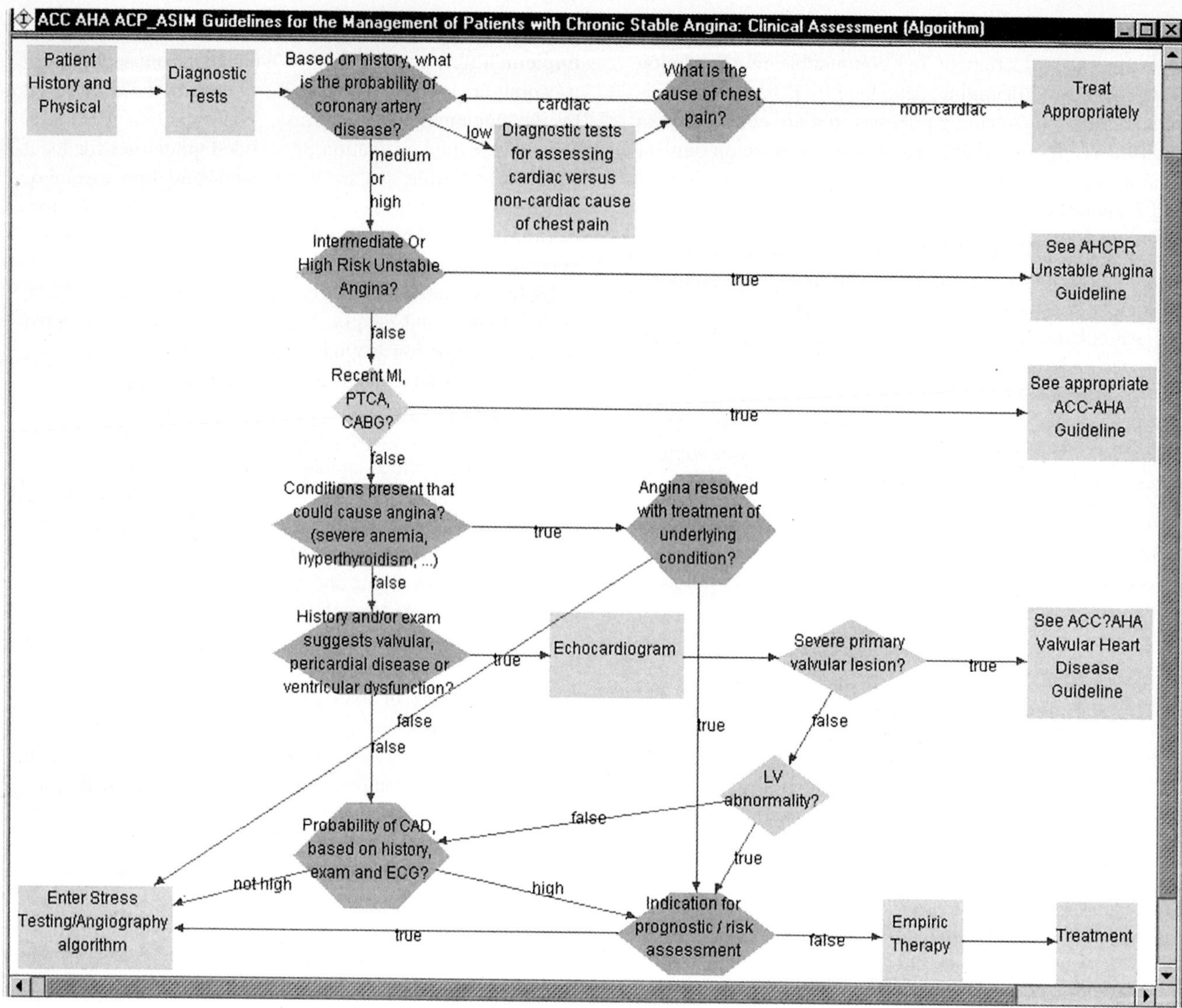



**FIG. 1.** A top-level view of the stable angina guideline, which includes evaluation of chest pain. Boxes represent action steps, diamonds represent automatic decision steps, and hexagons represent user decision steps.

of action specifications that guideline authors can use to model both programming-oriented actions (e.g., sending a message to a user) and medically oriented actions (i.e., actions that rely on medical concepts such as ordering a clinical test). Medical concepts and patient-data elements that need to be referenced by action and decision steps are specified in GLIF's **domain ontology**, which contains the clinical meaning of the concepts (i.e., by referencing controlled medical vocabularies, such as SNOMED) as well as the data model of patient data. Defining medical concepts in relation to standard medical vocabularies allows the guideline encoding to reference concepts that are institution-independent.

Mapping to institution-dependent EMR codes and procedures can therefore be specified in another level.

The default medical data model, used by GLIF's domain ontology, is based on HL7's Reference Information Model (RIM) [23]. The clinical part of HL7's RIM version 1.0 (http://www.hl7.org/library/data-model/RIM/C30100/rim0100h.htm#EL10003) can model medical knowledge and patient data uniformly. All clinical data are specified as *Act* objects, or *Acts*. Acts have attributes that provide information about the clinical concepts they represent and their timing. Relationships are used to model the Act circumstances and allow grouping the Acts and reasoning about them. Acts are specialized into procedures performed on a patient, observations about the patient, medications given to the patient, and other kinds of services. Subclasses contain additional attributes that help characterize an Act. For example, Observation has a *value* attribute, whereas Medication has attributes about dosage and route of administration. Act objects have a *mood* that distinguishes the ways in which they can be conceived: as an event that occurred, an intent, an order, etc.

When decision or eligibility criteria are used, they are specified in GEL, and can reference medical concepts and data that are defined in the domain ontology. These refinements turn the *conceptual* specification into a *computable* specification. An example of a refinement is the following GEL *criterion* that refines the abstract decision "Conditions present that can cause angina? (severe anemia, hyperthyroidism, . . .)" that was stated in text at the top-level view of the guideline specification (Fig. 1).

(SevereAnemia *is in* ProblemList) OR (Hyperthyroidism *is in* ProblemList). . . . *ProblemList* is a list of *concepts* that represent all of the known current problems, retrieved from the EMR. The GEL operator *"is in"* checks for membership of the left argument in the right argument, which is a list. Unlike the Arden Syntax's *"is in"* operator, the GEL operator can work with complex objects, such as Concept, which has three attributes: the concept name; the concept's unique identifier, taken from a controlled vocabulary; and the unique identifier that represents the controlled vocabulary itself. In this example, we check whether the concepts *SevereAnemia* or *Hyperthyroidism* occur within the list of current problems that are associated with this patient.

At the *implementable* (third) level, the guideline is mapped onto procedures and data that are used by the implementing institution and local interpretation of high-level guideline recommendations is performed. For example, the stable-angina guideline addresses the evaluation of chest pain, but does not specify which tests should be ordered for a patient judged to be low-risk based on history, physical examination, and initial diagnostic testing. One institution may decide that the relevant test should be serial-troponin levels, whereas another institution may prefer that physicians order either creatine phosphokinase (CPK) or immediate stress testing. Other local implementation considerations may include how guideline advice should be delivered to the user (e.g., alert versus interactive session).

GLIF includes constructs for modeling events, logical criteria, and actions. Therefore, GLIF can represent alerts and reminders. For ease of authoring, modelers who are familiar with the Arden MLM can model alerts and reminders using a special GLIF construct, *MLM macro step*. A **macro step** in GLIF3 is a special class that has attributes that define the information required to initiate a set of underlying GLIF steps. Those underlying steps represent a pattern that appears in clinical guidelines [24]. In this way, macro steps provide a means to specify declaratively a procedural pattern in a single construct that is realized by a set of GLIF steps. An *MLM macro step* represents a particular pattern of GLIF components: a GLIF *event* (MLM evoke slot), followed by a GLIF *decision criterion* (MLM logic slot), followed by a GLIF *action specification* that can be a *Message__Action, Assignment__Action*, or *Event__Action* (MLM action slot). The guideline author fills in evoke, logic, and action slots of the MLM macro. As shown in Fig. 2, the MLM macro step can be replaced by a sequence of two GLIF guideline steps that do not include macros. The first of these two steps is a decision step that references instances of two GLIF classes: *event* class and *criterion*, which correspond to the evoke and logic slots of the MLM macro. The decision step is followed by an action step that references instances of the GLIF Action__Specification class that correspond to the action slot of the MLM macro.

Figure 1 shows that, after a history and physical examination have been obtained, the action step "Diagnostic tests" should be executed. A possible implementation of this action is first ordering tests and then notifying the physician when the test results are back. The notification can be modeled as an MLM macro step, as shown in Fig. 3. The action slot of the MLM uses a GLIF Message__Action to specify the message to be sent and the destination. The Message__Action is adapted from the Arden Syntax's write statement (i.e., WRITE ⟨message⟩ AT ⟨destination⟩).

Note that the guideline does not specify which diagnostic tests should be performed to assess the risk of coronary artery disease (CAD). Therefore, we would like to define the evoking event of the MLM macro as "storage in the medical record of diagnostic results of tests for assessing the risk of CAD." By this event definition we mean that, regardless of which tests are chosen, when the result of one of them is stored in the EMR, the MLM macro step is evoked. Mapping this kind of event in a standard and portable manner to an institutional EMR is difficult, and has not yet been defined by either GLIF or the Arden Syntax. Therefore, the example in Fig. 3 assumes that performing the diagnostic test consists of obtaining serum hemoglobin, fasting glucose, and fasting lipid panel (total cholesterol, HDL cholesterol, triglycerides, and calculated LDL cholesterol).

The alert, shown in Fig. 3, is evoked when the results of any of these laboratory tests are recorded in the EMR. Then, a logic criterion is evaluated to determine that all the tests were performed within the past 12 h, and that the results are of numeric type. These requirements are imposed to

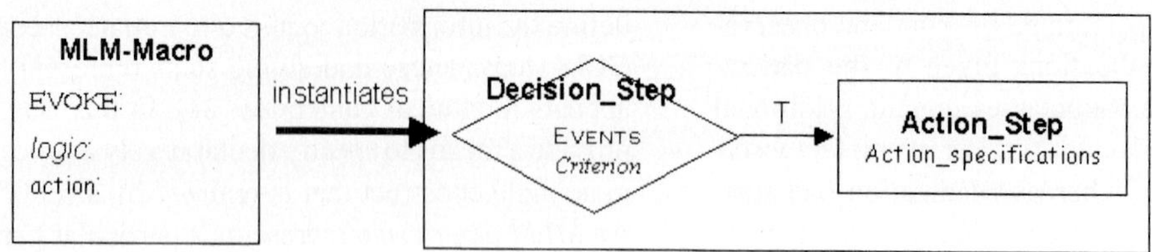

FIG. 2. An MLM macro and its mapping to GLIF steps.

ensure that the measurements are current and have legal values (nonempty numeric results). For simplification, (1) no checks were written to verify that the results are within an acceptable range (e.g., *6 < Hemoglobin < 20*), and (2) the units of measurement were not considered. Note that although all of these tests are needed for the alert to be sent, the MLM is triggered when any of these results are recorded in the EMR. This is because the MLM evoke slot can contain a disjunction of events but not a conjunction.

The *logic criterion* of the MLM macro step is expressed in GEL. The Arden Syntax operators "is number," "latest," "where," "time of," and "it" are used by GEL. The value TRUE is returned by "is number" if the latter's argument is a number. The operator "latest" acts on a **query-result**—a list of elements that have data values and primary times (i.e., the time of occurrence)—and returns the query result element that has the latest primary__time. The operator

"where" allows expression of a criterion that is applied to every element in the query result. In this example, only elements for which the primary time occurred within the past 12 h are selected. The "where" clause uses the "time of" and "it" operators. The operator "it" iterates over the elements of the query result. The "time of" operator returns the primary time of a query result element. The *logic criterion* of the MLM macro step uses the GEL function "select-Attribute" to access attributes of a complex object (a legal value type in GEL). In this example, selectAttribute selects the "value" attribute of a query-result element.

The criterion shown in Fig. 3 refers to variables that represent query results extracted from records of the laboratory-test results (*Hemoglobin, FastingGlucose, FastingTotalCholesterol, FastingHDLCholesterol, Fasting-Triglycerides*, and *CalculatedFastingLDLCholesterol*). The *CalculatedFastingLDLCholesterol* query result is shown in

```
                    Alert: Tests results for CAD risk assessment are back (MLM-macro)
    evoke:  Event:
                    event_name: Hemoglobin              event_type: patient_data_availability
                    Event:
                    event_name: FastingGlucose          event_type: patient_data_availability
                    Event:
                    event_name: FastingLipids           event_type: patient_data_availability
    logic:  Criterion:
                is number (selectAttribute ("value", latest Hemoglobin where time of it >= (now – 12 hours))) and
                is number (selectAttribute ("value", latest FastingGlucose where time of it >= (now – 12 hours))) and
                is number (selectAttribute ("value", latest FastingTotalCholesterol where time of it >= (now – 12 hours))) and
                is number (selectAttribute ("value", latest FastingHDLCholesterol where time of it >= (now – 12 hours))) and
                is number (selectAttribute ("value", latest FastingTriglycerids where time of it >= (now – 12 hours))) and
            is number (selectAttribute ("value", latest CalculatedFastingLDLCholesterol where time of it >= (now – 12hours)))

    action:     Message_Action
                    message: "Tests results for CAD risk assessment are back."
                destination: mail_dest;
```

FIG. 3. Mapping of the guideline encoding to procedures used by the implementing institution. The institution uses an MLM macro step to create an alert when certain laboratory-test results become available.

Fig. 4a. Each element of the query result holds a value, which is a number that represents the LDL cholesterol level, and the primary time at which each measurement was made. The values and primary times are taken from *data items*. **Data items**, defined by GLIF's *medical ontology*, refer to codes from controlled medical vocabularies, and to data structures defined by medical data models. As was noted, the default medical data model is HL7's Reference Information Model (RIM). As shown in Fig. 4b, the data item *Calculated-FastingLDLCholesterolDataItem* refers to a vocabulary code, taken from UMLS [25], and to an HL7 RIM observation.

Because GLIF builds on other standards for the medical data model (HL7 RIM) and expression language (GEL, based on the Arden Syntax logic grammar), we had to reconcile incompatibilities among these standards. These incompatibilities include the Arden Syntax's lack of support for complex data types and time intervals that are part of the HL7 RIM. In addition, there is a mismatch between Arden Syntax's single primary time and the multiple time attributes of the HL7 RIM [21]. The solution was to allow GEL to support Arden Syntax's data types as well as complex data values. Thus, GEL's *query results* and *lists* are like Arden Syntax's corresponding types, but their values can be complex types. To map from GLIF's default data model, the HL7 RIM, to GEL's data model, we defined the *Get_Data_Action* construct. *Get_Data_Action* retrieves patient data from the EMR as lists of HL7 RIM objects of the patient that correspond to a single medical concept (e.g., LDL cholesterol values) and transforms them to results of type *query result*, which is supported by GEL [21]. A guideline author can use Get_Data_Action to specify that an attribute of a complex HL7 RIM class is the source of data values for the *query result*, and that values of another attribute serve as the primary time in the *query result*. The Get_Data_Action that is used to retrieve the *Calculated FastingLDLCholesterol* query result is shown in Fig. 4c. In this case, the values of the query-result elements are numbers that represent the LDL cholesterol level in mlligrams/deciliter.

## 4. DISCUSSION

When the paper describing GLIF2 was published (1998), some observers expressed concern as to whether GLIF was a competitor to the Arden Syntax. As we have shown, GLIF and the Arden Syntax are not competing methodologies, but rather are related, complementary methodologies for the expression and sharing of medical knowledge. Arden Syntax is useful for sharing medical knowledge that can be expressed as individual MLMs that can be used, for example, for generating warnings about drug interactions or alerts regarding abnormal laboratory-test results. GLIF, in contrast, is designed to specify multistep guidelines that unfold over time. Although GLIF can also encode simple decisions, the overhead (i.e., the machinery necessary to use GLIF-encoded knowledge) is much greater than that required for the Arden Syntax. Therefore, if the task can be modeled as a single medical decision, Arden MLMs, rather than GLIF, should be used. Even in the context of a single institution, it is possible, that both Arden MLMs and GLIF-encoded guidelines could be implemented at the same time. GLIF would be used to execute multistep guidelines, while MLMs could be used to implement alerts and reminders that involve single decisions. In relation to guidelines, MLMs can be used to alert physicians of patients that are potentially eligible for guidelines and protocols. MLMs can also be used as safety monitors that check the interactions among several GLIF-encoded guidelines that are applied to a single patient. For example, MLMs can alert a physician if an application using GLIF-encoded guideline issued a recommendation for a test or medication, whereas another application recommended a similar or conflicting order for the same patient. This way, these safety monitors could be reused for any guideline interaction and would not need to be embedded within the logic of each guideline.

Its developers did not originally intend the Arden Syntax to be used for encoding complex guidelines that involve multiple decisions. However, encoding of multistep guidelines using the Arden Syntax is possible albeit clumsy, as demonstrated by the implementation of a care plan for the postoperative management of patients following coronary-artery bypass graft surgery [26]. Nevertheless, there is no support in the Arden Syntax specification to aid human understanding of the way MLMs interact with one other. Therefore, the authoring and implementation of multistep guidelines, although possible, is difficult and awkward. Another aspect of guidelines that is not well supported by MLMs is decisions for which a guideline provides guidance, but not deterministic choice (i.e., choices that cannot be represented by if . . . then . . . else rules. GLIF can model such decisions by listing rules for and against each of the decision's options. For example, a decision regarding the appropriate treatment of CAD can be modeled as a user choice that has several alternatives (decision options). One such decision option is pharmacological treatment. A rule

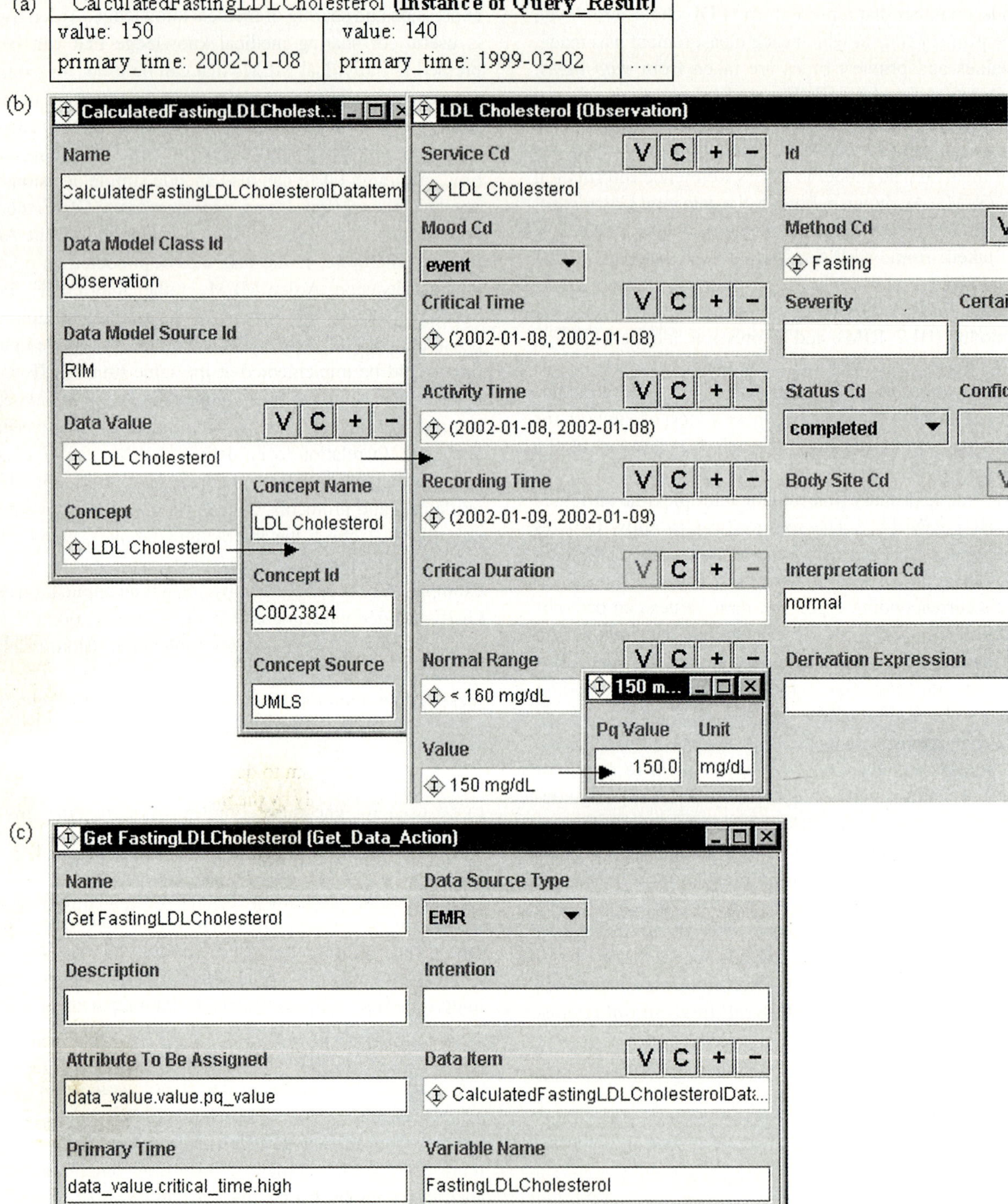



**FIG. 4.** The Get__Data__Action and its query result, which holds CalculatedFastingLDLCholesterol data values and their primary times. (a) The CalculatedFastingLDLCholesterol query result. (b) The CalculatedFastingLDLCholesterolDataItem from which the query result was extracted. (c) The Get__Data__Action used to retrieve the query result.

in favor is "if the patient is at high risk for surgical complications, consider pharmacological treatment"; a rule against it is "If the patient has severe three-vessel disease, do not consider pharmacological treatment." Guideline developers, who are using GLIF, can represent decisions without committing to the way in which the recommendations should be delivered to a user (e.g., ranking the options by the number of favorable rules that they satisfy, or simply presenting to the user the rules for each option). Unlike GLIF, the Arden Syntax has no special constructs for representing such non-if … then … else decisions in a way that is independent from implementation choices. An MLM can present, to a user, recommendations that are based on nondeterministic choices by specifying a message whose content is tailored to these rule-in and rule-out arguments, thus committing to some delivery choice.

Because the Arden Syntax has been accepted as a mature standard for delivering alerts and reminders and has been implemented and tested by multiple academic groups and commercial vendors, developers of GLIF wanted to leverage the years of work that have gone into the development of the Arden Syntax. GLIF3 draws on the modeling approaches taken both by GLIF2 and by the Arden Syntax for MLMs. GLIF3 extends GLIF2 models, which represented guidelines in a way that is not computable (i.e., did not support computer-based interpretation involving automatic inference), by defining a formal expression language, GEL, based on the Arden Syntax. GEL, together with formal definitions of medical concepts and data items, action specifications, and control flow, enables GLIF3 specifications to be *computable*. The computable specification reconciles differences between the Arden Syntax's data model and GLIF's object-oriented medical data model. Although GEL supports complex data types, it is deficient in specifying expressions that relate to more than one of an object's attributes (e.g., getting the latest LDL cholesterol value in milligrams/deciliter that was measured after fasting for 12 h. This expression needs to access the primary time, value, value__unit, and method by which an LDL cholesterol value was obtained (see Fig. 4b) [21]. We are exploring the possibility of designing an object-oriented expression language to overcome this problem.

Guideline authors can use the three layers of representation in GLIF to develop computer-interpretable guidelines in a top–down manner, specifying the abstract flowchart of the clinical decision and actions first, then defining formally the guideline's logic, and, finally, concentrating on implementation details. MLM developers can also carry out a top–down development process. A medical domain expert can create a documentation-level specification by entering the *maintenance* and *library* categories of an MLM. Based

on the narrative description of the MLM's function, found in the *purpose* and *explanation* slots of the library category, an informatician can then define the MLM's logic by formally specifying the *evoke, logic*, and *action* slots of the knowledge category in the Arden Syntax's grammar. Then, implementers in local institutions can define the data slot, thus mapping data items and events used by the MLM's knowledge category into institutional EMR codes and procedures. Note that this mapping has not yet been standardized. Even though the top–down modeling process is similar, GLIF3 and MLMs differ in the granularity of the entity they try to model. When a guideline is more complex than a single medical decision, the Arden Syntax does not provide support for maintaining a conceptual view of a guideline that is implemented as multiple interacting MLMs.

Both the Arden Syntax and GLIF try to solve the problem of creating a computer-interpretable specification of medical knowledge that could be adapted to local health-care settings and integrated into local clinical systems. When MLMs are locally adapted, the codes of data items, events, and message destinations that are defined in curly braces, within the data slot, are changed. In GLIF, guideline authors can model a guideline on the textual *conceptual*-level and on the formal *computable-level* without making any commitments on the way the recommendations will be delivered to the user. As in Arden MLMs, guidelines encoded at the conceptual or computable levels can be shared among different institutions, each of which has the freedom to adapt the guideline to their needs at the implementation level. GLIF can use the macro-step mechanism to delineate specific procedures that should be done locally by the implementing institution. Then each local institution must map these procedures in its own clinical information system's functions. We are still developing these mapping mechanisms.

To adapt a guideline to a particular health-care setting, the implementing institution must modify the guideline in accordance with availability of resources and expertise, local workflow, practice preferences, and differences in patient population. Adaptation may simply involve a refinement of generic instructions into concrete procedures, but may also require changes in the guideline's logic [27]. For example, certain decision options may be eliminated because they involve procedures that cannot be performed at the institution; such deletions change the guideline's logic. A generic instruction, such as "perform diagnostic tests for assessing the risk of CAD," can be refined into procedures such as performing specific tests and notifying the physician when the test results are back. As we explained in Section 3, the notification can be done through GLIF's *macro-step* mechanism.

Another mechanism that GLIF offers for refining actions is *nesting*. Nesting enables expansion of action and decision steps in a high-level flowchart through the use of subguidelines. Thus, the nesting mechanism, like the macro step, is useful in managing the complexity of large and multi-branched guidelines. Nesting also facilitates model extensibility and reuse of part of a guideline, which is encapsulated as a subguideline. Nesting may also be useful in showing the relationship of a guideline to other guidelines by creating a top-level view that makes such relationships explicit.

Achieving an *implementable* specification entails mapping of guideline variables onto institutional data elements and methods. We designed GLIF's *medical ontology* to facilitate mapping of concepts, data items, and medically oriented action specifications to institutional data items and procedures in order-entry systems. The Arden Syntax, on the other hand, does not provide a standard way to map MLM variables to institutional data elements. GLIF's medical ontology structures data items by referring to (1) codes from controlled medical vocabularies, and (2) data structures defined by medical data models. GLIF's default medical data model is HL7's RIM. In the future, we will structure the medical ontology further to represent mapping between its terms and institutional data elements (i.e., institutional term dictionaries or procedures used to obtain the corresponding data elements) and methods (e.g., order-entry methods). Currently, GLIF's medical data model abstracts concepts and data based on their medical characteristics (e.g., what are the characteristics of a medication prescription). We are considering changing the data model to reflect the different categories commonly used in EMRs (e.g., coded note entries, laboratory-test results).

GLIF-encoded guidelines might be implemented in a variety of ways, among which could be compiling or interpreting the guidelines into executable actions, or translating them into sequences of MLMs, thus taking advantage of the software tools that already exist for implementing MLMs. For the latter, we stress that the process of generating a set of MLMs from a GLIF-encoded guideline depends on many decisions that must be made along the way, not all of which are technical in nature. For example, we might not want to convert GLIF decision steps intended to be made by users into MLMs because the Arden Syntax does not have special constructs for representing them, as was explained earlier in this section. Also, translating parallel execution in GLIF into a set of interacting MLMs may be difficult. Even when the guideline developer decides that certain guideline steps should be mapped into MLMs, more decisions are required. For example, a guideline may specify that "the patient's body temperature must be measured every 2 hours," but will not tell you how the information (that the collection is to take place) should be given the user. Should care providers be reminded *before* this action needs to take place? Alternatively, should care providers be reminded only if they fail to perform the action on time? The local institutions must make these decisions to implement the guideline. Then, they can add MLM macro steps to the GLIF-encoded guideline.

Because an MLM macro step contains slots that are analogous to the MLM evoke, logic, and action slots, automatically translating MLM macro steps into Arden MLMs should be easier than translating sequences of GLIF action and decision steps that contain information that is not easily mapped into MLM slots. For example, it is not easy to translate GLIF's iteration specifications into part of an MLM's logic slot, or to translate the variety of GLIF action specifications (e.g., Get_Data_Action) into MLM actions. Although, by converting MLM macro steps into Arden MLMs, we have the advantage of using existing Arden Syntax tools for MLM implementation, we lose information during the translation process. The main loss is GLIF's structured definition of complex data items, which can aid in mapping the data items onto the institutional patient data elements, and also assists in encapsulating related data items, such as a medication dose, route, and time of administration. In the translation process, we would have to convert GEL expressions into expressions in the Arden Syntax's logic grammar that lack complex data items and GEL functions. We would also need to break each complex data item into items that each have a single value and a single (primary) time stamp.

Although GLIF and the Arden Syntax are not code compatible (i.e., we cannot execute Arden MLMs using GLIF machinery), GLIF constructs such as the MLM macro facilitate the transition from the Arden Syntax to GLIF should such transition be necessary. However, converting simple MLMs into a GLIF specification may not be worthwhile because GLIF has a much more complex model than is necessary for representing simple rules.


## 5. CONCLUSION

The Arden Syntax represents efficiently individual decision rules, but makes difficult the representation of multistep algorithms that unfold over time. We specifically designed GLIF to enable representation of large, complex guidelines. GLIF may be cumbersome, however, for the expression of individual medical decisions leading to an action, usually an alert or reminder. Recognizing that the Arden Syntax is an established standard that can model medical decisions, GLIF3 builds on Arden's development by basing its expression language and several other constructs on the Arden Syntax, while creating constructs that are suitable for representing multistep guidelines. GLIF's expression language diverges from the Arden Syntax's logic grammar because of the need to support complex medical data structures, such as those of the HL7 RIM. Developers of both GLIF and the Arden Syntax are involved in the Clinical Decision Support Technical Committee of HL7. Together, we are exploring the possibility of developing an expression language that is consistent with the HL7 RIM.

## REFERENCES


1. Hripcsak G, Ludemann P, Pryor TA, Wigertz OB, Clayton PD. Rationale for the Arden Syntax. Comput Biomed Res 1994; 27(4):291–324.

2. Clinical Decision Support & Arden Syntax Technical Committee of HL7, inventor Arden Syntax for Medical Logic Systems, version 2.0. Draft revision. U.S.A. July 7, 1999.

3. Jenders R. Arden Syntax Web site. In: http://www.cpmc.columbia.edu/resources/arden/. Jenders R, editor. 2000.

4. Lobach DF, Gadd CS, Hales JW. Structuring clinical practice guidelines in a relational database model for decision support on the Internet. Proc AMIA Annu Fall Symp 1997; 158–62.

5. Fox J, Rahmanzadeh A. Disseminating medical knowledge: the PROforma approach. Artif Intell Med 1998; 14:157–81.

6. Shahar Y, Miksch S, Johnson P. The Asgaard project: a task-specific framework for the application and critiquing of time-oriented clinical guidelines. Artif Intell Med 1998; 14:29–51.

7. Tu SW, Musen MA. A flexible approach to guideline modeling. Proc AMIA Symp 1999; 420–4.

8. Peleg M, Boxwala A, Ogunyemi O, Zeng Q, Tu S, Lacson R, *et al*. GLIF3: the evolution of a guideline representation format. Proc AMIA Annu Symp 2000; 645–9.

9. Kuperman GJ, Gardner RM, Pryor TA. HELP: a dynamic hospital information system. New York: Springer-Verlag, 1991.

10. Jenders RA, Dasgupta B. Assessment of a knowledge-acquisition tool for writing medical logic modules in the Arden Syntax. Proc AMIA Annu Fall Symp 1996; 567–71.

11. Bang M, Eriksson H. Generation of development environments for the Arden Syntax. Proc AMIA Annu Fall Symp 1997; 313–7.

12. Musen MA, Tu SW, Eriksson H, Gennari JH, Puerta AR. PRO-TEGE-II: an environment for reusable problem-solving methods and domain ontologies. International Joint Conference on Artificial Intelligence; 1993; Chambery, Savoie, France; 1993.

13. Hripcsak G, Cimino JJ, Johnson SB, Clayton PD. The Columbia-Presbyterian Medical Center decision-support system as a model for implementing the Arden Syntax. Proc Annu Symp Comput Appl Med Care 1991; 248–52.

14. Kuhn RA, Reider RS. A C++ framework for developing medical Logic modules and an Arden Syntax compiler. Comput Biol Med 1994; 24(5):365–70.

15. Ohno-Machado L, Gennari JH, Murphy S, Jain NL, Tu SW, Oliver DE, *et al*. The GuideLine Interchange format: a model for representing guidelines. J Am Med Inform Assoc 1998; 5(4):357–372.

16. Bernstam E, Ash N, Peleg M, Tu S, Boxwala AA, Mork P, *et al*. Guideline classification to assist modeling, authoring, implementation and retrieval. Proc Am Med Inform Assoc Annual Symposium; 2000, 66–70.

17. Peleg M, Boxwala AA, Tu S, Greenes RA, Shortliffe EH, Patel VL. Handling expressiveness and comprehensibility requirements in GLIF3. Proc Med Inform 2001. In press.

18. Grosso WE, Eriksson H, Fergerson R, Gennari JH, Tu SW, Musen MA. Knowledge modeling at the millennium (the design and evolution of Protege-2000). In: Gains BR, Kremer R, Musen M, editors. The 12th Banff Knowledge Acquisition for Knowledge-Based Systems Workshop.; 1999; Banff, Canada; 1999, 7-4-1–7-4-36.

19. Greenes RA, Boxwala A, Sloan WN, Ohno-Machado L, Deibel SR. A framework and tools for authoring, editing, documenting, sharing, searching, navigating, and executing computer-based clinical guidelines. In: Proc AMIA Symp 1999; 1999; 261–5.

20. Boxwala AA, Greenes RA, Deibel SR. Architecture for a multipurpose guideline execution engine. In: Proc AMIA Symp 1999; 701–5.

21. Peleg M, Ogunyemi O, Tu S, Boxwala AA, Zeng Q, Greenes RA, *et al*. Using features of Arden Syntax with object-oriented medical data models for guideline modeling. Proc AMIA Annu Symp 2001. In press.

22. American College of Cardiology/American Heart Association/American College of Physicians-American Society of Internal Medicine. Guidelines for the management of patients with chronic stable angina. J Am Col Cardiol 1999; 33:2092–197 (http://www.acc.org/clinical/guidelines/june99/pdf/jun99.pdf).

23. Schadow G, Russler DC, Mead CN, McDonald CJ. Integrating medical information and knowledge in the HL7 RIM. Proc AMIA Annu Symp 2000; 764–8.

24. Boxwala AA, Mehta P, Peleg M, Lacson R, Ash N, Bury J, *et al*. Modeling guidelines using domain-level knowledge representation components. AMIA Annu Symp 2000; 645.

25. Lindberg C. The Unified Medical Language System (UMLS) of the National Library of Medicine. J Am Med Rec Assoc 1990; 61(5):40–2.

26. Starren J, Hripcsak G, Jordan D, Allen B, Weissman C, Clayton PD. Encoding a post-operative coronary artery bypass surgery care plan in the Arden Syntax. Comput Biol Med 1994; 24(5):411–7.

27. Fridsma DB, Gennari JH, Musen MA. Making generic guidelines site-specific. Proc AMIA Annu Fall Symp 1996; 597–601.

# Risk-Adjusted Monitoring of Binary Surgical Outcomes

STEFAN H. STEINER, PhD, RICHARD J. COOK, PhD, VERN T. FAREWELL, PhD

A graphical procedure suitable for prospectively monitoring surgical performance is proposed. The approach is based on accumulating evidence from the outcomes of all previous surgical patients in a series using a new type of cumulative sum chart. Cumulative sum procedures are designed to "signal" if sufficient evidence has accumulated that the surgical failure rate has changed substantially. In this way, the chart rapidly detects deterioration (or improvement) in surgical performance while not overreacting to the expected fluctuations due to chance. Through the use of a likelihood-based scoring method, the cumulative sum procedure is adapted so that it adjusts for the surgical risk of each patient estimated preoperatively. The procedure is therefore applicable in situations where it is desirable to adjust for a mix of patients. Signals of the chart lead to investigations of the cause and to the timely introduction of remedial measures designed to avoid unnecessary future failures. **Key words:** cumulative sum; monitoring performance; patient mix; risk factors; surgical outcomes. **(Med Decis Making 2001;21:163–169)**

The need to formally monitor surgical outcomes has been brought to the forefront in some recent well-publicized cases[1,2] where undesirably high rates of surgical complications remained undetected for an undue length of time. In such cases, the rapid detection of deterioration in surgical performance is critical since it should result in prompt investigation of the cause and procedural changes.

A number of methods for surgical monitoring have recently been described. Lovegrove and others[3] and Poloniecki and others[4] suggest simple monitoring schemes based on a plot of the difference between the cumulative expected number of deaths and cumulative observed deaths. These charts provide valuable visual aids that show how the current surgical performance compares with past performance. However, the charts do not specify how much variation in the plot is expected under good surgical performance and hence how large a deviation from the expected should be a cause for concern.

de Leval and others[5] and Steiner and others[6] propose an alternative surgical monitoring procedure based on a cumulative sum (CUSUM) chart that uses a methodology borrowed from an industrial context where process monitoring has been extensively studied.[7] In the industrial setting, CUSUM charts have been shown to be ideally suited to detecting relatively small persistent changes in the event rate over time.[8] Traditional CUSUM approaches, however, make no adjustment for different risk profiles because machine inputs are usually relatively homogeneous, and such adjustments are not required in industrial settings. In contrast, patients undergoing a particular surgical intervention are often very heterogeneous in their clinical presentation and physiology. This means that even for a surgeon with an acceptable overall complication rate, the probability of a successful outcome may vary considerably across patients.

We propose the use of a CUSUM chart to monitor surgical outcomes, where the CUSUM procedure is adapted to address the level of preoperative risk. The procedure is illustrated with sample data kindly supplied by Professor M. de Leval from a United Kingdom study of neonatal arterial switch operations for transposition of the great arteries. In

Received 10 August 1999 from the Department of Statistics and Actuarial Sciences, University of Waterloo, Waterloo, Ontario, Canada N2L 3G1 (SHS, RJC); and the Department of Statistical Sciences, University College, London, United Kingdom (VTF). Revision accepted for publication 12 December 1999. This research was supported, in part, by the Natural Sciences and Engineering Research Council of Canada and the Medical Research Council of Canada. R.J. Cook is a Scholar of the Medical Research Council of Canada.

Address correspondence and reprint requests to Dr. Steiner: Department of Statistics and Actuarial Sciences, University of Waterloo, Waterloo, Ontario, Canada N2L 3G1; telephone: (519) 888-4567 x6506; e-mail: shsteine@uwaterloo.ca.

the example, patient survival status constitutes the response and gender and the arterial pattern or diagnosis are the 2 risk factors of primary interest that characterize the patient mix. The data set is based on 230 operations from a number of surgical centers over a 3-year period. To illustrate the methodology, we use a random ordering of the observations and monitor the postoperative mortality rate of this artificially ordered series of 230 surgeries as if they came from 1 center over a 3-year period.

## Standard CUSUM Procedure

A CUSUM procedure is a monitoring scheme that may be used to accumulate evidence regarding the recent level of surgical performance.[6] The idea is to monitor surgical performance prospectively to detect as quickly as possible if the level of performance has changed. The cumulative sum is a sum of scores where each patient contributes a score. The sum is taken over all patients operated on from the start of monitoring until the point of observation. Mathematically, a CUSUM chart involves plotting $X_t$ versus $t$, where

$$X_t = \max(0, X_{t-1} + w_t), \qquad (1)$$

$t = 1, 2, 3, \ldots, X_0 = 0$, and $w_t$ is the score assigned to patient $t$. In the standard CUSUM, a patient's score is based on his or her surgical outcome (success or failure), the acceptable overall death rate, and a change in the death rate deemed to be important. The acceptable death rate could be estimated from previous data, or a desired rate could be obtained from other surgical centers. See de Leval and others[5] and Steiner and others[6] for examples. When designing the chart to detect increases in the surgical failure rate, we define scores associated with failures to be positive whereas successes receive a negative score. We assume that at any point in time the surgical performance may change (improve or deteriorate). As such, although individual scores may be negative, the CUSUM is restricted to nonnegative values to make the CUSUM sensitive to recent runs of poor performance.

The CUSUM value (equation 1) has accumulated the information from all previous surgeries. It will become large if the surgical performance level has deteriorated, but it will fluctuate close to 0 for a long time if no change has occurred. The surgical process is assumed to be acceptable as long as the CUSUM remains below a predetermined value, denoted $h$, called the *control limit*. When the CUSUM exceeds the control limit, we conclude enough evidence of a change in surgical failure rate has accumulated, and we say the CUSUM *signals*. Signals from the CUSUM chart should trigger a review of surgical procedures, including possible retraining.[5]

A CUSUM is designed to continually monitor the surgical performance until a signal occurs. The procedure will theoretically always eventually signal even if the surgical performance has not changed due to chance. This implies that the usual criteria for the evaluation of test procedures, such as false positive error rates and power, are not appropriate for assessing the performance of CUSUMs. In a sense, for a CUSUM, both the false alarm rate and power can be thought of as equal to 1 because, if the procedure has not signaled yet, we continue to monitor (i.e., take a larger sample size) until a signal occurs. The number of patients seen before the CUSUM first exceeds the control limit is called the *run length* of a CUSUM. We evaluate CUSUMs based on aspects of the run length distribution such as the average run length. Ideally, if the surgical failure rate has not changed (and is acceptable), the run length is long because signals represent false alarms. On the other hand, if the failure rate has increased substantially, short run lengths are desirable to ensure remedial action is brought about in a timely fashion. When evaluating a CUSUM, we consider the run length a random variable whose distribution represents all the possible values of the run length that may arise given a particular mortality rate and the effects of chance. Thus, when the failure rate is acceptable, the average run length is similar in some ways to the type I error rate of a traditional statistical test. Likewise, the average run length of the CUSUM when the surgical failure rate has increased substantially is somewhat analogous to the power of a traditional statistical test. Determining the average run length of a CUSUM at the design stage is computational intensive since it is based on all possible outcomes for a long series of surgeries; however, they may be closely approximated.[6] An appropriate value for the control limit, $h$, in any specific example is based on the desired average run length of the CUSUM while the failure rate is acceptable. Note that we should always react to a CUSUM signal even if that signal follows a long run length, since the signal may be evidence of a recent change in the surgical performance.

## Risk-Adjusted CUSUM Procedure for Cardiac Surgery

Unlike a traditional CUSUM procedure, with our new procedure, the magnitude of the scores, given by $w_t$ in equation 1, depends on each patient's surgical risk estimated preoperatively. Thus, the score depends on 4 factors: the current acceptable level of surgical performance, a chosen level of surgical performance deemed undesirable, the patient's surgical risk estimated preoperatively, and the actual surgical outcome for the patient. The scores ($w_t$) are derived based on the log likelihood ratio of the current risk compared to a specified change in risk (see equation 2, below). For example, we may decide we wish to optimize the chart to detect a doubling in the odds of failure. Assuming patient $t$ has a surgical risk of death equal to $p_t$, the likelihood for patient $t$ is given by $p_t^y (1-p_t)^{1-y}$, where $y$ = unity if a surgical failure occurs and 0 otherwise. The surgical risk for each patient may be determined preoperatively using a rating method such as Parsonnet risk factors[3,4] or may be based on a logistic regression model fit to some sample data. Given an estimated risk of failure equal to $p_t$, the odds of failure equal $p_t/(1 - p_t)$. The CUSUM is a formal sequential procedure for assessing the null hypothesis $H_0$: odds ratio = 1, versus the alternative hypothesis $H_A$: odds ration = $OR_A$. To detect increases, we set $OR_A > 1$. The choice of $OR_A$ affects the patient scores, but the ability of the procedure to quickly detect changes in actual odds ratios is relatively insensitive to $OR_A$. For patient $t$, assuming an odds ratio of $OR_A$, the odds of failure equal $OR_A p_t/(1 - p_t)$, which corresponds to a probability of failure under $H_A$ equal to $OR_A p_t/(1 - p_t + OR_A p_t)$ Then, the 2 possible log-likelihood ratio scores for patient $t$ are

$$w_t = \begin{cases} \log\left[\dfrac{OR_A}{(1 - p_t + OR_A p_t)}\right] & if\ y = 1 \\[2ex] \log\left[\dfrac{1}{1 - p_t + OR_A p_t}\right] & if\ y = 0 \end{cases} \qquad (2)$$

## Characteristics of the Procedure

To illustrate the characteristics of the risk-adjusted CUSUM, we use the arterial switch example discussed above. In the data set a total of 15 deaths occurred, giving an overall death rate of 6.5%. The risk of death as a function of the explanatory variates was estimated through a logistic regression model. The estimated risk varied significantly with gender and the preoperative arterial pattern or diagnosis and effectively classified patients into 10 risk groups. The lowest-risk patients in the group were estimated to have a risk of death of just 1.8% following surgery, whereas the patients with the highest risk had a mortality rate of 46%. This suggests that some adjustment for the patient mix is necessary. We designed the CUSUM chart to detect a doubling of the odds of death from the preoperative risk. In this example, a doubling of the odds results in a death rate of 3.5% and 63% for the lowest- and highest-risk groups, respectively. Based on the likelihood ratio statistic, this leads to the following possible patient scores: 0.68 and −0.02 for the lowest-risk patient, and 0.31 and −0.38 for the highest-risk patients, where the positive score is assigned in the case of death and the negative score is assigned in the case of survival. These scores are derived using equation 2 with $OR_A = 2$ and $p_t$ either 0.018 or 0.46. Note that the scores reflect the surgical risk assessed preoperatively, since the "penalty" for death of a low-risk patient is more severe than for a high-risk patient. Setting the control limit $h$ at 2 gives an average run length of around 460 patients when the surgical performance is acceptable. Given the frequency of surgery in this artificial example, this implies a positive signal from the monitoring procedure, on average once every 6 years, even if no true changes in the death rate have occurred. If surgical procedures were more frequent, it might be desirable to select a longer average run length while the surgical mortality rate is acceptable. We add a similarly designed CUSUM chart to detect decreases in the odds of death ($OR_A = 0.5$). The CUSUM designed to detect improvements (decreases) in the surgical failure rate is useful because, if it signals, it suggests that the currently acceptable failure rate should be reestimated. This may happen if either the actual failure rate has decreases or if our initial estimate of the acceptable failure rate was too high.

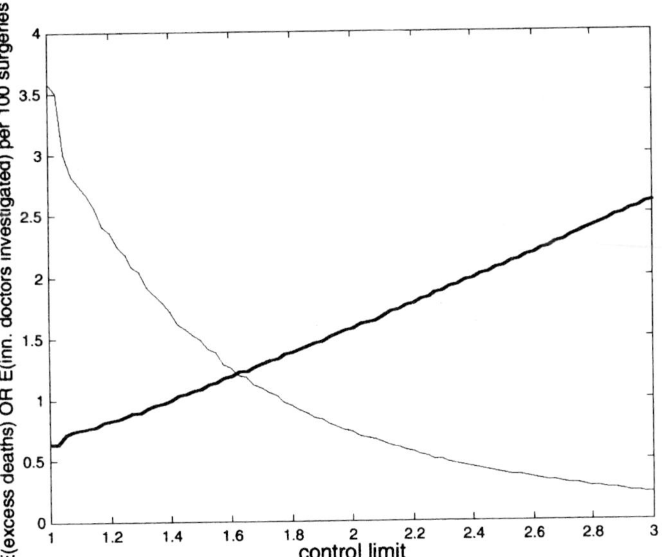

FIGURE 1. Trade-off inherent in the choice of control limit ($h$). The solid line indicates 100 times expected number of innocent doctors investigated. The dashed line gives the expected excess deaths.

The choice of the control limit ($h$) involves an inherent trade-off based on the in-control versus out-of-control average run length of the proposed procedure. Figure 1 illustrates the trade-off by showing the expected "excess deaths" that would result before a doubling of the odds of failure signals and the expected number of "innocent doctors investigated" due to false alarms as we change $h$. To create Figure 1, we assume the CUSUM scores, patient mix, and so on, of the example problem. The expected number of innocent doctors investigated is proportional to 1 over the average run length when the odds of failure have not changed. To put the quantities on a similar scale, we plot the expected number of innocent doctors investigated per 100 surgeries. The expected excess deaths that result if the failure rate changes to $OR_A$ equals $(p_1 - p_0)ARL[OR_A]$, where $p_1$ is the overall failure rate when $OR = OR_A$, $p_0$ is the current overall failure rate, and $ARL[OR_A]$ is the average run length when $OR = OR_A$. Figure 1 allows us to quantify the effects of the choice of control limit in terms of the medical context. In the example, we chose a control limit equal to 2 for the CUSUM to detect increases in the odds of failure. From Figure 1, this results in an average of 0.73 innocent doctors investigated per 100 surgeries and an average of 1.57 excess deaths if the odds ratio of failure doubles.

The CUSUM is designed to prospectively monitor the surgical performance; that is, we would use the logistic equation for death rate estimated from the current data together with equations 2 and 1 to monitor our future performance. However, to illustrate the procedure, we create a CUSUM plot using the current data ignoring the fact that we used the series to design the CUSUM. This analysis corresponds to a check of whether the surgical performance was stable over the 230 patients. Figure 2 shows 2 examples of the resulting pair of CUSUM charts designed to detect either increases or decreases in the mortality rate. For ease of presentation, the CUSUM to detect decreases in odds of mortality accumulates negative values when there are surgical successes. Thus, on each plot in Figure 2 we see 2 CUSUM charts. The top pair of CUSUM charts is the result from the randomly ordered set of 230 operations and shows no signals. The bottom plot shows the resulting CUSUM charts when all the 9 deaths that previously occurred between patients 100 to 230 are concentrated (but randomly distributed) between patients 100 to 150. This corresponds to a surgeon's having an odds ratio of approximately 3.5 for the series of patients numbered 100 to 150. The bottom pair of CUSUM charts signals an increase in the death rate at around patient number 115. This suggests unstable surgical performance over time since there is a run of poor performance.

To quantify how the proposed CUSUM adjusts for preoperative risk, we consider the extreme case where we observe a number of deaths in a row. Given the scores and the control limit for the

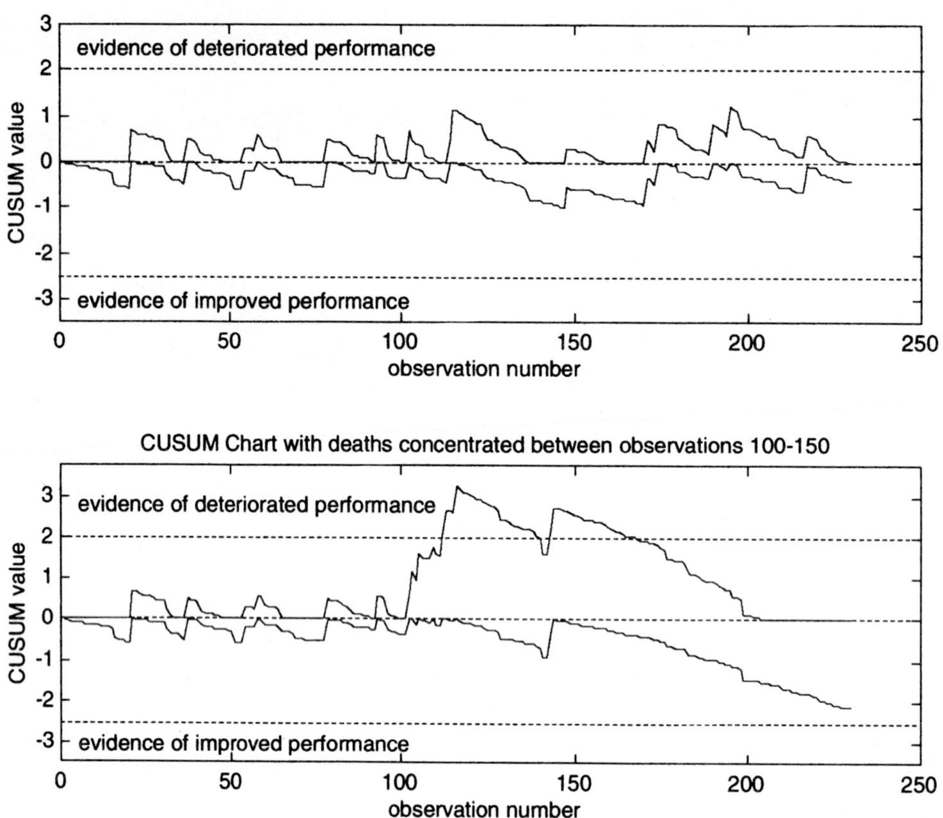



FIGURE 2. Cumulative sum (CUSUM) charts designed to detect increases or decreases in performance. *Top*, chart showing no evidence of a change in death rate; *bottom*, chart showing a string of deaths not likely caused by chance.

example problem as defined previously, and assuming the CUSUM starts at 0, 3 low-risk deaths in a row would trigger a signal, whereas it would take 6 high-risk deaths in a row. Note that the procedure is very flexible and that by changing the control limit and/or the alternate hypothesis $(OR_A)$, monitoring schemes with a wide variety of operating characteristics are possible.

We may also quantify the ability of the CUSUM procedure to quickly detect increases in the odds of death. More generally, Figure 3 shows plots of the average run length versus a measure of the actual surgical performance (given in terms of the odds ratio) for different patient mixes. The acceptable level of surgical performance is given by an odds ratio equal to unity, whereas increases in the odds ratio signifies a deterioration of performance. The solid line gives the results for the current mix of high- and low-risk patients. For this particular example, extreme changes in patient mix substantially change the run length properties of the procedure when monitoring the death rate, as shown by the plot on the left. This suggests that, when monitoring the death rate, if patient mix changes dramatically the control limit of the monitoring procedure should be adjusted. This sensitivity is due to the large difference in risk of death between the lowest- and highest-risk patients. In other situations where the preoperative risks are more similar, the run length curve is much less sensitive to the patient mix. As an example, the plot on the right of Figure 3 shows the average run length curves when monitoring for either a death or the need to reinstitute cardiopulmonary bypass after a trial period of weaning, called a *near miss* in de Leval.[5] When using death or near miss as the response, the estimated rates of failure for the lowest- and highest-risk categories are 19% and 52%, respectively.

To focus attention on the performance of the monitoring procedure under $H_0$ and $H_A$, we may examine a plot of the approximate cumulative run length distribution. Figure 4 shows the cumulative probability of a signal for the in-control condition

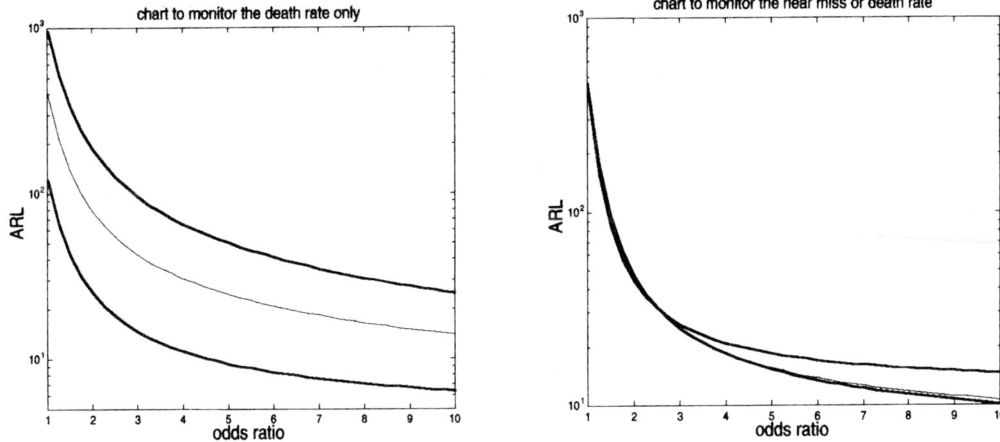



FIGURE 3. Average run length for different actual odds ratios. The solid lines indicate performance with current patient mix. The dotted lines indicate all lowest-risk patients. The dashed lines indicate all highest-risk patients.

(OR = 1) and when the odds ratio has doubled. The figure shows that even with no increased rate of failure, the CUSUM would signal around 51.4% of the time by 100 surgeries. Although this seems like a high rate of false positive signals, we must remember that in our example this represents around 15.5 months' worth of surgeries from a number of surgical centers. Also, through our choice of the control limit $h$, the in-control run length distribution can be changed to satisfy whatever CUSUM design characteristics are desirable. Similarly, we can see from Figure 4 that if the odds of a failure have doubled, the CUSUM will signal around 89% of the time within 50 patients. A caution in the interpretation of Figure 4 is necessary: Assume our CUSUM signals after a long run length of, say, 500 patients. We may be tempted to conclude that this must correspond to a false signal because, if the odds ratio had actually doubled, the CUSUM would likely have signaled much earlier based on Figure 4. But this rationale may well be incorrect. Recall that Figure 4 is based

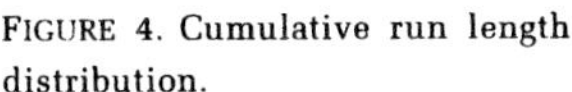

FIGURE 4. Cumulative run length distribution.

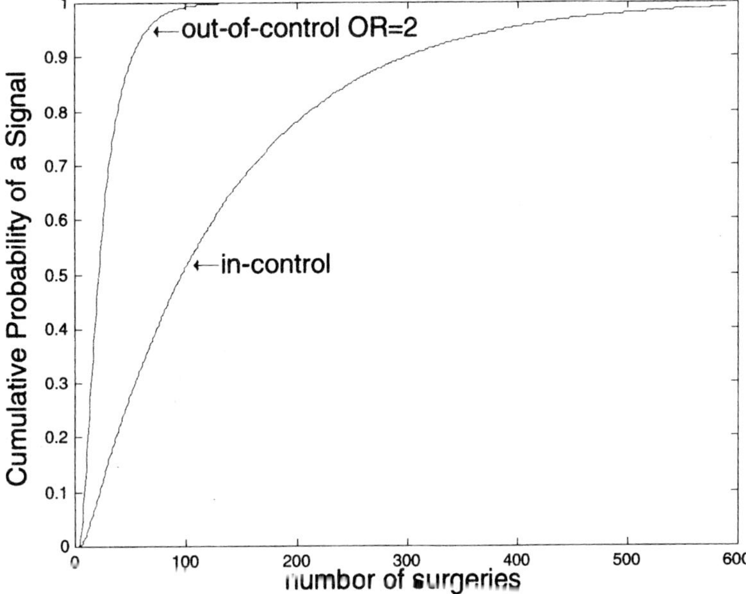

on the assumption that the rate of failure (through the odds ratio) stays constant. The observed CUSUM signal may be due to the rate of failure's changing somewhere in the series of 500 patients. For example, perhaps only for the last 50 patients has the odds ratio been 2. The purpose of a CUSUM chart is to quickly detect any changes in the failure rate no matter when they occur.

## Conclusions

The use of a CUSUM chart with scores adjusted to reflect the estimated surgical risk of the patients is proposed to monitor surgical performance. This approach provides a logical way to accumulate evidence over many patients while adjusting for patient characteristics that significantly affect the risk. This is particularly important when monitoring outcomes of surgery at referral centers, where referral patterns may change over time. Through use of the CUSUM procedure, the sensitivity of the chart can be set so that false alarms do not happen very frequently but substantial changes in the failure rate are quickly detected. This approach is appealing because the ability of the chart to detect specific changes can be easily quantified. Note that the CUSUM method- ology is also applicable when the covariates are continuous or a mix of continuous and categorical variables.

In summary, the proposed CUSUM chart is a valuable tool in the assessment and monitoring of surgical outcomes since it allows the early detection of problems such as an increased failure rate. Evidence of any problems would lead to a review of surgical procedures and possibly some remedial measures, such as retraining, that could prevent unnecessary future failures.

## References


1. Waldie P. Crisis in the cardiac unit. The Globe and Mail, Canada's National Newspaper 1998 Oct 27;Sect A:3(col. 1).

2. Treasure T, Taylor K, Black N. Independent Review of Adult Cardiac Surgery—Unite Bristol. Bristol, UK: Health Care Trust, 1997.

3. Lovegrove J, Valencia O, Treasure T, Sherlaw-Johnson C, Gallivan S. Monitoring the results of cardiac surgery by variable life-adjusted display. Lancet. 1997;18,350(9085): 1128–30.

4. Poloniecki J, Valencia O, Littlejohns P. Cumulative risk adjusted mortality chart for detecting changes in death rate: observational study of heart surgery. British Medical Journal. 1998;316:1697–1700.

5. de Leval MR, François K, Bull C, Brawn WB, Spiegelhalter D. Analysis of a cluster of surgical failures. J Thorac Cardiovasc Surg. 1994;March:914–24.

6. Steiner S, Cook R, Farewell V. Monitoring paired binary surgical outcomes using cumulative sum charts. Stat Med. 1999;18:69–86.

7. Montgomery DC. Introduction to Statistical Quality Control. 2nd ed. New York: John Wiley and Sons, 1991.

8. Hawkins DM, Olwell DH. Cumulative Sum Charts and Charting for Quality Improvement. New York: Springer, 1998.

# *Section 7:*

## *Computer-Supported Education*

*Reprinted by kind permission of:*
*American Chemical Society (591)*
*Elsevier Science (607), Kluwer*
*Academic Publishers (583),*
*Radiologcial Society*
*of North America (599)*

**Ch. Daetwyler**

Interactive Media Lab
Dartmouth College Medical School
Lebanon, NH, USA

# Synopsis

# *Computer-Supported Education*

## Introduction and framing

I am a medical Doctor, not a computer scientist. The reason, why I was asked to write this synopsis, I guess, is my long lasting interest in the application of information technology for medical education. This interest resulted in several learning programs – and even in a publication about the "Use of computers in medical education"[1] where I brought 16 authors, among them pioneers like Florian Eitel (President of the GMA: German Association for Medical Education), Joe Henderson (Director of the IML: Interactive Media Lab at Dartmouth College Medical School), Rolf Schulmeister (Director of the Interdisciplinary Center for Didactics at the University of Hamburg) and Vic Spitzer (Creator of the Visible Human Project, UCHSC in Denver, CO) together. Hence, in this synopsis I will try to synthesize what I learned during the last 9 years, and on the other hand emphasize on my background as a physician with an interest in philosophy and medical history – hopefully that this approach may expand the view of computer scientists, and so contributes to a more comprehensive understanding of this very interesting matter.

In ancient times, many believed that good health was a divine gift given by the gods: good people were rewarded with good health [2]. Back then it was obvious that spirituality and health care were hand in hand [3]. Nowadays masses are held in churches to pray for health, a proof that this correlation is still in place[4] - and there is good evidence that people who are religious cope better with serious illness than people who do not: a religious faith can be a very good medication in many cases [5]. This spiritual correlation needs to be considered as we now switch our focus from the "supernatural roots" of medicine to the role of Informatics for the quality of health care.

In Informatics, Computer scientists are in charge of the action.
And because computer scientists have to rely on quantitative facts, they are more likely to measure "objective" data than indefinable facts like "happiness" or "the ability to tell well ones story of life". This tendency to rely on "countable facts" is to a certain extend understandable because it is assumed to be "objective", however, it can lead to a very narrow view of the world if we exclude what is not easily measurable. A good example of this unhealthy balance is the "Guinness Book of Records" [6]. In the pages of this book, one can learn about the fastest ascent of to the top of Mount Everest or how Peter Dowdeswell consumed a pint of Guinness stout in 2.1 seconds [7] This book contains many other unnecessary and often very unhealthy achievements of mankind. And I am not afraid to admit that this quest for records did not stop in front of hospital doors...

When it then comes to the question, "how to measure," many computer scientists enter the field of demographic and epidemiological data [8], trying to analyze and to visualize this. Let me show this with an example from Edward Tufte's Book "Visual Explanations"[9]. The chapter entitled "Visual and Statistical Thinking" is based on analyses of the London cholera epidemic of 1854. While investigation the epidemic, John Snow M.D. began counting the number of deaths directly related to Cholera and plotting the location of outbreaks on a map of London. This process enabled him to pinpoint one of the major sources of causation of the disease: the handle of the Broad Street Pump. When the pump then was sealed, the epidemic was contained. This is an example of where the display of the data, not the data itself, resulted in some important conclusions. It is also an example, how the intelligent display of data can trigger understanding.

## Education of Health Care Professionals

Modern Western Medicine is the product of several hundred years of experience and investigation, brought together by thousands of ingenious individuals. The field has grown far too complex to be understood by any single mind. Therefore, a modern medical curriculum does not attempt to teach all medicine, but rather a core of basic medical concept and skills [10,11,12]. This is often done in a "Problem Based Learning" setting which encourages students to first study a problem, then to define learning goals, collect relevant information – using the Internet and other sources – and to synthesize this into knowledge. This process usually takes place in a teamwork setting. The paradigm is about hunting gathering: if you provide a beggar with fish, he will have food for a day – if you teach him how to fish, he may won't starve any more. However, do not forget to teach how to figure out which fish are edible and which are not (more important if it were about mushrooms). In the case of the medical literature: it has to be carefully taught how to detect if such information is valid or not. To perform this task, we get help from Evidence Based Medicine (EBM):

"This paradigm shift [towards EBM] is manifested in a number of ways. There has been a profusion of articles instructing clinicians on how to access, evaluate, and interpret the medical literature. Proposals to apply the principles of clinical epidemiology to day-to-day clinical practice have been put forward. A number of major medical journals have adopted a more informative structured abstract format which incorporates issues of methods and design into the portion of an article the reader sees first." [13]

Learning how to use the Internet or medical library to find accurate primary medical literature is important. However, this procedure is often far too time consuming as if it could become the primary source of medical learning. There is simply too much valid information out there as if a student could condense this down to what is needed for the primary understanding of a matter. This is where I like to come up with the need for computer-supported education.

## The role of computers in Medical Education

People often talk about computer-supported education as if it were a term describing a method and not a tool. They couldn't be more wrong. The fact, that a computer is used, does not offer any clue about what a program is like – and what it can be used for. But it implies the use of the computers capabilities, which are: display of audiovisual content including movies, providing feedback and allowing the fast access to information using the Internet. What is done with these premises is up to the creators of educational programs. And like the fact that only a few people know how to paint with artistry – nevertheless the fact that brushes, paint and paper are accessible to all of us – there are many programs out there, but only a few that are done with real artistry (which is one of these indefinable terms mentioned in the introduction to this synopsis).

Let me go on with a discussion of the most important models that came to my attention. I will exemplify each model with several award-winning programs:

## Models for Problem Based Learning (PBL)

### CASUS [14] / CAMPUS [15] / DxR [16]

When Howard S. Barrows noticed that "medical students and residents, for the most part, did not seem to think at all" [17], he introduced as a consequence the "Problem Based Learning" in order to "..allow all students to learn the way good students always learn." [18]

There are quite a few programs out there that are based on the principles of problem-based learning. Because of the assumption made by PBL that knowledge has to be worked out in an active process, some of these programs are not addressing an active thinking alone but allow even an active authoring of cases (CASUS, CAMPUS).

Though all of these programs apply Barrows PBL algorithms for clinical decision-making, they differ in some aspects:

CASUS allows the learner to draw the reasoning process as a semantic net – and then to compare this with the "ideal" one provided by a specialist.

CAMPUS shows always the users progress on a graphic representing the PBL algorithm.

DxR is to a high grade complete in simulating possible responses to the learner's actions and provide the learner as well with accurate feedback. This allows "explorative" learning to a certain extent, which makes it the link to the next topic.

## Models for Case Based Learning (CBL)

### LAENNEC [19] / NEUROLOGY INTERACTIVE [20] / HEADACHE INTERACTIVE [21]

Most of the PBL programs for clinical education are case based, but case based learning does not necessarily rely on PBL algorithms.

Case based learning is mainly build on the fact that the patient is the center of a physician's world. Many students like the feeling of being in the position of a physician and having the chance to interact meaningfully with a patient. When the cases are carefully done, they can become quite natural – and then the learner can enter a continuum where he/she is driven by feelings similar to those occurring in real encounters: empathy, care and responsibility – to name a few. In such a continuum, the primary information that the learner obtains consists of symptoms and signs presented by the simulated patient. The goal of the learner is then to understand the causes of an illness – and the specific situation of the individual patient. To achieve this, the programs allow the learner to perform virtual history taking (HEADACHE INTERACTIVE), virtual physical exams (LAENNEC, NEUROLOGY INTERACTIVE) and virtual further investigations.

## Models to train specific skills

ECHO EXPLORER [22] / HEMO-SURF [23] / HEART SOUNDS AND MURMURS [24]

The learning of medical skills plays an important rule in the formation of a physician. Some skills like the manual examination of an abdomen in surgery are not likely to be taught on a computer screen because it's about haptic, invisible and inaudible informations. But many skills base on audiovisual information – like the auscultation of heart sounds (cardiology) or the interpretation of skin lesions (dermatology) - and therefore can be demonstrated, explained and trained using computers capable of displaying multimedia contents. Besides, modern methods like MRT and Ultrasound result in a shift from "other" towards visual information when it comes to diagnostics.

ECHO EXPLORER enables the learner to understand in depth the ultrasonographic imaging of the heart using sophisticated interactive visualization and animation techniques.

HEMOSURF teaches how to interpret blood smears. This is mainly achieved with exposing the learner to a lot of pictures depicting hematological conditions - and make so "pattern recognition" happen.

HEART SOUND AND MURMURS explains the physiological origins of heart sounds and murmurs using audio, visualization and animation.

---

## Complete models bringing together most of the above... adding even more to it

THE VIRTUAL PRACTICUM [25]

In the "Virtual Practicum" model, a mentor guides the student through a simulated clinic. There learning takes place in an idealized setting where carefully scripted simulated patients make learning by experience happen, case discussions explain about clinical decision making, lectures provide the theoretical background and interviews with "real patients" make the personal dimension of being affected with a condition understandable.

This is all done with intense use of high quality multimedia. In the simulated cases, actors behave as patients who act directly towards the learner. The stories they tell are very realistic and made to trigger the learner's interest for a medical condition. But the learner is not left as a passive listener - the simulated patients are demanding participation quite often by asking for clarification of medical terms and by demanding medical decisions concerning their case. That is where the learner experience how "swampy" clinical medicine is, because there is often more than one "solution" – and sometimes there is none at all.

Another very important element of the "Virtual Practicum" model is that the best specialists are asked to do case discussions on the simulated patients (expository learning). This creates an opportunity for providing the learner with priceless "pearls" of medical expertise.

Joe Henderson, the creator of the "Virtual Practicum" model, emphasizes on..

"..the application of technology to promote more comprehensive clinical education in the biopsychosocial aspects of primary care. Comprehensive refers to the inclusion, in addition to scientific and technical knowledge, of knowledge that is less easily characterized, quantified, and taught: empathy, intuition, the demonstration of artistry." (Henderson 1997)

---

## Papers presented in this section

"Do Computers Teach Better? A Media Comparison Study for Case-based Teaching in Radiology" compares the outcome of using problem-based teaching in radiology with and without computers and/or interactive elements. The models used are Problem Based and Case Based Learning.

"Enhancing Social Problem Solving in Children with Autism and Normal Children Through Computer-Assisted Instruction" shows how problem-solving skills in autistic children can be improved using computer-aided instruction. The model to train specific skills is used to achieve this goal.

"Design and Development of Computer-Aided Chemical Systems: Virtual Labs for Teaching Chemical Experiments in Undergraduate and Graduate Courses" presents a model for the construction of virtual experiments in chemistry.

---

"DiasNet – A Diabetes Advisory System for Communication and Education via the Internet" describes a method to use the Internet for patient empowerment in dealing with diabetes.

## Closing remarks

I hope that you enjoyed reading this synopsis – and that it did contribute some aspects to a comprehensive understanding of the many faces of Computer Supported Education in Medicine.

Last but not least I would like to thank Raphael Bonvin MD (Université de Lausanne, Switzerland), Joe Henderson MD (IML Dartmouth Medical School, USA) and Bill Tishler BA (IML Dartmouth Medical School, USA) for their contributions to this synopsis.


## References

1. Daetwyler C, editor. Use of computers in medical education. Innsbruck: Studienverlag; 2001. online at http://www.aum.iawf.unibe.ch/did/zsfhd.htm
2. Porter R. The greatest benefit to mankind: A medical history of humanity. New York: W.W. Norton & Company; 1 Amer Ed edition; April 1998.
3. Diamandopoulos A. Exorcisms Used for Treatment of Urinary Tract Diseases in Greece during the Middle Ages and Renaissance. Am J Nephrol 1999;19:114-24.
4. Walach H, Bosch H, Haraldsson E, Marx A, Tomasson H, Wiesendanger H, et al. Efficacy of Distant Healing - a Proposal for a Four-Armed Randomized Study (EUHEALS). Forsch Komplementarmed Klass Naturheilkd 2002;9:168-76.
5. Pettus MC. Implementing a medicine-spirituality curriculum in a community-based internal medicine residency program. Acad Med 2002;77 (7):745.
6. Guinness Book of Records. http://www.guinnessworldrecords.com/
7. Guinness Book of Records. http://www.guinnessworldrecords.com/content_pages/record.asp?recordid=56408
8. Descriptive Statistics and Exploratory Data Analysis (Multimedia Software). http://www.fernuni-hagen.de/STATISTIK/Neu/Lernsoftware/Statistik_e.html
9. Tufte E. Visual Explanations, Envisioning Information, The Visual Display of Quantitative Information, and Data Analysis for Politics and Policy. http://www.edwardtufte.com/
10. Master of Medical Education at the University of Illinois in Chicago, USA and at the University of Berne, Switzerland. http://www.uic.edu/ and http://www.iawf.unibe.ch/mme/mmeex.htm
11. The curriculum at the University of Maastricht, Netherlands. http://www.unimaas.nl/
12. The new curriculum at the Charité in Berlin, Germany. http://www.charite.de/rv/reform/english /Structure_of_the_Berlin_reformed_curriculum.html
13. Evidence-Based Medicine: A New Approach to Teaching the Practice of Medicine Users Guides of Evidence Based Medicine, published by JAMA 1992 Nov 4;268(17):2420-5. online at http://www.cche.net/usersguides/ebm.asp
14. AG Instruct (Fischer et al). http://www.promediweb.de/index_en.html
15. http://www.mi.fh-heilbronn.de/interna/campus_bericht2002.pdf
16. Hurley Myers. http://www.dxrgroup.com/
17. Barrows HR, Twomblyn RM. Problem-Based Learning – An Approach to Medical Education. Springer Series on Medical Education Vol.1. New York: Springer; Publ. Comp.; 1980. p. xi (Preface).
18. Barrows HR. How to design a problem-based curriculum for the preclinical years. Springer series on medical education Vol. 8. New York: Springer Publ. Comp.; 1985.
19. Bonvin. http://www.hospvd.ch/public/chuv/cemcav/HTMLLaennec/Laennec.html
20. Daetwyler. http://www.aum.iawf.unibe.ch/prod/cd/Neuro_Projekt.htm
21. Daetwyler. http://www2000.easa-award.net/comp/winners2000/headache.html
22. Grunst. http://www.aum.iawf.unibe.ch/did/ZfHD_Papers/GRUNST.doc
23. Woermann. http://www.aum.iawf.unibe.ch/vlz/BWL/HemoSurf/Index.htm
24. Criley. http://www.blaufuss.org
25. Henderson JV. Comprehensive, Technology-Based Clinical Education: The "Virtual Practicum". Int J Psychiatry Med 1998;28(1):41-79. online at http://www.iml.dartmouth.edu/education/pubs/index.html



Address of the author:
Christof Daetwyler MD
Interactive Media Laboratory
Dartmouth College Medical School
Colburn Hill, One Medical Center Drive
Lebanon, NH 03756, USA
E-mail: christof.j.daetwyler@dartmouth.edu

# Enhancing Social Problem Solving in Children with Autism and Normal Children Through Computer-Assisted Instruction

Vera Bernard-Opitz,[1,2] N. Sriram,[1] and Sharul Nakhoda-Sapuan[1]

Children with autism have difficulty in solving social problems and in generating multiple solutions to problems. They are, however, relatively skilled in responding to visual cues such as pictures and animations. Eight distinct social problems were presented on a computer, along with a choice of possible solutions, and an option to produce alternative solutions. Eight preschool children with autism and eight matched normal children went through 10 training sessions interleaved with 6 probe sessions. Children were asked to provide solutions to animated problem scenes in all the sessions. Unlike the probe sessions, in the training sessions problem solutions were first explained thoroughly by the trainer. Subsequently these explanations were illustrated using dynamic animations of the solutions. Although children with autism produced significantly fewer alternative solutions compared to their normal peers, a steady increase across probe sessions was observed for the autistic group. The frequency of new ideas was directly predicted by the diagnostic category of autism. Results suggest young children with autism and their normal peers can be taught problem-solving strategies with the aid of computer interfaces. More research is required to establish whether such computer-assisted instruction will generalize to nontrained problem situations in real-life contexts.

**KEY WORDS:** Autism; social problem solving; computer-assisted instruction.

## INTRODUCTION

Problem solving, conflict resolution and empathy are core components of "emotional intelligence," a construct popularized in recent years by Goleman (1997, 1998). He presented a body of research implying that, in addition to cognitive inputs, effective learning is powerfully modulated by variables in the social and emotional domains. Various child development projects and school centers in the Western world have emphasized social competence or self-science in their curricula (Elias, 1992). These skills are taught to children as

young as 4 years old and form the basis for books, training programs, and videotapes for children (Berry, 1995).

Children with autism show significant problems in the domains of communication, emotion recognition, empathy, and social skills (Happé, 1994; Wing, 1990). They often fail to process subtle transient stimuli such as expressed emotions and are overwhelmed by the complexity of social settings (Hobson, Ouston, & Lee, 1989; Prior & Ozonoff, 1998; Volkmar, Cohen, Bergman, Hooks, & Stevenson, 1989). If conflict arises, inappropriate coping strategies such as withdrawal or severe tantrum behaviors have been observed. Lack of understanding the emotional states of others, and a deficient Theory of Mind, has been identified as one of the deep-rooted problems that need to be tackled for this population (Baron-Cohen, Leslie, & Frith, 1985; Howlin & Baron-Cohen, 1999; Ozonoff & Miller,

[1] Department of Social Work and Psychology, National University of Singapore.

[2] Address all correspondence to Vera Bernard-Opitz, Department of Social Work and Psychology, National University of Singapore, 11 Law Link, Singapore, 117570; e-mail: swkberna@nus.edu.sg

1995). Some of these children manage to achieve normal academic standards in mainstream educational settings. However, their poor social awareness, low flexibility, and awkwardness in social settings have limited the success of their integration into mainstream schools.

On the other hand, children with autism demonstrate relatively good skills in responding to fixed visual cues such as pictures or written words (Quill, 1997). Parents, too, report fascination and good learning rates through watching videos or computers. Research has supported these reports by effectively teaching communication skills and specific social scripts through computer programs (Heiman, Nelson, Tjus, & Gilberg, 1995).

These findings suggest that an appropriately designed computer program could be an effective aid for teaching problem-solving skills to children with autism. A program was developed to present everyday conflicts and elicit solutions. For example, two children would be fighting over their turn to use a slide in the playground. This was followed by icons representing animated alternative problem solutions such as making a polite request versus throwing a tantrum. Children were also requested to produce alternative solutions; these were reinforced by short clips of a satisfactory resolution to the conflict and access to any one of eight reinforcing scenes. We hypothesized that exposure to animated solutions and the reinforcement of alternative solutions would jointly enhance the production of the latter. Based on the finding that sensory reinforcers enhance the learning rate of young children with autism (Rincover, 1978), participants could choose among sensory (e.g., dynamic spirals) or natural reinforcement, animation related to the problem setting (e.g., after having bargained for a toy bus, boy is shown driving happily around with the bus). We hypothesized that both normal children as well as children with autism would show generalization by producing alternative solutions on nontrained problems. We also wanted to contrast the learning rates of children with autism and normal children in nontrained problem situations.

## METHOD

### Procedure

In collaboration with a Singaporean computer firm, IT 21, a computer program presenting eight conflict settings was developed to be run from the CD-ROM on Windows 95 based PCs (Table I). Some of the conflicts were modeled after the training program

**Table I.** Settings on Social Problem Solving

| Easy level | Difficult level | Targets |
|---|---|---|
| 1. Boat | 5. Slide | Taking turns |
| 2. Rambutans | 6. Bicycle | Requesting for help/objects |
| 3. Fish | 7. Eggs | Giving in |
| 4. Bus | 8. Money | Negotiating |

by Shure on "I can Problem-Solve" (Shure, 1992). Others were tailored to reflect the contextual knowledge of Singaporean children (e.g., not being able to reach the rambutan fruits on a tree). Four easy and four difficult problems were pictured with cueing options for various possible solutions. Eight distinct social problems were presented, along with a choice of possible solutions, and an additional option (indicated by a light bulb) for producing alternative solutions. Problems differed in level of difficulty to assure that participants of various levels could be successful as well as challenged by them. In easy conflicts, the child had to find solutions to everyday problems such as not getting his turn or not being able to reach an item. By contrast, difficult conflict settings illustrated higher level social problems such as not having sufficient money to buy a desired item or being scolded for breaking an object. The distinction between "easy" and "difficult" problem settings was based on consensus among the program designers.

Problem settings were illustrated by animations that also incorporated recorded speech using children's voices. Children were cued by a computer voice to solve the problem (e.g., "What would you do?"). Pictures presenting two appropriate and two inappropriate options were given. While these pictures were static and only briefly described by the trainer during baseline sessions, they were animated and explained by the trainer during training. Participants were also prompted by a light bulb to verbally produce ideas. ("Do you have any good ideas?"). Novel ideas not shown in the pictured alternatives were reinforced, if they were appropriate to the problem. Inappropriate solutions were ignored. Upon the production of an innovative idea, a computer voice praised the child with a "happy end" to the conflict, such as the animation of children taking turns, and sharing toys or food. After this scene, the child could select from eight pictures, leading to additional reinforcement. Four sensory conditions (such as spirals or lines) and four natural conditions (such as a child jumping on a trampoline or rabbits coming out of a magician's hat) were included. Once a child had seen the reinforcing component, he returned to the orig-

**Table II.** Baseline Settings Across Participants

| Autistic children | | | Normal children | | |
|---|---|---|---|---|---|
| Name | Baseline | | Name | Baseline | |
| A4 | Fish | Bicycle | N4 | Fish | Slide |
| A5 | Bus | Eggs | N6 | Bus | Money |
| A1 | Fish | Money | N8 | Rambutans | Slide |
| A3 | Bus | Bicycle | N3 | Rambutans | Bicycle |
| A2 | Rambutans | Money | N7 | Fish | Bicycle |
| A7 | Bus | Slide | N1 | Bus | Bicycle |
| A6 | Fish | Eggs | N2 | Fish | Eggs |
| A8 | Boat | Slide | N5 | Boat | Bicycle |

inal problem setting and was requested to give additional ideas. When the child stopped producing new ideas on a particular problem, the trainer activated a new problem setting. In a session, children went through two easy and two difficult problem situations. The assignment of situations was randomized across children and sessions (Table II). Overall each child participated in ten training sessions.

Prior to and during the training each child was assessed for his responding to four nontrained conflict situations. The first and fourth probe session coincided with the first and ninth learning sessions while the two other probes were randomly chosen to coincide with two in-between sessions. In the probe sessions, children were not given explanations of possible solutions nor were they shown animations illustrating these solutions. The number of good ideas was checked for reliability in 87% of the video samples. The interobserver agreement on production of good ideas was .97 for normal children and .94 for children with autism.

## Participants

Out of a group of 176 children with autism 15 verbal children were considered as possible candidates for the study. Participants were selected if they had an autism score above 65 and an IQ in the normal range. All children were diagnosed using the Autism Behavior Checklist (ABC: Krug, Arick, & Almond, 1979). Eight children with autism and eight normal preschool children participated in the experiment (Table III). All the children came from middle class, English-speaking Singaporean families, and were of Chinese ethnicity. Originally 10 children were planned for each group, but participants dropped out due to illness and other unforeseen circumstances. Children with autism ranged

**Table III.** Cognitive Functioning and Language Comprehension[a]

| Participant | Sex | Autism scores | Age (years:months) | K-Bit Composite standard score | K-Bit Vocabulary standard score | BPVS Standard score | BPVS Age equivalent |
|---|---|---|---|---|---|---|---|
| Autism | | | | | | | |
| A1 | M | 68 | 8:1 | 108 | 79 | 69 | 5.0 |
| A2 | M | 70 | 7:1 | 103 | 92 | 79 | 5.0 |
| A3 | M | 68 | 8:5 | 108 | 109 | 88 | 5.0 |
| A4 | M | 69 | 8:5 | 98 | 89 | 68 | 5.2 |
| A5 | M | 72 | 7:4 | 102 | 92 | 77 | 5.1 |
| A6 | F | 70 | 5:8 | 109 | 100 | 88 | 4.7 |
| A7 | F | 70 | 5:8 | 110 | 102 | 89 | 4.8 |
| A8 | M | 70 | 7:4 | 93 | 87 | 71 | 4.6 |
| Average | | | 7:1 | 104 | 94 | 79 | 4.9 |
| Normal | | | | | | | |
| N1 | F | | 4:4 | 127 | 124 | 102 | 4.4 |
| N2 | M | | 4:0 | 109 | 111 | 106 | 4.4 |
| N3 | F | | 4:5 | 126 | 112 | 99 | 4.3 |
| N4 | M | | 4:9 | 97 | 89 | 97 | 4.6 |
| N5 | F | | 4:9 | 103 | 100 | 92 | 4.1 |
| N6 | M | | 4:9 | 97 | 107 | 94 | 4.3 |
| N7 | M | | 4:4 | 128 | 117 | 100 | 4.2 |
| N8 | M | | 4:6 | 122 | 119 | 101 | 4.5 |
| Average | | | 4:6 | 114 | 110 | 99 | 4.4 |

[a] K-Bit = Kaufman Brief Intelligence Test, BPVS = British Picture Vocabulary Test.

in age from 5.8 years to 8.5 years with a mean of 7.1 years. The normal preschool children were a more homogeneous and significantly younger group with a mean of 4.56 years (range: 4.0 to 4.9). An attempt was made to match normal and autistic children on their general cognitive functioning using the Kaufman Brief Intelligence Test (K-BIT; Kaufman & Kaufman, 1990) and on their language comprehension using the British Picture Vocabulary Scale (BPVS, Dunn, Dunn, Whetton, & Pintilie, 1981).

The groups did not differ significantly in their overall composite standard score, ($M_{\text{autistics}}$ = 103.9, $M_{\text{normal}}$ = 113.6), $t(14)$ = 1.8 $p$ > .05, (see Table III), but autistic children showed significantly lower standard scores on comprehension (BPVS) compared to the normal children ($M_{\text{autistics}}$ = 76.4, $M_{\text{normal}}$ = 98.9) $t(14)$ = 6.9, $p$ < .001. Note, however, that the age equivalence BPVS scores were higher for children with autism ($M_{\text{autistics}}$ = 4.93, $M_{\text{normal}}$ = 4.35), $t(14)$ = 6.2, $p$ < .001 (see Table III). In absolute terms, performance of the autistic children on BPVS and K-BIT was comparable to the normal children; however, as they were older, their standard, age-corrected scores were considerably lower than the normals.

## RESULTS

The principal dependent measure was the number of novel ideas produced during the probe and training sessions. Repeated-measures ANOVA was conducted for the data from the two session types with autism as a between-groups variable. The mean number of novel ideas across sessions was used in another repeated-measures ANOVA contrasting the two session types. The efficacy of autism in predicting production of novel ideas was contrasted with individual differences in unstandardized scores on IQ and comprehension using multiple regression.

### Training Sessions

Compared to normal children, children with autism had a significantly lower number of novel ideas produced in the training sessions ($Ms$ = 2.25 vs. 6.9), $F(1, 14)$ = 27.3, $p$ < .001. There was a trend of greater productivity as the sessions progressed, $F(9, 126)$ = 5.3, $p$ < .01. Figures 1 and 2 reveal that this trend differed across the two groups, $F(9, 126)$ = 2.1, $p$ < .05. The effect of training was more consistent for normal children (see Fig. 3); after 4 to 6 computer sessions these children showed rapid improvement of produced ideas, usually doubling the number of ideas from the initial sessions. For children with autism this trend was variable. An increasing trend was evident for five children whereas three children did not increase their productivity of ideas (Fig. 4). All three subjects (A6, A7, & A8) had the lowest verbal age equivalent (<5 years). They started out with the lowest number of solutions during the baseline sessions.

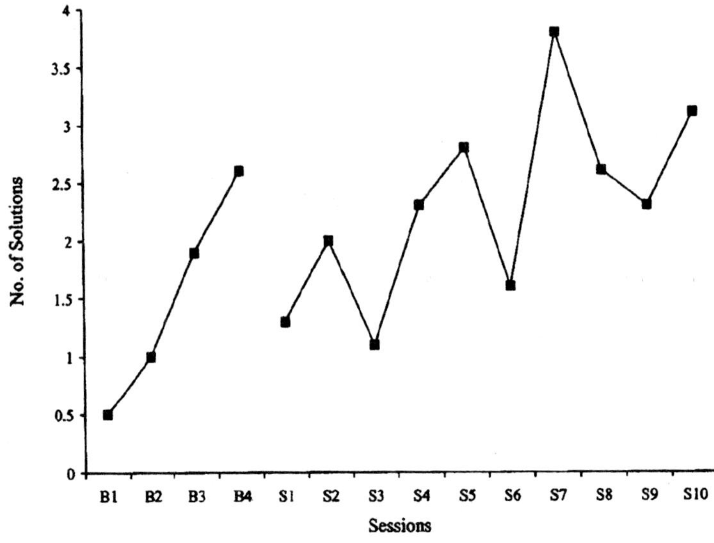


**Fig. 1.** Problem solutions of children with autism.

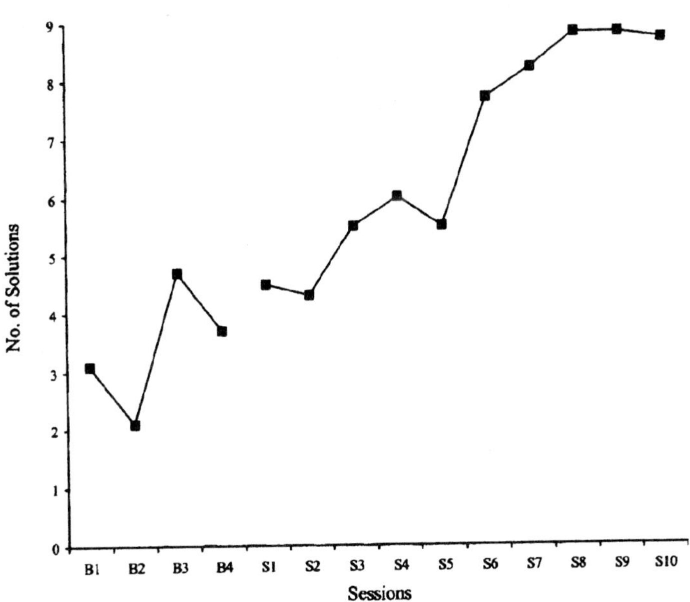

**Fig. 2.** Problem solutions of normal children.

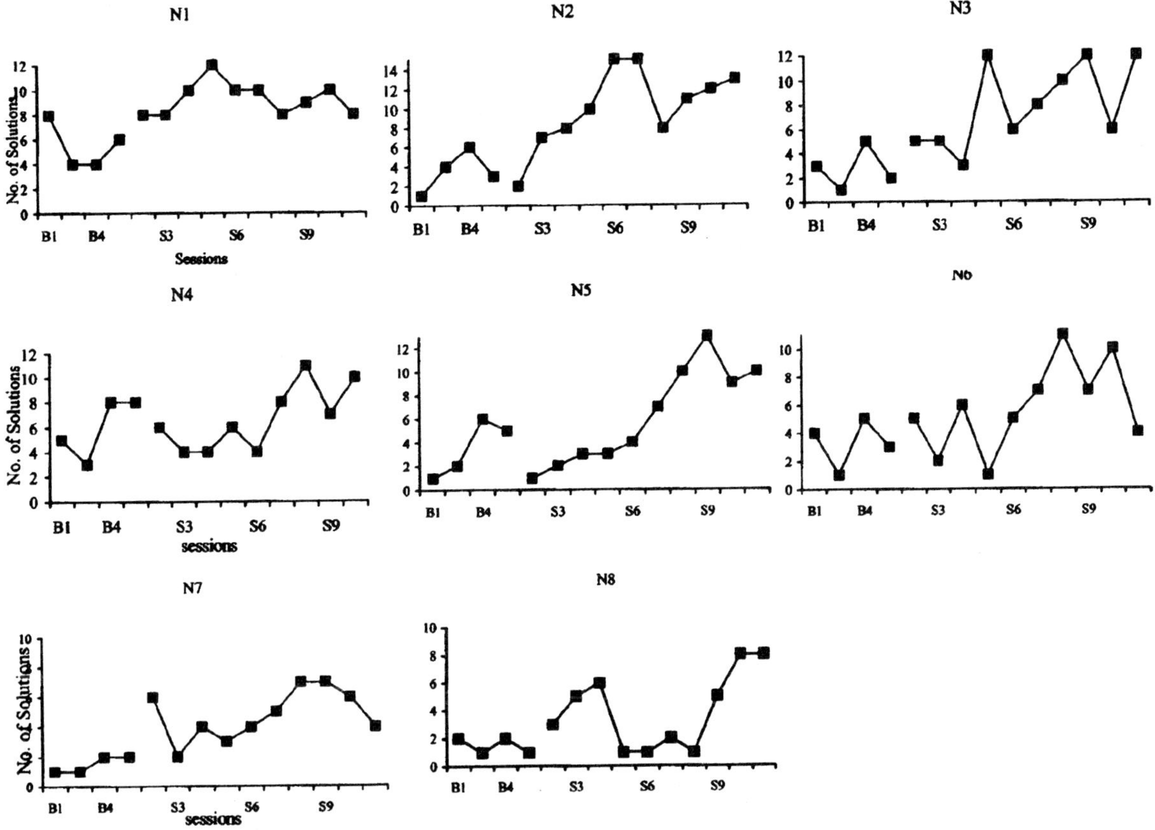

**Fig. 3.** Normal children on producing appropriate solutions

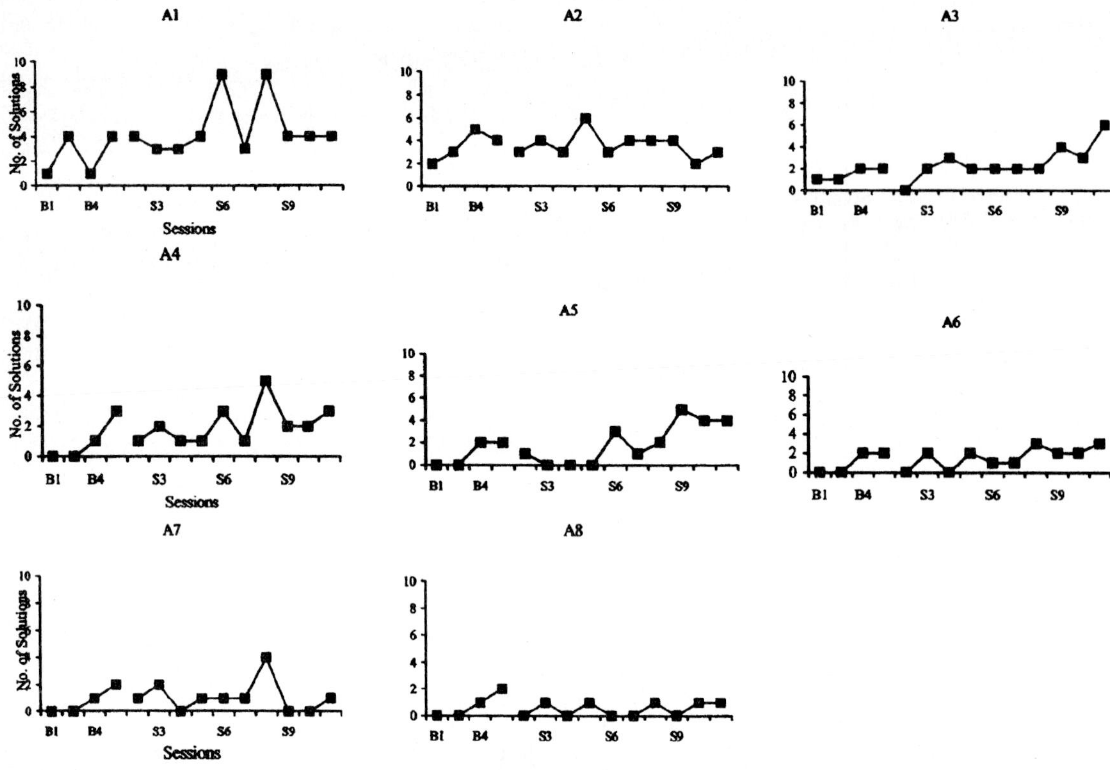

**Fig. 4.** Children with autism on producing appropriate solutions.

### Probe Sessions

A repeated-measures ANOVA revealed that performance in the probe sessions was markedly lower than that in learning sessions (2.47 vs. 4.57), $F(1, 14) = 39.7, p < .001$. The lower productivity of children with autism was also evident in the probe sessions (1.5 vs. 3.4), $F(1, 14) = 8.2, p < .05$. Performance increased across the four probes, $F(3, 42) = 8.9, p < .001$, indicating that the improvement in the training sessions was also reflected by the probes. Even though the number of solutions given during baselines was small (2 to 5 solutions), an increase across probes was observed for seven out of the eight autistic participants (see Fig. 1). This may be considered to be preliminary evidence for the generalization of problem-solving strategies to untrained conflicts for young children with autism.

### Predictors of Productivity

In addition to autism, it is plausible that individual differences in receptive and expressive vocabulary might account for the variability in the production of novel ideas. To test this possibility, we carried out a multiple regression wherein the production of novel ideas was predicted from three variables; autism and unstandardized values of expressive and receptive vocabulary. This regression model accounted for over 70% of the variance ($R^2 = .702$). The productivity of new ideas was solely predicted by autism ($\beta = 1.08$, $t = 3.48, p < .005$); it was unrelated to the absolute values of expressive and receptive vocabulary ($\beta$'s = .153 and .229, $ts = -.41, 1.2, ps > .20$). These results suggest that, in this sample, the productivity of novel ideas was directly related to the diagnostic category of autism. If the regression model excluded autism, the adjusted $R^2$ dropped to .31 from .62 and both the regression coefficients failed to reach significance.

### Comparing Reinforcer Choices for Autistic and Normal Children

Children with autism showed a significant preference for sensory reinforcers over natural reinforcers, which they selected in 61% of the cases. The normal peers preferred them only in 40% of the cases. More important, only one normal child had a value that was in the range of preference for children with autism (Table IV).

## DISCUSSION

The above results affirm that normal and autistic preschool children can be taught social problem solving using animated models of problem solutions presented by a computer. Although the dramatic increase in novel ideas produced by normal preschool children is not surprising, the results also give hope for young autistic children. They complement recent findings on teaching autistic children social skills through video modeling and pictured time schedules (Quill, 1997). Using predictable animation of real life problem settings not only enhanced the production of increasing numbers of solutions but also influenced performance on untrained problems. The improvement in production across probe sessions was present in both groups but was clearer for autistic children. In comparison to normal preschoolers, children with autism favored sensory over natural reinforcement, supporting previous research on sensory stimulation (Rincover, 1978).

Care must be taken in interpreting the data because of limitations regarding the subject sample, the definition of the dependent variable, and the restricted array of trained and tested problem settings. The sample was drawn from autistic children with normal intelligence, a population that constitutes only about 25% of the general population of children with autism. Although participants with autism learned to produce novel ideas, their productivity of problem solutions was significantly lower than that of normal children. Using predictable animation of real life problem settings not only enhanced the production of increasing numbers of solutions but also influenced performance on untrained problems.

The developed software package encompassed conflicts in taking turns, communicating, and bargaining, which have been described in the problem-solving program by Shure (1992). Although these problems seemed important for the included children, they are just a small selection from the vast array of potential conflict situations.

The dependent variable was the number of appropriate problem solutions. This might not necessarily be an appropriate indicator of adequate problem solving even though this criterion is also adopted by problem-solving programs that require the generation of alternative solutions (Camp & Bash, 1985).

Our study focused only on the children's responding during a computer program and did not assess generalization to real life settings or other tests on problem solving. A recent study in our laboratory indicates that generalization of problem solving to real life settings critically depends on the similarity between the simulated and in vivo problems. In a crossover multiple baseline design across four children with autism, the computer-presented problem of getting help to reach the rambutan fruits on a tree generalized to the real setting of a helium balloon out of reach, but did not generalize to a bargaining situation, which had not been trained (Tan, 2000).

Observational data indicated that the autistic children enjoyed the programs, while the normal preschool children showed signs of boredom in the later sessions of the study. Objective enthusiasm assessment and social validity measures would serve as useful collateral data in future studies.

There are several implications of our research. Simulating social problem solving with the aid of computer programs might be a possible new avenue to enhance social problem solving for normal children as well as high-level children with autism. Whether behavior learned in the computer setting generalizes to the real setting might depend on the similarity of the trained problem to the untrained problem (Tan, 2000). Further research is necessary to identify problem

**Table IV.** Percentage of Recognized and Sensory Choices

| Participant | Recognized problems (%) | Sensory choices (%) |
| --- | --- | --- |
| **Autism** | | |
| A1 | 100 | 50 |
| A2 | 100 | 50 |
| A3 | 100 | 72 |
| A4 | 90 | 47 |
| A5 | 100 | 87 |
| A6 | 100 | 66 |
| A7 | 100 | 62 |
| A8 | 100 | 57 |
| Total | 98 | 61 |
| **Normal** | | |
| N1 | 100 | 41 |
| N2 | 100 | 41 |
| N3 | 95 | 43 |
| N4 | 97 | 43 |
| N5 | 97 | 15 |
| N6 | 97 | 56 |
| N7 | 93 | 38 |
| N8 | 100 | 40 |
| Total | 97 | 40 |

settings relevant for the development of social skills in people with autism across the life-span. It also seems important to compare teaching methods aimed at standard social scripts and the development of cognitive sets such as the set in our study to have another "good idea." Further exploration is required to determine whether brainstorming skills acquired through computer programs can lead to general increases in flexible thinking. Teaching of cognitive sets regarding "good/new ideas" or "try a new way" might be a relevant pivotal skill (Koegel & Frea, 1993) to counter the rigidity of people with autism in social interactions, communication, play, or insistence on sameness.

Properly designed, computer programs can assist the teaching of conflict solutions, brainstorming, and consequential thinking to young children, from age 4 years onwards. Such programs exemplify the possibility of teaching components of emotional intelligence to parents and teachers. Since self-help books and books on emotions for young children have sold in the millions (Berry, 1995), computer programs with this focus might also have a similar potential. They also might give parents and educators a demonstration of alternative thinking strategies in conflict situations, self-management methods, and the power of reinforcement (Meichenbaum, 1976).

In the Asian context, parents and teachers seem more accepting of computer programs than role-play, think-aloud strategies, or self-control exercises that have similar goals. While the local education system increasingly recognizes the need to incorporate thinking skills, creativity, and emotional intelligence into the curriculum, parents and teachers continue to place high priority on reading, writing, and arithmetic. About 50% of all Singaporean children receive tuition, starting from kindergarten, targeting the 3 Rs. This bias in favor of literacy and numeracy ignores findings suggesting that school success depends crucially on emotional and social variables rather than hinging entirely on factual knowledge and reading skills (Head Start, 1992).

For children, adolescents, and adults with autism, computer programs modeling everyday conflicts and their solutions might be a possible avenue to reduce problem behavior in real-life settings, teach divergent and consequential thinking, and appropriate social scripts. Multidisciplinary approaches, involving educational specialists, psychologists, programmers as well as parents and their child with autism, could be useful. Although real-life practice remains the most important part of social problem solving, computer-based simulations might be a nonthreatening starting point for individuals with autism, contributing to the facilitation of better social and communicative competence.

## ACKNOWLEDGMENTS

This article is based on research made possible by a grant (RP981007) from the National University of Singapore. We very much appreciate the thoughtful comments of the reviewers.

## REFERENCES

Baron-Cohen, S., Leslie, A. M., & Frith, U. (1985). Does the autistic child have a "Theory of Mind"? *Cognition, 21*, 37–46.

Berry, J. (1995). *Let's talk about saying "no" feeling angry/feeling afraid etc.* New York: Scholastic.

Camp, B. W., & Bash, M. A. (1985). *Think aloud: Increasing social and cognitive skills.* Champaign, IL: Research Press.

Dunn, L. M., Dunn, L. M., Whetton, C., & Pintilie, D. (1981). *British Picture Vocabulary Test.* CITY: NFER-Nelson.

Elias, M. J. (1992). *Social decision making in the middle school.* Gaithersbury, MD: Aspen.

Goleman, D. (1997). *Emotional intelligence.* CITY: Deutscher Taschenbuch Verlag.

Goleman, D. (1998). *Working with emotional intelligence.* New York: Boston Books.

Happé, F. G. E. (1994). An advanced test of theory of mind: Understanding of story characters' thoughts and feelings by able autistics, mentally handicapped and normal children and adults. *Journal of Autism and Developmental Disorders, 24*, 129–154.

Head Start. (1992). *The emotional foundations of school readiness.* CITY: National Center for Clinical Infant Programs.

Heiman, M., Nelson, K. E., Tjus, T., & Gilberg, C. (1995). Increasing reading and communication skills in children with autism through an interactive multimedia program. *Journal of Autism and Developmental Disorders, 25*, 459–480.

Hobson, R. P., Ouston, J., & Lee A. (1989). Naming emotion in faces and voices: Abilities and disabilities in autism and mental retardation. *British Journal of Developmental Psychology, 7*, 237–250.

Howlin, P., & Baron-Cohen, S. (1999). *Teaching children with autism to mindread.* New York: Wiley.

Kaufman, A. S., & Kaufman, N. L. (1990). *Kaufman Brief Intelligence Test.* Circle Pines, MN: American Guidance Service.

Koegel, R. L., & Frea, W. D. (1993). Treatment of social behavior in autism through the modification of pivotal social skills. *Journal of Applied Behavior Analysis, 26*, 369–377.

Krug, D. A., Arick, J. R., & Almond, P. G. (1979). Autism screening instrument for educational planning: Background and development. In J. Gilliam (Ed.), *Autism: Diagnosis, instruction, management and research.* Austin, TX: University of Texas Press.

Meichenbaum, D. H. (1976). Self-instructional methods. In F. Kanfer & A. Goldstein (Eds.), *Helping people change.* New York: Pergamon.

Ozonoff, S., & Miller, J. N. (1995). Teaching theory of mind: A new approach to social skills training for individuals with autism. *Journal of Autism and Developmental Disorders, 25*, 415–433.

Prior, M., & Ozonoff, S. (1998). Psychological factors in autism. In F. R. Volkmar (Ed.), *Autism and pervasive developmental disorders.* CITY: Cambridge University Press.

Quill, K. A. (1997). Instructional considerations for the young children with autism: The rationale for visually cued instruction. *Journal of Autism and Developmental Disorders, 27*, 697–714.

Rincover, A. (1978). Variables affecting stimulus fading and discriminative responding in psychotic children. *Journal of Abnormal Psychology, 87*.

Shure (1992). *I can problem solve: An interpersonal cognitive problem-solving program for children.* Champaign, IL: Research Press.

Tan Hey Li J. (2000). *Teaching children with autism social problem-solving skills through computer-assisted instruction.* Academic Exercise, Dept. of Social Work & Psychology, National University of Singapore.

Volkmar, F. R., Cohen, D. J., Bergman, J. D., Hooks, M. Y., & Stevenson, J. M. (1989). An examination of social typologies in autism. *Journal of the American Academy of Child and Adolescent Psychiatry, 28*, 82–86.

Wing, L. (1990). What is Autism? In K. Ellis (Ed.), *Autism: Professional perspectives and practice* (Chap. 1). London: Chapman & Hall.

# Design and Development of Computer-Aided Chemical Systems: Virtual Labs for Teaching Chemical Experiments in Undergraduate and Graduate Courses

I. Luque Ruiz,* E. López Espinosa, G. Cerruela García, and M. A. Gómez-Nieto

Department of Computing and Numerical Analysis, University of Córdoba, Campus Universitario de Rabanales, Edificio C2, Planta-3, E-14071 Córdoba, Spain

Received February 28, 2001

An environment for the construction of virtual chemistry experiments is presented. This environment is based on the $E(V) = M + m$ model—*Experiment (Virtual) = Materials + method*—proposed and described herein, which allows the representation and subsequent building of chemistry experiments in virtual 3D worlds to any degree of complexity. The object-based nature of the environment not only allows its use on the Internet but also facilitates integration with other systems, while enabling the system to represent and organize knowledge in such a way that it is available to any teaching environment dealing with chemical laboratory experiments.

## 1. INTRODUCTION

While problems arising in the teaching of chemistry at high school, graduate, and undergraduate level may not be vastly different from those of other experimental disciplines, they are still specific to the practical teaching of chemistry and require a directed approach, as described in other studies. The need exists for an adaptation of methods and teaching media to the new computer technologies since students are well-aware of and influenced by the latest developments in computer technology at a practical or sociocultural level and will also be required to work in computer-oriented environments.[1-6]

The efforts of the chemical community to adopt these new technologies may be clearly seen in the great number of studies published, particularly in the past decade, and in the vast amount of information, which is today available on the Internet.[7-18] Public and private organizations, high schools, universities, and professionals in the private sector have been producing—for general or restricted access—an ever-increasing stream of teaching material of varying degrees of complexity for the use of students and professionals in the world of chemistry teaching.

This published material may be grouped as follows:

**Tutorials**: teaching material dealing with specific aspects of chemistry and found as hypertext documents (html) or formatted for one of the standard word processors.[20,21]

**Support software**: small-to-mid-sized software programs aimed at both teaching and enabling the student to solve chemical problems, or storage, retrieval and processing of chemical information. This software is mainly directed at areas such as periodic table information, balancing reactions, detailed composition, calculation of molecular masses, viewing molecular structures, interpretation of spectra, etc. In many cases, the software is accompanied by tutorials that "explain" the basics and the chemical, mathematical, and deductive processes to follow in order to solve the given problem.[21-26]

In this group and closely related to the foregoing we have intelligent tutorial systems (ITS), including such categories as simulations (the prevailing category), learning systems and knowledge-based systems.[27-30]

**Laboratory software**: software designed to simulate teaching lab experiments. Such products have recently come much to the fore, with teaching and research centers investing great effort in development owing to reasons discussed in the next section of this paper. Applications in this category would include the following: *Chemlab*, an excellent computer-based lab simulator that includes a wide range of experiments such as acid−base titration, precipitation, manipulation of materials, gravimetric analysis, calorimetry, and reaction kinetics and comes with utilities that would otherwise be classed within the other aforementioned groups, *Electro-Chemical Cells Pro*, which allows the performance of redox experiments in a 2D environment, and the *IrYdium Project*, software developed by the University of Massachusetts, which comprises a 2D virtual lab developed in Java and where lab experiments can be designed and carried out. Further commercial programs are listed in the literature.[31-33]

As interest in the development of virtual labs soars, there arises a series of issues with respect to chemistry teaching and found in a great number of recent programs, namely the following:

1. They are developed for a fixed platform or operating system, which reduces the number of possible users.

2. Some require local installation for their use and will only run on that local model, while others may be run solely on the World Wide Web.

3. In some cases one (or a small set) of the experiments is predefined, together with parameters, materials, and all the physicochemical items required to run it, leaving the user unable to modify, much less expand, the experiment.

4. The user interface does not present the user with a virtual lab environment; at best there is a classical 2D

---

* Corresponding author phone: +34-957-212082; fax: +34-957-218630; e-mail: ma1lurui@uco.es.

interface, although some systems do provide a 3D view of molecular structures.

5. Only occasionally do these systems present a global approach to the teaching of experiments, providing the user with teaching material (tutorials), exercises, and observations, alongside experimental procedures and a dialogue system to assist in learning.

Furthermore, the bulk of this developed material is either privately held or cannot be reused by other systems due to being written in different languages or operational modes and sometimes to different standards, all of which means that educators are forced to expend effort in the redundant construction of teaching materials using the new technologies.

The present study describes the $E(V) = M + m$ model—*Experiment (Virtual) = Materials + method)*—for the building of chemistry lab experiments in a virtual environment. The model is suitable for use in the construction of an ITS, as it offers the following features: (1) inclusion of the teaching component, since content may be ordered and sequentialized for adaptation to both the student and the experiment; (2) simple representation of the domain of the problem (the experiment), specialized in blocks ordered according to the teaching process; (3) easy integration of other modules forming part of the ITS, such as that of the student, as well as the integration of other refinements; and (4) a communication interface created in line with current standards (based in windows interface), which facilitates user-system interaction.

This paper first describes the objectives of the study and then in section 3 provides a description of the proposed paradigm. The description includes specification of the structure and content of experiments in an object-oriented model, allowing both the classification of knowledge in learning blocks and its sequencing in the teaching process. Section 4 describes the operating prototype and its static operational architecture, closing with a discussion of the work that mentions future projects and enhancements currently under development.

## 2. OBJECTIVES AND BASIS OF THE MODEL

The present project aims to tackle certain of the problems reported in the teaching of chemistry lab experiments; as with other researchers, the present authors believe that the new technologies may contribute toward a solution.[4,6-8,10,30-33]

Generally speaking, these teaching problems may be broken down as follows:

**1. Cost**: the high cost to educational centers incurred by practical classes, where substantial investment in instruments, apparatus, reagents, and so on may frequently result in fewer lab sessions, often determined by expenditure.

**2. Safety**: especially in the case of high school students, the risk involved in manipulating chemicals and certain instruments and materials leads to the avoidance of dangerous experiments and cuts down on practice time.

**3. Time**: the shortage of time allocated to practical work in current curricula means that very few experiments can be performed; equally, the student will have little or no chance of repeating the task for greater understanding and learning.

**4. Space/Size**: lab space and the size of student groups attending practice sessions, in addition to the abovementioned factors, will sometimes mean that not all students may be involved in the manipulation of materials involved in the experiment.

**5. Lack of motivation**: the 21st century student requires motivational techniques adapted to the present day. These should encourage the use of modern technology in the same way the student uses this technology to carry out everyday social activities. The teaching of practical chemistry through traditional lab sessions does not, however, greatly promote student participation, perhaps then calling for the introduction of modern technology.

All these issues present a complex situation for teaching centers relying on conventional techniques and procedures; the introduction of modern methods and procedures should, however, provide an answer for at least some of these problems, while increasing student motivation.[1,2,8-10]

In the foregoing section, reference was made to ongoing studies aimed at tackling these problems; great effort has been made to adapt the new technologies to the teaching of chemical knowledge—theory, concepts, techniques, and procedures.

Clearly then, many teachers and researchers believe that use of the computer, and particulary Internet, can motivate the student, while reducing attendance requirements and thus the cost, risks, and so on involved in the teaching of chemistry. However, the form in which such knowledge is placed at the disposal of the student and how it is used may have a direct effect on its success.

The present study is based on a solution that, making use of the latest technology, allows the interactive transference of knowledge, making the most of resources in an environment of shared experiments and results and should lead to greatly increased student motivation.

To achieve these objectives, the authors propose the following:

1. Chemistry practical work should be split between traditional, hands-on teaching (where possible), and computer-based virtual experiments performed on the Internet (again, where possible).

2. Teaching resources employed should be available in the public domain. In other words, both the required software resources and the theoretical and practical content should be available for use by anyone with Internet access.

3. The technological or virtual teaching content should permit the reuse of software applications and their content.

4. The online aspect of teaching should be enacted using virtual laboratories where any kind of chemistry experiment could be performed, from any location or computer.

5. Chemistry experiments should be able to be performed at varying levels of complexity, in line with different educational grades.

6. Experimental content should be reusable, allowing its partial or complete use in the building of new experiments.

7. The performance of such practical work should involve the technical training of the student in line with the complexity of carrying out the experiment.

Thus, virtual labs may be viewed as another type of ITS where a suitable ontological model is used to build system components based on "chunks" of knowledge.[28-30,34,35]

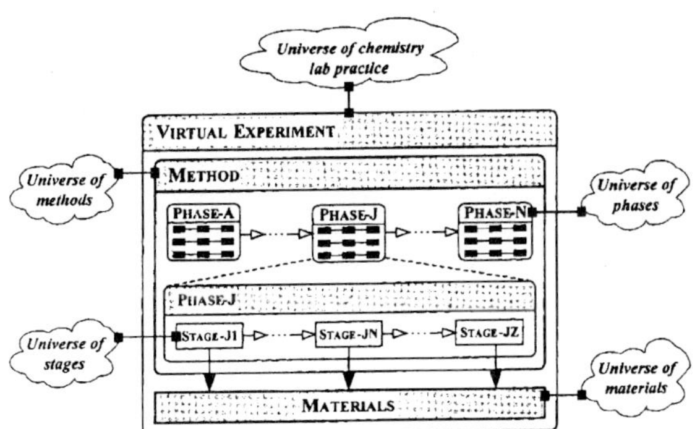

**Figure 1.** Context diagram of the $E(V) = M + m$ paradigm.

## 3. THE $E(V) = M + m$ PARADIGM

The paradigm $E(V) = M + m$—*Experiment(Virtual) = Materials + method*—which we propose in this paper is based on the concept that a virtual experiment may be described by a method which uses a set of materials.

The paradigm employed is based on the supposition that a virtual experiment may be described by a method which uses a set of materials.

Running a virtual experiment, performed in an interactive computer environment using a system of dialogues, the user may experience a 3D presentation simulating a chemistry experiment. Each experiment takes place in a virtual environment containing all the materials with which the user might interact—the virtual laboratory. Labs may be shared by multiple experiments and may also be built using different technologies and software, so user interaction will depend on the technology employed to build them.

Each virtual experiment has an objective and is thus accompanied by descriptive content aimed at delivering knowledge for the user to learn. While the nature and extent of the experimental content may be highly varied, presentation and user interaction is independent of the experiment.

This standardization of presentation and user interaction facilitates assimilation and leads to the user easily adapting to the virtual learning model.

Each experiment has a unique associated method. A method is a precise description of the tasks and resources used in the experiment.

Each method comprises structure and content. The structure of the method lists the processes to be carried out during the experiment, while the content includes all necessary information and the way in which this is manipulated therein.

The method's structure is made up of a sequence of phases. Each phase involves a global task or activity performed during the experiment, which may be broken down into further elementary tasks called stages.

The level of abstraction for the method's structure is independent of the method and thus of the experiment, thus allowing any experiment to be described at various levels of complexity.

This structural breakdown of an experiment, in which different knowledge blocks are organized chronologically in a working network, is a key factor in user learning.[5,35]

Figure 1 shows a context diagram of the paradigm $E(V) = M + m$. It may be seen that a virtual experiment represents the knowledge of a laboratory experiment through a method structured in phases, which in turn are divided into

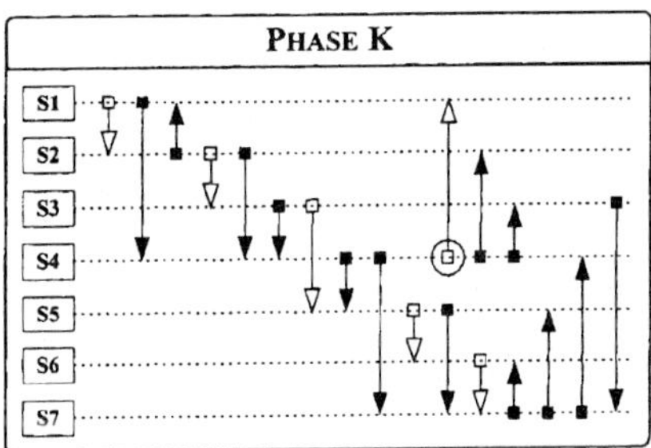

**Figure 2.** Diagram showing permitted transitions for phase-k.

stages where the materials are manipulated. These structural elements of experiments are extracted from a general universe, enabling them to be reused in the same or indeed in a different experiment.

**3.1. Structure of the $E(V) = M + m$ Paradigm.** Let us now examine the structural elements of the model using a bottom-up approach, according to complexity.

**3.1.1. Stages.** Stages are basic tasks in the structural description of an experiment. Depending on the level of detail required for the description of an experiment, a task may vary from a simple manipulation such as "Obtain a pipet" to one like "Obtain a pipet, fill it, and empty the contents into an Erlenmeyer flask".

Stages imply manual or automated processes carried out in the lab and involving some laboratory material.

They are distributed throughout the experiment, grouped in *Phases*. Within a phase, stages comprise a sequence of tasks that may be described by one or more directed graphs.

Take a *phase-j* consisting of "Pour 10 mL HCl from the stock bottle into an Erlenmeyer flask". This phase may be defined by the following stages:

| | |
|---|---|
| **PJS1** | Obtain a 10 mL pipet from the rack. |
| **PJS2** | Pipet 10 mL HCl from the bottles. |
| **PJS3** | Empty the pipet's contents into the Erlenmeyer flask. |

Clearly the only possible order to carry out the stages from *phase-j* would here be **PJS1, PJS2, PJS3**.

Suppose now that we wish to represent the same process in greater detail—*phase-k*:

| | |
|---|---|
| **PKS1** | Obtain a 10 mL pipet from the rack. |
| **PKS2** | Open the bottle of concentrated HCl. |
| **PKS3** | Pipet 10 mL HCl from the bottle. |
| **PKS4** | Take the Erlenmeyer flask from the shelf and place on the bench. |
| **PKS5** | Empty the pipet's contents into the Erlenmeyer flask |
| **PKS6** | Place the pipet in the sink. |
| **PKS7** | Close the bottle of concentrated HCl. |

Figure 2 contains a transition diagram[36] showing the different routes that could be taken to perform *phase-k* (for a clearer description, the user is assumed to be reasonably skilled). Again in Figure 2, stages are represented by labeled boxes: shaded boxes show stages that could be the start of *phase-k* (*S1, S2, S4*), and the arrows indicate the transitions allowed between stages. If when performing *phase-k* the user chose to begin at stage *S1*, the next permissible stage would be *S2* or *S4*. If the user opted to follow the transition to *S2*, the next stage could be either *S3* or *S4*.

If the transition to *S3* were chosen, the next move would have to be to *S4*, since getting to *S5* would suppose a transition prior to *S3*, that is, an Erlenmeyer flask must be present.

Alternatively, if the user had decided upon a transition to *S4*, the next move must be to *S3*, since moving on to *S5* would require a transition prior to stage *S3*, that is, the pipet has to be filled, and moving to *S7* would mean that not all the transitions to all the stages of *phase-k* could be completed by any of the existing routes.

Thus, if *phase-k* is started at *S1* it can be performed suitably or correctly by the system using any of the following routes:

| | | | |
|---|---|---|---|
| **R1**: | S1, S2, S3, S4, S5, S6, S7 | **R2**: | S1, S2, S3, S4, S5, S7, S6 |
| **R3**: | S1, S2, S3, S4, S7, S5, S6 | **R4** | S1, S2, S4, S3, S5, S6, S7 |
| **R5**: | S1, S2, S4, S3, S5, S7, S6 | **R6**: | S1, S2, S4, S3, S7, S5, S6 |
| **R7**: | S1, S4, S2, S3, S5, S6, S7 | **R8**: | S1, S4, S2, S3, S5, S7, S6 |
| **R9**: | S1, S4, S2, S3, S7, S5, S6 | | |

White arrows in Figure 2 show the permitted route that is considered, on defining *phase-k*, as the most recommendable and which will be taken into account by the system for the automatic execution of this phase without user intervention.

At each stage at least one **Material** is required for manipulation. The use of a material on occasion implies the presence of other materials, as shown by **PKS3** where a pipet is used—thus implying the existence of the bottle of concentrated HCl. Manipulation of material implies the following: (1) the presence of the material as well as those materials thereby affected and (2) a condition where the material manipulated and any other intervening material are in such a state that the manipulation may be successfully performed.

In the same foregoing example of **PKS3** the bottle of HCl must be open to allow the pipetting of 10 mL (a prior transition to **PKS2** has taken place) and the pipet has already been obtained (a prior transition to **PKS1** has occurred).

Thus, Figure 2 shows all the possible transitions that represent manipulation processes involving *phase-k*. However, from any given stage only some of these transitions will be allowed for the performance of *phase-k*, depending on the transitions previously carried out and therefore on the current state of the material.

The permitted routes for the user to perform a generic phase *n* will be those that (1) run through, with no repetition, all of the stages comprising *phase-n* and (2) for any given stage perform only those transitions that do not violate the priorities existing between the stages of *phase-n*, as defined by the state of the material.

**3.1.2. Phases.** Phases are global elements in the task network that detail a method and group together stages, amounting to a general task. Regarding an experiment, a phase is an activity that leads to an elementary step in the experiment and in which a recognizable, measurable result is produced.

Like stages, phases may be defined to varying degrees of abstraction and thus represent experimental activity at different levels of complexity. For example, an experiment to titrate 0.1 M NaOH with 0.1 N HCl may be either described as a single phase consisting of the titration process or said to comprise the following sequence of phases:

| | |
|---|---|
| P1 | Prepare a 0.1 M NaOH solution. |
| P2 | Prepare a 0.1 N HCl solution. |
| P3 | Titrate 0.1 M NaOH with 0.1 N HCl. |

Again in the same way as stages, phases are laid out in a time-ordered route throughout a **Method** that describes a virtual experiment.

**3.1.3. Methods.** Methods describe the structure and chronological route of activities as occurring in the course of an **Experiment**. A method is an abstract sequence of procedures representing the tasks to be carried out, the material to be used and its manipulation in order to successfully perform a chemistry experiment.

Since phases and stages may be described at various levels of abstraction, one laboratory experiment can be described by different methods at various levels of complexity, but as shall be seen in the next section (description of content), the user may carry out an experiment using a method at various levels of interaction according to the level of detail and complexity sought for the interaction.

**3.1.4. Experiments.** The term "experiments" is used to describe practical laboratory experiments whose operational technique and underlying knowledge are to be passed on to the student through a virtual environment.

In the $E(V) = M + m$ paradigm, an experiment is defined as the use of a method to manipulate a set of **Materials**. Thus each experiment has an associated method that is described by the phases and stages in which the materials are employed.

Furthermore, an experiment has an associated virtual world containing the materials to be used and where the activities described in its associated method are carried out.

**3.1.5. Materials.** Materials represent the physical elements recognized in the virtual world or laboratory associated with an experiment and which can be used therein.

The materials category embraces a great variety of laboratory items, differentiated by their properties and associated functionalities.

Hence, the context of material includes such diverse items as chemicals (e.g. existing products), furniture (e.g. lab benches), material (e.g. glassware), or instruments (e.g. pH meters).

**3.2. Content of the $E(V) = M + m$ Paradigm.** Modeling of the $E(V) = M + m$ paradigm was performed using the object-oriented paradigm, and complies with the UML standard.[37,38] Using the object model, a system can be described by a set of objects listing the properties and behavior of the system and each of its component parts.

The class diagram in Figure 3 shows the main entities of the static model representing the $E(V) = M + m$ paradigm, as follows:

A *Component* is considered to be any object existing in the system and may in turn be formed by other components.

The *Component* class is an abstract generalization class. By the term "abstract" we mean that objects belonging to the generalization class must be refined to one of the specialization classes of which it is composed.[38] The dynamic keyword shown in Figure 3 is a UML stereotype. When a stereotype is applied to an element such as a node or a class, new elements related to the vocabulary of a domain are being introduced; these are like primitive building blocks. Each stereotype may provide its own set of labeled values, semantics, notation, and so on.

Here, the stereotype enables us to indicate that the generalizations may be updated for a given object. When a

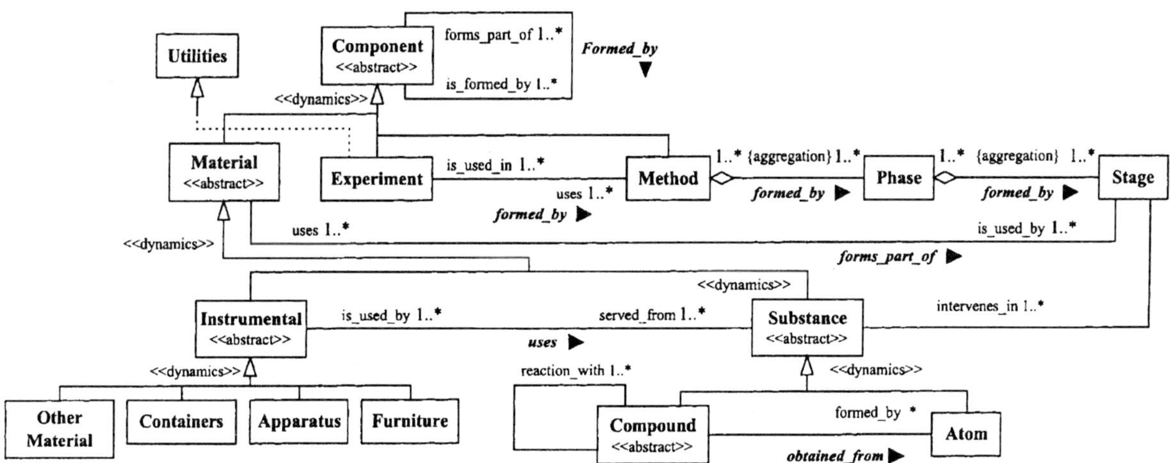



**Figure 3.** Class diagram of the proposed model.

relationship has been marked as nondynamic, nontransferable in ERD notation (*Entity-Relationship Diagram*), once the object has been refined its type cannot be changed.[38]

A series of components is constructed, stored in a library, and then used by a determined method, in a determined form and following a fixed timeline for the performance of an experiment, which in itself may be another component. A few examples of the objects included in this class would be the following: a decanting method, a precipitation flask, an experiment for the titration of NaOH with HCl, filter paper, a funnel, lab scales, etc.

The *Method* class is a dynamic specialization of the *Component* class and as such inherits all the attributes and methods of the *Component* generalization class. Each object contained in this class represents a procedure through which tasks are carried out in a determined order so that an experiment may be performed, thus describing a time-based view of phases, each of which comprises a series of stages in which a task is performed.

The *Phase* class is a dynamic specialization of the *Method* class. Each of the objects contained in this class represents the different parts or global steps to be completed in the course of an experiment. A phase will include one or a set of stages, its structure being determined by the level of abstraction employed in the representation.

The *Stage* class is a dynamic specialization of the *Method* class. Each object contained in this class represents the elementary functions or activities carried out in the various steps or phases employed in a given experiment following a given method. The activity represented will be as complex as the level of abstraction or detail used to represent an operation performed in the lab.

The *Experiment* class is a dynamic specialization of the *Component* class and therefore inherits all its attributes and methods. Each object from this class represents the basic lab operations which permit the discovery, checking, and demonstration of the most common chemistry phenomena, situations, or scientific principles, within a virtual environment.

The *Material* class is a dynamic specialization of the *Component* class while in turn acting as an abstract generalization class (objects belonging to the class must be refined

to one of the specialization classes) of the *Instrumental* and *Substance* classes.

A Material object is characterized by its properties and functionality. Properties distinguish one material from another, in turn characterizing and identifying it. Its functionality determines how the material may be used in experiments.

The *Instrument* class is a dynamic specialization of the *Material* class and in turn acts as an abstract generalization of the *Other Material, Containers, Apparati*, and *Furniture* classes. Each object from this class represents materials commonly used in the lab.

The *Substance* class is a dynamic specialization of the *Material* class and in turn acts as an abstract generalization of the *Atom and Compound* classes. Each object contained in this class represents the basic elements of which the material is formed and which intervene in the chemical processes, mainly in reactions.

The *Utilities* class is an interface which is implemented by *Experiment* class. The *Utilities* class is in charged to represent information and methods used in the development of experiments (e.g. to obtain the molecular weight, concentration of compounds in different magnitudes, etc.).

**3.2.1. Classes in the $E(V) = M + m$ Paradigm.** The object classes shown in Figure 3 allow the representation of the proposed paradigm. These classes include in their definition the properties and behavior that each of the system components may exhibit through the methods.

Properties characterizing these classes may be divided into the following groups:

**Identifiers**: responsible for the unique identification of each of the objects from the class, both by the system at runtime and storage and by the user when accessing and loading data. For example, the identifier and name of each stage.

**Descriptors**: responsible for the concise description of particular class objects. The aim here is to provide the user with quick, concise, and accurate information about objects accessed. For instance, the description of a stage, danger warnings, theoretical content, and information on the material employed.

**Definers**: responsible for the representation of information (distinct from the foregoing kind) characterizing class objects. Their function is to store any relevant information for the characterization of the objects employed to deliver knowledge and/or perform the virtual experiment. For example, information dealing with the obligatory nature of a step or phase, whether it is to be viewed or only used for internal operations, the dimensions and capacity of material, its location, or the composition and properties of a substance.

**Executors**: these represent the runtime characteristics of the objects. Designed to inform the system how each object will behave in its interaction with the user, they might include information on how to manipulate materials or valid timelines for the performance of experiments (the sequence of stages and phases, calculation of physicochemical parameters, etc.)

**Visualizers**: these store and show visual data for the virtual process that will accompany objects. For instance, images of the material, visual effects for the stages and phases, the appropriate virtual world, and so on.

**Documentation**: description of both the chemistry knowledge and the manual or automatic process accompanying the class objects. This covers the storage of aspects such as the chemistry concepts required, the experimental process, expected results, material required, or the operational process to be followed. For example: information about material, chemical substances, reactants, theoretical basis, or the extent and purpose of the experiment.

Likewise, the methods describing class behavior may be grouped as follows:

**constructors**: responsible for the generation of new class objects when the user defines and/or builds a new component.

**destroyers**: for the removal of objects that are no longer required.

**modifiers**: to modify object properties.

**browsers**: to allow access to the objects present. The aim here is to provide the user with a wide range of ways to access both the object database and memory during runtime.

**executors**: to perform the tasks specified in the processes defining the experiments. They should be able to run an experiment automatically as well as checking and ensuring the user carries out the tasks required of an experiment by following one of the ways defined in the experiment's task network. Executors are also responsible for object management in the virtual world using the information stored by objects in their properties along with that gained by user interaction.

Figure 4 shows, by way of example, a (partial) definition of the Stage class, indicating the various types of properties and methods described above.

## 4. CONSTRUCTION OF THE SYSTEM

An operational prototype of the proposed model has been built and is currently undergoing tests. It has been developed using the Java programming language, which is platform-independent and should run on any computer. The user interface has been created using Java applets that can be instantiated on most of the currently available browsers.

Information is handled by the Oracle 8i.X database manager. The object-relational features of Oracle 8i.X permits the correct implementation of the class model described in the previous section. Moreover, this DBMS allows the storage of Java and VRML procedures in the very nucleus of the database alongside SQL procedure, in addition to storing media attributes such as images and files in the

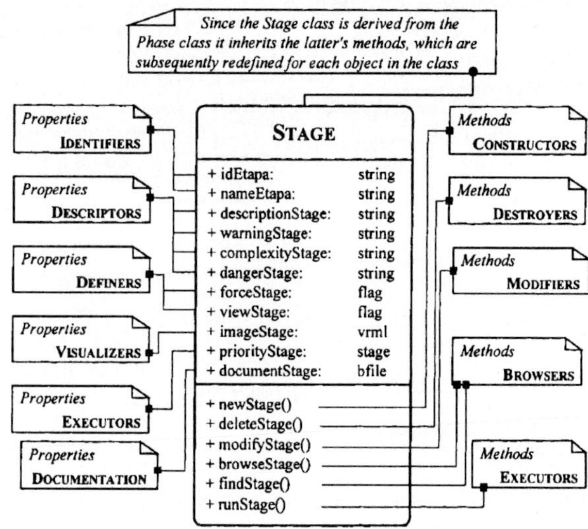


**Figure 4.** Property and method types in the model classes.

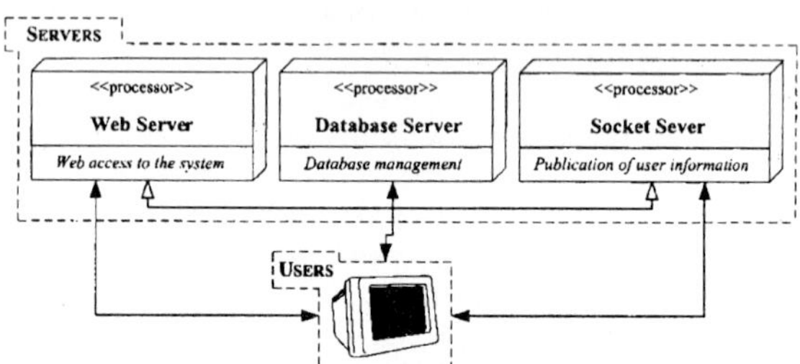


**Figure 5.** Deployment diagram of system statics.

definition of the table structure, which facilitates and enhances the development and performance of procedures.[39,41]

The virtual world (the labs) and its components (materials) were developed under VRML 2.0, along with utilities to permit the graphical construction of these elements and their generation in VRML format.[42,43]

**4.1. System Architecture.** Figure 5 shows a deployment diagram of the system statics. It may be seen that there are three differentiated layers for user interaction via any computer with a graphical interface, Java, and a VRML plug-in.[44,45]

The *Web Server* provides access to the system and its working environment; it contains the entire hierarchy of directories comprising the website.

Closely related to the *Web Server* we have the *Socket Server*, running on the same machine, and this is responsible for publishing, in the directory hierarchy of the *Web Server*, any information fed in by the user, which might be accessed by other users (e.g. VRML images of components, explanatory documentation for an experiment, etc.) The *Socket Server* is constantly listening to its clients (users) and must translate and publish on the *Web Server* relevant files that are physically resident on users' computers.

Finally, the *Database Server* is the home of all the information about lab components (containers, apparati, etc.) and of the experiments, methods, phases, and steps that have been defined. This server provides all the information required for the creation of new experiments or the running of existing ones.

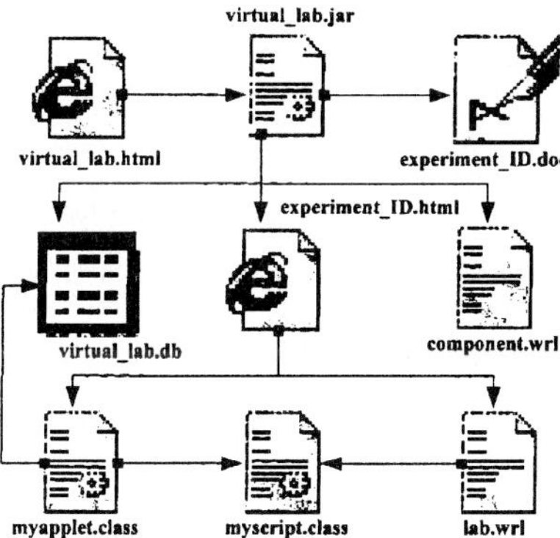

**Figure 6.** Deployment diagram of system dynamics.

When the user introduces a new component into the system, the corresponding information is stored on the *Database Server*, while other information connected with the component is published, via the *Socket Server*, on the *Web Server*.

A working version of the system is shown in the component diagram in Figure 6. The system starts up from a web page (*virtual_lab.html*) that contains an applet that requests user identification then runs the actual application.

All the Java classes making up the system are held in the file *virtual_lab.jar* on the *Web Server*. On managing any kind of component the user will access the system database (*virtual_lab.db*), and if the component in question has a VRML image assigned to it, this is displayed (*component.wrl*).

When a predefined experiment is run, the system launches a web page (*experiment_ID.html*), which contains an embedded VRML file containing the virtual lab associated with the experiment (*lab.wrl*). This VRML file has an associated compiled Java script listing the specific sequence of steps to be taken in order to perform the associated experiment (*myscript.class*).

Communication between the user and the virtual world is achieved through an applet (*myapplet.class*) that displays a toolbar allowing operations to be performed on the system. This applet retrieves information from the database and sends messages to the experiment's Java script detailing the actions the user wishes to carry out. The script must then control the correct execution of the experiment or show the user an error message if things go wrong.

All the documentary information connected with the experiment is linked to the *experiment_ID.html* page; links can be made automatically or manually by the user. Furthermore, this information may be accessed globally through the *experiment_ID.doc* file.

## DISCUSSION

Practical chemistry teaching is in great need of further effort on the part of professionals to adapt to the present-day teaching situation, especially in undergraduate and graduate courses. Such an effort might involve the use of the new technologies and the introduction of software systems that could lead to enhanced student learning, surmounting the obstacles present in the current school environment.

The proposal detailed in this paper is based on the use of virtual laboratories to provide extra support in the teaching of chemistry laboratory experiments. The proposal is based on an $E(V) = M + m$ paradigm that permits the structuring of knowledge in chunks of information describing basic stages in laboratory usage. The grouping of these stages in phases—both stages and phases are held in a set of permitted sequences—allows definition of the method or protocol for a lab experiment to be performed.

This structure, defined using a set of transitions that are allowed on the basis of the state of the materials employed, offers the possibility of the user carrying out an experiment in any permissible order of phases and stages and is thus not restricted to just one preset sequence, as is the case with other existing systems; moreover, the system can "advise" on the most suitable sequence and give feedback on the user's errors, a feature that adds greatly to its educational value.

The model has been implemented in an operational object-oriented prototype using the latest software technology (Oracle 8i, Java, and VRML), bestowing the system with the set of properties required by authoring systems for the construction of intelligent tutorial systems; among these features are the reuse of software, easy integration of other components, and a user-machine interface suited to the needs of assisted learning.

The authors are currently working to improve and expand several of the components of the subsystems that should form part of an ITS. In particular, other systems already developed by the authors are being integrated, such as a formulator[46,47] and a balancing system for inorganic reactions.[48,49] Additionally, work is underway on the definition of a suitable ontology for the construction of a dialogue system between the user (student) and the system, such that through the use of an explanatory system running in parallel with the experiment, the student may both learn and be given explanations of conceptual and procedural aspects of the task in hand. In the present system this aspect is managed by static explanations held in.doc and.html files that are delivered to the user either on request or automatically, as might happen when some kind of exception arises.

Moreover, work is being carried out toward enhancement of the virtual world employed. Further effort is being applied to the construction of new VRML components (e.g. materials) and also to evaluating different software such as Java3D and image soundrounding for building the virtual world, hopefully reducing hardware requirements.

## ACKNOWLEDGMENT

The authors would like to thank Messrs. Manuel Cachinero Olmo and Francisco Gabriel Muñoz Rodríguez for their invaluable assistance in the construction of the system, as part of their degree course at the University of Córdoba, Spain.

## REFERENCES AND NOTES

(1) *Changing University Teaching: Reflections on Creating Educational Technologies*; Evans, T., Nation, D., Eds.; Kogan Page: London, 2000.

(2) Gagné, R. *The Conditions of Learning and Theory of Instruction*; New York, 1985.

(3) *Sci/Tech Librarianship: Education and Training*; Hallmark, J., Seidman, R., Eds.; Haworth Press: New York, 1998.

(4) Judson, P. N.; Fox, J.; Krause, P. J. Using New Reasoning Technology in Chemical Information Systems. *J. Chem. Inf. Comput. Sci.* **1998**, *36*(4), 621−624.

(5) Moen, E.; Boersman, K. The Significance of Concept Mapping for Education and Curriculum Development. *J. Interactive Learning Res.* **1997**, *8*(3), 487−502.

(6) Tissue, B. M. The Costs of Incorporating Information Technology in Education. http://www.chem.vy.edu/archive/chemconf97/paper04.html.

(7) Cloete, E. Electronic Education System Model. *Comput. Educ.* **2001**, *36*(2) 151−170.

(8) Lagowski, J. J. Chemical Education: Past, Present, and Future. *J. Chem. Educ.* **1998**, *75*(4), 425−436.

(9) Murray-Rust, P.; Rzepa, H. S.; Whitaker, B. J. The World Wide Web as a Chemical Information Tool. *Chem. Soc. Rev.* **1997**, *27*, 1−10.

(10) Seal, K. C.; Przasnysk, Z. H. Using The World Wide Web for Teaching Improvement. *J. Chem. Inf. Comput. Sci.* **2001**, *36*(1), 33−40.

(11) Somerville, A. N. Chemical Information Instruction in Academe: Recent and Current Trends. *J. Chem. Inf. Comput. Sci.* **1998**, *38*(6), 1024−1030.

(12) Warr, W. A. Communication and Communities of Chemistry. *J. Chem. Inf. Comput. Sci.* **1998**, *38*, 966−975.

(13) The Internet Journal of Chemistry. http://www.ijc.com.

(14) Wiggins, C. Chemistry on the Internet: The Library on your Computer. *J. Chem. Inf. Comput. Sci.* **1998**, *38*, 956−965.

(15) Borchardt, J. K. Improving the General Chemistry Laboratory. www-chenweb.com/alchem2000/news/nw-000922-edu.html.

(16) Jurs, P. C. *Computer Software Application in Chemistry*, 2nd ed.; John Wiley & Sons Inc.: New York, 1996.

(17) Rzepa, H. S. Internet-Based Computational Chemistry Tools. In *Encyclopedia of Computational Chemistry*; Wiley: London, 1998.

(18) Tonge, A. P.; Rzepa, H. S.; Yoshida, H. Authentication of Interned-Based Distributed Resources in Chemistry. *J. Chem. Inf. Comput. Sci.* **1999**, *39*(3), 483−390.

(19) Csizmadia, F. JChem: Java Applets and Molecules Supporting Chemical Database Handling from Web Browsers. *J. Chem. Inf. Comput. Sci.* **2000**, *40*(2), 323−324.

(20) (a) marian.creighton.edu/~ksmith/tutorials.html. (b) www.emory.edu/CHEMISTRY/pointgrp. (c) www.chem.uwimona.edu.jm: 1104/chemprob.html. (d) www.chemsoc.golbook.

(21) (a) chem.lapeer.org/Chem1Docs/Index.html. (b) www.geocities.com/CapeCanaveral/9687/index.html. (c) www.lanzadera.com/qgeum. (d) www.scripps.edu/~nwhite/B/Download/. (e) jchemed.chem.wisc.edu/JCEsoft/Issues/ Series_SP/SP8/abs-sp8.html. (f) chem-www.mps.ohio-state.edu/~lars/ moviemol.html.

(22) Barna, N.; Dori, Y. J Computerized Molecular Modeling as a Tool to Improve Chemistry Teaching. *J. Chem. Inf. Comput. Sci.* **1998**, *36*(4), 629−634.

(23) Ivancinc, O. ChemPlus for Windows. *J. Chem. Inf. Comput. Sci.* **1996**, *36*(4), 919−921.

(24) Ivanov, A. S.; Rumgantsev, A. B.; Archakov, A. I. Education Program for Macromolecules Structure Examination. *J. Chem. Inf. Comput. Sci.* **1996**, *36*(4), 660−663.

(25) Parril, A. L. Periodi 2.0 fro Macintosh. *J. Chem. Inf. Comput. Sci.* **1997**, *37*(4), 820−820.

(26) Yoshida, H.; Mausura, H. MOLDA for Windows. A Molecular Modeling and Molecular Graphics Program using a VRML Viewer on Personal Computers. *J. Chem. Software* **1997**, *3*(4), 147−156 (cssj.chem.sci.hiroshima-u-ac.jp/molda/download.html).

(27) Arruarte, A.; Fernández-Castro, I.; Ferrero, B. The IRIS Shell: How to Build ITSs from Pedagogical and Design Requisites. *Intl. J. Artificial Intelligence Educ.* **1997**, *8*, 341−381.

(28) Jonassen, D.; Reeves, T.; Hong, N.; Harvey, D.; Peters, K. Concept Mapping as Cognitive Learning and Assessment Tools. *J. Interactive Learning Res.* **1997**, *8*(3), 289−308.

(29) Murray, T. Expanding the Knowledge Acquisition Bottleneck for Intelligent Tutoring Systems. *Intl. J. Artificial Intelligence Educ.* **1997**, *8*(3), 222−234.

(30) Nussbaum, M.; Rosas, R.; Peisano, I.; Cardenas, F. Development Intelligent Tutoring Systems Using Knowledge Structures. *Comput. Educ.* **2001**, *36*(1), 15−32.

(31) Borman, S. Lab Systems Embrace the Web. *Chem. Eng. News.* January 27, **1997**, 25−27.

(32) (a) www.modelscience.com/products.html. (b) www.chemnews.com. (c) website/lineone.next/~chemie/reviews.html. (d) www2.acdlabs.com/ilabs. (e) www.chemsw.com/10202.html. (f) www.compuchem.com/dldref/formdem.html. (g) www.ir.chem.cmu.edu/irProject/applets/virtuallab/applet_wPI.asp.

(33) Rzepa, H. S.; Tonge, A. P. VchemLab: A Virtual Chemistry Laboratory. The Storage, Retrieval and Display of Chemical Information Using Standard Internet Tools. *J. Chem. Inf. Comput. Sci.* **1998**, *36*(6), 1048−1053.

(34) Sowa, J. F. *Knowledge Representation: Logical, Philosophical and Computational Foundations*; Brooks/Cole: 1999.

(35) Luger, G. F.; Stubblefield, W. A. *Artificial Intelligence: Solutions and Strategies for Complex Problem Solving*; Addison-Wesley: Reading, MA, 1992.

(36) Jacobson, I.; Booch, G.; Rumbaugh, J. *The Unified Software Development Process*; Addison-Wesley Longman Inc.: U.S.A., 1999.

(37) Booch, G.; Rumbaugh, J.; Jacobson, I. *The Unified Modeling Language. User Manual*; Addison-Wesley Longman Inc.: U.S.A., 1999.

(38) Rumbaugh, J.; Jacobson, I.; Booch, G. *The Unified Modeling Language. Reference Manual*; Addison-Wesley Longman Inc.: U.S.A., 1999.

(39) Cary Anderson, J.; Loy Stone, B. *Manual de Oracle JDeveloper*; McGraw-Hill/Oracle Press: Madrid, 1999.

(40) Dorsey, P.; Hudicka, J. R. *Oracle8 Principios de Diseño de Base de Datos Usando UML*; McGraw-Hill: Madrid, 1999.

(41) Roehl, B.; Couch, J.; Reed-Ballreich, C. et al. *Late Night VRML 2.0 with Java*; Ziff-Davis Press: EmeryVille, CA, U.S.A., 1997.

(42) Guerrero, J. *VRML 2.0, El Lenguaje 3D de Internet*; Abeto, Madrid, 1998.

(43) Jamsa, K.; Schmauder, P.: Yee, N. *VRML, Biblioteca del Programador*; McGraw-Hill: Madrid, 1998.

(44) Lea, R.; Matsuda, K.; Miyashita, K. *Java for 3D and VRML Worlds*; New Riders: Indianapolis, U.S.A., 1996.

(45) (a) java.sun.com/products/jama-media/3D. (b) www.rtzvirtual.es. (c) www. VRML.org/Specification/VRML97. (d) www.wmaestro.com/web3d/docs/ portada.html.

(46) Luque Ruiz, I.; Cruz Soto, J. L.; Gómez-Nieto, M. A. Computer Translation of Inorganic Chemical Nomenclature to a Dynamic Abstract Data Structure. *J. Chem. Inf. Comput. Sci.* **1994**, *34*, 4(3), 526−533.

(47) Luque Ruiz, I.; Cruz Soto, J. L.; Gómez-Nieto, M. A. Error Detection, Recovery, and Repair in the Translation of Inorganic Nomenclatures. 1. A Study of the Problem. *J. Chem. Inf. Comput. Sci.* **1996**, *36*, 6(1), 7−15. 2. A Proposed Strategy. *J. Chem. Inf. Comput. Sci.* **1996**, *36*, 6(1), 16−24. 3. An Error Handler. *J. Chem. Inf. Comput. Sci.* **1996**, *36*(3), 483−490.

(48) Luque Ruiz, I.; Martínez Pedrajas, C.; Gómez-Nieto, M. A. Design and Development of Computer-Aided Chemical Systems: Representing and Balance of Inorganic Chemical Reactions. *J. Chem. Inf. Comput. Sci.* **2000**, *40*(3), 744−752.

(49) Luque Ruiz, I.; Gómez-Nieto, M. A. Solving Incomplete Inorganic Chemical Systems through a Fuzzy Knowledge Frame. *J. Chem. Inf. Comput. Sci.* **2001**, *41*(1), 83−99.

CI010015W

# Do Computers Teach Better? A Media Comparison Study for Case-based Teaching in Radiology[1]

*Martin Maleck, MD[2] • Martin R. Fischer, MD[2] • Birgit Kammer, MD*
*Claudius Zeiler, MD • Eugen Mangel, MD • Franz Schenk, MD*
*Klaus-Juergen Pfeifer, MD*

A prospective study was performed to better define the role of computers in teaching radiology to medical students. Two hundred twenty-five 3rd-year students were randomly assigned to one of four groups and exposed to 10 radiology cases as well as to a voluntary weekly radiology lecture. Group A used computer-based cases with interactive elements; group B used computer-based cases without interactive elements; group C used paper-based cases with interactive elements; and group D was not exposed to the cases and served as a control group. On a multiple-choice question test, groups A, B, and C showed significant improvement (+11.2%, +15.1%, and +13.0%, respectively), whereas group D did not (+0.6%). On an image interpretation test, group A showed the most improvement (+15.7% [$P < .001$]), followed by group B (+15.1% [$P < .01$]) and group C (+10.2% [$P < .05$]); group D showed no significant improvement (+8.5%). No significant differences in the learning outcome were found between the two interactive groups (computer based and paper based). Computer-based teaching with case studies (with or without interactivity) improves students' problem-solving ability in radiology.

**Index terms:** Computers, educational aid • Education

**RadioGraphics 2001;** 21:1025–1032

[1]From the Departments of Medicine (AG Instruct) (M.M., M.R.F.), Diagnostic Radiology (M.M., B.K., E.M., F.S., K.J.P.), and Surgery (C.Z.), Klinikum Innenstadt, Ludwig Maximilians University, Ziemssenstrasse 1, 80336 Munich, Germany. Received April 21, 2000; revision requested June 20; final revision received October 19; accepted December 1. **Address correspondence to** M.M. (e-mail: *martin.fischer@medinn.med.uni-muenchen.de*).

[2]Both authors contributed equally to the work.

## Introduction

Research on computer-assisted instruction tools started at the beginning of the 1970s (1), but the practicality of their use in radiology is still unclear. There seems to be a discrepancy between the rich availability of software and computer technologies and the poor integration of these new tools into clinical teaching. Early reports on computer-assisted instruction in radiology were focused mainly on describing a new learning program or tool (2,3) or related to improvements in computer technology (4–6).

Early on, only a few studies explored the possibilities of embedding the computer into medical curricula (7,8). Computer-assisted instruction was evaluated by groups of users, mostly medical students, for acceptance and motivational aspects (9,10). It is now evident that this method of subjective self-evaluation would provoke much criticism from experts in education; however, it identified a gap in educational research (11–13).

Within the general discussion about "the way in which we teach" and the movement toward problem-based learning (14), the discussion about the best way to use computers in medical education became more and more important and led to studies that compared computer use with use of textbooks or traditional lectures (15–19). However, previous media comparison studies were limited by confounding factors (20). Some articles explained how to develop computer-assisted instruction tools yet ignored didactic developments (21,22).

With the rapid growth of the Internet community, computer-assisted instruction holds great promise for providing high-quality teaching materials that are readily available anywhere at any time. Distribution and updating of educational data should be easier, faster, and more economical. But can all students handle the technology adequately? Is the learning outcome at least as good as with the well-established traditional teaching approaches?

We performed a study that compared use of different versions of a computer-assisted instruction program with use of a paper-based version of the same teaching material. Factors for successful integration of computer-assisted instruction into clinical teaching in radiology should be identified and described.

## Materials and Methods

We created 10 cases for the computer with the CASUS authoring system (23) (Fig 1) and a paper-based traditional version with copies of the original radiographs; the cases were created as an extension to the radiology lecture in the second clinical year at Ludwig Maximilians University. The cases were developed with contributions from experts in the fields of radiology, surgery, and internal medicine. Five cases focus on typical problems seen on chest radiographs (adult respiratory distress syndrome, lung carcinoma, tuberculosis, atelectasis, and pneumothorax). The other five cases cover problems seen at bone imaging (benign tumor, malignant tumor, fracture, bone infection, and degenerative bone disease). The structure of each case includes two screens (pages) of medical history and physical examination results. In the second part, four or five screens (pages) deal with the related imaging studies and a final screen refers to therapy and follow-up. In addition, hypertext links, graphics, audio, and a mapping tool to illustrate the differential diagnostic process are included. The time users spent on each case varied from 20 to 30 minutes.

All 225 students from the 1998 summer term participated in the study. The case studies were a mandatory part of the curriculum; the students were required to participate as a prerequisite for the surgery course in the next term. Selection bias could thus be excluded. The students had the options of attending radiology lectures (lecture duration, 45 min/wk) on a voluntary basis and of using textbooks. Students were randomly assigned to one of four instructional groups by using random selection based on radioactive decay numbers. The teaching content was identical for all groups.

Group A used the computer-based cases along with interactive elements, which included multiple-choice and free-text questions and a drag-and-drop mapping tool for the differential diagnostic process. Group B used the computer-based cases but without the interactive elements. Group C used the paper versions of the cases together with the original film radiographs. Group D was not exposed to the cases and served as a control group. (The students from group D were offered the opportunity to learn with the cases after the end of the term.)

The control group was important to avoid the negative effects of confounding factors. The exposition on learning cases deals only with groups A–C. Owing to organizational problems (overlapping courses), 20 students could not be included in group A, B, or C and had to be assigned to group D. A subgroup analysis showed no statistical differences between those 20 students and the students in the four study groups.

The 10 cases for the intervention groups were offered in two blocks of five cases. Each student had to work through five cases on Tuesday and five cases on Wednesday of the same week (Fig

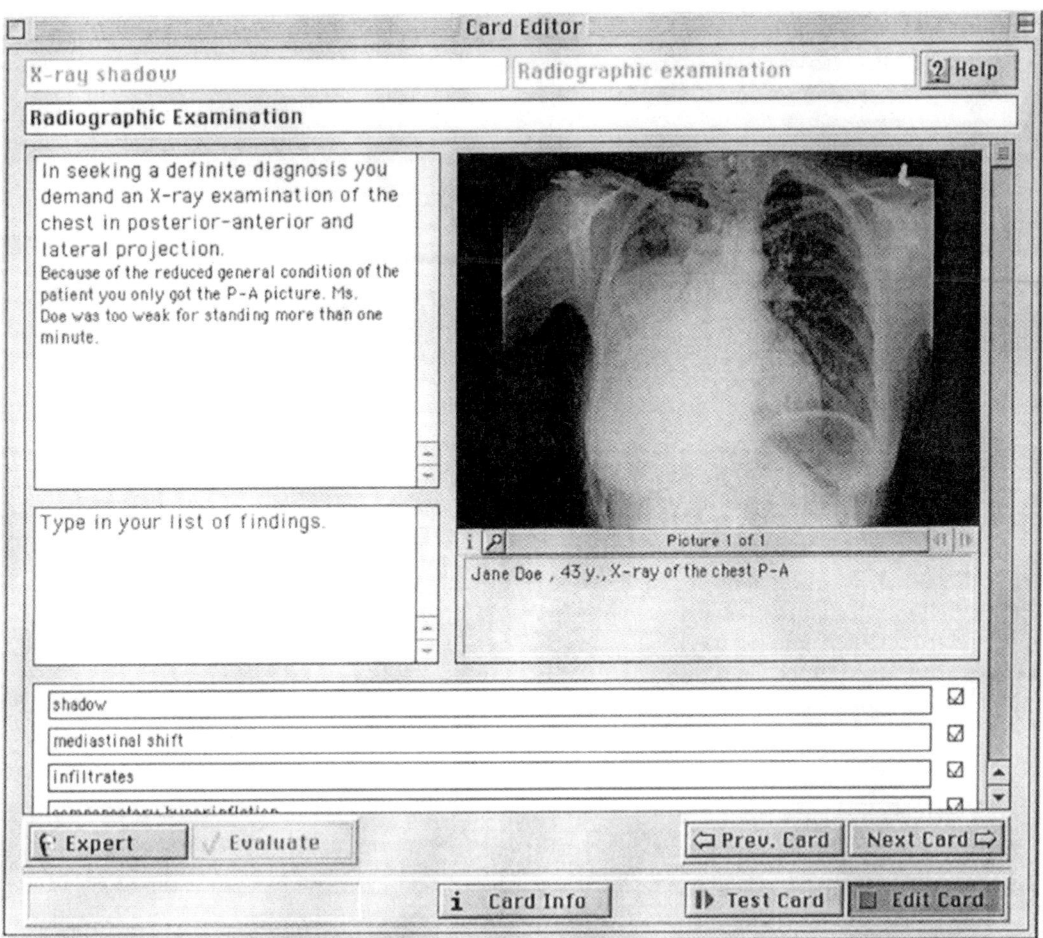


**Figure 1.** Sample card from the cases in the CASUS system.

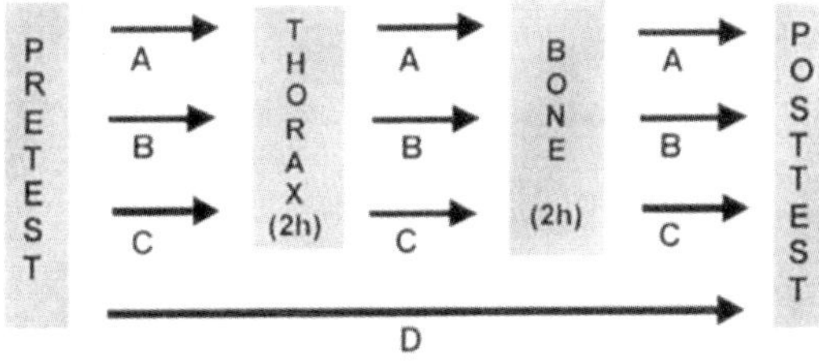


**Figure 2.** Design of the study.

2). We changed the case order and rotated the groups during the term to minimize confounding effects related to case order, time between case studying, and the posttest. The same tutor gave an introduction to all students on each course day. The students worked on the cases in groups of two or three.

All students took a pretest at the beginning of the semester and a posttest at the end of the semester; both the pretest and the posttest contained 14 multiple-choice questions originally used for part II of the National Boards Examination ("2. Staatsexamen") and four free-text questions related to interpretation of radiographs, which were projected with a slide projector. An answering time of 90 seconds was allowed for each multiple-choice question; an answering time of 2 minutes was allowed for each free-text question. The radiographs used in the tests were not the same as those used in the cases. To determine success-pressure effects, the students were told that they must take part only in the posttest and that they would not fail. We normalized the results of the multiple-choice questions and of the free-text questions to a 100% standard to exclude variations between the pretest and the posttest. The standard of reference for the multiple-choice questions was the score of the national examination. For the free-text questions, it was the interpretation of a radiology professor (K.J.P.). Before taking each test, the students had to fill out an evaluation form with about 35 items so that we could collect individual and subjective data related to motivational aspects.

For groups A and B, we used our Computer Learning Center, which has nine workstations

**Table 1**
**Group Characteristics Based on Information from a Questionnaire**

| Group | Teaching Approach | No. of Students | Mean Age (y) | Sex M (%) | Sex F (%) | Prior Profession (%) | Prior PBL Knowledge (%) |
|---|---|---|---|---|---|---|---|
| A | Computer-based, interactive | 47 | 26.3 | 47 | 53 | 20.0 | 10.0 |
| B | Computer-based, noninteractive | 38 | 25.2 | 38 | 62 | 15.6 | 0.0 |
| C | Paper-based, interactive | 42 | 25.5 | 55 | 45 | 11.8 | 9.0 |
| D | None (control group) | 65 | 25.5 | 45 | 55 | 20.0 | 11.5 |
| All | ... | 192 | 25.6 | 47 | 53 | 17.5 | 8.3 |

Note.—The questions "I have a prior profession?" and "I have prior knowledge of problem-based learning [PBL]?" could be answered with "yes" or "no." There was no significant difference between the groups for any item in the $\chi^2$ table test.

(Macintosh Power PC 8200/120 [Apple Computer, Cupertino, Calif]). The computers were placed in a row and were divided by opaque walls, and all had multiple headphones. The computer cases were saved on a server and were used by the students in client-server mode. The paper-based group was placed in the appointment rooms of the outpatient clinic next door to the Computer Learning Center. Each group of two or three students had its own room with a radiographic viewing device. For all groups, the same student tutor was present at all times and gave the same standardized introduction before starting the course. No commentaries or help related to the cases was given outside of technical advice on use of the computers or software.

We used the F test for same variances and contingency tables to analyze the evaluation data and the Wilcoxon signed rank test for nonparametric data to evaluate the pre- and posttest results (categorical data).

## Results

Nineteen students were physically not present for the whole semester for individual reasons like failed examinations, studies abroad, or illness. Thus, the total number of participants was 206 (92% of all students). Only students who completed the pretest and posttest (groups A–D) and at least one of the two course days (groups A–C) were included in the evaluation. The reasons why students did not complete the posttest are not known. The students who completed only half of the cases had to select atypical courses for individual reasons. Therefore, the number of students included in the study was 192 (85%). Group comparison ($\chi^2$ table test) showed no significant differences between the groups for age, sex, prior

**Table 2**
**Results of Evaluation of Program-related Items Performed Directly after Course Participation**

| Item | A | B | C | All |
|---|---|---|---|---|
| Concentration | 4.1 | 3.6 | 4.4 | 4.1 |
| Difficulty of content | 4.0 | 3.6 | 4.0 | 3.9 |
| Enough time | 3.4 | 4.8 | 2.6 | 3.8 |
| Fun factor | 4.4 | 4.1 | 5.0 | 4.5 |

Note.—Items were rated on a scale from 1 (lowest) to 6 (highest). Results of significance testing between the groups are given in the text.

profession, or prior knowledge of problem-based learning (Table 1), nor differences in computer skills. This information was requested on the questionnaire the students had to fill out before they took the pretest.

### Subjective Student Self-Evaluation

Self-evaluation forms filled out directly after each learning session showed a significant difference in the level of concentration while working on the cases between group B and groups A and C ($P <$ .05 [contingency table analyses, which were used for all self-evaluation data]) (Table 2). The students in group C rated their concentration as highest, followed by groups A and B. In addition, group B rated the difficulty of the cases significantly lowest in comparison with groups A and C ($P <$ .05). The adequacy of the available time for working on the cases was judged very differently by the three groups: Group B thought that there was enough time, whereas groups A and C mentioned time constraints as a major problem ($P <$ .0001). Groups A and C rated the benefits from

**Table 3**
**Results of Evaluation of the Different Learning Facilities**

| Method of Knowledge Improvement | Group | | | | |
|---|---|---|---|---|---|
| | A | B | C | D | All |
| Lecture | 3.3 | 2.9 | 2.7 | 3.5 | 3.2 |
| Textbook | 2.5 | 3.1 | 2.3 | 2.8 | 2.7 |
| Case-based course | 3.2 | 3.5 | 3.7 | ... | 3.4 |

Note.—Items were rated on a scale from 1 (lowest) to 6 (highest). Results of significance testing between the groups are given in the text.

**Table 4**
**Results of Testing with 14 State Examination Multiple-Choice Questions**

| Group | Score on Pretest (%) | Score on Posttest (%) | Change (%) |
|---|---|---|---|
| A | 80.1 | 91.3 | +11.2* |
| B | 80.9 | 96.0 | +15.1† |
| C | 76.0 | 89.0 | +13.0† |
| D | 80.2 | 80.8 | +0.6 |

Note.—Test results were correlated with the results of the examination candidates; the range for the students was between four and 13 correct answers.
*$P < .05$.
†$P < .01$.

**Table 5**
**Results of Testing with Four Typical Radiographs**

| Group | Score on Pretest (%) | Score on Posttest (%) | Change (%) |
|---|---|---|---|
| A | 19.6 | 35.3 | +15.7* |
| B | 22.8 | 37.9 | +15.1† |
| C | 22.0 | 32.2 | +10.2‡ |
| D | 22.5 | 31.0 | +8.5 |

Note.—Test results were correlated with the number of findings identified by a chief radiologist; the range for the students was between one and 11 points versus the 18 points of the radiologist.
*$P < .001$.
†$P < .01$.
‡$P < .05$.

interactivity as high (89%), whereas 42% of the students in group B missed interactivity. The degree of "fun" while working on the cases was rated highest in group C, followed by groups A and B with significant differences (group A vs group C, $P < .05$; group B vs group C, $P < .001$).

At the end of the semester, use of a radiology textbook was rated low (mean of 1.7 on a scale from 1 to 6) by all of the groups, as was lecture attendance (1.9). However, lectures, textbooks, and the case-based radiology course subjectively played a different, supportive role for the improvement of knowledge in the different groups (Table 3). There was no significant difference between the groups concerning subjective improvement of knowledge. There was a large variance in all of the groups in evaluating the role of the textbook. We asked the students whether they would recommend the course to peers. Group A answered this question positively (mean of 4.5 on a scale from 1 to 6), as did group B (4.4) and group C (5.0). There was a significant difference only between groups B and C ($P < .05$).

## Objective Outcome Measures

The scores for the multiple-choice questions showed a significant increase in knowledge in groups A–C and a nonsignificant one in group D (Wilcoxon signed rank test) (Table 4). The highest improvement was found in group B.

The scores for the free-form radiographic interpretation questions also showed a significant increase in groups A–C, with the highest improvement in group A (Table 5). Group D again showed no significant improvement.

## Discussion

Many studies on educational interventions in radiology demonstrate limitations with respect to the number of students evaluated, bias due to low voluntary participation rates, and heterogeneous measuring tools (15–17). Owing to our ability to make the curricular intervention of this study compulsory for all students, a selection bias could be avoided: The 85% of the students ($n = 192$) included in our evaluation represents a high number and allows a powerful interpretation of the results. Nevertheless, we are aware of some limitations of our methodologic approach: We did not track the interpersonal communications between students in front of the screen or the light box, which might have been essential for a successful learning experience. All three intervention groups had the same chance for small-group interactions; therefore, the results of our measures should be equally biased in this respect. Furthermore, it seems ethically problematic, in general, to primarily exclude a group of students from an educational opportunity. We decided to make this sacrifice to obtain an adequate control group for comparison. Finally, since we conducted a short-term study over only 3 months, we were not able to answer questions on long-term effects like National Boards Examination results in radiology and organizational problems of curriculum planning. Long-term studies are even more difficult to control for confounding factors (15,24).

## Media Comparison

Media comparison studies raise some general methodologic questions: It is quite difficult to control for confounding variables (25). Furthermore, the hypothesis for such a comparison should be clearly defined and not only a justification of the use of new media technology (20).

The design of our study does not allow comparison of case-based learning (interactive or non-interactive) with traditional learning by means of lectures and textbooks. We wanted to explore the effects of a small intervention with case-based learning performed with different technical approaches on acceptance, motivation, and learning success. We are not aware of any study on case-based learning in radiology in which an interactive computer-based approach was compared with a noninteractive computer-based approach. The studies of Erkonen et al (15) and D'Alessandro et al (24) compared a printed and a multimedia version of a radiology textbook in a non–case-based teaching scenario.

## Motivation and Learning Success

The level of acceptance of case-based learning with or without computers was very high, as in many other studies (26): Ninety percent of all students recommended the cases to their peers. The noticeably high correlation between the self-evaluated improvement in knowledge of the students and the objective test results gives us a strong argument for the validity of student evaluations. The validity of student evaluations is a controversial issue in the discussion of curricular evaluation.

We conclude that interactivity was highly valued by the students to whom it was offered. The fact that only 42% of the students in group B missed interactivity may be due to the fact that there was no crossover between groups and therefore no direct comparison between the interactive and noninteractive approaches. The interactivity between learners in front of the screen may have

affected the data and was not analyzed. The interpretation of these results is therefore difficult, and a direct controlled comparison with a crossover design should be performed in the future.

The case-based approach should teach the ability to connect clinical findings with imaging findings as an essential learning objective in radiology (27). Since it is generally difficult to evaluate learning success in problem-solving environments, we decided on a twofold testing scenario. Surprisingly, results from both the image interpretation test and the multiple-choice questions showed that the control group did not significantly improve its scores during the semester. On the other hand, all groups who were exposed to the cases showed significant improvement in both measures. Although no significant differences between the three intervention groups were detected (score differences; Wilcoxon signed rank test), it is noteworthy that the interactive computer-based group performed better in image interpretation and performed worse on the multiple-choice questions than did the noninteractive computer-based group. One might speculate that this observation becomes more prominent with a more fundamental intervention. For teaching the key ability of image interpretation in an applicable way, the interactive case-based format seems to offer clear advantages concerning the learning outcome. Multiple-choice questions on image interpretation seem to be less adequate to prepare students for clinical work.

Some well-appreciated studies from instructional psychology on case-based learning suggest that interactive teaching is superior to noninteractive teaching with respect to medical practice (28–31). The observation that the control group did not improve on the multiple-choice question test but showed a tendency toward improvement on the image interpretation test can be attributed to an internal medicine course in the same semester, which includes bedside radiographic interpretation and was attended by all students. The radiology lecture was obviously attended by only a small proportion of the students. The students who attended the lecture rated it subjectively as high as the case-based course. All groups used radiology textbooks with a relatively low level of intensity. Therefore, what was the reason for the significant differences in the test results? We conclude that the case-based intervention was the main reason, despite all of the confounding factors. The 3-hour intervention with 10 mini-cases on chest and bone radiology led to a significant increase in knowledge of radiology.

## Implementation of Case-based Learning for Radiology

One can only speculate about the effects of a more complete radiology case library to support all key topics of the lecture. As more cases are being authored (including nuclear medicine objectives), we will soon be able to evaluate this scenario. On the basis of this study, one can confidently speculate that the effects will be positive.

The high usability of the CASUS authoring system (23) contributed to the efficacy of case creation. This interactive radiology case library can be used for easy dissemination on compact disk, read-only memory (CD-ROM) or via an intranet or the Internet. Our study did not include evaluation of the case-authoring process. However, the initial results of an ongoing evaluation are available. It seems to be advantageous to support the content experts with a student tutor (32).

The creation of paper cases used up more resources, including the costly generation of hundreds of film radiographs. When the respective computing infrastructure is available, we therefore recommend the more flexible and affordable computer-based use of cases.

Our cases were used in a self-study mode with the technical advice of a student tutor. We did not investigate the potentially beneficial effect of a radiologist who could answer further questions related to the case content. We believe that such a setting could make our approach even more useful (33).

In conclusion, the results of our study support the integration of computer-based cases for teaching radiology into the clinical medical curriculum as a supplement to lectures and practical courses. The continuation of implementation efforts may not need to focus on controlled comparisons. Instead, improvement of the integration process and development of content (20) will require special attention.

## References


1. Patton DD. Computer-assisted instruction in the radiological sciences using a desk-top computer. Radiology 1971; 100:553–559.
2. Skinner JB, Knowles G, Armstrong RF, Ingram D. The use of computerized learning in intensive care: an evaluation of a new teaching program. Med Educ 1983; 17:49–53.
3. Pickell GC, Medal D, Mann WS, Staebler RJ. Computerizing clinical patient problems: an evolving tool for medical education. Med Educ 1986; 20:201–203.
4. Costaridou L, Panayiotakis G, Sakellaropoulos P, Cavouras D, Dimopoulos J. Distance learning in mammographic digital image processing. Br J Radiol 1998; 71:167–174.
5. Sinha S, Sinha U, Kangarloo H, Huang HK. A PACS-based interactive teaching module for radiologic sciences. AJR Am J Roentgenol 1992; 159:199–205.
6. Desch LW. Use of commercial "authoring systems" for medical education. Med Educ 1986; 20:417–423.
7. Murray TS, Barber JH, Dunn WR. Attitudes of medical undergraduates in Glasgow to computer-assisted learning. Med Educ 1978; 12:6–9.
8. Brown DW, Groome DS, Niehoff RD, Cleaveland JD. Computer-assisted instruction in nuclear medicine. JAMA 1968; 206:1059–1062.
9. Kuszyk BS, Calhoun PS, Soyer PA, Fishman EK. An interactive computer-based tool for teaching the segmental anatomy of the liver: usefulness in the education of residents and fellows. AJR Am J Roentgenol 1997; 169:631–634.
10. Morin FD, Dubreuil B, Dussault RG, DiCori S, Bret PM. The radiographic signs of arthritis: a computer teaching module. RadioGraphics 1995; 15:703–708.
11. Keane DR, Norman GR, Vickers J. The inadequacy of recent research on computer-assisted instruction. Acad Med 1991; 66:444–448.
12. Armstrong R. Interactive computer programs. J Rheumatol 1999; 26(suppl 55):56–57.
13. Jaffe CC, Lynch PJ. Computer-aided instruction for radiologic education. RadioGraphics 1993; 13:931–937.
14. Schmidt HG, Dauphinee WD, Patel VL. Comparing the effects of problem-based and conventional curricula in an international sample. J Med Educ 1987; 62:305–315.
15. Erkonen WE, D'Alessandro MP, Galvin JR, Albanese MA, Michaelsen VE. Longitudinal comparison of multimedia textbook instruction with a lecture in radiology education. Acad Radiol 1994; 1:287–292.
16. D'Alessandro MP, Galvin JR, Erkonen WE, et al. An approach to the creation of multimedia textbooks for radiology instruction. AJR Am J Roentgenol 1993; 161:187–191.
17. Chew FS, Stiles RS. Computer-assisted instruction with interactive videodisc versus textbook for teaching radiology. Acad Radiol 1994; 1:326–331.
18. Brown RL, Carlson BL. Early diagnosis of substance abuse: evaluation of a course of computer-assisted instruction. Med Educ 1990; 24:438–446.
19. Mangione S, Nieman LZ, Gracely EJ. Comparison of computer-based learning and seminar teaching of pulmonary auscultation to first-year medical students. Acad Med 1992; 67(10 suppl): S63–S65.
20. Friedman CP. The research we should be doing. Acad Med 1994; 69:455–457.
21. Calhoun PS, Fishman EK. Developing a computer-assisted instruction program: a process overview for the radiologist. RadioGraphics 1997; 17: 1277–1291.
22. Mammone GL, Holman BL, Greenes RA, Parker JA, Khorasani R. Inside BrighamRAD: providing radiology teaching cases on the Internet. RadioGraphics 1995; 15:1489–1498.

23. Fischer MR, Schauer S, Grasel C, et al. CASUS model trial: a computer-assisted author system for problem-oriented learning in medicine. Z Arztl Fortbild 1996; 90:385–389. [German]

24. D'Alessandro DM, Kreiter CD, Erkonen WE, Winter RJ, Knapp HR. Longitudinal follow-up comparison of educational interventions: multimedia textbook, traditional lecture, and printed textbook. Acad Radiol 1997; 4:719–723.

25. Clarke R. Dangers in the evaluation of instructional media. Acad Med 1992; 67:820–821.

26. Jelovsek FR, Adebonojo L. Learning principles as applied to computer-assisted instruction. MD Comput 1993; 10:165–172.

27. Norman GR, Brooks LR, Coblentz CL, Babcook CJ. The correlation of feature identification and category judgments in diagnostic radiology. Mem Cognit 1992; 20:344–355.

28. Norman GR, Brooks LR, Cunnington JP, Shali V, Marriott M, Regehr G. Expert-novice differences in the use of history and visual information from patients. Acad Med 1996; 71(10 suppl):S62–S64.

29. Regehr G, Norman GR. Issues in cognitive psychology: implications for professional education. Acad Med 1996; 71:988–1001.

30. Mennin SP, Friedman M, Skipper B, Kalishman S, Snyder J. Performances on the NBME I, II, and III by medical students in the problem-based learning and conventional tracks at the University of New Mexico. Acad Med 1993; 68:616–624.

31. Schmidt HG, Machiels-Bongaerts M, Hermans H, ten Cate TJ, Venekamp R, Boshuizen HP. The development of diagnostic competence: comparison of a problem-based, an integrated, and a conventional medical curriculum. Acad Med 1996; 71:658–664.

32. Maleck M, Fleissner S, Fischer MR. Drag and drop authoring of cases for clinical teaching with CASUS. Do clinicians manage the technology and didactics alone? Med Teacher (in press).

33. Schmidt HG, Moust JH. What makes a tutor effective? A structural-equations modeling approach to learning in problem-based curricula. Acad Med 1995; 70:708–714.

# DiasNet—a diabetes advisory system for communication and education via the internet

Søren Plougmann [a], Ole K. Hejlesen [a,*], David A. Cavan [b]

[a] *Department of Medical Informatics and Image Analysis, Aalborg University, Fredrik Bajersvej 7 D1, DK-9220, Aalborg, Denmark*
[b] *Bournemouth Diabetes and Endocrine Centre, Bournemouth, UK*

## Abstract

Intensive diabetes treatment can lead to a substantial reduction of the rate of the complications associated with diabetes. However, a number of patients may have poor control despite specialist care, and this along with devolution of care to non-specialists suggests that alternative interventions should be developed. The present paper describes an Internet based system where more emphasis is put on patient empowerment, the keywords being education and communication. The DiasNet system is based on a well documented decision support system, Dias, designed for use by clinicians. The scope of DiasNet has been widened from being used by clinicians to give advice on insulin dose, to also being used by patients as a tool for education and communication. Patients can experiment with their own data, adjusting insulin doses or meal sizes. In this way different therapeutic and dietary alternatives can be tried out, allowing the patient to gain experience in achieving glycaemic control. DiasNet is implemented in *JAVA* according to the client/server principle, enabling a new way of communication between patient and clinician: in case of any problems, the patient simply phones the clinician, who immediately, using his or her office PC, can take a look at the data the patient has entered. © 2001 Published by Elsevier Science Ireland Ltd.

*Keywords:* Diabetes; Decision support; Internet; Patient empowerment; Communication; Education

## 1. Introduction

In both developed and developing countries diabetes is one of the major chronic diseases and a growing public health problem [1]. Diabetes' direct costs in the USA in 1992 is estimated to represent 5.8% of total personal health-care expenditures, which again represented over 14% of the GDP, and the indirect costs were even higher [2,3]. The considerable loss of quality of life connected with the disease is primarily due to the late complications: blindness, kidney failure, circulatory diseases etc. Although studies have shown that intensive diabetes treatment with the goal of maintaining blood glucose concentrations close to the normal range can lead to a substantial reduction of the rate of

* Corresponding author. Tel.: +45-9635-8808; mobile: +45-2045-9779; fax: +45-9815-4008.
*E-mail address:* okh@mi.auc.dk (O.K. Hejlesen).

the complications, this can be difficult to achieve using conventional means.

Even though decision support systems may provide a possible answer to some of the problems, none of the numerous systems developed during the last two decades have, up till now, gained widespread use or acceptance [4–20].

One reason for this apparent lack of success might be the problems in handling the interpatient and intrapatient variability, and other reasons might be the uncertainties in the data involved and the fact that the blood glucose control in diabetes is influenced by numerous factors like stress, fever, exercise etc. Still other reasons for the lack of acceptance might be associated with the evaluation of the systems [21,22]. We believe that a decision support system in the classical sense is not enough, and that more emphasis should be put on patient empowerment. We believe that the keywords in such a strategy should be *education* and *communication*.

## 2. Background

The core of Dias is a compartment model of the human carbohydrate metabolism, and the model has two associated state variables: one state variable keeps track of the amount of carbohydrate in the gut compartment, and another keeps track of the amount of glucose in the blood compartment. The state variables are functions of process variables which model the processes in various organ systems: muscles, kidneys, brain, liver etc. The model is implemented as a Bayesian network (CPN or causal probabilistic network), which gives it the ability to handle the uncertainty, for example, in blood glucose measurements [23,24].

Dias is operated in two modes: the learning mode and the prediction mode. In the learning mode data on blood glucose measurements, insulin regime and meals from one or more days are used to estimate patient specific parameters. In this way the system is tuned to fit each individual patient. In the prediction mode the system uses the estimated parameters to make predictions of the blood glucose, given information on meals and insulin. This mode can be used to predict the effect on the blood glucose of suggested changes in the insulin or meals.

In addition to studies verifying the ability of the model to accurately predict blood glucose, Dias has been evaluated in five small controlled clinical studies. In these studies Dias was used to give advice on insulin dose, and the results are summarised in Table 1. The study in 1993 in London was mainly focused on the safety of using Dias and did not include HbA1c measurements, but in the other four studies a meta-analysis shows that the mean reduction in HbA1c for the patients

Table 1
Outline of the results from the controlled clinical studies

| Clinical site | London UK | Sønderborg Denmark | Aalborg Denmark | Portsmouth UK | Foligno Italy |
|---|---|---|---|---|---|
| Year | 1993 | 1993–94 | 1994–95 | 1997–98 | 1998 |
| Number of patients | 20 | 12 | 13 | 20 | 17 |
| Reduction in HbA1c (%) Dias vs. control group | N/A | 1.9 vs. 0.9 | 0.6 vs. 0.3 | 1.5 vs. 0.8* | 0.8 vs. −0.5* |

Significant differences ($P < 0.05$) are denoted by a*.

using Dias was 1.2% compared to 0.3% for the patients in the control groups, who used advice from experienced clinicians. The mean reduction in hypoglycaemia (inappropriately low blood glucose) was approximately 0.3 episodes per day in the Dias group. Some studies have indicated that a 1.2% reduction in HbA1c corresponds to a reduction in the risk of complications of approximately 30–40% [1].

In addition to the formal results outlined in Table 1, some of the studies, where the patients were sitting in front of the computer, while the system was used to analyse their data, showed a clear benefit from using Dias to explain, for example, the rationale behind changing insulin regimen to the patients. It was striking to see the remarkable interest from many patients when confronted with their own data being used to generate and illustrate their own personal advice.

## 3. DiasNet

Based on the experience from the clinical studies, a new web based system, DiasNet, has been implemented. The scope of this Internet version of the system has been widened; from being used by clinicians to give advise on insulin dose, to also being used by patients as a tool for education and communication.

An essential part of education of diabetes patients is learning how to achieve good glycaemic control. Using the system, patients can experiment with their own data, adjusting insulin doses or meal sizes, and thereby learning how to cope with various situations. In this way different therapeutic and dietary alternatives can be tried out, allowing the patient to gain experience in achieving glycaemic control, without the risk of actually experiencing hypoglycaemic or hypergly-

caemic (inappropriately high blood glucose) episodes. The effect of increased carbohydrate intake during, for example, weekends can be simulated and appropriate countermeasures found. Likewise, patients can immediately see the effect of a missed insulin injection, and benefits or disadvantages from shifting to a different insulin type can be predicted. Compared with traditional educational material, the major benefit from using the system is that it uses the patients own data to improve the patients understanding of the disease.

In addition to the educational aspect, the system enables a new way of communication between patient and clinician. It is implemented in *JAVA* according to the client/server principle and can run both as an ordinary application on a standard PC, and as an Internet *JAVA* applet using a standard browser. Fig. 1 illustrates the physical integration of the patient–clinician environment.

The patient can sit at home entering his data into the system running on his home PC, and in case of questions or problems he can phone (or email) the clinician, who can use a web browser on his office PC to view the data that the patient just entered. This will allow newly diagnosed patients to be regularly monitored remotely, and as a routine part of the ambulatory visits, clinicians can use DiasNet to get a clear overview of the patient's data without having to spend time deciphering a hand written patient diary.

### 3.1. Screen presentation

To demonstrate the use of DiasNet, a specific patient scenario will be presented in which the different system functionalities will be explained. During the development of the graphical user interface (GUI) strong emphasis has been put on creating a very simple and

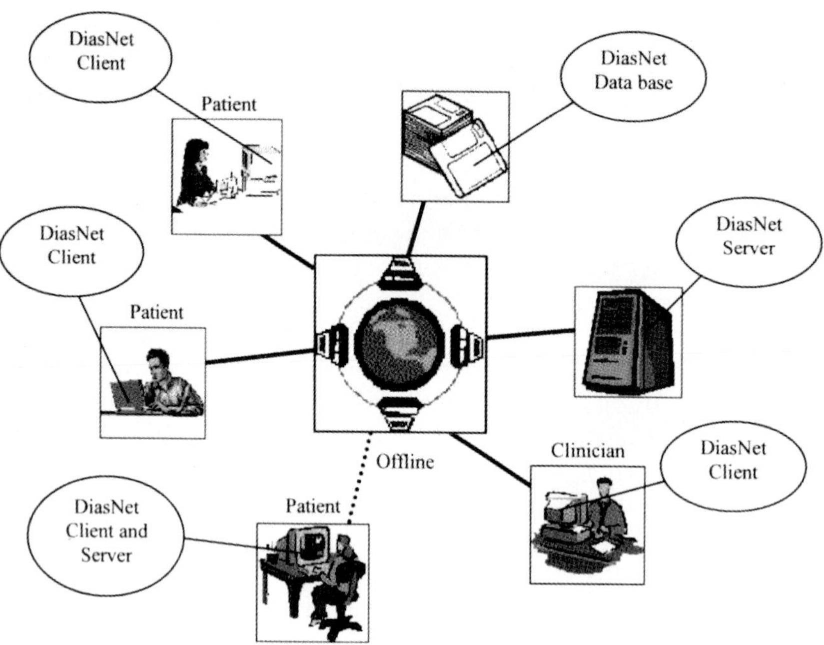



Fig. 1. The different physical parts of the DiasNet system. Utilising the client/server principle a server is used for central data storage and model computations allowing relatively thin clients. The patient and clinicians can access the DiasNet via Internet from a platform supporting *JAVA*. In case of no Internet connection a virtual server can be executed on the client computer.

user friendly interface in order to increase the acceptance of the system as a tool for patients. The DiasNet GUI consists of four main parts, a Data section for entering meal, insulin and blood glucose data, a Simulation section for graphical display of data and simulations, a Future section for experimenting with therapeutic and dietary alternatives and an Advanced section which displays advanced model information. As shown in Fig. 2, the Simulation section is always displayed in the top half to give a clear overview of data and the bottom half can via tabs be toggled between the Data, Future and Advanced sections. This provides simplicity and all functionalities are only one click away.

### 3.2. Data section

As the first step in using the system, blood glucose, meal and insulin data have to be entered. This is done via the Data section which besides providing functionality for entering the daily data, also displays patient information such as age, weight, height, sex and individual notes. Experience from the previous versions of the system identified entering of data as a bottleneck as it was very time consuming clicking through various popup windows for the different data types. The Data section part of DiasNet which has sought to solve this problem, is shown in Fig. 3.

As it can be seen, simplicity has been stressed in the design, and to enter data the following routine is adviced:

1. By clicking, select the data type; either Meal, BG (blood glucose measurement) or a specific insulin type.
2. Click in the date field, enter the date and press Return—the cursor now automatically moves to the time field.

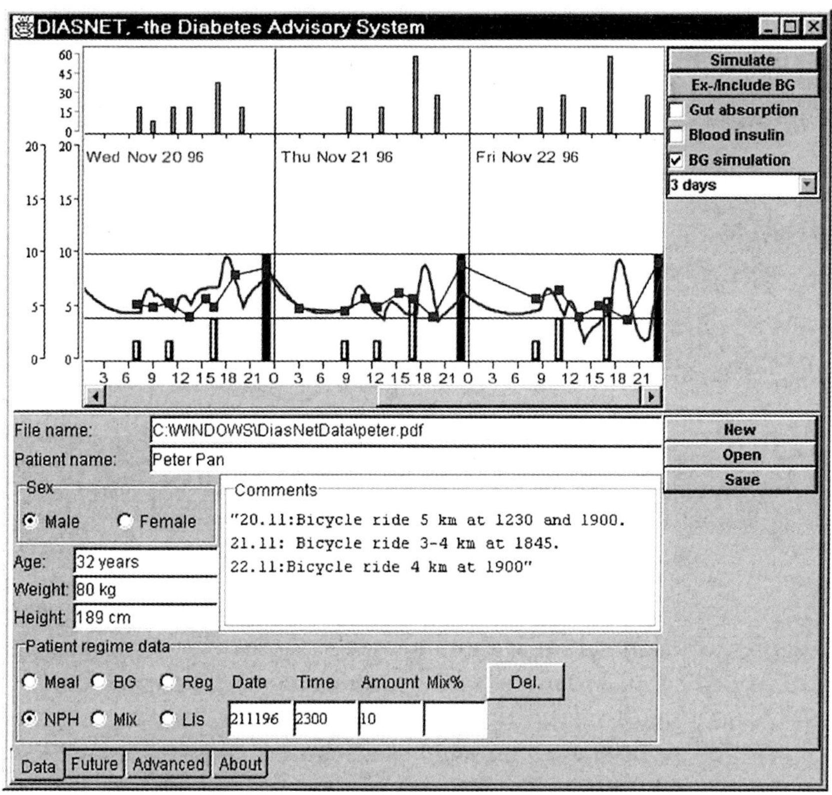



Fig. 2. Overview of the layout of the DiasNet GUI. The GUI is divided into two halfs, where the top half always displays the Simulation section. The bottom half can be toggled between the Data, Future and Advanced sections. This is done via the tabs in the bottom left corner. In the figure the Data section is diplayed in the bottom half.

3. Enter the time and press Return—the cursor now automatically moves to the amount field.

4. Enter the amount and press Return—the cursor now automatically moves back to the time field.

5. Continue entering the selected data type for this day (assisted by the cursor automatically moving in the step 3 and 4 loop) or select a different data type.

6. Pressing Return again without entering new data will automatically advance the date in the date field one day.

In this way, when Return is pressed, the input focus is automatically moved to the next logical component. Clicking in the Simulation section on a specific day will automati-

cally insert the corresponding date in the date field, and clicking on a specific data item in the Simulation section will insert its data for editing. Placing the mouse on the different data entry fields displays a help text: as shown in Fig. 3, the accepted formats for the time field are shown, and as it can be seen,

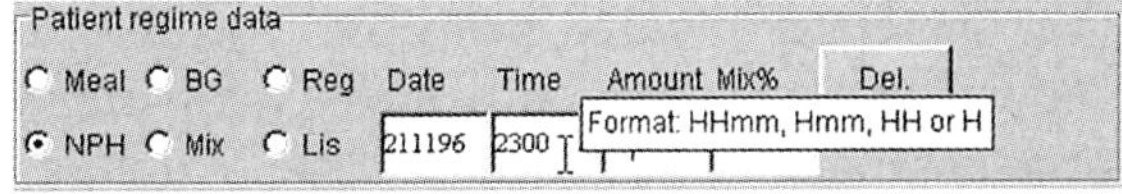



Fig. 3. The data enetering part of the Data section. On the left the different data types are shown. In the middle the textboxes for entering data are shown. All components have a help text, which is displayed when the mouse is positioned on the component, as shown for the time field.

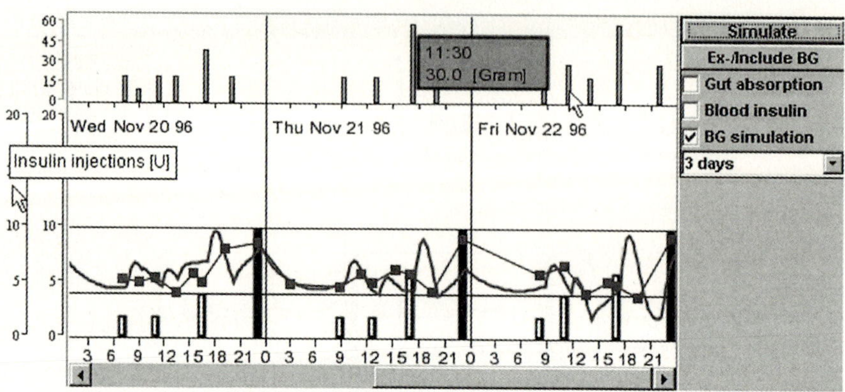

Fig. 4. The Simulation section. The figure shows 3 days of patient data on carbohydrate content in meals (grey bars in upper section), regular and NPH insulin injections (lower white bars with black outline and black bars, respectively) and blood glucose measurements (grey squares connected by straight lines). Blood glucose 4 and 10 mmol/l is indicated by horizontal lines. The bold grey curve shows the blood glucose prediction generated by the system.

several formats can be used. As data are entered, the display in the Simulation section is automatically scrolled so that the last entered item is simultaneously displayed in the middle of the Simulation section, enabling an easy continous visual monitoring of the data entry. A prototype module which interfaces blood glucose meters has been developed thereby reducing the need for keying in data.

### 3.3. Simulation section

Once data has been entered, the patient, by pressing the Simulate button, can perform a simulation (prediction) of the blood glucose based on the entered data: as step one, the model parameters are automatically adjusted to the specific patient data and, as step two, the predicted blood glucose profile is shown—to the user, however, step one is transparent. Fig. 4 shows 3 days of patient data on carbohydrate content in meals (grey bars in upper section), regular and NPH insulin injections (lower white bars with black outline and black bars, respectively) and blood glucose measurements (grey squares connected by straight lines). The typical in-

terval for good glycaemic control (blood glucose values between 4 and 10 mmol/l) is indicated by horizontal lines. The bold grey curve shows the blood glucose prediction generated by the system. Placing the mouse cursor on a data point, as shown for the lunch on November 22, will display the exact time and amount. Likewise, pointing at the axes, as shown to the left in the figure, will display their labels.

In addition to the blood glucose prediction, the predicted glucose absorption from the gut and the predicted blood insulin concentration can also be displayed. This is done via the check boxes in the right side of the Simulation section, where also the so-called active view, instead of the 3 days of data in Fig. 4, can be set to display, for example, data for a week. Questionable blood glucose measurements can be excluded by activating the Ex-/Include BG button. For example, due to an insufficient amount of blood applied to the blood glucose meter strip, there may be false measurements, which, preferably, should be excluded before estimating model parameters and calculating blood glucose predictions. Furthermore, the facility also serves as a tool in the detection of long-term hypoglycaemic counter regulations described by Hejlesen et al. [25].

A closer look at the measured blood glucose data displayed in Fig. 4 indicates fairly good glycaemic control, i.e. all measurements are between 4 and 10 mmol/l. However, on November 22, the system predicts severe hypoglycaemia around 14:00, which, due to the pre lunch regular insulin being increased (relative to the previous day), seems plausible. In fact, the patient had reported cases of symptomatic hypoglycaemia at that time of the day. Later that same day around 22:00 an additional hypoglycaemic episode is predicted by the system, which can be explained by the shift in time of the evening snack, compared to the previous days. In this way, potential problems are highlighted to the patient, and the patient can then experiment with the data in the Future section:

### 3.4. Future section

To experiment with data the patient simply clicks in the Simulation section on the day of interest, and this day is then automatically inserted in the Future section for further experiments. The layout of the Future section is identical to the Simulation section with the axes to the left, data in the middle and various buttons to the right. In Fig. 5 the data for November 22, where the system predicted hypoglycaemic episodes, is displayed.

In the Future section meals and insulin injections can be changed by simply using the mouse to drag the bars, and immediately seeing the resulting blood glucose prediction. As an example, the problem on November 22 has been addressed by increasing the meal at lunch time (from 30 to 50 g, as shown in the figure) and decreasing regular insulin at 17:00. The thin grey and bold grey curves show the blood glucose prediction before and after these adjustments, respectively. The original values of the meals and insulin injections are displayed as empty boxes with shadows.

Other therapeutic experiments can also be performed. Utilising the 'New item' functionality shown to the right in Fig. 6, the patient can illustrate the effect of various insulin types: for example using ultra-short acting insulin (Lispro) instead of short acting (regular) insulin.

The thin grey curve shows the resulting blood glucose profile that was found in Fig. 5

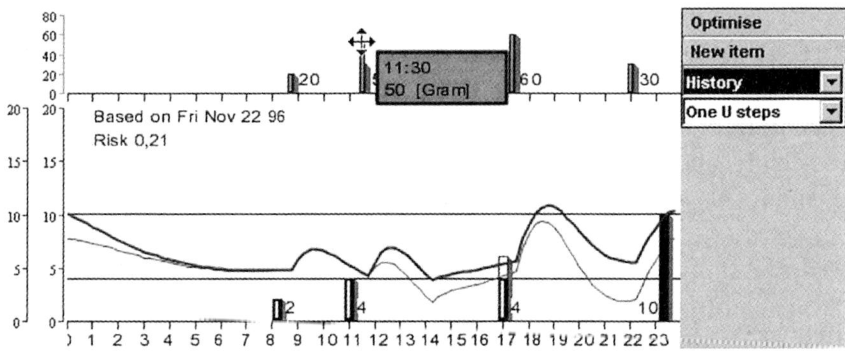



Fig. 5. The Future section. The figure shows a window, which allows the patient to change meals or insulin doses by simply using the mouse to drag the bars, as shown for the meal at 11:30, and immediately seeing the resulting blood glucose prediction. The lower thin grey and upper bold grey curves show the blood glucose prediction before and after these adjustments, respectively.

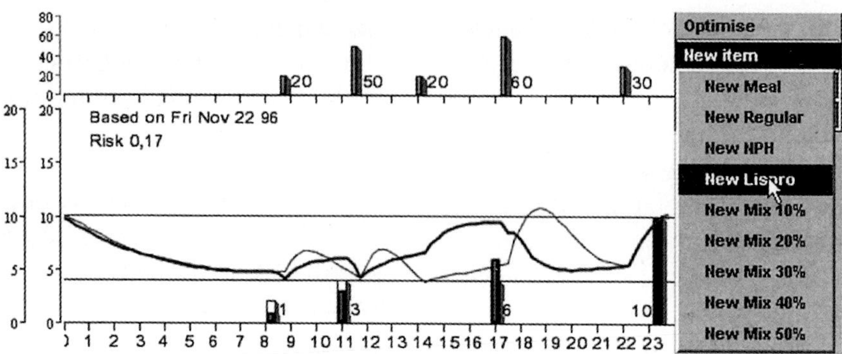



Fig. 6. The Future section. All three bolus insulin injections have been changed from regular insulin to Lispro. On the right the 'New item' menu displays the different insulin types available. Lispro injections are displayed as grey bars with black outline and the bold grey curve corresponds to the new regime with Lispro injections.

after increasing the meal at lunchtime and decreasing regular insulin at 17:00. The bold grey curve shows the blood glucose prediction after replacing regular (short acting) insulin injections by Lispro (ultra-short acting) injections. It can be seen how the elevating effect on the blood glucose of the meals is faster neutralised when using Lispro. However, at 14:00 the effect of the Lispro injection at 11:00 is almost gone and the snack at 14:00 therefore elevates the blood glucose. This illustrates that on a Lispro regime the patient probably should not have the between meals snacks, which, due to the longer absorption profiles, were necessary when the patient was on the regular insulin regime. Furthermore it can be seen that the Lispro injection probably should be taken at the beginning of the meals and not, as shown in the figure and as recommended with regular insulin, 30–45 min before the meal.

As can be seen, the thin grey curve and the empty boxes with shadow provide a History functionality that helps the patient track the changes, when experimenting with data. The patient can at any time reset the History functionality to store the current regime. To match various types of insulin pens, the system can operate in either one or two unit steps for the insulin injections.

Instead of the patient manually adjusting meals and insulin injections, the system can also perform an automatic optimisation of the insulin regime, given a fixed timing of meals and insulin. The principle is described in detail by Hejlesen et al. [26]. Fig. 7 shows the data from November 22, illustrating the result of an automatic optimisation.

When performing an automatic optimisation the patient can choose to optimise all insulin injections, or only the short or ultra-short acting injections (bolus injections) i.e. not changing the long acting injection (basal or NPH type insulin). Where the latter option should be used by the patient in most cases, the former might be more useful to the clinician. As shown on the right of Fig. 7 the basal injection was fixed, and the result of automatic optimisation was a relatively small reduction of all three bolus injections elevating the predicted blood glucose profile above the critical 4 mmol/l.

In the automatic optimisation, described in more detail by Hejlesen et al. [26], the system utilises a lopsided U-shaped utility or penalty function which penalises blood glucose values outside the 4–10 mmol/l interval. Values be low 4 mmol/l are penalised greater than values above 10 mmol/l as the potential harm of a hypoglycaemic episode is much greater than that of a hyperglycaemic episode—i.e. the lower arm of the U-shaped utility or penalty function is steeper than the upper arm.

As already mentioned and as described by Hejlesen et al. [23,26], the system also utilises patient specific parameters, the most important being the so-called insulin sensitivity. The parameters are automatically estimated based on the specific insulin regime, the meals and the blood glucose measurements, and in this way the model is tuned to fit each specific patient. The insulin sensitivity parameter is given by a discrete distribution, and therefore the resulting blood glucose profile, shown in the Simulation and the Future sections, is in fact, only the median of a distribution of blood glucose profiles. Fig. 8 shows two different insulin sensitivity distributions.

In Fig. 8, the distribution to the left is estimated from the patient data shown in Fig. 4 and used by the system in all simulations shown above. Given the unlikely assumption that the model was perfect and that there was no patient variation (i.e. noise) in the data, the insulin sensitivity distribution would be one thin peak with zero standard deviation, and accordingly the model blood glucose prediction would pass directly through all blood glucose measurements. The distribution to the right in Fig. 8 has been generated from the same data as the distribution to the left, using the Exclude functionality to remove blood glucose measurements representing the largest patient variation before performing the parameter estimation, thereby giving approximately the same median and a smaller standard deviation of the insulin sensitivity parameter.

A combination of the lopsided utility or penalty function and the blood glucose prediction distribution in the optimisation yields relatively good performance of the system: for patients with a large standard deviation of the insulin sensitivity parameter (corresponding to a larger variation in the patient data, i.e. more 'noise' in the patient data) the system, due to the steeper lower arm in the lopsided penalty curve, aims at higher blood glucose levels corresponding to lower insulin levels, which again implies a smaller risk of hypoglycaemia. For patients with a small standard deviation (less 'noise' in the patient data) the system 'dares' to suggest a more aggressive insulin therapy, i.e. aims at higher

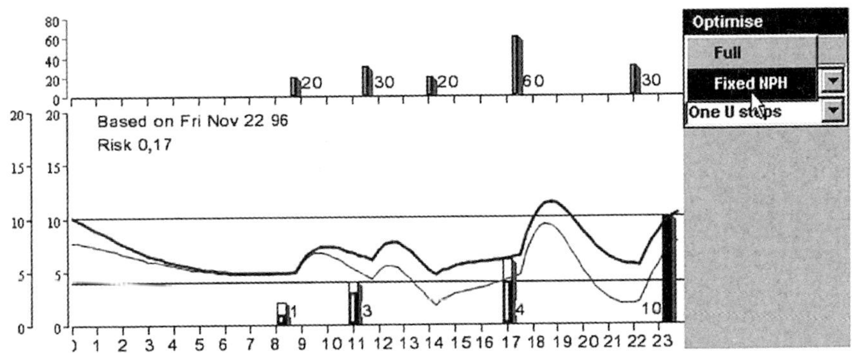


Fig. 7. The Future section. The system has performed an automatic optimisation on the insulin regime. As shown to the right both a full optimisation including all injections and an optimisation with fixed NPH (basal) insulin type injections is available.

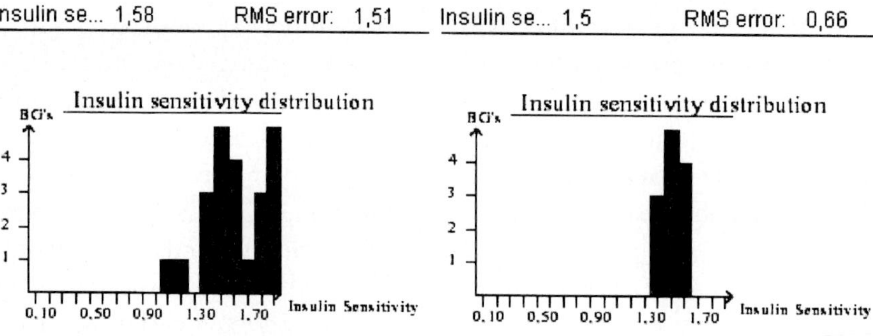



Fig. 8. Insulin sensitivity distributions from the Advanced section.

insulin doses resulting in a lower blood glucose predictions—which due to the lower variation in the blood glucose measurements seems justified. This effect is illustrated in Fig. 9 which shows the result of an optimisation with fixed NPH type insulin and using the distributions displayed in Fig. 8. It can be seen that because of the relatively small standard deviation of the insulin sensitivity distribution, the system has greater confidence in the accuracy of the blood glucose prediction and thereby positions the bold grey prediction curve (small standard deviation) closer to the bottom 4 mmol/l line, as compared with the thin grey prediction curve (larger standard deviation). It should be noted that the estimation of parameters and usage of distributions described above is completely transparent for the user.

## 4. Discussion

Dias is a decision support system based on a physiological model of human carbohydrate metabolism. The system has been evaluated in five small controlled clinical studies, which indicated a significant benefit from using the system to give advice on insulin dose.

DiasNet, which is an Internet version of Dias implemented in *JAVA* according to the client/server principle, is based on the experience from the clinical studies. It can run both as an ordinary application on a standard PC, and as an Internet application using a standard browser. The scope of this Internet version of the system has been widened; from being used by clinicians to give advise on insulin dose, to also being used by patients as a tool for education and communication.

Using the system, patients can experiment with their own data, adjusting insulin doses or meals sizes, and thereby learning how to cope with various situations. In this way different therapeutic and dietary alternatives can be tried out, allowing the patient to gain experience in achieving glycaemic control, without the risk of actually experiencing hypoglycaemic or hyperglycaemic episodes.

Both the database and the engine generating the blood glucose predictions can run both on the client, i.e. on the patients PC or handheld computer, and on a central server located at, for example, the hospital. This means that a new way of communication between patient and clinician is possible: In case of any problems, the patient simply phones the clinician, who immediately, using his or her office PC, can take a look at the data the patient has entered.

DiasNet is now being tested on a small group of patients with insulin dependent diabetes in Bournemouth, UK. To begin with, the patients had a training session where a nurse and a doctor first explained DiasNet to

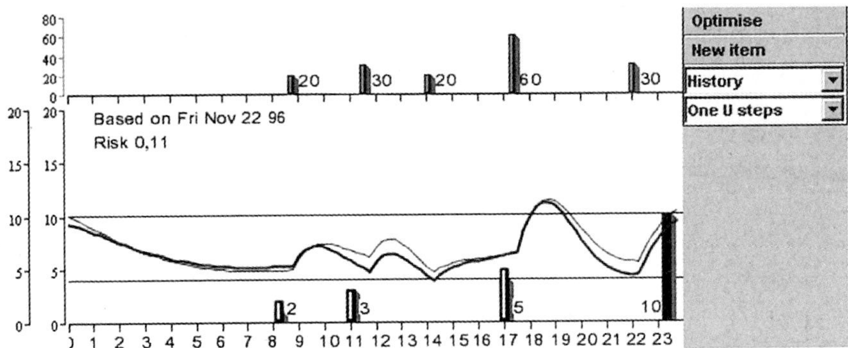


Fig. 9. The Future section. The figure shows the automatic optimisations using the two distributions in Fig. 8. The thin grey curve corresponds to the left distribution and the bold grey curve to the right distribution. It can be seen that the bold grey blood glucose prediction is positioned lower than the thin grey prediction.

the patients, and the patients then had time to experiment with the system on their own. Patients were then usernames and passwords enabling them to access DiasNet over the Internet. Preliminary results are promising.

The DiasNet system is part of ongoing research in different areas: a prototype module for integration of data from a subcutaneous glucose sensor into the DiasNet system has been developed. This gives a clear presentation of the sensor profile, in contrast to the relatively raw presentation of the data provided by the manufacturer. This would allow, for example, data from the sensor to be used to verify the metabolic model in DiasNet and to study various physiological phenomena [27]. Further developments include an interface for patients on continuous infusion pumps and a prototype DiasNet model which simulates the effects of alcohol ingestion on blood glucose concentration [28].

## Acknowledgements

The authors appreciate the financial contributions received from various national and international funds: from Nordjyllands Udviklingsfond (The Development Foundation of North Jutland), from the International Doctoral School at Aalborg University, from Novo Nordisk, from Lifescan and from the European Commission: The Dias Value Project, the DiabStyle Project, the MFIT Concerted Action and the TANDEM Project.

## References

[1] The Diabetes Control and Complications Trial Research Group, The effect of intensive treatment of diabetes on the development and progression of long-term complications in insulin-dependent diabetes mellitus, The New England Journal of Medicine 329 (1993) 977–986.

[2] American Diabetes Association, Direct and Indirect Costs of Diabetes in the United States in 1992, 1993.

[3] K. Black Jr., H.D. Skipper Jr., Life Insurance, Prentice Hall Business Publishing, 1993.

[4] G.W. Swan, An optimal control model of diabetes mellitus, Bull. Math. Biol. 44 (1982) 793–808.

[5] L.C. Schafer, R.E. Glasgow, K.D. McCoul, Adherence to IDDM regimens: relationship to psycosocial variables and metabolic control, Diabetes Care 6 (1983) 493–498.

[6] L.H. Chanoch, L. Jovanovic, C.M. Peterson, The evaluation of a pocket computer as an aid to insulin dose determination by patients, Diabetes Care 8 (1985) 172–176.

[7] A. Schiffrin, M. Mihic, B.S. Leibel, M. Albisser, Computer assisted insulin dosage adjustment, Diabetes Care 8 (1985) 545–552.

[8] F.E. Harvey, E.R. Carson, Diabeta—an expert system for the management of diabetes, in: D.D. Tsiftsis (Ed.), Objective Medical Decision-Making: Systems Approach in Disease, Springer-Verlag, Berlin, 1986, pp. 166–174.

[9] J. Schneider, K. Piwernetz, R. Engelbrecht, R. Renner, DIACONS—a consultation system to assist in the management of diabetes, in: O. Reinhoff, U. Piccolo, B. Schneider (Eds.), Expert Systems and Decision Support in Medicine, Springer-Verlag, Berlin, 1988, pp. 44–49.

[10] S.C. Chao, A.M. Albisser, The diabetes simulator, in Decision Support for Patient Management: Measurement, Modelling and Control (British Medical Informatics Society, London, 1989) 86–88.

[11] T. Deutsch, E.R. Carson, F.E. Harvey, E.D. Lehmann, P.H. Sonksen, G. Tamas, G. Whitney, C.D. Williams, Computer-assisted diabetic management: a complex approach, Comput. Methods Programs Biomed. 32 (1990) 195–214.

[12] E. Salzsieder, G. Albrecht, U. Fischer, A. Rutscher, U. Thierbach, Computer-aided systems in the management of type I diabetes: the application of a model-based strategy, Comput. Methods Programs Biomed. 32 (1990) 215–224.

[13] M.P. Berger, R.A. Gelfand, P.L. Miller, Combining statistical, rule-based and physiologic model-based methods to assist in the management of diabetes mellitus, Comput. Biomed. Res. 23 (1990) 346–357.

[14] M.S. Leaning, M.A. Boroujerdi, A system for compartmental modelling and simulation, Comput. Methods Programs Biomed. 35 (1991) 71–92.

[15] E.D. Lehmann, T. Deutsch, A.V. Roudsari, E.R. Carson, J.J. Benn, P.H. Sonksen, A metabolic prototype to aid in the management of insulin treated diabetic patients, Diabetes Nutr. Metab. 4 (Suppl. 1) (1991) 163–167.

[16] A. Ryff-de Leche, H. Engler, E. Nutzi, M. Berger, W. Berger, Clinical application of two computerized diabetes management systems: comparison with the log-book method, Diabetes Res. 19 (1992) 97–105.

[17] M.A. Boroujerdi, A.M. Umpleby, R.H. Jones, P.H. Sonksen, A simulation model for glucose kinetics and estimates of glucose utilization rate in type 1 diabetic patients, Am. J. Physiol. 268 (1995) E766–E774.

[18] G. Bleckert, U.G. Oppel, E. Salzsieder, Mixed graphical models for simultaneous model identification and control applied to the glucose–insulin metabolism, Comput. Methods Programs Biomed. 56 (1998) 141–155.

[19] L.F. Meneghini, A.M. Albisser, R.B. Goldberg, D.H. Mintz, An electronic case manager for diabetes control, Diabetes Care 21 (1998) 591–596.

[20] U. Bott, S. Bott, D. Hemmann, M. Berger, Evaluation of a holistic treatment and teaching programme for patients with Type 1 diabetes who failed to achieve their therapeutic goals under intensified insulin therapy, Diabetes Med. 17 (2000) 635–643.

[21] J. Wyatt, D. Spiegelhalter, Evaluating medical expert systems: what to test and how?, Med. Inform. 15 (1990) 205–217.

[22] J. Wyatt, C. Friedman, D. Spiegelhalter, Evaluating medical decision-aids, in: S. Uckun (Ed.), State-of-the-Art and Future Directions in AI in Medicine, Elsevier, Amsterdam, 1994.

[23] O.K. Hejlesen, S. Andreassen, R. Hovorka, D.A. Cavan, DIAS—the Diabetes Advisory System: an outline of the system and the evaluation results obtained so far, Comput. Methods Programs Biomed. 54 (1997) 49–58.

[24] O.K. Hejlesen, S. Andreassen, N.E. Frandsen, T. Brandt Sørensen, S.H. Sandø, D.A. Cavan, R. Hovorka, Using a double blind controlled clinical trial to evaluate the diabetes advisory system: a feasible approach?, Comput. Methods Programs Biomed. 56 (1998) 165–173.

[25] O.K. Hejlesen, S. Andreassen, D.A. Cavan, R. Hovorka, Analysing the hypoglycaemic counterregulation: a clinically relevant phenomenon?, Comput. Methods Programs Biomed. 50 (1996) 231–240.

[26] O.K. Hejlesen, S. Andreassen, S.K. Andersen, Implementation of a learning procedure for multiple observations in a Diabetes Advisory System based on causal probabilistic networks, in: S. Andreassen, R. Engelbrecht, J. Wyatt (Eds.), Artificial Intelligence in Medicine, IOS Press, Amsterdam, 1993, pp. 63–74.

[27] O.K. Hejlesen, S. Plougmann, E. Cheyne, J. Kentish, D. Kerr, D.A. Cavan. Using the Dias metabolic model to identify patients with unrecognised hypoglycaemia, Diabetic Medicine 18(Suppl 2) (2001) 34.

[28] O.K. Hejlesen, S. Plougmann, A Nielsen, B Turner, D.A. Cavan. A metabolic model of the effect of alcohol on the blood glucose level in insulin dependent diabetes, Proceedings of the World Congress on Medical Physics and Biomedical Engineering, Chicago, USA, July 23–28, 2000.

# *Section 8:*



Recommended additional readings by the Managing Editor:
- Achard F, Vaysseix G, Barillot E: XML, bioinformatics and data integration.
  Bioinformatcs Review 2001; 17(2):115-25.
- Foster JA. Evolutionary Computation.
  Nat Rev Genet 2001; 2:428-36.
- Vidal M. A biological Atlas of Functional Maps.
  Cell 2001; 104:333-9.


*Reprinted by kind permission of:*
*Oxford University Press (625),*
*Elsevier Science (632, 639, 652),*
*Henry Stewart Publications (663)*

**H. Tanaka**

Department of Bioinformatics
Medical Research Institutes
Tokyo Medical and Dental University
Japan

# Synopsis

# *Computational approach towards challenges in the post-genomic era*

In this section, articles which reflect current post-genomic trends in bioinformatics are collected. Here we overview the various post-genomic challenges and, in relation to them, we briefly introduce the contents of the collected articles.

## 1. Bioinformatic studies in the post-genomic era

Since the human genome project is almost finished [1,2], main interests in the life science community are now moving to post-genomic challenges, such as functional genomics, comparative genomics, proteomics, metabolomics, pathway analysis, systems biology. In bioinformatics analysis, although sequence analyses have been and are still the most common tasks in the routine analyses, new topics in bioinformatics studies have appeared to tackle post-genomic challenges. We briefly overview several study fields below.

### (1) Whole genome informatics

Now that whole genome sequences of more than 100 species are finished to read, though most are prokaryotes, the study of the whole genome structure becomes possible. Comparative genomics [3] is a new branch of genome sciences which compares whole genome sequences between different species to find genome-wide common structure and its evolutionary change. One of the classical examples in comparative genomics is to infer the minimum gene set of life from the comparison among the genomes of the primitive microbial organisms [4, 5]. Other typical studies are related to the evolutionary trace of large-scaled change of genome structures, such as chromosome duplication in the course of evolution concerning the gene cluster [6].

In the whole of genome informatics, effective usage of genome databases is a prerequisite. There are many well-known databases for whole genome such as GDB (Genome DataBase), LocusLink/ReqSeq, FlyBase and WormBase. To ensure usability and accessibility of the database, it becomes important to eliminate the factors militating against the full exploitation of the genomic information.

In the paper by Coppel, a Malaria genome database (Plasmodium DB) is taken and discussed with regards to several problems related to ensuring the full exploitation of whole genome sequences. The paper presents several lessons learned which would be of use to other organism-specific databases.

### (2) Transcriptome analysis and microarray data processing

Transcriptome, comprehensive information of gene expression (mRNA) at the whole cell level, can now be observed by DNA chip and cDNA microarray. Whereas the genome is a possible repertory of biological function in terms of gene set and the proteome is the currently expressed whole set of functional protein, the transcriptome reflects the current production rate of functional protein in each cell, so that it shows, so to speak, intentions of living cells under the imposed cell conditions, which are not found in the information of the genome and the proteome.

A great deal of new bioinformatics studies related to microarray data have emerged over the years. There are mainly two sub fields in microarray information processing. One is phenomenological processing of gene expression data in micro-arrays such as the classification of the expression profile through clustering methods to make groups both for genes and subjects, or to identify the differentially expressed genes under the two comparative conditions of micro-arrays [7, 8].

The other is to identify structural relations among expressions of each gene. Along this line of the study, a typical study is to identify genetic (regulation) networks from the expression profiles of micro-arrays [9,10]. Many models are used for representing the genetic network; for example the Boolean genetic network model where, though its connected path, a gene facilitates or suppresses the other's expression is a simple deterministic model of the genetic network. On the other hand, there are also probabilistic models where the interactions between connected genes are random.

In the paper by Reis et al., temporal slopes of the expression level of each gene are determined based on the sequential observations of mRNA expression pattern of *Saccharomyces cerevisiae* and correlation coefficients are calculated between these temporal slopes of all genes. By random permutation of expression data, they estimated the variation of the correlation coefficients when there is no significant correlation between genes, and determined the thresholds over which we judge the existence of significant correlation. By connecting pairs of genes having over-threshold correlation, so to speak dynamically correlated pattern ("relevance network") among the genes can be obtained. They show high association in this dynamic correlation well agrees with functional and regulatory relationships between genes.

### (3) Other areas

The bioinformatics field related to proteins, called "Protein Informatics" has also drastically progressed recently. This field includes (1) structural genomics where structural prediction of protein or classification of representative structure of basic protein folds is a main topic, (2) proteomics which is related to the comprehensive observation and characterization of functional proteins in the cell and (3) functional genomics which predicts protein function from the sequences and structures such as to estimate binding sites or reaction sites.

## 2. Pathway analysis and systems biology

Other important new areas of bioinformatics research are those which aim to understand life as a whole functional organization from comprehensive bio-information. This area ranges from the more confined topic called "pathway analysis", to more generally proposed disciplines of "systems biology".

### (1) Pathway analysis

In the pathway analysis, metabolic pathway or protein-protein networks such as signal transduction cascade are of main interests. We have already several well known pathway DBs, for example, KEGG (Kyoto encyclopedia of Genes and Genomes), an online database for metabolic and regulatory pathways, ExPASy molecular biology server, a scanned map of Boehringer-Mannheim 'Biochemical Pathways', EcoCyc, a comprehensive database for metabolic and regulatory pathways of E. Coli. TRANSPATH and CNSDB (Cell signaling Network Database) are databases especially for signal transduction cascades.

In these pathway DBs, pathways are visualized in graph format but mostly in a static way. It would be preferable that graph representation of the pathways can be automatically and dynamically updated when new components are incorporated. In the paper by M. Becker, a new algorithm is presented to draw the metabolic pathway by combination of circular, hierarchic and force-directed graph layout. This automatic drawing of the metabolic network is of great use to promote the feasibility of pathway DBs.

### (2) Systems biology
#### 1) Concept

Although Kitano coins the word "systems biology", it is now widely accepted as a generic term. The field and purpose of systems biology [11] is not new in bioinfomatics. So far, similar disciplines have been called "integrative biology" or "biological system analysis". One of the typical and established research areas for this sort of analysis has been in the area of "metabolic control analysis" [12] where traditional control system theory is applied to the metabolic pathway to investigate the system performance or sensitivity of rate-limiting path in the metabolic system.

Prior to the post-genomic era, there had been no largely organized comprehensive biological data ("–omic" data) to be utilized in the model analysis. These studies were therefore forced to be theoretical using only simple mathematical models and few experimental data. Now, many kinds of comprehensive biological data are available and the studies dealing with the integrative behavior of life are gradually changing with regard to study style. They use large-scaled data obtained by genome-wide measurement such as whole gene expression profile by cDNA micro-array, and the modeling becomes more comprehensive and realistic in dealing with whole cells, though modeled organisms are primitive microbes. The following topics are now being studied currently in systems biology:

(1) Comprehensive simulation of large-scale pathways of metabolism, including a whole cell metabolism

(2) System analysis of the metabolic pathway or genetic regulatory network

(3) System identification of the metabolic pathway or genetic regulatory network from comprehensive experimental data such as the cDNA expression profile.

(4) System design of the artificial organism or artificial bacteria having preferable characteristics.

(5) Pathway databases and signal transaction cascade databases

(6) Tools and software to support the system biology such as the cell

simulation package and standard documentation language for cell modeling.

### 2) Projects

In the last several years, systems biology has become one of the nation-wide projects in the post-genomic era. In the United States, NIH/NIGMS supports the Alliance for the Cellular Signaling (AFCS) project which aims at examining the signal transduction inside cells, by analyzing mouse's G-protein coupled signaling system where 1000 proteins work cooperatively. They also support a cellular communication and cell migration consortium and many other groups conducting the quantitative analysis of complex biological systems.

The Department of Energy (DOE) is also conducting a "Genome to Life" project mainly aiming to model the microbial "virtual cell", especially its metabolic system organization and its migration. The biomedical engineering projects in NIH called physiome projects also have a strong relation to systems biology. In EU, Model of Life (MOL) projects are now being conducted.

In Japan, E-Cell, a simulator for virtual cells with minimal gene set (127 genes) was developed by Tomita which is used as a base model for a human red blood cell [13].

### 3) Related areas – Biological modeling, complex systems, dynamical network theory

From a slightly different perspective, another stream also attracts interests in the systems biology community. This stream is nonlinear modeling or the complex systems approach to biological systems. So far in the field of theoretical biology, complex systems approaches were adopted because biological systems are always nonlinear. In the complex systems approach, the whole system is considered more than the sum of its parts and emerging properties of biological systems are well recognized in the origins of life, biological evolution, and development process. So far, as often seen in the Kauffman theory [13], for modeling those essential phenomena of life, Erdos random network theory has been ordinarily used for the base model of biological relations. For example, random reaction networks of autocatalytic sets of biopolymers are used for modeling the origin of life, random epigenetic interaction networks among the genes are used for calculating the integrative fitness landscape of multiple genes of evolution, and random Boolean networks are utilized to describe the regulation of cell types in biological development.

But recently random networks haven't been seen as the appropriate model for real networks, instead "scale free" networks [15] in which the frequency distribution of number of edge connecting to the nodes has a long tail obeying power-law (straight line in log-log plot) or otherwise "small world" networks [16] are used. It was shown that the metabolic pathway [17] and protein-protein interaction network of Yeast Two Hybrid [18] is a scale-free network. Hence, with comprehensive biological information and a new dynamical network theory, system level organization of biological networks will drastically be clarified in theory.

In the paper by Yates, by taking the immunological system as an example, techniques and the issues in building "good" biological modeling are discussed, where nonlinear threshold effects and bifurcation or emerging phenomena in immunological response are investigated by a phase plain method about the immunological cytokine (TNF) network and T helper T cell differentiation. Monte Carlo simulation is described for stochastic simulation for cross talk for T cell receptors.

# 3. Clinical bioinformatics

## (1) Polymorphism of the human genome

Comprehensive approaches for biological information also begin to exert important influences on clinical medicine. Various polymorphisms of the human genome sequence characterize the individual specificity of the patient genome, such as restriction enzyme polymorphism, VNTR (variable number of tandem repeat), SINE, LINE and SNP (single nucleotide polymorphism). Especially SNPs are recently the main target of comprehensive surveys in relation to drug discoveries. SNPs are found on average every one thousandth nucleotide, so that three million SNPs are supposed to characterize the haplotype of the patient genome, which would be related to the disease and drug response. Hence it would be of main interest for clinical application of genome to realize "Personalized medicine".

## (2) System theoretic approach to diseases – disease modeling

Disease might be due to the defect of a single gene (mono-genic disease) or caused by defects of more than one gene (polygenic disease). Since mono-genic diseases seem to be mostly explored, polygenic diseases, which cover most "common diseases" such as hypertention, diabetes and ischemic heart diseases, are now attracting more attention. In the polygenic common diseases, diseases are thought to form themselves in the combined manner of the various gene defects and the environment. For example, more than 20 genes are related to the occurrence of diabetes. So like systems biology for normal biosystems, a systems-pathological approach or systematic disease modeling would be of great value to comprehensive understanding of polygenic diseases.

One of the promising approaches in disease modeling is the "Virtual

Patient". Entelos Inc. has developed the virtual patient system that is used to model obesity, diabetes and asthma. The virtual patient model involves various levels of knowledge, such as related to the genetic, pathophysiologic and life-style factors and both top-down and bottom-up approach between genetic level to symptomatologic level are employed. The day will come soon when we use these virtual patient models for clinical decision making.

In the paper by Sreekumar et.al, they show the many examples wherein by using comparative genomics and computational sequence analysis, especially for domain analysis of functional protein, many human disease-related genes can be identified and the etiology is accessed. It could be considered as a preliminary trial of "systems pathology" or "disease modeling".

## 4. Conclusions

In the bioinformatics field, new research topics to solve post-genomic challenges are emerging. In this synopsis, whole genome informatics (comparative and functional genom-ics), pathway analysis, systems biology and clinical bioinformatics were especially discussed. Collected papers have strong relation to these topics.

## References


1. International Human Genome Sequencing Consortium. Initial sequencing and analysis of the human genome. Nature 2001;409:860-921.
2. Venter JC, Adams MD, Myers EW, Li PW, Mural RJ, Sutton GG, et al. The sequence of the human genome, Science 2001;291:1304-51.
3. Koonin.EV. The emerging paradigm and open problems in comparative genomics. Bioinfomatics 1999;15(4):265-6.
4. Hutchison CA, Peterson SN, Gill SR, Cline RT, White O, Fraser CM, et al. Global transposon mutagenesis and a minimal mycoplasma genome. Science 1999;286:2165-9.
5. Koonin EV, Mushegian AR. Complete genome sequences of cellular life forms. Curr opin genet dev 1996;6(6):757-62.
6. Koonin EV, Aravind L, Kondrashov AS. The impact of comparative genomics on our understanding of evolution. Cell 2000;101(6):573-6.
7. Quackenbush J. Computational analysis of microarray data. Nat Rev Genet 2001 Jun;2(6):418-27.
8. Raychaudhuri S, Sutpin PD, Chang JT, Altman RB. Basic micro array analysis:grouping and feature reduction. Trends Biotechnol 2001;19(5):189-93.
9. Liang S, Fuhrman S, Somogyi R. REVEAL, a general reverse engineering algorithm for inference of genetic network architectures. Pac Symp Biocomput 1998:18-30.
10. D'haeseleer P, Liang S, Somogyi R. From co-expression clustering to reverse engineering. Bioinfomatics 2000;16(8): 707-26.
11. Kitano H. Systems biology: a brief overview. Science 2002; 295:1662-4.
12. Fell D, Snell K, editors. Understanding the Control of Metabolism. Portland Press;1997.
13. Tomita M. Whole cell simulation: a grand challenge of 21$^{st}$ century. Trends Biotechnol 2001;19(6):205-10.
14. Kauffman S. Origins of Life. Oxford;1994.
15. Babarasi A. Linked. Perseus; 2002.
16. Watts D. Small Worlds. Princeton; 1999.
17. Jeong H, Tombor B, Albert R, Oltavi ZN, Barabasi AL. The large-scale organization of metabolic networks. Nature 2000; 407(6804):651-4.
18. Jeong H, Mason SP, Barabasi AL, Oltavi ZN. Centrality and lethality of protein networks. Nature 2001;411(6833):41-2.



Address of the author:
Hiroshi Tanaka
Department of Bioinformatics
Medical Research Institutes
Tokyo Medical and Dental University
1-5-45, Bunkyo
Tokyo 113-8510, Japan
Tel:        0081/3-5803-5839
Fax:        0081/3-5684-3618
E-mail:     tanaka@cim.tmd.ac.jp

# A graph layout algorithm for drawing metabolic pathways

*Moritz Y. Becker* and Isabel Rojas*

*Scientific Databases and Visualization Group, European Media Laboratory, Schloss-Wolfsbrunnenweg 33, D-69118 Heidelberg, Germany*

Received on September 9, 2000; revised on December 6, 2000; accepted on January 16, 2001

## ABSTRACT

**Motivation:** A large amount of data on metabolic pathways is available in databases. The ability to visualise the complex data dynamically would be useful for building more powerful research tools to access the databases. Metabolic pathways are typically modelled as graphs in which nodes represent chemical compounds, and edges represent chemical reactions between compounds. Thus, the problem of visualising pathways can be formulated as a graph layout problem. Currently available visual interfaces to biochemical databases either use static images or cannot cope well with more complex, non-standard pathways.

**Results:** This paper presents a new algorithm for drawing pathways which uses a combination of circular, hierarchic and force-directed graph layout algorithms to compute positions of the graph elements representing main compounds and reactions. The algorithm is particularly designed for cyclic or partially cyclic pathways or for combinations of complex pathways. It has been tested on five sample pathways with promising results.

**Availability:** On request from the authors.

**Contact:** mywyb2@cam.ac.uk

## INTRODUCTION

Today, a large amount of information on metabolic pathways is available in various databases. Pathways are typically modelled as complex networks of chemical compounds and reactions. It is evident that a graphical representation of such networks is useful for managing the intrinsic complexity of the data. Powerful research tools could be built which dynamically query a database and visualise the resulting pathway. The visualised pathway could be used to refine the query and to navigate through the database.

An example of such a system is KEGG (Kyoto Encyclopaedia of Genes and Genomes), an online database system for querying information on metabolic and regulatory pathways and genome sequences (Kanehisa and Goto, 2000). As in most currently available systems, KEGG visualises pathways in a static way. Pathway diagrams are manually drawn and stored as bitmap image files. These diagrams are displayed as interactive image maps with links to additional information on enzymes and to adjacent pathways.

Another example for static visualisation of pathways is the ExPASy Molecular Biology Server (Appel *et al.*, 1994) which gives online access to the scanned-in version of the Boehringer Mannheim 'Biochemical Pathways' map (Michal, 1993). The map is partitioned into 115 rectangular pieces. Keywords entered by the user are matched against entries on the map, and the corresponding pieces of the map can be displayed.

As Brandenburg *et al.* (1998) pointed out, static visualisation has many severe disadvantages. Whenever the data has been updated, the corresponding images have to be edited manually to reflect the changes. Furthermore, there is no way to specify the amount of detail to be displayed or to hide parts of the pathway. Finally, when it comes to visualising user defined or novel pathways, static visualisation is not applicable at all.

Therefore the visualisation process should be performed dynamically at runtime, based on the information provided by the database. Dynamic visualisation in contrast to static visualisation provides high flexibility, which is necessary for complex queries and the construction of novel pathways.

Metabolic pathways are commonly modelled as directed graphs. A pathway is a collection of interconnected biochemical reactions. Main reactants and products (the compounds that constitute the 'backbone' of the pathway) are represented as nodes and the reactions as edges of the graph. Usually the enzymes catalysing the reaction are displayed as edge labels. Side substrates are drawn near the edge, connected to the edge by curved arcs. Therefore, the problem of dynamically drawing a pathway is a graph layout problem. Given as input a combinatorial description of a graph, a graph layout algorithm should compute geometric positions for the graph elements

---

*To whom correspondence should be addressed at: Trinity College, University of Cambridge, Cambridge CB2 1TQ, UK.

according to a set of rules.

There are a number of standard graph layout algorithms. Examples include algorithms for circular, orthogonal or planar drawing, and force-directed layout heuristics (Di Battista *et al.*, 1994, 1999; Brandenburg *et al.*, 1997). However, none of these algorithms give satisfactory results when applied to pathway networks.

Little previous work has been done on developing graph layout algorithms for drawing biochemical networks. Karp and Paley (1994) have pointed out that rather than searching for one single, all-purpose graph layout algorithm, different algorithms should be applied to parts of the pathway with different topologies. They devised an algorithm for drawing metabolic pathways which breaks the graph into cyclic, linear and tree-structured components and then applies different layout methods to each of these individually. Their algorithm has been implemented in the EcoCyc system, an electronic encyclopaedia that allows scientists to visualise a collection of biochemical information (Karp *et al.*, 2000).

Takai-Igarashi and Kaminuma (1998) developed a Cell Signalling Network Database (CSNDB) with an interface for dynamic visualisation of pathway data. A new system, PaF-CSNDB, also allows users to find and construct novel pathways (Takai-Igarashi and Kaminuma, 1999). Pathway diagrams are constructed dynamically by a modified version of an algorithm first implemented in the ACEDB software (A. C. elegans database) (Durbin and Mieg, 1991). The original algorithm (S.Letovsky, personal communication) is very similar to the one by Karp and Paley. Acyclic and cyclic components of the graph are identified and laid out using a hierarchic and a circular algorithm, respectively.

PathDB, a pathway database focused on plant metabolism, takes a similar approach. The information stored in the database is converted into a graph structure. If the structure contains cycles, the visualisation front-end lets the user choose between a hierarchical or a circular layout method to calculate the co-ordinates of the nodes (J.Blanchard, personal communication).

In this paper we propose a new algorithm for drawing graphs representing metabolic pathways. Based on the one proposed by Karp and Paley, it takes into account the topological structure of the graph. The algorithm is supplemented by a special force-directed layout algorithm and additional layout heuristics.

We will concentrate on the placement of the graph nodes and edges representing main reactants and products only. The problem of placement of labels that contain information on enzymes and other information related to the biochemical reactions is also being addressed by our research group and will be the topic of a publication currently in preparation. Readers interested in this topic are encouraged to contact the authors for more information.

## SYSTEM AND METHODS

The algorithm was implemented in Java 1.3 and executed on a Pentium II workstation running Windows NT. The Java-based graph library YFiles (Wiese *et al.*, 2000) was used to create, manipulate, and view the graph. YFiles provides Java classes representing data structures for graphs, nodes, and edges. These data structures do not only contain information about the abstract graph but also graphical information such as location, sizes and labels of nodes and edges. The library also offers a number of standard graph layout modules, in particular for circular and hierarchic layout, both of which are used in the presented algorithm. The YFiles graphical user interface provides functions for viewing, navigation and interactive editing.

The algorithm does not depend on the choice of the underlying graph library. There are many other packages which could have been used for implementation instead of YFiles. For example, Automatic Graph Drawing (AGD) from Algorithmic Solutions Software, the Graph Drawing Toolkit from Integra Sistemi or the Graph Layout Toolkit from Tom Sawyer Software all offer features which are similar to YFiles.

## AESTHETIC GOALS

Common graph layout algorithms draw a graph in such a way that it satisfies certain well-defined aesthetic criteria and constraints such as planarity, minimal edge crossings (edges intersecting with other edges or nodes), minimal drawing area, and maximal symmetry. In the case of metabolic pathways it is difficult, if not impossible, to state such a set of clear cut constraints. Apart from meeting the aesthetic criteria stated above it seems to be important to adhere to well-established, albeit not well-defined, conventions as can be found in relevant biochemistry textbooks (Michal, 1999).

In the figures of such textbooks one can identify two different structures that are used noticeably frequently: directed, hierarchic components and circular components. Whenever such a circular subgraph exists the remaining components are laid out around the circle in such a way that the components are near the nodes of the circle to which they are connected. Sufficiently small components which are connected to the circle by a relatively large number of edges are often placed inside the circle in order to avoid edge crossings. Our algorithm is based on these observations.

## ALGORITHM

Some chemical reactions have more than one main reactant or product. In these cases the reaction has to be represented as a hyperedge, i.e. an edge with multiple source and target nodes. The YFiles library does not

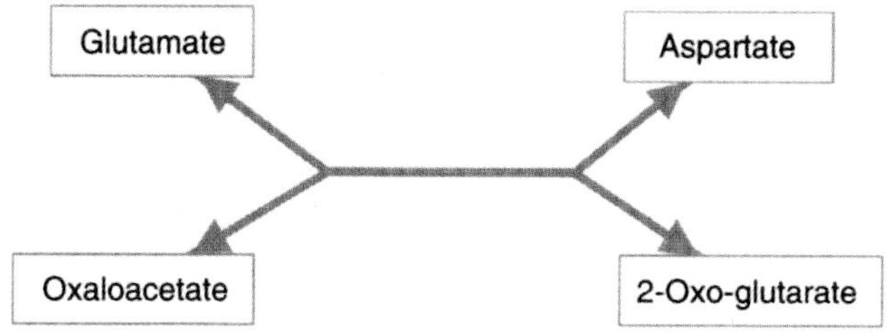


**Fig. 1.** Hyperedges model chemical reactions with multiple main reactants or products. Zero size dummy nodes are inserted at the forking positions.

support hyperedges, so hyperedges were simulated by inserting a dummy node at the front of an edge which forks out to the multiple target nodes. Similarly, a dummy node is inserted at the back of the edge which is connected to all source nodes. The sizes of the dummy nodes were set to zero (Figure 1).

A simple cycle is a cyclic path in which each node of the path is visited exactly once. The algorithm starts by traversing the directed connected graph to look for the longest simple cycle contained in the graph. The cycle is found by breaking the graph into strongly connected components (subgraphs in which every two nodes are reachable from each other) and then using a depth first search on these components.

### Base cases

Two trivial base cases can now be identified: if no cycle could be found at all, the top-to-bottom hierarchic layout algorithm provided by the graph library is applied. The hierarchic layout algorithm partitions the nodes into layers such that nodes in one layer can only be connected to nodes in adjacent layers. If this is not possible, edges crossing several layers are split into several shorter edges, and dummy nodes are inserted. Then the nodes within a layer are permuted to minimise edge crossings. Finally the nodes are positioned to give a balanced layout (Sugiyama *et al.*, 1981; Eades and Sugiyama, 1990).

The other base case applies when the longest cycle is in fact the entire graph. In this case the circular layout algorithm provided by the graph library is used.

### General case

If none of the two base cases apply, a longest cycle must have been found, and this cycle must be a proper subgraph of the given graph, so there exist nodes which do not belong to the cycle. These nodes are now grouped into connected components, i.e. sets of connected nodes. The resulting components are by definition not connected to each other. Since the original graph was a connected graph, each of the components must have at least one

connection to the cycle. We can distinguish two kinds of components. The *inner components* are those consisting of only one node and that are connected to the cycle by at least two edges, and will be placed inside the circle. All other components are *outer components*, and will be placed around the circle. The choice of one node as threshold for the inner components was made in a somewhat arbitrary manner, since it appeared to be aesthetically the best value. There can be more than one inner node in a cycle but only if they are not connected to each other.

Next, the circular layout algorithm is applied to the cycle, and the minimum radius is chosen such that the resulting circle is large enough to accommodate all inner components.

The outer components are then laid out by recursively applying the same algorithm to each of them individually. The recursion is guaranteed to terminate since one of the two base cases will eventually hold. After that, each component is collapsed into a supernode. The supernode is set to the same location and extent as the subgraph it represents. The supernode–subgraph relationship is stored in a hash table so that later the supernodes can be expanded quickly.

A customised spring embedding layout algorithm (Quinn and Breuer, 1979; Eades, 1984) is applied to the remaining graph, now consisting of the circular cycle, the inner components and the outer supernodes. The spring embedding algorithm places the inner components inside and the supernodes around the circle. The placement is done in such a way that the inner components and the supernodes lie near the circle nodes they are connected to but without overlapping each other. The details of this algorithm are discussed in the next section.

Finally, the supernodes are expanded and replaced by the corresponding subgraphs.

## THE CUSTOMISED SPRING EMBEDDING ALGORITHM

The purpose of this sub-algorithm is to lay out the inner components inside the given circle and the supernodes outside the circle. We add the further constraints that nodes must not overlap and that nodes not belonging to the circle are positioned near the nodes on the circle to which they are connected. A force-directed approach seems to be the most natural solution to this problem. Force-directed layout algorithms model the graph as a system of particles with forces acting on them and attempt to find a minimum energy configuration of this system. The spring embedding algorithm is the best known force-directed layout algorithm (Quinn and Breuer, 1979; Eades, 1984). Each edge acts as a spring with a preferred length and exerts a repulsive or attractive force on the nodes connected by it. Nodes are considered as mutually repulsive charges. The total energy of the system is minimised by iteratively letting the nodes move in direction of the forces exerted on them, starting from their initial positions.

The YFiles library implements a version of the spring embedding algorithm. However, it was found to be unsuitable for our purpose, mainly because it does not consider node sizes. We developed a customised implementation with additional heuristics.

As in the original algorithm, the force strength is dependent on the distances between two nodes, but now the distance is computed not as the distance between the centres of the two nodes but rather as the distance between the boundaries of the nodes, thus taking node sizes into account. This is essential because the size of a supernode is the extent of the bounding box of the corresponding subgraph.

Furthermore, each supernode in the system can be assigned a *centre of mass* location. We define the centre of mass of a supernode to be the average position of those nodes inside the supernode which are connected to the circle. In the original spring embedding algorithm, the mutually repulsive charge forces act as if the entire charge was concentrated at the geometric centre of the node. In our model the charge is concentrated at the centre of mass. Also, the ends of the springs are modelled as if they were attached not to the geometric centre of a supernode but to its centre of mass. Using the centre of mass location rather than the geometric centre takes into account the internal structure of a supernode without adding too much overhead.

Each node is associated with a value for its inertia, i.e. its resistance to move, and each edge with an individual preferred length. Clearly the nodes of the circular subgraph should be fixed, hence these nodes are assigned an infinite inertia.

The energy configuration of the system may have multiple local minima, and depending on the initial placement of nodes the algorithm will converge to one of these minima. Therefore care must be taken to compute appropriate initial positions for the nodes.

## Computing initial positions

The inner components can simply be placed at the centre of the circle initially. The spring embedding algorithm will automatically find appropriate positions for these nodes within the circle.

For the outer supernodes we can define a *preferred radial angle* relative to the circle. This angle is the average of radial angles of those nodes of the circle to which the supernode is connected.

Suppose the centre of mass of a supernode lies in its upper region. That means that the edges connecting

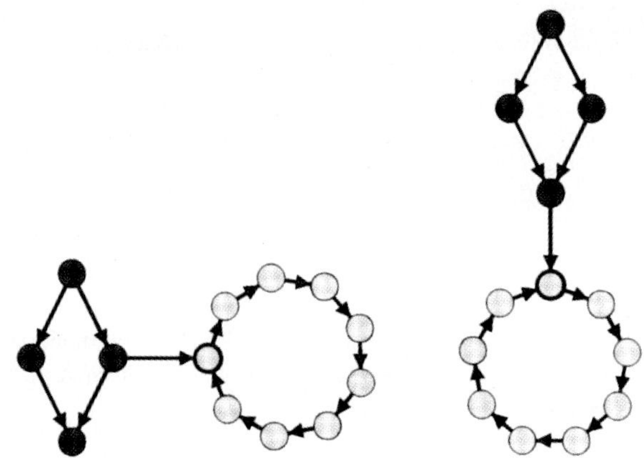

**Fig. 2.** In the left-hand panel the only node of the outer supernode (darkly shaded) which is connected to the circle lies on the right, so the centre of mass of the supernode lies on the right, hence the preferred orientation is west. The circle is rotated such that the supernode lies west of the circle. Similarly, in the right-hand panel, the centre of mass of the outer supernode is at its bottom, hence the preferred orientation is north of the circle.

it to the circle are incident with internal nodes of the supernode which are located mainly in the upper region of the supernode. So if the supernode is initially positioned such that its centre of mass is south of the circle (at $-90°$ relative to the circle) and if the circle is then rotated in such a way that the resulting preferred radial angle of the supernode is $-90°$, it is likely that fewer edge crossings occur. In this case we say that the *preferred orientation* of the supernode is South. Note that the preferred orientation of a supernode depends only on the displacement of its centre of mass relative to its geometric centre.

Similarly, the preferred orientation of a supernode is North if the centre of mass lies in its bottom region, East if the centre of mass lies on its left-hand side and West if it lies on its right-hand side (Figure 2).

It is clear that this preference cannot be satisfied for all supernodes simultaneously. In our algorithm the circle is initially rotated in such a way that at least the largest supernode has its preferred orientation.

After the rotation has been performed, the preferred radial angle is computed for all other supernodes, and each supernode is placed around the circle accordingly (Figure 3). The preferred edge lengths are set to the actual current lengths of the supernode edges. This ensures that the radial angles are conserved during the spring embedding layout process, if possible.

The customised spring embedding algorithm is then applied to the circle nodes, the inner components and the outer supernodes.

For each outer supernode, its new position is analysed, and it is checked whether its centre of mass can be

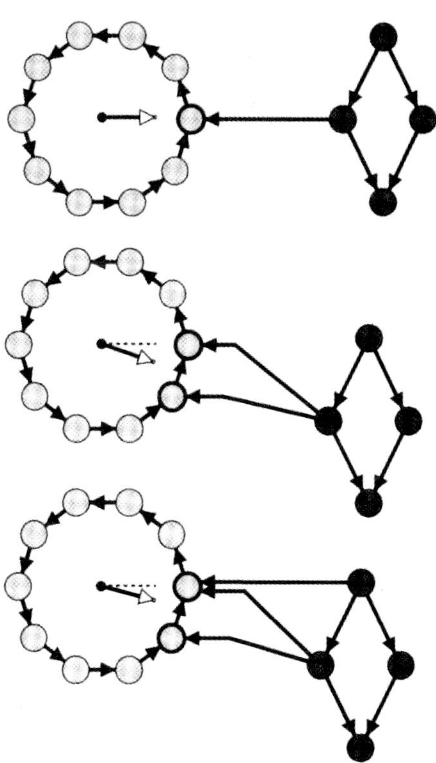

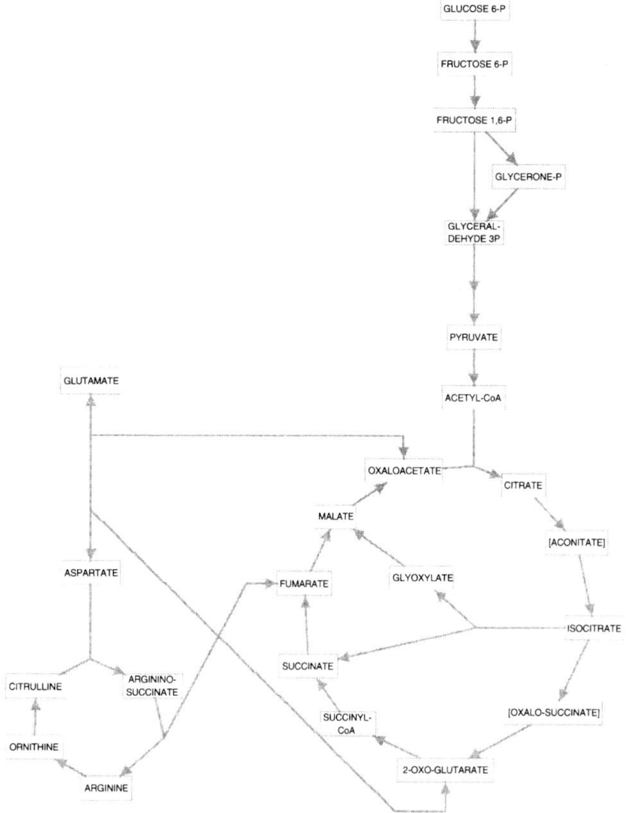



**Fig. 3.** The preferred radial angle of the centre of mass of an outer supernode (darkly shaded) is computed by taking the weighted average over the angles of the connected circle nodes (bold borders). The preferred angle ($0°$, $-18°$ and $-12°$, respectively) is indicated by the arrow in the centre of the circle.

**Fig. 5.** Combination of TCA cycle, Glycolysis and Urea cycle.

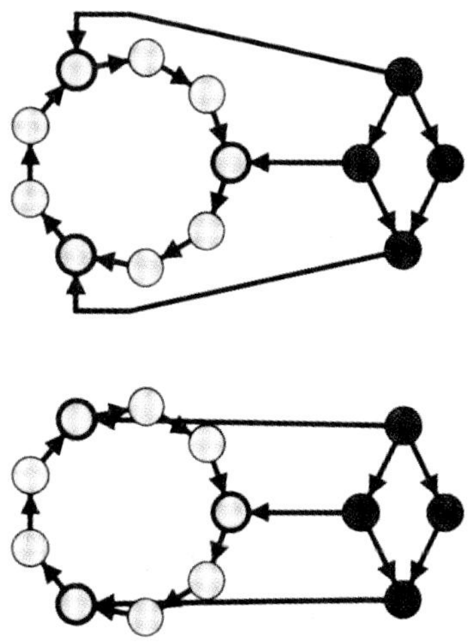

**Fig. 4.** In the top panel, bends are inserted at the edges connecting the circle to the outer supernode (darkly shaded) in an attempt to avoid edge crossings with the circle. In the bottom panel, the same graph without bends. The edges clearly intersect with the circle.

brought closer to the circle by mirroring or flipping it. This heuristic attempts to further reduce the number of edge crossings.

Finally, bends are attached to edges connecting the circle to outer components so that the edges emerge orthogonally from the circle. This is done in an attempt to reduce edge crossings with the circle (Figure 4).

## EXPERIMENTAL RESULTS

The algorithm has been tested on five different pathways or combinations of pathways.

The tested pathways were all relatively complex in that they contain cyclic as well as hierarchical components. In all five cases good results were produced. The layout is clear and easy to understand because it emphasises the topological structures of different parts of the graph and keeps logically connected units together. The algorithm managed well to avoid overlapping components and to reduce the required drawing area and unnecessary edge crossings.

Due to space limitations we only show two of the resulting images. Figure 5 shows the TCA cycle connected to Glycolysis and the Urea cycle. The TCA cycle is

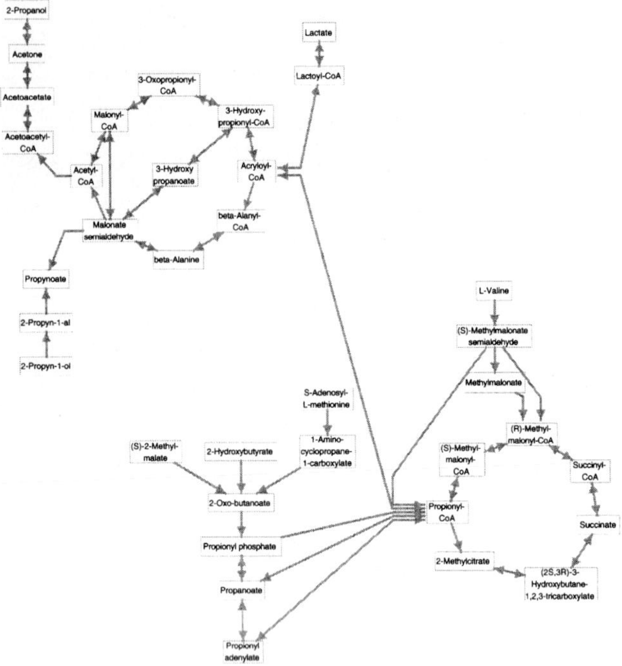

**Fig. 6.** Propanoate metabolism.

the longest cycle found and has two outer components: Glycolysis, and the Urea cycle together with Aspartate and Glutamate. Glyoxylate is the only inner component of the TCA cycle and hence placed inside the circle. The hierarchical layout algorithm is applied to Glycolysis since it does not contain a cycle. The second outer component, the Urea cycle connected to Aspartate and Glutamate, is laid out recursively. The Urea cycle is found as the only cycle of the subgraph, and Glutamate and Aspartate as the only outer component of the cycle.

Figure 6 shows the Propanoate metabolism. Here the longest cycle is the one containing Acetyl-CoA, having one inner component and four outer components, only one of which requires the recursive step.

The results of the other experiments, images depicting the Pentose phosphate cycle, the Urea cycle together with the metabolism of amino groups, and Phenylalanine, Tyrosine and Tryptophan biosynthesis can be found on the web at the EML research site (http://www.eml.villa-bosch.de).

## DISCUSSION AND CONCLUSION

Potentially, the most time-consuming part of the algorithm is the search for the longest cycle since the corresponding decision problem is NP-complete. However, we observed that the depth first search algorithm has good performance if the displayed graph is sparse and not too large (a few hundred nodes and an edge to node ratio of less than 1.5) as it is usually the case with metabolic pathway

networks for display purposes. For larger or more highly connected graphs the search for the longest cycle becomes the major bottleneck, and heuristic methods will be necessary. The customised spring embedding algorithm has a time complexity quadratic in the number of nodes to be laid out and linear in the number of edges. Since it can be assumed that the number of distinct connected components outside the longest cycle in the graph is small, the spring embedding algorithm is efficient enough for our purposes. Furthermore, it worked well with a relatively low maximum iteration bound of less than 500. The overall performance of the pathway layout algorithm is good enough for use in interactive applications.

The algorithm proposed by Karp and Paley (1994) does not only compute positions for main compounds but also deals with the problem of placing side substrates and enzymes. This last point has been left out in our algorithm, where we concentrated on the placement of the main compounds. Apart from that, their algorithm differs from ours mainly in that they use a special tree layout algorithm in which nodes are packed as compactly as possible (Karp *et al.*, 1994), whereas in our case a customised spring embedding algorithm is used. Our algorithm gives better results for topologically more complex graphs, e.g. if a combination of different pathways is to be visualised simultaneously. The heuristic computation of initial positions of nodes and the subsequent spring embedding process helps to reduce the number of edge crossings and to place interconnected components at more appropriate locations.

It should be noted that the results produced by the algorithm often differ in many aspects from the conventional drawings in biochemistry textbooks. For instance, in some cases a sequence of reactions is conventionally not drawn as a circle although a cycle exists. In large pathways, it is often the case that individual compounds have a high degree of connectivity. If the algorithm is given such data as input, 'unconventional' cycles will be discovered and presumably many edge crossings will occur. This problem can be avoided if highly connected compounds are allowed to appear in multiple instances of graph nodes, thereby reducing the edge to node ratio. In fact, this is what is usually done in conventional manual drawings.

Details such as the relative placement of well-known pathways in a bigger pathway map or the traditional orientation of specific hierarchical structures (e.g. left-to-right or top-to-bottom) also belong to the established conventions in biochemistry.

In order to comply with the above-mentioned conventions the algorithm would need additional layout information that is specific to the pathway or reactions to be drawn. We assumed that such information is not available to the algorithm, which is the case if the graphs to be drawn are novel or computer generated pathways, or the results of complex queries, and not only historically important pathways.

In the future, work has to be done to develop graph libraries and graph layout algorithms tailored to graphs with hyperedges. Simulating hyperedges by inserting dummy nodes did not always give optimal results because the current algorithms treat them like normal nodes.

The presented algorithm appears to be an attractive choice for visualising metabolic pathways. It produces good results, even in complex cases where cyclic pathways are to be visualised in the context of connected pathways. Thus, the algorithm could well be used to enhance existing and to build new graphical user interfaces to access biochemical databases.

## ACKNOWLEDGEMENTS

We would like to thank Ulrike Wittig and Andreas Kohlbecker for assistance with the acquisition of data sets. The work presented in this paper was carried out thanks to the support of the German Ministry for Education and Sciences (BMBF) (Project Bioregio 0312212) and the Klaus Tschira Stiftung (KTS).

## REFERENCES

Appel,R., Bairoch,A. and Hochstrasser,D. (1994) A new generation of information retrieval tools for biologists: the example of the ExPASy WWW server. *Trends Biochem. Sci.*, **19**, 258–260.

Brandenburg,F.-J., Jünger,M. and Mutzel,P. (1997) Algorithmen zum automatischen Zeichnen von Graphen. *Informatik Spektrum*, **20**, 199–207.

Brandenburg,F.-J., Gruber,B., Himsolt,M. and Schreiber,F. (1998) Automatische Visualisierung biochemischer Information. In *Proceedings of the Workshop Molekulare Bioinformatik, GI Jahrestagung*, pp. 24–38.

Di Battista,G., Eades,P., Tamassia,R. and Tollis,I.G. (1994) Annotated bibliography on graph drawing algorithms. *Comput. Geom.-Theor. Appl.*, **4**, 235–282.

Di Battista,G., Eades,P., Tamassia,R. and Tollis,I.G. (1999) *Graph Drawing: Algorithms for the Visualization of Graphs*. Prentice Hall, New Jersey.

Durbin,R. and Mieg,J.T. (1991) A C. elegans Database. Documentation, code and data available from anonymous FTP servers at lirmm.lirmm.fr, cele.mrc-lmb.cam.ac.uk and ncbi.nlm.nih.gov.

Eades,P. (1984) A heuristic for graph drawing. *Congr. Numer.*, **41**, 149–160.

Eades,P. and Sugiyama,K. (1990) How to draw a directed graph. *J. Inform. Proc.*, **13**, 424–437.

Kanehisa,M. and Goto,S. (2000) KEGG: Kyoto encyclopedia of genes and genomes. *Nucleic Acids Res.*, **28**, 27–30.

Karp,P.D. and Paley,S. (1994) Automated drawing of metabolic pathways. In Lim,H., Cantor,C. and Robbins,R. (eds), *Third International Conference on Bioinformatics and Genome Research*.

Karp,P.D., Lowrance,J.D., Strat,T.M. and Wilkins,D.E. (1994) The Grasper-CL graph management system. *LISP Symb. Comput.*, **7**, 251–290.

Karp,P.D., Riley,M., Saier,M., Paulsen,I.T., Paley,S. and Pellegrini-Toole,A. (2000) The EcoCyc and MetaCyc databases. *Nucleic Acids Res.*, **28**, 56–59.

Michal,G. (1993) *Biochemical Pathways* (poster). Boehringer Mannheim GmbH.

Michal,G. (1999) *Biochemical Pathways*. Spektrum Akadem., Heidelberg.

Quinn,N.R., Jr and Breuer,M.A. (1979) A force directed component placement procedure for printed circuit boards. *IEEE Trans. Circuits Syst.*, CAS **26**, 377–388.

Sugiyama,K., Tagawa,S. and Toda,M. (1981) Methods for visual understanding of hierarchical systems. *IEEE Trans. Syst. Man Cybern.*, **11**, 109–125.

Takai-Igarashi,T. and Kaminuma,T. (1998) A database for cell signaling networks. *J. Comput. Biol.*, **5**, 747.

Takai-Igarashi,T. and Kaminuma,T. (1999) A pathway finding system for the cell signaling networks database. *In Silico Biol.*, **1**, 129–146.

Wiese,R., Eiglsperger,M. and Schabert,P. (2000) The Y-files graph library: documentation and code available at http://www-pr.informatik.uni-tuebingen.de/yfiles.

Review

# Bioinformatics and the malaria genome: facilitating access and exploitation of sequence information

Ross L. Coppel *

*Department of Microbiology and the Victorian Bioinformatics Consortium, P.O. Box 53, Monash University, Melbourne, Victoria 3800 Australia*

## Abstract

The torrent of sequence information unleashed by the various genome sequencing projects, including that of *Plasmodium falciparum*, will lead to an unprecedented increase in the data available for research purposes. The scientific community is struggling to develop ways to assimilate this information and ensure that it is fully analysed in a way that enables rapid development of new therapeutic and diagnostic advances. This is particularly so for the field of tropical medicine where many of the scientists have had limited training in the area of Bioinformatics and may be further hampered by poor access to the sequence data. A number of collections of malaria genome sequence are available, each with their own advantages and disadvantages, however further improvements in these information resources are needed. In particular, there would be great benefit in integrating genomic sequence and functional genomics results with the large amount of pre-existing knowledge related to parasite biology and immunological interactions with the host. Attempts to achieve this include the PlasmoDB database, and the lessons learned in this effort could be of great utility to other organism-specific databases. © 2001 Elsevier Science B.V. All rights reserved.

*Keywords: Plasmodium falciparum*; Genome project; Bioinformatics; Genome databases; Annotation; Curation

## 1. Introduction

The biological sciences are entering a period of enormous change in which the scale of experimentation has increased in an unprecedented manner, and this in turn is altering the way experiments are performed and reported. The amount of data being generated by automated sequencing projects and various functional genomics projects such as microarrays and proteomics is so large that analysis defies traditional methods. The requirement for computer-assisted methods has spawned the discipline of Bioinformatics. Bioinformatics can be viewed as the intersection of information technologies and applied mathematics with molecular biology and genetics, and it provides the tools to collect, store and analyse the vast amount of new information. It is clear that those with the skills to use this new discipline will have a large competitive advantage in

---
* Tel.: + 61-3-9905-4822; fax: + 61-3-9905-4811.
*E-mail address:* ross.coppel@med.monash.edu.au (R.L. Coppel).

using this new data to perform experiments aimed at the discovery of new knowledge and the development of new treatment modalities and diagnostic tests.

The *Plasmodium falciparum* genome project was initiated subsequent to the completion of a successful chromosome mapping project funded by the Wellcome Trust. By 1996 scientists were actively debating the feasibility of sequencing the entire genome of *P. falciparum*. An international consortium was established comprising three sequencing centres: the Institute for Genomic Research (TIGR, Rockville, MD, USA), the Sanger Centre (Hinxton, UK) and Stanford University (Stanford, CA, USA). Funding was supplied by the Burroughs Wellcome Fund, the National Institutes of Health and the Department of Defence. The purpose of the consortium was to completely sequence the genome and to annotate it, with a target completion date by 2002–2003. The 14 chromosomes were divided between the three centres and sequencing began [1,2].

At the time of its inception in the mid 1990s, it was not clear whether the sequencing of an organism with such an A–T rich genome was technically feasible, given the numerous reports of difficulties that had bedevilled the sequencing of individual genes [3]. As is now clear, these fears proved largely to be groundless, although there are some gaps in the sequence which are proving quite difficult to close. It is likely that the project will be largely completed by the end of 2001, with essentially all genes discovered by that time. This 'first draft' of the genome will be available to all, for further exploitation. It should not be forgotten that the announcement of the genome project was attended by some controversy and scepticism. One common criticism was that tropical medicine was so starved for funds that big science of this magnitude was not appropriate and diverted money from control projects, or other uses of funds that were more practical. Such arguments have lost a great deal of force, not the least because the sources of funding would not have supported such alternative uses, but rather used the money to sequence other organisms. However, one point that is still valid is that the genome sequence in itself is of no particular value. Rather, the ultimate success of the Genome Project will depend on how readily and easily the data is made available to the scientific community and on how widely it is used.

## 2. Factors militating against full exploitation of genomic information

So if effective utilization of the genome sequence will be the ultimate criterion of success for the project, it becomes important to ensure that these goals of enhancing usability and accessibility of the sequence data are met. What factors militate against full exploitation of the genome? An initial problem was due to the fragmented nature of the sequencing project itself. With three separate centres generating sequence information, the data was available on three individual web sites, each with their own peculiarities of navigation and format. A BLAST search against all available data became a time consuming and often frustrating exercise. Updates in data could occur at one site independent of the others with no method of alerting users of the availability of new information. Fortunately, this problem has now been eliminated and at least four sites have collated all the available *P. falciparum* sequence and made it available, including the NCBI malaria genetics and genomics site, the TDR malaria database, the MR4 site and PlasmoDB. BLAST searches against the entire genome sequence are available at NCBI, MR4 and PlasmoDB (Table 1). There remains a problem in that updating these collating sites with newly available sequence is not instantaneous. Thus one sequencing centre may have unique information, but typically this is only the case for a few days at most.

A second problem was the data release policy and the differing ways that has been interpreted by members of the malaria community. The policy stated that use of the sequence data to enable analysis of individual genes was acceptable, but that whole chromosome or whole genome analyses must await the primary publication of the data by members of the sequencing centres. Consequently a degree of controversy has attended publications that have examined multiple *P. falciparum* genes in a single publication [4,5]. This seems to have arisen in part because of difficulties in interpreting what is meant by the data release policy, and a degree of antagonism has arisen between some in the sequencing centres and some members of the research community. On the one hand is the natural desire of those engaged in sequence acquisition to realise the fruits of their work and report in the scientific literature. Against this is juxtaposed a desire to fully utilise the sequence data as early as possible to advance individual lines of research. Indeed it has been argued that the sequencing centres are not involved in the normal processes of scientific research but rather as industrial entities performing a contracted service. Thus the argument goes, the normal considerations of data ownership by scientists do not apply, but the data is really the property of the malaria community. Considerable ill feeling has been generated and quite strong opinions have been voiced [6,7]. My own opinion is that the sequencing project was undertaken under a set of conditions agreed to by the funding agencies, the sequencing centres and the malaria community. To vary those conditions retrospectively seems somewhat unfair. At the same time, the sequencers are obligated to complete the genome in a timely manner, as the data release restriction should not be allowed to apply indefinitely. A settlement along these lines is anticipated in the near future, and it is likely that use of the data will be unrestricted by early 2002, when the 'first draft' of the malaria genome is likely to be published.

One of the problems specific to the field of tropical diseases research is that a significant fraction of the scientists studying these problems are situated in the developing world, where Internet access may be problematic. There are large volumes of information associated with genome projects and the bandwidth and reliability of access are not sufficient in many countries. Indeed given the explosion in use of the Internet such problems are confronted by scientists even in relatively prosperous countries at times of peak Net usage. The issue of poor Internet services has been recognized as a significant impediment to scientists in the developing world and a number of schemes have begun to address this. For example, the Health Internetwork is a consortium of groups who aim to boost access by researchers and health workers to reliable information via the Internet and to improve global public health by facilitating the flow of information. A pilot programme is underway involving four centres in Africa and five centres in central Asia and Eastern Europe. The consortium partners include the WHO, the Open Society Institute and a number of information providers. Centres will receive hardware, wide band connectivity and full access to a number of databases and online medical journals. It may be some time before all malaria researchers in the developing world are in a similar position, but the programme intends to extend these facilities to 13 000 access points in some 40 countries by the end of 2003. Another solution to this problem is through the TDR Malaria Database CD-ROM Distribution scheme in which subscribers receive the collated genome sequences on CD-ROM at regular intervals.

Further problems in utilization of the genome data relate to the relative newness of the discipline and the techniques involved. Bioinformatics analysis requires a particular set of skills and a knowledge base that has not traditionally been part of standard biological teach-

Table 1
Malaria genome resources available on the web

| Web Resource | URL | Features | Comments |
| --- | --- | --- | --- |
| Sanger Centre | http://www.sanger.ac.uk/Projects/P_falciparum/ | BLAST, Search of annotated genes | Focus is portion of the genome sequenced at Sanger |
| TIGR | http://www.tigr.org/tdb/edb2/pfal/htmls/ | BLAST, Search of annotated genes | Focus is portion of the genome sequenced at TIGR |
| Stanford University | http://sequence-www.stanford.edu/group/malaria/index.html | BLAST, Sequence retrieval and search of annotated genes | Chromosome 12 only. Community annotation of this chromosome may be done here |
| NCBI Malaria Genomics And Genetics | http://www.ncbi.nlm.nih.gov/Malaria | BLAST, microsatellites, genome data collection, optical mapping, ESTs | Tool to map candidate genes using genetic cross |
| WHO TDR Malaria Database | http://www.wehi.edu.au/MalDB-www/who.html | Genome data collection, bibliographies, sequence alignments, SRS query engine, malaria discussion group | Annotated sequences may be searched in a nomenclature independent manner. Best site to collect multiple alleles of a single gene |
| PlasmoDB | http://www.plasmodb.org | BLAST, chromosome maps | Under continuous development to meet community needs. Should become the most useful genome site. |
| Malaria Parasite Metabolic Pathways | http://sites.huji.ac.il/malaria/ | KEGG style pathway maps and useful bibliography, links to Expasy | Not linked to sequence data at present. Some attempts to look at more complex phenomena such as transport, cytoadherence and rosetting |
| MR4 | http://www.malaria.mr4.org/mr4pages/index.html | Access to research reagents, BLAST and sequence retrieval facility planned | Malaria Research Protocols available |
| Parasite Proteome Server | http://www.ebi.ac.uk/parasites/proteomes.html | Classification of proteins of *P. falciparum* into functional categories | Attempt at placing genes in functional categories. Minimally curated. Will be more useful as genome project is completed |
| Pedant Analysis of Chromosome 2 | http://pedant.mips.biochem.mpg.de/cgi-bin/wwwfly.pl?Set = PfalciparumII&Page = index | Complete automated annotation of 205 proteins on chromosome 2 | Riddled with errors due to the automated nature of the process, including mistakes in localisation and similarity. |
| SANBI Plasmodium | http://www.sanbi.ac.za/malaria-genesearch/ | Assemblies and BLAST comparisons of sequences from *P. falciparum*, *P. vivax* and *P. berghei* | In its present incarnation, it is difficult to navigate and hard to extract information. Likely to become more useful when genome data is completely available |
| Malaria Full Length cDNA project | http://fullmal.ims.u-tokyo.ac.jp/ | Sequencing runs taken from a library of putative full length cDNA clones | Needs further data before it becomes truly useful |
| Gene Sequence Tag Project | http://parasite.vetmed.ufl.edu/ | *P. berghei* and *P. vivax* gene sequencing projects | Useful early information on these genomes. Forthcoming genome projects will provide more complete data elsewhere |

This is not an exhaustive listing but describes some features of the more important sequence and genome resources available. Many are being continuously updated and features will change with time.

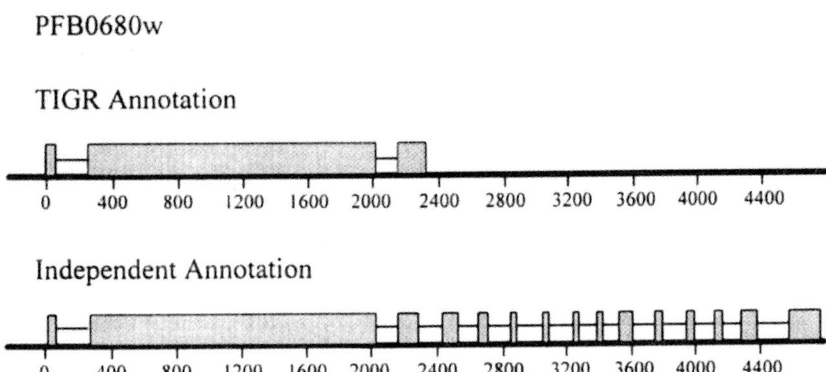


Fig. 1. Comparison of the results between different gene prediction programmes on a region of chromosome 2. The exons are represented by rectangles with the greyed rectangles identifying exons predicted to have identical boundaries by both approaches and the hatched rectangles identifying exons predicted to have differing boundaries. In this case the prediction by the method of Huestis and Fischer [17] was proven to be correct by RTPCR analysis of asexual stage mRNA.

ing and practice. Although new courses in Bioinformatics are appearing, few practicing scientists have other than a passing familiarity with this area. It may be difficult for scientists unskilled in this area to fully appreciate how the genome may be valuable in advancing their own field of interest. There is much more to Bioinformatics than performance of BLAST searches and fairly sophisticated analyses can give insights into parasite metabolism or phylogeny that are of great value. Widely disparate levels of user competence in Bioinformatics are particularly noticeable in fields such as tropical medicine. This problem can be ameliorated to some extent by collaborations with specifically trained Bioinformaticians who can contribute their skills to a shared project. However, a large percentage of the research base working in malaria are situated in endemic countries and they may have relatively little access to trained Bioinformaticians at their institutions or even in their country. Many scientists working in biology have rudimentary skills in mathematics, and have abandoned instruction in these areas early in their educational life. It is a cruel joke to see the resurgence of a need for these skills after so many years of refuge from the mysteries of maths. However, studies in Bioinformatics may only need relatively low cost computing resources and thus are suitable for endemic country scientists who may not have access to expensive biological apparati involved in functional genomics such as microarrayers.

Finally, we do not yet know to what level of completion the genome data will be taken. For chromosomes 2 and 3 it has proved possible to produce a single contiguous sequence extending across the whole chromosome [8,9]. It is unknown if sequencing will be equally successful for the other chromosomes and some such as the BLOB offer major technical challenges. Thus it may be that for some time, we will not be able to completely search the genome. This is not likely to be too much of a problem, except for the rare gene, perhaps within a metabolic pathway, that is thought to be absent from the genome.

## 3. Current resources

There are several repositories of genomic sequence information and a number of these are listed in Table 1. The primary sites are of course the sequencing centres at TIGR, the Sanger Centre and Stanford University. These sites concentrate on the data generated at each respective centre and are supplemented by varying degrees of analysis and annotation, both manual and automated. The gene finding algorithms that are utilised for other genomes such as fruit fly or human are less successful when confronted with the high AT rich sequence of *P. falciparum* in particular. Retraining of the gene finders on malaria sequence has yielded improvements, such as the improved performance of GlimmerM over Glimmer [9]. Although the sequencing centres view these models as provisional, there is a tendency among scientists to accept them as correct, and base their experiments on this information. Thus a search for exported genes in asexual stages, looking for genes that have a 2-exon structure would have examined a fairly large number of false positives based on the initial chromosome annotations, as well as missing some 2 exon genes not properly identified. It must be remembered that the current annotations are predictions and must be verified by experiment. Some *P. falciparum* genes can be quite unusual in structure, being composed of multiple small exons and current prediction software do not easily predict these genes. An example of this is shown in Fig. 1, taken from a paper appearing elsewhere in this issue and shows an example of this type of difficult gene which was not predicted by the semi-automated gene finders, but by other manual methods and subsequently proven by experiment. It is difficult to get such corrections incorporated into the public record at Genbank, as any corrections to a record must be submitted by the originator of the record, in this case TIGR. Even with the best will in the world, such corrections may be a long time coming, and there needs to be a better mechanism for incorporating these changes into the public databases. A set of alternative gene predictions are maintained at the TDR malaria sequence database and will ultimately appear on PlasmoDB.

Detailed descriptions of the genome various sites will not be given; rather the interested readers are encouraged to investigate them for themselves. Each has some particular feature of worth or some specific dataset. For example, the NCBI has a unique set of software tools for linkage analysis and provides information about the microsatellite markers that may be employed in this endeavour. Similarly, the TDR Malaria Database has annotated the sequences stored there to improve searching. It is an unfortunate complication in malaria research that gene nomenclature has been somewhat haphazard. Thus the 195 kDa merozoite surface protein 1 (MSP1) [10] has appeared in the literature under many names including the polymorphic schizont antigen (PSA) [11], the precursor to the major merozoite surface antigen (PMMSA) [12] and merozoite surface antigen 1, both with and without a hyphen [13,14]. Searching for allelic forms of this protein will lead to differing results depending on what name is used. In many cases, unless care is taken, many additional sequences from other organisms are returned. The SRS engine at the TDR Malaria Database site overcomes this problem returning an identical and complete set of allelic sequences for any alternative gene term (Table 2).

One important question about many of these existing resources is what mechanism is in place to ensure that the data is continually updated and vetted for correctness. There are already orphan information resources such as the malaria antigen database at http://ben.vub.ac.be/malaria/mad.html. This database, established by the European Commission, the World Health Organization and the United States Agency for International Development had useful information about vari-

ous vaccine candidates. Unfortunately, the data has not been kept current and the database has not been updated since 1995. A mechanism needs to be developed to ensure that such information is incorporated into databases that continue to be actively curated.

## 4. Improving existing genome resources

Several factors mandate the need for improved databases. The fragmented nature of the genome project itself and the existence of individual sequences at the three sequencing centres absolutely required the design of a single repository for those sequences in the longer term. Once the centres complete their sequencing tasks, it is unlikely that significant resources will be allocated to maintenance and ongoing curation and annotation of this particular genome. However, it is essential that the genome continues to be annotated over time, as experimental verification will be required for many gene models. The results will need to be incorporated into the databases in a timely manner, as will the results from many other forms of experimentation. This responsibility will fall to the malaria community, which must support ongoing development and curation of the genome database.

I commented about how the unusual nature of the sequencing consortium initially led to a situation where the accumulating data was held in several different sites, and searching the entire sequence was difficult. Although this problem is now solved, this issue of fragmented data appears in another form. The study of malaria did not commence with the genome sequence. There is a considerable amount of important information already available on various malaria proteins, their stage specificity and location, structural properties, their functional role, immunological interactions and protein–protein interactions. There is information about the epidemiology of malaria as an infection and a disease, its pathophysiology and the entomology of the mosquito vector. Metabolic pathways have been mapped, antigenic diversity and variation documented and the effect of many drugs studied. It is important that this information be integrated with the genome sequence, and functional genomics results. Similarly,

Table 2

Comparative search results using terms describing MSP1 in the nucleotide sections of Genbank, EMBL and the TDR Malaria Database

| Search Term | MSP-1 | MSP1 | MSA-1 | MSA1 | PMMSA | PSA |
|---|---|---|---|---|---|---|
| Entrez at Genbank | 483[a] | 348 | 54 | 137 | 8 | 0 |
| SRS at EBI | 78 | 276[b] | 13 | 36 | 11 | 0 |
| TDR Database | 472 | 472 | 472 | 472 | 472 | 472 |

[a] The MSP-1 query through Entrez in Genbank returns more than a hundred AMA1 sequences.

[b] The MSP1 query through SRS at EBI returns 276 additional sequences unless the query is restricted to 'Plasmodium'.

many reagents of various sorts have been generated as a result of these experiments, and appropriate pointers to such reagents should be built into the database. Finally, *P. falciparum* is only the first malaria species to be sequenced. There are projects that are in various stages of planning and execution to sequence at least an additional eight malaria species and strains. In the near future, we will see attempts at improving these databases, so that information is more readily obtained and the types of queries that can be readily answered made more powerful. This is not a problem for malariologists alone, and is being faced by all scientists coming to grips with this next phase of biology. Thus it is likely that there will be new developments in databases in other systems that can be usefully applied to malaria.

One interesting approach to the problem of integrating genomic information with other biological information is that of the Gene Ontology™ Consortium whose goal is to produce a dynamic controlled vocabulary that can be applied to all eukaryotes to describe the role of genes and protein products in cells. The classification of genes is based on properties such as their molecular function, involvement in biological processes and in the formation of cellular components. Clearly, for organisms such as *Plasmodium*, there will need to be modification of the vocabulary to apply to specialised processes and structures, such as for example red cell invasion, the rhoptries and the apicoplast. However, adoption of such a general classification scheme could allow malaria information to be placed into a general database, or queried in a way that allows direct comparison of a number of organisms. Interested readers are referred to the appropriate web site: http://www.geneontology.org/.

As the best way to construct such an integrated database is not clear cut, it is important to try different approaches. One of the new information resources is PlasmoDB, which is funded by the Burroughs Wellcome Fund for 3 years and commenced its work in February 2000. Developed at the University of Pennsylvania, Philadelphia and Monash University, Melbourne, this site offers several querying facilities, including BLAST and motif searches. One of the newer tools is an attempt to offer a more powerful way of searching the genome for complex properties of genes. For example, it is possible to frame a query asking for all predicted genes containing a signal and an anchor sequence, or that are composed of two exons with specific size limits. This enables researchers to quickly assemble lists of candidates for surface molecules or exported proteins. Augmenting such search facilities will be an important step in making the genome more accessible.

The integration of other malaria information into a genome database is not rapidly done. It is a laborious process, as it requires capturing information from the literature, critically analysing it and incorporating it in an expert manner. Such an approach is not easily automated, and it must be continually updated. Thus it is really only worth starting if there is a long term commitment from the malaria community and the funding agencies. It is important that such databases are able to demonstrate their utility and not be mere academic exercises. Thus it is important that there be a continuous process of evaluation, comment and database improvement in response to community feedback, so that a useful informatics tool is developed.

Finally, no database can provide all the information that scientists may require. A number of the analyses, such as analyses of transmembrane regions or similarity searches, require a choice of parameters with different results being obtained using different parameter choices. The general Bioinformatics skills of malariaologists will need improvement. To this end it is gratifying to see the efforts of the MR4, TDR and other organizations which are organising training programmes in Bioinformatics. These, together with web-based training courses should help raise the general levels of expertise in this discipline and improve exploitation of the genome data.

## 5. Conclusions

There is little doubt that the availability of genome sequences will form an essential underpinning of biology over the next century and will influence the direction of scientific studies. Already the first studies that build on the genome sequence to augment our arsenal of anti-malarial strategies are appearing [15]. Recognition of enzymes involved in the mevalonate-independent pathway of isoprenoid synthesis within the genome data enabled scientists to focus in on a potentially vulnerable pathway. Indeed, inhibitors of this pathway have already been found and two compounds identified that block the pathway and cure mice of experimental malaria infection. Scanning of the genome data has revealed potential candidate vaccine molecules including another merozoite surface protein that contains two epidermal growth factor-like domains, a structure similar to that found in MSP1 [16]. It is likely that other insights of this sort will come, but such insights will come more rapidly if scientists are assisted in their access to and analysis of the genome data. The issues that the malaria community will grapple with, such as improved training, better databases and integration with other forms of data are likely to be mirrored throughout the biological field. Solutions will be developed in different arenas and we must make use of them as rapidly and completely as we can. Finally, it must be emphasised that the tools of Bioinformatics represent another approach of value to biologists, but the predictions coming out of this form of analysis will need to be verified by experiment.

## Acknowledgements

R.L.C. is supported by the Australian National Health and Medical Research Council, the UNDP/ World Bank/WHO Special Programme for Research and Training in Tropical Diseases, the Howard Hughes Medical Institute International Scholars in Infectious Diseases and Parasitology Program and the Burroughs Wellcome Fund. I would like to thank Peter Hallowes for his work on the malaria database and Robert Huestis for useful comments and provision of unpublished results.

## References

[1] Carucci DJ, Gardner MJ, Tettelin H, Cummings LM, Smith HO, Adams MD, Hoffman SL, Venter JC. The Malaria Genome Sequencing Project. Exp. Rev. Mol. Med. 1998; 5 May: http://www-ermm.cbcu.cam.ac.uk/dcn/txt001dcn.htm.

[2] Gardner MJ. The genome of the malaria parasite. Curr Opin Genet Dev 1999;9:704–8.

[3] Coppel RL, Black CG. Malaria Parasite DNA. In: Sherman IW, Sherman IW, editors. Malaria: Parasite biology, pathogenesis and protection. New York: ASM Press, 1998;185–202.

[4] van Dooren GG, Waller RF, Joiner KA, Roos DS, McFadden GI. Traffic jams: protein transport in *Plasmodium falciparum*. Parasitol Today 2000;16:421–7.

[5] Waller RF, Keeling PJ, Donald RG, Striepen B, Handman E, Lang-Unnasch N, Cowman AF, Besra GS, Roos DS, McFadden GI. Nuclear-encoded proteins target to the plastid in *Toxoplasma gondii* and *Plasmodium falciparum*. Proc Natl Acad Sci USA 1998;95:12352–7.

[6] Hyman RW. Sequence data: posted vs. published. Science 2001;291:827.

[7] Macilwain C. Biologists challenge sequencers on parasite genome publication. Nature 2000;405:601–2.

[8] Bowman S, Lawson D, Basham D, Brown D, Chillingworth T, Churcher CM, Craig A, Davies RM, Devlin K, Feltwell T, Gentles S, Gwilliam R, Hamlin N, Harris D, Holroyd S, Hornsby T, Horrocks P, Jagels K, Jassal B, Kyes S, McLean J, Moule S, Mungall K, Murphy L, Barrell BG, et al. The complete nucleotide sequence of chromosome 3 of *Plasmodium falciparum*. Nature 1999;400:532–8.

[9] Gardner MJ, Tettelin H, Carucci DJ, Cummings LM, Aravind L, Koonin EV, Shallom S, Mason T, Yu K, Fujii C, Pederson J, Shen K, Jing JP, Aston C, Lai ZW, Schwartz DC, Pertea M, Salzberg S, Zhou LX, Sutton GG, Clayton R, White O, Smith HO, Fraser CM, Adams MD, Hoffman SL, et al. Chromosome 2 sequence of the human malaria parasite *Plasmodium falciparum*. Science 1998;282:1126–32.

[10] Holder A, Blackman M, Burghaus P, Chappel J, Ling I, Mccallumdeighton N, Shai S. A malaria merozoite surface protein (MSP1)-structure, processing and function. Mem Inst Oswaldo Cruz 1992;87:37–42.

[11] McBride JS, Newbold CI, Anand R. Polymorphism of a high molecular weight schizont antigen of the human malaria parasite *Plasmodium falciparum*. J Exp Med 1985;161:160–80.

[12] Burns JM Jr, Majarian WR, Young JF, Daly TM, Long CA. A protective monoclonal antibody recognizes an epitope in the carboxyl- terminal cysteine-rich domain in the precursor of the major merozoite surface antigen of the rodent malarial parasite, *Plasmodium yoelii*. J Immunol 1989;143:2670–6.

[13] Cheng Q, Stowers A, Huang TY, Bustos D, Huang YM, Rzepczyk C, Saul A. Polymorphism in *Plasmodium vivax* MSA1 gene—The result of intragenic recombinations? Parasitology 1993;106:335–45.

[14] Deleersnijder W, Hendrix D, Hamers R. Analysis of MSA-1 diversity in *Plasmodium chabaudi* chabaudi strains. Mol Biochem Parasitol 1991;46:315–8.

[15] Jomaa H, Wiesner J, Sanderbrand S, Altincicek B, Weidemeyer C, Hintz M, Turbachova I, Eberl M, Zeidler J, Lichtenthaler HK, Soldati D, Beck E. Inhibitors of the nonmevalonate pathway of isoprenoid biosynthesis as antimalarial drugs. Science 1999;285:1573–6.

[16] Black CG, Wu T, Wang L, Hibbs AR, Coppel RL. Merozoite surface protein 8 of *Plasmodium falciparum* contains two epidermal growth factor-like domains. Mol Biochem Parasitol 2001;114:217–26.

[17] Huestis R, Fishcher K. Prediction of many new exons and introns in *Plasmodium falciparum* chromosome 2. Mol Biochem Parasitol 2001;118:187–199.

# Extracting Knowledge from Dynamics in Gene Expression

Ben Y. Reis,* Atul S. Butte,† and Isaac S. Kohane‡,[1]

*Harvard–MIT Division of Health Science Technology, Cambridge, Massachusetts 02139;
†Children's Hospital Informatics Program & MIT Division of Health Science Technology, Boston,
Massachusetts 02115; and ‡Children's Hospital Informatics Program, Boston, Massachusetts 02115*

*Received December 22, 2000; published online March 15, 2001*

Most investigations of coordinated gene expression have focused on identifying correlated expression patterns between genes by examining their normalized static expression levels. In this study, we focus on the *dynamics* of gene expression by seeking to identify correlated patterns of changes in genetic expression level. In doing so, we build upon methods developed in clinical informatics to detect temporal trends of laboratory and other clinical data. We construct relevance networks from *Saccharomyces cerevisiae* gene-expression dynamics data and find genes with related functional annotations grouped together. While some of these associations are also found using a standard expression level analysis, many are identified exclusively through the dynamic analysis. These results strongly suggest that the analysis of gene expression dynamics is a necessary and important tool for studying regulatory and other functional relationships among genes. The source code developed for this investigation is freely available to all non-commercial investigators by contacting the authors.   © 2001 Academic Press

*Key Words:* gene expression; clustering; dynamics; bioinformatics; clinical informatics; trends.

## INTRODUCTION

To understand a system fully, one must study its dynamics. With the sequencing of the human genome completed last

year, the focus of the research community is shifting toward a functional understanding of the roles of and relationships between different genes. With advances in genetic expression profiling techniques [1, 2] enabling detailed genomic scale measurements of genetic activity, it is important for the purposes of knowledge discovery to extract all the meaningful information present in the data. To date, most analyses [3, 4] have focused on clustering genes based simply on correlated patterns of genetic expression, ignoring other relationships present in the data. In this report we propose that further identifying correlated patterns of gene expression *dynamics* reveals additional meaningful information in the data.

In pursuing the investigation of gene dynamics, we are recapitulating and building on a large body of work in clinical informatics dealing with the identification of temporal abstractions and trend analysis. The literature is replete with reports of the limitations of performing diagnosis or planning with atemporal data [5] and the leverage obtained by capturing the dynamics of biomedical processes [6–11]. Until recently, the application of these techniques in bioinformatics has been relatively limited, particularly in the analysis of gene expression, in part because of the paucity of data sets with sufficient time points. Those analyses that have been published have focused primarily on the use of signal processing techniques using the Fourier transform [12, 13].

Many techniques have been used in functional genomics

[1] To whom correspondence should be addressed at Children's Hospital Informatics Program, Harvard Medical School, 300 Longwood Avenue, Boston, MA 02115. Fax: (617) 355-3456. E-mail: isaac_kohane@harvard.edu.

for clustering, including phylogenetic trees [4], self-organizing maps [14, 15], and relevance networks [16, 17]. These clustering techniques have relied on a variety of association metrics such as Euclidean distance, correlation coefficients, and mutual information. These different techniques and association measures have, to varying degrees, all proved successful in clustering genes known to be related in function. While many differences among these various approaches exist, all of them cluster according to the absolute level of genetic expression. In this study, we propose an alternate approach involving the dynamics of genetic expression, and formulate a methodology for clustering genes according to changes in genetic expression level.

### Clustering Genes According to Expression Dynamics Has Important Advantages

We use the term *dynamics* to refer to the rate of change of genetic expression over time, calculated as the first-order difference of the genetic expression levels ($E_{t2}$-$E_{t1}$, $E_{t3}$-$E_{t2}$). This is different from the simple temporal pattern of genetic expression ($E_{t1}$, $E_{t2}$, $E_{t3}$) that we refer to as *statics*.

The primary motivation for studying gene expression dynamics is that existing static techniques may not identify all the important relationships. Some genes may have associated dynamic behaviors but may not have associated static expression behaviors. A hypothetical example is shown in Fig. 1: Gene A codes for an enhancer protein that regulates the expression of gene B—a high level of gene A causes an up-regulation of expression in gene B. Since gene B can be at many possible expression levels before being affected by gene A, the enhancer-type relationship between the two genes cannot be noticed by simply examining the correlation of static expression patterns. Instead, one needs to examine the dynamics of gene expression—the way in which the expression level of gene A leads to a change in gene B—in order to detect the underlying dynamic relationship. We therefore hypothesize that this dynamic approach has the potential to discover relationships between genes that are not detectable using existing static techniques. It is the goal of this study to formulate, validate, and evaluate this dynamic approach for knowledge discovery in functional genomics.

## METHODS

### Experimental Data

We studied the *Saccharomyces cerevisiae* (Table 1) mRNA-expression data aggregated from several experiments reported by Eisen *et al.* [3] in which the response of

the yeast cells to several different stimuli is recorded. The data contain 79 data points in 10 time-series measured under different experimental conditions, shown in Table 1. Of over 6000 genes in the yeast genome, Eisen included only 2467 genes that had functional annotations. We analyze the same subset of genes.

### Representing Gene Expression Dynamics

Slopes are calculated between each adjacent pair of expression data points, $Et_n$ and $Et_{n+1}$:

$$\text{Slope}(n,n + 1) = \frac{\text{expression_level}_{n+1} - \text{expression_level}_n}{(\text{time}_{n+1} - \text{time}_n)}. \quad (1)$$

Since slopes are only calculated between data points within the same time series, the 79 data points in 10 time series are reduced to only 69 slope measurements. The units of the slope measurements are in normalized expression level units per minute.

### Data Visualization and Analysis

Relevance networks are constructed for the purposes of analysis and visualization of the data. Relevance networks are reviewed briefly here and have been described in full previously [16–18].

Relevance networks help identify groups of interrelated genes. A metric of association is chosen for comparing patterns of genetic expression between genes. After all pairwise gene–gene association strengths are calculated, a statistically significant threshold level of association is determined. All connections weaker than this threshold are removed, leaving small interconnected islands of significantly related genes called relevance networks. The method for determining this threshold is outlined below, but as described in prior work [16–18] it involves permuting the entire original data set, to preserve the distribution of gene expression values, but breaking the link between expression value and a particular condition or tissue. The pairwise association strengths are recalculated for each permutation and the largest value of association obtained in the pairwise associations is recorded. After a large number of permutations, this maximum value becomes the minimum threshold value for any association in the unpermuted data sets.

For this study, we use a linear correlation coefficient as a measure of association. Slopes are calculated as described

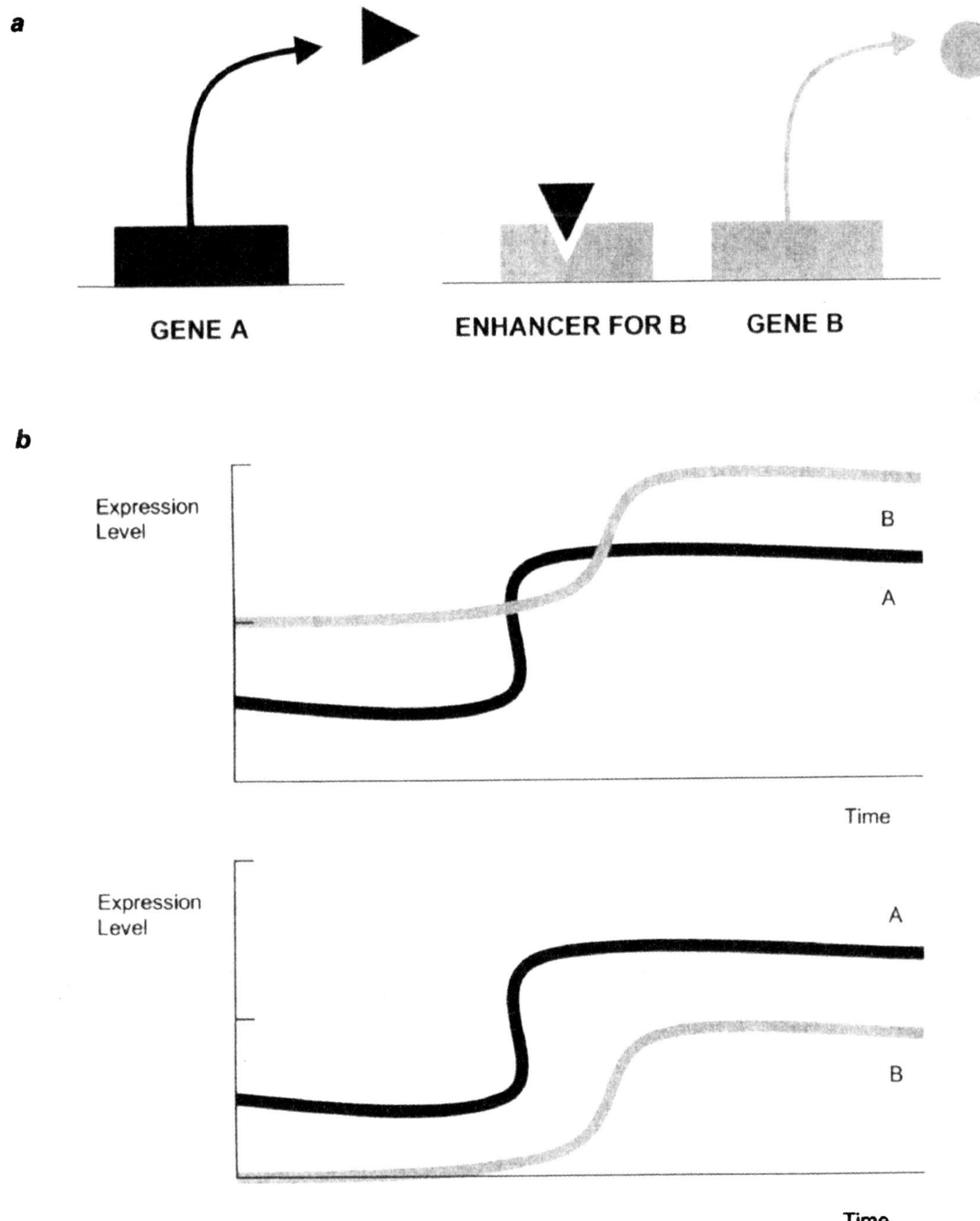


**FIG. 1.** Dynamic relationships between genes. (a) The expressed product of gene A binds an enhancer region that increases transcription of gene B (b) B's initial expression level before being affected by A can vary throughout the experiment. As a result, measuring the correlation between the absolute levels of genes A and B will not reveal the underlying enhancement relationship between the two. Instead, this can only be done by analyzing the expression dynamics—the change in expression level of gene B in relation to the expression level of gene A.

TABLE 1

Experimental Conditions

| Number of time points | Conditions |
| --- | --- |
| 18 | Cell cycle after Alpha factor arrest and release. |
| 14 | Cell cycle after elutriation. |
| 15 | Cell cycle for cdc 15 mutants after temperature-sensitive arrest and release. |
| 6 | Sporulation, Experiment 1. |
| 3 | Sporulation, Experiment 2. |
| 2 | Sporulation, Experiment 3. |
| 6 | Response to high-temperature shock. |
| 4 | Response to reducing shock. |
| 4 | Response to low-temperature shock. |
| 7 | Response to diauxic shift. |

*Note.* The experimental conditions under which the gene expression measurements reported by Eisen *et al.* [4] were taken.

above, yielding a dataset where each row is the time series of a particular gene's expression dynamics. Pairwise Pearson correlation coefficients are then calculated between all possible combinations of two rows. These are squared to yield the $R^2$, after which the original sign is reappended to conserve the information of whether the genes are positively or negatively correlated [7]. We call this final signed value $R^2$.

Correlation coefficients are sensitive to outlying values, which can bias downstream data analysis. Two symmetric outlying values may artificially raise the correlation coefficient of an otherwise nonlinear distribution. That is, in all except one or two microarrays, a gene will have a scatter within a small range and then due to an artifact of the hybridization process, the one or two microarrays will have a very high value for that gene. This is all the more striking in the data set on which this analysis has been performed where each data point belongs to a time series of a given stimulus and where the rest of the time series shows much smoother changes. We have had to apply the filter for these outlier values also in prior studies for the same reason [17]. It should be pointed out, nonetheless, that we will necessarily miss those few occasions where outlier values do represent quantum and dramatic change in expression. Consequently, an entropy-based filter is used to remove genes with outlying values in their distributions from the analysis. First, the individual entropies of the dynamics time series are calculated for each gene, with the entropy H(A) defined as:

$$H(A) = \sum_n - p(A_n)\log_2 p(A_n). \qquad (2)$$

The genes are ranked according to their entropies, and the bottom 5% (entropy threshold $<2.1464$) are excluded from the analysis.

*Issues Specific to Dynamics*

The inclusion of dynamics in the methodology introduces a number of important issues that will be addressed in turn. First, the issue of stasis: we observe that most genes do not change their expression levels most of the time. Figure 2 shows the distribution of slopes taken from all the points in the data set. The widespread stasis in the data can lead to seriously misleading analyses, as genes that remain stationary together can lead to an artificially high measure of association.

To address this issue, we filter out the stationary data points, including only the more dynamic ones in the analysis. This involves setting an exclusion range, or hole, around the zero slope range. We choose thresholds of $\pm0.02$ normalized slope units per minute, for a total hole size of 0.04. This approach removes approximately 70.0% of the original data points, and allows us to study the genes that *change* in a coordinated fashion, while avoiding the misleading identification of genes that simply remain stationary together. We automatically evaluated a range of hole sizes and picked the value of 0.04 based on maximizing the number of retained data points and minimizing the threshold association level in the permuted data (described below).

This solution leads to the second complication: Since many data points are removed, the remaining data can be very sparse. To ensure that all correlation coefficient calculations are based on enough points to avoid too many spurious associations (as defined by our permutation analysis, below), we set a threshold requiring a minimum of five data points for a calculation to be valid: any pairwise distribution having fewer data points than this threshold is excluded from the analysis. This thresholding approach is similar to the one used in work on clinical data relevance networks [18].

The last step in the relevance networks methodology involves determining a threshold association level that represents a likely nonspurious association between genes. We determine this level by permuting the time points within each gene and obtaining the distribution of pairwise correlation coefficient values. We perform this permutation 100 times and then compare the average permuted distribution with the distribution obtained from the original data set. It is clear from Fig. 3 that much stronger correlations are present in the original dataset. We comfortably place the threshold

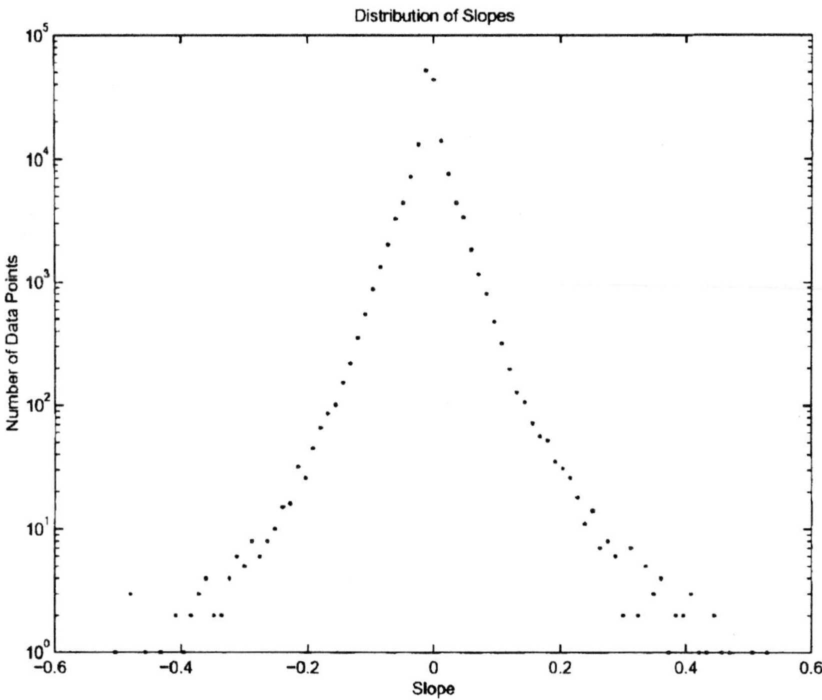



**FIG. 2.**  Slope measurements of gene expression. A semilog plot of the distribution of slopes derived from the yeast genetic expression dataset reported by Eisen *et al.* Almost all of the slopes are near zero, illustrating that most genes remain stationary most of time. The complications caused by this widespread stasis must be addressed with in analyzing gene expression dynamics data, as described in the text.

level of significance at $\pm 0.78$, as no permuted data points are able to achieve an $R^2$ value greater than that.

## RESULTS

The relevance networks generated from the dynamics analysis are presented first. These are then evaluated in the context of the networks generated from a static analysis below.

### Dynamic Relevance Networks

Using a threshold of $R^2 = 0.78$, the dynamic analysis yields 71 relevance networks consisting of 348 nodes (Fig. 4). Of the 3,041,811 possible gene–gene connections, only 371 (0.012%) are above this threshold. A box labeled with the gene name represents each gene. The width of each box represents its indegree—the number of other genes connected to it.

There are far too many associations to discuss each one individually. We therefore present the strongest associations found, as well as some of the more interesting negative associations. The full dataset and analysis are available at http://www.chip.org/chip/people/kohane/papers/dynamics/readme.html.

Of the 71 networks, the largest one contains 154 nodes with 238 links and consists mostly of ribosomal proteins and related genes, such as RNA helicases, RNA polymerases, translation initiation proteins, and other translational regulators. All of these genes are directly related in function to protein synthesis. A smaller network, with 14 nodes and 19 links, also consists of mostly ribosomal proteins.

The gene with the highest indegree is *RRP4*, a $3' \rightarrow 5'$ exoribonuclease involved in a diverse array of RNA processing [19]. It is linked with 12 other genes, including RNA helicases, RNA polymerases, and other translational regulators. Its high connectivity suggests that it is coregulated with many of the genes involved in protein synthesis and appears to interact with these genes in a dynamic manner.

Of all the dynamic associations found, Table 2 shows the 10 with the highest $R^2$ values. The gene pairs found are

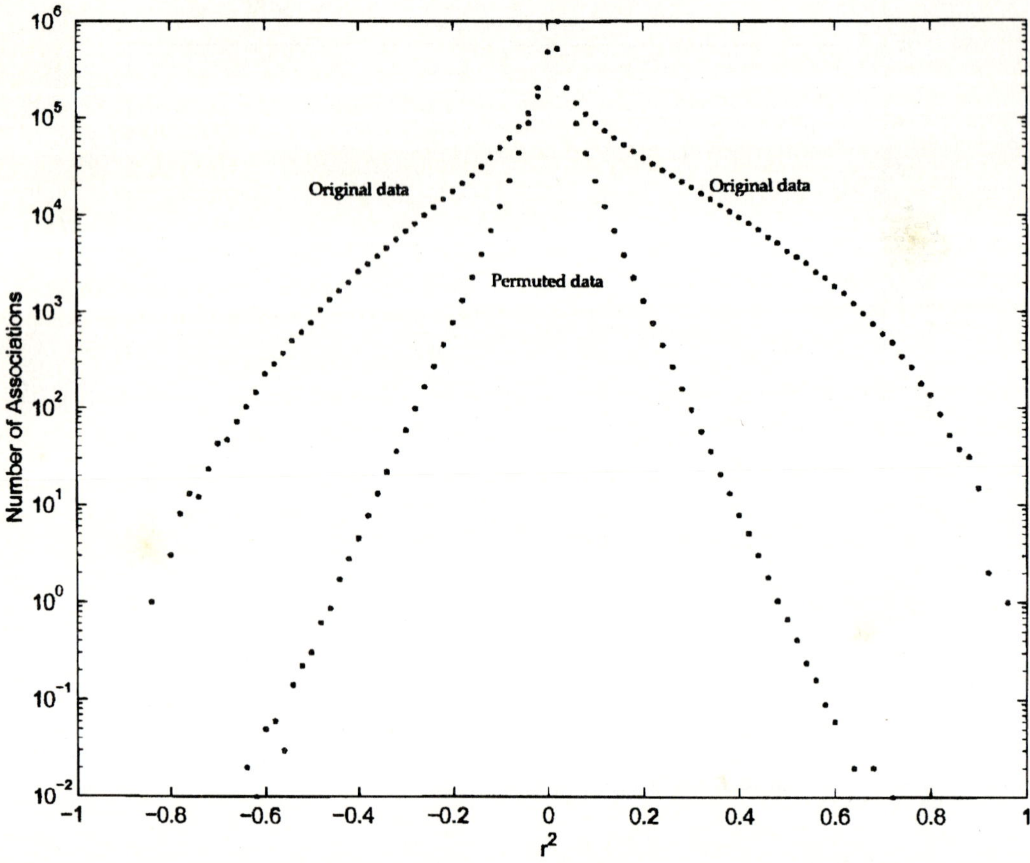



**FIG. 3.** Dynamic correlations of gene expression. A semilog plot of the distribution of $R^2$ calculated from the pairwise comparisons of the dynamic expression patterns of all the yeast genes. Plotted are the permuted and the unpermuted data. The permuted data points represent the average $R^2$ distribution derived from 100 permutations of the dataset. It is clear from the graph that the original data are able to achieve high $R^2$ values that are not achieved in any of the permuted runs.

closely related in function, including the four occurrences of *ASP3* (L-asparaginase II), which are redundantly present on the microarray used for making the measurements. These associations are shown graphically in Fig. 5A.

### Negative Associations

We also examine two negative associations of interest. First, we look at *EXM2* and *MAD3* (Fig. 6A). *EXM2* is a protein involved in allowing cells to exit mitosis, while *MAD3* is a spindle–assembly checkpoint protein that *prevents* certain cells from leaving mitosis [20]. These two counteracting genes appear as negatively correlated in their dynamics with an $R^2$ of $-0.797$. Meanwhile, they are/are not found to be strongly associated in the static analysis.

Figure 6B shows the distribution of slopes between *RAD6*

and *MET18*. *RAD6* is a ubiquitin-conjugating enzyme concentrated in the nucleus that is essential for mediating the degradation of amino-end rule-dependent protein substrates [21]. *MET18*, also known as *MMS19*, is a protein concentrated in the nucleus that affects RNA polymerase II transcription [22]. These are inversely related in their dynamics, with an $R^2$ of $-0.791$. It is not surprising that a gene responsible for protein degradation has an inverse relationship to a gene responsible for RNA transcription leading to protein synthesis.

The circles in Fig. 6B represent the static data points that we filter out to avoid direct the analysis to finding correlated changes in gene expression. If these static points are included in the analysis, the $R^2$ shifts from $-0.79$ to $-0.58$, far below the determined level of significance. This illustrative example highlights the methodological utility of the filtering

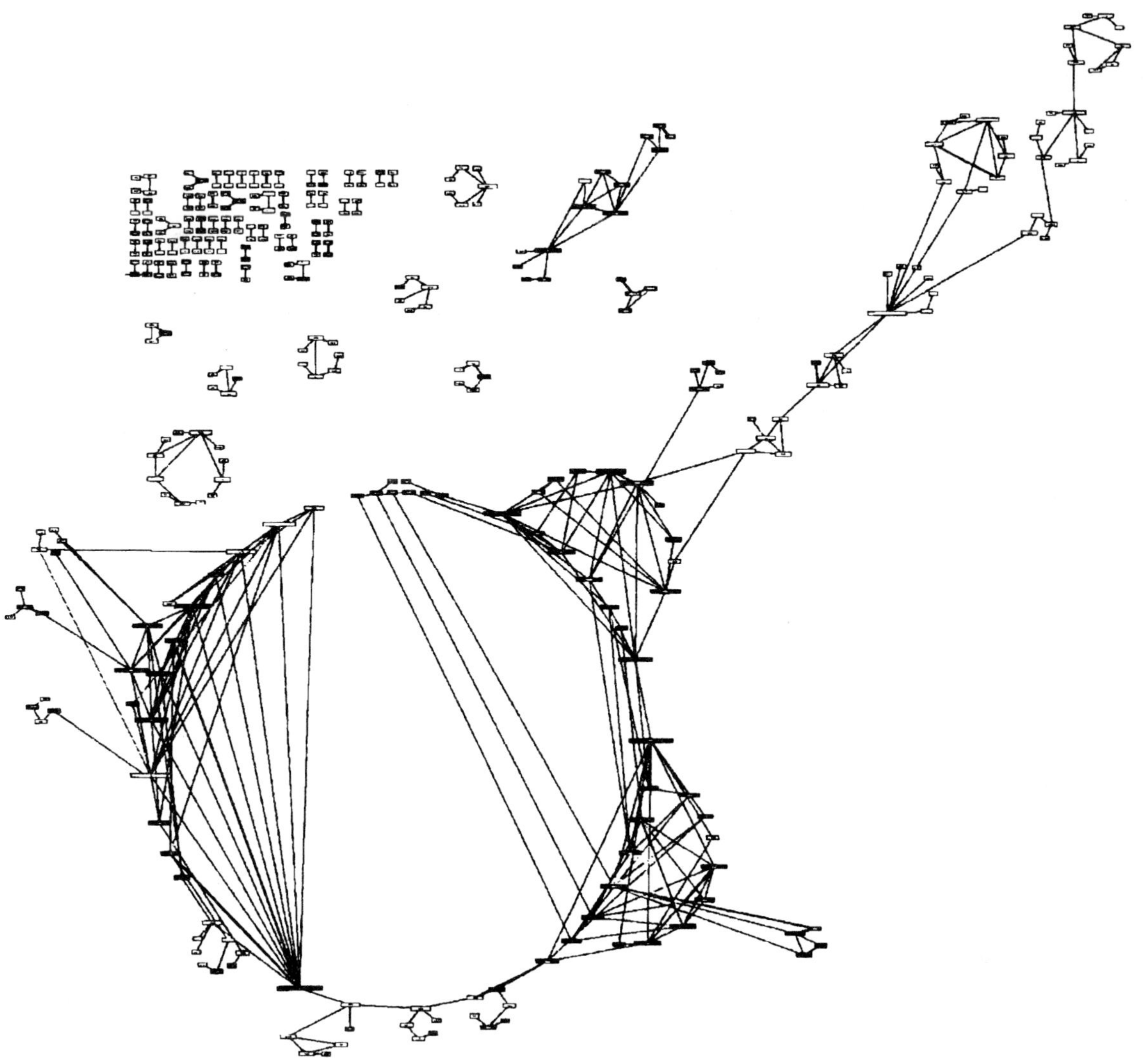

**FIG. 4.** Dynamic relevance networks. The relevance networks generated using the dynamics methodology proposed in this study. Each box represents a gene, labeled with its alphanumeric identification tag. The width of each box is determined by how many other genes it is connected to. The various groups of interconnected genes are called relevance networks. The shaded genes are those that are also found in the static analysis.

out the stationary data points when clustering according gene expression dynamics.

As shown in Fig. 3, there are far more strong positive associations than strong negative associations. Figure 7 shows the distribution for the strongest positive association (two ribosomal proteins *RPL42* and *RPS24*, $R^2 - 0.957$), and for the strongest negative association (two RNA polymerase genes *RPO31* and *SRB8*, $R^2 = -0.854$). In general, the distributions with an extremely tight linear fit are all positive. It could be argued that these tight correlations represent more direct relationships between genes, such as two genes occurring in the same step of a biological pathway—two

ribosomal proteins that are always up-regulated or down-regulated together. It could further be argued that there are no extremely strong negative correlations because negative feedback in biological systems occurs mostly through multistep signal cascades. These are by definition more indirect and thus result in less tight linear relationships between negatively correlated genes.

### Comparison of Dynamics and Static Analyses

In this work we have formulated a methodology for clustering genes according to gene expression dynamics. To

TABLE 2

Dynamic Associations

| Gene name | Category | Gene description | $R^2$ |
|---|---|---|---|
| RPL42B | Protein synthesis | Ribosomal protein L42b | 0.957 |
| RPS24B | Protein synthesis | Ribosomal protein L24B | |
| ASP3 | Asparagine utilization | L-Asparaginase II | 0.910 |
| ASP3 | Asparagine utilization | L-Asparaginase II | |
| RRP4 | rRNA processing | Exoribonuclease / rRNA processing | 0.905 |
| SUA5 | Protein synthesis | Translation initiation protein | |
| LOS1 | tRNA splicing | Involved in tRNA splicing | 0.900 |
| NIP1 | Nuclear protein targeting | Subunit of translation initiation | |
| RPL5 | Protein synthesis | Ribosomal protein | 0.897 |
| RPS0A | Protein synthesis | Ribosomal protein | |
| NMD3 | mRNA decay | Required for stable ribosomal subunit formation | 0.897 |
| NSR1 | Nuclear targeting protein | NLS binding protein/rRNA processing | |
| RPL9A | Protein synthesis | Ribosomal protein | 0.894 |
| RPS8B | Protein synthesis | Ribosomal protein | |
| HHF2 | Chromatin structure | Histone H4 | 0.894 |
| HTB1 | Chromatin structure | Histone H2B | |
| ASP3 | Asparagine utilization | L-Asparaginase II | 0.893 |
| ASP3 | Asparagine utilization | L-Asparaginase II | |
| IMG1 | Protein synthesis | Mitochondrial ribosomal protein | 0.893 |
| RSC6 | Chromatin structure | Chromatin remodeling complex subunit | |

*Note.* The strongest associations between genes found using the dynamics analysis.

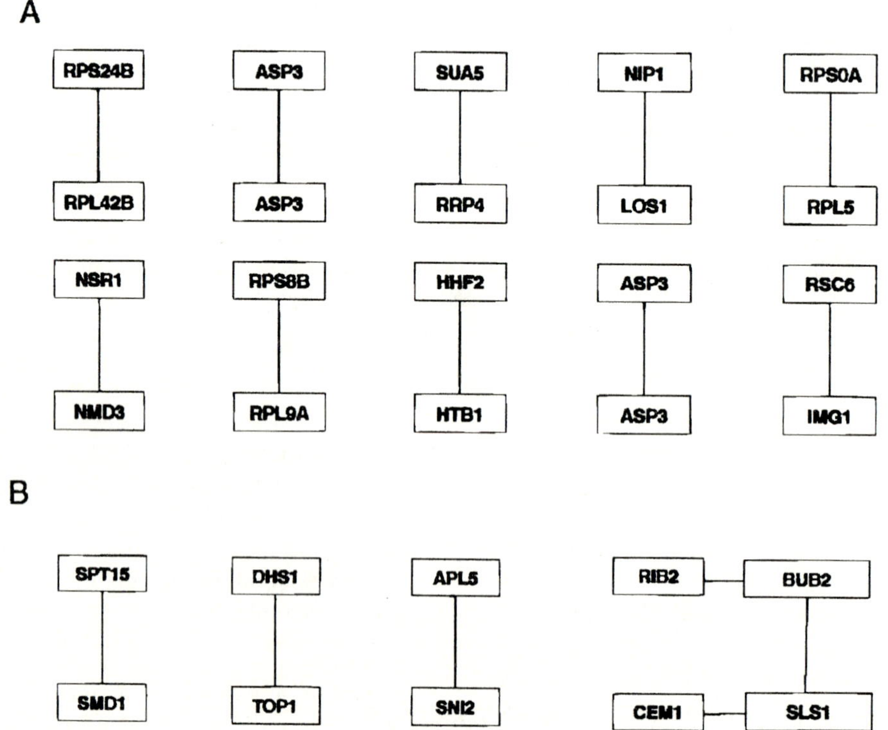


**FIG. 5.** (A) The strongest associations found using the dynamics analysis. (B) Selected networks found using the dynamics analysis, but not the static analysis.

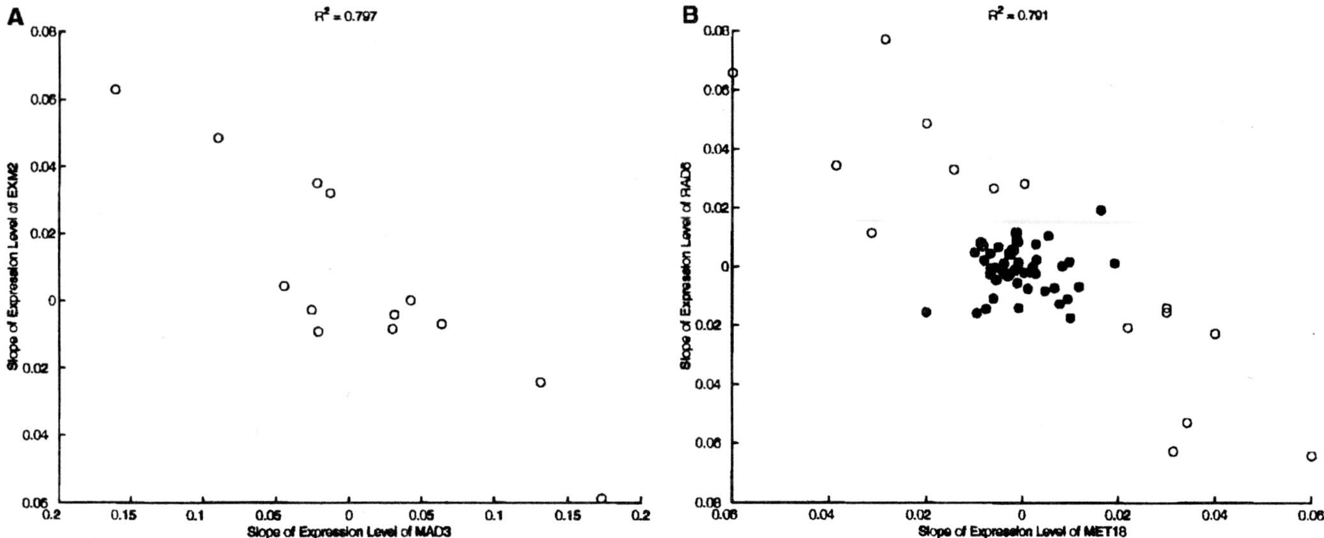

**FIG. 6.** Negative dynamic correlations. (A) The distribution of slopes of MAD3 and EXM2 plotted one against another. (B) The distribution of slopes of MET18 and RAD6 plotted one against another. The filled points in the middle are those static points excluded in the analysis to ensure identification of only truly dynamic relationships between genes.

evaluate this methodology in the context of existing techniques, we construct a second set of relevance networks based on a static analysis of the same dataset.

The static analysis is performed as above, with a few key differences. First, we use the original gene expression data, and not the first difference of gene expression. Second, while the genes are still ranked by entropy value and the bottom 5% (entropy threshold <2.2187) are removed, there is no need to filter out any "stationary" data points since this is a static analysis.

For purposes of comparison, we set the threshold $R^2$ to 0.70, creating a set of relevance networks with a similar number of genes as that seen in the dynamic analysis (356 static vs 348 dynamic). Of the 3,041,811 possible gene–gene connections, 4872 (0.16%) are found to be above this threshold.

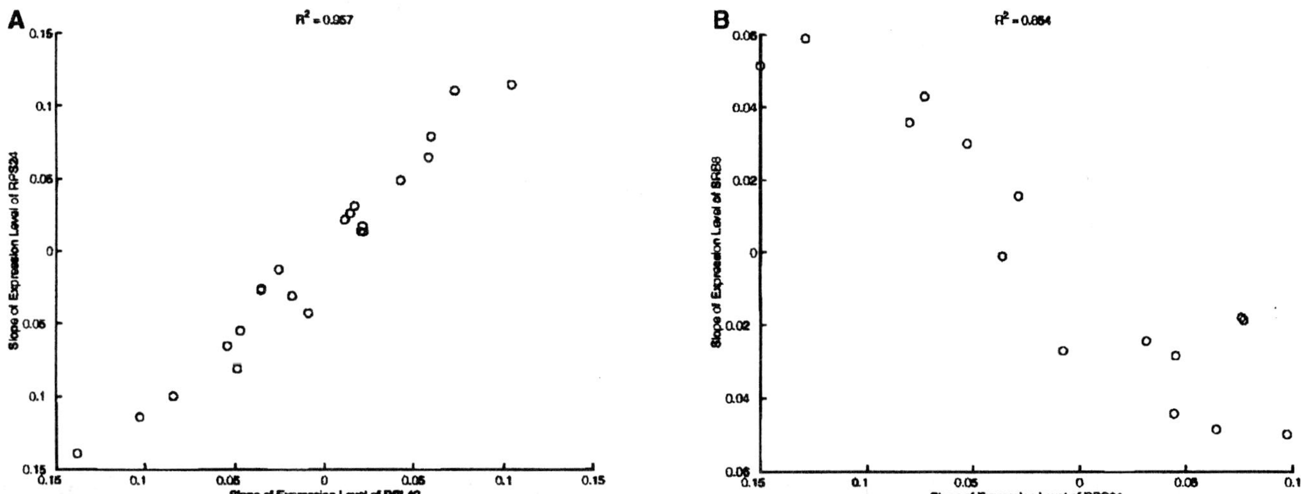

**FIG. 7** Positive and negative correlations. Slope–slope distributions of the strongest positive correlation (A) and the strongest negative correlation (B). On the whole, the strongest positive correlations were more tightly linear than the strongest negative ones, as explained in the text.

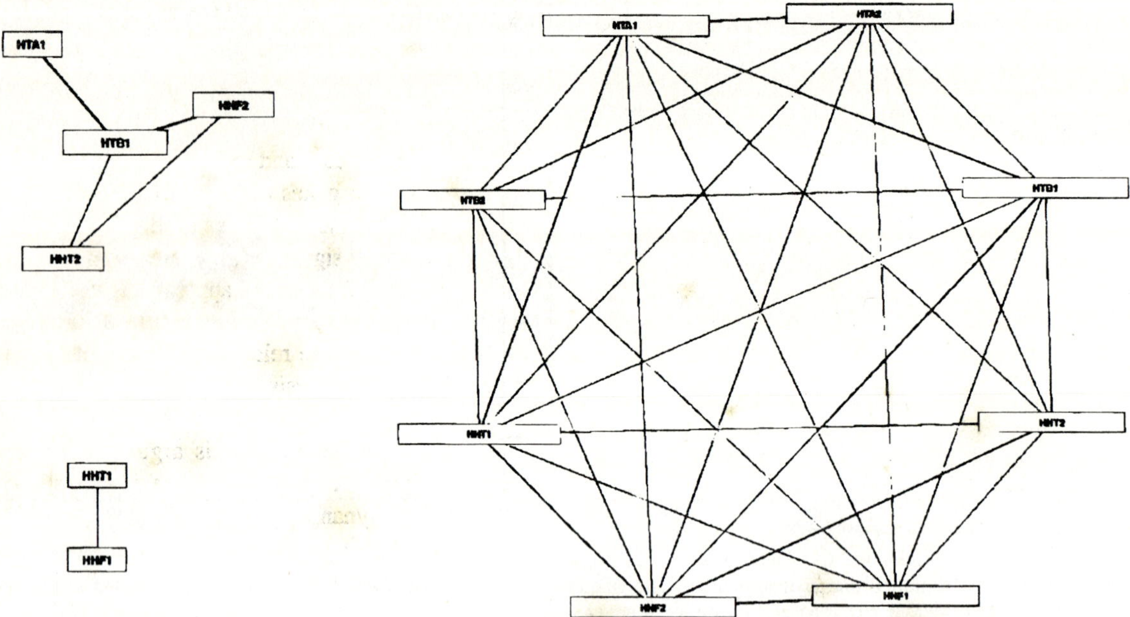

**FIG. 8** Comparison of networks. A group of histone genes grouped together by both the static and dynamic analyses. The dynamics analysis (left) found few dynamic connections compared to the almost fully connected clique formed by the static analysis.

Although both analyses contain a similar number of genes, there are more individual networks generated from the dynamics analysis (71 separate networks vs 45 in the static), while there are far more interconnections between genes in the static analysis (4872 links vs 371 in the dynamic). These results may indicate that slope–slope associations are less common biologically, or that they are more difficult to detect with this methodology than static associations.

We find that 133 genes appear in both the static and dynamic analyses, leaving 215 genes that are exclusive to the dynamics analysis. However, only about half of the 133 shared genes appear linked to the same genes in both analyses—most appear linked to other genes.

*Relationships Appearing in Both Analyses*

A number of links are found identically in both analyses, some of which are shown in Table 3. A large interconnected network of histone genes responsible for chromatin structure found by the static analysis appears broken up into two networks in the dynamics analysis (Fig. 8). This may indicate that certain associations are inherently more dynamic than others.

Some genes are found in both analyses, but appear associated with different genes. One particularly interesting example is discussed here. In the dynamic analysis, three genes involved in protein synthesis are groups into a single network: *PRS1* is involved making PRPP, required for making amino acids [23]; *SIK1* is a nucleolar protein necessary for ribosomal subunit assembly [24]; *SUI2* codes for a subunit of a translation initiation factor [25]. All three of these genes appear in the static analysis as well, but none are linked to each other. In fact, while *PRS1* and *SIK1* do appear indirectly related in the same network in the static analysis, they are not found to be strongly directly linked to each other. These examples illustrate how using both static and dynamic approaches can attain a complementary view of gene–gene relations.

*Associations Found Exclusively in the Dynamics Analysis*

Most of the genes appearing in the dynamics analysis are not found using the static analysis. A selection is reviewed here (Fig. 5B).

One network grouped *SMD1*, involved in mRNA splicing [26], with *SPT15*, a gene involved in transcription [27].

TABLE 3

Shared Associations

| Name | Category | Description |
| --- | --- | --- |
| POL30 | Replication | DNA polymerase processivity factor |
| RFA1 | Replication | Replication factor A, 69 kDa subunit |
| RPN12 | Protein degradation | 26S proteasome regulatory subunit |
| RPN9 | Protein degradation | 26S proteasome regulatory subunit |
| CUP1 | $CU^{2+}$ Ion homeostasis | Metallothionenein |
| CUP1 | $CU^{2+}$ ion homeostasis | Metallothionenein |
| ASP3 | Asparagine utilization | L-Asparaginase II |
| ASP3 | Asparagine utilization | L-Asparaginase II |
| APT1 | Purine biosynthesis | Adenine phosphoribosyltransferase |
| None | Protein synthesis | Tryptophan–TRNA ligase |
| HHF1 | Chromatin structure | Histone H4 |
| HHT1 | Chromatin structure | Histone H3 |
| HTB1 | Chromatin structure | Histone H2B |
| HHF2 | Chromatin structure | Histone H4 |
| HHT2 | Chromatin structure | Histone H3 |
| HTA1 | Chromatin structure | Histone H2A |
| RPS25B | Protein synthesis | Ribosomal protein S25B |
| RPS31 | Protein synthesis | Ribosomal protein S31 |
| RPL18A | Protein synthesis | Ribosomal protein L18A |
| RPL8B | Protein synthesis | Ribosomal protein L8B |
| RPL1B | Protein synthesis | Ribosomal protein L1B |
| RPS19B | Protein synthesis | Ribosomal protein S19B |

*Note.* Selected associations found by both the dynamic and static analyses.

Another network grouped *TOP1*, involved in DNA replication [28], with *DHS1*, involved in DNA repair and recombination [29]. Yet another network grouped *APL5*, involved in vacuolar protein targeting [30], with *SNI2*, a gene involved in secretion [31].

Another interesting network consists of one cell cycle gene *BUB2* [22] and three genes localized in space in the mitochondria: *SLS1* is integral membrane protein involved in mitochondrial metabolism [32]; *CEM1* is a mitochondrial protein involved in fatty acid metabolism [33]; *RIB2* is involved in riboflavin synthesis, also localized to the mitochondria [34].

The intuitive nature of many of these relationships suggests that the dynamics analysis can identify meaningful associations that are not found using a statics analysis.

## DISCUSSION

### Summary of Results

We have formulated and evaluated an analytic methodology for clustering genes according to gene expression dynamics. The relevance networks produced from the dynamics analysis reveal significant and meaningful relationships, indicating that the dynamics approach is useful for knowledge discovery in functional genomics. Furthermore, the fact that most of these relationships are not found using a comparable static analysis further suggests that the dynamic approach is actually necessary for a more complete picture of gene–gene interactions. It is argued that the inherent dynamic nature of certain gene–gene relationships requires this inherently dynamic approach for knowledge discovery.

A sizable number of associations are found using both the static and dynamic analyses. The similarity between the results of the dynamic analysis and those of the already established static analysis serves to further validate the proposed dynamic methodology.

There were clearly also relationships found with the static approach that were not found using the dynamic approach. From these results we conclude that to extract all the valuable information from gene expression measurements, one needs a full set of complementary analysis methodologies that capture the dynamics of these systems. With continuing work in this emerging and important area of research, and the continued decreased cost of massively parallel expression measurements, the dynamics approach is ready to take its place amidst the growing set of tools for knowledge discovery in functional genomics. We anticipate that many more of the techniques developed to handle "noisy" dynamic processes in clinical informatics will find ready and immediate application to functional genomics.

### Future Work

The slope measurements reported here were measured between adjacent data points. Longer-term effects can be studied by measuring slopes between time points that are more distant from one another. The associations reported here were measured between simultaneous slopes. We are currently studying possible time-lagged associations between slopes, allowing for signal propagation times and other delays. This phase generalization expands the analysis methodology to extract even more information from the gene expression data.

## REFERENCES


1. Cheung VG, Morley M, Aguilar F, Massimi A, Kucherlapati R, Childs G. Making and reading microarrays. Nat Genet 1999; 21(1 Suppl):15–19.

2. Botwell D. Options available—from start to finish—for obtaining expression data by microarray. Nat Genet 1999; 1 (Suppl):25–32.

3. Eisen MB, Spellman PT, Brown PO, Botstein D. Cluster analysis and display of genome-wide expression patterns. Proc Natl Acad Sci USA 1998; **95**(250):14863–8.

4. Michaels G S, Carr D B, Askenazi M, Fuhrman S, Wen X, Somogyi R. Cluster analysis and data visualization of large-scale gene expression data. Pac Symp Biocomput 1998; 42–53.

5. Schwartz WB, Patil RS, Szolovits P. Artificial intelligence in medicine: where do we stand? N Engl J Med 1987; 316(11): 685–688.

6. Haimowitz I J, Le P P, Kohane I S. Clinical monitoring using regression-based trend templates. Artificial Intelligence Med 1995; 7:471–472.

7. Russ TA. Reasoning with time dependent data [PhD]: Massachusetts Institute of Technology; 1992.

8. Kohane IS. Temporal reasoning in medical expert systems. In: Salomon R, Blum B, Jørgensen M, editors. MEDINFO 86/Fifth World Congress on Medical Informatics; 1986; Washington, DC: Elsevier Science, 1986; 170–174.

9. Rutledge G, Thomsen G, Farr B, Tovar M, Sheiner L, Fagan L. VentPlan: a ventilator-management advisor. In: Clayton PD, editor. Symposium on Computer Applications in Medical Care, 1991. Washington, DC, 1991; 869–871.

10. Shahar Y, Tu S, Musen M. Knowledge acquisition for temporal abstraction mechanisms. Knowledge Acquisition 1992; 1(4): 217–236.

11. Kahn MG, Fagan LMB, Sheiner L. Model-based interpretation of time-varying medical data. In: Proceedings Symposium Computer Applications in Medical Care, 1989; 1989. 28–32.

12. Spellman PT, Sherlock G, Zhang MQ, Iyer VR, Anders K, Eisen MB, et al. Comprehensive identification of cell cycle-regulated genes of the yeast *Saccharomyces cerevisiae* by microarray hybridization. Mol Biol Cell 1998; 9(12):3273–97.

13. Chen T, He HL, Church GM. Modeling gene expression with differential equations. Pac Symp Biocomput 1999; 29–40.

14. Toronen P, Kolehmainen M, Wong G, Castren E. Analysis of gene expression data using self-organizing maps. FEBS Lett 1999; 451(2):142–6.

15. Tamayo P, Slonim D, Mesirov J, Zhu Q, Kitareewan S, Dmitrovsky E, et al. Interpreting patterns of gene expression with self-organizing maps: methods and application to hematopoietic differentiation. Proc Natl Acad Sci USA 1999; 96(6):2907–12.

16. Butte A, Kohane I. Mutual information relevance networks: functional genomic clustering using pairwise entropy measurements. In: Altman R, Dunker K, Hunter L, Lauderdale K, Klein T, editors. Pacific Symposium on Biocomputing 2000; Hawaii: World Scientific, 2000; 418–429.

17. Butte AJ, Tamayo P, Slonim D, Golub TR, Kohane IS. Discovering functional relationships between RNA expression and chemotherapeutic susceptibility using relevance networks [In Process Citation]. Proc Natl Acad Sci USA 2000; 97(22):12182–6.

18. Butte A, Kohane IS. Unsupervised Knowledge Discovery in Medical Databases Using Relevance Networks. In: Lorenzi N, editor. Fall Symposium, American Medical Informatics Association; 1999; Washington, DC: Hanley and Belfus, 1999; 711–715.

19. Mitchell P, Petfalski E, Shevchenko A, Mann M, Tollervey D. The Exosome: A conserved eukaryotic RNA processing complex containing multiple $3' \rightarrow 5'$ exoribonucleases. Cell 1997; 91: 457–466.

20. Hwang LH, Lau LF, Smith DL, Mistrot CA, Hardwick KG, Hwang ES, et al. Budding Yeast Cdc20: A Target of the Spindle Checkpoint. Science 1998; 279:1041–4.

21. Watkins JF, Sung P, Prakash S, Prakash L. The extremely conserved amino terminus of RAD6 ubiquitin-conjugating enzyme is essential for amino-end rule-dependent protein degradation. Genes Dev 1993; 7(2):50–61.

22. Lauder S, Bankmann M, Guzder SN, Sung P, Prakash L, Prakash S. Dual requirement for the yeast MMS19 gene in DNA repair and RNA polymerase II transcription. Mol Cell Biol 1996; 16:6783–93.

23. Carter AT, Beiche F, Hove-Jensen B, Narbad A, Barker P, Schweizer LM, Schweizer M. PRS1 is a key member of the gene family encoding phosphoribosylpyrophosphate synthetase in *Saccharomyces cerevisiae*. Mol Gen Genet 1997; 254:148–56.

24. Gautier T, Berges T, Tollervey D, Hurt E. Nucleolar KKE/D repeat proteins Nop56p and Nop58p interact with Nop1p and are required for ribosome biogenesis. Mol Cell Biol 1997; 17:7088–98.

25. Cigan AM, Pabich EK, Feng L, Donahue TF. Yeast translation initiation suppressor sui2 encodes the alpha subunit of eukaryotic initiation factor 2 and shares sequence identity with the human alpha subunit. Proc Natl Acad Sci USA 1989; 86:2784–8.

26. Rymond BC. Convergent transcripts of the yeast PRP38-MSD1 locus encode two essential splicing factors, including the D1 core polypeptide of small nuclear ribonucleoprotein particles. Proc Natl Acad Sci USA 1993; 90:848–52.

27. Cormack BP, Struhl K. The TATA-binding protein is required for transcription by all three nuclear RNA polymerases in yeast cells. Cell 1992; 69:685–96.

28. Christman MF, Dietrich FS, Fink GR. Mitotic recombination in the rDNA of *S. cerevisiae* is suppressed by the combined action of DNA topoisomerases I and II. Cell 1988; 55:413–25.

29. Tishkoff DX, Boerger AL, Bertrand P, Filosi N, Gaida GM, Kane MF, Kolodner RD. Identification and characterization of *Saccharomyces cerevisiae* EXO1, a gene encoding an exonuclease that interacts with MSH2. Proc Natl Acad Sci USA 1997; 94: 7487–92.

30. Cowles CR, Odorizzi G, Payne GS, Emr SD. The AP-3 adaptor complex is essential for cargo-selective transport to the yeast vacuole. Cell 1997; 91:109–118.

31. Lehman K, Rossi G, Adamo JE, Brennwald P. Yeast homologues of tomosyn and lethal giant larvae function in exocytosis and are associated with the plasma membrane SNARE, sec9. J Cell Biol 1999; 146:125–40.

32. Rouillard JM, Dufour ME, Theunissen B, Mandart E, Dujardin G, Lacroute F. SLS1, a new *Saccharomyces cerevisiae* gene

involved in mitochondrial metabolism, isolated as a syntheticlethal in association with an SSM4 deletion. Mol Gen Genet 1996; 252:700–8.

33. Harington A, Herbert CJ, Tung B, Getz GS, Slonimski PP. Identification of a new nuclear gene (CEM1) encoding a protein homologous to a $\beta$-keto-acyl synthase which is essential for mitochondrial respiration in *Saccharomyces cerevisiae*. Mol Microbiol 1993; 9:545–55.

34. Pallotta MLBC, Fratianni A, DeVirgilio C, Barile M, Passarella S. *Saccharomyces cerevisiae* mitochondria can synthesise FMN and FAD from externally added riboflavin and export them to the extramitochondrial phase. FEBS Lett 1998; 428(3):245–9.

# Computational analysis of human disease-associated genes and their protein products
## Kodangattil R Sreekumar, L Aravind and Eugene V Koonin*

The complete genome sequences for human, *Drosophila melanogaster* and *Arabidopsis thaliana* have been reported recently. With the availability of complete sequences for many bacteria and archaea, and five eukaryotes, comparative genomics and sequence analysis are enabling us to identify counterparts of many human disease genes in model organisms, which in turn should accelerate the pace of research and drug development to combat human diseases. Continuous improvement of specialized protein databases, together with sensitive computational tools, have enhanced the power and reliability of computational prediction of protein function.

**Addresses**
National Center for Biotechnology Information, National Library of Medicine, National Institutes of Health, Bethesda, Maryland 20894, USA
*e-mail: koonin@ncbi.nlm.nih.gov

**Current Opinion in Genetics & Development** 2001, **11**:247–257

0959-437X/01/$ – see front matter


**Abbreviations**
| | |
|---|---|
| **BIR** | baculovirus inhibition of apoptosis protein repeats |
| **CARD** | caspase recruitment domain |
| **CBD** | carbohydrate-binding domain |
| **FRDA** | Friedreich's ataxia |
| **IAP** | inhibitor of apoptosis |
| **MALT** | mucosa-associated lymphoid tissue |
| **MKKS** | McKusick–Kaufman syndrome |
| **PTP** | protein tyrosine phosphatase |
| **TFPP** | type-4 prepilin peptidase |
| **VEGFR-3** | vascular endothelial growth factor receptor-3 |

## Introduction

Inherited diseases are caused by mutation(s) in one or more genes. Diseases that are due to defect(s) in a single gene are called monogenic diseases; polygenic diseases are caused by defect(s) in more than one gene, with all those genes individually contributing to the development of the disease. In some diseases, such as Lafora's (see below), the defect in proteins implicated in the disease can be directly related to the specific pathological state, whereas in others the link between the disease manifestation and the apparent defect observed at the level of the nucleotide or deduced amino-acid sequence may not be obvious. Irrespective of whether there is an obvious relationship between a defective gene and the pathological state, once a disease-associated gene (or a 'disease gene', in a common, if not precise, parlance) is identified, computational analysis of the gene is a critical step that can provide clues to the molecular basis of pathogenesis and invaluable insights for further experimental analysis.

Computational sequence analysis draws its strength from the conservation of critical features of a gene/protein in phylogenetically divergent sources. This branch of biology has greatly benefited from the finished and continuing genome-sequencing projects, as well as sequencing efforts undertaken on a smaller scale. Genome sequencing of three eukaryotic organisms — the fruitfly *Drosophila melanogaster*, the thale cress *Arabidopsis thaliana* and (in a draft form) *Homo sapiens* — has been completed in the past two years [1••–4••]. Table 1 lists some of the genes implicated in human disorders during the past year, and some of the previously identified human disease genes for which computational analysis in the same time frame has produced important new findings.

Procedures for undertaking rigorous sequence analysis, certain pitfalls in such analysis, methods to circumvent these problems, and the predictive power of computational analysis have been described previously [5–7]. Selected tools and databases that are currently available and are widely used in sequence and structure analysis are listed in Table 2. Here we focus on recent insights obtained by computational analysis of disease genes, and in particular how defects in one or more protein domains affect the cellular function of the encoded protein. The work that we discuss serves only to illustrate how computational analysis of disease genes can provide important clues about molecular basis of pathogenesis (we apologize to those researchers whose important contributions to this burgeoning field are not be cited owing to space limitations).

## Conserved globular domains and their defects

Most proteins consist of one or more evolutionarily conserved domains, each with a distinct structure and function. An alteration of the amino-acid sequence of a domain is likely to hamper its proper functioning, especially if the alteration is in a highly conserved region and/or involves a non-conservative replacement of an amino-acid residue. Several tools are available for the automatic detection of protein domains to aid in function prediction (Table 2); however, the existing domain databases are still far from comprehensive, and the detection methods have limited sensitivity. It is therefore critical to analyze protein sequence in detail, on a case-by-case basis, by using several tools and methods and by assessing the relevance of the results obtained by computational approaches in the context of the available experimental data. Below, some recent discoveries of defects in proteins that result in human disorders are discussed with a view to relate a defective domain/motif to specific biological consequences.

### Bcl10 and mucosa-associated lymphoid tissue lymphoma

A frameshift mutation in Bcl10, resulting in truncation distal to the caspase recruitment domain (CARD), is

**Table 1**

**Protein products of some genes mutated in human diseases.**

| Disease | Protein | Domain(s)* | Other sequence features/motifs | Demonstrated or predicted protein function | Effect of mutation(s) | Reference |
|---|---|---|---|---|---|---|
| **Soluble, globular proteins** | | | | | | |
| MALT lymphoma | Paracaspase | DEATH+ 2(IG) + paracaspase | – | Predicted protein oligomerization, interaction with other proteins and protease activity potentially involved in apoptosis | Translocation produces a chimericprotein that might be an inhibitor of apoptosis. | [13] |
| MALT lymphoma | Bcl10 | CARD | Serine/ Threonine-rich region | The Ser/Thr-rich domain may be involved in regulatory phosphorylation. The CARD domain mediates specific protein-protein interactions in the apoptotic system | Frameshift and truncation beyond the CARD domain might renderthe protein unstable or disruptSer/Thr phosphorylation | [8,9] |
| Fukuyama type CMD | Fukutin | Predicted phosphoryl-sugar/choline transferase | Signal peptide | Similarity to bacterial proteins suggests a role in modifying cell-surface glycoproteins or glycolipids | Transposon insertion disrupts the predicted enzymatic domain | [27,29] |
| Friedreich's ataxia | Frataxin | Frataxin | Mitochondrial import peptide | Nuclear-encoded mitochondrial protein with a key role in the regulation of energy conversion | Several point mutations affect conserved amino-acid residues | [30,33] |
| Parkinson's disease | Parkin | Ubiquitin+ PARKIN_finger + RING | – | E3 ubiquitin-protein ligase | Mutations in ubiquitin domain affect binding to target proteins; mutations in RING prevent recruitment of E2 | [55,56•] |
| Giant axonal neuropathy | Gigaxonin | POZ+IVR+ kelch repeats | – | POZ-kelch domain combination suggests a role in cytoskeleton structure–assembly | Mutations that disrupt POZ or Kelch domains might disrupt protein–protein interactions causing in cytoskeleton defects | [57] |
| Retinitis pigmentosa | MERTK | Ig-like+ Fn3-like+ Tyr-kinase | – | Fn3 and Ig-like modules indicate ligand-binding ability; Tyr-Kinase domain implies protein phosphorylation; MERTK may be a receptor for a specific extra-cellular ligand | Mutations affecting Tyr-kinase domaindisrupt the phosphorylation cascade activated by it. | [58] |
| Laterality defects | CFC1 | EGF+ CFC | Signal peptide and membrane-associating region | Extracellular signal molecule | Mutations in the conserved residuesin EGF domain could disrupt inter-actions with its receptor | [59] |
| Macular corneal dystrophy | CHST6 | Sulfo-transferase | Signal peptide | Transfers sulfate groups from PAPS to various substrates | R50C mutation in the conserved region encompassing the sulfate donor binding site may prevent PAPSbinding | [60] |
| Dominant optic atrophy | OPA1 | Dynamin-like GTPase | Mitochondrial import signal | Possible role in maintenance and inheritance of mitochondria | R290Q, G300E, deletion of invariant I432 and a nonsense mutation in the dynamin GTPase domain | [45,46] |
| X-linked congenital SNB | nyctalopin | LRR-NT+ 15(LRR)+ LRR-CT | Signal peptide, GP anchor | Predicted LRR–containing glyco-protein of extracelluar matrix mediating protein–protein interactions | Missense mutations cause truncation, insertion and deletions affecting LRRs and/or loss of GPI–anchor | [61,62] |
| X-linked mental retardation | ARHGEF6 | CH+SH3+ RhoGEF+ PH | – | Signal transduction via the RhoGTPase cycle (RhoGEF domain); predicted to interact with actin filaments proline-rich peptides in proteins and inositol phosphate. | Intronic mutation resulting in exon 2 skipping, affects CH domain | [63] |
| Lafora's disease | EPM2A | CBD-4 +tyrosine phosphatase (PTP) | Signal peptide | Binds polysaccharides via CBD-4; phosphatase domain may signal the catabolism of Lafora bodies. | W32G mutation in CBD, T194I in the PTP domain | [23] |

**Table 1 (continued)**

**Protein products of some genes mutated in human diseases.**

| Disease | Protein | Domain(s)* | Other sequence features/motifs | Demonstrated or predicted protein function | Effect of mutation(s) | Reference |
|---|---|---|---|---|---|---|
| Usher syndrome type 1c | Harmonin | 2(PDZ)+bZIP+ PDZ | Proline/Serine/ Threonine-rich region; leucine zipper | Predicted to dimerize via leucine zipper and mediate protein-protein interactions via PDZ domain. The P/S/T-rich region might serve as binding site for SH3 and WW domain-containing proteins | Mutations resulting in loss of most orall of the globular domains. | [64] |
| Familial segmental glomerulo-sclerosis | ACTN4 | 2(CH)+ 4(SPEC) + 2(EF) | – | Predicted actin-binding and cross-linking protein (CH domains) and Ca-binding (EF hands) protein. Probable component of the cyto-skeletal network (SPEC domain) | K228E, T232I, and S235P mutations in the 2nd CH domain cause increased affinity for actin | [65] |
| May-Hegglin anomaly and Fechtner and Sebastian syndromes | MYH9 | Myosin + IQ | – | Nonmuscle myosin heavy chain 9; predicted to bind calmodulin (IQ motif) | N93K predicted to destabilize the 2nd helix of myosin catalytic domain, R702C predicted to alter helical stability and ATPase activity. | [66] |
| Mulibrey nanism | MUL | RING+ B-box + BBC + MATH | – | Predicted nuclear protein, may participate in ubiquitin-mediated protein degradataion as a E3 ubiquitin ligase (RING) and possibly in apoptosis (MATH) | Deletions (splice site and lcoding) ead to truncation, with the loss of MATH domain in two cases | [41•] |
| McKusick-Kaufman syndrome | MKKS | Group II chaperonin | – | Facilitates correct protein folding in conjunction with ATP hydrolysis | One mutation predicted to affect intermolecular interaction based on structural modeling | [34••] |
| combined pitutary hormone deficiency | LHX3 | 2(LIM) + HOX | – | Predicted transcriptional regulator via DNA-binding homeodomain protein–protein interaction via LIM domain | A conserved Y replaced by C in LIM domain; frameshift leading to loss of homeodomain | [67] |
| Netherton syndrome | SPINK5 | 15 (KAZAL) | Signal peptide | Potential extracellular adhesion molecule | Insertions and deletions leading to frameshift and protein truncation | [68] |
| familial cylindro-matosis | CYLD | 3(CAP-GLY)+ B-BOX+ UCH-2 | Proline-rich region | Predicted to coordinate attach-ment of cellular organelles to microtubules via CAP-GLY domain and down-regulate protein degradation via the ubiquitin hydrolase via UCH-2 domain | Nonsense and splice site mutations leading to truncation of the C-terminal 2/3 of the protein | [69] |
| Type 2 diabetes | MAPK8IP1 | SH3 + PTB | N-terminal low-complexity region, probably non-globular | Regulation of JNK signaling pathway by mediating protein–protein interactions via the SH3 and PTB domains | S59N mutation outside the two globular domains, not fully penetrant | [70] |
| Cranio-synostosis and enlarged parietal foramina | MSX2 | Homeobox | | DNA-binding protein, transcription factor | P148H enhances DNA-binding affinity of homeobox; R172H and deletion of RK159-160 cause low DNA-binding affinity of homeobox | [15,16] |
| Tricho-rhino-phalangeal syndrome type 1 | TRPS1 | 8 (C2H2) + GATA + 2(C2H2) | – | Multiple DNA-binding domains predict a transcription factor | 3 nonsense and 3 frameshift mutations cause loss of 2–4 Zn-fingers | [71] |

**Membrane proteins**

| Disease | Protein | Domain(s)* | Other sequence features/motifs | Demonstrated or predicted protein function | Effect of mutation(s) | Reference |
|---|---|---|---|---|---|---|
| Wolcott–Rallison syndrome | EIF2AK3 | β-propeller + TMS TM + S/T protein kinase | Signal peptide | ER membrane-associated translation initiation factor elF-2α kinase | Mutations in kinase domain or truncations N-terminal to the kinase domain. β-propeller domainin the N-terminus was previouslyundetected | [72] |

**Table 1 (continued)**

**Protein products of some genes mutated in human diseases.**

| Disease | Protein | Domain(s)* | Other sequence features/motifs | Demonstrated or predicted protein function | Effect of mutation(s) | Reference |
|---|---|---|---|---|---|---|
| Endotoxin hypo-respon-siveness | TLR4 | 11(LRR) + LRRCT + TMS + TIR | Signal peptide | Intracellular signaling (TIR domain), cell adhesion and LRRs interaction with protein ligands (extracellular LRRs) | Mutations A290G and T399I within the LRRs | [73] |
| Diastrophic dysplasia | DTD | 8(TMS) + STAS | – | Sulfate transporter | Impaired sulfate transport across cell membrane cause low sulfate content of cartilage | [39,74, 75] |
| Pendred syndrome | Pendrin | 10(TMS) + STAS | – | Potential iodide-chloride trans-porter | Mutation in predicted phosphate-binding loop. Also deletions, missense and splice site mutations | [38,39•] |
| congenital chloride diarrhoea | DRA | 10(TMS) + STAS | – | Chloride–NaHCO3 exchanger | Missense and deletion mutations | [39•,76] |
| X-linked mental retardation | TM4SF2 | 4(TMS) | Signal peptide | Member of the tetraspanin family that potentially interact with β-1 integrins. | Translocation removing 4th TMS | [77] |
| Stargardt disease, age-related macular degeneration | ABCA4 | 5(TMS) + ABC+ 7(TMS) + ABC | – | Membrane-associated, ATP-dependent transporter | Mutations in the NTP-binding motifs (nearly) abolish ATP binding | [78] |
| Presenile dementia | TYROBP | TMS | Signal peptide and ITAM motif | Predicted transmembrane protein involved in signal transduction via the ITAM motif | Large deletion, and single base pair deletion cause truncation in TM segment and loss of ITAM motif | [79] |
| Niemann–Pick C1 disease | NPC1 | 13(TMS) + sterol-sensing domain | Signal peptide | Lysosomal protein involved in sequestering sterols in lysosomes | Glu20stop: truncation, perhaps null; another truncation results from frameshift in exon2 | [80,81] |
| Spondylo-costal dysostosis | DLL3 | DSL + 11(EGF) + TMS | Signal peptide | Predicted Ca$^{2+}$-binding membrane protein involved in signal transduction | Insertion leading to truncation in DSL domain; deletion in 4th EGF repeat and G385D mutation in 5thEGF repeat | [82] |
| Brachy-dactyly type B | ROR2 | IGc2 + Frizzled + Kringle + TMS + TyrKinase | Serine/ Threonine-rich region | Predicted protein tyrosine kinase involved in signal transduction and ligand-binding | Y755stop, W749stop, and a deletion leading to frameshift beyond G750, perhaps affect interaction with an SH3 domain | [83] |
| Hailey–Hailey disease | ATP2C1 | 8(TMS) + P-type ATPase | | ATP-powered Ca$^{2+}$ pump that transports Ca$^{2+}$ into Golgi bodies | Large deletion, missense and splice site mutations cause truncation | [84] |
| Primary lympho-edema | VEGFR-3 | 2(IG) + IGc2 + IG + IGc2 + 3(IG) + IGc2 + IG + IGc2 + TMS+TyrKinase | Signal peptide | Class III receptor Tyr kinase; binds ligands and is involved in signal transduction | G857R mutation in kinase motif; R1041P, R forms H-bonds with substrate OH- and aspartic acid that is involved in phosphotransfer | [36••,85] |
| Alzheimer's disease | Presenilin 1 | 9(TMS) | – | Apparently a membrane aspartyl protease, with two aspartate required for activity | G384A mutation, next to the critical D385, causes higher levels of residues amyloidogenic Aβ42 production | [14••,86] |

*Domain name abbreviations are as in the SMART database. The number of domains of a particular type is indicated (for example, 2IG denotes two consecutive immunoglobulin domains). Consecutive domains are connected with '+'. Abbreviations: CMD, congenital muscular dystrophy; PAPS, phosphoadenosine phosphosulfate; TM, transmembrane; SNB, stationary night blindness.

associated with mucosa-associated lymphoid tissue (MALT) lymphomas that have the translocation t(1;14)(p22;q32) [8,9]. The CARD domain was first identi-fied in a comparison of the sequences of several apoptotic proteins [10]; this CARD domain comprises six antiparallel α helices and mediates homotypic interactions between proteins involved in apoptosis [11]. Besides caspase recruitment, which is a critical step in the chain of events leading to apoptosis, protein–protein interactions mediated by CARD contribute to activation of the transcription factor NF-κB. The mutated Bcl10 protein seen in MALT lymphomas has lost its pro-apoptotic functions but retains the ability to activate NF-κB [12].

In a different MALT lymphoma translocation, t(11;18(q21;q21), a fusion of the inhibitor of apoptosis (IAP)-2 gene to the MLT1/MALT1 locus generates a chimeric protein comprising BIR repeats of IAP-2 and the caspase-like predicted protease domain of the protein designated paracaspase [13••]. The paracaspase family of caspase homologs has been identified recently, along with the metacaspase family, in a detailed computational analysis of the caspase-like protease superfamily [13••].

Paracaspases contain a predicted caspase-like proteolytic domain, a Death domain capable of mediating specific protein–protein interactions and, in certain cases, including the human representative immunoglobulin domains. In the MALT lymphoma translocation t(11;18)(q21;q21), the prodomain of human paracaspase is replaced with BIR repeats that might function as inhibitors of apoptosis. The BIR–paracaspase fusion has been found to activate NF-κB in a manner dependent on the predicted catalytic cysteine of the paracaspase, thus supporting the computational prediction [13••]. Notably, the prodomain of human paracaspase interacts with Bcl10, which suggests that the two translocations associated with MALT lymphomas affect the same apoptotic pathway.

### Alzheimer disease – presenilins
Familial Alzheimer disease is associated with mutations in genes that encode the paralogous integral membrane proteins presenilin 1 and presenilin 2. Presenilins are required to cleave several other integral membrane proteins, including the β-amyloid precursor proteins Notch and Ire1 that are central to the pathogenesis of Alzheimer disease. It has been shown that two aspartate residues of presenilin 1 — one located in the intracellular loop between helices 6 and 7 and the other one located in helix 7 — are required for these proteolytic events, leading to the hypothesis that presenilins themselves belong to a distinct class of membrane proteases called γ-secretases [14••].

Sequence database searches using all available methods, including different types of profile analysis, have failed to detect similarity between presenilins and any known proteases. However, a pattern search carried out by Steiner et al. [14••] revealed that the signature [G/A]xGDh (where x is any residue, h is a bulky hydrophobic residue, and alternative residues are shown in brackets) is shared by presenilins and bacterial type-4 prepilin peptidases (TFPP), and includes one of the functionally critical aspartates of both protein families.

Presenilins and TFPPs have similar membrane topology, with eight transmembrane helices present in each family, but show no appreciable sequence similarity beyond the above signature. Therefore, although Steiner et al.'s [14••]

observation reinforces the hypothesis that presenilins are the catalytically active γ-secretases, rather than cofactors of a still unidentified protease, it remains unclear whether they are homologs of TFPPs or whether the similarity in the (predicted) active sites is due to convergence. Given the relatively relaxed functional constraints that are typical of membrane proteins, with selection preserving mainly the membrane topology rather then sequence, common origin cannot be ruled out despite the absence of sequence conservation.

### MSX1 and MSX2
Craniosynostosis and enlarged parietal foramina are caused by mutations in the homeodomain — a highly conserved DNA-binding domain containing three helical regions — of the MSX2 protein [15,16]. A mutation (P148H) that leads to craniosynostosis enhances the DNA-binding affinity of this protein, whereas another mutation (R172H) that results in parietal foramina has the opposite effect of lowering the protein's affinity for DNA. Similarly, a mutation in the MSX1 gene (R31P) that affects the second helix of the homeodomain [17], and a nonsense mutation that leads to a truncation at position 104 and a peptide lacking the entire homeodomain [18] are implicated in tooth agenesis.

Other examples of diseases caused by mutations in homeodomains include microphthalmia [19], amegakaryocytic thrombocytopenia and radio-ulnar synostosis [20]. The paired (PAX) domain, another DNA-binding module involved in transcription regulation, is defective in certain individuals diagnosed with oligodontia [21]. An enhanced or diminished DNA-binding capacity of a transcription factor is likely to result in altered level of protein(s) encoded by genes under its control, which in turn might lead to pathogenesis.

### Laforin
The presence of polyglucosan inclusion bodies in the brain is characteristic of progressive myoclonus epilepsy or Lafora's disease. The EPM2A product, laforin, which is defective in patients suffering from this disease, was initially designated as a protein tyrosine phosphatase (PTP) because of the presence of a consensus sequence characteristic of the catalytic site of PTPs [22]. Minassian et al. [23••] have carried out a detailed computational analysis resulting in significant insights about this protein and its probable link to the accumulation of polyglucosan inclusions. Analysis of protein domains in laforin using the Pfam database [24] revealed the presence of the carbohydrate-binding domain (CBD)-4 at the amino (N) terminus of the protein, in addition to the dual-specificity phosphatase domain, which belongs to a distinct subfamily of PTPs, at the carboxyl (C) terminus. Furthermore, two sequence motifs characteristic of the glucohydrolase family as documented in PROSITE [25] were detected.

On the basis of these findings and the mutations detected in the EPM2A gene, Minassian et al. [23••] proposed that normal laforin prevents the accumulation of polyglucosan

**Table 2**

**Selected tools and databases useful in sequence analysis, with an emphasis on those dedicated to disease genes*.**

| Tools/database | Comments | URL | Reference |
|---|---|---|---|
| **Tools and databases for functional annotation** | | | |
| SignalP | Predicts location of signal peptide and cleavage site in proteins. | http://www.cbs.dtu.dk/services/SignalP/ | [87] |
| TopPred | Predicts location and orientation of TM segments. | http://www.sbc.su.se/~erikw/toppred2/ | [88] |
| CDD | Collection of protein domains with links to structures if available. CDD uses a library of PSSMs that is searched by Reverse Position-Specific BLAST to match a protein query. | http://www.ncbi.nlm.nih.gov./Structure/cdd/cdd.shtml | [89] |
| COG | Phylogenetic classification of proteins from complete genomes that groups orthologous proteins; useful for functional annotation of newly sequenced genomes. COGNITOR can be used to place a protein into one of the COGs. | http://www.ncbi.nlm.nih.gov./COG/ | [52•] |
| Pfam | Collection of protein domains and families consisting of multiple alignments and hidden Markov models generated in a semi-automatic manner. | http://www.sanger.ac.uk/Pfam/ | [24] |
| SMART | Searchable collection of protein domains for detecting and analysing domain architecture. | http://smart.embl-heidelberg.de/ | [90] |
| BLOCKS | Database of highly conserved regions of proteins derived automatically and represented in the form of ungapped multiple alignments. Also tools to detect and verify protein sequence conservation. | http://www.blocks.fhcrc.org/ | [91] |
| PRINTS | Database of protein fingerprints (group of motifs distributed in the sequence characteristic of a family). | http://bmbsgi11.leeds.ac.uk/bmb5dp/prints.html | [92] |
| PROSITE | Database of biologically significant sites, patterns and profiles in proteins that helps in function prediction. | http://www.expasy.ch/prosite/ | [25] |
| **Tools for sequence similarity search** | | | |
| BLAST | Programs for rapid sequence similarity searches for protein and DNA sequences. Also provides searches for nucleotide sequences translated in all six frames. | http://www.ncbi.nlm.nih.gov/BLAST/ | [28] |
| HMMER | Programs for constructing multiple protein sequence alignments and performing database searches using the HMM approach. | http://hmmer.wustl.edu | [93] |
| PSI-BLAST | An implementation of BLAST capable of detecting distantly related proteins by creating a PSSM from the significant matches detected in one round and using that PSSM as the query in the next iteration. | http://www.ncbi.nlm.nih.gov./blast/psiblast.cgi | [28] |
| **Tools for protein structure prediction and comparison** | | | |
| PHD | Neural network dependent secondary structure prediction. | http://dodo.cpmc.columbia.edu/pp/predictprotein.html | [94] |
| PSI-PRED | Prediction of secondary structure using PSI-BLAST derived scoring matrices. | http://insulin.brunel.ac.uk/psipred | [95] |
| Hybrid fold recognition | Combined algorithm for fold recognition using both sequence-based evolutionary information and secondary structure predictions. | http://www.cs.bgu.il/~bioinbgu | [96] |
| FSSP/DALI | Automatic structural classification of protein domains with the DALI search facility for structure comparisons. | http://www2.ebi.ac.uk/dali/fssp/ | [97] |
| SWISS-PDB Viewer and Swiss Model | Powerful structure visualization and homology modeling system for personal computers. | http://www.expasy.ch/spdbv/ | [98] |
| VAST | Structure similarity search tool based on the definition of the threshold of statistically significant structural similarity. | http://www.ncbi.nlm.nih.gov/Structure/ | [99] |
| **Databases for disease genes** | | | |
| Genes and Disease | Information on selected human diseases with links to genes, chromosomes, scientific literature and OMIM. | http://www.ncbi.nlm.nih.gov./disease/ | |
| OMIM | Catalog of human genetic disorders and associated phenotypic and genetic information. | http://www.ncbi.nlm.nih.gov./entrez/query.fcgi?db=OMIM | [100] |

**Table 2 legend**

*The number of tools and databases for computational analysis of genes and proteins that are available online has been rapidly growing during the past few years. Inevitably, this is an arbitrary selection of those we have used extensively and found to be useful. HMM, hidden marker model; PSI-BLAST, position-specific iterating BLAST; PSSM, position specific scoring matrix.

inclusion bodies in neurons by binding polyglucosan through the CBD and cleaving the β-linkages through the putative glucohydrolase domain. A more detailed examination of the sequence and domain architecture of laforin shows, however, that the putative glucohydrolase domain largely overlaps with the confidently predicted dual-specificity phosphatase domain, which suggests that the presence of the glucohydrolase motifs in this protein is spurious (KR Sreekumar, L Aravind, EV Koonin, unpublished data).

The dual-specificity phosphatase activity of laforin has been confirmed experimentally [26]. The CBD domain of laforin probably targets the protein to polyglucosan inclusion bodies, whereas the phosphatase domain might activate a protein dephosphorylation pathway that triggers its destruction through a still unknown mechanism. This example illustrates both the utility of computational analysis of protein domains for function prediction and the need for caution in interpreting computational results.

### Fukutin

Fukuyama type congenital dystrophy is caused by retroposon insertions in the gene encoding a protein called fukutin [27]. Extensive database searches using the PSI-BLAST program [28] detected moderate, but statistically significant similarity between fukutin and a family of bacterial and eukaryotic enzymes that catalyze phosphoryl-ligand transfer. Additional multiple alignment analysis showed that fukutin shares with these proteins the predicted catalytic residues [29].

The combination of these observations with the prediction of a signal peptide in fukutin, and the experimental data on its localization in the endoplasmic reticulum and secretory granules [27] has led to the prediction that fukutin modifies cell-surface molecules, most probably through the attachment of phosphoryl-sugar moieties [29].

### Frataxin

Friedreich's ataxia (FRDA) is an autosomal recessive disease characterized by progressive ataxia, hypertrophic cardiomyopathy and diabetes mellitus. Gibson *et al.* [30] have carried out computational analysis of the FRDA gene product, frataxin, and shown that it has homologues in bacteria of the γ subdivision of the Proteobacteria, but not in any other prokaryotes, and also that it possesses a non-globular N-terminal domain predicted to function as a mitochondrial targeting peptide [30]. They predicted a distinct fold, consisting of a β sheet flanked by two long α helices, on the basis of a multiple alignment of the frataxin homologs, and further proposed that frataxin is anuclear encoded, and, accordingly, that FRDA is a 'mitochondrial disease'.

Both the mitochondrial localization and the αβ sandwich structure predictions, which were based on computational analysis of frataxin, have been confirmed experimentally [31,32], and more recent studies have shown that frataxin is a key regulator of mitochondrial energy conversion [33*].

### McKusick–Kaufman syndrome

Mutations in a gene on chromosome 20 have been shown to cause McKusick–Kaufman syndrome (MKKS) and Bardet–Biedl syndrome (see also review by Sheffield *et al.*, this issue, pp 317–321) — developmental anomalies that involve hydrometrocolpos, postaxial polydactyly and congenital heart disease [34**,35]. Sequence database searches show that the predicted protein encoded by the MKKS gene belongs to a family of group II chaperonins that promote protein folding in an ATP-dependent manner.

The three-dimensional structural model of the MKKS protein predicts that the Y37C mutation lies in the highly conserved loop region between helix 1 and strand 2 which is involved in interaction among subunits [34**]. Another mutation, H84Y, is predicted to lie in a region responsible for ATP hydrolysis. This appears to be the first description of a disease caused by a defect in a molecular chaperone — a finding that complements the data on the role of defects in transcription regulators in several diseases, as discussed above.

### Vascular endothelial growth factor receptor-3

Another example of a human disease for which sequence analysis and three-dimensional structure modeling has provided insights into pathogenesis is primary lymphoedema caused by mutations in vascular endothelial growth factor receptor-3 (VEGFR-3) [36**]. The VEGFR-3 protein consists of six classical immunoglobulin domains, four immunoglobulin C2 domains, a signal peptide, a single transmembrane segment and an intracellular tyrosine kinase catalytic domain.

Four mutations that co-segregate with lymphoedema phenotype map within the tyrosine kinase domain. Finegold and co-workers [36**] have built a three-dimensional model of VEGFR-3, based on the crystal structure of VEGFR-2, from which functional implications of mutations observed in VEGFR-3 can be inferred. For example, the model shows that the G857R mutation (the last glycine of the conserved GXGXXG kinase motif) lies in a critical turn between β strands 1 and 2 and is expected to affect ATP-binding and catalysis severely.

### DTD, Pendrin and congenital chloride diarrhoea

Diastrophic dysplasia/achondrogenesis type IB (DTD), Pendred's syndrome and congenital chloride diarrhoea are caused by malfunctions of anion transporters of the sulfate transporter family [37,38]. Unexpectedly, it has been shown that the C-terminal cytoplasmic portion of these proteins shares a conserved domain named STAS (after sulfate transporter anti-sigma) with bacterial anti-sigma-factor antagonists, and this connection provides clues for the regulation of anion transporters [39•]. (Anti-sigma factors prevent formation of active RNA polymerase holoenzyme by trapping the sigma factor. Anti-sigma antagonists bind the anti-sigma factors and prevent the formation of sigma-antisigma complex.) The STAS domain of the antisigma-factor antagonist binds GTP and has a weak GTPase activity [40], leading to the prediction that the cytoplasmic domain of the anion transporters might regulate transport through NTP binding [39•].

### Mulibrey nanism

Muscle–liver–brain–eye (Mulibrey) nanism is an autosomal recessive disorder that affects several tissues of mesodermal origin, which suggests that a highly pleiotropic gene is involved in this disease. The complex multidomain architecture of the recently cloned MUL gene product is compatible with this notion [41•]. The MUL protein comprises a RING-finger domain, a B-box domain, a coiled-coil domain and a MATH domain. Avela *et al.* [41•] suggest that MUL is likely to be involved in various protein–protein interactions that might be important in development regulation; however, the combination of domains present in this protein calls for more specific functional predictions.

There is growing evidence that the primary function of the RING domain is as the E3 component of the ubiquitin ligase cascade that facilitates the transfer of ubiquitin from the E2 protein to target proteins [42]. MATH is a versatile adaptor domain that mediates specific protein–protein interactions in the programmed cell death system, chromatin remodeling and other functional contexts [43]. Thus, MUL can be predicted to function as an E3 ubiquitin ligase, with additional regulatory interactions, possibly related to apoptosis, mediated by the MATH domain.

## Mutations outside functional protein domains

Mutations that lie outside globular domains and transmembrane segments of proteins, or outside the protein-coding part of a gene altogether often affect gene expression. Such mutations may be located in untranslated regions, promoters, introns and sequences encoding signal peptides. The effect of these mutations may manifest itself as a defective globular or transmembrane domain, however, owing to exon skipping, aberrant splicing and abnormal cellular localization.

### Untranslated and non-coding regions

Sequence analysis can provide hints as to the molecular basis of defects caused by mutations in untranslated regions. For example, in individuals with severe protein C deficiency, who suffer from massive disseminated intravascular coagulation or neonatal purpura fulminans, promoter mutations in the protein C (PROC) gene have been identified. These mutations alter the consensus sequence for the transcription factor HNF-3-binding, resulting in reduced PROC promoter activity, and accordingly a reduced level of protein C [44].

A splice-site mutation in intron 9 of the OPA1 gene, which has been detected in individuals with autosomal dominant optic atrophy, leads to either exon-10 skipping or a frameshift with a premature stop codon [45]. The OPA1 product is a mitochondrial protein comprising an N-terminal mitochondrial localization signal and a dynamin GTPase domain. The defective protein produced by the mutant gene lacks a part of the GTPase domain [45,46].

### Signal peptides

Duplications in exon 1 of the TNFRSF11A (RANK) gene that segregates with familial expansile osteolysis have been identified recently [47]. These mutations are short in-frame insertions in the hydrophobic core region of the RANK signal peptide, and affect proper cleavage of the signal peptide.

The RANK protein consists of four tumor-necrosis factor repeats and a transmembrane segment, besides the signal peptide that directs the protein to the secretory pathway. Failure to cleave the signal peptide might result in higher intracellular accumulation of defective RANK in compartments of the secretion pathway that could lead to a higher incidence of receptor self-association and increased RANK signal transduction [47]. An NF-κB responsive reporter assay of transfected cells has indeed suggested that mutations occurring in familial expansile osteolysis result in increased constitutive RANK signaling [47].

## Conclusions and future directions

The examples of disease genes discussed here and in previous publications [6,48–50] illustrate the importance of sequence and structure analysis in predicting the molecular basis of pathogenesis, in guiding further work and in understanding the biology of the respective functional systems. Proteins for which predictions based on sequence analysis have been experimentally verified include frataxin and the MALT-associated paracaspase. Using the complete genome sequences, efforts are being made to assemble databases of orthologous genes from diverse organisms, and these databases are already proving to be valuable in functional annotation of genes [51,52•].

The presence of orthologs for many of the human disease genes in model organisms such as mouse, fruitfly, nematode and yeast enable experimental verification of the predictions. In particular, apparent counterparts for 178 of 287 analyzed human disease genes have been identified in fruitfly by large-scale comparative genomics [53••,54••]. At present, some of the human disease genes do not seem to have an ortholog in other organisms, but the anticipated availability in the next several years of the complete genome sequences of primates and other mammals should drastically reduce the number of 'orphan' disease genes.

The predictive power of sequence and structure analysis, combined with the wealth of genome sequence data, should not only enhance our understanding of the biology that underlies the effect of mutations in disease genes, but also enable the identification of many new drug targets and accelerate the process of drug design and the development of therapeutic strategies.

## References and recommended reading


Papers of particular interest, published within the annual period of review, have been highlighted as:

* of special interest
** of outstanding interest

1. Adams MD, Celniker SE, Holt RA, Evans CA, Gocayne JD,
** Amanatides PG, Scherer SE, Li PW, Hoskins RA, Galle RF *et al.*: **The genome sequence of *Drosophila melanogaster*.** *Science* 2000, **287**:2185-2195.
The second (nearly) complete genome of a multicellular eukaryote to be sequenced, after the nematode *Caenorhabditis elegans*. The completion of the fly genome is particularly important: first, because the enormous wealth of genetic data available for this organism can be systematically correlated with gene and protein sequences; and second, because an in-depth comparison of two animal genomes has become possible for the first time.

2. The *Arabidopsis* Genome Initiative: **Analysis of the genome
** sequence of the flowering plant *Arabidopsis thaliana*.** *Nature* 2000, **408**:796-815.
Sequencing of the first complete plant genome is fundamentally important as it sets the stage for a comparative study of genomes representing the three major lineages of the eukaryotic crown group – animals, fungi and plants.

3. Lander ES, Linton LM, Birren B, Nusbaum C, Zody MC, Baldwin J,
** Devon K, Dewar K, Doyle M, FitzHugh W *et al.*: **Initial sequencing and analysis of the human genome.** *Nature* 2001, **409**:860-921.
This paper reports the results of the public effort on human genome sequencing. A preliminary analysis of the predicted human proteome performed with a variety of computational techniques, with particular emphasis on the 'Interpro' collection of protein domains, is presented. The major conclusions are that human proteins consistently have more complex domain architectures compared to their homologs from other eukaryotes and domain rearrangements have a prominent role in eukaryotic evolution. Over 1300 apparent orthologs common to human, fly, worm and yeast have been identified.

4. Venter JC, Adams MD, Myers EW, Li PW, Mural RJ, Sutton GG,
** Smith HO, Yandell M, Evans CA, Holt RA *et al.*: **The sequence of the human genome.** *Science* 2001, **291**:1304-1351.
The report of the human genome sequence from the private company Celera Genomics. In the preliminary analysis of the predicted human proteome, molecular functions for ~60% of the proteins have been assigned by automatic means utilizing the protein family databases such as Pfam and SMART. The authors have also identified a partial set of human–fly and human–worm orthologs. A preliminary survey of the differences between the human genome and other sequenced eukaryotic genomes is also presented.

5. Altschul SF, Boguski MS, Gish W, Wootton JC: **Issues in searching molecular sequence databases.** *Nat Genet* 1994, **6**:119-129.

6. Bork P, Koonin EV: **Predicting functions from protein sequences – where are the bottlenecks?** *Nat Genet* 1998, **18**:313-318.

7. Baxevanis AD, Francis Ouellette BF: **Bioinformatics: a practical guide to the analysis of genes and proteins.** In *Methods of Biochemical Analysis*, vol 39. New York: John Wiley; 1998:1-370.

8. Willis TG, Jadayel DM, Du MQ, Peng H, Perry AR, Abdul-Rauf M, Price H, Karran L, Majekodunmi O, Wlodarska I *et al.*: **Bcl10 is involved in t(1;14)(p22;q32) of MALT B cell lymphoma and mutated in multiple tumor types.** *Cell* 1999, **96**:35-45.

9. Du MQ, Peng H, Liu H, Hamoudi RA, Diss TC, Willis TG, Ye H, Dogan A, Wotherspoon AC, Dyer MJ, Isaacson PG: **BCL10 gene mutation in lymphoma.** *Blood* 2000, **95**:3885-3890.

10. Hofmann K, Bucher P, Tschopp J: **The CARD domain: a new apoptotic signalling motif.** *Trends Biochem Sci* 1997, **22**:155-156.

11. Hofmann K: **The modular nature of apoptotic signaling proteins.** *Cell Mol Life Sci* 1999, **55**:1113-1128.

12. Zhang Q, Siebert R, Yan M, Hinzmann B, Cui X, Xue L, Rakestraw KM, Naeve CW, Beckmann G, Weisenburger DD, Sanger WG, Nowotny H *et al.*: **Inactivating mutations and overexpression of BCL10, a caspase recruitment domain-containing gene, in MALT lymphoma with t(1;14)(p22;q32).** *Nat Genet* 1999, **22**:636-638.

13. Uren AG, O'Rourke K, Aravind L, Pisabarro MT, Seshagiri S, Koonin EV,
** Dixit VM: **Identification of paracaspases and metacaspases. Two ancient families of caspase-like proteins, one of which plays a key role in MALT lymphoma.** *Mol Cell* 2000, **6**:961-967.
This example of combining computational analysis and experimental verification reveals the molecular basis of a class of MALT lymphoma translocation. Computational analysis using sensitive tools for sequence-profile analysis was critical for the identification of two new families of caspase-related proteases, which produce a new perspective on the evolution of this important class of enzymes.

14. Steiner H, Kostka M, Romig H, Basset G, Pesold B, Hardy J, Capell A,
** Meyn L, Grim ML, Baumeister R *et al.*: **Glycine 384 is required for presenilin-1 function and is conserved in bacterial polytopic aspartyl proteases.** *Nat Cell Biol* 2000, **2**:848-851.
Reports the site-directed mutagenesis of presenilin 1 and detection of the similarity between its putative catalytic site and that of bacterial type-4 prepilin peptidases. A functional and possibly evolutionary connection, revealed by computer analysis of protein sequences and structures, is plausible despite the absence of significant sequence similarity.

15. Ma L, Golden S, Wu L, Maxson R: **The molecular basis of Boston-type craniosynostosis: the Pro148→His mutation in the N-terminal arm of the MSX2 homeodomain stabilizes DNA binding without altering nucleotide sequence preferences.** *Hum Mol Genet* 1996, **5**:1915-1920.

16. Wilkie AO, Tang Z, Elanko N, Walsh S, Twigg SR, Hurst JA, Wall SA, Chrzanowska KH, Maxson RE Jr: **Functional haploinsufficiency of the human homeobox gene MSX2 causes defects in skull ossification.** *Nat Genet* 2000, **24**:387-390.

17. Vastardis H, Karimbux N, Guthua SW, Seidman JG, Seidman CE: **A human MSX1 homeodomain missense mutation causes selective tooth agenesis.** *Nat Genet* 1996, **13**:417-421.

18. van den Boogaard MJ, Dorland M, Beemer FA, and van Amstel HK: **MSX1 mutation is associated with orofacial clefting and tooth agenesis in humans.** *Nat Genet* 2000, **24**:342-343.

19. Ferda Percin E, Ploder LA, Yu JJ, Arici K, Horsford DJ, Rutherford A, Bapat B, Cox DW, Duncan AM, Kalnins VI *et al.*: **Human microphthalmia associated with mutations in the retinal homeobox gene CHX10.** *Nat Genet* 2000, **25**:397-401.

20. Thompson AA, Nguyen LT: **Amegakaryocytic thrombocytopenia and radio-ulnar synostosis are associated with HOXA11 mutation.** *Nat Genet* 2000, **26**:397-398.

21. Stockton DW, Das P, Goldenberg M, D'Souza RN, Patel PI: **Mutation of PAX9 is associated with oligodontia.** *Nat Genet* 2000, **24**.18-19

22. Minassian BA, Lee JR, Herbrick JA, Huizenga J, Soder S, Mungall AJ, Dunham I, Gardner R, Fong CY, Carpenter S *et al.*: **Mutations in a gene encoding a novel protein tyrosine phosphatase cause progressive myoclonus epilepsy.** *Nat Genet* 1998, **20**:171-174.

23. Minassian BA, Ianzano L, Meloche M, Andermann E, Rouleau GA,
** Delgado-Escueta AV, Scherer SW: **Mutation spectrum and predicted function of laforin in Lafora's progressive myoclonus epilepsy.** *Neurology* 2000, **55**:341-346.
This paper underscores both the potential of computational analysis of protein domains and the need to be cautious in interpreting such results. Computational analysis of laforin reveals the presence of a carbohydrate-binding domain and a dual specificity phosphatase domain; however, the apparent glucohydrolase motifs detected in this protein are likely to be spurious.

24. Bateman A, Birney E, Durbin R, Eddy SR, Howe KL, Sonnhammer EL: **The Pfam protein families database.** *Nucleic Acids Res* 2000, **28**:263-266.

25. Hofmann K, Bucher P, Falquet L, Bairoch A: **The PROSITE database, its status in 1999.** *Nucleic Acids Res* 1999, **27**:215-219.

26. Ganesh S, Agarwala KL, Ueda K, Akagi T, Shoda K, Usui T, Hashikawa T, Osada H, Delgado-Escueta AV, Yamakawa K: **Laforin, defective in the progressive myoclonus epilepsy of lafora type, is a dual-specificity phosphatase associated with polyribosomes.** *Hum Mol Genet* 2000, **9**:2251-2261.

27. Kobayashi K, Nakahori Y, Miyake M, Matsumura K, Kondo-Iida E, Nomura Y, Segawa M, Yoshioka M, Saito K, Osawa M, Hamano K *et al.*: **An ancient retrotransposal insertion causes Fukuyama-type congenital muscular dystrophy.** *Nature* 1998, **394**:388-392.

28. Altschul SF, Madden TL, Schaffer AA, Zhang J, Zhang Z, Miller W, Lipman DJ: **Gapped BLAST and PSI-BLAST: a new generation of**

protein database search programs. *Nucleic Acids Res* 1997, 25:3389-3402.

29. Aravind L, Koonin EV: **The fukutin protein family — predicted enzymes modifying cell-surface molecules.** *Curr Biol* 1999, 9:R836-R837.

30. Gibson TJ, Koonin EV, Musco G, Pastore A, Bork P: **Friedreich's ataxia protein: phylogenetic evidence for mitochondrial dysfunction.** *Trends Neurosci* 1996, 19:465-468.

31. Koutnikova H, Campuzano V, Foury F, Dolle P, Cazzalini O, Koenig M: **Studies of human, mouse and yeast homologues indicate a mitochondrial function for frataxin.** *Nat Genet* 1997, 16:345-351.

32. Dhe-Paganon S, Shigeta R, Chi YI, Ristow M, Shoelson SE: **Crystal structure of human frataxin.** *J Biol Chem* 2000, 275:30753-30756.

33. Ristow M, Pfister MF, Yee AJ, Schubert M, Michael L, Zhang CY, Ueki K,
• Michael MD 2nd, Lowell BB, Kahn CR: **Frataxin activates mitochondrial energy conversion and oxidative phosphorylation.** *Proc Natl Acad Sci USA* 2000, 97:12239-12243.
Experimental validation of the role of frataxin in mitochondrial energy conversion that corroborates with the computational prediction.

34. Stone DL, Slavotinek A, Bouffard GG, Banerjee-Basu S, Baxevanis AD,
•• Barr M, Biesecker LG: **Mutation of a gene encoding a putative chaperonin causes McKusick–Kaufman syndrome.** *Nat Genet* 2000, 25:79-82.
This paper illustrates how DNA sequence data obtained form positional cloning experiments can be subjected to computational analysis and further structure modeling to provide insights into biology of the system. On the basis of sequence analysis, MKKS is predicted to be a chaperonin. The structure of MKKS is modeled to explain the loss of function associated with mutations in this gene.

35. Slavotinek AM, Stone EM, Mykytyn K, Heckenlively JR, Green JS, Heon E, Musarella MA, Parfrey PS, Sheffield VC, Biesecker LG: **Mutations in MKKS cause bardet-biedl syndrome.** *Nat Genet* 2000, 26:15-16.

36. Karkkainen MJ, Ferrell RE, Lawrence EC, Kimak MA, Levinson KL,
•• McTigue MA, Alitalo K, Finegold DN: **Missense mutations interfere with VEGFR-3 signalling in primary lymphoedema.** *Nat Genet* 2000, 25:153-159.
Homology-based structure modeling of VEGFR-3 predicts that a mutation implicated in primary lymphoedema eliminates ATP binding by the serine/threonine protein kinase domain of this protein.

37. Scott DA, Wang R, Kreman TM, Sheffield VC, Karnishki LP: **The Pendred syndrome gene encodes a chloride-iodide transport protein.** *Nat Genet* 1999, 21:440-443.

38. Everett LA, Green ED: **A family of mammalian anion transporters and their involvement in human genetic diseases.** *Hum Mol Genet* 1999, 8:1883-1891.

39. Aravind L, Koonin EV: **The STAS domain — a link between anion
• transporters and antisigma- factor antagonists.** *Curr Biol* 2000, 10:R53-R55.
This paper describes an NTP-binding STAS domain common to anion transporters and bacterial antisigma-factor antagonists, providing clues to the regulation of anion transporters. This finding illustrates the potential of sequence analysis to reveal completely unexpected connections between domains contained in proteins that are not considered to be evolutionarily or functionally related.

40. Najafi SM, Harris DA, Yudkin MD: **The SpoIIAA protein of *Bacillus subtilis* has GTP-binding properties.** *J Bacteriol* 1996, 178:6632-6634.

41. Avela K, Lipsanen-Nyman M, Idanheimo N, Seemanova E, Rosengren S,
• Makela TP, Perheentupa J, Chapelle A, Lehesjoki AE: **Gene encoding a new RING-B-box-coiled-coil protein is mutated in mulibrey nanism.** *Nat Genet* 2000, 25:298-301.
Identification of a disease gene coding for a protein with a complex domain architecture. It appears that even more specific predictions than described in this paper are possible on the basis of the combination of domains present in the MUL protein.

42. Jackson PK, Eldridge AG, Freed E, Furstenthal L, Hsu JY, Kaiser BK, Reimann JD: **The lore of the RINGs: substrate recognition and catalysis by ubiquitin ligases.** *Trends Cell Biol* 2000, 10:429-439.

43. Aravind L, Dixit VM, Koonin EV: **The domains of death: evolution of the apoptosis machinery.** *Trends Biochem Sci* 1999, 24:47-53.

44. Millar DS, Johansen B, Berntorp E, Minford A, Bolton-Maggs P, Wensley R, Kakkar V, Schulman S, Torres A, Bosch N, Cooper DN: **Molecular genetic analysis of severe protein C deficiency.** *Hum Genet* 2000, 106:646-653.

45. Delettre C, Lenaers G, Griffoin JM, Gigarel N, Lorenzo C, Belenguer P, Pelloquin L, Grosgeorge J, Turc-Carel C, Perret E *et al.*: **Nuclear gene OPA1, encoding a mitochondrial dynamin-related protein, is mutated in dominant optic atrophy.** *Nat Genet* 2000, 26:207-210.

46. Alexander C, Votruba M, Pesch UE, Thiselton DL, Mayer S, Moore A, Rodriguez M, Kellner U, Leo-Kottler B, Auburger G *et al.*: **OPA1, encoding a dynamin-related GTPase, is mutated in autosomal dominant optic atrophy linked to chromosome 3q28.** *Nat Genet* 2000, 26:211-215.

47. Hughes AE, Ralston SH, Marken J, Bell C, MacPherson H, Wallace RG, van Hul W, Whyte MP, Nakatsuka K, Hovy L, Anderson DM: **Mutations in TNFRSF11A, affecting the signal peptide of RANK, cause familial expansile osteolysis.** *Nat Genet* 2000, 24:45-48.

48. Koonin EV, Altschul SF, Bork P: **BRCA1 protein products... Functional motifs.** *Nat Genet* 1996, 13:266-268.

49. Madej T, Boguski MS, Bryant SH: **Threading analysis suggests that the obese gene product may be a helical cytokine.** *FEBS Lett* 1995, 373:13-18.

50. Mushegian AR, Bassett DE Jr, Boguski MS, Bork P, Koonin EV: **Positionally cloned human disease genes: patterns of evolutionary conservation and functional motifs.** *Proc Natl Acad Sci USA* 1997, 94:5831-5836.

51. Tatusov RL, Koonin EV, Lipman DJ: **A genomic perspective on protein families.** *Science* 1997, 278:631-637.

52. Tatusov RL, Natale DA, Garkavtsev IV, Tatusova TA, Shankavaram UT,
• Rao BS, Kiryutin B, Galperin MY, Fedorova ND, Koonin EV: **The COG database: new developments in phylogenetic classification of proteins from complete genomes.** *Nucleic Acids Res* 2001, 29:22-28.
An evolutionary classification of proteins from sequenced genomes based on the notion of orthologous relationships. This new version includes proteins from *C. elegans* and *Drosophila* that have homologs in Archaea and/or Bacteria.

53. Fortini ME, Skupski MP, Boguski MS, Hariharan IK: **A survey of
•• human disease gene counterparts in the *Drosophila* genome.** *J Cell Biol* 2000, 150:F23-F30.
A careful analysis of human disease genes with the goal of identifying counterparts of disease genes in fruitfly — an approach that is applicable to other model eukaryotic organisms as well.

54. Rubin GM, Yandell MD, Wortman JR, Gabor Miklos GL, Nelson CR,
•• Hariharan IK, Fortini ME, Li PW, Apweiler R, Fleischmann W *et al.*: **Comparative genomics of the eukaryotes.** *Science* 2000, 287:2204-2215.
A comparative analysis of the predicted proteomes of three eukaryotes — yeast, worm and fly — that reveals unity and diversity of protein families and domain architecture of proteins in these organisms. Being the first attempt of such systematic comparative analysis, many of the conclusions need further refinement, but some of the approaches used in this study have general application in comparative genomics.

55. Morett E, Bork P: **A novel transactivation domain in parkin.** *Trends Biochem Sci* 1999, 24:229-231.

56. Shimura H, Hattori N, Kubo S, Mizuno Y, Asakawa S, Minoshima S,
• Shimizu N, Iwai K, Chiba T, Tanaka K, Suzuki T: **Familial Parkinson disease gene product, parkin, is a ubiquitin-protein ligase.** *Nat Genet* 2000, 25:302-305.
Experimental confirmation of the predicted function of a protein containing the RING domain.

57. Bomont P, Cavalier L, Blondeau F, Hamida CB, Belal S, Tazir M, Demir E, Topaloglu H, Korinthenberg R, Tuysuz B *et al.*: **The gene encoding gigaxonin, a new member of the cytoskeletal BTB/kelch repeat family, is mutated in giant axonal neuropathy.** *Nat Genet* 2000, 26:370-374.

58. Gal A, Li Y, Thompson DA, Weir J, Orth U, Jacobson SG, Apfelstedt-Sylla E, Vollrath D: **Mutations in MERTK, the human orthologue of the RCS rat retinal dystrophy gene, cause retinitis pigmentosa.** *Nat Genet* 2000, 26:270-271.

59. Bamford RN, Roessler E, Burdine RD, Saplakoglu U, dela Cruz J, Splitt M, Towbin J, Bowers P, Marino B, Schier AF *et al.*: **Loss-of-function mutations in the EGF-CFC gene CFC1 are associated with human left-right laterality defects.** *Nat Genet* 2000, 26:365-369.

60. Akama TO, Nishida K, Nakayama J, Watanabe H, Ozaki K, Nakamura T, Dota A, Kawasaki S, Inoue Y, Maeda N *et al.*: **Macular corneal dystrophy type I and type II are caused by distinct mutations in a new sulphotransferase gene.** *Nat Genet* 2000, 26:237-241.

61. Bech-Hansen NT, Naylor MJ, Maybaum TA, Sparkes RL, Koop B, Birch DG, Bergen AA, Prinsen CF, Polomeno RC, Gal A *et al.*:

Mutations in NYX, encoding the leucine-rich proteoglycan nyctalopin, cause X-linked complete congenital stationary night blindness. *Nat Genet* 2000, **26**:319-323.

62. Pusch CM, Zeitz C, Brandau O, Pesch K, Achatz H, Feil S, Scharfe C, Maurer J, Jacobi FK, Pinckers A *et al.*: The complete form of X-linked congenital stationary night blindness is caused by mutations in a gene encoding a leucine-rich repeat protein. *Nat Genet* 2000, **26**:324-327.

63. Kutsche K, Yntema H, Brandt A, Jantke I, Gerd Nothwang H, Orth U, Boavida MG, David D, Chelly J, Fryns JP *et al.*: Mutations in ARHGEF6, encoding a guanine nucleotide exchange factor for rho GTPases, in patients with X-linked mental retardation. *Nat Genet* 2000, **26**:247-250.

64. Verpy E, Leibovici M, Zwaenepoel I, Liu XZ, Gal A, Salem N, Mansour A, Blanchard S, Kobayashi I, Keats BJ *et al.*: A defect in harmonin, a PDZ domain-containing protein expressed in the inner ear sensory hair cells, underlies usher syndrome type 1C. *Nat Genet* 2000, **26**:51-55.

65. Kaplan JM, Kim SH, North KN, Rennke H, Correia LA, Tong HQ, Mathis BJ, Rodriguez-Perez JC, Allen PG, Beggs AH, Pollak MR: Mutations in ACTN4, encoding alpha-actinin-4, cause familial focal segmental glomerulosclerosis. *Nat Genet* 2000, **24**:251-256.

66. Mutations in MYH9 result in the may-hegglin anomaly, and fechtner and sebastian syndromes. *Nat Genet* 2000, **26**:103-105.

67. Netchine I, Sobrier ML, Krude H, Schnabel D, Maghnie M, Marcos E, Duriez B, Cacheux V, Moers A, Goossens M, Gruters A, Amselem S: Mutations in LHX3 result in a new syndrome revealed by combined pituitary hormone deficiency. *Nat Genet* 2000, **25**:182-186.

68. Chavanas S, Bodemer C, Rochat A, Hamel-Teillac D, Ali M, Irvine AD, Bonafe JL, Wilkinson J, Taieb A, Barrandon Y, Harper JI, de Prost Y, Hovnanian A: Mutations in SPINK5, encoding a serine protease inhibitor, cause Netherton syndrome. *Nat Genet* 2000, **25**:141-142.

69. Bignell GR, Warren W, Seal S, Takahashi M, Rapley E, Barfoot R, Green H, Brown C, Biggs PJ, Lakhani SR, Jones C, Hansen J *et al.*: Identification of the familial cylindromatosis tumour-suppressor gene. *Nat Genet* 2000, **25**:160-165.

70. Waeber G, Delplanque J, Bonny C, Mooser V, Steinmann M, Widmann C, Maillard A, Miklossy J, Dina C, Hani EH *et al.*: The gene MAPK8IP1, encoding islet-brain-1, is a candidate for type 2 diabetes. *Nat Genet* 2000, **24**:291-295.

71. Momeni P, Glockner G, Schmidt O, von Holtum D, Albrecht B, Gillessen-Kaesbach G, Hennekam R, Meinecke P, Zabel B, Rosenthal A, Horsthemke B, Ludecke HJ: Mutations in a new gene, encoding a zinc-finger protein, cause tricho- rhino-phalangeal syndrome type I. *Nat Genet* 2000, **24**:71-74.

72. Delepine M, Nicolino M, Barrett T, Golamaully M, Lathrop GM, Julier C: EIF2AK3, encoding translation initiation factor 2-alpha kinase 3, is mutated in patients with Wolcott-Rallison syndrome. *Nat Genet* 2000, **25**:406-409.

73. Arbour NC, Lorenz E, Schutte BC, Zabner J, Kline JN, Jones M, Frees K, Watt JL, Schwartz DA: TLR4 mutations are associated with endotoxin hyporesponsiveness in humans. *Nat Genet* 2000, **25**:187-191.

74. Hastbacka J, de la Chapelle A, Mahtani MM, Clines G, Reeve-Daly MP, Daly M, Hamilton BA, Kusumi K, Trivedi B, Weaver A *et al.*: The diastrophic dysplasia gene encodes a novel sulfate transporter: positional cloning by fine-structure linkage disequilibrium mapping. *Cell* 1994, **78**:1073-1087.

75. Superti-Furga A, Rossi A, Steinmann B, Gitzelmann R: A chondrodysplasia family produced by mutations in the diastrophic dysplasia sulfate transporter gene: genotype/phenotype correlations. *Am J Med Genet* 1996, **63**:144-147.

76. Hoglund P, Haila S, Socha J, Tomaszewski L, Saarialho-Kere U, Karjalainen-Lindsberg ML, Airola K, Holmberg C, de la Chapelle A, Kere J: Mutations of the Down-regulated in adenoma (DRA) gene cause congenital chloride diarrhoea. *Nat Genet* 1996, **14**:316-319.

77. Zemni R, Bienvenu T, Vinet MC, Sefiani A, Carrie A, Billuart P, McDonell N, Couvert P, Francis F, Chafey P *et al.*: A new gene involved in X-linked mental retardation identified by analysis of an X;2 balanced translocation. *Nat Genet* 2000, **24**:167-170.

78. Sun H, Smallwood PM, Nathans J: Biochemical defects in ABCR protein variants associated with human retinopathies. *Nat Genet* 2000, **26**:242-246.

79. Paloneva J, Kestila M, Wu J, Salminen A, Bohling T, Ruotsalainen V, Hakola P, Bakker AB, Phillips JH, Pekkarinen P *et al.*: Loss-of-function mutations in TYROBP (DAP12) result in a presenile dementia with bone cysts. *Nat Genet* 2000, **25**:357-361.

80. Naureckiene S, Sleat DE, Lackland H, Fensom A, Vanier MT, Wattiaux R, Jadot M, Lobel P: Identification of HE1 as the Second Gene of Niemann-Pick C Disease. *Science* 2000, **290**:2298-2301.

81. Davies JP, Levy B, Ioannou YA: Evidence for a Niemann-pick C (NPC) gene family: identification and characterization of NPC1L1. *Genomics* 2000, **65**:137-145.

82. Bulman MP, Kusumi K, Frayling TM, McKeown C, Garrett C, Lander ES, Krumlauf R, Hattersley AT, Ellard S, Turnpenny PD: Mutations in the human delta homologue, DLL3, cause axial skeletal defects in spondylocostal dysostosis. *Nat Genet* 2000, **24**:438-441.

83. Oldridge M, Fortuna AM, Maringa M, Propping P, Mansour S, Pollitt C, DeChiara TM, Kimble R B, Valenzuela DM, Yancopoulos GD, Wilkie AO: Dominant mutations in ROR2, encoding an orphan receptor tyrosine kinase, cause brachydactyly type B. *Nat Genet* 2000, **24**:275-278.

84. Hu Z, Bonifas JM, Beech J, Bench G, Shigihara T, Ogawa H, Ikeda S, Mauro T, Epstein EH Jr: Mutations in ATP2C1, encoding a calcium pump, cause Hailey–Hailey disease. *Nat Genet* 2000, **24**:61-65.

85. Irrthum A, Karkkainen MJ, Devriendt K, Alitalo K, Vikkula M: Congenital hereditary lymphedema caused by a mutation that inactivates VEGFR3 tyrosine kinase. *Am J Hum Genet* 2000, **67**:295-301.

86. Wolfe MS, Xia W, Ostaszewski BL, Diehl TS, Kimberly WT, Selkoe DJ: Two transmembrane aspartates in presenilin-1 required for presenilin endoproteolysis and γ-secretase activity. *Nature* 1999, **398**:513-517.

87. Nielsen H, Engelbrecht J, Brunak S, von Heijne G: A neural network method for identification of prokaryotic and eukaryotic signal peptides and prediction of their cleavage sites. *Int J Neural Syst* 1997, **8**:581-599.

88. Claros MG, von Heijne G: TopPred II: an improved software for membrane protein structure predictions. *Comput Appl Biosci* 1994, **10**:685-686.

89. Wheeler DL, Church DM, Lash AE, Leipe DD, Madden TL, Pontius JU, Schuler GD, Schriml LM, Tatusova TA, Wagner L, Rapp BA: Database resources of the national center for biotechnology information. *Nucleic Acids Res* 2001, **29**:11-16.

90. Schultz J, Copley RR, Doerks T, Ponting CP, Bork P: SMART: a web-based tool for the study of genetically mobile domains. *Nucleic Acids Res* 2000, **28**:231-234.

91. Henikoff JG, Greene EA, Pietrokovski S, Henikoff S: Increased coverage of protein families with the blocks database servers. *Nucleic Acids Res* 2000, **28**:228-230.

92. Attwood TK, Croning MD, Flower DR, Lewis AP, Mabey JE, Scordis P, Selley JN, Wright W: PRINTS-S: the database formerly known as PRINTS. *Nucleic Acids Res* 2000, **28**:225-227.

93. Eddy SR: Profile hidden Markov models. *Bioinformatics* 1998, **14**:755-763.

94. Rost B, Sander C, Schneider R: PHD — an automatic mail server for protein secondary structure prediction. *Comput Appl Biosci* 1994, **10**:53-60.

95. McGuffin LJ, Bryson K, Jones DT: The PSIPRED protein structure prediction server. *Bioinformatics* 2000, **16**:404-405.

96. Fischer D: Hybrid fold recognition: combining sequence derived properties with evolutionary information. *Pac Symp Biocomput* 2000, 119-130.

97. Holm L, Sander C: Touring protein fold space with Dali/FSSP. *Nucleic Acids Res* 1998, **26**:316-319.

98. Guex N, Peitsch MC: SWISS-MODEL and the Swiss-PdbViewer: an environment for comparative protein modeling. *Electrophoresis* 1997, **18**:2714-2723.

99. Madej T, Gibrat JF, Bryant SH: Threading a database of protein cores. *Proteins Struct Funct Genet* 1995, **23**:356-369.

100. Antonarakis SE, McKusick VA: OMIM passes the 1,000-disease-gene mark. *Nat Genet* 2000, **25**:11.

# An approach to modelling in immunology

*Andrew Yates, Cliburn C. W. Chan, Robin E. Callard, Andrew J. T. George and Jaroslav Stark*

Date received (in revised form): 5th June 2001


**Andrew Yates**
held postdoctoral positions in theoretical physics before coming to ICH/UCL to model cytokine networks in the immune system. He now holds a Wellcome Trust research training fellowship in Mathematical Biology.

**Cliburn C. W. Chan**
qualified as a medical doctor from Singapore, and is currently at UCL completing a PhD on mathematical models of T-cell activation.

**Robin E. Callard**
is an experimental immunologist and Head of Infection and Immunity at ICH. He is joint director of the CoMPLEX 4 year PhD programme in modelling biological complexity at UCL.

**Andrew J. T. George**
held postdoctoral fellowships in Southampton and the NIH, following which he went to the RPMS (now Imperial College) where he is now Reader in Molecular Immunology.

**Jaroslav Stark**
is a mathematician specialising in the theory and applications of non-linear dynamics. Within the past few years, he has developed a particular interest in modelling cell-cell signalling especially within the immune and reproductive systems.

*Keywords:* immunology loop, non-linearity, mathematical modelling

Andrew Yates,
CoMPLEX (Centre for Mathematics and Physical Sciences in the Life Sciences and Experimental Biology),
University College London,
Gower Street,
London WC1E 6BT, UK

Tel: +44 (0) 20 7905 2317
Fax: +44 (0) 20 7813 8494
E-mail: ayates@ich.ucl.ac.uk


## Abstract


Like most other fields in biology, immunology has been revolutionised by the techniques of molecular biology and the resulting explosion in available experimental data. It is argued that efforts to integrate the data to gain insight into how various subsystems in the immune system interact and function require mathematical modelling and computer simulation in close collaboration with experimentalists. This paper illustrates some of the techniques available for modelling immune systems, and highlights the issues that should be borne in mind by anyone starting down the modelling path.


## INTRODUCTION

The human immune system is enormously complex and the battle to understand it has presented problems that pre-date those being faced now by geneticists and molecular biologists dealing with genomic data: abundant information within a theoretical framework that is relatively underdeveloped. Mammalian immune systems show a high degree of evolutionary conservation and through studies of both humans and other species, a great deal of the molecular mechanisms at work and the interactions at the intercellular level that drive immune responses have been uncovered. However, our understanding of the properties of the immune system *as a whole* is still limited, and this in turn constrains therapeutic approaches. This is apparent, for example, in autoimmune diseases or in the case of HIV infection.

In order to put the current challenges into context, we can divide the development of the biological sciences, and immunology in particular, into three stages:

- *Cell biology/physiology era.* This was largely an experiment-driven whole animal or cellular black box approach in which inputs were compared to outputs without much understanding of the genetic or molecular events that linked them. Great insights into system behaviour were gained with relatively simple discriminative experiments.

- *Molecular biology era.* This has been characterised by the recent 'data explosion' from high-throughput molecular biology techniques, the development of advanced experimental techniques and information management, leading to genome sequencing, extensive cataloguing of the structure and function of gene products and the description of metabolic and signalling pathways. However, insight into system behaviour has lagged behind data acquisition, partly due to the reductionist approach that is frequently employed.

- *Post-genomic era.* We are currently faced with the difficult but exciting task of integrating huge experimental data sets with new theoretical frameworks to produce useful models of system behaviour.

It is increasingly being realised that the properties of whole biological systems cannot be deduced by intuition alone, nor deduced directly from the data being provided by the molecular biology approach. This is due to a number of factors:

- *Combinatorial complexity*. The number of potential interactions between individual elements (eg proteins) in a system grows extremely rapidly with the number of elements. There is increasing evidence that this network of interactions cannot be ignored. The action of every protein will be modulated and affected by the presence of many other proteins. This is not addressed using current experimental technique. One can attempt to determine the function of every gene by knocking them out individually in an animal (a massive job that has been completed for *Drosophila* but not for the mouse). However, to understand the function of a gene it would be necessary to knock out every pair, triplet, etc. of genes. This is clearly not feasible.

- *Feedback* loops appear to be ubiquitous in physiological systems, and these operate at various levels in the immune system. For example, antigen stimulates the formation of the appropriate antibody, which then results in the clearance of the antigen, a classical negative feedback loop. A similar example at the intracellular level is that of NF-$\kappa\beta$ which activates the transcription of I$\kappa\beta$, which binds to NF-$\kappa\beta$ and inactivates it. Positive feedback loops are also seen, for example, when the presence of active TNF-$\alpha$ results in the recruitment of immune cells which then release more TNF-$\alpha$, as described in the TNF-$\alpha$ model below. Although the effects of a single feedback loop can probably be understood intuitively, this is no longer the case when several feedback loops begin to interact.

- *Delays*. Similarly, most biological effects involve a delay. Thus for instance when a T cell receives a proliferative signal, it first needs to

synthesise DNA and undergo the biochemical changes required for cell division. Delays, especially when combined with feedback loops introduce many unforeseen effects into a system, for instance oscillations (eg Haurie *et al.*[1]).

- *Non-linearity*. A system is called non-linear if its response is not always proportional to the stimulus. Non-linearity is all-pervasive in biological systems, and indeed is essential for their functioning. Examples include saturation of signalling pathways or the ability of some signalling molecules to switch on different genes at different concentrations (eg Shimizu and Gurdon[2]). It is well known that even simple non-linear feedback systems can exhibit complex and counter-intuitive behaviour (eg Callard *et al.*[3]).

It is therefore clear that more rapid data acquisition and more sophisticated information management are insufficient by themselves to understand the complexities of the immune system. Our belief is that increasingly mathematical modelling is becoming an essential tool to complement experimental and conventional bioinformatical techniques in immunology. Together, such approaches offer the possibility of gaining new insights into the behaviour of the immune system, of providing new frameworks for organising and storing data and performing statistical analyses, of suggesting new hypotheses and new experiments, and even of offering a 'virtual laboratory' to supplement *in vivo* and *in vitro* work.

However, mathematical modelling in immunology, and in the life sciences more generally, is far from straightforward, and suffers from a number of potential pitfalls:

- *Mathematically sophisticated but biologically useless models*. These can arise because of a lack of biological input, leading to models that are biologically unrealistic, or address a question of little biological importance. The latter, more insidious, problem often arises because the reasons for constructing the model have not been clearly articulated.

- *Biologically realistic but mathematically intractable models.* The converse problem usually arises because biologists unfamiliar with the limitations of mathematical analysis want to include every known biological effect in the model. Even if it were possible to produce such models they would be of little use since their behaviour would be as complex to investigate as the experimental situation.

**Formulating the question**

In our experience, the single most important factor in avoiding either of these is to formulate clear *explicit biological goals* before attempting to construct a model. This will ensure that the resulting model is biologically sound, can be experimentally verified and will generate biological insight, or new biological hypotheses. We stress that the aim of a model should not simply be to reproduce the biological data, and indeed often the most useful models are those that exhibit discrepancies from experiment. Such

deviations will typically stimulate new experiments or hypotheses. Our ideal is therefore an iterative approach, starting with a biological problem, developing a mathematical model, and then feeding back into the biology (Figure 1). Once established, this *collaborative loop* can be traversed many times, leading to ever-increasing understanding. There are many potential benefits for the biological side of the collaboration. As well as indicating new experimental directions, developing the mathematical formulation of a system may focus thinking and clarify definitions. At the same time it will frequently motivate new mathematical questions and lead to unexpected pay-offs for the mathematical side. It is crucial that both sides benefit in this way and the collaboration is conducted between equals. If either the mathematician is simply seen as providing a service to the biologist, or conversely the mathematician fails to be interested in solving the biological problem (rather than a mathematical one), then it is unlikely that the collaboration will survive, or produce any worthwhile results. It is therefore essential that there is good communication between the disciplines, and this can take a long time

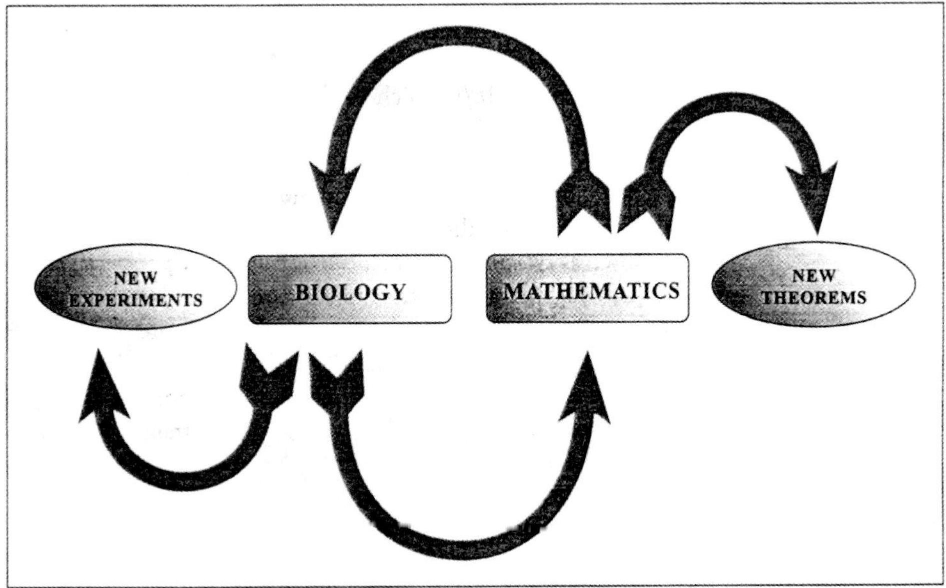


**Figure 1:** The collaborative loop

to establish. Our experience has been that it may be several years for a collaboration to become productive, and often several rounds of discussion before experimentalist and theorist can agree on a common question and methodology. On the other hand we are convinced that such an investment to build an effective collaboration is then repaid many-fold.

It can obviously be difficult for an immunologist unfamiliar with mathematical modelling to know how to start in this area. Our experience has been that mimicking existing role models can be valuable. In this paper, we therefore illustrate a number of modelling issues and approaches using examples developed over the last few years at the Centre for Mathematics and Physics in the Life Sciences and Experimental Biology (CoMPLEX) at University College London.

## A BRIEF TOUR OF THE IMMUNE SYSTEM

Adaptive immune responses in vertebrates are generated following exposure to a foreign *antigen*, generally an infectious microorganism such as a virus or bacteria. The infected individual responds rapidly by the production of specific antibodies made by B lymphocytes and by the expansion and differentiation of effector and regulatory T lymphocytes. This response aimed at clearing the infectious agent is coordinated by a network of highly specialised cells that communicate through cell surface molecular interactions and through a complex set of intercellular communication molecules known as *cytokines* and *chemokines*. Following clearance of the infectious agent, the individual is able to respond more rapidly and more vigorously to a second exposure to the same infection (antigen). This is known as immunological *memory*. Induction of immune memory is the basis for long-term immunity to pathogens we have already encountered, either through infection or vaccination. The adaptive immune response is highly specific, and

antibodies and T cells generated in response to one pathogen generally fail to respond to antigens from unrelated pathogens. In addition, the immune system is able to discriminate between self and foreign antigens. The processes involved in this tolerance to self-antigens include deletion, anergy and active regulation. Failure of these safety mechanisms can result in autoimmunity, in which the immune response is directed towards the host tissue.

One of the most intriguing features of the immune system is its multi-functionality. Its cellular components are complex, context-sensitive agents that respond in a non-linear fashion to an enormously diverse set of signals from cytokines, chemokines and direct cell–cell interactions. Further, the messenger molecules are typically expressed by several cell types and are themselves multi-functional. Laboratory experiments tend to isolate and study one or two interactions at a time, but this approach alone will not shed light on the interacting whole. Our understanding of the immune system has reached a level such that mathematical modelling is becoming a useful and powerful investigative tool. The abundance of experimental information has led to a situation in which higher levels of description are needed to integrate the data.

The immune system can often be viewed as operating in isolation from other physiological subsystems. This allows us, at least in principle, to describe it from both top-down and bottom-up perspectives. Some authors have prescribed 'goals' to the immune system in order to construct models of its behaviour (see, for example, Segel and Lev Bar-Or[4]). Others have tried to demonstrate how properties may have emerged or evolved by considering optimal solutions to trade-offs (eg selection of T-cell receptor repertoires[5]). Another modelling philosophy is to build dynamical models based on experimental data and attempt to understand the emergent behaviour of complex interacting systems of cells and/or molecules. The latter approach is the one we have pursued to date. Some of the questions we have started to tackle are the following:

- How can the immune system effectively distinguish between self and foreign antigens? Under what situations does tolerance to self break down?

- How does a coherent immune response emerge from the multiple interactions of the cytokine network?

- How is immune memory maintained in the face of multiple serial infections throughout the life of an individual?

**Background reading**

We describe these below. There are obviously many other areas that merit investigation. For further background, the reader is advised to consult one of the many good immunology textbooks, eg Paul[6] and Janeway and Travers.[7] A good mathematical introduction to modelling in biology is Murray,[8] though unfortunately there does not appear to be a comparable text suitable for those with a biological background. Other reviews of the application of modelling to immunology are Perelson and Weisbuch[9] and Morel.[10]

## MODELLING ISSUES
### Level of detail

As indicated above, attempting to incorporate every single known interaction rapidly leads to an unmanageable model. Further, parameter determination in such models can be a frightening experience. Estimates come from diverse experiments, which may be elegantly designed and well executed but can still give rise to widely differing values for parameters. Data can come from both *in vivo* and *in vitro* experiments and results that hold in one medium may not always hold in the other. Further, despite the many similarities between mammalian immune systems, significant differences

**Using experimental data**

do exist and so results obtained from experiments using animal and human tissue may not always be consistent. Given the mathematical tools currently available to us and uncertainty in the data, then, any modelling approach is obliged to be coarse-grained to some extent. How does one decide which are the crucial components? Typically the temptation is to include a multitude of factors. In most immunological contexts, many of the interactions, components or parameter values are ill defined, and even for well-characterised systems a thorough exploration of parameter space for exhaustively detailed models is effectively impossible. The experimentalists' insight into which interactions are important is the first resource.

### Robustness

Robustness is another important guiding principle: the cellular components of the immune system operate in noisy media, with significant environmental and genetic variation among individuals, and yet immunity to most pathogens is maintained. Realistic models of biological systems may need to be insensitive to changes in kinetic parameters or concentrations of mediators, eg Barkai and Liebler.[11] This is something we have tried to explore in our models to date. Rather than set out to construct models with these properties, however, robustness can be used as a means of evaluating or comparing models that have been developed purely with the biological data in mind.

### Modularity

Despite its complexity, it seems likely that hierarchical or modular descriptions of the immune system are possible. The most obvious example is that of the inter-/ intracellular split, in which we consider cells to be 'black boxes' with complicated but nonetheless calculable input/output characteristics. This has certainly been the implicit assumption in many successful models. An excellent review of modularity in biological systems can be found in Hartwell *et al.*[12]

Another aspect of modularity is the repetition of common motifs or components in molecules involved in cellular interactions or communication. For example, cytokine receptors are typically constructed from several components, some of which may be common to several distinct receptor types. Many cytokine interactions may have arisen from a small set of precursors that duplicated and diversified over time, resulting in repeated units with similar structure but different functions. This modularity can simplify aspects of modelling as it both allows individual parts of the whole system (modules) to be initially considered in isolation and allows the application of common approaches to different aspects of the same system.

## Anatomical and spatial considerations

The immune system does not operate in a well-stirred chamber with no structure. The cells move between different anatomical compartments and molecules on the cell surface can be organised into particular spatial patterns that are important for their function. For example, germinal centres are highly organised, temporary structures in lymph nodes within which B cells pass through repeated rounds of antibody mutation, proliferation and selection. This results in the generation of antibodies of high affinity during an immune response, eg Oprea *et al.*[13] Similar spatial compartmentalisation is seen in the thymus, an organ in which newly generated T cells that are both viable and not overly reactive to self are selected and exported to the periphery. At the cellular level, when T cells recognise their antigen there is a reorganisation of molecules on the surface of both the T cell and the antigen-presenting cell (APC) to form the immunological synapse, which has a distinct spatial and temporal organisation.[14]

## Stochasticity

One of the major tools in modelling is the use of simple differential equations. When dealing with large, well-mixed populations of cells and relatively long time-scales it is reasonable to use this approach. However, many processes in the immune system are probabilistic or have stochastic elements (see, for example, Borghans *et al.*[5] and van den Berg *et al.*[15]). Examples are the recognition of foreign antigen by T-cell receptors amid a noisy background of self-peptides, the generation of an effective and safe T-cell repertoire, and somatic hypermutation of B cells. We discuss our approach to the first example in the section on 'Cross-talk between T-cell receptors' below.

Many processes, particularly intracellular reactions, involve small numbers of molecules and stochastic effects are likely to be very important. This is an area of research that has received very little attention.

## MODELLING EXAMPLES

We now present four examples from our own work illustrating the points developed above. A common theme running through these is the presence of non-linear effects and both negative and positive feedback loops. These are often thought of as simply damping down and amplifying mechanisms respectively. We show that they have a role to play in cellular differentiation, as a rapid response mechanism, as well as in preserving diversity in the memory pool and enhancing the specificity of the immune response. These varied roles of feedback are not intuitively obvious, and become apparent only through modelling.

## TNF oscillations

Our first example shows how even extremely simple control systems in immunology can exhibit unexpected behaviour. Motivated by experimental results demonstrating oscillations in the level of the inflammatory cytokine tumour necrosis factor $\alpha$ (TNF-$\alpha$) in the

**Activator inhibitor model**

aqueous humour of rabbits receiving corneal allografts,[16] we developed a simple ordinary differential equation model[17] for these oscillations, based on the regulatory interactions between TNF-$\alpha$ and its inhibitors (IL-10, TGF-$\beta$, soluble TNF-$\alpha$ receptor). The model is illustrated in Figure 2. Such an intuitive model is then converted into coupled ordinary differential equations, using the simple principle of balancing rates for each cytokine:

rate of change of cytokine concentration

= rate of formation − rate of clearance

This leads to the coupled pair of equations:

$$\frac{dx}{dt} = \nu_1 \frac{(x^n + \varepsilon_1^n)}{(x^n + \alpha^n)} \frac{\beta}{(\gamma + \beta)} - d_1 x \tag{1}$$

$$\frac{d\gamma}{dt} = k_2 + \nu_2 \frac{(x + \varepsilon_2)}{(x + \gamma)} - d_2 \gamma \tag{2}$$

where $x$ is the concentration of TNF so that $dx/dt$ represents the rate of change of cytokine concentration. The concentration of the inhibitor is given by $\gamma$. The first term on the right of equation (1) models the positive feedback loop shown in Figure 2 (and so is dependent on $x$, the concentration of TNF). The parameter $\nu_1$ is the maximal rate of TNF production, set by the strength of

antigenic stimulus. The parameters $\varepsilon_1$ and $\alpha$ represent, respectively, a baseline level of TNF-$\alpha$ production and the threshold value of the TNF concentration at which positive feedback on its own production becomes apparent. The second term incorporates the negative feedback (dependent on $\gamma$, the concentration of the inhibitor), where $\beta$ sets the threshold inhibitor concentration for negative feedback on TNF production. The final term represents the clearance (or catabolism) of the cytokine, which is considered to be dependent only on the concentration of TNF. The equation describing the rate of change of inhibitor concentration is similar, though the rate of formation of the inhibitor is dependent only on $x$, as there is no positive feedback loop. In all cases the interactions of $x$ and $\gamma$ are given by Hill functions, which are a mathematical representation of a standard sigmoid dose response curve.

For given parameter values, a plot of the time evolution of TNF concentration against inhibitor concentration results in a phase diagram, which reveals the long-term qualitative behaviour of the system. Such plots can be easily generated using general computer algebra software packages (eg Maple[TM] or Mathematica[TM]) as well as software written for analysis of non-linear dynamical systems (eg DsTool[18]). We can also systematically vary each parameter value and see how this affects the system behaviour. This is known as *bifurcation analysis* and is generally done numerically using dedicated software (eg Auto[19] or Content[20]), though unfortunately such packages are probably not easily used by non-specialists. A list of dynamical systems software is available at Dynamical Systems Software.[21]

In this particular case, bifurcation analysis was used to characterise the qualitatively different solutions of the model. It revealed that even such a simple two-component network could show a rich set of behaviours under quantifiable conditions, including excitability, oscillations (Figure 3), hysteresis,

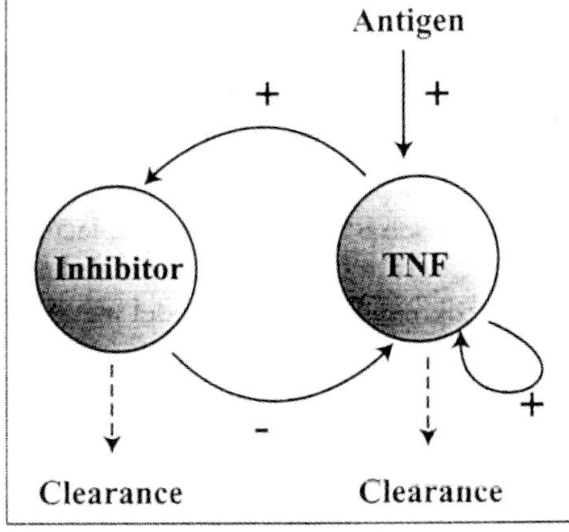


**Figure 2:** Regulation of TNF-$\alpha$ by both negative and positive feedback. After illustration in Chan *et al.*[17]

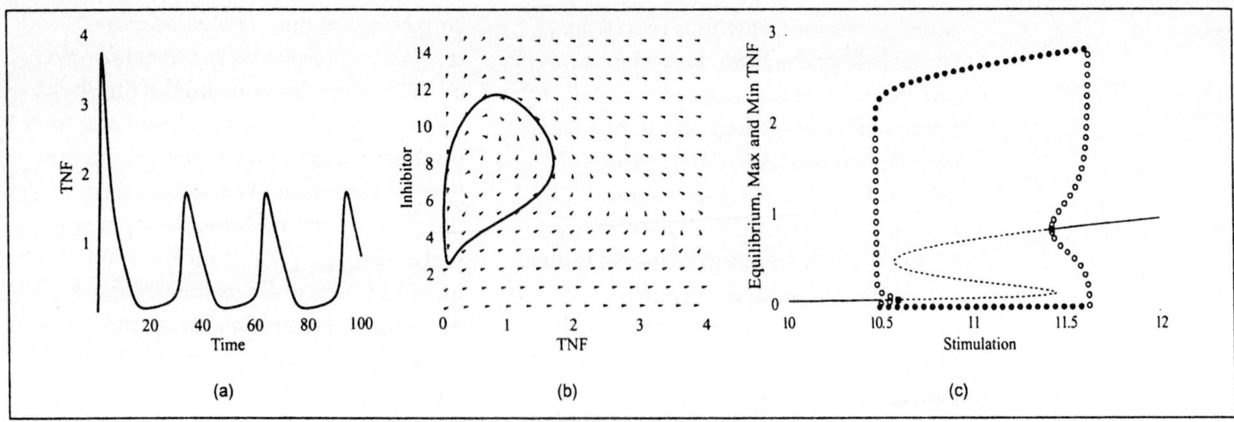

**Figure 3:** Oscillations arising from feedback interactions between TNF and inhibitors. (a) and (b) The time series and phase diagram representations of the oscillations; (c) bifurcation diagram showing the range of values of the parameter $v_1$, the strength of antigenic stimulation, over which oscillations occur. Reproduced from Chan *et al.*,[17] copyright Royal Society of London

threshold behaviour and bistability. One of the interesting predictions of the model is that oscillations exist only for an intermediate degree of antigenic driving, and both increasing and decreasing the antigen load can abolish these oscillations. The possibility of such counter-intuitive behaviour should obviously be borne in mind by those attempting to perturb 'real' cytokine networks for therapeutic purposes, for example, in the use of anti-TNF monoclonal antibodies to treat rheumatoid arthritis.[22]

## Th1/2 differentiation

**Reducing complexity**

Although real cytokine networks are highly complex, it is sometimes possible to reduce the complexity drastically by separating time-scales so that a lower dimensional system is obtained. Then the tools mentioned above (eg phase plane analysis) can be used to analyse this reduced system. Such an approach is described next.

Complex networks of cytokine interactions pervade the immune system but there are a few subsystems that are sufficiently isolated and well studied to be amenable to modelling. One such area is T-helper cell differentiation. After encountering foreign antigen in the periphery, APCs migrate to lymph nodes and display antigen fragments to T cells.

APC–T cell encounters of sufficient specificity lead to activation, proliferation and differentiation of T cells into clones with effector functions. An important subset of T cells, CD4+ T helper cells, can be further subdivided into Th1 cells that are involved in cellular immunity and inflammation, and Th2 cells that interact with B cells and are associated with antibody production and isotype switching. The immune system 'decides' which T-helper response is the most appropriate for a given pathogen, based on both signals from the innate immune system (costimulatory signals from APCs and cytokines produced by other cell types), the antigen dose and the cytokines produced by the proliferating T cells themselves.

We developed an ordinary differential equation model of T-helper cell differentiation[23] in order to determine the essential factors determining the Th1/2 outcome of an immune response. The model was simplified significantly by making the assumption that the rates of cytokine production and consumption were much faster than the rates of cell proliferation, allowing us to make quasi-steady state assumptions and hence treat the various cytokine concentrations as simple functions of Th1 and Th2 cell numbers. In other words, fast dynamics drive cytokine concentrations to steady states, which then track slow parameter changes (ie cell numbers). The cytokine concentrations are then eliminated as dynamical variables. This 'slaving' principle reflects, to some extent, the hierarchical structure in the immune system. By separating time-scales we reduce the need to consider the dynamics in full. The interactions we included in the model are illustrated in Figure 4.

**Th1/Th2 asymmetries**

The model generated a number of interesting results, most of which were rooted in asymmetries in Th1 and Th2 regulation. One feature of particular interest was the induction of switches in the immune response by external means. The model predicted that to switch from a Th2 to a Th1 response required both addition of pro-Th1 cytokines and a reduction in antigen load, which is borne out by data in the literature. Further, it highlighted differences in the regulation of Th1 and Th2 responses: Th1 through apoptosis induced by cell−cell contact, Th2 by negative feedback of the proliferating cells on the APCs. Dynamical switches from Th1 to Th2 responses were also predicted in chronic infections. Interestingly, we also found that under a wide range of parameters,

varying the antigen dose induced a switch between two stable states (Th1 and Th2 responses) through an intermediate oscillatory phase, similar to that observed in the TNF model described above. Whether this is a generic feature of cytokine networks is under investigation.

This model did not mimic in full the detailed dynamics of a real T-cell response. Rather, the two-dimensional representation of the system reproduced many of its features and predicted more. These encouraging results reinforce the idea that rather than building detailed dynamical models of systems from scratch, a more coarse-grained approach may be preferable or even necessary in many situations.

## Maintaining T-cell memory

In this final example of an ordinary differential equation model, rate equations for the number of resting and cycling memory T-cell pools were derived by balancing proliferation and clearance rates as before. The model was then extended to accommodate different T-cell clones (basically by giving each clone its own set of ordinary differential equations), resulting in a model that could take into account the heterogeneity of the T-cell

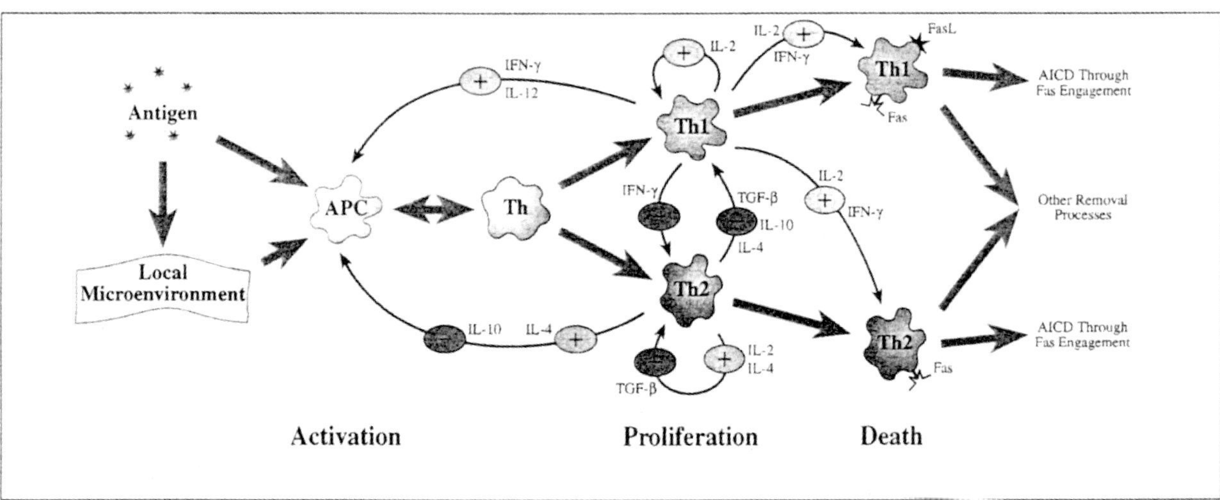



**Figure 4:** Schematic representation of the interactions governing Th1/2 differentiation, proliferation and death. Arrows labelled with (+) or (−) reflect positive or negative feedback respectively, mediated by cytokines as indicated. AICD is an acronym for activation-induced cell death. Reproduced from Yates *et al.*,[23] with permission from Academic Press

**Homeostatis and immune memory**

memory population that develops as the organism is successively challenged by different antigens.

Our immune memory is carried in part by a population of T cells that remains approximately constant in number from puberty onwards. This memory T-cell pool is a diverse collection of clones (a clone is a number of cells derived from the same ancestor), each of which is specific for a particular antigen. These cells are ready to respond rapidly upon re-encountering their specific antigen and form the basis of lasting immunity. We maintain memory to many pathogens for years or even our lifetime, and yet the lifetimes of the cells that make up our immune memory may be as short as a few weeks.

The mechanisms that maintain our T-cell pools at a constant size are largely unknown. Experiments suggest that memory can persist in the absence of repeated exposure to antigen or cross-reactive stimulation. Other workers have shown that cytokines produced by other cell types may be sufficient to drive the low levels of proliferation necessary to balance cell loss in the memory compartment. Data from patients with depleted T-cell pools (for example, those who have undergone chemotherapy followed by bone marrow transplantation)

show that normal homeostatic numbers of T cells can be reconstituted after a year or two.[24] What is the mechanism at play here? In a recent paper[25] we used the observation that proliferating cells, which make up a small minority of memory cells at any time, are susceptible to programmed death or apoptosis by a mechanism dependent on contact between cells (known as activation-induced cell death, or AICD). Proposing a simple model of the memory pool including resting and cycling cells (Figure 5), we predict that the homeostatic level is insensitive to the lifetime of resting memory cells (which may partly account for the diverse experimental estimates of this quantity) and that the dynamics of the memory pool are determined largely by the properties of the minority of dividing cells. Reconstitution times agree well with the data in the literature. Further, individuals with genetic defects in the AICD pathways have greatly increased numbers of memory T cells, also in agreement with the model.

When we extend this simple model to include the multi-clonal structure of memory it predicts that clonal proportions are preserved under fluctuations in the pool size. This appears to be intuitively the simplest solution to the problem of ensuring the preservation of the full range of clones under various perturbations, including the introduction of new clones (caused by infection by hitherto unencountered pathogens) into a memory pool already full to capacity.

These results highlight a recent shift in our perception of cell dynamics. The rate of turnover of many cell types in mammals is relatively high, particularly in the blood: surely there is an energy cost associated with this apparent continual over-production and removal of cells? The answer may be that it allows us to respond rapidly to changes in our environment or to trauma. Regulation of apoptosis may allow rapid expansion or contraction of cell numbers, while rates of proliferation are constrained by the time it takes cells to divide.

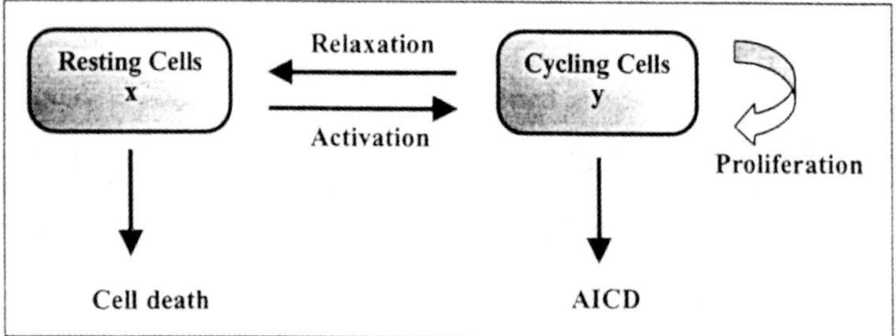


**Figure 5:** The proposed model for T-cell memory homeostasis, after Yates and Callard.[25] Resting cells become activated by cytokines or other environmental stimuli at rate $a$, degrade at rate $d$ and are replenished by cells leaving cycle at rate $r$. Cycling cells divide at rate $c$ and die through contact with other cycling cells at rate $f$. This leads to the simple rate equations $dx/dt = ry - ax - dx$ and $dy/dt = ax + cy - fy^2 - ra$

**Monte Carlo models**

## Cross-talk between T-cell receptors

Sometimes, the system we are interested in is too complex to easily capture in the form of an ordinary differential equation model. For example, the behaviour of individual agents may be highly complex, or there may be stochastic or heterogeneous spatial elements not easily modelled using differential equations. In such a case, we may still obtain insight into the system using a Monte Carlo simulation. The next model, which has both stochastic and spatial elements, attempts to understand the problem of how T cells discriminate between ligands accurately, and simulates individual T-cell receptors (TCRs) as a Markov chain, with the transition probability between states determined by ligand binding and modifier signals from neighbouring receptors.

**Antigen presentation and TCR sensitivity**

During an infection, antigen from an infectious organism is captured by an APC, and presented on the cell surface in the peptide groove of major histocompatibility molecules (MHC). The recognition of the peptide–MHC ligand complex by TCR is responsible for maintaining the specificity of the immune response. It is known that 10–200 foreign antigens mixed with perhaps 100,000 self-antigens on the APC are sufficient to trigger T-cell proliferation and effector response.[26] This requires an astonishing degree of accuracy from the TCR which must rapidly discriminate between self and foreign antigens. Even more surprisingly, the TCR discriminates almost exclusively on the basis of the duration of ligand engagement,[27] which is a stochastic event. Previous models of how the T cell achieves its exquisite sensitivity and specificity rely on the concept of kinetic proofreading to explain how TCRs discriminate ligands based on their dissociation time,[28] and the idea of multiple serial encounters by the peptide–MHC complex with different TCR to explain its sensitivity.[29] However, a problem with this scenario is that owing to the stochastic nature of ligand

dissociation, the T cell will be very sensitive to both the duration of ligand engagement and the ligand concentration, and it is difficult to see how the T cell can avoid being swamped by false positive signals from the myriad self-antigens presented by the APC.

Recent experiments have documented both positive and negative feedback regulating the response of TCR to ligand.[30] Surprisingly, these feedback effects were not confined to the particular TCR encountering ligand, but appeared to affect neighbouring receptors as well. Encounters of TCR with antagonist ligands (which bind for an intermediate duration) result in recruitment of inhibitor molecules to the receptor's local neighbourhood. Encounters with agonist ligands (which bind for a long duration) result in recruitment of protective molecules to the neighbourhood, which prevent docking of the inhibitor molecules. When we included these neighbour feedback effects in a Monte Carlo simulation of the T cell–APC interface,[31] the model T cell could reliably detect the presence of low densities of foreign peptide with high specificity. Cross-talk between TCR effectively allows the T cell to make more accurate decisions about the nature of the ligands on the APC by pooling information about ligands encountered by different TCR. This observation, coupled with alterations in the degree of receptor cross-talk (especially inhibition) during T-cell maturation, also provides possible solutions to several puzzles in developmental T-cell biology, including how T cells can respond differently to a similar set of antigens presented at different stages, how a single ligand can generate a large T-cell repertoire and why the sensitivity to weak ligands is reduced several hundredfold during T-cell maturation, but the sensitivity to strong ligands remains unchanged. More generally, this study shows how modelling the interactions of the molecules involved in negative and positive feedback with the TCR complex helped reveal its role in the emergent T-cell properties of sensitivity and specificity.

## CONCLUSIONS

**Current and future work**

There are many avenues still to explore in the projects described above. For example, our models of Th1/2 differentiation are now focusing on the information transferred from infected tissues via APCs to T cells, and how this, along with the dynamics of cytokine and transcriptional factors, influences T helper cell polarisation. In the model of TCR cross-talk, we are exploring the consequences of a more realistic distribution of both self and foreign peptides on the APC; incorporating spatial and mobility constraints governing the interaction of peptide–MHC with TCR; and studying the implications of the model for how altered peptide ligands work. We have found that one has to be prepared to rebuild models from scratch or change focus when new experimental information comes to light, and be rigorous in pursuit of well-defined biological problems.

In summary, our approach is one of close collaboration with experimentalists (ideally with the mathematician actually working in the laboratory) to develop models that can accommodate our uncertainty in our knowledge of the systems we are studying. A good mathematical model will shed light on experimental phenomena and point the way to new experiments. In turn this leads to refinement of the model and the cycle continues.

**Acknowledgements**
AY is supported by EPSRC/BBSRC Joint Initiative in Mathematical Modelling, Simulation and Prediction of Biological Systems award to RC and JS, grant reference 39/MMI09771. CCWC is supported by a UK Overseas Research Support award and a UCL Graduate School postgraduate scholarship.

## *References*

1. Haurie, C., Dale, D. C. and Mackey, M. C. (1998), 'Cyclical neutropenia and other periodic hematological diseases: A review of mechanisms and mathematical models', *Blood*, Vol. 92, pp. 2629–2640.

2. Shimizu, K. and Gurdon, J. B. (1999), 'A quantitative analysis of signal transduction from activin receptor to nucleus and its relevance to morphogen gradient interpretation', *Proc. Natl Acad. Sci. USA*, Vol. 96, pp. 6791–6796.

3. Callard, R., George, A. J. T. and Stark, J. (1999), 'Cytokines, chaos and complexity', *Immunity*, Vol. 11, pp. 507–513.

4. Segel, L. A. and Lev Bar-Or, R. (1998), 'Immunology viewed as the study of an autonomous decentralised system', in Dasgupta, D., Ed., 'Artificial Immune Systems and their Applications', Springer-Verlag, Berlin, pp. 65–88.

5. Borghans, J. A., Noest, A. J. and de Boer, R. J. (1999), 'How specific should immunological memory be?', *J. Immunol.*, Vol. 163, pp. 569–575.

6. Paul, W. E. (1999), 'Fundamental Immunology', 4th edn, Lippincott-Raven, Philadelphia.

7. Janeway, C. and Travers, P. (2001), 'Immunobiology', 4th edn, Garland, New York.

8. Murray, J. (1993), 'Mathematical Biology', 2nd edn, Springer-Verlag, Berlin.

9. Perelson, A. S. and Weisbuch, G. (1997), 'Immunology for physicists', *Rev. Mod. Phys.*, Vol. 69, pp. 1219–1267.

10. Morel, P. A. (1998), 'Mathematical modelling of immunological reactions', *Frontiers Biosci.*, Vol. 3, pp. 338–347.

11. Barkai, N. and Liebler, S. (1997), 'Robustness in simple biochemical networks', *Nature*, Vol. 387, pp. 913–917.

12. Hartwell, L. H., Hopfield, J. J., Leibler, S. and Murray, A. W. (1999), 'From molecular to modular cell biology', *Nature*, Vol. 402, pp. C47–C50.

13. Oprea, M., van Nimwegen, E. and Perelson, A. S. (2000), 'Dynamics of one-pass germinal center models: Implications for affinity maturation', *Bull. Math. Biol.*, Vol. 62, pp. 121–153.

14. Grakoui, A., Bromley, S. K., Sumen, C. *et al.* (1999), 'The immunological synapse: a molecular machine controlling T-cell activation', *Science*, Vol. 285, pp. 221–227.

15. van den Berg, H. A., Rand, D. A. and Burroughs, N. J. (2001), 'A reliable and safe T cell repertoire based on low-affinity T cell receptors', *J. Theor Biol.*, Vol. 209, pp. 465–486.

16. Rayner, S. A., King, W. J., Comer, R. M. *et al.* (2000), 'Local bioactive tumour necrosis factor (TNF) in corneal allotransplantation', *Clin. Exp. Immunol.*, Vol. 122, pp. 109–116.

17. Chan, C. C. W., Stark, J. and George, A. J. T. (1999), 'Analysis of cytokine network dynamics in corneal allograft rejection', *Proc. R. Soc. B*, Vol. 266, pp. 2217–2223.

18. DsTool (1998), URL: ftp://cam.cornell.edu/pub/dstool/

19. Auto (1997), URL: http://indy.cs.concordia.ca/auto/

20. Content (1997), URL: http://www.can.nl/Systems_and_Packages/Per_Purpose/Special/DiffEqns/Content/GCbody.html

21. Dynamical Systems Software (1997), URL: http://www.maths.ex.ac.uk/~hinke/dss/

22. Feldmann, M. and Maini, R. N. (2001), 'Anti-TNF-$\alpha$ therapy of rheumatoid arthritis: What have we learned?', *Annu. Rev. Immunol.*, Vol. 19, pp. 163–196.

23. Yates, A., Bergmann, C., van Hemmen, J. L. *et al.* (2000), 'Cytokine-modulated regulation of helper T-cell populations', *J. Theor. Biol.*, Vol. 206, pp. 539–560.

24. Godthelp, B. C., van Tol, M. J., Vossen, J. M. and van den Elsen, P. J. (1999), 'T-Cell immune reconstitution in pediatric leukemia patients after allogeneic bone marrow transplantation with T-cell-depleted or unmanipulated grafts: evaluation of overall and antigen-specific T-cell repertoires', *Blood*, Vol. 94, pp. 4358–4369.

25. Yates, A. and Callard, R. (2001), 'Cell death and the maintenance of immunological memory', *Discrete and Continuous Dyn. Sys. B*, Vol. 1, pp. 43–60.

26. Harding, C. V. and Unanue, E. R. (1990), 'Quantitation of antigen-presenting cell MHC class II/peptide complexes necessary for T-cell stimulation', *Nature*, Vol. 346, pp. 574–576.

27. Matsui, K., Boniface, J. J., Steffner, P. *et al.* (1994), 'Kinetics of T-cell receptor binding to peptide/I-Ek complexes: Correlation of the dissociation rate with T-cell responsiveness', *Proc. Natl Acad. Sci. USA*, Vol. 91, pp. 12862–12866.

28. McKeithan, T. W. (1995), 'Kinetic proofreading in T-cell receptor signal transduction', *Proc. Natl Acad. Sci. USA*, Vol. 92, pp. 5042–5046.

29. Valitutti, S., Muller, S., Cella, M. *et al.* (1995), 'Serial triggering of many T-cell receptors by a few peptide–MHC complexes', *Nature*, Vol. 375, pp. 148–151.

30. Germain, R. N. and Stefanova, I. (1999), 'The dynamics of T cell receptor signalling: Complex orchestration and the key roles of tempo and cooperation', *Annu. Rev. Immunol.*, Vol. 17, pp. 467–522.

31. Chan, C., George, A. J. T. and Stark, J. (2001), 'Cooperative enhancement of specificity in a lattice of T-cell receptors', *Proc. Natl Acad. Sci. USA*, Vol. 98, pp. 5758–5763.

# Authors' Index of Selected Articles

# MeSH Index of Selected Articles